For Tif Loehnis

To whom I owe my career
and by consequence
much else besides

CONTENTS

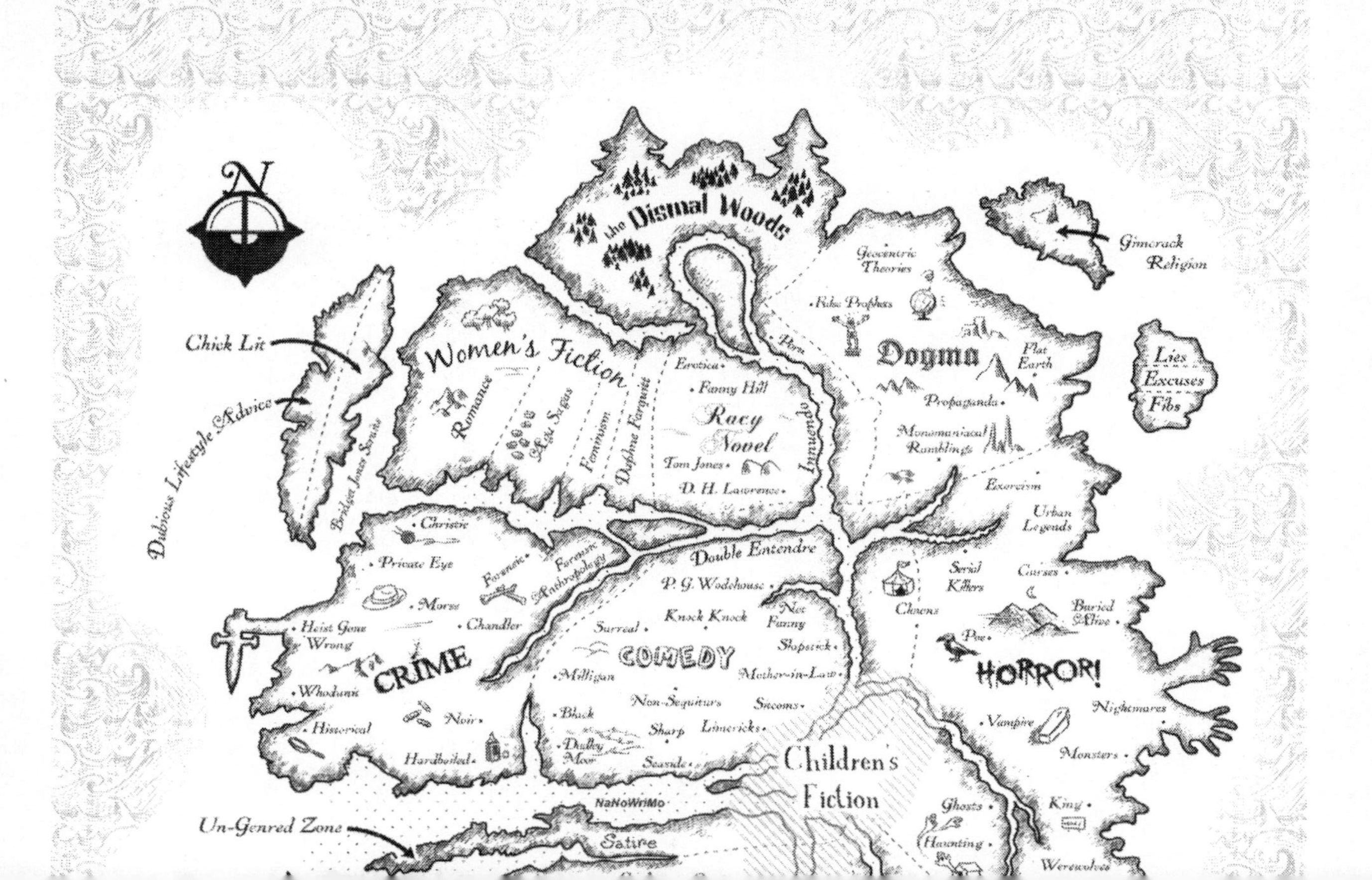

N
the Dismal Woods
Gimcrack Religion
Lies
Excuses
Fibs
Geocentric Theories
Fake Prophets
Dogma
Flat Earth
Propaganda
Monomaniacal Ramblings
Porn
Chick Lit
Dubious Lifestyle Advice
Bridget Jones Sequels
Women's Fiction
Romance
Aga Sagas
Feminism
Daphne Farquitt
Erotica
Fanny Hill
Racy Novel
Tom Jones
D. H. Lawrence
Innuendo
Exorcism
Urban Legends
Christie
Private Eye
Forensic
Forensic Anthropology
Morse
Chandler
Heist Gone Wrong
CRIME
Whodunit
Historical
Noir
Hardboiled
Double Entendre
P. G. Wodehouse
Knock Knock
Not Funny
Surreal
COMEDY
Slapstick
Milligan
Mother-in-Law
Non-Sequiturs
Sitcoms
Black
Sharp
Limericks
Dudley Moor
Seaside
Serial Killers
Clowns
Curses
Buried Alive
Poe
HORROR!
Vampire
Nightmares
Monsters
Children's Fiction
Ghosts
Haunting
King
Werewolves
NaNoWriMo
Un-Genred Zone
Satire

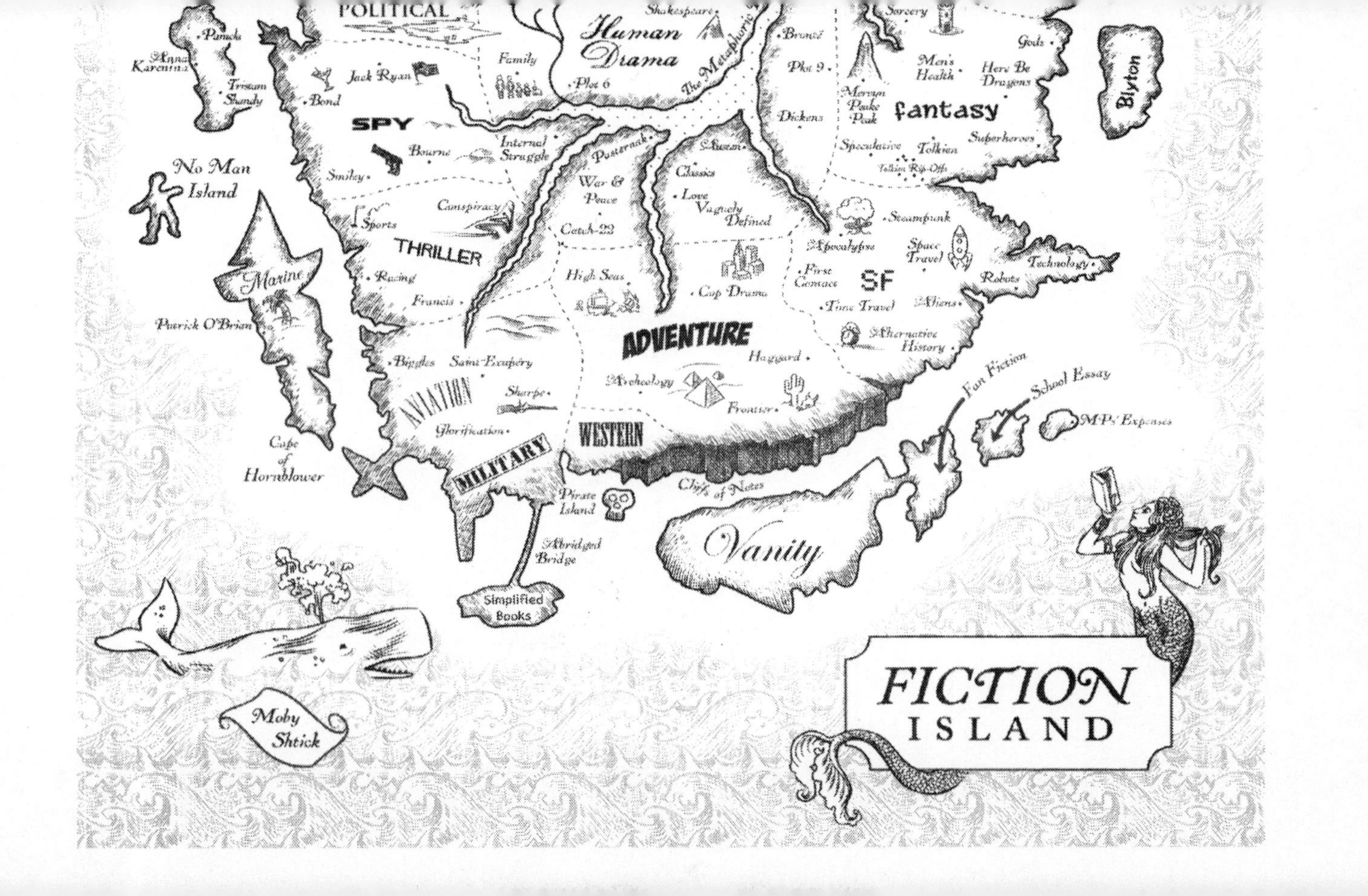
FICTION
ISLAND
POLITICAL
Human Drama
Shakespeare
Plot 6
The Metaphorical
Family
Jack Ryan
Bond
SPY
Bourne
Smiley
Internal Struggle
Conspiracy
Sports
THRILLER
Racing
Francis
Pamela
Anna Karenina
Tristram Shandy
No Man Island
Marine
Patrick O'Brian
Cape of Hornblower
Biggles
Saint-Exupéry
AVIATION
Sharpe
Glorification
MILITARY
Pirate Island
Abridged Bridge
Simplified Books
Moby Shtick
Pasternak
War & Peace
Catch-22
High Seas
WESTERN
ADVENTURE
Archeology
Haggard
Frontier
Cliffs of Notes
Vanity
Austen
Classics
Love Vaguely Defined
Cop Drama
Brontë
Plot 9
Dickens
Sorcery
Mervyn Peake Peak
Men's Health
Here Be Dragons
Gods
fantasy
Speculative
Tolkien
Tolkien Rip-Offs
Superheroes
Blyton
Steampunk
Apocalypse
Space Travel
First Contact
SF
Time Travel
Aliens
Robots
Technology
Alternative History
Fan Fiction
School Essay
MPs' Expenses

1.
The BookWorld Remade

The remaking was one of those moments when one felt a part of literature and not just carried along within it. In less than ten minutes, the entire fabric of the BookWorld was radically altered. The old system was swept away, and everything was changed forever. But the group of people to whom it was ultimately beneficial remained gloriously unaware: the readers. To most of them, books were merely books. If only it were that simple. . . .

Bradshaw's BookWorld Companion
(2nd edition)

Everyone can remember where they were when the BookWorld was remade. I was at home "resting between readings," which is a polite euphemism for "almost remaindered."

But I wasn't doing nothing. No, I was using the time to acquaint myself with EZ-

Read's latest Laborsaving Narrative Devices, all designed to assist a first-person protagonist like me cope with the strains of a sixty-eight-setting five-book series at the speculative end of Fantasy.

I couldn't afford any of these devices — not even Verb-Ease™ for troublesome irregularity — but that wasn't the point. It was the company of EZ-Read's regional salesman that I was interested in, a cheery Designated Love Interest named Whitby Jett.

"We have a new line in foreshadowing," he said, passing me a small blue vial.

"Does the bottle have to be in the shape of Lola Vavoom?" I asked.

"It's a marketing thing."

I opened the stopper and sniffed at it gingerly.

"What do you think?" he asked.

Whitby was a good-looking man described as a youthful forty. I didn't know it then, but he had a dark past, and despite our mutual attraction his earlier misdeeds could only end in one way: madness, recrimination and despair.

"I prefer my foreshadowing a little less pungent," I said, carefully replacing the stopper. "I was getting all sorts of vibes about you and a dark past."

"I wish," replied Whitby sadly. His book had been deleted long ago, so he was one of the many thousands of characters who eked out a living in the BookWorld while they waited for a decent part to come along. But because of his minor DLI character status, he had never been given a backstory. Those without any sort of history often tried to promote it as something mysterious when it wasn't, but not Whitby, who was refreshingly pragmatic. "Even having no backstory as my backstory would be something," he had once told me in a private moment, "but the truth is this: My author couldn't be bothered to give me one."

I always appreciated honesty, even as personal as this. There weren't many characters in the BookWorld who had been left unscathed by the often selfish demands of their creators. A clumsily written and unrealistic set of conflicting motivations can have a character in therapy for decades — perhaps forever.

"Any work offers recently?" I asked.

"I was up for a minor walk-on in an Amis."

"How did you do?"

"I read half a page and they asked me what I thought. I said I understood every word and so was rejected as being overqualified."

"I'm sorry to hear that."

"It's okay," he said. "I was also offered a four-hundred-and-six-word part in a horror last week, but I'm not so sure. First-time author and a small publisher, so I might not make it past the second impression. If I get remaindered, I'd be worse off than I am now."

"I'm remaindered," I reminded him.

"But you were *once* popular," he said, "so you might be again. Do you know how many characters have high hopes of a permanent place in the readers' hearts, only to suffer the painful rejection of eternal un-readfulness at the dreary end of Human Drama?"

He was right. A book's life could be very long indeed, and although the increased leisure time in an unread novel is not to be sniffed at, a need to be vigilant in case someone *does* read you can keep one effectively tied to a book for life. I usually had an understudy to let me get away, but few were so lucky.

"So," said Whitby, "how would you like to come out to the smellies tonight? I hear *Garden Peas with Mint* is showing at the Rex."

In the BookWorld, smells were in short supply. *Garden Peas with Mint* had been the best release this year. It only narrowly beat *Vanilla Coffee* and *Grilled Smoked Bacon* for the prestigious Noscar™ Best Adapted Smell award.

"I heard that *Mint* was overrated," I replied, although I hadn't. Whitby had been asking me out for a date almost as long as I'd been turning him down. I didn't tell him why, but he suspected that there was someone else. There was and there wasn't. It was complex, even by BookWorld standards. He asked me out a lot, and I declined a lot. It was kind of like a game.

"How about going to the Running of the Bumbles next week? Dangerous, but exciting."

This was an annual fixture on the BookWorld calendar, where two dozen gruel-crazed and indignant Mr. Bumbles yelling, "More? MORE?!?" were released to charge through an unused chapter of *Oliver Twist.* Those of a sporting or daring disposition were invited to run before them and take their chances; at least one hapless youth was crushed to death every year.

"I've no need to prove myself," I replied, "and neither do you."

"How about dinner?" he asked, unabashed. "I can get a table at the Inn Uendo. The maîtred' is missing a space, and

I promised to give her one."

"Not really my thing."

"Then what about the Bar Humbug? The atmosphere is wonderfully dreary."

It was over in Classics, but we could take a cab.

"I'll need an understudy to take over my book."

"What happened to Stacy?"

"The same as happened to Doris and Enid."

"Trouble with Pickwick again?"

"As if you need to ask."

And that was when the doorbell rang. This was unusual, as random things rarely occur in the mostly predetermined BookWorld. I opened the door to find three Dostoyevskivites staring at me from within a dense cloud of moral relativism.

"May we come in?" said the first, who had the look of someone weighed heavily down with the burden of conscience. "We were on our way home from a redemption-through-suffering training course. Something big's going down at Text Grand Central, and everyone's been grounded until further notice."

A grounding was rare, but not unheard of. In an emergency all citizens of the BookWorld were expected to offer hospitality to those stranded outside their books.

I might have minded, but these guys were from *Crime and Punishment* and, better still, celebrities. We hadn't seen anyone famous this end of Fantasy since Pamela from *Pamela* stopped outside with a flat tire. She could have been gone in an hour but insisted on using an epistolary breakdown service, and we had to put her up in the spare room while a complex series of letters went backwards and forwards.

"Welcome to my home, Rodion Romanovich Raskolnikov."

"Oh!" said Raskolnikov, impressed that I knew who he was. "How did you know it was me? Could it have been the subtle way in which I project the dubious moral notion that murder might somehow be rationalized, or was it the way in which I move from denying my guilt to eventually coming to terms with an absolute sense of justice and submitting myself to the rule of law?"

"Neither," I said. "It's because you're holding an ax covered in blood and human hair."

"Yes, it is a bit of a giveaway," he admitted, staring at the ax, "but how rude am I? Allow me to introduce Arkady Ivanovich Svidrigailov."

"Actually," said the second man, leaning

over to shake my hand, "I'm Dmitri Prokofich Razumikhin, Raskolnikov's loyal friend."

"You are?" said Raskolnikov in surprise. "Then what happened to Svidrigailov?"

"He's busy chatting up your sister."

He narrowed his eyes.

"My sister? That's Pulcheria Alexandrovna Raskolnikova, right?"

"No," said Razumikhin in the tone of a long-suffering best friend, "that's your mother. Avdotya Romanovna Raskolnikova is your sister."

"I always get those two mixed up. So who's Marfa Petrovna Svidrigailova?"

Razumikhin frowned and thought for a moment.

"You've got me there."

He turned to the third Russian.

"Tell me, Pyotr Petrovich Luzhin: Who, precisely, is Marfa Petrovna Svidrigailova?"

"I'm sorry," said the third Russian, who had been staring at her shoes absently, "but I think there has been some kind of mistake. I'm not Pyotr Petrovich Luzhin. I'm Alyona Ivanovna."

Razumikhin turned to Raskolnikov and lowered his voice.

"Is that your landlady's servant, the one who decides to marry down to secure her future, or the one who turns to prostitution in order to stop her family from descending into penury?"

Raskolnikov shrugged. "Listen," he said, "I've been in this book for over a hundred and forty years, and even I can't figure it out."

"It's very simple," said the third Russian, indicating who did what on her fingers. "Nastasya Petrovna is Raskolnikov's landlady's servant, Avdotya Romanovna Raskolnikova is your sister who threatens to marry down, Sofia Semyonovna Marmeladova is the one who becomes a prostitute, and Marfa Petrovna Svidrigailova — the one you were *first* asking about — is Arkady Svidrigailov's murdered first wife."

"I knew that," said Raskolnikov in the manner of someone who didn't. "So . . . who are you again?"

"I'm Alyona Ivanovna," said the third Russian with a trace of annoyance, "the rapacious old pawnbroker whose apparent greed and wealth led you to murder."

"Are you *sure* you're Ivanovna?" asked Raskolnikov with a worried tone.

"Absolutely."

"And you're still alive?"

"So it seems."

He stared at the bloody ax. "Then who

did I just kill?"

And they all looked at one another in confusion.

"Listen," I said, "I'm sure everything will come out fine in the epilogue. But for the moment your home is my home."

Anyone from Classics had a celebrity status that outshone anything else, and I'd never had anyone even remotely famous pass through before. I suddenly felt a bit hot and bothered and tried to tidy up the house in a clumsy sort of way. I whipped my socks from the radiator and brushed off the pistachio shells that Pickwick had left on the sideboard.

"This is Whitby Jett of EZ-Read," I said, introducing the Russians one by one but getting their names hopelessly mixed up, which might have been embarrassing had they noticed. Whitby shook all their hands and then asked for autographs, which I found faintly embarrassing.

"So why has Text Grand Central ordered a grounding?" I asked as soon as everyone was seated and I had rung for Mrs. Malaprop to bring in the tea.

"I think the rebuilding of the BookWorld is about to take place," said Razumikhin with a dramatic flourish.

"So soon?"

The remaking had been a hot topic for a number of years. After Imagination™ was deregulated in the early fifties, the outburst of creative alternatives generated huge difficulties for the Council of Genres, who needed a clearer overview of how the individual novels sat within the BookWorld as a whole. Taking the RealWorld as inspiration, the CofG decided that a Geographic model was the way to go. How the physical world actually appeared, no one really knew. Not many people traveled to the RealWorld, and those who did generally noted two things: one, that it was hysterically funny and hideously tragic in almost equal measure, and two, that there were far more domestic cats than baobabs, when it should probably be the other way round.

Whitby got up and looked out the window. There was nothing to see, quite naturally, as the area *between* books had no precise definition or meaning. My front door opened to, well, not very much at all. Stray too far from the boundaries of a book and you'd be lost forever in the interbook Nothing. It was confusing, but then so were *Tristram Shandy, The Magus* and Russian novels, and people had been enjoying them for decades.

"So what's going to happen?" asked Whitby.

"I have a good friend over at Text Grand Central," said Alyona Ivanovna, who had wisely decided to sit as far from Raskolnikov and the bloody ax as she could, "and he said that to accomplish a smooth transition from Great Library BookWorld to Geographic BookWorld, the best option was to close down all the imaginotransference engines while they rebooted the throughput conduits."

This was an astonishing suggestion. The imaginotransference engines were the machines that transmitted the books in all their subtle glory from the BookWorld to the reader's imagination. To shut them down meant that reading — *all* reading — had to stop. I exchanged a nervous glance with Whitby.

"You mean the Council of Genres is going to shut down the entire BookWorld?"

Alyona Ivanovna nodded. "It was either that or do it piecemeal, which wasn't favored, since then half the BookWorld would be operating one system and half the other. It's simple: All reading needs to stop for the nine minutes it requires to have the BookWorld remade."

"But that's insane!" exclaimed Whitby.

"People will notice. There's always someone reading *somewhere.*"

From my own failed experience of joining the BookWorld's policing agency, I knew that he spoke the truth. There was a device hung high on the wall in the Council of Genres debating chamber that logged the Outland ReadRate — the total number of readers at any one time. It bobbed up and down but rarely dropped below the 20-million mark. But while spikes in reading were easier to predict, such as when a new blockbuster is published or when an author dies — always a happy time for their creations, if not their relatives — predicting slumps was much harder. And we needed a serious slump in reading to get down to the under-fifty-thousand threshold considered safe for a remaking.

I had an idea. I fetched that morning's copy of *The Word* and turned to the week's forecast. This wasn't to do with weather, naturally, but trends in reading. Urban Vampires were once more heavily forecast for the week ahead, with scattered Wizards moving in from Wednesday and a high chance of Daphne Farquitt Novels near the end of the week. There was also an alert for everyone at Sports Trivia to "brace themselves," and it stated the reason.

"There you go," I said, tapping the newspaper and showing it to the assembled company. "Right about now the Swindon Mallets are about to defend their title against the Gloucester Meteors, and with live televised coverage to the entire planet there is a huge potential fall in the ReadRate."

"You think that many people are interested in Premier League croquet?" asked Razumikhin.

"It *is* Swindon versus Gloucester," I replied, "and after the Malletts' forward hoop, Penelope Hrah, exploded on the forty-yard line last year, I would expect ninety-two percent of the world will be watching the game — as good a time as any to take the BookWorld offline."

"Did they ever find out *why* Hrah exploded?" asked Whitby.

"It was never fully explained," put in Ivanovna, "but traces of Semtex were discovered in her shin guards, so foul play could never be ruled out entirely. A grudge match is always a lot of fu—"

Her voice was abruptly cut dead, but not in the way one's is when one has suddenly stopped speaking. Her voice was clipped, like a gap in a recording.

"Hello?" I said.

The three Russians made no answer and were simply staring into space, like mannequins. After a moment they started to lose facial definition as they became a series of complex irregular polyhedra. After a while the number of facets of the polyhedra started to lessen, and the Russians became less like people and more like jagged, flesh-colored lumps. Pretty soon they were nothing at all. The Classics were being shut down, and if Text Grand Central was doing it alphabetically, Fantasy would not be far behind. And so it proved. I looked at Whitby, who gave me a wan smile and held my hand. The room grew cold, then dark, and before long the only world that I knew started to disassemble in front of my eyes. Everything grew flatter and lost its form, and pretty soon I began to feel my memory fade. And just when I was starting to worry, everything was cleansed to an all-consuming darkness.

#shutting down imaginotransference engines, 46,802 readers

#active reader states have been cached

#dismounting READ OS 8.3.6

#start programs

#check and mount specified dictionaries

#check and mount specified thesauri

#check and mount specified idiomatic database

#check and mount specified grammatical database

#check and mount specified character database

#check and mount specified settings database

Mount temporary ISBN/BISAC/duodecimal book category system

Mount imaginotransference throughput module

Accessing "book index" on global bus

Creating cache for primary plot-development module

Creating /ramdisk in "story interpretation,"

default size=300

Creating directories: irony

Creating directories: humor

Creating directories: plot

Creating directories: character

Creating directories: atmosphere

Creating directories: prose

Creating directories: pace

Creating directories: pathos

Starting init process

#display imaginotransference-engine error messages

#recovering active readers from cache

System message=Welcome to Geographic Operating System 1.2

Setting control terminal to automatic

System active with 46,802 active readers

"Thursday?"

I opened my eyes and blinked. I was lying on the sofa staring up at Whitby, who had a concerned expression on his face.

"Are you okay?"

I sat up and rubbed my head. "How long was I out?"

"Eleven minutes,"

I looked around. "And the Russians?"

"Outside."

"There is no outside."

He smiled. "There is now. Come and have a look."

I stood up and noticed for the first time that my living room seemed that little bit more realistic. The colors were subtler, and the walls had an increased level of texture. More interestingly, the room seemed to be brighter, and there was light coming in through the windows. It was *real* light, too, the sort that casts shadows and not the pretend stuff we were used to. I grasped the handle, opened the front door and stepped outside.

The empty interbook Nothing that had separated the novels and genres had been replaced by fields, hills, rivers, trees and forests, and all around me the countryside opened out into a series of expansive vistas with the welcome novelty of *distance.* We were now in the southeast corner of an island perhaps a hundred miles by fifty and bounded on all sides by the Text Sea, which had been elevated to "Grade IV Picturesque" status by the addition of an azure hue and a soft, billowing motion that made the text shimmer in the breeze.

As I looked around, I realized that whoever had remade the BookWorld had considered practicalities as much as aesthetics. Unlike the RealWorld, which is inconveniently located on the *outside* of a sphere, the new BookWorld was anchored on the *inside* of a sphere, thus ensuring that horizons worked in the opposite way to those in RealWorld. Farther objects were higher in the visual plane than nearer ones. From anywhere in the BookWorld, it was possible to view anywhere else. I noticed, too, that we were not alone. Stuck on the inside of the sphere were hundreds of other islands very similar to our own, and each a haven for a category of literature therein.

About ten degrees upslope of Fiction, I could see our nearest neighbor: Artistic Criticism. It was an exceptionally beautiful island, yet deeply troubled, confused and suffused with a blanketing layer of almost impenetrable bullshit. Beyond that were Psychology, Philately, and Software Manuals. But the brightest and biggest archipelago I could see upon the closed sea was the scattered group of genres that made up Nonfiction. They were positioned right on the other side of the inner globe and so were almost directly overhead. On one side of the island the Cliffs of Irrationality were slowly being eroded away, while on the opposite shore the Sands of Science were slowly reclaiming salt marsh from the sea.

While I stared upwards, openmouthed, a steady stream of books moved in an endless multilayered crisscross high in the sky. But these weren't books of the small paper-and-leather variety that one might find in the Outland. These were the collected *settings* of the book all bolted together and connected by a series of walkways and supporting beams, cables and struts. They didn't look so much like books, in fact, but more like a series of spiky lumps. While some one-room dramas were no bigger than a double-decker bus and zipped across the sky, others moved slowly enough for us to wave at the occupants, who waved back. As we stood watching our new world, the master copy of *Doctor Zhivago* passed overhead, blotting out the light and covering us in a

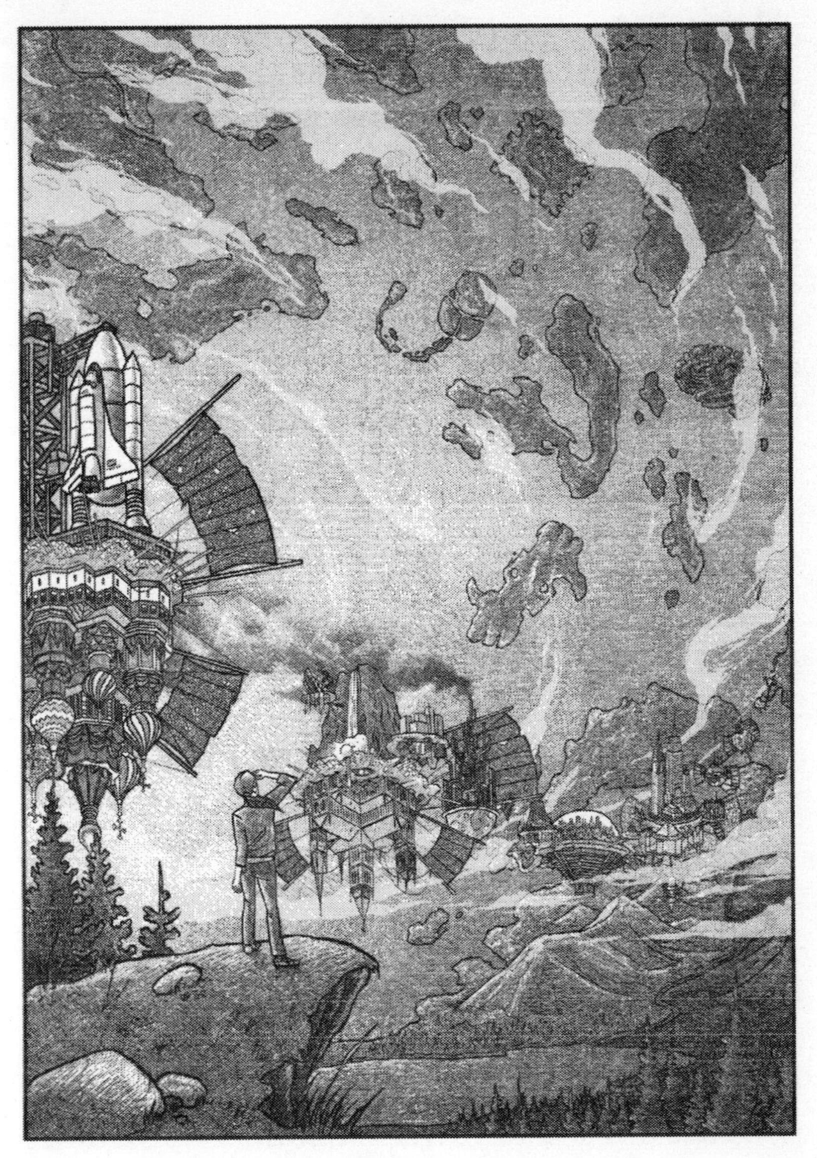

"O brave new world, that has such stories in't!"

light dusting of snow.

"What do you think?" asked Whitby.

"O brave new world," I whispered as I gave him a hug, "that has such stories in't!"

2.
A Woman Named Thursday Next

A major benefit of the Internal Sphere model of the remade BookWorld is that gravitational force diminishes with height, so it is easier to move objects the higher you go. You have to be careful, though, for if you go too high, you will be attracted to the gravitational dead spot right in the center of the sphere, from where there could be no return.

Bradshaw's BookWorld Companion
(6th edition)

My father had a face that could stop a clock. I don't mean that he was ugly or anything; it was a phrase that the Chrono-Guard used to describe someone who had the power to arrest time to an ultraslow trickle — and that's exactly what happened one morning as I was having a late breakfast in a small café quite near where I worked. The world flickered, shuddered and stopped. The barman of the café froze to a halt in midsentence, and the picture on the television stopped dead. Outside, birds hung motionless in the sky. The sound halted, too, replaced by a dull snapshot of a hum, the world's noise at that moment in time paused indefinitely at the same pitch and volume.

"Hello, Sweetpea."

I turned. My father was sitting at a table behind me and rose to hug me affectionately.

"Hi, Dad."

"You're looking good," he told me.

"You, too," I replied. "You're looking younger every time I see you."

"I am. How's your history?"

"Not bad."

"Do you know how the Duke of Wellington died?"

"Sure," I answered. "He was shot by a French sniper early on during the Battle of Waterloo — why?"

"Oh, no reason," muttered my father with feigned innocence, scribbling in a small notebook. Once done, he paused for a moment.

"So Napoléon *won* at Waterloo, did he?" he asked slowly and with great intensity.

"Of course not," I replied. "Field Marshal Blücher's timely intervention saved the day.

This is all high school history, Dad. What are you up to?"

"Well, it's a bit of — hang on," said Dad, or rather the character *playing* my book-father. "I think they've gone."

I tasted the air. He was right. Our lone reader had stopped and left us dangling in a narrative dead zone. It's an odd sensation: a combination of treading on a step that isn't there, someone hanging up the telephone midspeech without explanation and the feeling you get when you've gone upstairs for some reason but can't think why. Scientists have proved that spaniels spend their entire lives like this.

"I was *marvelous,*" intoned my book-father haughtily, the inference being that it was somehow my fault the reader didn't last until even the end of the first page. "You need to *engage* the readers more, darling. Project yourself. Make the character come *alive.*"

I didn't agree that I was at fault but wasn't going to argue. He had played my father longer in the series than I had played Thursday, so he had a kind of seniority, even if I was the protagonist, and first-person player to boot.

"Sometimes I yearn for the old days," he said to Hector, his dresser, but obviously intending for me to hear.

"What do you mean by that?"

He stared at me for a moment. "This: It was a lot better when we had the previous Thursday play Thursday."

"She was violent and immoral, Dad. How could that *possibly* be better?"

"She might have been a shit of the highest order, darling, but she brought in the readers. I'll be in my dressing room. Come, Hector."

And so saying, he swept from the café setting with his ever-present dresser, who pouted rudely at me as they left. My bookfather had a point, of course, but I was committed to promoting the type of Thursday the *real* Thursday wanted to see in the series. The series had originally been written to feature a violent and disorderly Thursday Next, who slept her way around the BookWorld and caused no end of murder, misery and despair. I was trying to change all that but had met with stiff resistance from the rest of the cast. They saw my attempt to depict reality as damaging to the overall readability — and for a character, the only thing worse than being read badly is to be badly unread.

I sighed. Keeping everyone within my series happy and fulfilled and focused was about as hard a job as acting in the book itself. Some books had a page manager to do all that boring stuff, but for financial reasons I had to do it myself with only a defective Mrs. Malaprop for assistance. Making us all readable was the least of my worries.

I walked slowly home through my book-version of Swindon, which was forty times more compact than the real one. Due to the limited number of locations mentioned in my series, I could go easily from the café to my mother's house to the GSD church and then on to the SpecOps Building in the space of a few minutes, something that would take the best part of an hour in the real Swindon. There were a few handy shortcuts, too. By opening a door at the back of Our Blessed Lady of the Lobster, I could find myself in the mockup of Thornfield Hall, and by taking the first door on the right past Jane's bedroom, I could be in the Penderyn Hotel in Wales. All told, the series covered about five acres on six levels and would have been larger if we hadn't doubled up the East facade of Thornfield with the front of Haworth Parsonage in Yorkshire, and the Gad's Hill Museum with the redressed lobby of the SpecOps Building. Economies like this were commonplace in remaindered books and helped us keep the cast at almost full strength. Doubling up characters *was* possible, but it caused problems when they were in scenes with themselves. Some characters could handle it, others could not. On one memorable occasion, Vronsky played *all* the parts in an abridged version of *Anna Karenina* whilst the rest of the cast were on strike for more blinis. When asked what it was like, he described it as "like, totally awesome, dude."

"Good morning, Pickwick," I said as I walked into the kitchen, which not only served as the command center of my series but also as the place where tea and toast could be made and eaten. "Good morning, Mrs. Malaprop."

"Cod Moaning, Miss Next," said the defective Mrs. Malaprop, bobbing politely.

"May I have a word?" asked Pickwick, in a not very subtle aside.

"Is it important?"

"It is vitally *crucial,*" said Pickwick, rolling her eyes oddly.

We moved out to the hallway.

"Okay, what's the problem?" I asked, since Pickwick *always* had a grievance of some sort — whether it was the cold or the heat or the color of the walls or a hundred and one other things that weren't quite right. Whitby and I referred to her as "Goldilocks without the manners" — but never to her beak.

"It's Mrs. Malaprop," said the dodo in an affronted tone. "She's becoming increasingly unintelligible. It would be okay if it were faintly amusing, but it isn't, and . . . well, quite frankly, there is the risk of infection, and it frightens me."

To a text-based life-form, unpredictable syntax and poor grammar is a source of huge discomfort. Ill-fitting grammar are like ill-fitting shoes. You can get used to it for a bit, but then one day your toes fall off and you can't walk to the bathroom. Poor syntax is even worse. Change word order and a sentence useless for anyone Yoda except you have.

"Now, then," I said, using an oxymoron for scolding effect, "it is totally unproven that malapropism is inflectious, and what did we say about tolerating those less fortunate than ourselves?"

"Even so," said Pickwick, "I want you to tell her to stop it. And her shoes squeak. And while we're on the subject, Bowden referred to me as 'that bird' again, the baobab in the back garden is cutting out the light from my bedroom, and I'm taking next Wednesday off to have my beak oiled, so you'll need to get a replacement — and not the penguin like last time. She didn't do justice to my dynamic personalty and poetic sensibilities. Played it all a bit . . . *fishcentric,* if you know what I mean."

"I'll do my best," I said, making a mental note to *definitely* rebook the penguin.

"Good," said Pickwick. "Have you the paper?"

We returned to the kitchen, and I found *The Word* for her.

"Hmm," she said thoughtfully, staring at the City pages. "Metaphor has risen by seventeen pounds a barrel. I should dump some metonym and buy into synecdoche futures."

"How are things going with Racy Novel?" I asked, since the political problems up in the North had been much in the news recently. A long-running dispute between Racy Novel, Women's Fiction and Dogma had been getting worse and was threatening to erupt into a genre war at the drop of a hat.

"Peace talks still on schedule for Friday," replied Pickwick, "as if that will do any good. Sometimes I think that Muffler nut-job wants nothing but a good scrap. By the way," she added, "did you hear about *Ra-*

phael's Walrus?"

"No."

"Got their eviction papers this morning."

This wasn't surprising. *Raphael's Walrus* was a book six doors down that hadn't been read for a while. I didn't know them well, but since we were located at the Speculative end of Fantasy, the real estate was valuable. We'd have a new neighbor almost the moment they left.

"I hope it's not Sword and Sorcery," said Pickwick with a shudder. "Goblins really drag down the neighborhood."

"Goblins might say the same about dodos."

"Impossible!" she retorted. "Dodos are cute and cuddly and lovable and . . . don't steal stuff and spread disease."

People often wondered why my written dodo was such a pain in the ass when the real Pickwick was so cute. The reason was simple: lack of choice. There are only three dodos in fiction. One was dangerously psychotic, the second was something big over in Natural History, which left only one: The dodo from *Alice* is the same bespectacled know-it-all in my series. Her name wasn't actually Pickwick — it was Lorina Peabody III, but we called her Pickwick, and she didn't much mind either way. She put down the paper, announced to the room that she would be taking her siesta and waddled off.

"Mrs. Malaprop," I said once Pickwick had left, "are you still attending your therapy sessions?"

Mrs. Malaprop arched a highbrow. She knew well enough who had complained about her.

"Eggs tincture is too good for that burred," she said in a crabby tone, "but isle do as Uri quest."

The average working life of a Mrs. Malaprop in *The Rivals* was barely fifty readings. The unrelenting comedic misuse of words eventually caused them to suffer postsyntax stress disorder, and once their speech became irreversibly abstruse, they were simply replaced. Most "retired" Mrs. Malaprops were released into the BookWorld, where they turned ferrule, but just recently rehoming charities were taking note of their plight. After they'd undergone intensive Holorime Bombardment Therapy to enable them to at least *sound* right even if they didn't *read* right, people like me offered them a home and a job. Our Malaprop was an early model — Number 862, to be precise — and she was generally quite helpful if a little tricky to understand. There was talk of using Dogberry stem cells to cure her, but we didn't hold our broth.

I stared at the diagnostics board that covered one wall of the kitchen. The number of readers on the Read-O-Meter was stuck firmly at zero, with thirty-two copies of my novels listed "bookmarked and pending." Of these, eighteen were active/resting between reads. The rest were probably lying under a stack of other unfinished books. I checked the RealWorld clock. It was 0842. Years ago I was read on the train, but that hadn't happened for a while. Unreadfulness was a double-edged sword. More leisure time, but a distinct loss of purpose. I turned to Mrs. Malaprop.

"How are things looking in the series?"

She stared at her clipboard.

"Toll rubble. Twenty-six care actors Aaron leaf or training courses; all can be covered by eggs Hastings characters. Of the settings, only Hayworth House is clothes bee coarse of an invest station of grammasites."

"Has Jurisfiction been informed?"

"We're low prior Tory, so they said a towers."

"How close is our nearest reader?"

"Nine teas heaven minutes' read time away."

It wasn't going to be a problem. He or

she wouldn't pickup the book again until this evening, by which time the problem would have resolved itself.

"If the reading starts early for any reason," I said, "we'll use the front room of Thornfield Hall as a stand-in. Oh, and my father has a flea in his ear about something, so keep an eye on him in case he tries to do his own lines. I got a letter last week from Text Grand Central about illegal dialogue flexations."

Mrs. Malaprop nodded and made a note. "Come harder hearing cold," she said.

"Sorry?"

"Comma DeHare ring cooled."

"I'm . . . still not getting this."

Mrs. Malaprop thought hard, trying to place the correct words in the correct place to enable me to understand. It was painfully difficult for her, and if Sheridan had known the misery that using acyrologia in a comedic situation would bring, he would possibly have thought butter of it.

"Come hander hair-in culled!" she said again in an exasperated tone, sweating profusely and starting to shake with the effort.

"Commander Herring called?" I said, suddenly getting it. "What about?"

"A naval antecedent," she said urgently, "in evasion."

She meant that a novel had met with an accident in Aviation.

"Why would he be calling me after I blew it so badly last time?"

"It sea reprised me, too. Here."

She handed me a scrap of paper. Commander James "Red" Herring was overall leader of the BookWorld Policing Agency. He was in command not only of the Fiction Police known as Jurisfiction but also of Text Grand Central's Metaphor Squad and at least eighteen other agencies. One of these was Book Traffic Control — and part of that was the Jurisfiction Accident Investigation Department, or JAID, a department I occasionally worked for. The overhead book traffic, despite its usefulness, was not without problems. Fiction alone could see up to two thousand book-movements a day, and the constant transportation of the novels across the fictional skies was not without mishap. I spent at least a day a week identifying sections that had fallen off books passing overhead, trying to get them returned — and, if possible, find out why they'd come unglued. Despite safety assurances, improved adhesives and updated safety procedures, books would keep on shedding bits. The loss of a pig out of *Animal Farm* was the most celebrated incident. It fell several thousand feet and landed inside a book of short stories by Graham Greene. Disaster was averted by a quick-thinking Jurisfiction agent who expertly sewed the pig into the narrative. It was Jurisfiction at its very best.

"Did Commander Herring say which book or why he was calling me?"

"A very spurious accident, Walsall he said. You're to to me, Tim, at this address."

I took the address and stared at it. Commander Herring's calling me *personally* was something of a big deal. "Anything else?"

"Your new-ender study is waiting to be interviewed in the front room."

This was good news. My book was first-person narrative, and if I wanted to have any sort of life outside my occasional readings — such as a date with Whitby or to have a secondary career — I needed someone to stand in for me.

I walked through to the front room. My potential understudy looked pleasant enough and had troubled to integrate herself into my body type and vague looks. She had a Thursday Next outfit on, too. She wanted this job badly.

"The written Thursday Next," I said, shaking her hand.

"Carmine O'Kipper," she replied with a

nervous smile. "ID A4-5619-23. Pleased to be here."

"You're an A-4, Miss O'Kipper?"

"Call me Carmine. Is that a problem?"

"Not at all."

An A-4 character was theoretically only three steps down from the Jane Eyres and Scout Finches. To be able to handle first person, you had to be an A-grade, but none of the other understudies had been higher than an A-9.

"You must be at least an A-2, yes?" she asked.

"Something like that," I replied as we sat. "Do you know of the series?"

"I used to keep a scrapbook of the *real* Thursday Next."

"If you're here to catch a glimpse of her, it's unlikely. She dropped in once soon after the remaking, but not since then."

"I'm really just after the work, Miss Next."

She handed me her CV. It wasn't long, nor particularly impressive. She was from an original manuscript sitting abandoned in a drawer somewhere in the Outland. She would have handled loss, love, uncertainty and a corkingly good betrayal. It looked like it might have been a good gig. But after fifteen years and not a single reader, it was time to move on.

"So . . . why do you want to work in my series?"

"I'm eager to enter a new and stimulating phase of my career," she said brightly, "and I need a challenging and engaging book in which I can learn from a true professional."

It was the usual bullshit, and it didn't wash.

"You could get a read anywhere," I said, handing back the CV, "so why come to the speculative end of Fantasy?"

She bit her lip and stared at me.

"I've only ever been read by one person at a time," she confessed. "I took a short third-person locum inside a *Reader's Digest* version of *Don Quixote* as Dulcinea two weeks ago. I had a panic attack when the read levels went over twenty-six and went for the Snooze."

I heard Mrs. Malaprop drop a teacup in the kitchen. I was shocked, too. The Snooze Button was reserved only for dire emergencies. Once it was utilized, a reverse throughput capacitor on the imaginotransference engines would cause the reader instantaneous yawning, drowsiness and then sleep. Quick, simple — and the readers suspected nothing.

"You hit Snooze?"

"I was stopped before I did."

"I'm very relieved."

"Me, too. Rocinante had to take over my part — played her rather well, actually."

"Did the Don notice? Rocinante playing you, I mean?"

"No."

Carmine was just what I was looking for. Overqualified understudies rarely stayed long, but what with her being severely readerphobic, the low ReadRates would suit her down to the ground. I was mildly concerned over her eagerness to hit Snooze. To discourage misuse, every time the button was pressed, one or more kittens were put to death somewhere in the BookWorld. It was rarely used.

"Okay," I said, "you're hired. One caveat: You don't get the Snooze Button access codes. Agreed?"

"Agreed."

"Excellent. How much reading time do you have?"

"Aside from my own book, I've got eighty-seven pages."

It was a lamentably small amount. A single quizzical reader hunting for obscure hidden meanings would have her in a stammering flat spin in a second.

"Get your coat and a notebook," I said.

“We’re going to go greet our new neighbors — and have a chat.”

3.
Scarlett O'Kipper

> Outland tourism was banned long ago, and even full members of Jurisfiction — the BookWorld's policing elite — were no longer permitted to cross over to the Real-World. The reasons were many and hotly debated, but this much was agreed: Reality was a pit of vipers for the unwary. Forget to breathe, miscalculate gravity or support the wrong god or football team and they'd be sending you home in a zinc coffin.
>
> *Bradshaw's BookWorld Companion*
> (17th edition)

After taking a pager off the counter so Mrs. Malaprop could reach me in case a reader turned up unexpectedly, we stepped out of the main gate and walked down the street. The remade Geographic BookWorld was as its name suggested — geographic — and the neighborhoods were laid out like those in an Outland housing estate. A single road ran down between the books, with sidewalks, grass verges, syntax hydrants and trees. To the left and right were compounds that contained entire novels with all their settings. In one was a half-scale Kilimanjaro, and in another a bamboo plantation. In a third an electrical storm at full tilt.

"We're right on the edge of Fantasy," I explained. "Straight ahead is Human Drama, and to your right is Comedy. I'll give you Wednesdays off, but I expect you to be on standby most of the time."

"The more first-person time I can put in," replied Carmine, "the better. Is there anything to do around here when I'm off-duty, by the way?"

"If Fantasy is your thing," I said, "plenty. Moving cross-genre is not recommended, as the border guards can get jumpy, and it will never do to be caught in another genre just when you're needed. Oh, and don't do anything that my dodo might disapprove of."

"Such as what?"

"The list is long. Here we are."

We had arrived on the top of a low rise where there was a convenient park bench. From this vantage point, we could see most of Fiction Island.

"That's an impressive sight," said Carmine.

There was no aerial haze in the Book-World, and because the island was mildly dished where it snuggled against the interior of the sphere, we could see all the way to the disputed border between Racy Novel and Women's Fiction in the far north of the island, and beyond that the unexplored Dismal Woods.

"That's the Metaphoric River," I explained, pointing out the sinuous bends of the waterway whose many backwaters, bayous, streams and rivulets brought narrative ambiguity and unnecessarily lengthy words to the millions of books that had made their home in the river's massive delta. "To the east of Racy Novel is Outdated Religious Dogma."

"Shouldn't that be in Nonfiction?" asked Carmine.

"It's a contentious issue. It was removed from Theology on the grounds that the theories had become 'untenable in a modern context' and 'were making us look medieval.' "

"And that island off the coast of Dogma?" she asked, pointing to a craggy island partially obscured by cloud.

"The smaller of the two is Sick Notes, and

the larger is Lies, Self-Delusion and Excuses You Can Use to Justify Poor Behavior. South of Dogma is Horror, then Fantasy, with Adventure and Science Fiction dominating the south coast."

"I'll never remember all that."

I handed her my much-thumbed copy of *Bradshaw's BookWorld Companion.* "Use this," I said, showing her the foldout map section and train timetables. "I've got the new edition on order."

Whilst we had been sitting there, the recently evicted book had been unbolted by a team of Worker Danvers.

"*Raphael's Walrus* has been unread for over two years," I explained, "so it's off to the narrative doldrums of the suburbs. Not necessarily permanent, of course — a resurgence of interest could bring it back into the more desirable neighborhoods in an instant."

"How come your series is still here?" she asked, then put her hand over her mouth. "Sorry, was that indelicate of me?"

"No, most people ask that. The Text Grand Central Mapping Committee keeps us here out of respect."

"For you?"

"No — for the *real* Thursday Next."

A smattering of soil and pebbles descended to earth as *Raphael's Walrus* rose into the air, the self-sealing throughput and feedback conduits giving off faint puffs of word vapor as they snapped shut. This was how the new Geographic BookWorld worked. Books arrived, books left, and the boundaries of the various genres snaked forwards and backwards about the land, reflecting the month-to-month popularity of the various genres. The Crime genre was always relatively large, as were Comedy, Fantasy and Science Fiction. Horror had gotten a boost recently with the burgeoning Urban Vampires sector, while some of the lesser-known genres had shrunk to almost nothing. Squid Action/Adventure was deleted quite recently, and Sci-Fi Horse Detective looked surely set to follow.

But the vacated area was not empty for long. As we watched, the first of many prefabricated sections of the new book arrived, fresh from the construction hangars in the Well of Lost Plots. The contractors quickly surveyed the site, pegged out strings and then signaled to large transporter slipcases that were hovering just out of sight. Within a few minutes, handling ropes were dropped as the sections moved into a hover thirty feet or so above, and the same small army of Worker Danvers, cheering and grunting, maneuvered the sections into position, and then riveted them in place with pneumatic hammers. The first setting to be completed was a semiruined castle, then a mountain range, then a forest — with each tree, rabbit, unicorn and elf carefully unpacked from crates. Other sections soon followed, and within forty minutes the entire novel had been hauled in piecemeal from the overhead, riveted down and attached to the telemetry lines and throughput conduits.

"It's a good idea to be neighborly," I said. "You never know when you might need to borrow a cupful of irony. Besides, you might find this interesting."

We walked up the drive and across the drawbridge into the courtyard. Notices were posted everywhere that contained useful directions such as THIS WAY TO THE DENOUEMENT or NO BOOTS TO BE WORN IN THE BACKSTORY and even DO NOT FEED THE AMBIGUITY. The contractors were making last-minute adjustments. Six were arranging the clouds, two were wiring the punctuation to the main distribution board, three were trying to round up a glottal stop that wasn't meant to be there, and two others had just slit a barrage balloon full of atmosphere. The ambience escaped like a swarm of tiny midges and settled upon the fabric of the book, adding texture and style.

"Hello!" I said to the cast, who were standing around looking bewildered, their heads stuffed unrealistically full of Best Newcomer prizes and a permanent place in every reader's heart. They were about to be published and read for the first time. They would be confused, apprehensive and in need of guidance. I was so glad I wasn't them.

"My name's Thursday Next, and I just dropped in to welcome you to the neighborhood."

"This is indeed an honor, Miss Next," said the king, "and welcome to *Castle of Skeddan Jiarg.* We've heard of your exploits in the BookWorld, and I would like to say on behalf of all of us —"

"I'm not that one," I replied, before it all got embarrassing. I had denied I was the *real* Thursday Next more times than I would care to remember. Sometimes I went through an entire week doing little else.

"I'm the *written* Thursday Next," I explained.

"Ah," said one of several wizards who seemed to be milling around. "So you're not Jurisfiction, then?"

"I got as far as a training day," I replied,

which was still a proud boast, even if I had been rejected for active service. It was annoying but understandable. Few make the grade to be a member of Fiction's policing elite. I wasn't tough enough, but it wasn't my fault. I was written to be softer and kinder — the Thursday who Thursday herself thought she wanted to be. In any event, it made me too empathetic to get things done in the dangerously dynamic landscape of the BookWorld.

They all returned my greeting, but I could see they had lost interest. I asked them if I could show Carmine around, and they had no objections, so we wandered into the grand hall, which was all lime-washed walls, flaming torches, hammerhead beams and flagstones. Some of the smaller props were only cardboard cutouts, and I noted that a bowl of fruit was no more than a Post-it note with "bowl of fruit" written on it.

"Why only a Post-it?" asked Carmine. "Why not a real bowl of fruit?"

"For economic reasons," I replied. "Every novel has only as much description as is necessary. In years past, each book was carefully crafted to an infinitely fine degree, but that was in the days of limited reader sophistication. Today, with the plethora of experience through increased media exposure, most books are finished by the readers themselves."

"The Feedback Loop?"

"Precisely. As soon as the readers get going, the Feedback Loop will start backwashing some of their interpretations into the book itself. Not that long ago, books could be stripped bare by overreading, but since the invention of the loop, not only do books suffer little internal wear but readers often *add* detail by their own interpretations. Was that a goblin?"

I had just seen a small creature with pixie ears and sharp teeth staring at us from behind a chair.

"Looks like it."

I sighed. Pickwick *would* have something new to complain about.

"What is Thursday like?" asked Carmine.

I got asked this a lot. "You've heard the stories?"

She nodded. Most people had. For over fifteen years, Thursday Next had worked at Jurisfiction, tirelessly patrolling the BookWorld like a narrative knight-errant, bringing peace and justice to the very edge of acceptable prose. She was head and shoulders above the other agents — giants like Commander Bradshaw, Emperor Zhark, Mrs. Tiggy-winkle or even the Drunk Vicar.

"Did she really take Hamlet into the Real-World?" asked Carmine, excited by my mentor's audaciousness.

"Among others."

"And defeat Yorrick Kaine?"

"That, too."

"What about the Great Samuel Pepys Fiasco? Did they *really* have to delete two weeks of his diary to make everything okay?"

"That was the least of her worries. Even Thursday had occasional failures — it's inevitable if you're at the top of your game. Mind you," I added, unconsciously defending my famous namesake, "if Samuel Pepys hadn't set Deb up in a pied-à-terre in the backstory of *Sons and Lovers* with Iago coming in for half-costs on alternate weekdays, it would never have escalated into the disaster it became. They could have lost the entire diaries and, as a consequence, anything in Nonfiction that used the journal as a primary source. It was only by changing the historical record to include a 'Great Fire of London' that never actually happened that Thursday managed to pull anything from the debacle. History wouldn't speak to the council for months, but Sir Christopher Wren was delighted."

We walked back out into the courtyard. The king and queen invited us around for a "pre-reading party" that evening, and I responded by inviting them around for tea and cakes the following day. Thus suitably introduced, we made our way out to the street again.

"So how do you want me to play you?" asked Carmine.

"You're not playing *me,* you're playing *her.* There's a big difference. Although I've been Thursday for so long that sometimes I think I am her, I'm not. I'm just the written her. But in answer to your question, I try to play her dignified. I took over from the *other* written Thursday — long story, don't ask — soon after the Great Samuel Pepys Fiasco was deleted — even longer story, still don't ask — and the previous Thursday played her a little disrespectfully, so I'm trying to redress that."

"I heard that the violent and gratuitous-sex Thursday had a lot more readers."

I glared at Carmine, but she simply stared back at me with big innocent eyes. She was making a statement of fact, not criticism.

"We'll get the readers back somehow," I replied, although I wasn't wholly convinced.

"Can I meet the real Thursday?" asked Carmine in a hopeful tone of voice. "For research purposes, naturally."

"She's very busy, and I don't like to

bother her."

I was exaggerating my influence. Despite overseeing my creation, the real Thursday didn't like me much, possibly for the very same reasons she thought she might be improved. I think it was a RealWorld thing: the gulf between the person you want to be and the person you are.

"Look," I said, "just play her dignified — the individual interpretation is up to you. Until you get into the swing of it, play her subtly different on alternate readings. Hamlet's been doing it for years. Of course, he has twenty-six different ways of playing himself, but then he's had a lot of practice. In fact, I don't think even he knows his motivation anymore — unless you count confusing readers and giving useful employment to Shakespearean scholars."

"You've met Hamlet?"

"No, but I saw the back of his head at last year's BookWorld Conference."

"What was it like?" asked Carmine, who seemed to enjoy celebrity tittle-tattle.

"The back of his head? Hairy," I replied cautiously, "and it might not have been him. In any event, keep your interpretation loose, and don't telegraph. Let the readers do the work. If you're going to explain *everything,* then we might as well give up and tell everyone to stick to television and movies."

"Were there any goblins?" asked Pickwick as soon as we walked back in.

"I didn't see any. Did you, Miss O'Kipper?"

"No, no, not a single one."

"Mrs. Malaprop," I said, "we'll be having royalty for tea tomorrow. Better bake some silver and have the buns cleaned."

"Very good, Mizzen Exe."

"Here," I said to Carmine, handing her the complete script for my part. "I have to go out for an hour. I'll test you on it when I get back."

She suddenly looked nervous. "What if someone starts to read us while you're away?"

"They won't," I replied, "and if they do, Mrs. Malaprop will point you in the right dictation. Just take it smooth and easy. The rest of the cast will help you along."

"What do I do with Skimmers?" she asked with a faint tinge of panic in her voice. All rookies feared Dippers, Skimmers and Last-Chapter-Firsters.

"There's no hard-and-fast rule. Skimmers move in a generally forward direction, and with experience you'll figure out where they're going to land next. But the main thing is not to waste time with the nuisance reader — in a word, *prioritize.* Find the stable, methodical, bread-and-butter readers and give them your best. Leave the Skimmers and Dippers high and dry if there's a crisis. When things die down later, you can pick them up then."

"And students?"

"A breeze. They'll pause at the end of each sentence to think quasi-intellectual deep thoughts, so as soon as a full stop looms, you can be off dealing with someone else. When you get back, they'll still be pondering about intertextuality, inferred narratives and the scandalously high price of the subsidized beer in the student union."

She was quiet and attentive, so I carried on.

"You should show no discrimination with readers. Treat the lip movers as you would the *New York Times* critic. You might not be able to distinguish between the two at first, but you soon will. Yossarian said that you can get to know individual readers by the *way* they read you. Mind you, he's been doing it a long time, and *Catch-22* gets reread a lot."

"You've met Yossarian?"

"He was just leaving the room after giving a talk. I saw his foot."

"Left or right?"
"Left."
"I met someone who was beaten about the head boy Sir John Falstaff," remarked Mrs. Malaprop in an attempt to show that she, too, hobnobbed with celebrities.
"I talked to someone who held Pollyanna's hat for three whole pages," added Carmine.
"Small fry," remarked Pickwick, eager to outdo us all. "Sam Spade *himself* actually spoke to me."
There was silence. This was impressive.
"What did he say?"
"He said, 'Get that stupid bird out of my way.' "
"Well, pretend to be a soldier and elope with my ward," remarked Mrs. Malaprop, her word choice rendered clean and clear by the sarcasm. "You can dine out on *that* one for years."
"It's better than your dumb Falstaff story."
"The thing to remember," I remarked, to stop the argument before it got to the next few stages, which were insults, crockery throwing and punches, "is that the more readers there are, the easier it becomes. If you relax, it actually becomes a great deal of fun. The words spring naturally to your lips, and you can concentrate on not just giving the best possible performance but

also dealing with any readers who are having problems — or indeed any readers who are trying to *cause* trouble for you and change the book. You'll be surprised by how strong the power of reader suggestion can get, and if you let readers get the upper hand, it'll be *Smilla's Sense of Snow* all over again."

Carmine looked thoughtful. The Sea Worms incident was a sobering lesson for everyone, and something that no one wanted to repeat.

"I'll be back as soon as I can," I said, preparing to leave. "I have to meet with Commander Herring. Mrs. Malaprop, will you show Carmine around the series and do the introductions? Start with the Gravitube and the Diatryma. After that it's all fairly benign."

4.
The Red-Haired Gentleman

> Despite the remaking of the BookWorld, some books remained tantalizingly out of reach. The entire Sherlock Holmes canon was the most obvious example. It was entirely possible that they didn't know there was a BookWorld and still thought they were real. A fantastic notion, until you consider that up until 11:06 A.M. of April 12, 1948, everyone else had thought the same. Old-timers still speak of "the Great Realization" in hushed tones and refer to the glory days when the possibility of being imaginary was only for the philosophers.
>
> *Bradshaw's BookWorld Companion*
> (4th edition)

I stepped out of the front door and walked the eight blocks to the corner of Adams and Colfer. A bus arrived in a couple of minutes — they always do — and after showing my pass to the driver, who looked suspiciously like a Dr. Seuss character on furlough, I took a seat between a Viking and a nun.

"I'm on my way to a pillage," said the Viking as he attempted to find some common ground on which to converse, "and we're a bit lean in the 'beating people to death with large hammers' department. Would you like to join us?"

"That's most kind, but it's really not my thing."

"Oh, go on, you might rather like it."

"No thank you."

"I see," said the Viking in a huffy tone. "Please yourself, then." And he lapsed into silence.

It was the nun's turn to speak.

"I'm collecting," she said with a warm smile, "for the St. Nancy's Home for Fallen Women."

"Fallen in what respect?"

"Fallen *readership.* Those poor unfortunate wretches who, through no fault of their own, now find themselves in the ignominious status of the less well read. Are you interested?"

"Not really."

"Well," said the nun, "how *completely* selfish of you. How would you like to be hardly read at all?"

"I *am* hardly read at all," I told her, mustering as much dignity as I could. There was an unfair stigma attached to those characters who weren't read, and making us into victims in need of saving didn't really help, to be honest.

The Viking looked at me scornfully, then got up and went to the front of the bus to pretend to talk to someone. The nun joined him without another word, and I saw them glance in my direction and shake their heads sadly.

I took the bus across the Fantasy/Human Drama border, then changed to a tram at Hemingway Central. In the six months since the BookWorld had been remade, its citizens had learned much about their new surroundings. It was easier to understand; we had usable maps, a chain of outrageously expensive coffee shops in which to be seen, known as Stubbs, and most important, a network of road, rail and river to get from one place to another. We now had buses, trams, taxis, cars and even paddlewheel steamers. Bicycles might have been useful, but for some reason they didn't work inside the BookWorld — no matter what anyone did, they just wouldn't stay up. Jumping directly from book to book had rapidly become unfashionable and was looked upon as hopelessly Pulp. If you really wanted to be taken seriously and display a sense of cool unhurried insouciance, you walked.

"So what do you think?" asked a red-haired, jowly gentleman who had sat next to me. He was dressed in a double-breasted blue suit with a dark tie secured by a pearl tiepin. His hair was long but combed straight, and there seemed rather a lot of it. So much, in fact, that he had gathered the bright red locks that grew from his cheeks into fine plaits, each bound with a blue ribbon. Aside from that, his deep-set eyes had a kindly look, and I felt immediately at ease in his company.

"What do I think about what?"

"This," he said, waving a hairy hand in the direction of the new BookWorld.

"Not enough pianos," I said after a moment's reflection, "and we could do with some more ducks — and fewer baobabs."

"I'd prefer it to be more like the Real-World," said the red-haired gentleman with a sigh. "Our existence in here is very much life at second hand. I'd love to know what a mistral felt like, how the swing and drift of fabric might look and what *precisely* it is about a sunset or the Humming Chorus that makes them so astonishing."

This was a sentiment I could agree with.

"For me it would be to hear the rattle of rain on a tin roof or see the vapor rise from a warm lake in the chill morning air."

We fell silent for a moment as the tram rumbled on. I didn't tell him what I yearned for above all, the most underappreciated luxury of the human race: free will. My life was by definition preordained. I had to do what I was written to do, say what I was written to say, without variance, all day every day, whenever someone read me. Despite conversations like this, where I could think philosophically rather than narratively, I could never shrug off the peculiar feeling that someone was controlling my movements and eavesdropping on my every thought.

"I'm sure it's not all hot buttered crumpets out there in the breathing world of asphalt and heartbeats," I said by way of balance.

"Oh, I agree," replied the red-haired gentleman, who had, I noticed, nut-brown hands with fingers that were folded tight along the knuckle. "For all its boundless color, depth, boldness, passion and humor, the RealWorld doesn't appear to have any clearly discernible function."

"Not that better minds than ours haven't tried to find one."

The jury had been out on this matter for some time. Some felt that the RealWorld was there only to give life to us, while others insisted that it *did* have a function, to which no one was yet party. There was a small group who suggested that the RealWorld was not real at all and was just another book in an even bigger library. Not to be outdone, the nihilists over in Philosophy insisted that reality was as utterly meaningless as it appeared.

"What is without dispute," said my friend once we had discussed these points, "is that the readers need us just as much as we need them — to bring order to their apparent chaos, if nothing else."

"Who are you?" I asked, unused to hearing such matters discussed on a Number 23 tram.

"Someone who cannot be saved, Miss Next. I have done terrible things."

I started at the mention of my name and was suddenly suspicious. Our chance meeting was no chance meeting. In fiction they rarely are. But then again, he might have thought I was the *other* Thursday Next.

"Sir, I'm not her."

He looked at me and smiled. "You're more alike than you suppose."

"Physically, perhaps," I replied, "but I

flunked my Jurisfiction training."

"On occasion, people of talent are kept in reserve at times of crisis."

I stared at him for a moment. "Why are you telling me this?"

"I don't have much time. I think they saw us talking. Heed this and heed it well: *One of our Thursdays is missing!*"

"What do you mean?"

"This: Trust no one but yourself."

"Which 'yourself'? I have several. Me, the real me and Carmine who is being me when I'm not me."

He didn't get to answer. The tram lurched, and with a sharp squeal of the emergency brakes we ground to a halt. The reason we had stopped was that two highly distinctive 1949 Buick Roadmaster automobiles were blocking the road, and four men were waiting for us. The cars and their occupants were among the more iniquitous features of the remaking. The Council of Genres, worried about increased security issues with the freedom of movement, had added another tier of law enforcement to the BookWorld. Shadowy men and women who were accountable only to the council and seemed to know no fear or restraint: the Men in Plaid.

The doors of the tram hissed open, and

one of the agents climbed inside. He wore a well-tailored suit of light green plaid with a handkerchief neatly folded in his top pocket.

I turned to the red-haired gentleman to say something, but he had moved across the aisle to the seat opposite. The Man in Plaid's eye fell upon my new friend, and he quickly strode up and placed a pistol to his head.

"Don't make any sudden movements, Kiki," ordered the Man in Plaid. "What are you doing so far outside Crime?"

"I came to Fantasy to look at the view."

"The view is the same as anywhere else."

"I was misinformed."

The red-haired gentleman was soon handcuffed. With a dramatic flourish, the Man in Plaid pulled out a bloodstained straight razor from the red-haired gentleman's pocket. A gasp went up from the occupants of the tram.

"This lunatic has been AWOL from his short story for twenty-four hours," announced the agent. "You are fortunate to have survived."

The red-haired gentleman was pulled from the tram and bundled into the back of one of the Buick Roadmasters, which then sped from the scene.

The Man in Plaid came back on the tram

and stared at us all in turn.

"A consummate liar, whose manipulative ways have seen two dead already. Did he say anything to anyone?"

The red-haired gentleman had admitted to me that he'd done terrible things, but that wasn't unusual. Out of their books, crazed killers could be as pleasant as pie.

"He murdered two women," continued the first Man in Plaid, presumably in order to loosen our tongues. "He cut the throat of one and strangled the other. Now, did he say anything to anybody?"

I remained silent, and so did everyone else. In the short time the Men in Plaid had been operational, people had learned they were simply trouble and best not assisted in any way.

"Are you a Man in Plaid?" asked one of the passengers.

The man stared at the passenger in a way you wouldn't like to be stared at. "It's not plaid. It's tartan."

The agent, apparently satisfied that the red-haired gentleman had not spoken to anyone, stepped off the tram, and the doors hissed shut. I shivered as a sudden sense of foreboding shuffled through the four hundred or so verbs, nouns and similes that made up my being. The red-haired gentleman had told me he thought that "one of our Thursdays is missing," and by that I took him to mean Thursday Next, the *real* Thursday Next. My flesh-and-blood alter-better ego. But I didn't get to muse on it any further, for a few minutes later we arrived at the border between Human Drama and Thriller.

5.
Sprockett

The logic of cog-based intelligences is unimpeachable. Unlike the inferior electronics-based intelligences, they cannot show error, for the constantly enmeshed cogs, wheels and drives never slip or jump. I think one can safely attest that there is no puzzle that Men of the Cog cannot solve, given sufficient oil, facts and winds.

Bradshaw's BookWorld Companion
(6th edition)

There was a queue to cross into Thriller, bookpeople either being permanently transferred or on a Character Exchange Program designed to stop characters from getting bored, restless and troublesome. There were a few traveling artisans, salesmen and a dozen or so tourists, apparently on a Get Beaten Senseless by Bourne package holiday, which had just overtaken the Being

Shot in the Leg by Bond break for popularity, much to the Fleming camp's disgust.

As little as two months ago, I would have been waved across with nary a glance, but the heightened security risk due to the potentially inflammable political situation up at Racy Novel had made everyone jumpy.

I took a TransGenre Taxi as far as the Legal part of Thriller, then continued on foot. I took a left turn by *The Firm* and picked my way along a weed-covered path and across a plank that spanned a ditch of brackish water, the best method to get into Conspiracy without being waylaid by deluded theorists, who always wanted to explain in earnest terms that President Formby was murdered by President Redmond van de Poste, that bestselling author Colwyn Baye was far too handsome and clever and charming to be anything other than an android or a reptile or an alien or all three.

I took a left turn at the Lone Gunman pub, and walked past a hangar full of advanced flying machines that all displayed a swastika, then entered a shantytown that was home to theories that lived right on the edge of Conspiracy due to a sense of overtired outrageousness. This was where the *Protocols* lived, along with alien abductions,

9/11 deniers and the notion that FDR somehow knew about the attack on Pearl Harbor. I had hoped I might tread unnoticed within the genre, but I was mistaken. Despite avoiding eye contact, I was spotted by a wild-looking loon with hair that stuck out in every direction.

"There's no such thing as time," he confided, with an unwavering sense of belief in his own assertions. "It's simply a construct designed by a cabal of financiers eager to sell us pensions, life insurance and watches in their pursuit of a global, timepiece-marketing agenda."

"Really?" I asked, which is probably the only answer to anything in Conspiracy.

"Definitely. And the seal is not a mammal — it's an insect. The truth has been suppressed by the BBC and Richard Attenborough, who want to promote a global mammalcentric agenda."

"Don't you mean *David* Attenborough?"

"So you agree?" he said, eyes opening so wide I was suddenly worried I might see his brain. "Would you like to stone a robot?"

"What?"

"Stone a robot. Just one of the first generation of mechanical men, designed to be placed amongst us in order to take over the planet and promote a clockwork, global cog-centric agenda."

"I'm not really into stoning anyone."

"Oh, well," said the theorist as he picked a rock off the ground. "Suit yourself."

And he walked off. Intrigued and somewhat concerned, I followed him to New World Order Plaza, where a small crowd had gathered. They were an odd bunch that comprised everything from small gray aliens to reptilian shape-shifters, Men in Black, Elvises, lost cosmonauts and a smattering of Jimmy Hoffa/Lord Lucan secret genetic hybrids. They were arranged in a semicircle around a tall man dressed in a perfectly starched frock coat, striped trousers and white gloves. Of his clockwork robotic origins there seemed little doubt. His porcelain face was bland and featureless, the only moving part his right eyebrow, which was made of machined steel and could point to an array of emotions painted in small words upon the side of his head. From the look of him, his mainspring was at the very last vestige of tension — he had shut down all peripheral motor functions, and if his eyes had not scanned backwards and forwards as I watched, I might have thought he had run down completely.

"They banish us here to Fiction," said a rabble-rousing gray alien, pointing his finger in the air, "when we should be up there, in Nonfiction."

The crowd agreed wholeheartedly with this sentiment and clacked their stones together angrily.

"And then," continued the alien, "they have the temerity to send robots amongst us to spy on our every movement and report back to a centralized index that holds the records of everyone in the BookWorld, all as a precursor to thought-control experiments that will rob us of our minds and make us into mere drones, lackeys of the publishing world. What do we say to the council? Do we politely say, 'No thank you,' or do we send their messenger home in a sack?"

The crowd roared. I didn't know much about Conspiracy, but I did know that its theorists were mostly paranoid and tended to value conviction above evidence.

I was just wondering what, if anything, could be done to stop the needless destruction of a finely crafted automaton when the mechanical man caught my eye, and with the last few ounces of spring pressure available to him, he moved his eyebrow pointer among an array of emotions in a manner that spoke of fear, loss, betrayal and hopelessness. The last plea from a condemned machine. Something shifted within me, and before I knew what I was doing, I had spoken up.

"There you are!" I said in a loud voice as I strode into the semicircle of stone-wielding conspirators. "I *knew* I should have given you an extra wind at lunchtime."

The aliens and Elvises and alien Elvises looked at one another suspiciously.

"Thursday Next," I said as I searched the automaton's pockets for his key. The crowd looked doubtful, and the alien ringleader blinked at me oddly, his large, teardrop-shaped eyes utterly devoid of compassion.

"Thursday Next is too important to trouble herself with the fortunes of a mechanical man," he said thinly, "and she told me personally she would rather kneel on broken glass than ever visit Conspiracy again."

This was doubtless true, and I could see why.

"You are an impostor," said the alien, "sent by the council as part of a plan to destabilize our genre and promote your own twisted evidence-centric agenda."

There was a nasty murmuring among the crowd as with fumbling hand I found the large brass key and inserted it into the socket located on the back of the automa-

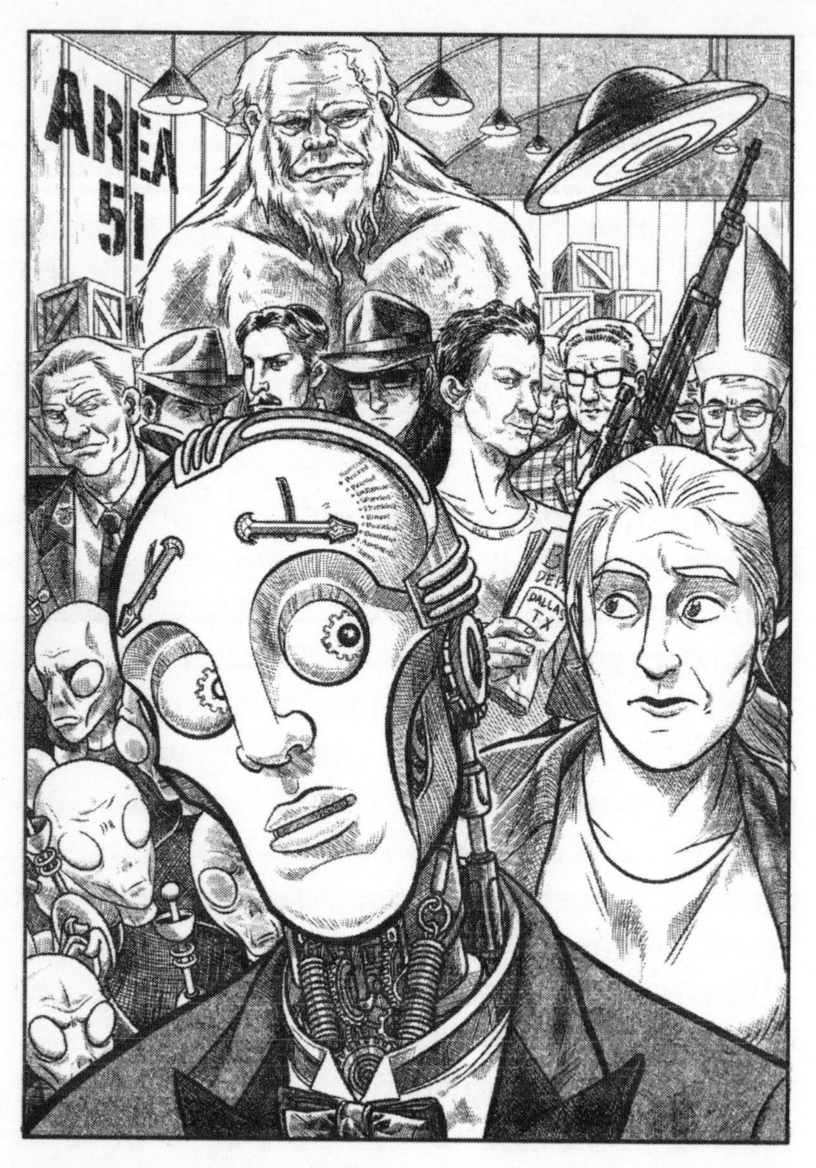

. . . and with the last few ounces of spring pressure available to him, he moved his eyebrow pointer among an array of emotions in a manner that spoke of fear, loss, betrayal and hopelessness.

ton's neck. I gave him a quick wind to get him started, and I felt his body shift slightly as the gyros, motors, cogs and actuators started to reboot his mechanical cortex.

"You're the *written* one," said someone at the back. "The dopey one who likes to hug a lot."

The situation had just taken a turn for the worse. But since this was Conspiracy and facts weren't necessarily the end of an argument, I thought I'd try a bluff. I reached into my pocket and held out my JAID shield. From a distance it might be confused with a Jurisfiction badge. I had to hope that no one would look too closely.

"Read it and weep," I said, swallowing down my nervousness. "Make a move on me and I'll have Jurisfiction dump forty tons of Intelligently Reasoned Argument right on your butt."

"So *you* say," said the small alien. "Elvis? Check her badge."

The two dozen Elvises looked at one another and began to squabble as they tried to figure out which Elvis the alien was talking to, and once this was established, I had half wound the mechanical man. If it came to a fight, I wouldn't be on my own.

"Steady on, lads," said the Elvis after looking at my badge. "She's not bluffing — it's her all right."

"I am?" I said, then quickly added, "Yes, I am. Now piss off."

The small group hurriedly made some excuse about having to view some reverse-engineered alien technology hidden in a hangar somewhere in a desert, and within a few moments the clockwork man and I were entirely alone.

"Permission to speak, madam?" said the automaton once I had wound him sufficiently to reboot his memory and thought processes. He spoke with the rich, plummy tones of the perfect gentleman's gentleman, but with a faint buzz — a bit like a bumble-bee stuck inside a cello.

"Of course."

"I am one of the older Duplex-5 models, so if madam would only wind me as far as twenty-eight turns, I would be most grateful. My spring will take a full thirty-two, but the last four winds have an *unpredictable* effect upon my central reasoning gears that render me unable to offer my best."

"I'll remember that," I said.

"And if I might be so bold," added the clockwork man, "I would highly recommend that you do not let me fall *below* two winds, as I fear I might become somewhat languorous in my movements and may stray unforgivably into short-tempered impertinence."

"Between two and twenty-eight it is."

I finished winding him but, as requested, was careful not to go beyond the red mark on the mainspring tension indicator just under his chin. Once I was done, he turned to face me, and his single expressive eyebrow quivered momentarily and then pointed to "Uncomfortable." I knew exactly what he meant: that the winding of a manservant is a mildly embarrassing undertaking, and to preserve both employer and employee's mutual respect, should not be commented upon again.

"That's a very useful eyebrow."

"It's a standard feature of the Duplex-5s. Since we have few genuine emotions, it helps to telegraph how we think we should be feeling, given the circumstances."

"It works for me, Mr. . . . ?"

"Sprockett," said Sprockett. "Ready and willing to enter your employ."

"I'm not sure I need a butler."

"In that you would be in error, ma'am. It has been long proved that *everyone* needs a butler. Besides, you saved my life."

It was complex, but I knew what he meant. Because I had saved him, he was indebted to me — and to refuse him an opportunity to reciprocate my kindness would leave him burdened by a favor unpaid. And if you had a potential life of a thousand years or more, you could be a long time fretting, and fretting increases wear on cogs. Clockwork life-forms could be annoyingly steadfast, but it was their saving grace, too.

"All right," I agreed, "but for a trial period only."

"Very good, ma'am. Would you care for a cocktail? I do a very good Tahiti Tingle — without the umbrella if you think they are a bit passé."

"Not now. I'm working."

"In Conspiracy, ma'am?"

I pointed at the book traffic that was moving constantly overhead.

"One of those came down last night, and I'm here to find out why."

"I see," said Sprockett, his eyebrow pointer nodding toward "Worried" as he looked upwards. "I will assist in whatever capacity I can."

We made our way toward the regional offices. Sprockett talked and thought well for an automaton, and aside from a slight limp, his empty features and a muted buzz when he moved or thought, he was reasonably lifelike. I asked him where he was from, and he told me he was from Vanity — in a pilot book for a series titled *The League of Cogmen,* about the many adventures that befall a series of mechanical men designed by an Edwardian inventor. Sprockett had been initially built as a butler but soon transcended his calling to become a dynamic machine of action. A mixture of *The Admirable Crichton, Biggles* and *The 1903 Watchmaker's Review.* When unemployment beckoned, he reverted to domestic service — butlers are more sought after than are action heroes.

"What was your book like?"

"Uneven," replied Sprockett. "A fine concept, but lacking in legs to carry it off. Sadly, I have too few emotions to be engaging as a principal character."

"Because you were designed as a butler?"

"Not at all — because I'm only a Duplex-5. The empathy escapement was never quite perfected before we went into production. I can indicate a range of emotions through my eyebrow pointer, but that's about it. I can recognize your sorrow and act accordingly — but I cannot feel emotions nor truly understand what 'emotion' or 'feel' actually means."

"But surely you felt danger when you were about to be stoned and relief when rescued?"

"Yes, but only in the context that to be destroyed would deny me the opportunity to serve cocktails — and that would contravene the second law of domestic robotics."

Sprockett told me that his books were hastily printed, had not been read once in seventeen years and now, aside from a few copies in the circulation of friends and family, were sitting unread in a cardboard box in the writer's garage in Cirencester.

"And becoming damp, too," he added. "Sometimes rain is blown under the garage doors. There is mold and damp seeping up the print run — look."

He rolled up a trouser leg to reveal a green patch of patination on his otherwise shiny bronze leg. His would be a long, lingering journey to unreadfulness. He would gradually look more tarnished and increasingly lost over the years until the last copy would be destroyed and — unless picked up in another book — he'd suddenly wink out of existence.

"What's it like living in Vanity?"

"May I be candid?"

"I'd welcome it."

"We tend not to use the term Vanity anymore. It sounds derogatory. We refer to it as Self-Published or Collaborative, and you'd be surprised just how much good prose is interspersed with that of an uneven nature."

This was true. Beatrix Potter, Keats and George Eliot had all been self-published, as was the first issue of *Alice in Wonderland.* I looked across to where the island of Vanity lay just off the coast beyond the Cliff of Notes. Even from here the high-stacked apartment buildings could clearly be seen. The turbulent waterway between Vanity and the mainland was swept with dangerous currents, whirlpools and tidal rips. Despite this, many Vanitarians attempted to make the perilous journey to brighter prospects on the mainland. Of those who survived, most were turned back.

"I'd like to come out and see the conditions for myself," I said, the unease in my voice setting Sprockett's eyebrow to flicker twice before pointing at "Worried."

"No, really," I said, "I would. You can't believe anything you read in *The Word* these days."

Sprockett demurred politely, but his eyebrow said it all — speaking of an entire genre kept marginalized, right on the edges of Fiction. The "Vanity Question" was one of many issues that had dogged the political elite since the remaking. The problem was, no published books liked anything self-published in the neighborhood. They argued — and quite eloquently, as it turned out — that the point of having similar books clustered in neighborhoods and genres was for mutual cross-fertilization of ideas, themes and topics. Having something from Vanity close by would, they claimed, "lower the tone of the prose." Liberal factions within the Council of Genres had attempted a cross-genre experiment and placed *The Man Who Died a Lot* right into the middle of McEwan on the basis that the localized erudition could only have a bettering effect on the Vanity book. It was a disaster. None of the characters within McEwan would talk to them and even claimed that some descriptive passages had been stolen. It was then that McEwan and the nearby Rushdie and Amis threatened to go on strike and lower their Literary Highbrow Index to a shockingly low 7.2 unless *The Man Who Died a Lot* was removed. The offending book was gone before teatime, and no one had tried anything since. Vanity's contribution to Fiction in general was an abundance of cheap labor and the occasional blockbuster, which was accepted onto the island with an apologetic, "Gosh, don't know how that happened."

We continued our walk through Conspiracy, past something odd that had been dug up on the Quantock Hills, and Sprockett asked me if I conducted many accident investigations.

"My last investigation was in a book-club edition of *Three Men in a Boat,* which had sprung a leak," I told him, "and lost forty thousand gallons of the river Thames as it passed across Crime Noir, where it fell quite helpfully as rain. My theory had been that it was a sticky pressure-relief valve on the comedy induction loops, probably as a result of substandard metaphor building up on the injectors. I penned an exhaustive report to Commander Herring, who congratulated me on my thoroughness but tactfully pointed out that comedy induction loops were not introduced until April 1956 — long *after* the book was built."

"Oh," said Sprockett, who perhaps had been expecting a story with a happier ending. "So what had *really* happened?"

I sighed. "Someone had simply left the plug out of the Thames and it had drained away."

We walked on in silence for a moment.

"Ma'am, if you would forgive the impertinence, might I place one small condition upon my employment?"

I nodded, so he continued.

"I have an overriding abhorrence for honey. No matter what happens, it always seems to end up in my insides, and it is the very devil to remove. In my last employ, my master insisted upon honey for breakfast, and a small quantity became lodged in my thought cogs. Until steam-cleaned, I became convinced I was the Raja of Sarawak."

"No honey," I said. "Promise."

And so, fully introduced, we talked about the much-heralded and much-delayed introduction of the advanced Duplex-6 clockwork automaton. And, after that, the relative merits of phosphor-bronze over stainless steel for knee joints. So it was that I arrived, thoroughly versed in the Matters of the Cog, at the regional Conspiracy offices a few minutes later.

6.
The Bed-Sitting Room

The ISBN security numbering system achieved little. Thieves simply moved into stealing and trading sections of older books. The members of the Out-of-Print Brigade were furious; after looking forward to a long and happy retirement, they instead found their favorite armchairs pinched from under them as they dozed. Entire books were stripped of all nouns, and in the very worst cases large sections of dramatic irony were hacked from the books and boiled down to extract the raw metaphor, rendering once-fine novels mere husks suitable only for scrapping.

Bradshaw's BookWorld Companion
(14th edition)

The local genre representative was sitting on a wicker chair on the veranda of his office, a clapboard affair that looked much ravaged by overreading. The rep was described as what we termed “UK-6 Aristocracy Dapper-12,” which meant that he had a fine pencil mustache and spoke as though he were from the Royal Academy of Dramatic Art. I told Sprockett to wait for me outside, which he unhesitatingly agreed to do.

The rep did not rise from his chair and instead looked me up and down and then said in a disparaging tone, “You’re a long way from Mind, Body and Soul, old girl.”

It’s true that I may have looked a bit New Agey, but I didn’t really need this. Bolstered by my earlier claim to be the real Thursday, I decided to try the same here.

“The name’s Thursday Next,” I said, waving my shield. The reaction was electric. He choked on his afternoon tea and crumpet and, in his hurry to get to his feet, nearly woke a large and very hairy Sasquatch who dozed in a wicker chair a little way down the veranda.

“Good gracious!” exclaimed the genre rep. “Please excuse me. The name’s Bilderberg. Roswell Bilderberg. My office is your office. Hey!” He kicked the foot of the Sasquatch, who opened one eye and stared at him indifferently. “Thursday Next,” hissed Roswell, nodding in my direction.

The Sasquatch opened his eyes wide and

jumped to his feet. "I was nowhere near the Orient Express that evening," he said hurriedly, "and even if I was, I had nothing against Mr. Cassetti — isn't that right, Roswell?"

"Don't drag me into your web of deceit," replied Roswell out of the side of his mouth, still smiling at me. "Now, how can we help you, Miss Next? Pleasure or business?"

"*Official* business," I said as the Sasquatch nonchalantly picked up a set of snowshoes and sneaked guiltily away.

"What sort of official business?" asked Roswell suspiciously. "We've heard that the Council of Genres was planning on moving us across to Juvenilia as part of a secret cross-BookWorld plan to marginalize those genres that don't toe the official line. And if we didn't comply, we would all be murdered in our sleep by government assassins who can drip poison into your ear down a thread — if such a thing is possible, or even likely."

As far as I knew, no such plans were afoot. But you didn't live in Conspiracy for long without imagining all sorts of nonsense. Not that Conspiracy always got it wrong. On the few occasions they *were* correct, a rapid transfer to Nonfiction was in order — which threw those who were left behind into something of a dilemma. Being in Fiction meant a wider readership, something that Nonfiction could never boast. Besides, a conspiracy theory that turned out to be real wasn't a theory anymore, and the loss of wild uncorroborated speculation could be something of a downer.

"I'm working with JAID — the Jurisfiction Accident Investigation Department."

"Ah!" he replied, suddenly realizing what I was here for. "The Lola incident. I believe that Commander Herring is already up there. Can I stress at this time that we will afford Jurisfiction's representatives all possible help and assistance?"

It was all he could say, really. No one wanted to fall afoul of Jurisfiction or the Council of Genres. This was Fiction. There were skeletons in everyone's closet.

"It came to earth nine hours ago," he said as we walked past two faked moon landings, three UFO abductions and a grassy knoll. "It bounced on a pamphlet regarding the notion that Diatrymas are being bred by the Goliath Corporation to keep people out of the New Forest, then landed on a book outlining the somewhat dubious circumstances surrounding the death of Lola Vavoom."

With Sprockett following at a discreet distance, we took a shortcut through a field of crop circles, passed a laboratory covertly designing infectious diseases for population control, moved aside as a white Fiat Uno drove after a black Mercedes, then entered the subgenre of Lola Vavoom Suspicious Death. Roswell pushed open the swinging doors of a concrete multistory car park that opened directly onto the tenth floor, and standing next to a large lump of tattered wreckage the size of a truck were two men. I didn't recognize the more disheveled of the two, but the older, wiser and clearly the boss was someone I did recognize: Regional Commander Herring of the BookWorld Policing Agency.

He was very much a hands-on type of administrator. He had no staff, carried all his notes in his head and was one of the few people who still jumped from book to book rather than taking a taxi or public transport. He was a BGH-87 character type. Male, persnickety and highly efficient, but seemingly without humor. He was about fifty and was dressed in a short-sleeved white shirt with an infinite quantity of pens in his top pocket and a garish tie. He wore spectacles, but only for effect. He was high up in the chain of command at the Council of Genres and had access, it was said, to Senator Jobsworth himself. He was the most powerful man I knew.

"About time," he said when I appeared. "Places to be, people to visit — wheels within wheels."

"Wheels within wheels," echoed the man next to him.

"This is Martin Lockheed," explained Herring. "You'll answer to him, as I am a busy man. After this meeting I do not expect us to meet again."

"Yes, sir."

"Your *Three Men in a Boat* investigation didn't really impress," he began.

"Yes, I'm sorry about that."

"Apologies don't really cut it, Next, but I am a man loyal to friends, and the real Miss Next has always intimated in the past that you may show promise one day."

"I'm very grateful to her . . . and you," I managed to stammer.

"So I look upon you as an investment," replied Herring, "and a long-standing favor to a valued colleague. Which is why we are here now. Do you understand?"

"I think so."

"Good."

"That's good," said Lockheed, as if I might not have heard what Herring said. The regional commander waved a hand at the wreckage.

"Easy one for you to cut your teeth on. It has all the signs of being another unprecedented event that despite all expectations has become repeatedly unrepeatable. Don't let me down, will you? Wrap it up nice and neat and don't get all showy or anything. Fiction has a 99.97 percent book-safety record, and the last thing we want is the residents of this fair island worried that the fabric of their world is prone to shredding itself at the drop of a participle, hmm?"

"I'll do my very best to discover that it's an unrepeatable accident," I told him, "and with indecent haste."

"Very good. Twenty-four hours should suffice, yes?"

"I'll see what I can do, sir, and I'd like to thank you for the opportunity."

"No need. Lockheed?"

"Yes, sir?"

Herring snapped his fingers impatiently, and the rather harassed Lockheed passed him a clipboard.

"These are the reported items of debris," Herring said, handing the clipboard straight to me without looking at it. "Not good, having narrative falling from the skies, so let's keep it simple, eh? Wheels within wheels, Thursday."

"Wheels within wheels," added Lockheed

earnestly.

"Wheels within wheels, sir. Would you thank Miss Next for me when you see her?"

"When next I see her. She's very busy."

He then looked at Sprockett, who was standing off from the group, being unobtrusive. "Who's that?"

"Sprockett," I replied, "my butler."

"I didn't know you had a butler."

"Everyone needs a butler, sir."

"I have no argument with that. Duplex-3, is he?"

"Duplex-5, sir."

"The Fives were prone to be troublesome without sufficient winding. I'll let you get on. You can call Lockheed anytime you want for guidance. Any questions?"

I thought of asking him if he had seen the real Thursday Next recently but decided against it. The red-haired gentleman had spoken of "being able to trust no one but myself," and besides, I didn't want to look a fool if the man on the tram really *was* a murderous nutjob.

"No questions, sir."

"Good luck, Miss Next."

He gave me a half smile, shook my hand and vanished.

"I'll be off, too," said Lockheed, handing me a business card and a folder full of health-and-safety literature. "Commander Herring is a great and good man, and you are lucky to have been given this opportunity to converse. He doesn't usually speak to people as low as you."

"I'm honored."

"And so you should be. I was his assistant for three years before he deigned to look me in the eye. One of my proudest moments. If you need me, the JAID offices are at Norland Park."

And he walked off. Eager not to waste the opportunity I had just been given, I turned my attention to the wreckage.

The chunk of book had splintered off the main novel as it broke up. But this wasn't pages or ink or anything; it was a small part of *setting.* Despite the ragged textual word strings that were draped across and the graphemes lying scattered on the floor nearby, the misshapen lump seemed to be a room from a house somewhere. It had landed on the asphalt covering of the car park and cracked the surface so badly that the textual matrix beneath the roadway was now visible. The battered section had landed upside down just behind Lola Vavoom's Delahaye Roadster, which had prevented her from reversing too quickly from her parking place, breaking through the barriers and falling eighty feet to her death. It had always been a suspicious accident, but nothing untoward was ever found to suppose it wasn't just that — an accident.

"Will this take long, dahling?" asked Lola, who was dressed in tight slacks and a cashmere sweater with a pink scarf tied around her hair. Her eyes were obscured by a pair of dark glasses, and she was casually sitting on the trunk of her car smoking a small Sobranie cigarette.

"As long as it must," I said, "and I'm sorry for the inconvenience."

"Do your best, dear," she intoned patronizingly, "but if I'm not dead in mysterious circumstances by teatime, someone is going to have some serious explaining to do."

I turned my attention to the wreckage. Spontaneous breakups were uncommon but not unheard of, and it was JAID's job to try to find the cause so that other books wouldn't suffer the same fate. Losing a cast of a thousand or more was not just a personal tragedy, but expensive. When a book-club edition of *War and Peace* had disintegrated without warning a few years ago as it passed over Human Drama, all those within the debris field were picking brass buttons and lengthy digressions out of their hair for a week. The JAID investigator assigned to the case painstakingly reconstructed the book, only to find that a batch of verbs had been packed incorrectly at the aft expansion joint and had overheated. Punctuation lock had no effect, and in a last desperate attempt to bring the book under control, the engineers initiated Emergency Volume Separation. A good idea, but undertaken too quickly. The smaller and lighter Epilogues could not alter course in time and collided with Volume Four, which in turn collided with Volume Three, and so forth. Of the twenty-six thousand characters lost in the disaster, only five survived. Verb quality control and emergency procedures were dramatically improved after this, and nothing like it had happened since.

"It seems to be a bed-sitting room of some variety," murmured Sprockett as he peered inside the large lump of scrap. "Probably ten pounds a week — furnished, naturally."

"Naturally."

"Are we looking for anything in particular?"

"An International Standard Book Number," I said, "an ISBN. We need to know what the book is and where it came from before we can start trying to figure out what went wrong. It's sometimes harder than it seems. The wreckage is often badly mangled, widely scattered — and there are a lot of books out there."

We stepped into the upside-down bed-sitting room, all its contents strewn around inside. It was well described, so it was either a popular book given depth and color by reader feedback, or pre-feedback altogether. The room hadn't been painted for a while, the carpets were threadbare, and the furniture had seen better days. It might seem trivial, but it was these sorts of clues that allowed us to pinpoint which book it was from.

"Potboiler?" I suggested.

"It's from HumDram if it is," replied Sprockett as he picked up a torn *Abbey Road* album. "Post-1969, at any rate."

We searched for half an hour amongst the debris but found no sign of an ISBN.

"This book could be any one of thousands," said Sprockett.

"Millions."

With nothing more to see here, we stepped back outside the bed-sitting room, and I laid a map of the BookWorld on the hood of Lola's car and marked where the section had been found. This done, I called in Pickford Removals, and within twenty minutes the bed-sitting room had been loaded onto the back of a flatbed for onward delivery to the double garage at the back of my house. This was ostensibly to allow the books in which they had landed to carry on unhindered. Not that a ton of tattered paragraph would necessarily be a problem. The entire cast of *A Tale of Two Cities* has steadfastly ignored a runaway pink gorilla that has evaded capture for eighty-seven years but, as far as we know, has not been spotted by readers once.

"I'm sorry to have troubled you," I said to Lola, who stubbed out her cigarette and climbed into her car. She stomped on the accelerator, and the Delahaye shot across the car park, drove straight through the wooden barrier behind her and landed with a crunch on top of the Mairzy Doats sandwich bar ten stories below.

"Come on," I said to Sprockett. "Work to be done."

The debris field extended across four genres, and we spent the next three hours listening to residents who claimed that falling book junk had "completely ruined their entrance," and on one rare occasion it actually had. There was a reasonable quantity of wreckage, but nothing quite as large as the bed-sitting room. We found a yellow-painted back axle, the remains of at least nine tigers, a few playing cards, some lengths of silk, a hat stand, sections of a box-girder bridge, nine apples, parts of a raccoon and a quantity of slate. There was a lot of unrecognizable scrap, too, much of it desyntaxed sentences that made no sense at all. We found only one piece of human remains — a thumb — except it might not have been a thumb at all but simply reformed graphemes.

"Graphemes?" asked Sprockett when I mentioned it.

"Everything in the BookWorld is constructed of them," I explained. "Letters and punctuation — the building blocks of the textual world."

"So why might that thumb not actually be a thumb?"

"Because once broken down below the 'word' unit, a grapheme might come from anywhere. The same *s* can serve equally well in a sword, a sausage, a ship, a sailor or even the sun. It doesn't help that under extreme pressure and heat, graphemes often separate out and then fuse back together into something else entirely. At Jurisfiction basic training, we were shown how a 'sheet of card,' once heated up white-hot and then struck with a blacksmith's hammer, could be made into 'cod feathers' and then back again."

"Ah," said Sprockett, "I see."

"Because of this, anything under a few words long found at an accident site can be disregarded as evidence — it might once have been something else entirely." Oddly enough, the process of graphusion and graphission, while occurring naturally in the Text Sea, was hard to do synthetically in the BookWorld but simplicity itself in the Outland. The long and short of it was that victims of extreme trauma in the BookWorld were rarely found. A sprinkling of graphemes was soon absorbed into the fabric of the book it fell upon and left no trace.

Once Sprockett and I had logged everything we'd found and dispatched it via Pickford's to my double garage, I called Mrs. Malaprop to check that all was well. It was, generally speaking. Pickwick was suspicious that there really might be goblins around, and Carmine was spending her time rehearsing with the various members of the cast. Whitby Jett had called to say that now that Carmine was there, he would be taking me out to Bar Humbug for a drink and nibbles at nine — and no arguments.

I'd known him for nearly two years, and I think I'd just come to the end of a very long trail of excuses and reasons that I couldn't go out on a date. I sighed. There was still one. Perhaps the *only* one I'd ever had. I told Mrs. Malaprop I would be home in half an hour, thought for a moment and then turned to Sprockett.

"Can I shut you down for a while?"

"Madam, that is a *most* improper suggestion."

"I'm about to do something illegal, and since you are incapable of lying, I don't want you in a position where you have to divide your loyalties between your duties as a butler and your duties to the truth."

"Most thoughtful, ma'am. Conflicting loyalties do little but strip teeth off my cogs. Shall I shut down immediately?"

"Not yet."

We hailed a cab at the corner of Heller and Vonnegut. The cabbie had issues with clockwork people — "all that infernal ticking" — but since Sprockett was, legally speaking, nothing more nor less than a carriage clock, he was consigned to the trunk.

"I don't mind being treated as baggage," he said agreeably. "In fact, I prefer it. Promise you'll restart me?"

"I promise."

And after he had settled back against the spare tire, I pressed the emergency spring-release button located under his inspection cover. There was a loud whirring noise, and Sprockett went limp.

I shut the trunk, settled into the cab and closed the door.

"Where to?"

"Poetry."

7.
The Lady of Shalott

Here in the BookWorld, the protagonists and antagonists, gatekeepers, shape-shifters, heroes, villains, bit parts, knaves, comedians and goblins were united in that they possessed a clearly defined motive for what they were doing: entertainment and enlightenment. As far as any of us could see, no such luxury existed in the unpredictable world of the readers. The Outland was extraordinarily well named.

Bradshaw's BookWorld Companion
(4th edition)

The taxi was the usual yellow-and-check variety and could either run on wheels in the conventional manner or fly using advanced Technobabble™ vectored gravitational inversion thrusters. This had been demanded by the Sci-Fi fraternity, who had been whingeing on about hover cars and jet packs for decades and needed appeasing before they went and did something stupid, like allow someone to make a movie based on the title of the book known as *I, Robot.*

The driver was an elderly woman with white hair who grumbled about how she had just given a fare to three Triffids and how they hadn't bothered to tip and left soil in the foot wells and were horribly drunk on paraquat.

"Poetry?" she repeated. "No worries, pet. High Road or Low Road?"

She meant either up high, dodging amongst the planetoid-size books that were constantly moving across the sky, or down low on the ground, within the streets and byways. Taking the High Road was a skillful endeavor that meant either slipstreaming behind a particularly large book or latching onto a novel going in roughly the same direction and being carried to one's destination in a series of piggyback rides. It was faster if things went well, but more dangerous and prone to delays.

"Low Road," I said, since the traffic between Poetry and Fiction was limited and one could orbit for hours over the coast, waiting for a novel heading in the right direction.

"Jolly good," she said, clicking the FARE ON BOARD sign. "Cash, credit, goats, chickens, salt, pebbles, ants or barter?"

"Barter. I'll swap you two hours of my butler."

"Can he mix cocktails?"

"He can do a Tahiti Tingle — with or without umbrella."

"Deal."

We took the Dickens Freeway through HumDram, avoided the afternoon jam at the Brontë-Austen interchange and took a shortcut through Shreve Plaza to rejoin the expressway at Picoult Junction, and from there to the Carnegie Underpass, part of the network of tunnels that connected the various islands that made up the observable BookWorld.

"How are you enjoying the new Book-World?" I asked by way of conversation.

"Too many baobabs and not enough smells," she said, "but otherwise enjoyable."

The baobabs *were* a problem, but it was hardly at the top of my list of complaints. After a few minutes with the cabbie telling me in a cheerful voice how she'd had Bagheera in the back of her cab once, we emerged blinking at the tunnel exit and the island of Poetry, where we were waved through by a border guard who was too busy checking the paperwork on a consignment of iambic pentameters to worry much about us.

We made our way slowly down Keats Avenue until we came to Tennyson Boulevard, and I ordered her to stop outside "Locksley Hall" and wait for me around the corner. I got out, waited until she had gone, then walked past "The Lotos-Eaters" and "The Charge of the Light Brigade" to a small gate entwined with brambles and from there into a glorious English summer's day. I walked up the river, past long fields of barley and rye that seemed to clothe the wold and meet the sky, then through the field where a road ran by, which led to many-towered Camelot. I walked along the river, turned a corner and found the island in the river. I looked around as aspens quivered and a breeze and shiver ran up and down my spine. I really wasn't meant to be here and could get into serious trouble if I was discovered. I took a deep breath, crossed a small bridge and found myself facing a square gray building with towers at each corner. I didn't knock, as I knew the Lady of Shalott quite well, and entered unbidden to walk the two flights of stairs to the tower room.

"Hullo!" said the lady, pausing from the tapestry upon which she was engaged. "I didn't expect to see you again so soon."

The Lady of Shalott was of an indeterminate age and might once have been plain before the rigors of artistic interpretation got working on her. This was the annoying side of the Feedback Loop; irrespective of how she had once looked or even *wanted* to look, she was now a Pre-Raphaelite beauty with long flaxen tresses, flowing white gowns and a silver forehead band. She wasn't the only one to be physically morphed by reader expectation. Miss Havisham was now elderly whether she liked it or not, and Sherlock Holmes wore a deerstalker and smoked a ridiculously large pipe. The problem wasn't just confined to the classics. Harry Potter was seriously pissed off that he'd have to spend the rest of his life looking like Daniel Radcliffe.

"Good afternoon, my lady," I said, curtsying. "I would like to conduct more research."

"Such adherence to duty is much to be admired," replied the lady. "How are your readings going?"

"Over a thousand," I returned, lying spectacularly. If I didn't pretend to be popular, she'd never have granted me access.

"That's wonderful news. Make good use of the time. I could get into a lot of trouble for this."

Satisfied, she left her tapestry and summoned me to the window that faced Camelot. The Lady of Shalott took great care not to look out of the window but instead gently stroked a mirror that was held in a large bronze hanger and angled it towards the windows, as if to see the view outside. But this mirror wasn't like other mirrors; the surface grew misty, turned the color of slate, then displayed an image quite unlike the reflection one might expect.

"Usual place?" she asked.

"Usual place."

The image coalesced into a suburban street in the Old Town of Swindon, and the Lady of Shalott touched me on the shoulder.

"I'll leave you to it," she told me, and quietly returned to her tapestry, which seemed to depict David Hasselhoff in various episodes from *Baywatch,* Series 2.

I stared into the mirror. The image flickered occasionally and was mildly desaturated in color, but it was otherwise clear and sharp.

"Left forty-five degrees."

The mirror shifted to look up the suburban road to the house where Thursday and Landen lived. But this wasn't a book somewhere, or a memory. This was the Real-World, the Outland. The Lady of Shalott uniquely possessed a window into reality and could see whatever she wanted, whenever she wanted to. Great lives, great events — even *Baywatch.* The images she saw were woven into a tapestry, and she couldn't look outside her own window on pain of death. It was all a bit weird, but that's Tennyson for you.

The view was live, and aside from the fact that it was mute, was almost as good as being there.

"Move forward six yards."

The viewpoint moved forward to a front door that was very familiar to me. I had a similar front door in my own book, but my version didn't have peeling paint or the random fine crackle that natural weathering brings. I sensed my heart beat faster.

"Go inside."

The viewpoint drifted through the door, where the hall was less familiar. Thursday and Landen's real house was only ever described briefly to the ghostwriter who wrote my series, so the interior was different. I jumped as someone moved past the mirror. It was a young girl aged no more than twelve, and she looked very serious for her years. This would have been Thursday and Landen's daughter, Tuesday, as brilliant as Uncle Mycroft but in the "confusing petulant" state of pubescence. Nothing was right and everything was wrong. If it wasn't problems over the revectoring of electrogravitational field theory, it was her brother, Friday, whom she regarded as a total loser and layabout.

"Advance two yards."

The viewpoint moved forward to the hall table. I could see that Thursday was not in, as her bag, keys, cell phone and battered leather jacket were absent. It didn't say she was missing; only that she wasn't at home right now.

"Advance six yards, rotate left twenty degrees."

The viewpoint moved into the kitchen, where a man was sitting at the table attempting to help Tuesday with her GSD uni-Scripture homework. He was graying at the temples and had a kindly face that was *very* familiar. This was Landen Parke-Laine, Thursday's husband. I blinked as my eyes moistened. They were talking, and he laughed. I couldn't hear him, but imagined as best I could how he might have sounded. Sort of like . . . *music.*

"One-twenty degrees to the right, pull out a yard."

The mirror did as I asked so I could see the family scene. I didn't have this. None of this. No husband, no children. Despite the real Thursday's wishes that Landen would be included in the series after I took over, he wasn't — and neither were any of the children. Thursday was overridden by a senator named Jobsworth over at the Council of Genres. So they reverted to the previous plan and had Landen continue to die in a house fire in the first chapter of *The Eyre Affair,* a clumsy attempt to give purpose to the written Thursday's fictitious crime fighting. The plot device might have been clunky, but the loss had been exceptionally well written; I felt it every minute of every day. Being fictional is a double-edged sword. You get to savor the really good times over and over, but the same is true of the bad. For every defeat of the Goliath Corporation, there is the loss of Miss Havisham, and for every moment in Mycroft's company there is a day in the Crimea. The delight at returning Jane Eyre to her book and thwarting Acheron is forever tempered by the inevitable loss of Landen, again and again forever.

So I stood there, staring at what should have been mine. I wanted to be with the children I should have been allowed to have and to spend my life expending time and energy in the glorious hope that I would one day become parentally redundant. In my bleaker moments, Pickwick and Mrs. Malaprop attempted to console me by explaining I had loss only to give relevance to what drove my character through the narrative, but it was meager consolation. I should have had a written Landen and written children to keep me company.

I watched Landen for several more minutes. Every movement, every nuance. I watched how he spoke to Tuesday with humor and infinite patience. I watched how he scratched his ear, how he laughed, how he smiled.

Friday joined them. My would-be son was a fine fellow — handsome like his father. Perhaps a bit rudderless at that age, but thought and function would eventually arrive in the fullness of time. I wanted to give him some guidance, but he had his mother for that. The real me. The real *her.* Besides, the mirror saw only in one direction. They had no idea that I was there, no idea that I felt as I did. I watched for a few more minutes, until Landen got up and walked to the sink, drew himself a glass of water and stared out the window.

"Pull out into the garden three yards, right

ninety degrees."

My viewpoint drifted through the kitchen wall, and after a brief glimpse of central-heating pipes and a bored-looking mouse, I was now outside looking at Landen, who was just on the other side of the window. Although he couldn't see me, we were staring into each other's eyes.

"Whitby has asked me out to the Bar Humbug," I whispered. "I wanted you to know that I'm going."

Landen couldn't hear me, but I knew I had to tell him. It was by way of apology. I blinked away tears but then frowned. Landen was blinking away tears, too. *Something had happened.* Thursday wasn't here, but for how long? An argument? Had she *died* in the Outland? I looked at the children, who were busy with homework. They seemed unconcerned.

Whatever it was, it was a burden shouldered by Landen alone.

"When did you last see Thursday?" I whispered.

Landen took a deep breath, wiped his eyes and returned to the children. I put out my hand to touch the mirror, but it simply rippled, like water in a pool.

"Left thirty degrees, three yards forward."

The mirror complied, and I found myself

close enough to the memo board above the telephone to read the notes. I peered amongst the receipts, pictures and old theater tickets before finding what I was looking for. A telephone message in Thursday's hand telling Landen that his sister wanted to talk to him. It was dated seven days ago. If Thursday *was* missing, it was for the maximum of a week.

"Did you see what you wanted?"

I jumped. The Lady of Shalott had returned and was standing just behind me.

"I think so," I replied hastily. "It was the . . . ah . . . state of her memo board I was looking at. You know what they say: 'A view into a woman's ephemera is a window to her soul.' "

"Do they say that?" asked the Lady of Shalott doubtfully.

"Frequently."

I made ready to leave. The visits to Shalott were as frequent as I could make them without arousing suspicion, the views they offered all too fleeting. I wanted to know where Thursday was, sure, but I had to see Landen and the kids, too. *Had* to.

I thanked her, and she walked me to the door. But this wasn't a favor, and she and I both knew it. I wasn't allowed to be in Poetry without just cause, and I certainly wasn't allowed to sneak-peek the Outland. She handed me a wooden box.

"You will look after them, won't you?"

"Of course," I replied, and placed the box in my shoulder bag. I walked outside the castle and returned to where the taxi was waiting to take me home. I was none the wiser as to where Thursday was, but I could reasonably surmise she was missing in the Outland, too. I took a deep breath. It had been, as always, *difficult.* I loved and hated seeing him, all at the same time. But it helped when it came to finally going on a date with Whitby. It lessened the sense of betrayal.

8.
The Shield

> The evidence for the existence of Dark Reading Matter remains obscure at best. Supposedly the vast amount of unread material either forgotten or deleted, DRM is also said to be home to the Unread: zombielike husks of former characters, their humanity sucked from their heads by continued unreadfulness. It is generally agreed that these stories belong to metamyth — stories within stories — and are used by drill sergeants at character college to frighten recruits into compliance.
>
> *Bradshaw's BookWorld Companion* (8th edition)

The queue to get out of Poetry was long, as always. The smuggling of metaphor out of the genre was a serious problem, and one that made the border guards extremely vigilant. The increased scarcity of raw metaphor in Fiction had driven prices sky-high, and people would take unbelievably foolish risks to smuggle it across. I'd heard stories of metaphor being hidden in baggage, swallowed, even dressed up to look like ordinary objects whose *meanings* were then disguised to cloak the metaphor. The problem at that point was trying to explain why you had a "brooding thunderstorm" or "broad sunlit uplands" in your luggage.

"Can we take the High Road?" I asked.

She turned around to look at me. Taking the High Road out of Poetry meant only one thing — that I wanted to avoid any entanglements with the border guards.

"My friend Jake was carrying a mule without realizing it last week," said the cabbie in a meaningful tone. "The mule had two kilos of raw metonym on him — hidden in the saddlebags."

Metonym wasn't as dangerous as smuggling raw metaphor, but the underworld would try anything to turn a buck and had set up labs to enrich variable forms of metaphor into the real McCoy. Extracting the "like" from simile was the easiest method, but the resulting metaphor was as weak as wet paper. Synecdoche was used in much the same way; the best minds in Jurisfiction were constantly trying to outwit them, and raided met labs on an almost daily basis.

"Did he get to keep his cab?" I asked. "Your friend Jake, I mean."

"His entire car was reduced to text with the metonym still in it."

"Reduced to text?" I echoed. "Sounds like a hammer to break a nut."

"Poeticals are like that," said the cabbie with a disrespectful snort. "Prone to fits of violent passion. I think it's all that absinthe. The point is this: I can get you out of Poetry, but it will cost."

"I'll lend you my butler for an afternoon."

"One afternoon and a garden party."

"A garden party."

"Done."

The cabbie flipped the vectored thrust nozzles, and in an instant we were climbing almost vertically upwards. It took less than a minute to reach the low-lying book traffic, and within a few seconds we had latched onto an academic paper moving from Physics to Biology. We stayed there for a few minutes and then detached, hovered for a moment and then reattached to the keel of an oil tanker that was part of a Bermuda Triangle book on its way to Fiction. We were under the massive rudder at the back, with one of the vast propellers looming over us.

"We'll ride this baby all the way into Fiction," said the cabbie as she took out some knitting, "about twenty minutes. We could fly the whole way, but we'd probably be picked up by the book-traffic controllers and get busted."

"Don't look now, but I think we just have."

The flashing red lights of a Jurispoetry squad car close by had alerted me to the fact that the cabbie wasn't quite as good as I thought she was. We could have detached there and then and dropped the mile towards the Text Sea before leveling out and making a run for the coast, but it was a risky undertaking. Cutting and running meant only one thing: guilty.

"Oh, crap," said the cabbie, dropping a stitch in surprise. "I hope you've got some friends in high places."

"Hullo," I said to the officer who was now standing outside the car. He was dressed in a baggy white shirt and smelled strongly of rhyming couplets. He stared at me with the supercilious look of someone who knew he had the upper hand and was certainly going to milk it.

"Oh, to sneak across the border, when it's plain you should not oughta?"

I had to think quickly. Unlike the Poetry government officials who conversed in rhyme royal, this was a lowly traffic cop who spoke only the gutter doggerel of the streets. He was using a soft-rhyming AA and so was probably not that bright. I hit him with some AABCCB.

"*Au contraire,* my friend, we did not intend to break any poetical code. We were waved through by others of your crew and simply took the upper road."

But he didn't go for it.

"I can see your little plan, but your stanzas barely scan. You, madam, I must nab, so get your butt from out the cab."

I climbed out and succumbed to a search. He soon found the box the Lady of Shalott had given me.

"Well, lookee here, what have we got? Is this metaphor or is it not?"

"Not one but other, I must confess, the situation's now a mess."

He opened the box and stared. It wasn't metaphor, but contraband nonetheless.

"You're in big trouble smuggling this junk. What else you got? Let's pop the trunk."

We did, and there was Sprockett. The officer stared at him for a moment.

"I'm sure you can explain away why a dead butler's in your trunk today?"

"He's a *clockwork* butler, Duplex-5, and even paused he's still alive."

The officer had seen enough and brought

out a report sheet to take down some details.

"Name?"

"Thursday Next."

The officer looked at me, then at my New Agey clothes, then at Sprockett.

"Now, which one could that be? The heroine or the one who likes to hug a tree?"

In for a penny, in for a pound. I had to hope that this guard could be fooled as easily as the Elvis back in Conspiracy.

"I am she, the Thursday proper. Those that cross me come a cropper."

"That seems likely, but before I yield, let me check your Jurisfiction shield."

I passed it across. The officer took one look at it, put away his report sheet and told his partner that they were leaving. He smiled and handed me back my badge.

"It's an honor, I'll be reckoned. Sorry to have kept you for even a second."

I signed my name in his autograph book and with growing confusion climbed back into the cab as the Jurispoetry car detached from the hull and fell away from the tanker, leaving us to continue our trip unmolested.

"You're Thursday Next?" said the cabbie, her attitude suddenly changed. "This ride is for free, kiddo. But listen, the next time you're in the RealWorld, can you find out why there have to be over a hundred different brands of soap? I'd really like to know."

"Okay," I muttered, "no problem."

The remainder of the journey was unremarkable, except for one thing: I spent the entire trip staring at the Jurisfiction shield that had allowed me not once but twice to squeak out of trouble. It wasn't my shield at all. It was Thursday's. The *real* Thursday's. *Someone had slipped it into my pocket that morning.* And the more I thought about the morning's events, the more I realized that I might have become involved — quite against my will — with a matter of some considerable consequence.

9.
Home

Rumor has it that undiscovered genres were hidden among the thick vegetation and impenetrable canopy in the far north of the island. Primitive, anarchic, strange and untouched by narrative convention, they were occasionally discovered and inducted into the known BookWorld, where they started off fresh and exciting before ultimately becoming mimicked, overused, tired and then passé. BookWorld naturalists argued strongly that some genres should remain hidden in order to keep the BookWorld from homogenizing, but their voices went unheeded.

Bradshaw's BookWorld Companion
(3rd edition)

"I had the most curious dream," mused Sprockett as soon as I had rewound him completely, "in which I was a full-hunter silent repeater. There was also this gramophone — you know, one of those windup varieties — and she was running overspeed and playing 'Temptation Rag.' And then there was this monkey hitting cymbals together, and I —"

He checked himself.

"I'm frightfully sorry, ma'am. My protocol gearing can become a bit gummy during deactivation. You are not offended by my drivel?"

"Not in the least. In fact, I didn't know machines *could* dream."

"I dream often," replied the butler thoughtfully. "Mostly about being a toaster."

"Dualit or KitchenAid?"

He seemed mildly insulted that I should have to ask.

"A Dualit four-slot, *naturally.* But perhaps," he added, his eyebrow pointer clicking from "Indignant" to "Puzzled," "I only *believe* I dream. Sometimes I think it is merely a construct to enable me to better understand humans."

"Listen, I should warn you about Pickwick," I said as we walked up the garden path.

"What is a Pickwick?"

"It's a dodo."

"I thought they were extinct."

"They may yet become so. She's trouble,

so be careful."

"Thank you, ma'am. I shall."

I pushed open the front door and was met by the sound of laughter. Carmine was sitting at the table with Bowden Cable and Acheron Hades, two of the other costars from the series. They were all sharing a joke, or at least they were until I walked in, when everyone fell silent.

"Hello, Thursday," said Bowden, whom I'd never really gotten along with, despite the fact that his counterpart in the RealWorld was one of Thursday's closest friends. "We were just telling Carmine the best way to play Thursday."

"The best way is the way I play her," I said in a firm yet friendly manner. "Dignified."

"Of course," said Bowden. "Who's your friend?"

"Sprockett," I replied, "my butler."

"I didn't know you needed a butler," said Bowden.

"Everyone needs a butler. He was going to be stoned, so I took him with me."

"What do cog-based life-forms get stoned with?" asked Bowden in an impertinent manner. "Vegetable oil?"

"Actually, sir," intoned Sprockett, "it's sewing-machine lubricant for a mild tipple.

Many feel that the exuberant effects of 3-in-One are worth pursuing, although I have never partaken myself. For those that have hit rock bottom, where life has become nothing more than a semiconscious slide from one partial winding to the next, it's WD-40."

"Oh," said Bowden, who had been put firmly in his place by Sprockett's forthrightness, "I see."

"Hmm," said Acheron, peering at Sprockett's data plate with great interest. "Are you the Duplex-6?"

"Five, sir. The Six's release has been delayed. A series of mainspring failures have put beta testing back several months, and now I hear the Six has pressure compensation issues on the primary ethical escapement module."

"What does that mean?"

"I have to admit I'm not entirely sure, sir. The main problem with clockwork sentience is that we can *never* understand the level of our own complexity — for to do so would require an even *greater* level of complexity. At present we can deal with day-to-day maintenance issues, but all we can ever know for sure is that we function. We tick, therefore we are."

Pickwick asked me how I thought we

could afford such an extravagance, but the real disapproval came from Mrs. Malaprop.

"Good afternoon, Mr. Sprockett," she said coldly. "I hope you are fully aquatinted with the *specific* roles of mousecreeper and butler?"

"Indeed, Mrs. Malaprop," replied Sprockett, bowing low. "And I don't require much space — I can easily fit in the cupboard under the stairs."

"You will knot," replied Mrs. Malaprop with great indignation. "*I* am resizing there. You may have the earring cupboard."

"Then with your permission I shall go and repack," announced Sprockett.

"You mean you're leaving?" I asked.

"Repack my knee bearings," he explained. "With grease. Knees, despite much design work, continue to be the Duplex-5's Achilles' heel."

And leaving us all to muse upon his odd choice of words, he departed.

"At least *try* to be nice to him," I said to Mrs. Malaprop when he had gone. "And I want you to order some oils of varying grades to make him feel welcome — and make sure all the clocks are kept wound. Cog-based life-forms take great offense at stopped clocks."

"As madam washes," replied Mrs. Malaprop, which was her way of telling me to get stuffed.

"If you don't need us, we're going to go and rehearse Acheron's death scene on the roof of Thornfield Hall," said Carmine.

"You'll need to unlock Bertha," I replied, handing her the key. "And don't forget to put the bite mask on her."

I watched them go with an odd feeling that I couldn't describe. Despite my being the protagonist, most of the characters were already here when I took over, and few of them were happy with my interpretation of Thursday, even though it was the one that Thursday herself had approved. They had all preferred the sex-and-violence Thursday who'd turned a blind eye to the many scams they had had cooking. Because of this, I hadn't really gotten on with any of them. In fact, the out-of-book relationship with the rest of the cast could best be described as barely cordial. Carmine seemed to get on with them a lot better. I shouldn't have minded, but I did.

"She's going to be trouble, that one," said Pickwick, who was doing the crossword while perched on the dresser.

"All she has to be is a good Thursday," I murmured. "Everything else is immaterial. Mrs. Malaprop?"

"Yes, madam?"

"Did you put anything in my pocket this morning? For a joke, perhaps?"

"*Joke,* madam?" she inquired in a shocked tone. "Malaprops always keep well clear of potentially hummus situations."

"I didn't think so. I'll be in my study. Will you have Sprockett bring in some tea?"

"Very good, madam."

"Pickwick? I need the paper."

"You'll have to wait," she said without looking up. "I'm doing the crossword."

I didn't have time for this, so I simply took the paper, ripped off the crossword section and handed it back to her. I ignored her expression of outrage and walked into my study and shut the door.

I moved quietly to the French windows and stepped out into the garden to release the Lost Positives that the Lady of Shalott had given me. She had a soft spot for the orphaned prefixless words and thought they had more chance to thrive in Fiction than in Poetry. I let the defatigable scamps out of their box. They were kempt and sheveled but their behavior was peccable if not mildly gruntled. They started acting petuously and ran around in circles in a very toward manner.

I then returned to my study and spent

twenty minutes staring at Thursday's shield. The only way it could have gotten into my pocket was via the red-haired gentleman sitting next to me on the tram. And if that was the case, he had been in contact with Thursday quite recently — or at least sometime in the past week. It didn't prove she was missing in the BookWorld any more than it proved she was missing in the RealWorld. I had only a telephone note, a husband's tears and the word of a murderer.

"Your tea and shortbread, ma'am," said Sprockett, placing the tray upon my desk. "A very comfortable house you have. I must confess that in a weak moment, and quite against your advice, I lent that odd-looking bird twenty pounds for her kidney operation."

"I warned you about Pickwick," I said with a sigh. "She doesn't need a kidney operation, and her mother isn't in 'dire straits,' no matter what she says."

"Ah," replied Sprockett. "Do you think I might be able to get my money back?"

"Not without a lot of squawking. Is Mrs. Malaprop causing you any trouble, by the way?"

"No, ma'am. We agreed to arm-wrestle for seniority in the house, and even though she attempted to cheat, I believe that we are all square now."

"I was given this by someone on a tram," I said, passing the real Thursday's shield across to Sprockett.

His eyebrow pointed to "Puzzled," then "Thinking," then "Worried."

"That would explain the ease by which I escaped the stoning in Conspiracy."

"And later, getting out of Poetry."

"I don't recall that."

"You were dreaming about gramophones. Can you call the Jurisfiction front desk and ask for Thursday Next? Tell them it's me and I need to speak to her."

Sprockett stood in the corner to make the calls. A request like this would be better coming from my butler.

"They tell me that she is 'on assignment' at present," replied Sprockett after talking quietly to himself for a few seconds.

"Tell them it's the written Thursday and I'll call again."

I wondered quite how she could be on assignment without her shield and idly turned over the newspaper. I stopped. The banner headline read, FAMED JURISFICTION AGENT TO LEAD PEACE TALKS. Thursday was due to table the talks on Friday, less than a week away. All of a sudden, her "absent" status took on a more menacing angle. If she was missing now, things could get very bad indeed.

For the past three years, Racy Novel and its leader, Speedy Muffler, had been causing trouble far in excess of his size, readership or importance. Sandwiched precariously between Women's Fiction and Outdated Religious Dogma, with Erotica to the far north and Comedy to the south, the large yet proudly anarchic genre had been troublesome ever since it was declared a member of the Axis of Unreadable along with Misery Memoirs and Celebrity Bio. Muffler, stung by the comparison to voyeuristic drivel or the meaningless nonadventures of celebrities, decided to expand his relevance within Fiction by attempting to push out his borders. The CofG responded to his aggression by transferring *Lady Chatterley's Lover* out of Racy Novel and into Human Drama, then moving *The History of Tom Jones* to Erotica. Sanctions soon followed that prevented anyone from supplying Racy Novel with good dialogue, plot or characterization. This did nothing to appease Speedy Muffler, and he claimed that the sanctions were preventing him from developing as a genre — quite against BookWorld law and the Character's Charter. The trouble was, Muffler and Racy Novel couldn't be ignored, since they were amongst the major exporters of metaphor. When Muffler claimed to possess a dirty bomb capable of hurling scenes of a gratuitously sexual nature far into Women's Fiction, the BookWorld finally took notice and the peace talks were set. Thursday Next would be the chief negotiator, and she had good form. When Scandinavian Detectives threatened to cede from Crime, it was she who brought them back.

"You seem perturbed," remarked Sprockett. "Is anything the matter?"

"I have reason to believe that the real Thursday Next might be missing," I replied guardedly. "And that's not good for all sorts of reasons."

"Has she gone missing before?" asked Sprockett.

"Many times."

"Then it's probably one of those . . . again."

I hoped he was right, but even if he wasn't, I wasn't quite sure what could be done about it. I was an underread A-8 character with no power and less influence. Besides, Jurisfiction was doubtless onto it. Commander Bradshaw, the head of Jurisfiction, was one of Thursday's closest friends.

There was a knock on the door, and Mrs.

Malaprop came in.

"Miss Next? Three awesome gentlemen to see you."

"Who are they?"

"They didn't give their gnomes."

The visitors didn't wait either, and strode in. They weren't the sort of people I wanted to see, but their presence might well reinforce my theories about Thursday. They were the Men in Plaid.

Several things seemed to happen at once. Sprockett's eyebrow quivered at Mrs. Malaprop, who got his meaning and knocked over an ornamental vase, which fell to the floor with a crash. The Men in Plaid turned to see what was going on, and at that very moment Sprockett grabbed Thursday's shield from the desk and threw it hard into the ceiling, where it stuck in the plasterboard. By the time the Men in Plaid looked back towards us, Sprockett was tidying my papers on the desk.

"Good afternoon, gentlemen," I said in a friendly tone. "What can I do for you?"

Like trousers, pear pips, twins and bookends, MiP always came in pairs. They were without emotion and designed to ensure that no personal ambiguity would muddy their operating parameters. MiP were designed to do what they were told to do, and nothing else.

"So," said the Man in Plaid, "you are Thursday Next A8-V-67987-FP?"

"Yes."

"Date of composure?"

"Third June, 2006. What is this about?"

"Routine, Miss Next," said the second MiP. "We are looking for some property stolen from a leading Jurisfiction agent, and we thought you might be able to help us. I won't mince my words. We think you have it."

I resisted the temptation to look up. The shield was in plain sight, embedded in the ceiling. "Do you want me to try to guess what you're after, or are you going to tell me?"

The MiP exchanged glances.

"It has come to our attention," said the taller of the two, "that someone's been waving the real Thursday Next's Jurisfiction shield around. That person used it to get out of Poetry an hour ago. Were you in Poetry today, Miss Next?"

I wasn't supposed to be there, so the answer had to be no. "No."

They stared at me. "The officers involved told us that someone of your description had a robotic butler in the trunk of a taxi. Do you still deny this?"

I looked at Sprockett, who stared impassively ahead.

"There are probably *hundreds* of robotic manservants in Fiction," I replied, "and all of them are technically luggage. But since automatons are incapable of misstatements, why don't you ask him yourself?"

They did, and Sprockett could answer without lying that he had absolutely no knowledge of the trip at all.

"Perhaps it was Thursday herself," I suggested. "Have you asked her?"

There was, perhaps, a subtle change in the Plaids' demeanor. But if she *was* missing, as I supposed, they weren't going to let on.

"How about Conspiracy?" asked the smaller Plaid. "We have a report from Elvis561 that someone looking a lot like Thursday and holding her Jurisfiction shield rescued a mechanical man from stoning."

"That was definitely me," I said. "I was on JAID business."

They both stared at me. It was highly uncomfortable.

"Then you *did* have her shield?"

"I used *my* JAID shield. Here."

I passed it across, and they stared at it. It was nothing like a Jurisfiction shield.

"The Elvis must have been mistaken," I

continued. "There is a certain degree of inbuilt hyperbole to the genre that might generate outrageous claims, wouldn't you agree?"

I stared at them intently as I tried to read their expressions, but their emotionless construction made them impossible to penetrate. They probably didn't do well at singles bars but would doubtless be able to play poker at tournament level.

"Very well," said the first Man in Plaid. "We will leave you for now. One more thing: A call to Thursday Next at Jurisfiction was traced to this book not ten minutes ago. Was there a reason for this?"

"I have a new understudy," I explained. "I thought Thursday might like to give her a few tips on how to play her. If you see her, will you pass my message along?"

"We're not messengers," said the second Plaid, and they left without another word.

There followed a moment of silence. I had just lied to the Men in Plaid, which was illegal, and even if they thought I was telling the truth, my being on their radar was probably not conducive to good health. But one thing that did cross my mind was this: If Thursday was missing, the Men in Plaid had been ordered to find her, and they didn't yet know of the connection between me and the red-haired gentleman.

But I didn't have any time to muse on it further, as I heard the Read Alarm go off. Somewhere in the Outland, a reader had picked up one of my books. Luckily for us, things can happen instantaneously in the BookWorld, so I dashed through to the kitchen to find Carmine already dressed and ready to go. I half thought of taking over, but I had to let her give it a whirl sooner or later.

"It's barely teatime in the Outland," I said, glancing at the clock. "Someone must be taking a break. Are you ready?"

Carmine nodded.

I turned to Mrs. Malaprop, who was monitoring the progress of all the readings on a circular screen that plotted in word-for-word detail which readers were where, and in what book.

"It's a slope oak," she said. "*Lost in a Good Book,* page 133, SpecOps Twilight Homes. I'll contract Granny Next."

She flipped a switch on the intercom, and her voice echoed around the series on the intercom.

"Hear this, hear this. Would Granny Next please pro-seed Toe-wads TN2, P133."

"An easy scene," I said, turning to Carmine. "How's your Ping-Pong?"

"Not bad."

"It doesn't matter. Granny Next will crush you anyway."

"What is a 'slope oak'?"

"She means 'a slow poke.' It's what we call readers who've been working their way through the series at a snail's pace. When they falter — which they often do — you should try to alter your dialogue for simplicity. You'll feel their ReadRate increase when you do, and we aim only to help. The reader is everything, yes?"

She looked up at me and bit her lip nervously.

"The reader is everything," she repeated. "But you'll step in if there are more than twenty concurrent reads, won't you?"

Being read simultaneously was often described as like trying to visit everywhere in Paris at the same time during rush hour. The simile was lost on me, but I made a point of never wanting to visit Paris, real or imaginary.

"Don't worry," I told her, "you'll be fine. We've got at least four hours before the other readers come onstream. Take a deep breath and repeat the first person's credo: 'Pace, Atmosphere, Plot, Prose, Character.' "

"Pace, Atmosphere, Plot, Prose, Character."

"Good. Give them hell."

And she gave me a wan smile and headed off towards the SpecOps Twilight Homes, which were cemented just between Thornfield Hall and the interior Skyrail set. With an odd feeling, I watched her go. I liked the time off, but I liked being Thursday, too — even if it was to an audience of only one.

"Here," I said, passing the Snooze access codes to Mrs. Malaprop. "Keep a close eye on her."

"This is a last resort, yes?" asked Mrs. Malaprop, who licked kittens probably more than most.

"Last resort. Call me and I'll come running."

I walked out of the kitchen. There was work to be done.

10.
Epizeuxis

Maps of the BookWorld are constantly updated as the genres snake back and forth in response to Outland trends and fads. The borders move so rapidly, in fact, that any notion of a fully updated map is considered laughable, and most maps are these days published with *average* borders that reflect reading trends of the past ten years.

Bradshaw's BookWorld Companion
(3rd edition)

Despite the unwanted attentions of the Men in Plaid, the warnings from the red-haired gentleman and the worrying possibility that Thursday might be missing, I spent a busy and anxious afternoon going through the heap of book junk in the garage. I was, to be honest, torn. Part of me wanted nothing better than to accede to Red Herring's wishes that this be an "unrepeatable" accident, and part of me was suspicious. The closer I examined the book junk, the worse it looked. It appeared that something, while not *exactly* rotten in the state of the BookWorld, was far from fresh.

At a little after five, and with a rising sense of foreboding, I called Sprockett into my study to compare notes.

"So what do you have?" I asked, letting him air his discoveries first.

He led me across to where the *Atlas of the BookWorld* lay open on my desk. He indicated the page that depicted the southeastern part of the island and showed me where he had plotted the crashed book's debris trail by a series of black crosses. Most sections of text would have pulverized into graphemes and simply absorbed, which explains why we rarely find anything when short stories or limericks come to grief, just a hollow concussion in the distance.

Almost all the debris had been strewn across the Aviation genre, with the notable exception of the bed-sitting room already discovered inside Conspiracy and a Triumph motorcycle within Thriller (Spy) that narrowly missed George Smiley as it traveled through an early draft of *Tinker, Tailor, Soldier, Hatmaker.* The book seemed to have disintegrated somewhere above Deighton and then strewn objects in a roughly straight line north, in the direction of the Great Library and the Ungenred Zone.

"What would tigers and a macaroon be doing in an Aviation novel?" asked Mrs. Malaprop, who was cleaning with a feather duster but actually wanted to be part of the investigation.

"They might be scrambled graphemes and not actually in the book at all. Best ignored."

"There doesn't seem to be any curve to the debris trail at all," added Pickwick, who had entered unseen and jumped onto the table to look more closely. I wouldn't have minded so much if she hadn't upset the ink-well and then stood clumsily in the ink.

"You're right," I said. "Mind your feet. And that means either a rapid breakup or that the book — whatever it was — was not from the Aviation genre."

"Look here," said Pickwick as she pointed with one of her claws. "If we extend the debris-field line backwards, we come out of Aviation, across Military, and end up right here in Adventure — somewhere around *King Solomon's Mines.*"

"Which might explain the tigers."

"But not the macaroon."

"Or the box-girder bridges — and the Triumph Bonneville motorcycle."

"I didn't say it *was* Haggard," said Pickwick, "only that it came from Adventure."

Unusually, Pickwick was being helpful. Probably because she'd taken Sprockett for some cash, had already had her nap but was not yet ready for her afternoon snack and was thus in an atypically good temper.

"I have an idea," said Sprockett. "Could we try unscrambling the letters of the items we found, and thereby find tantalizing clues as to what the book might be about?"

"To an outside observer, that would seem entirely logical," I replied, "but for one thing: Anagram-related clues were outlawed six years ago by the NCU."

"NCU?"

"Narrative Clunker Unit. Villains haven't been allowed to be albinos for years, identical twins as plot devices are banned, and double negatives are a complete no-no. Forget anagrams."

"Isn't there a black box data reorder in every book?" asked Mrs. Malaprop. "We could analyze the tea lemon tree."

"Usually," I replied, "but engineering contracts have to be spread around the BookWorld, and the construction of Book Data Recorders was subcontracted to James McGuffin and Co. of the Suspense genre, so they have a tendency to go missing until dramatically being found right at the end of an investigation. It's undoubtedly suspenseful, but a little useless. Want to see what I found?"

We walked out through the French windows and the garden to my double garage, which was another example of the inverted physics of the BookWorld. The more you filled it, the emptier it appeared. But it could never be *entirely* empty, as that would require an infinite amount of stuff — or in the case of a double garage, *twice* an infinite amount of stuff.

All the sections of crashed book were laid out on the concrete floor, ostensibly so we could try to find a reason for the accident, or even to figure out a rough plot of the mystery book. We had a few page numbers, but nothing attached to any dialogue. It was a mess. I walked past the yellow-painted back axle, pushed aside a fridge/freezer and beckoned them to one particular piece of wreckage.

"What do you make of this?" I asked.

We were standing over the bent Triumph motorcycle, and I told them to be quiet. There was a whisper in the air, and if you leaned close to the damaged motorcycle, you could hear it:

The works that built the cycle worked;
The cycle's labor labored on.
And workers sought and workers bought
The managers out and managed 'owt
Until the cycle's cycle cycled round.
But markets moved and markets shifted,
To Eastern trade that Eastern made.
Loans were pleaded, loans were needed,
The workers' workers worked their last.
But ruin didn't do as ruin does,
For Triumph's collapse led to Triumph's
triumph.

"I don't get it," said Pickwick, who had always favored Harley-Davidson.

"It's a poem that charts the fall and rise of the Triumph motorcycle company in the late seventies and early eighties," I said. "It's seeped out of the descriptive flux of the motorcycle — a glowing afterember of the accident."

"That's not unusual," replied Pickwick. "Poetry and prose are different facets of the same basic element. When prose breaks down, it often spontaneously rhymes. Poetry is prose in another form, and prose is simply poetry waiting to happen."

"Epizeuxis," murmured Sprockett, "a rhetorical device that repeats the same word in the same sentence for increased dramatic

effect. This book was almost certainly destroyed by a rhetorical worm."

I had come to the same conclusion myself. The worm would attempt to restructure sentences, and when that failed, it would take words from other sentences, leaving dangerous holes in the narrative. Once there were no more complete words to be taken, the worm would start to harvest letters to make up the shortfall, weakening the structure until the entire book disintegrated. In RealWorld terms it would be like instantaneously removing every rivet from an aircraft that was in flight.

"The problem," I said slowly, "is that rhetorical worms don't occur naturally. They're used in the demolition business to tear apart sections of scrapped books. It's cheaper and safer than chains, hooks and crowbars. A well-placed worm can burrow into prose, dissolve away tired exposition and leave description and dialogue untouched. Either the book was carrying unlicensed worms that were accidentally activated or it was —"

"Sabotage!" hissed Mrs. Malaprop, and I felt myself suddenly go quite cold. Such a device would require a level of sophistication utterly outside the realm of ordinary citizens. There were stories of the Council

of Genres' Men in Plaid using rhetorical devices to cause injury or death, but that was mostly conjecture — drummed up by Conspiracy, no doubt.

"Okay," I said, "we have the *possibility* of skulduggery — but it's not the only explanation. Epizeuxis is often used as a rhetorical device."

"But so blatantly? And in a poem to describe the failure of a motorcycle-manufacturing cooperative?" exclaimed Pickwick. "What kind of nut would try something like that?"

"We still need to find out what the book was called," I said as we walked back into the house. "We need an ISBN. Did we check the thumb we found for fingerprints?"

"Not a single one."

"That's annoying. Those severed hands we found a few weeks ago had fingerprints all over them."

"What about DNA evidence?" asked Sprockett.

"DNA fingerprinting is still under a blanket ban," I explained. "Forensic Procedural is allowed to use it, but you know how tight the Crime genre can be."

Sadly, this was true. The Guild of Detectives had argued that although DNA fingerprinting had a use in the RealWorld, such annoyingly precise and utterly noncerebral detection methods really had no place in Fiction. And because the Crime lobby represented such a huge part of Fiction, the Council of Genres had reluctantly agreed. Mind you, detection rates hadn't suffered as a result, so everyone was happy.

I looked up at the Read-O-Meter. There were twelve simultaneous readings going on, and Carmine hadn't hit the panic button, so she was doing fine. I had a look at the clock and then went upstairs to have a bath and change. Despite all that was going on, what with sabotaged books, worms and missing Jurisfiction agents, I still had a date with Whitby Jett. I tried a call to Jurisfiction myself and was told that Thursday Next was still unavailable. I dried, then tried on several dresses but didn't like any of them. I had just dismissed the sixth and was rummaging in the bureau for a yellow top I remembered buying last time I was in Chick Lit, when I came across a photograph. It was one I had wanted to throw away but had pushed to the back of a drawer instead. It was a backstory snap of me and Landen, taken when we were in the Crimea, before Landen had lost a leg and I'd lost a brother. Happy days. I stared at it for a long time, then rang for Sprockett.

"Ma'am?"

"Is Whitby downstairs?"

"Yes, ma'am. He's waiting in the kitchen with a bunch of flowers the size of the Amazonian Basin."

"Would you send him my apologies and ask him to leave? Politely, of course."

"Ma'am?"

"I need to keep an eye on Carmine. It's her first day, and I need to stand by in case of mishaps."

"Miss Carmine is doing very well, by all accounts, ma'am, and Mr. Jett seems happily effusive over the prospect of an evening with you. I believe that his conduct has all the hallmarks of . . . love, ma'am."

"Sprockett," I said, "just do this for me, would you? Tell him I'm busy and I'll meet him for lunch tomorrow."

"Very good, ma'am. Where shall I say you will be meeting him?"

"I'll call him."

I came downstairs twenty minutes later to find the flowers on the hall table. I sighed at my own foolishness, then walked into the book and found Carmine about to play the croquet match in *The Well of Lost Plots.* I told her my date was canceled and that I'd take over from her. I think she was secretly relieved.

"Don't forget there's a party tonight at *Castle of Skeddan Jiarg,*" I told her. "The queen said to drop in anytime."

"I think I might just do that," she said with a smile. "I could get hyphenated, let my hair down and chat up a goblin or something."

I didn't like the sound of this.

"I don't mean to seem judgmental. Actually, come to think of it," I said, changing my mind, "I *do* mean to seem judgmental. You mustn't bring goblins home. Quite apart from the hygiene and theft issues, Pickwick can be a real prude. She'll be plocking on about it for months, and frankly, I could do without her endless complaints."

She winked.

"I will be *most* discreet. Why don't you join me when you're done? I know goblins aren't everyone's cup of tea, but what they lack in physical beauty they make up for in endurance."

I told her I didn't really feel like going to a party or dancing all night, and she gave me a hug before skipping off.

Reading-wise, it wasn't such a bad evening. The Ph.D. student gave up pretty soon to watch *Deal or No Deal,* a popular woodworking program in the Outland, and the new readers were for the most part forgiving, with only a few of them requiring extra attention to get them over some of the more wayward plot points. As for the rereads, they pretty much looked after themselves and added a useful amount of feedback, too — the curtains had never looked brighter, and Pickwick positively shone.

11.
Plot Thickens

Minor narrative changes were often ignored, but major variations were stomped on without mercy. Perpetrators would be rounded up and banished to a copy of *Bunty* or *Sparky* until suitably contrite. Repeat offenders were suspended, and after three strikes were erased — usually without warning. Some thought it worth the risk. After all, being unread was arguably no different from erasure. Some put it this way: Better dead than unread.

Bradshaw's BookWorld Companion
(7th edition)

I was up and about while everyone else in the book was still sleepily inactive. There had been no readings at all since 2:00 A.M., and I wanted to be in costume and ready on the off chance that anyone read a few pages before breakfast. It paid to keep at a state of readiness, just in case. There had been trouble inside *Captain Corelli's Mandolin* when a sudden reinterest in the book caught everyone napping — the first hundred pages or so have yet to fully recover.

I walked about the settings of the series, checking to make sure everything was ready to go. My tour wasn't just a technical housekeeping exercise either — it was about a sense of pride. Despite the lack of readers and a certain "dissatisfaction" from particular members of the cast who suggested that I might improve the readability by spicing up the prose with a bit more sex and violence, I still wanted to keep the books going as well as I could — and to win Thursday's approval, which was more important than the author's.

Once I had made sure that everything was to my satisfaction, I called Whitby to apologize for standing him up. He took it better than I had expected, but I could sense he was annoyed. I told him I would *definitely* be free for lunch, suggested the expensive and needlessly spacious Elbow Rooms, then pretended that Pickwick had broken something, so I could end the conversation.

I drew a deep breath, cursed myself for being so stupid, took a pager with me and walked down the road to Stubbs, the outrageously expensive coffee shop on the corner.

"Could I not have a coffee?" I said, meaning I wanted an empty cup. Stubbs had become so expensive that no one could afford the coffee, but since the ambience in the café was so good and the establishment so fashionable, it was always full.

"What would you not like?" asked Paul, who wore a black gown and a wig due to a syntactical head cold that made him unable to differentiate himself between a barista and a barrister.

"Better not give me a latte," I replied, "and better not make it a large one."

"How did the date with Whitby go?"

"So-so."

Paul raised an eyebrow, made no comment and handed me an empty cup. I went to a booth at the back of the store and sat down. I came here most mornings and usually read the paper over my noncoffee. I scanned the headlines of *The Word,* but if Thursday was missing, they didn't know about it. Oversize Books had gained a victory at the council. Constantly irked by snide comments about taking more than their allotted shelf space, they had sought to have their own genre and succeeded. A representative for Oversize Books had praised "common sense" and said that they looked forward to "moving to their own island as soon as one big enough was made available."

There was more about Racy Novel, with Speedy Muffler claiming that troop movements near his borders were "an act of aggression." In rebuttal, Senator Jobsworth of the Council of Genres reiterated that there would be no troop movements ahead of the peace talks on Friday.

"If Thursday is missing," I said to myself, "there won't be any peace talks."

"Mumbling to yourself?"

I looked up. It was Acheron Hades, the designated evildoer and antagonist from *The Eyre Affair.* Inside the book he was a homicidal maniac who would surgically remove people's faces for fun, but outside the book he collected stamps and wrote really bad poetry.

"Peace talks," I said, showing him the paper.

"I'm not going to hold my breath," he remarked. "Speedy Muffler is the master of brinksmanship. Any deal on the table will be unraveled the following morning — military intervention is the only thing that will stop him."

Acheron's attitude was not atypical. There were few who didn't think an all-out genre war between Women's Fiction and Racy

Novel was pretty much inevitable. The more absorbing question was, Will it be broadcast live? And then, Will it involve me or damage my own genre?

"Dogma will almost certainly be dragged into the fray," I said gloomily.

"And Comedy to the south," added Acheron, "and they won't like it. I don't think they were joking when they said they would defend their land to the last giggle."

The door opened, and the king and queen walked in. They looked a little worse for wear. I nodded a greeting, and they ordered a cappuccino each, which placed Paul in something of a panic — I don't think he'd ever made one before.

"By the way," said Acheron, "I think Lettie is the best understudy yet."

"Carmy?"

"Carmine. *Great* interpretation. Are you going to keep her?"

"I've . . . not decided yet."

"Just so you know, I approve," he said. "She can vanquish me any day of the week." He stared into his empty cup for a moment. "Can I talk to you about something?"

"Is it about your poetry?"

"It's about Bertha Rochester."

"Biting again?"

Acheron showed me his hand, which had

nasty tooth marks on it.

"Painful," I agreed. "I told you to keep the bite mask on until the last moment. But you do throw her to her death. She's allowed to struggle a *bit.*"

"That's another thing," he said as he pulled a pained expression. "Does she have to look at me in that accusatory way when I chuck her off the roof? It makes me feel all funny inside."

Unlike Acheron, who differed wildly from his in-book persona, Bertha really *was* bonkers. She had come to us after a grueling forty-six-year stint as Anne Catherick in *The Woman in White* and was now quite beyond any form of rehabilitation. In a cruel and ironic twist, Grace Poole kept our version of Bertha Rochester locked securely up in the attic. It was safer for everyone that way.

"I'll have a word," I said, then asked after a pause, "So . . . why do you think Carmine is so good?"

"Her interpretation is respectful, but with an edginess that is both sympathetic and noir."

"And you think that's better than my interpretation?"

"Not better," replied Acheron diplomatically, "different. And there's nothing wrong with *that,*" he added cautiously, finding a piece of invisible fluff on his jacket. "Carmine just plays her in a way that is . . . well, how shall I put it?"

"More readable?"

"She's an A-4 — you're an A-8. You'd *expect* her to exhibit a bit more depth."

"Thanks for that."

"Don't sweat it. Carmine can't handle quantity, and when and if she can, she'll be off to the bright lights of HumDram/Highbrow. Your job is assured. Besides," he added in a lighter tone, "if it *did* come to a vote, I'd go with you."

"I'm grateful for that at the very least," I replied despondently. "So you prefer the real Thursday Next to a more marketable one?"

"Well, yes — and the free time. Poetry is a *most* absorbing pastime."

It wasn't what I really wanted to hear, and after chatting for a few more minutes he left. I finished the paper and wandered back to the book. I had a brief chat with the series prop master on the way. He was the technician responsible for all the interactive objects in the series — items that could be handled or manipulated in some way.

"We've managed to repair your car," he said, "but go easy on it during the car chase.

If you could just pull up sharply rather than slewing sideways, I'd really appreciate it."

We were working to a budget these days. The remaking of the BookWorld had sneakily reorganized its budgetary systems. Instead of the "single-book payment," we now earned a "reader stipend" for every reading, with a labyrinthine system of bonuses and extra payments for targets. It wasn't universally liked. Any book that fell below the hundred-readers-a-week level could find itself hit by a double whammy: not enough funds to maintain the fabric of the novel, yet not enough Feedback Loop to hope the readers would do it for you.

I got back to the house at midmorning to find Pickwick already laying the table for lunch. She often picked up fads and trends from the BookWorld and just recently had caught the "reality bug" and insisted we sit for every meal, even though there was nothing to eat and we didn't need to. She also insisted that we play parlor games together in the evenings. This would have been fine if she didn't have to win at everything, and watching a dodo cheat badly at KerPlunk was not a happy spectacle.

I found Scarlett in the kitchen looking a little green about the gills and with an ice pack on her head.

"Problems?" I asked.

"N-n-n-none at all," groaned Carmine. "I j-j-just think I hit the hyphens a little t-t-t-too hard last n-n-night."

She groaned, closed her eyes and pressed the ice pack more firmly to her head.

"If you're hyphenated while working you'll be in serious trouble," I said in my most scolding voice. "And as your mentor, so will I."

"Yeah, yeah," murmured Carmine, eyes firmly closed. "I'll be fine. B-b-but can you p-p-p-please get the b-b-birdbrain over there to shut up?"

"I'm sorry," said Pickwick haughtily, "but was the drunken tart addressing me?"

"Why, is there *another* b-b-birdbrain present?"

"Okay, okay," I said, "calm down, you two. What's the problem?"

"That b-birdbrain insists on staring at m-me and sighing."

"Is this true?"

Pickwick ruffled her feathers indignantly. "She brought a goblin home, and they're nothing but trouble. What's more, I think she is *entirely* unsuitable for carrying on the important job of being Thursday. We all like a hyphen from time to time, but consorting with pointy-eared homunculi is *totally out of order!*"

She squawked the last bit, and Carmine rolled her eyes.

"I didn't b-bring a g-goblin home."

"He followed you home. It amounts to the same thing."

"You're j-just sour because you're not g-g-getting any," sneered Carmine. "And anyway, Horace is n-n-not like other g-g-goblins."

"Hang on," I said. "So you *did* bring a goblin home?"

"He g-g-got locked out of his b-b-book. What was I supposed to d-d-do?"

I threw up my arms. "Carmine!"

"D-don't you be so j-judgmental," she replied indignantly. "Look at yourself. F-f-five books in one s-series, and each by a different g-g-ghostwriter."

"Your private life is your own," I replied angrily, "but goblins can't help themselves — or rather they *can* help themselves — to anything not nailed down."

I ran upstairs to find that my bedroom had been ransacked. Anything of even the slightest value had been stolen. Inviting a goblin to cross your threshold was a recipe for disaster, and certainly worse than doing the same with a vampire. With the latter all you got was a nasty bite, but the company, the extraordinarily good sex and the funny stories more than made up for it — apparently.

"That was dumb," I said when I'd returned. "He's taken almost everything."

Carmine looked at me, then at Pickwick, then burst into tears and ran from the room.

"Goblins!" said Pickwick with a snort. "They're just trouble with a capital *G*. By the way," she added, now cheerier since she'd been proved correct, "Sprockett wanted to show you something. He's in your office."

I walked through to my study, where Sprockett was indeed waiting for me. He wasn't alone. He had his foot on top of a struggling goblin, and a burlap sack full of stolen possessions was lying on the carpet.

"Your property, ma'am?" he asked. I nodded, and he took the letter opener from the desk, held the goblin tightly by one ear and placed the opener to its throat. His eyebrow twitched. It was clearly a bluff. I decided to play along.

"No," I said, "you'll ruin the carpet. Do it outside."

The goblin opened his eyes wide and stared at me in shocked amazement, then started to babble on about an "influential uncle" who would "do unpleasant things" if he "went missing."

"Just kidding," I added. "Let him go."

"Are you sure?" asked Sprockett. "I can make it look like a shaving accident."

"Yes, I'm sure. You," I said, jabbing a finger at the goblin, "are a disgrace. Place a single toe in my series again and I'll make you wish you'd never been written."

Sprockett took his foot off the goblin, and it ran to the window, paused on the sill for a moment, made an obscene gesture and then ran off. That was the trouble with being stuck in Fantasy — too many goblins, spells, ogres, wizards, elves and warlocks. I reckoned it frightened readers off.

"So," I said, locking the window after the goblin, "what's the deal?"

"I was reappraising the condition of the wreckage from the debris field."

He showed me the Triumph Bonneville's exhaust pipe. It had been folded almost in half by the impact. He pointed to a small patch on the chrome. There was a slight mottling about four inches long and an inch wide.

"A fault in the manufacturing?" I suggested.

"But it wasn't manufactured," said Sprockett. "It was *written.* It should be perfect — better than any real motorcycle."

"You asked me in here to show me an imperfection on a Bonneville exhaust?"

"There's more. I found this orange inside the bed-sit. Here."

He tossed the orange across, and I noticed that this *also* had a slight mottling on the side. He then showed me similar imperfections on a Polaroid camera, a toaster, a half-eaten sandwich and a plastic bath duck. Then I got it.

"The mottling," I said slowly. "They are — *were* — ISBNs. Are you trying to tell me someone has *removed* all identification marks from this book?"

He didn't answer, which was answer enough. All doubts were off. *This wasn't an accident.* Someone had hacked into the novel's source code to delete the ISBN in order to cover his tracks and ensure that no one found out which book had been destroyed or why. The epizeuxis worm and now this. We didn't have a crashed book, we had a crime scene. But it wasn't *quite* that simple.

"Only Text Grand Central or the Council of Genres would have the power to scrub ISBNs and put together a rhetorical device," I said. "And while I'm not one to use coarse idioms, someone would have to be connected up the wazoo to pull this off. Have you attempted to find out what the ISBN actually was?"

Sprockett placed a series of photographs on the desk. "I took the liberty of subjecting the marks to a complex series of photographic techniques, which while appearing to have the veneer of scientific reality actually just sounded good. Do you want the full two pages of dull exposition or just the results?"

"Better just give me the results," I said, looking at my watch. "Whitby will be here any moment for a lunch date."

"Might I inquire where you are going, ma'am?"

"We thought we'd try the Elbow Rooms."

"A fine establishment. I meet up with the Hartzel chess player every two weeks there to discuss Matters of the Cog. I'd avoid the lobster."

"Food poisoning?"

"No, no, not on the menu — at the bar. *Very* opinionated and apt to lapse into unspeakably dull arthropod-related digressions. But see here."

He handed me a photograph that was many images superimposed on top of one another. The revealed ISBN was indistinct but legible. I jotted down the number in my notebook.

"Thank you, Sprockett. You're a star."

"Madam is most kind."

I fetched the unimaginatively titled *Cheshire Cat's Complete Guide to All Books Ever Written Everywhere* and looked up the ISBN. Our crashed book was from Self-Publishing and titled *The Murders on the Hareng Rouge,* by Adrian Dorset. I'd never heard of him. But it was Vanity, so I'd hardly be expected to. There was no other information. The ISBN database held only titles, authors, publishers' details, three-for-two offers, that kind of thing. I looked at the map we had pinned on the wall that charted the book's final journey. If you extended the line back through Adventure and past the Cliff of Notes, it made landfall in Vanity. We'd never considered such a thing. It must have lifted off there and proceeded in an almost straight line to where the Council of Genres was located, but it had come down over Conspiracy.

I sat, leaned back in my chair and ran through the likely scenarios. It was possible *The Murders on the Hareng Rouge* was a potential world beater on its way to being published. Jealousies ran deep in the Book-World, and the possibility of someone in HumDram/Highbrow nobbling the potential competition was quite real. It had happened before; bad Vanity was universally disliked but tolerated in a condescending "yes, well done, jolly good" kind of way, but good Vanity was reviled as the worst kind of upstart.

"Blast," I said, as a more personal note added itself to the mix. "It explains why I was asked to handle the investigation. No one expected me to find anything."

Sprockett's eyebrow pointed to "Bingo."

"The thought had occurred to me, ma'am. In fact, the precise reason you were selected for this investigation, given your lack of adequacy, has been troubling me for some time."

I thought about Acheron's comments with regard to the fact that Carmine was an A-4.

"I so need that sort of comment right now."

His eyebrow clicked from "Bingo" to "Apologetic."

"Merely the facts as I see them, ma'am."

I thought carefully. Part of me — the Thursday part — was outraged over the crime, but the rest of me was more realistic. There were some things that were simply not worth meddling with, and anyone willing to engineer the destruction of an entire book wouldn't think twice about eliminating me. There were few — if any — characters who couldn't be replaced.

"Have you told anyone about this?" I asked, and Sprockett shook his head.

"Keep it that way," I murmured. "I think all we've found is what Red Herring wanted me to find: an unprecedented event that is unrepeatable."

"If asked for an opinion, ma'am," said Sprockett in an unusually forceful turn of phrase, "I should like to find out who asked Commander Herring to allocate you to this investigation."

I stared at him. I should like to know, too, but I couldn't think of a way to frame the question that wouldn't have me in the trunk of a car heading towards the traditional place to dump bodies, the New Jersey area of Crime.

"This was never meant to be reported," I said. "This was meant for looking the other way and carrying on with life as though nothing had happened. There was a good reason I was asked to do this, and I will not impugn my lack of competence by being irresponsibly accurate. I have a reputation to uphold."

It was a hopelessly poor argument, and he and I both knew it. I sat down at my desk and drew a sheet of writing paper from my stationery drawer.

"Permission to speak openly?" he asked.

I took a deep breath. "I don't want to hear what you have to say, but I should."

"It's not what Thursday Next would have done."

"No," I replied, "but then Thursday could deal with this sort of stuff. She *enjoyed* it. A woman has to know her limitations. If Herring had wanted this accident to be investigated properly, he would have given it to someone else. Maybe it's for the best. Maybe there really *are* wheels within wheels. Maybe some stuff has to be left, for the good of all of us. We leave crime to the authorities, right?"

"That would certainly seem to be the safe and conventional option, ma'am."

"Exactly," I replied. "Safe. Conventional. Besides, I have a series to look after and dignity to be maintained for Thursday. If anything happened to me, as likely as not Carmine would take over, and I'm not convinced she'd uphold the standards quite as I do, what with the goblins and the hyphenating and such."

I looked away as I said it and began to rearrange the objects on my desk. I suddenly felt hot and a bit peculiar and didn't want to look Sprockett in the eye.

"As madam wishes."

Sprockett bowed and withdrew, and I spent the next hour writing up a report for Herring. It wasn't easy to write. Try as I might, I couldn't make the report longer than forty words, and it deserved more than that. I managed at one point to write a hundred words, but after I'd taken out the bit about the epizeuxis worm and the scrubbed ISBN, it was down to only thirty-seven again. I decided to ask Whitby his hypothetical opinion and finish the report after lunch.

I called the Jurisfiction offices again to see if Thursday was available to talk.

"She's still unavailable," I reported as I trotted into the kitchen. "I might try to speak to her when I go over to deliver the report to Commander Herring this afternoon. Do you think I'm dressed okay for Whitby or should I . . ."

My voice had trailed off because something was wrong. Sprockett and Mrs. Malaprop were looking at me in the sort of way I imagine disgruntled parents might.

"You tell her," said Mrs. Malaprop.

"It's Whitby," said Sprockett.

I suddenly had a terrible thought. This being fiction, long-unrequited romances often end in tragedy just before they finally begin, inevitably leading to a lifetime's conjecture of what might have happened and all manner of tedious and ultimately overwritten soul-searching. The scenario was almost as hideous as actually losing Whitby.

"He's dead?"

"No, ma'am, he's not dead. At least he was still alive two minutes ago."

"He was here? Why isn't he here now?"

Sprockett coughed politely. "I am sorry to say, ma'am, that I had to send Mr. Jett away."

I stared at him, scarcely believing what I was hearing. "Why would you do something like that?"

"I feel, ma'am, that he is *unsuitable.*"

"What?"

He showed me a newspaper clipping that was about two years old. "I exhort you to read it, ma'am, no matter how painful."

So I did.

"It is the painful duty of this journalist," went the article, "to report an act of such base depravity that it causes the worst excesses of Horror to pale into insignificance. Last Tuesday an unnamed man, for reasons known only to himself, set fire to a busload of nuns who were taking their orphaned puppies to a 'How cute is your puppy?' competition. Unfortunately, the perpetrator of this vile and heartless act is still at liberty, and . . ."

I stopped reading as a sense of confusion and disappointment welled up inside me. There was a picture accompanying the article, and even though the piece did not mention Whitby by name, there was a photograph of a man whom "Jurisfiction wanted to question." It was Jett, without a doubt — holding a two-gallon gasoline can and chuckling. I didn't really know what was worse — Whitby killing the busload of nuns or me having finally plucked up the courage to have lunch at the Elbow Rooms, only for the rug to be pulled from under my feet.

"Is this true?"

"I'm afraid so. I'm sorry, ma'am. Was I wrong to send him away?"

"No, you were right."

I sighed and stared at the report I was carrying. "Better call a cab. I'm going to tell Herring what he wants to hear. At least that way someone gets to be happy today. You can come, too."

It took me twenty minutes to coax Carmine out of her bedroom. I assured her it wasn't so bad, because Sprockett had caught the goblin and recovered the swag, so he wasn't *technically* a thief. I had to tell her that he wasn't *that* unhandsome — for a goblin — and that no, I was sure he wasn't just saying nice things to her so he could be invited across the threshold. I told her she was now on book duty, as I would be out for a while, and she replied, "Yes, okay, fine," but wouldn't look at me, so I left her staring angrily at the patterned wallpaper in the front room.

12.
Jurisfiction

Budgetary overruns almost buried the remaking before the planning stage, until relief came from an unexpected quarter. A spate of dodgy accounting practices in the Outland necessitated a new genre in Fiction: Creative Accountancy. Shunned by many as "not a proper genre at all," the members' skills at turning thin air into billion-dollar profits were suddenly of huge use, and the remaking went ahead as planned. Enron may have been a pit of vipers in the Outland, but they quite literally saved the BookWorld.

Bradshaw's BookWorld Companion
(16th edition)

I took the bus to Le Guin Central and then the first train to HumDram/Classics. As the train slowly steamed from the station, I sat back and stared out the window. I was mildly interested to learn that Heathcliff was on the same train, although we didn't see him — just a lot of screaming and fainting girls on the platform whenever we stopped. We halted briefly at Gaiman Junction before steaming on a wide arc to Shakespeare Terminus. There was a delay leaving the platform, as security was being taken a little more seriously than usual. A group of heavily armed Men in Plaid were scrutinizing everyone's IDs.

"Do you think this is about the Racy Novel peace talks?" I asked a French Wilkins Micawber who was there on an exchange trip.

"*Mais oui.* But I think ze CofG is being a leetle jittery 'bout Racy Novel," he explained in a pointlessly overblown French accent. "Zey think zat zere may be fizz columnists eager to cause — 'ow you say? — mischief. I'd not like to be without shirt and medallion while Barry White plays in ze background right now, I can tells you."

"Reason for visit?" asked the Plaid on guard duty.

"I have to report to Mr. Lockheed regarding a crashed-book investigation."

"Very well," said the Plaid. "And what's with the mechanical butler?"

"To lend tone to the proceedings."

This was enough for the Man in Plaid,

and with a gruff "Welcome to the Classics, have an eloquent day," I was allowed to pass. On our way out of the station, I noticed a small group of characters who had been pulled aside. Some of the women wore miniskirts, tube tops and stilettos, and the men had shirts open to the navel. It seemed as though anyone even remotely resembling someone from Racy Novel was immediately under suspicion. They were protesting their innocence and complaining bitterly about the unfair character profiling, but to little avail.

We took a tram along Austen Boulevard and got out just outside the gates to *Sense and Sensibility.* This was a large compound, and a high wall topped with barbed wire surrounded the many settings that made up the book. On each corner were watchtowers, from which armed Plaids kept a constant lookout. Such tight security wasn't just to protect the Dashwoods — the residence of Norland Park within *Sense and Sensibility* was also the headquarters of Jurisfiction, Fiction's policing agency.

Waiting at the gates was a group of characters with day passes, ready for the tour. For some reason those in Sci-Fi had a thing about the classics, so of the twenty or thirty characters waiting, at least two-thirds were aliens. Since most of them hailed from the poor end of the genre, they had a lot of tentacles and left sticky trails after themselves, which caused no end of cleaning up.

"No clockwork automatons," said one of the guards on duty. "You should know better than that, Miss Next."

I had to explain that I wasn't *that* Miss Next, and the guard peered closer at me, grunted and then explained that a Duplex-4 had suffered a mainspring failure several months before and killed eight bystanders, so all cog-based life-forms below the Duplex-6 had been banned.

"The Six has been released?" asked Sprockett, who had a vested interest in the competition. To sentient machines the primary cause of worry was obsolescence, closely followed by metal fatigue and inadequate servicing.

"It was launched just after the remaking," said the guard, "but I've not seen one yet."

"They must have rushed them into production," murmured Sprockett. "A risk, if they're still at the beta-test stage."

I suggested to Sprockett that he nip into the local Stubbs and not have a coffee or two until I returned, to which he gratefully acquiesced.

After signing the visitors' book and a risk

assessment that included "erasure, swollen ankles and death by drowning," I was issued a visitor's pass and allowed to walk up the graveled path towards the house. Since we were now actually *within* the backstory of *Sense and Sensibility,* the view upwards was not of the rest of the BookWorld — the curved inside of the sphere and books moving about — but of clouds and a clear blue sky. The trees gently rustled as though in a breeze, and the herbaceous borders were alive with a delicate symphony of color. This was one of the better attributes of the Reader Feedback Loop. When readers imbue a book with their own interpretations, the weather always comes first, then colors, symmetry, trees, architecture, fixtures and fittings and finally texture. Birdsong, however, is generally not something brought alive by the reader's imagination, so the birds still have to be provided. Since we were now in the unread zone of the novel, the birds were either off-duty or populating another book elsewhere. There is a certain degree of economics within the BookWorld; Austen birds are the same as Brontë ones — listen carefully and you'll hear.

I stopped at the front door to Norland Park and gave my name to the footman, who looked as much like a frog as you can without actually being one. He gazed at me for a long time and opened his eyes so wide I thought for a moment they might fall out, and I readied myself with a pocket handkerchief in case they did. But they didn't fall out, and after another minute's thought he relaxed and said, "You do look like her, don't you?"

I thought of telling him that he looked very much like a frog but thought better of it.

"You're the first person not to confuse me with her for a while," I remarked. "How did you know?"

"The real Thursday always ignored me," he replied, "walked past without a word. But never in a bad way — she always did it respectful like."

"Do you get ignored a lot?"

"I do, and not just by ordinary citizens. I've been ignored by some of the greats, you know." He then proceeded to list twenty or so major characters who hadn't acknowledged his existence on a regular basis. He had a particular fondness for David Copperfield, whom he had escorted almost three hundred times "without a glance in my direction."

"That must be quite upsetting."

"I'm a footman," he explained. "We're trained to be not-there-but-there. Being ignored is the yardstick of a footman's professional abilities. My father was sixty-seven years in the employ of the first Lord Spongg and wasn't acknowledged once. He went to his grave a fulfilled man. If you want to be ignored by the movers and shakers of the BookWorld," concluded the frog-footman proudly, "this is the place to do it."

"You've very fortunate," I said, humoring him. "Some people don't get to be ignored at all."

"Don't I know it," he replied, licking the end of his pencil and consulting his clip-board. "Now, reason for visit?"

"I'm to see Mr. Lockheed at Accident Investigation."

"Correct. This way."

The entrance hall was large and empty except for a round mahogany table in the middle, upon which stood a vase of flowers. The way to Herring's office took us past the ballroom, from which Jurisfiction's agents were given their instructions and posted to all corners of the BookWorld to face adversaries so dangerous that it was truly astonishing that anyone ever survived. I had been in there a few times when I'd been a trainee of the real Thursday, but I hadn't visited since I failed my training day. I slowed my pace as we passed, for the door was open and I could see Jurisfiction's elite talking and laughing. I recognized Emperor Zhark and a large hedgepig that could only be Mrs. Tiggy-winkle. The Red Queen was there, too, and several others.

The frog-footman coughed his disapproval, and we made to move on. But at that moment a short man in late middle age and dressed as a big-game hunter stepped out of the open door. He was wearing a pith helmet and a safari suit, and across his body was slung a Sam Brown belt and holster, with the outfit finished off by a pair of brown leather riding boots. Since Thursday's disappearance, he was probably the third-most-important person in the BookWorld after Senator Jobsworth and Red Herring. His name was Commander Bradshaw, and his expert guidance at Jurisfiction had kept the agency at the top of its game for almost as long as anyone could remember — his exploits ensured that he was hardly ever off the front page of *The Word,* and his much-updated *BookWorld Companion* was the definitive work on the BookWorld, both before and after the remaking.

He was deep in conversation with a youngish agent. I felt out of place, so I looked straight ahead and quickened my pace. But he noticed me and without pausing for a second took me firmly by the arm and steered me to an alcove.

"Thursday," he hissed in an agitated manner, "why are you dressed in those ridiculous clothes, and where in heaven's name have you been?"

"I'm not her, sir. I'm the one who looks after her series. I'm actually A8-V-67987-FP."

He frowned, then stared at me for a moment. "You're telling me you're the *written* one?"

I nodded, and he burst into laughter.

"Well, strike me pink!" he said. "You gave me a turn and no mistake. I was . . . ah, expecting Thursday to be here any moment," he added, looking at his watch in an unsubtle manner. "I suspect she has been delayed."

His explanation didn't ring true at all. Thursday was *definitely* more missing than he would like me to know. We returned to where Bradshaw's companion was waiting for us. He was studiously ignoring the frog-footman, who for his part was accepting the snub with quiet dignity.

"I'd forgotten just how identical you looked," he said. "Are you keeping well?"

"I am, sir," I managed to mumble. "I trust you are well read?"

It was a stupid gaffe; Bradshaw's brand of jingoistic Imperialist fiction hadn't been read for a half century. But he took no offense.

"Not read anymore, and quite right, too," he said laughingly, then stared at me for a while before saying to his companion, "You've met the other Thursday, the real one?"

"Sure have," he replied. "One helluva goddamn fine operative."

"Look alike, don't they? Apart from the clothes, of course."

"Like two peas in a pod."

Bradshaw thought for a moment. "Has Thursday been down to see you recently?" he asked me with an air of feigned nonchalance.

"Not since the remaking, sir," I replied. "May I ask a question?"

"Of course."

"Am I to understand that Thursday Next is . . . *missing?*"

"She's currently on leave in the RealWorld," he said in a dismissive manner, "enjoying some time off with her family before the peace negotiations on Friday."

"Are you sure about that? I saw —"

I checked myself. I could get into big trouble for sneak-peeking the RealWorld, and the Lady of Shalott could get into bigger trouble for letting me.

"What did you see?" asked Bradshaw.

"Nothing. I must have . . . dreamt it. I'm very sorry to have wasted your time, sir."

He looked at me for a long while, trying to divine what, if anything, I knew. Finally he said, "You are keeping the Thursday Next series dignified, I trust?"

"Yes, sir — even at the expense of readability."

"Being read isn't everything. Some of the best people are hardly read at all. Listen," he said thoughtfully, staring at me with his intelligent blue eyes, "would you do something for me?"

"Of course."

Right then a man draped in the white linen robes of the most senior senatorial office walked briskly through the front doors of Norland Park and into the entrance hall in which we stood.

"Oh, crap," said Bradshaw under his breath. "Just what we need: Jobsworth."

If he was over here in person, it would be for a very good reason — probably about the Racy Novel peace talks.

I thought of dropping to one knee and

averting my eyes as the frog-footman had done, but for some reason I didn't. The Thursday part of me, I suppose. Jobsworth was not alone. As well as the usual phalanx of staff, hangers-on and deputies, there was Barnes, Jobsworth's executive assistant; Colonel Barksdale, the head of the Avoiding War Department; and Commander Herring, who was busy reading a report and hadn't yet seen me.

"Good morning, Bradshaw," said Jobsworth. Bradshaw wished the senator good morning, then the same to Commander Herring and Colonel Barksdale. Barnes was too far down the pecking order to be greeted, as were all the other members of Jobsworth's staff. The senator began to speak, then saw me. His eyes opened wide.

"Great Panjandrum!" he said. "Thursday?"

Bradshaw looked at me, then at the senator. I opened my mouth to reply, but Bradshaw held up a hand. In such company it was *strictly* speak-when-spoken-to. Protocol in the BookWorld was like grammatical rules — rigidly structured, arcane and fiercely defended by librarians wielding wooden rulers with painful accuracy.

"No, Senator, it's the *written* version."

"Truthfully?" asked Jobsworth. "She looks

an awful lot like her."

"If she *were* the real one, do you think she would be here accompanied by that . . . that — what's your name?"

The frog-footman looked startled at being spoken to. "Wesley," he said in a quiet voice.

"Right," said Bradshaw, not really listening, "being shown around by frog guy? If this *were* the one, she'd be in the office discussing the peace talks and the metaphor crisis."

"I'll vouch that she's the written one," said Herring, who had just looked up. "Are you here on JAID business, Next?"

"I am, sir."

"Then you can take your findings direct to Lockheed."

It seemed a good moment to leave, so I bobbed politely and began to withdraw.

"Wait," said the senator. "Bradshaw, why were you speaking to her if she's just the copy?"

For a fleeting moment, Bradshaw looked uncomfortable.

"I was asking her if . . . she could ask Lorina Peabody to head up the Talking Animal Division of Jurisfiction."

"Who the hell's Lorina Peabody?"

"She's a dodo," I said.

Jobsworth stared at Bradshaw suspiciously,

then me. "Introduce us," he said after a pause.

"Very well," said Bradshaw with a sigh. "Senior Senator Giles Jobsworth, head of Fiction and emissary to the Great Panjandrum, the written Thursday Next."

"Hello," he said, shaking me by the hand and giving me the smile of somebody who was considering how best one could be exploited.

"Honored, Senator, sir," I replied dutifully.

Jobsworth was perhaps sixty or sixty-five, graying at the temples and with the look of someone weighed down heavily by responsibility. He stepped forward and put a finger under my chin. I should have been more overawed in his presence, but I wasn't. In fact, I had every reason to dislike him. When the senior senator was merely a senator, he had blocked my series from having Landen in it. He had said having no Landen was "as the author intended," but that didn't really help, to be honest.

"It looks *exactly* like her," he breathed.

"Like two goddamn peas in a pod," agreed Bradshaw's companion.

"I'm mirrored with her, Senator," I explained. "The books were built using H-29 biographical architecture before they were moved to Nonfiction, so my looks are directly linked to hers. I age at the same rate and even grow the same scars in sympath—"

"Fascinating. Does it have skills and an intellect to match, Commander Bradshaw?"

"It does not — nor any dress sense. What's your interest in an A-8 copy of Thursday Next, Senator?"

"The interests of the council are not necessarily the interests of Jurisfiction, Bradshaw."

They stared at each other for several seconds. I expect this happened quite a lot. Jurisfiction was a policing agency, working under the council, who were wholly political. I can't imagine they *ever* got on.

"Sir?" said Barnes, gently coaxing the senator to stick to his schedule. "You have a meeting."

"Very well," said the head of Fiction, and he strode off into the Jurisfiction offices with Herring, Barksdale and his entourage. Bradshaw stared at me for a moment, then told me I was excused. I needed no further bidding, and curtsied politely before hurrying off with the frog-footman.

"Well, thanks for that," said the frog-footman sarcastically. "You just ruined my six-year 'being ignored by Commander

Bradshaw' record."

"He didn't remember your name," I said, trying to be helpful, "and was horribly insensitive when he called you 'frog guy.' "

"Well, okay," said the frog-footman, "that does take the sting out a little bit. But tell me," he said, staring at me with his large, protruding eyes and broad mouth, "why did he call me 'frog guy'?"

"I was up for Jurisfiction once," I said, quickly changing the subject, "but it didn't work out."

"Me, too," sadly replied the frog-footman, whose mind didn't seem to pause on any one subject for long. "I didn't make it past the 'What is your name?' question. You?"

"Training day. Froze when the going got tough. Nearly got my mentor killed."

"To fail spectacularly is a loser's paradise," said the frog-footman wistfully. "This way."

14.
Stamped and Filed

Distilling metaphor out of raw euphemism was wasteful and expensive, and the euphemism-producing genres on the island were always squeezing the market. Besides, the by-product of metaphor using the Cracked Euphemism Process liberates irony-238 and dangerous quantities of alliteration, which are associated with downright dangerous disposal difficulties.

Bradshaw's BookWorld Companion
(9th edition)

We walked down the seemingly endless corridors, every door placarded with the name of the department contained within. One was labeled OLD JOKES and another NOUN-TO-VERB CONVERSION UNIT. Just past the offices of the Synonym Squad and the Danvers Union headquarters was a small office simply labeled JAID.

"Right. Well," I said, "I'll see myself out

when I'm done."

"I'm afraid not," replied the frog-footman. "I am instructed to escort you both in *and* out."

So while the frog-footman sat on a chair in the corridor opposite, I knocked on the door.

"Commander Herring told me you would be stopping by," said Lockheed as I entered. "Do come in. Tea?"

"No thank you."

I looked around. The office was roomy, had a large window and was paneled in light pine. The pictures that decorated the walls all depicted a book disaster of some sort, mostly with Lockheed featured prominently in the foreground, grinning broadly. There was little clutter, and the single filing cabinet probably contained nothing but a kettle and some cookies. Jurisfiction had finally managed to commit itself to a paperless office — all files were committed to the prodigious memory of Captain Phantastic, just down the hall.

"Impressive office, eh?" said Lockheed. "We even have a window — with a view. Come and have a look."

I walked over to the window and looked out. All I could see was a brick wall barely six feet away.

"Very nice," I murmured.

"If you lean right out with someone hanging on to your shirttails, you can almost see the sky, but not quite. Would you like to try?"

"No thanks."

"So," said Lockheed, sitting down on his swivel chair and motioning me to a seat, "something to report to Commander Herring about the accident?"

I swallowed hard. "It was simply that," I said, an odd leaden feeling dropping down inside me. "An accident."

Lockheed breathed a visible sigh of relief. "Commander Herring will be delighted. When he hears bad news, he usually likes to hit someone about the head with an iron bar, and I'm often the closest. Are you *sure* there is nothing to report?"

I wondered for a moment whether to report the epizeuxis worm, scrubbed ISBN and the Vanity roots of *The Murders on the Hareng Rouge.* Not necessarily because it was the right thing to do, but simply to watch the eye-popping effect it might have on Lockheed.

"Nothing, sir."

"Unprecedented and unrepeatable?"

"Exactly so."

I felt the curious leaden feeling again. I

didn't know what it was; I patted my chest and cleared my throat.

"Little cog, big machine," said Lockheed as he filled out a form for me to sign. "We are here to facilitate, not to pontificate. If we can sew this whole incident shut, the sooner we can get on with our lives and maintain our unimpeachable hundred-percent dealt-with rate. Wheels within wheels, Thursday."

"Wheels within wheels, sir."

"Did you find out what the book was, by the way?"

"Not a clue," I lied. "I didn't find a single ISBN, so I thought 'Why bother?' and decided to simply give up."

I didn't know why I was suddenly being sarcastic. It might have been something to do with the odd leaden feeling inside. Lockheed, however, missed the sarcasm completely. Most D-3s did.

"Splendid!" he said. "I can see that you and Commander Herring will be getting on very well. You can expect a few more incidents heading your way with this kind of flagrant level of inspired disinterest. Sign here . . . and *here.*"

He handed the form over, and I paused, then signed on the dotted line. This isn't what Thursday would have done, but then I wasn't Thursday.

"Excellent," he said, rising from his seat. "I'll take this along to Captain Phantastic for memorizing."

"Why don't I take it?" I suggested. The odd leaden feeling in me had released a sense of purpose, but of what I was not sure. "You can stay here and have some tea and cookies or something."

I nodded my head in the direction of the filing cabinet.

"Goodness me, that is so *very* kind," replied Lockheed, condemning the lost souls in the unknown book to eternal anonymity with a ridiculously large rubber stamp before handing me the form. "Fourth door on the left."

"Right you are."

I opened the door, thanked him again and found the frog-footman waiting for me in the corridor. I told him I had some filing to do, and he led me past the doors marked PIANO DIVISION, ITALICS, and PEBBLES (MISCELLANEOUS) before we got to a door marked RECORDS. The frog-footman told me he'd wait for me there, and I stepped inside.

The room was small and shabby and had a half dozen people waiting to be seen, so I sat on a chair to wait my turn.

"Thursday Next," I said to the gloomy-looking individual sitting next to me, who was reading a paper and appeared to have a toad actually *growing* out of the top of his head. The pink skin of his balding pate seemed to merge with the browny-green of the toad. "The copy," I added, before he asked. But the man ignored me. The toad growing out of his head, however, was more polite.

"Ah," said the toad. "A good copy?"

"I do okay."

"Humph," said the toad before adding, "Tell me, do I look stupid with a human growing out of my bottom?"

"Not at all," I replied politely. "In fact, I think it's rather fetching."

"Do you really?" said the toad with a smile.

"Who are you talking to?" asked the man, looking up from his paper.

"The toad."

The man looked around. "What toad?"

"What did the man just say?" asked the toad.

"I like your books," said the woman on the other side of me. "When are we going to see some more?"

"Five is all you'll get," I said, happy to get

away from the man-toad. "What are you seeing Captain Phantastic for?"

"I'm head of the Metaphor Allocation Committee," she explained. "Once we move to the Metaphor Credit Trading System, those books with excess metaphor will be able to trade it on the floor of the Narrative Device Exchange. Naturally, more complex figurative devices such as hypothetical futures and analogy and simile trust funds will have to be regulated; we can't have hyperbole ending up as overvalued as it was — the bottom dropped out of the litotes market, which, as anyone will tell you, was most undesirable."

"*Most* undesirable," I remarked, having not understood a word. "And how will Captain Phantastic help with all this?"

She shrugged. "I just want to run the idea past him. There might be a historical precedent that could suggest collateralized metaphor obligations might be a bad idea. Even so," she added, "we might do it anyway — just for kicks and giggles. Excuse me."

While we'd been talking, Captain Phantastic had been dealing with each inquiry at lightning speed. This wasn't surprising, as the Records Office relied on nothing as mundane as magnetic storage, paper filing or even a linked alien supermind. It had in its possession instead a single elephant with a prodigiously large memory. It was efficient and simple, and it required only buns, hay and peanuts to operate.

When it was my turn, I walked nervously into his office.

"Hello," said the elephant in a nasally, trumpety, blocked-nose sort of voice. I noticed he was dressed in an unusual three-piece pin-striped suit, unusual in that not only did it have a watch fob the size of a saucepan in the waistcoat pocket, but the pinstripes were running horizontally.

"So how can I help?"

"Jurisfiction Accident Investigation Department," I said, holding up my shield. I paused as a sudden thought struck me. Not about elephants, or even of a toad with a man growing out of its bottom, or of the volatile metaphor market. I suddenly thought about *lying.* Of subterfuge. It was wrong, but in a *right* kind of way, because I had finally figured out what the leaden feeling was. It was a deficiency of Right Thing to Do — and I needed to remedy the shortfall, and fast.

"We're investigating a crashed book out in Conspiracy," I said, tearing up the accident report behind my back, "and we need some background information on *The Murders on the Hareng Rouge* by Adrian Dorset."

"Of course," trumpeted the elephant. "Take a seat, Miss . . . ?"

"Next. *Thursday* Next. But I'm not —"

"It's all right," he said, "I know. I know everything. More even than the Cheshire Cat. And that's saying something. I'm Captain Phantastic, by the way, but you can call me 'the Captain.' You and I haven't met, but the real Thursday and I go back a ways — even partnered together during the whole sorry issue surrounding *The Cat in the Hat III — Revenge of the Things.* Did you hear about it?"

"I'm sorry, I didn't."

"No matter." And he sniffed at me delicately for a moment with his trunk.

"Do you have a chicken living in your house?"

"A dodo."

"Would that be Lorina?"

"We call her Pickwick these days, but yes."

"Tell her that Captain Phantastic is still waiting for that date she promised."

I wasn't aware that Pickwick dated elephants — or anyone, come to that.

"Did she promise you recently?"

"Eighty-six years, three months, and two days ago. Would you like me to relate the conversation? I can do it word for word."

"No thanks. I'll give her the message."

The Captain leaned back on his chair and closed his eyes.

"Now, *The Murders on the Hareng Rouge.* I try to read most books, but for obvious reasons those in Vanity I delegate. So many books, so little time. Listen, you don't have a bun on you, do you? Raisins or otherwise, I'm not fussy."

"I'm afraid not."

"Shame. Okay, well, there's not much to tell, really. *The Murders on the Hareng Rouge* was a junker on its way to be scrapped."

I wasn't expecting this. "I'm sorry?"

"It was a stinker. One of the very worst books ever written. Self-published by one Adrian H. Dorset, who as far as we know has not written anything else. He printed two copies and spiral bound them in his local print shop. Semiautobiographical, it was the story of a man coming to terms with the death of his wife and how he then immersed himself in work to try to take revenge on the person he thought responsible. Flat, trite and uninspiring. The author burned it as a form of catharsis. By rigid convention, the version here in the BookWorld has to be scrapped before sundown. Did it hurt anyone?"

"Only the people in it."

"It should have been empty," said the elephant. "Scrapped books always have the occupants reallocated before the book is torn apart."

"We found the remains of *someone*."

"How much?"

"A thumb."

The elephant shrugged. "A hitchhiker, perhaps? Or reformed graphemes?"

"We thought the same."

"In any event," concluded Phantastic, "that's all I have."

"You're sure it was a junker?" I asked, trying to figure out why anyone would risk almost certain erasure by deleting the ISBN and then using demolition-grade epizeuxis to destroy an unreadable book from Vanity that was destined to be scrapped anyway.

"Completely sure."

I thanked Captain Phantastic for his time, promised to bring some buns next time and walked out of his office, deep in thought.

"You were in there a while," said the frog-footman as he escorted me from the building.

"The Captain likes to talk," I said. " 'Hannibal said this, me and Dumbo did that, Horton's my best friend, I was Celeste's first choice but she took Babar on the rebound' — you know what it's like."

"After Madame Bovary," said the frog-footman, rolling his eyes, "the Captain is the worst name-dropper I've ever been ignored by."

I went and found Sprockett in the local Stubbs. He had got chatting to a Mystical Meg Fortune-Telling Automaton and discovered that they were distantly related.

"I've got you a fortune card, ma'am," said Sprockett. "Archie was a great-great-uncle to us both, and Meg's father-in-law is Gort."

"Nice chap?"

"So long as you don't get him annoyed."

I looked at the small card he had given me. It read, "Avoid eating oysters if there is no paycheck in the month," which is one of those generic pieces of wisdom that Mechanical Mystics often hand out, along with "Every chapter a new beginning" and "What has a clause at the end of the pause?"

Sprockett hailed a cab, and we were soon trundling off in the direction of Fantasy.

"Did all go as planned, ma'am?" he asked as we made our way back out of the genre on the Dickens Freeway.

I paused. It was better if Sprockett didn't know that the investigation was covertly still running. Better for me, and better for him. Despite being a cog-based life-form, he could still suffer at the hands of inquisitors, and he needed deniability. If I was going to go down, I'd go down on my own.

In ten minutes I had told him everything. He nodded sagely, his gears whirring as he took it all in. Once I was done, he suggested that we not tell anyone, as Carmine might tell the goblin and Pickwick was apt to blurt things out randomly to strangers. Mrs. Malaprop we didn't have to worry about — no one would be able to understand her. Besides, she probably already knew.

"The less people who know, the better."

"Fewer. The *fewer* people who know, the better."

"That's what I meant."

"That's what *who* meant?"

"Wait — who's speaking now?"

"I don't know."

"You *must* know."

"Damn. It must be me — you wouldn't say 'damn,' would you?"

"I might."

We both paused for a moment, waiting for either a speech marker or a descriptive line. It was one of those things that happened every now and again in BookWorld — akin to an empty, pregnant silence in the middle of an Outland dinner party.

"So," said Sprockett once we had sorted ourselves out, "what's the plan?"

"I don't know our next move," I said, "but until I do, we do nothing — which is excellent cover for what we should be doing — nothing."

"An inspired plan," said Sprockett.

The taxi slowed down and stopped as the traffic ground to a halt. The cabbie made some inquiries and found that a truckload of "their" had collided with a trailer containing "there" going in the opposite direction and had spread there contents across the road.

"Their will be a few hiccups after that," said the cabbie, and I agreed. Homophone mishaps often seeped out into the RealWorld and infected the Outlanders, causing theire to be all manner of confusion.

"I know a shortcut through Comedy," said the cabbie, who was, purely as an irrelevant aside, an anteater named Ralph. "It shouldn't be too onerous — the risibility is currently at thirty yards and the mirthrate down to 1.9."

"What about puns?"

"Always about, but they're not funny, so the chance of unbridled hysteria is low."

Trips through Comedy were usually avoided, as the giggling could be painful and sometimes fatal, but the comedy in Comedy had been muted of late. I told him to go ahead, and we pulled out of the traffic and drove off in the opposite direction.

"What kind of man sets fire to a busload of nuns?" I asked, Whitby still annoyingly on my mind.

"I cannot answer that, ma'am, but I suspect one who is neither kind nor considerate."

There was a pause.

"May I ask a question regarding the subject of empathy, something I am at a loss to understand?"

"Of course."

"Since I have set neither a nun nor a puppy on fire nor gleefully pushed an old lady downstairs, does that make me kind and compassionate?"

"Not really," I replied. "It makes you normal, and respectful of accepted social rules."

"But not compassionate?"

"To be compassionate you have to demonstrate it in some sort of act that shows you care for someone."

"Care for someone? Care as in how a butler cares for someone?"

"More than that."

"I'm not sure I can envisage any greater care than that which a butler can offer."

And he sat and buzzed to himself in such

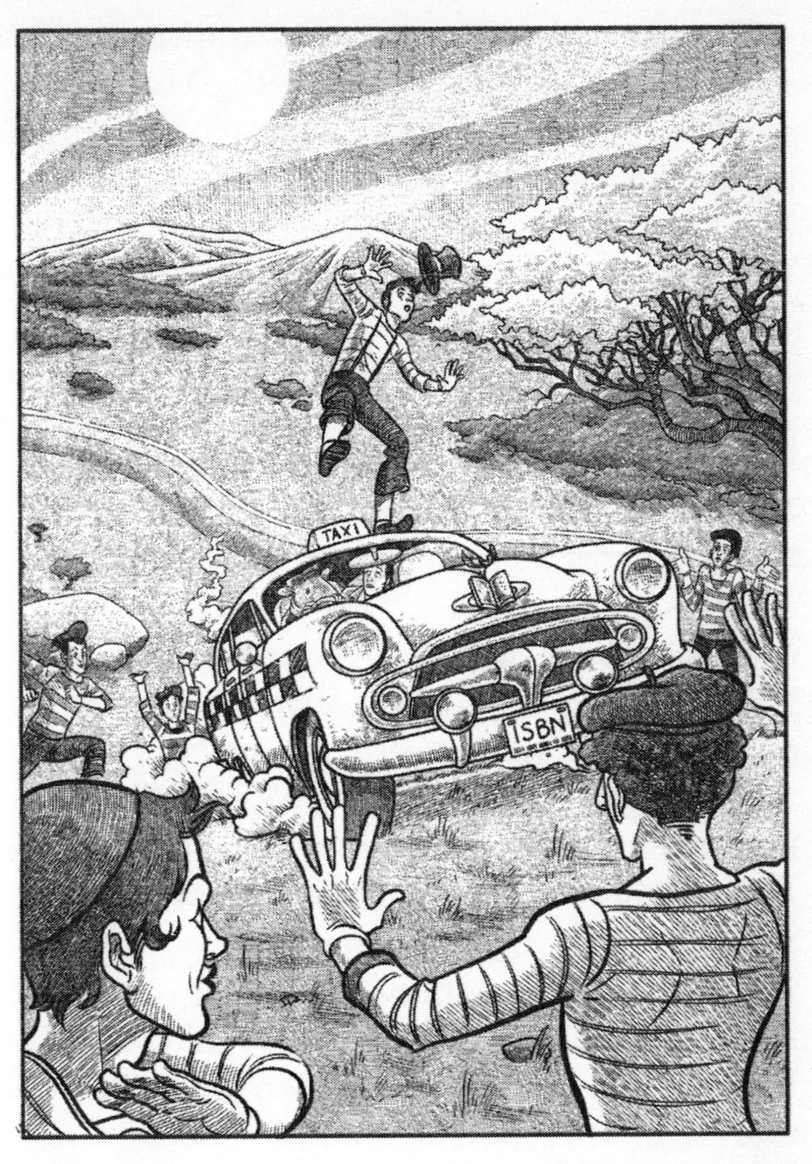

"Don't anyone move. . . . I think we've driven into a mimefield."

deep thought that I had to give him two extra winds, much to the cabbie's sniffy disapproval.

We entered Comedy a few miles farther on by way of the Thurber Freeway, then took a funny turn at Bad Joke and bumped along a back road of compacted mother-in-law one-liners. We passed the Knock-Knock? Quarry, where we were held up for a few minutes while they did some blasting, then continued on past Limericks, Amusing Anecdotes and Talking-Horse Gags to the empty wilderness known as the Burlesque Depression. The huge influx of stand-up comedians in the RealWorld had overjoked the stocks of natural glee, and the stony comedic landscape was now almost barren. As an emergency measure, unfunny comedy sneakily branded "alternative" was now flooding the RealWorld until the natural stock of jokes had replenished itself. The lack of comedy in Comedy was no laughing matter.

Almost from nowhere a car shot past us at speed and, as it did so, swerved violently. The cabbie attempted to avoid a collision and spun the wheel hard to the left. He overcorrected, slewed sideways and hit the fence at the side of the road. There was a crunch as splintered wood flew everywhere, the windscreen crazed, and the taxi thumped down the short embankment, ran across some rough ground and came to rest with a clatter and a hiss against a tree.

"Are you okay?" I asked.

Sprockett nodded, even though I could see he had a crack in his porcelain face. The cabbie looked a bit shocked and was about to open his door when I placed a hand on his shoulder.

"Wait. Don't anyone move. . . . I think we've driven into a mimefield."

15.
The Mimefield

Books' moving from Nonfiction to Fiction was uncommon, but it did happen. The most recent immigrant was *I Got Beaten Every Day for Eight Years by My Drunken Father* from Misery Memoirs, when it was discovered the author had made most of it up. By all accounts *Eight Years* had to leave in disgrace, tail between bruised legs, but I think secretly delighted. There is nowhere more depressing than Misery Memoirs, and the few visitors it has are usually characters-in-training who have a tricky scene to do in Human Drama and need some inspiration.

Bradshaw's BookWorld Companion
(10th edition)

Sprockett and the cabbie looked outside. Surrounding the car were five hundred or so mimes, all dressed uniformly in tight black slacks, a stripy top, white greasepaint and a large hat with a flower stuck in the crown. They were miming in the most terrifying fashion, their hideous faces contorted with exaggerated expressions, their bodies moving in a frighteningly sinuous movement that defied written description. The cabbie panicked and started the engine. It burst into life, and he popped the car into reverse.

"Hold it," I said, looking out the rear window. "You can't go backwards — there's a mime stuck inside a pretend glass cube just behind you. Wait — he's out. No, hang on, there's another, bigger pretend glass cube outside the smaller one."

The cabbie started to sob.

"Calm down," I said. "Panic is the mind killer. We can get out of this alive if we keep our heads straight. Turn the engine off."

We glanced around as the mimes, now curious, moved closer. I almost cried out as one peered into the car while doing a routine with a balloon that was heavy, then light, then immovable.

"What are they doing?" asked the cabbie, his voice tremulous with rising fear. "I don't understand."

Comedy was one of those genres that while appearing quite jolly was actually highly dangerous. In order to generate new jokes, the custodians of the genre had tried to use nonwritten and nonverbal comedy as a growing medium. Mimes had no real home in a written or spoken canon, but some of their movements and actions could cross-pollinate with others that did. Slapstick was used for the same effect, as was as a well-timed look, a comical pause and silly expressions, voices and walks.

"Don't move," said Sprockett. "Mimes don't generally attack unless they are threatened."

"How do you threaten a mime?"

"By sighing during a performance, looking away, rolling your eyes — that sort of thing. Mimes hate being ignored or having their performance interrupted. In that respect they're almost as touchy as poets."

We did as I suggested and watched as the mimes continued their strange movements, and we laughed and applauded at the right moments. Some of the mimes appeared hardly to move at all and adopted poses like statues, and others seemed to be walking against the wind. There was also a lot of going in and out of doors that weren't there, canoeing and pretending to walk up and down stairs. It was all *very* mystifying. Mind you, I was worried just how long we could laugh and applaud. Every moment we paused, they became dangerously aggressive once more.

After another five minutes of this odd posturing, the cabbie couldn't take it anymore. He flung open his door and made a run for it. We watched with growing horror as the unfortunate taxi driver was suddenly copied in his every movement and expression. Two mimes walked close behind him, while another engaged in some curiously expressive banter. Within half a minute, it was all over, and the cabbie's tattered clothes were all that remained upon the ground.

I looked at Sprockett, whose eyebrow flicked up to "Doubtful," which meant he was out of ideas. Now that they had been blooded, the mood of the mimes seemed to have changed. A minute ago their features had been ridiculously smiley, but now they wore doleful expressions of exaggerated sadness. They also seemed to be approaching the car. Once they got in, it would be all over. Or at least it would be for me.

"Lean forward."

"Might I inquire as to why, ma'am?"

"I'm going to press your emergency spring release," I said. "You'll be nothing but an inert box of cogs to them — they'll not touch you. Someone will chance across you in a few months, and you can be rewound. You can tell them what happened."

He looked at me and buzzed for a moment. "Would that be a compassionate act on your behalf, ma'am?"

"I suppose so. Only one of us need die."

Sprockett thought about this for a moment. "I'm sorry, ma'am, but I may have to politely decline your offer. A butler never leaves his position and is loyal until death."

I made a grab for the access panel on the back of his left shoulder, but he caught my hand with surprising speed.

"In this matter, ma'am," he said firmly, "my cogs are made up."

I relented, and Sprockett let go of my arm as several mimes improvised a trampoline routine on the back bumper.

"Okay," I said as a sudden thought struck me, "here's the plan: I need you to act like a robot."

"How do I do that?"

"You tell me. *You're* the robot, after all."

"Agreed. But the whole point of the Duplex series is that we *act* human in order to function more seamlessly with our masters. 'More human than the dumbest human' is the Duplex Corporation's motto. I don't know the first thing about actually *being* a robot."

"You're going to have to give it your best shot."

Sprockett raised his eyebrow as a shower of broken glass erupted from the rear window. The mimes had become markedly more aggressive when we weren't laughing and applauding hard enough during a not-very-amusing routine where they pretend to sculpt a statue out of clay.

"Very well," said Sprockett. He opened the car door and stepped out. His gait was sporadic and clumsy, and at the end of each movement there seemed to be a slight "spring" to his actions that gave the impression of increased mass. The effect upon the mimes was instantaneous and dramatic. They all took a step back and gazed in wide-eyed astonishment as Sprockett lumbered from the car with me close behind. A few of them dropped to their knees, and others fell into paroxysms of exaggerated crying.

"What do I do?" whispered Sprockett. "I can't keep this up for long."

"Head back towards the road."

So he did, and I followed him. The mimes stayed with us, their grief and sadness changing to anger and surprise. Sprockett continued his overblown movements, but it wasn't working. The mimes closed in, and just when their white gloves were upon us, they suddenly paused and exhibited the sort of mock surprise you can feign by opening your mouth wide and placing both hands on your cheeks.

The reason for this was soon apparent. One of their number had started to *copy* Sprockett in a series of similar robotic moves. Uncertain at first, the moves soon gained fluidity until his gestures exactly matched Sprockett's. Within a few seconds, the "robot" idea had spread amongst them like a virus, and the field was full of five hundred or so mimes acting like robots. As soon as they were all distracted in this fashion, I yelled "Run!" and we sprinted back to the road.

"Well," said Sprockett, stretching the barbed-quip wire back across the hole in the fence to keep the five hundred or so mimes from escaping, "I think that was a close-run thing, ma'am. Might I congratulate you on your quick thinking?"

"Let's just say it was a team effort."

He bowed politely, and I sat on a rock by the side of the road to regain my composure. I looked around. The dusty track was empty in both directions, and aside from the books drifting silently overhead and the now-robotic mimes, the only signs of life were corralled Jokes of Questionable Taste sitting silently in fenced-off areas a little way distant.

"Did you get a good look at that car that passed us?" I asked.

"Yes, ma'am. I believe it was a 1949 Buick Roadmaster."

"Men in Plaid?"

"So it would appear. Their capacity for causing us harm and annoyance seems not to be abating."

I saw it simpler: *They had just tried to kill us.* The only question that remained was, Why? And more worryingly, How much longer before they succeeded?

Just then a rattly pickup stopped opposite us. The bearded driver was staring at us with an amused twinkle in his eye. He was a Funnster, one of a hardy breed of crusty old men and women who spent their days trapping gags and taking them to market.

"Have an accident?" he asked.

It was the height of bad manners in Comedy to decline a feed line when offered, so I had to think quickly.

"No thanks," I replied, "I've already had one."

The Funnster laughed, took off his hat and mopped the sweat from his brow. He looked awhile at the mimes, who had evolved their new robot idea into robots going downstairs, robots canoeing, robots getting stuck inside glass cubes and robots walking against the wind.

"Looks like you may have started something," said the Funnster with a chuckle, climbing out of the cab and rummaging for a net and a baseball bat in the flatbed. "Wait here."

A few moments later, we were bowling down the road towards the local railway station, sitting in the back of the flatbed. On one side of us there was a mime who was miming a robot being trapped inside a net while *actually* being trapped inside a net, and on the other side of us a mature Austrian gentleman with a beard, a small hat and the look of someone who was trying to figure out what we were thinking and why we were thinking it.

After considering us for a moment, he leaned forward and said, "How many Sigmund Freuds does it take to change a lightbulb?"

"I don't know," I said. "How many?"

"Penis," said the Freud, then quickly corrected himself. "I mean father. No, wait! One. One Sigmund Freud. All it takes. Yes. *Verflucht und zugenäht!*" He added gloomily, *"Wenn ich nur bei der Aalsektion geblieben wäre!"*

16.
Commander Bradshaw

Perils for the Unwary #231: literalism. Usually a result of substandard wiring in the synonym-distribution box or a ripple in the contextual flux, the literalism can appear randomly, without warning. Example: One of the loan sharks inside *Get Shorty* turned out to be a three-ton great white with HERTZ SHARK RENTAL stamped on the side, and it was all the cast could do to keep a straight face and carry on as though nothing had happened. Peril Rating: medium-high. Action: walk away.

Bradshaw's BookWorld Companion (5th edition)

We were dropped off at Cooper Central, thanked the Funnster and said farewell to Freud, who had become all wobbly and tearful. We bought some tickets and then gave them to the fez-wearing inspector who hailed us with the customary "Just like that" before directing us to our carriage. Within a few minutes, the train was steaming out of the station and towards Fantasy.

We weren't the only people in the compartment eager to get out of Comedy. A small man who wore the off-duty fatigues of a foot soldier enlisted in the Clown Army was looking about anxiously and sweating. You could tell he was off-duty because he wasn't wearing his bright red nose and his long shoes were carefully strapped to his duffel bag.

"What's your unit?" I asked.

"Sixth Clown," he said nervously, "Supply and Gigglistics. We deploy next week to Bawdy Romp, the buffer zone between Comedy and Racy Novel. Purely as a precaution, you understand. I'm on leave and certainly not stealing military equipment, no, ma'am."

And he stared at his feet, leaving Sprockett and me to wonder what he *was* stealing and whether it was hazardous. The Clown Army's Supply division was notoriously porous, and sneeze and itching powder often found its way into the wrong hands, such as Blyton separatists — always an angry mob.

"I hope your deployment goes well."

"Thank you," said the clown, staring out

the window.

We sat in silence for a while.

"Ma'am?" asked Sprockett, who had been buzzing quietly to himself in the corner.

"Yes?"

"Why do you think we were attacked?"

"Because of what we know."

"But who knows what we know? Others have to *know* that we know. Just *us* knowing it isn't enough — unless we attacked ourselves, which isn't likely."

I thought carefully. There were at least half a dozen people who might have had an idea that the investigation wasn't totally open and shut, all the way from Captain Phantastic to Pickwick/Lorina. But it was also possible we were being silenced for some other reason entirely, an accident or even a textual glitch, such as happens from time to time in the BookWorld.

"The attempt on our life *might* have been a lexicographical literalism," I said. "After all, comedians often 'kill' their audiences or 'die' onstage, and the phrases 'You'll be the death of me' or 'It was so funny I could have died' might all have colluded to cause us harm."

I was fooling myself. Although Buick Roadmasters *did* exist independently of the Men in Plaid, it seemed too suspicious to ignore. Besides, running people off the road was something that occurred in Crime, where it would be unusual to drive five miles without having it happen at least twice. It was much more unlikely in Comedy. Or at least not without a punch line. But then again, maybe my "No thanks, I've already had one" *was* the punch line. Comedy was never straightforward. When all the good jokes had left, only the dubiously amusing stuff remained. Was the mimefield funny or not? To us I think not. But it might have been funny to *someone.*

I stared out the window, thinking about my current predicament. I had a junker on its way to the scrap yard from Vanity that someone had destroyed and then tried to cover his tracks in case of discovery. The accident had been handed to the least skilled accident investigator for a quick and easy resolution, and I had almost been murdered by the Men in Plaid. I had compounded my difficulties by lying to Lockheed, gaining intelligence from Captain Phantastic on false pretenses, and I had not only failed to deliver a legal accident report but destroyed it. If I was found out, I would be confined to my series and as likely as not lose Carmine and possibly Sprockett, too. It was a good moment to pack it all in, accept the level of my own incompetence and start concentrating on what should be my primary goal: increasing readership in the Thursday Next series. Thursday, after all, could take care of herself — she had done so on numerous occasions. If I shared my plans with Sprockett, I reasoned, it would be an affirmation of my resolve, and harder to go back on.

"Sprockett?"

He started out of standby mode with a buzz.

"A cocktail, ma'am?"

"No thank you. It's just that I've decided to . . ." I sighed and rubbed my temples.

"Decided to what, ma'am?"

"Nothing."

And I slumped down into my seat, cursing the Thursday in me.

The train slowed to a halt at the border between Fantasy and Comedy and the off-duty clown started fidgeting.

"Identification, please." One of the border guards was standing at the doorway, and we all rummaged for our identification papers.

"I'll deal with this," said a familiar voice, and Commander Bradshaw appeared in the corridor. He flashed his own ID at the border guard, who saluted smartly and moved on.

Sprockett and I both stood up politely, as did the clown, who didn't want to be left out.

"Please," said Bradshaw, "sit down. What's this, a joke?" he asked, indicating the clown once we had all sat and Sprockett had offered Bradshaw a cocktail.

"A lance corporal in the Sixth Clown," I said, "Supply and Gigglistics."

"Oh, yes?" said Bradshaw with a smile. "And what would you be smuggling across the border?"

The clown sighed resignedly and opened his duffel bag to reveal boxes of military-grade custard pies. He wasn't a very good smuggler. Few were.

"It's jail for you, my lad," said Bradshaw sternly. "CPs are banned in every genre outside Comedy. I'd turn you in, but I'm busy. If you can dispose of them all before we get to Gaiman Junction, I'll overlook it."

"How would I do that?"

"Do you have a spoon in your bag?"

So while the off-duty clown began to eat his way through four dozen custard pies, Bradshaw explained what he was there for.

"*Please* don't ask Lorina to contact me," he said. "That was just for Jobsworth to hear."

"I figured."

"Is she still a colossal pain in the butt, by the way?"

"Getting worse, if anything."

Bradshaw looked at Sprockett, who took the cue and shimmered from the compartment with the clown, who was already on his ninth custard pie and groaning quietly to himself. Sprockett returned momentarily with the Chicago Fizz he had mixed for Bradshaw, then departed again.

Bradshaw leaned forward, looked left and right and whispered, "Are you her? The real one, I mean?"

"No."

He stared at me for a while. "Are you sure? You're not doing some sort of deep-cover double bluff or something?"

"Yes, quite sure. I think I know who I am."

"Prove it."

"I can't. You'll have to take my word for it. Believe me, I wish I were."

Bradshaw seemed satisfied with this and stared at me some more for quite some time. He wasn't here on a social visit.

"What can I do for you, sir?"

"The thing is," he began, taking a sip from his Chicago Fizz, "we're in a bit of a pickle here in the BookWorld, what with Speedy Muffler and the whole Racy Novel debacle. Add to that the dwindling metaphor issue, the e-book accelerators using a disproportionate amount of Text Grand Central's throughput capacity and all the other day-to-day whatnot we have to handle, and I'm sure you'll appreciate that we need the real Thursday now more than ever. Do we agree?"

"We do."

He sighed and ran his fingers through his hair. "She was due to be the Jurisfiction delegate at the Racy Novel peace talks on Friday. I'll have to send Emperor Zhark instead, and his negotiating skills are more along the lines of annihilate first, ask questions later, but without the 'ask questions later' part."

"She may turn up."

He shook his head. "I knew she was going undercover, but she said she'd check in two days ago without fail. She didn't. That's not like her. She might be stuck in a book somewhere, lost in a book somewhere — even held against her will. The possibilities are endless."

"If she *was* lost, wouldn't she have a TextMarker™ homing beacon on her?"

"True — but Textual Sieve coverage is patchy even in Fiction, and absent entirely across at least two-thirds of the BookWorld. We've sent unmanned probes into the most impenetrable tomes at Antiquarian and dispatched agents into almost every genre there is — nothing. The BookWorld is a big place. We've even considered that she might be in the DRM."

I raised an eyebrow. If they were considering this, they really were desperate. The DRM was the Dark Reading Matter — the unseeable part of the BookWorld.

"It's been almost two weeks," continued Bradshaw, "and I fear that something dreadful might have happened."

"Dead?"

"Worse — retired back to the RealWorld."

He stopped and stared at me. It wasn't just Thursday's absence from Jurisfiction that he was worried about; he had lost a good friend, too. Thursday trusted Commander Bradshaw implicitly. I thought I should do likewise.

"I sneak-peeked the Outland yesterday," I said. "I realize it was wrong. But it seemed to me that Landen was missing her, too."

Bradshaw raised an eyebrow. "Truthfully?"

"Yes, sir."

He took a sip of the cocktail, set it down and strode about the compartment for some minutes.

"Look here," he said, "desperate situations

call for desperate measures. I want you to talk to Landen and see if you can find out anything. Perhaps locate her in time for the peace talks."

"Talk to Landen? How can I do that?"

"By traveling to the RealWorld."

My heart nearly missed a beat.

"You're joking."

"No joke, Miss Next. In fact, I'll *tell* you a joke so you'll know the difference. How many Sigmund Freuds does it take to change a lightbulb?"

"I've heard it."

"You have? Blast. In any event, you look *exactly* like Thursday — the best cover in the world. And what could possibly go wrong?"

There was actually quite a lot, but before I could itemize the first sixteen, Bradshaw had moved on.

"Splendid. All transfictional travel has been strictly banned this past eighteen months, so you'll be doing this covertly. If anyone finds out, I'll deny everything. Most of all, you can't tell anyone from the Council of Genres. If Jobsworth or Red Herring finds I've been breaking the transfictional travel embargo, they'll want to send their own. And I can't have that. Do you understand?"

"Yes, but —"

"Then that's all agreed," said Bradshaw, rising from his seat and handing me a signed authorization. "This will give you access to Norland Park to see Professor Plum on the pretext of adding e-book accelerators to your series. He'll know why you're there. I'll also contact my deep-cover agents to offer you every assistance in the Outland. Any questions?"

I had several hundred, but didn't know where to start. Bradshaw took my silence to mean I didn't have any, and he shook me by the hand.

"Good to have you on board. Twelve hours in the RealWorld isn't long, but enough to at least get an idea of what's happened to her. I could send you out for longer, but Thursday has many enemies in the RealWorld, and they'll be onto you pretty quick. If you die in the RealWorld, you die for real, and I'm not having that on my conscience. Shall we say tomorrow morning? Oh, and officially speaking, I was never here."

"You were never here."

"Good show. Appreciate a girl who knows she wasn't somewhere. Oh, and thank your man for the Chicago Fizz, will you? But next time a little less gherkin. Cheerio."

And without another word, he opened the outside door, a motorcycle drew alongside the train, Bradshaw hopped onto the pillion and was gone.

"Might I inquire of madam what that was all about?" asked Sprockett, who returned with a very ill-looking clown.

"A little too much gherkin in the Chicago Fizz."

"He came all the way over here just to tell you that?"

"No — I'm going to the RealWorld to look for Thursday so we can get her to the peace talks on Friday."

"In that case," said Sprockett, "I'd better lay out your things. Will madam be staying long?"

"Twelve hours."

"I'll pack you a toothbrush, a scrunchie and some clean socks."

"I'd be grateful."

I spent the rest of the journey fretting about my trip to reality. It was only a twelve-hour trip — barely a flash in and out — but that wasn't important. What *was* important was that I would meet Landen in person, and although the notion of that filled me with a tingly sensation of anticipation, his rejection of me when he found out I wasn't his wife would be . . . well, not pleasant —

for him and for me. I almost thought of not going. Bradshaw couldn't exactly punish me for not doing something he hadn't told me to do. But then there was the possibility that I might help to find Thursday, and that filled me with the same sense of purpose I'd felt when I lied to Lockheed and Captain Phantastic. I sighed inwardly. Life was easier when I was just a character in a book, going from Preface to Acknowledgments without a care in the world. Within another twenty minutes, the train steamed into Gaiman Junction, and we took the bus home.

"You're back," said Pickwick, who liked to open any conversation by pointing out the obvious.

"Yes indeed," I replied. "What's the news?"

"My water dish is empty."

"That's because you just trod in it."

Pickwick looked at her foot. "I have a wet foot . . . and my water dish is empty."

"Anything else?"

"I saw Carmine with that goblin again. Sitting in the *niche d'amour* at the bottom of the garden, they were."

"As long as she doesn't invite him over the threshold again, I'm not bothered."

"You should be. Goblins. *Nasty.* Full of

diseases."

"That's Carmine's problem. I told you, I'm not bothered."

Actually, I was. I had tried to give Carmine a dressing-down for her poor choice in men, but she'd just stared at me and retorted that yes, Horace *might* be a thief, but at least he hadn't set fire to a busload of nuns.

"Any news of Whitby?" I asked.

"Being questioned in custardy," replied Mrs. Malaprop, who had walked in with a clipboard full of reports that all needed my signature. "His pasta is catching up with him. How were things at Jurisfiction?"

I didn't tell them what had happened as it was safer that way.

"Captain Phantastic mentioned you owed him a date," I said to Pickwick.

"The Captain?" she said with a fond smile. "I'm amazed he remembers — it was a long time ago. We were both young and foolish, and I'd do anything for a dare. Ah, Frederic — so many cats, so little recipes."

"*Few* recipes."

"What?"

"So many cats, so *few* recipes," I said, pleased that I had figured out who'd been talking earlier.

Pickwick looked at me disdainfully, muttered "amateur" and marched out.

"The investigation is still on," I said to Mrs. Malaprop as soon as Pickwick had gone, "but keep it under your hat, will you?"

"Squirtainly, ma'am. I found this note pinned to the newel post."

Gone to find Horace, back in half an hour.
P.S.: I don't care what Pickwick thinks.

"Horace?"

"The goblin."

I wasn't particularly annoyed with Carmine for chasing after the goblin — as long as he wasn't invited back in again — but I *was* very annoyed that she had gone AWOL. It meant that for the past ten minutes there'd been no one here to play Thursday. If word had gotten out, there might have been a panic from the other characters, and it was against at least nine regulations that I could think of.

"Do we report her as absinthe without leaf?" asked Mrs. Malaprop.

I scrunched up the note. Reporting her as missing would get Jurisfiction involved, and Carmine would probably be shipped off to spend the next decade in *Roger Red Hat.*

"No," I said, "but let me know the moment she gets back so I can give her a ticking off."

Sprockett knocked and entered, his eyebrow pointing firmly at the "Worried" mark.

"Excuse me, ma'am, but the Men in Plaid are back."

"So soon? You better admit th—"

"Thursday Next?" said the first of the MiP as he walked in the door.

"Yes?"

"You're coming with us," said the second.

"I can't leave the series," I said. "My understudy is at lunch."

"That's not what the board says," observed the first, pointing at Carmine's status on the indicator board, which was now blinking an orange "at readiness" light, despite the fact that she was out looking for Horace. "Is she AWOL?"

"No," I lied.

"Then she's in?"

"Yes," I lied again.

"Then you can come with us."

I looked at Malaprop and Sprockett. They knew what needed to be done — find Carmine at the earliest opportunity.

The Man in Plaid who seemed to be in charge jerked a thumb in the direction of the front door, and we walked outside. Predictably, there was a Buick Roadmaster, but that wasn't the end of the story. The left-hand mudguard was dented and streaked with yellow paint — the sort of yellow paint that taxis are finished in. This was the car that had forced us off the road and into the mimefield.

"Am I in some sort of trouble?"

"You are if you don't come with us."

17.
The Council of Genres

The Council of Genres is the administrative body that looks after all aspects of BookWorld regulation, from policy decisions in the main debating chamber to the day-to-day running of ordinary BookWorld affairs, supply of plot devices and even the word supply coming in from the Text Sea. It controls the Book Inspectorate, which governs which books are to be published and which to be demolished, and also manages Text Grand Central and Jurisfiction.

Bradshaw's BookWorld Companion
(11th edition)

I sat between the Men in Plaid in the back, which was uncomfortable, as they seemed to have a plethora of weapons beneath their suits, all of which poked me painfully in the ribs.

"So," I said brightly, doing what I hoped

Thursday would do — showing no fear. "How long have you been in plaid?"

"It's not plaid. It's tartan."

"Right," said the second one, "tartan."

And despite more questions of a similar nature, they declined to talk further. I hoped to goodness that Mrs. Malaprop and Sprockett managed to hunt down Carmine in time for the early-evening readers.

We drove past Political Thriller on the Ludlum Freeway and made our way towards the towering heights of the Great Library, and I guessed where we were headed. On the twenty-sixth floor would be the Council of Genres and Senator Jobsworth, the man from whom the Men in Plaid ultimately drew their authority. Like Bradshaw, he must have figured out a way in which a Thursday Next look-alike could be used.

The security was even tighter here, and the Roadmaster slowed to negotiate the concrete roadblocks and high anti-bookjump mesh. We were waved through with only a cursory glance and drove across a narrow bridge and into the Ungenred Zone. This was an area of independent, narrative-free space where the governing body of the BookWorld could exist free from influence and bias. Or at least that was the theory. I'd been a few times to the

Council of Genres, but only with the real Thursday. Ordinary citizens didn't come here unless strictly on business. If we wanted to pretend we had influence, we could take any grievances to our genre representatives, and they would intercede on our behalf — or so the theory went.

"Where are you taking me?" I asked.

"Right to the very top."

"That high, huh?"

Having the Great Library and the Ungenred Zone on Fiction Island was not without problems. Theoretically speaking, if it was located here, then it must be potentially readable by the RealWorld population, something about which the CofG was not happy. If it became common knowledge that there was a text-based realm on the other side of the printed page, hacking into the BookWorld would be a far bigger problem than it was already. The Outlander corporation known as Goliath had been attempting to find a way in for decades, but aside from their transfictional tour bus, quaintly named the Austen Rover and the occasional bookhacker, the independent existence of the BookWorld remained secret.

Even so, council officials were taking no chances, and the entire Ungenred Zone was rendered invisible to potential bookhackers by the simple expedient of not being written about. At least not directly. The adventures in my own series hinted at a BookWorld but these were heavily fictionalized, since the ghostwriter had no collaboration from Thursday when writing them. There was only the vaguest reference to the Great Library, and nothing about Jurisfiction or the Council of Genres. Despite this, some of the more talented readers in the Outland had managed to hack into the zone by exploiting a hole in the defenses that allowed one to "read between the lines." To counter this, the CofG had all the borders covered in soporific paint the shade of young lettuces, which worked like a charm. Every attempted incursion into the Ungenred Zone was met by drowsiness followed by an almost instantaneous torpor on the part of the potential hacker. It had exactly the same effect as the emergency Snooze Button, except that no kittens were ever hurt or injured.

The Roadmaster drove up to the BookWorld's main port, where the Metaphoric River joined the Text Sea by a series of locks, weirs, traps and sluices. The port was large, and several hundred scrawl trawlers rode gently in the swell, grammasites wheeling above the mast tops, hoping to dart down and snatch a dropped article. On the dockside was the day's catch. Most scrawlers simply netted the words that basked upon the surface for a quick and easy sale to the wordsmiths, while others deep-trawled for binary clause systems, whereby a verb and a noun had clumped together in a symbiotic relationship to form a protosentence. But even these hardened scrawlers were in awe of those who hunted fully formed sentences. These weather-beaten sea dogs would sail far across the Text Sea in search of an entire paragraph, a descriptive zinger or even an original comedy monologue — the elusive Moby-Shtick that legends speak of.

Facing the docks and beyond the coils of ropes, nets, harpoons and infinitive splitters were several rows of single-story workshops where the words and letters were crocheted, knitted, sewed, glued, riveted or nailed together into sentences, depending on the softness of the prose to which they were destined. The completed sentences were either rough-sorted into bundles and sold direct to the Well of Lost Plots or woven into standard paragraphs on power looms, the nouns, verbs and adjectives left loose so the end users could make their own choices.

The Buick pulled to a stop outside the

main entrance of the Great Library, and we climbed out. The library was housed in a towering Gothic skyscraper that stood as a reminder of the BookWorld before it was remade. Back then the area below the Great Library had been simply unexplored jungle. All that was swept away in the nine minutes of the remaking. The BookWorld may be slow when it comes to changing fashions and storytelling conventions, but it can rebuild itself in a flash if required.

I paused for a moment. It was impossible not to be impressed by the Great Library, and this in a world noted for its superlative structures, settings and depth. Just by way of example, the landscape inside *Lord of the Rings* was *so* stunning and *so* stupendous that it could be absorbed as a form of nourishment. The huge tourism opportunities within the trilogy had been long understood and exploited, and even though the battles were exciting and fun to watch, most people went only for the valleys, rivers, waterfalls, crags, trees and moss.

I stepped into the lobby of the library and paid my respects to those names on the Boojumorial — a marble tablet that commemorated Jurisfiction agents from both the RealWorld and the BookWorld who had lost their lives in the protection of the written word. They may have been carbon- or text-based, but here they were equal; no preference was given to the real over the imaginary. My companions, however, due either to indifference or to long acquaintance with the "Honored Erased," paid it no heed at all. We walked towards the circular void that ran through the building, and I looked up. Twenty-six floors above us, the glazed roof was just visible. Twenty-six floors of every book that had ever been written, and here logged faithfully in alphabetical order for mostly serial-continuity purposes. It wasn't necessary to have the library anymore, but it paid to have a backup in case something went wrong. And something always *did* go wrong. Although infuriating, it was unavoidable. With all the drama at hand, it was inevitable that the BookWorld would spontaneously erupt into intrigue, which would then set off a chain reaction of unexpected consequence. If the BookWorld were itself a book, it would be self-writing.

I glanced down. Below me were the twenty-six basements that made up the Well of Lost Plots — the place where all books are built. As I looked, I could see flashes of light as inspiration fired off in small bursts of energy. A really good idea could burn brightly for many months and give nearby books-in-progress much-needed warmth.

We entered the elevator, and I felt myself grow increasingly apprehensive as the ancient lift slowly clanked its way to the top. The senator's summons might have been related to Bradshaw's recent request, to our chance meeting in Norland Park or to something else entirely — I had no idea. The lift doors opened, and the CofG spread out in front of us, a seething mass of offices, desks, meeting rooms and people scurrying back and forth in a ceaseless quest to keep the BookWorld running as efficiently as possible. The chamber was bigger in here than it appeared from the outside, but nothing was particularly linear or even logical within the BookWorld; the fabric of imagination is elastic, and that reflected itself within the Council of Genres.

I passed the big viewing windows, where I had stood with the real Thursday when she was my mentor, and peered out at a BookWorld that appeared deceptively orderly. Because I was quite high and the island dished to fit snugly on the inside face of the sphere, I could clearly see every part of it, from the volcanoes in the far north all the way down to Vanity Island off the southern tip. I could even see my own series as a dark smudge in the distance.

I was escorted away from the viewing windows and walked past the public gallery above the debating chamber. There was a session in progress, and although it was being conducted in **Courier Bold,** the antiquated yet universal language of the BookWorld, I could make out that it was a discussion about the possibility of Text Sea levels rising due to the advent of e-books. I'd heard about this issue. The argument went that because e-books were composed almost entirely of electrons and barely any ink and paper at all, the scrawl trawlers' work would be cut by 90 percent overnight, and there was a possibility for inundation of the low-lying areas of the BookWorld — essentially Maritime and Disaster. This argument was countered by a delegate who maintained that e-books were the way of the future, and since the power of a book is undiminished irrespective of the carrier medium, no such panic was necessary. Still another delegate suggested that the advent of e-books might actually *increase* the demand for new material and thus cause a shortage of words — something for which the BookWorld must be prepared by the construction of more scrawl trawlers and the training of extra scrawlermen. All three were experts, and all three had conflicting views. I was reminded of Clarke's Second Law of Egodynamics: "For every expert there is an equal and opposite expert."

"Come on," said one of the Plaids. "We're not bleeding tour guides."

We walked down a corridor, past more security, then arrived at an opulent antechamber with expansive views across the BookWorld.

"Miss Next?" said a friendly clerk holding a clipboard. "The senator will see you now."

18.
Senator Jobsworth

Dark Reading Matter: the hypothetical last resting place of books never published, ideas never penned and poems held only in the heart by poets who died without passing them on. Theoretical bibliologists have proved that the Background Story Radiation was appreciably more than the apparent quantity of STORY in the Book-World. No one had any idea where it might be or how you could reach it. DRM's existence remained theoretical, at best.

Bradshaw's BookWorld Companion
(4th edition)

The senator was sitting behind his desk as I was ushered into his office. Several men and women dressed in the uniform of almost every military conflict there was were in attendance, as well as a couple of high-ranking generals, Colonel Barksdale and Commander Herring, the chief of staff.

"Would you excuse us?" said the senator, and everyone except Red Herring and Colonel Barksdale filed out, looking at me suspiciously as they did so. I stood in front of Jobsworth's desk while he finished what he was doing. I didn't know which book he had come from, but wagging tongues suggested he was an illegal immigrant from Quackery, a subgenre within Lies & Self-Delusion, just off the north coast. I don't think anyone ever raised it with him, or if they did, no answer was forthcoming. It didn't really much matter, since Jobsworth had been the overall leader of the Council of Genres for as long as it had been in existence, and his unassailable position as head of the council looked set to continue far into the future. He had the ear, apparently, of the Great Panjandrum himself, who could fix almost everything when he had a mind to.

"They say she's dead, you know," said Jobsworth, striding to the large window in his office that looked out over the BookWorld, the islands of the various categories of books patches of verdant green against the dark slatey gray of the Text Sea. "Killed in the Outland, killed in the BookWorld — who knows? What do you think?"

"I have no opinion on the matter, sir. I

just play her in the series."

"You must have *some* idea."

I looked across at the chief of staff, who was gazing at me intently. "No."

Jobsworth stared at me for a long while, then grunted and looked outside his office again. Yet this time he wasn't looking at the larger BookWorld, but rather at the island of Fiction below him. The Ungenred Zone was on the west coast about halfway up. Crime was just to the north, but the areas I knew best — Adventure, Fantasy and Sci-Fi — were situated in the southeast, out of sight. It was Herring who spoke next.

"Ever been up-country?"

"I've been to Crime."

"Farther. Towards Racy Novel."

"No."

"So there is a good chance they haven't seen you up there? Or even know about you?"

I suddenly had a very unpleasant feeling and turned back to Jobsworth. "What is it you want me to do, Senator?"

"A small favor. I wouldn't ask you if it wasn't important. And if you do this for us, I'm sure it will be to your benefit if you reapply to join Jurisfiction."

I was right. If that was the carrot, I could be in for some serious stick.

"It's nothing too onerous," added Colonel Barksdale, who had so many campaign medals on his chest that he was probably bulletproof. "It simply requires you to take Thursday's place at the peace talks on Friday."

I was momentarily at a loss for words. I should have tried to extricate myself, but I had paused too long.

"Splendid," said Jobsworth, crossing to a scale model of the island that was built upon a large oak table. "Let me give you some background."

"Would you excuse me?" said Herring. "I have to revise the upcoming Linguistic Hygiene Bill if we're to have any chance of rejecting it."

"Thank you, Red."

Herring wished me good day, thanked me for my selfless adherence to duty and walked from the room. Jobsworth beckoned me closer to the large model of the island, where the topography was perfectly realized in miniature, including the individual genres along with their borders, railway networks, major rivers and capital novels. He swept his hand in the direction of the Northern Genres.

"You've heard about Speedy Muffler's threats and the peace talks on Friday?"

I said that I had.

"Speedy Muffler claims to have developed a dirty bomb," announced Jobsworth with a grimace, "a loosely bound collection of badly described scenes of a sexual nature. The detonation of such a bomb could cause untold damage, flinging wholly gratuitous sex scenes as far as *Mrs. Dalloway.*"

"But has he really?" I asked, since the possession of the bomb was only conjecture, much like Comedy's claim to be experimenting with a fifty-megaton-yield deep satire device.

"Do you know," said Jobsworth, "it doesn't matter. Feminism and Dogma are taking the threat seriously and are massing armies on the border ready to take preemptive action ahead of the peace talks. And we can't have that."

"Invasion?" I said. "What would Feminism and Dogma do with Racy Novel?"

"They'll simply push the rogue genre up north towards Porn and De Sade. *Fanny Hill, The Story of O* and *The Adventures of Tom Jones* will be annexed back into Classics, and the territory shared between them. Comedy will still insist upon the buffer zone of Bedroom Farce, and since Comedy is regarded with a certain sense of reluctant admiration by Romance and Dogma, they'll not want to go any farther."

He took a deep breath.

"But we can't risk that kind of disruption. The genres might take months to rebuild to current strength, and the prose will suffer terribly. With the advent of e-books in the Outland, this is not a good time to have a cross-genre war. The battle between Sci-Fi and Horror all those years ago has still left its mark; their reputations as serious literature have still to recover completely — and the civil war inside Fantasy has left the reading public with an entirely unwarranted dismal view of the genre. I can't have Romance and Female Crime marginalized in the same way — they're 43.9 percent of our readership."

"I'm not sure what I can do," I said. "I'm not much good at negotiating. I tend to want everyone to simply hug and make up."

"I'm not asking you to *do* anything, you little fool. We're putting it about that you — the *real* Thursday — has irritable vowel syndrome and can't speak, so Emperor Zhark will be doing the talking. You'll just sit there and nod and look serious. Muffler might be a troublemaker, but even he will knuckle under if he thinks Thursday Next might be annoyed if he shouts too loudly. How about it?"

He was asking too much. No, it was more than that — *insane,* even by Council of Genre standards. If Muffler found out I wasn't her, things might get even worse, and I wasn't going to have a cross-genre war on my conscience.

"I may have to politely decline," I said.

He stared at me for a moment, then opened a manila folder on his desk.

"Hmm," he said, "looks like we have a lot of illegal narrative flexations in your series, doesn't it?"

"I'm playing Thursday as Thursday wants me to."

"We have only your word for that. There is also a possible charge of your understudy consorting with undesirables and, most seriously, your harboring an illegal alien from Vanity."

He meant Sprockett.

"We call it Self-Publishing these days."

"Immaterial. We'll be taking the Metaphoric River route up-country via paddle steamer. I'll have a car pick you up Friday morning at 0700. Are we agreed?"

I took a deep breath. "Yes, sir."

"Excellent!"

He pressed a button on his desk.

"Miss Next, you must also understand that in matters of BookWorld politics like this, it is essential you do not speak of this to anyone, *especially* that busybody Bradshaw. Jurisfiction has a twisted vision of the good work we do at the council, and I don't want him to get the wrong idea. Do you understand?"

If there was any lingering doubt that the CofG and Jurisfiction distrusted each other, it was dispelled. Neither wanted the other to know what it was asking me to do. The clerk came back in, and I was escorted from the building by the same two Men in Plaid who had brought me there.

In a very short time, I was deposited back at my front door, and the Roadmaster pulled silently away. Sprockett was waiting for me in the hall, his single eyebrow pointer clicking alternately between "Quizzical" and "Uncomfortable."

But he knew what to do.

"Can I interest ma'am in a Ludlow Scorcher?"

I told him a cocktail would go down very well so long as he went easy on the parsley, and then I related what had just happened with Jobsworth. I decided not to mention the threats he'd made regarding Sprockett and Carmine, but I *did* mention that I would be going up-country on Friday — and also the dent and the streak of yellow paint on the Men in Plaid's Buick Roadmaster.

"The fact that they haven't tried to kill us again tends to indicate that they believe we have abandoned the investigation," said Sprockett, handing me the cocktail. "Are you sure it was *our* yellow paint on the side of their Roadmaster?"

"What else is painted yellow in the BookWorld?"

As soon as I said it, I suddenly remembered something. I stood up and quickly walked to the garage at the bottom of the garden, Sprockett close behind.

"Ma'am?" he said as I swung up the double doors and started to poke amongst the book junk for what I was looking for. I found it easily enough: the back axle that had once been painted yellow. There was no sign of an ISBN, scrubbed or otherwise.

"It wasn't from *The Murders on the Hareng Rouge,*" I said excitedly. "It's from a Trans-Genre Taxi. I rode back from Poetry stuck onto the side of an ocean tanker, part of a book about the Bermuda Triangle. There was a taxi attached to *Murders* when it went down, piggybacking from one part of the BookWorld to another. The sabotage might not have been aimed at the book at all — *it might have been aimed at whoever was in the cab!"*

"Or both," said Sprockett, annoyingly muddying the waters.

"Or both," I agreed.

"Where *is* the rest of the cab?" asked Sprockett.

"Who knows? Either vaporized or embedded somewhere in the unread backwaters of Thriller. Here's the deal: You're going to call the TransGenre Taxi offices and find out about any missing cabs, and I'm going to find out more about *The Murders on the Hareng Rouge* and Adrian Dorset."

"But where, ma'am? If Captain Phantastic doesn't know, it's unknowable."

"In the RealWorld, Sprockett. Cheers."

I tried the Scorcher. It wasn't too bad. A bit loamy for my taste, but otherwise good.

I went upstairs and packed a small tote bag. A few clothes and some spare underwear — I'd heard all the scare stories — then worried about taking my pistol or not, but eventually I did. After that I dithered over taking ammunition and decided to, but only one cartridge and of the armor-piercing variety. I argued to myself that I would be too scared to use it, so I wouldn't. I gave Carmine some last-minute instructions in case of emergencies, ignored her protestations about "having to face more readers than she was happy with" and then ordered a cab. "If I have to press the Snooze Button," said Mrs. Malaprop as I waited, "it's on your conch séance, not mine."

"Agreed."

"Where to?" asked the cabbie when he pulled up ten minutes later.

"Norland Park," I said, "*Sense and Sensibility.* Any route you like."

But at that moment someone else got into the cab by way of the opposite door. He was wearing a large floppy hat that partially obscured his features.

"Sorry," I said, "cab taken."

The other passenger lifted the brim of the hat so I could see his face. It was Whitby.

"It's okay," I said to the cabbie, and we moved off.

"Holy cow!" I said, turning to Whitby, "you've got a nerve. When were you going to tell me about setting fire to that busload of nuns? Two years I spent building myself up to a date, and then I find that you're a homicidal maniac."

"*Lots* of people are homicidal maniacs," he replied. "Throw a stick into Crime and you'll hit six of them."

"But we're not in Crime, are we?"

He stared at me for a moment. "I've done lots of good in my life, Thursday — helped people to narrative independence, coached Generics through entrance exams, was EZ-Read's Employee of the Month three months running, and I even helped little old ladies across the road — some when they actually wanted to go. Do I get credit for that? No. All you want to think about is the nuns."

"*Orphaned* nuns," I reminded him.

"Actually, it was the puppies who were orphaned," he said petulantly. "Let's stick to the facts here."

"Does it matter?"

"Not really. But I don't think that one teensy-weensy incident with a small busload of nuns and puppies should taint a man's life."

"I think it does, Whitby. You might have told me."

"I couldn't."

"Why?"

He sighed. "You remember Dermot McGruber? EZ-Read's rep over in Hum-Dram?"

"Yes."

"He wanted to impress a girl. But he'd done some seriously bad shit when he was a character in Crime."

"The nuns?"

"Right. With a backstory like that hanging around his neck and guilt consuming his every moment, he couldn't even *begin* to get a date. So I said I'd look after his backstory for the weekend so he could ask her out, guilt-free and with an easy heart."

"That was generous of you."

He shrugged. "He helped me out once when I over-ordered some EZ-Read PlotHoleFiller. I owed him. A weekend of all-consuming guilt seemed easy enough. I could keep myself to myself, get totally hyphenated, and no one need ever know."

"Let me guess," I said. "He's legged it."

Whitby nodded as the cabbie changed down a gear and moved onto the Dickens Freeway.

"I don't know where Dermot's gone. In fact, I think he might have been planning this for a while. I feel such an idiot — and what's more, I think he put Jurisfiction onto me. You won't tell them, will you?"

"Not yet, but I will. You can't set fire to people — nuns or otherwise — and expect to get away with it."

"I know," he said sadly. "It weighs heavily on my conscience. The yapping, oh, the *yapping*."

I sat in silence for a moment. The thing

about backstories is that once you've taken one on, they're true and real, irrespective of who owned them before you. You could pass it on, of course, but it was understandably tricky. Who wants a busload of burning nuns and puppies on his conscience?

"So what do you want?" I asked.

"I just wanted to see you," he said simply, "and hear your voice."

"Well, now you have," I replied, a bit more harshly than perhaps I should have. "Maybe we should say good-bye."

"I'm living over in Hemingway if you need anything," he said, not wanting to give up on the slimmest chance a date was still possible. "Page 127, *To Have and Have Not.* If you need anything, just whistle. You can drop me on this corner, driver."

The cabbie pulled up, and Whitby got out. He told me to take care and then hurried off around a street corner. The taxi moved on, and I slumped back into my seat as we turned onto Austen Boulevard. I thought of turning him in, then of not turning him in. It was a tricky call, but luckily the least of my worries.

I wasn't feeling that good about the trip, to be honest. A nervy, sickly feeling was festering in the pit of my stomach — and not just from the difficulty of making the move across, or what I might find there or the truth about *The Murders on the Hareng Rouge.* Notwithstanding the recent developments with Whitby, I was most worried about meeting Landen. He was the man I was written to love and never meet. And now I was going to meet him.

19.
JurisTech, Inc.

> The JurisTech Museum is open Monday to Friday, a half day on Wednesday. A whole range of technologies both past and present is on display, including an impressive array of BookWorld weaponry, grammasite traps, word dams, Eject-O-Hats, TextMarkers, grapheme splitters and noun-to-verb alchemical technologies. On Tuesdays there is a technical demonstration of the Textual Sieve (not to be missed).
>
> *Bradshaw's BookWorld Companion*
> (3rd edition)

I turned up at the front gate of *Sense and Sensibility* and showed the guards the authorization given to me by Bradshaw. The guards rang through and spoke briefly to JurisTech before I was once more issued a docket and ushered in. I met the frog-footman at the front door, who was surprised to see me again so soon.

"You again?" he said, staring at the docket. "What do you want with JurisTech?"

Fortified by the mission entrusted to me by Bradshaw, I was no longer so frightened of him.

"None of your business," I replied, and his face lit up. This was more how he liked it.

"Labs or office?"

"Labs."

He guided me through the long corridors of Norland Park, down several flights of steps and an elevator or two before we stopped outside an inconspicuous door with a pair of milk bottles outside.

"The JurisTech Labs," announced the frog-footman. "My instructions are to wait for you."

"It'll be a long wait. Pick me up in twelve hours. Here," I said, handing him a Rubik's Cube. "See if you can figure this out."

The frog-footman stared at the cube curiously. All six faces were quite naturally the same color, and all was orderly and neat.

"You have to try to make it random," I said, "by twisting the faces."

The frog-footman twisted the faces in a fairly haphazard manner, but try as he might, every face remained the same color. For a BookWorld puzzle, it was a classic.

The lack of randomness within the orderly structure of the BookWorld tended not to permit disorder. As far as I knew, no one had yet managed to scramble a Rubik's, but I thought it might pass the time for him.

"Thank you," replied the frog-footman, and he sat cross-legged on the floor, twisting the cube this way and that as he tried to scramble the faces.

I knocked on the door, and it was soon answered by a small man in a brown boiler suit that was liberally covered in oil stains, food and science merit badges.

"Good Lord!" he said when he saw me. "Thursday? Come inside quick."

Once safely away from the prying ears of the frog-footman, I explained who I was — or, more important, who I wasn't — and showed Professor Plum the authorization from Bradshaw.

"Did he give you a code word?"

"What?"

"A code word."

"The commander didn't say anything about a code word."

"Correct. There is no code word — but only Bradshaw would know that. Follow me."

The basement was twice the size of a cathedral and quite full to capacity with machinery. An army of technicians scurried around looking purposeful while lights blinked on and off as arcs of electricity discharged into the air at regular intervals.

"That's mostly for effect," explained Plum as we moved among the machines. "It's sometimes of equal importance to have a machine's form and function in equilibrium. Who wants an italicizer that can be carried around in the pocket? Much better to have a large device that flashes lights randomly and occasionally goes bzzz."

I agreed, even if I'd never *seen* an italicizer, much less *used* one.

"All this technology," I mused. "Is there any limit to what you can do?"

"If there is, we haven't found it," replied Plum. "We can figure out most technologies, and those that we can't are subcontracted to Technobabble™ Industries, which can usually cobble something together. The good thing about being in the BookWorld is that we aren't hampered by anything as awkward as physical laws. The RealWorld must be hideously annoying to do science in, but given how difficult it is, I suppose breakthroughs are of greater value. In here, for example, perpetual-motion machines are quite feasible."

"What's stopping us from using them?"

"Finding a way to make them *stop.* Once we've figured that out, we'll have perpetual engines in every minicab and bus in the BookWorld."

He paused while I stared at a machine that could transform dark humor to sarcasm and then back again with no loss of narrative mass.

"As you know," continued Plum, "the Council of Genres permits us to suspend the rules of physics in order that we can develop the somewhat unique technologies that the BookWorld requires. See this?"

We had stopped next to a large machine that seemed to be nothing but a riveted tube about a yard thick running through the entire length of the workshop. It appeared through one wall and then vanished out the other. If I hadn't known any better, I would have thought it a throughput pipe or a footnoterphone conduit.

"This is just a small part of the Large Metaphor Collider."

"What does that do?"

Professor Plum stopped for a moment at the control panel. "You know we've got a serious metaphor deficit at present?"

I nodded. The problem was well documented. Most of Fiction's rhetorical power, dramatic irony and pathos were brought naturally by the mighty Metaphoric River that snaked about the island. But the huge influx of novels in the past century had exacted a burden on the waterway as the much-needed metaphor was abstracted on a massive scale, and these days it was no longer considered possible that the river could supply all of Fiction's requirements, hence the trade in raw metaphor and JurisTech's attempts to synthesize it.

"This collider," continued Professor Plum, "will take depleted metaphor — simile, in effect — and accelerate it in a circular trackway over eighteen miles long to a velocity approaching ninety-five percent of absurd, at which point it will be collided with indisputable fact. There is a brief flash of energy as the two different modes of communication are fused together and then explode in a burst of high-energy subcomprehension particles. We then record the event as traces on a sheet of onionskin paper."

"The flimsy blue variety?"

"*Exactly.* In this manner we hope not only to figure out the individual building blocks of STORY in order to have a better understanding of how it all works but also to use it as a way of extracting usable quantities of metaphor from even the most prosaic, tired or clumsily constructed simile."

"Does it work?"

"I was just about to test it. You can help if you want."

I said I would be delighted, and Plum pointed me in the direction of a lidded crucible that was steaming gently to itself.

"You'll find some tongs and gloves over there — I need that simile in the accelerator chamber."

He carried on with his measurements. The crucible was steaming not from heat but from cold. Liquid nitrogen was keeping a raw simile in an inactive state. So much so that I couldn't tell what it was, as the meaning and illusion were all contracted and frozen into one lump. I put on the glove and, using the wooden pincers, placed the simile in the acceleration chamber.

"Excellent," said Plum, who closed the door and spun a wheel on the front to effect a secure lock. He then pressed a button, and there was a low humming noise, which gradually increased in pitch as the simile started to move around the accelerator. There was a dial marked "Absurd Velocity," and the needle began to rise as the simile zipped round at ever-increasing speeds.

"The Council of Genres is very keen to

have this up and running as soon as possible," he said, staring at the dials carefully. "Synthesizing metaphor is the holy grail of the BookWorld, if you don't count finding the Holy Grail, which confusingly is *also* the holy grail of the BookWorld."

The Large Metaphor Collider had by now wound itself up to a whine so high-pitched that I couldn't hear it, and all the equipment on the desk was vibrating. As the needle nudged up to .95 Absurd, Plum took a deep breath and pressed the red button, which instantaneously brought indisputable fact into the path of the absurdly fast simile.

It is difficult to describe what happened next. The machine changed from being something akin to an engine with a throttle stuck wide open to that of a Brave New Dawn. I saw the Clouds Open and the Rain Stop. The Lark Ascended, and I saw Saint John on the island of Patmos, and a New Heaven and a New Earth. I saw — But in another second, those feelings had vanished, and all we were left with was the collider, humming down to speed.

"What was that?" I asked.

"A sudden flash of pure metaphor," replied Plum excitedly. "This kind of event usually liberates about a hundred and twenty PicoMets."

"Is that safe?"

"Don't worry," he said with a smile. "The background metaphor level is about fifty PicoMets, and a fatal dose is up around the forty-MilliMet mark. You'd have to do something daft for that to happen, although there have been accidents. A few years ago, a colleague of mine was experimenting with a few grams of dead metaphor when it went critical. He was bathed in almost a hundred MilliMets and started barking on about Prometheus stealing fire from the gods before he exploded into a ball of fire and ascended into the night sky, where he could be seen for many weeks, a salutary lesson of the dangers of playing with metaphor. Wrecked the laboratory, too. Let me see."

Professor Plum pulled the single sheet of onionskin from the annihilation chamber and looked at it, brows knitted. The paper had recorded the subword particles. Some were dotted, others colored, some hatched. There was even a legend at the bottom explaining what each one meant. Fiction has no time for lengthy and potentially confusing data analysis, so experimentation is always followed by easily interpretable and generally unequivocal results.

"That's alliteration," said Plum, tracing the various paths with his finger. "Anaphora, epistrophe, epanalepsis, analepsis, hyperbole and polyptoton."

In all, he could list twenty-nine submeaning particles, but of pure metaphor there was no evidence at all.

"You felt it, though, didn't you?"

I answered that I had. A feeling of a new dawn and old things being swept away.

Plum stared at the paper for a long time. So long, in fact, that I thought he might have gone to sleep standing up and might need catching when he fell over.

"Well," he said at last, "back to the drawing board."

"But we felt something, didn't we?" I said.

"Without proof we've got nothing," he said in a resigned voice. "Perhaps metaphor has no mass. If so, I'm very surprised — although it might explain why Dark Reading Matter is undetectable. It could be mostly metaphorical. Come on. Let's get you real."

The professor led me to the back of the workshop, past the entrance to a scrubbing device for declichéing otherwise healthy idioms and down a corridor to a door obscured by several discarded packing cases and a stack of unread copies of the almost fatally dull *JurisTech Review.*

"We haven't used the Jumper for over

eighteen months," he explained, struggling with a padlock that had grown rusty with age. "Not since the imaginatively titled 'RealWorld Travel Ban' banned all travel to the RealWorld."

"Why the ban?"

"I didn't ask, and neither should you. If anyone at the CoG gets wind of this, you and I are nothing but text."

I didn't like the sound of this.

"But Bradshaw —"

"Bradshaw is a good man," interrupted Plum, "but in matters like this he'd deny he even knew you. And me. And himself, it it came to that. I agree with him. To maintain the integrity of Jurisfiction, I would accept being reduced to a bucket of graphemes. And so should you."

He left me thinking about this and pulled opened the door. He paused, the interior of the lab a dark hole.

"You can leave now if you want to."

"No, I'm okay," I said, even if I wasn't. "Let's just get on with it, yes?"

He turned on the light to reveal a large room that was musty and hung with cobwebs. Occasionally there was a low rumble, and dust trickled from the ceiling.

"The Carnegie Underpass," explained Plum. "It runs directly overhead."

In the middle of the room was a large machine that looked like a collection of sieves, each lined up one in front of the other. The sieves began with one that might have been designed to make chips, so long as you could hurl a potato at it fast enough, and the rest were of rapidly decreasing mesh, until the penultimate was no more than a fine wire gauze. The last of all was a thin sheet of silver that shimmered with the microscopic currents of air that moved around the workshop. Beyond this was the wide end of a copper funnel with the sharp end finishing in a point no bigger than a pin — and beyond this a small drop of blue something-or-other within a localized gravitational field that kept it suspended in the air. Around the room was an array of computers covered with more dials, levers, switches and meters than I had ever seen before.

"What exactly is it?" I asked, not unnaturally and with a certain degree of trepidation.

"It's the Large Textual Sieve Array," he explained. "Although the construction and methodology of Textual Sieves remain generally unexplained, they can be used for a number of functions. Cross-triangulation searches, the 'locking' of text within books

— and, more controversially, for making fictional people real, even if for only a short period."

"How long?"

"I can send you out for forty-eight hours, but Bradshaw insisted you go for only twelve. As soon as that time is up, you'll spontaneously return. We'll send you in at midday, and you'll be out at midnight — pumpkin hour. If you want to stay longer, you'll have to Blue Fairy, but then you're there for good and you'll have to suffer the worst rigors of being real — aging, death and daytime television.

The twelve-hour pumpkin option suited me fine, and I told him so. I'd heard many stories about the RealWorld, and although it sounded an interesting place to visit, you'd not want to live there.

"So how does it work?" I asked.

"Simplicity itself. You see this howitzer?"

He pointed at a large-caliber cannon that was pointed directly at the sieves. It was mounted on a small carriage and was gaily decorated with red stars and had THE FLYING ZAMBINIS painted on the side.

"You are placed in this cannon and then fired into the array at .346 Absurd speed. The mesh of the first sieve is quite broad, to break down your base description into individual words. The next breaks the words down into letters, and then the letters are divided further into subcalligraphic particles, until you hit the silver sheet, which has holes in it one-tenth the size of a polyptoton. After that," he concluded as he tapped the large funnel, "your descriptive dust is compressed in the Pittmanizer to a concentrated pellet of ultradense prose, where the several thousand words of your description take up less space than one-millionth of a period. Put it another way: If all Fiction were compressed to the same degree, it would take up the space of an average-size rabbit."

"I like comparative factoids like that."

"Me, too. This tiny speck of you is then injected at speed into a drop of AntiBook, where your essence is rebuilt into something closely resembling human. By controlling the Sieve Array, I can drop you wherever you want in the RealWorld."

"Does it hurt?"

"Quite a lot, actually," he admitted, "but only fleetingly. You'll barely have enough time to scream before it will be over. The return is not so dramatic. You'll simply find yourself in our arrivals suite, which is just behind that door."

"Do you have any advice?"

"I've never been there myself," confessed Plum, "but they say if you can handle the first ten minutes, you're good for the whole twelve hours. If you can't hack it, then just find a quiet wardrobe in which to hide until the free return brings you back."

I found his comments disconcerting.

"What is there that one might not be able to handle?"

Professor Plum made a clicky noise with his tongue. "It's highly disorderly," he explained, "not like here. There is no easily definable plot, and you can run yourself ragged wondering what the significance can be of a chance encounter. You'll also find that for the most part there is no shorthand to the narrative, so everything happens in a long and painfully drawn-out sequence. Apparently the talk can be confusing — for the most part, people just say the first thing that comes into their heads."

"Is it as bad as they say it is?"

"I've heard it's worse. Here in the BookWorld, we say what needs to be said for the story to proceed. Out there? Well, you can discount at least eighty percent of chat as just meaningless drivel."

"I never thought the percentage was *that* high."

"In some individuals it can be as high as

ninety-two percent. The people to listen to are the ones who don't say very much."

"Oh."

"There are fun things, too," said Plum, sensing my disappointment. "You'll get used to it in the end, but if you go out there accepting that seventy-five percent of talk is utter twaddle and eighty-five percent of people's lives are spent dithering around, you won't go far wrong. But above all don't be annoyed or distracted when random things happen for absolutely no purpose."

"There's always a purpose," I said, amused by the notion of utter pointlessness, "even if you don't understand what it is until much later."

"That's the big difference between here and there," said Plum. "When things happen after a randomly pointless event, all that follows is simply unintended consequences, not a coherent narrative thrust that propels the story forward."

I rolled the idea of unintended consequences around in my head. "Nope," I said finally, "you've got me on that one."

"It confuses me, too," admitted Plum, "but that's the RealWorld for you. A brutal and beautiful place, run for the most part on passion, fads, incentives and mathematics. A *lot* of mathematics."

"That's it?" I asked, astonished by the brevity in which Plum could sum up the world that had, after all, made us.

"Pretty much," he replied glumly. "And some very good cuisine. And the smells. You'll like those, I assure you. And real sex — not like the oddly described stuff we have to make do with in here."

"I assure you I'm not going to the RealWorld for the sex."

"When tourism was permitted, many visitors used it for little else. Anything that is impossible to describe adequately in the BookWorld was much sought and, coincidentally, usually beginning with *c:* cooking, copulation, Caravaggio, coastlines and chocolate. Will you do me a favor and bring some back? I adore chocolate. As much as you can carry, in fact. And none of that Lindt or Nestlé muck — Cadbury's the thing."

I promised him I would, and he opened the hatch at the back of the cannon.

"Good luck," he said. "Don't worry if it seems a bit odd to begin with. You're made in the image of the flesh-and-bloods, so there's nothing you can't figure out as long as you keep your wits about you. It helps if you crouch tight, like a hedgehog. It's why

Mrs. Tiggy-winkle was so good at moving across."

I crawled inside and crunched myself up into the fetal position. Plum instructed me to hold my breath when he reached the count of two, as it helped to have a breath in you when you arrived, since breathing out can give a good indication of how breathing actually works. I thanked him for the advice, and he closed the hatch. I looked along the barrel of the cannon to the muzzle, and beyond that to the series of textual sieves that would chop me into the smallest component parts imaginable. I admit it, I was nervous. I waited for about a minute in the gloom, and then, when nothing had happened, I called out.

"Sorry!" came Plum's voice. "I'm just winding her up to speed. If I don't get you to *exactly* .346 of Absurd Speed, all you'll be is a tattered mass of text caught in the sieves. If I fire you too fast, you'll be embedded in the back of the laboratory."

"What would happen then?"

"Paper over you, I suppose."

I wasn't particularly reassured by this but waited patiently for another half minute until I heard a faint whine that grew in pitch as Plum counted down from ten. When he got to five, the whine had grown so loud I could hardly hear him, so I guessed when two would be and took a deep breath. I was just thinking that perhaps this wasn't such a great idea after all and I should really be getting back to my series and staying there for a sensible period of time — such as forever — when there was a noise like a thousand metallic frogs all croaking at the same time and my body was suddenly skewered by a thousand hot needles. Before I could cry out, the pain passed, and after a low hum and a sensation of treacle, Klein Blue and Wagner all mixed together but not very well, there was a brilliant flash of light.

20.
ALIVE!

The "Alive" simulator at the BookWorld Conference is one of those devices that all characters should try at least once. The experience of being real has two purposes: firstly, to assist characters in their quest for a greater understanding of people and, secondly, to discourage characters from ever attempting to escape to the Real-World. Most customers last ten minutes before hitting the panic button and being led shaken from the simulator.

Bradshaw's BookWorld Companion
(8th edition)

I heard a gurgling sound, a heavy thumping and something odd in my nose that generated backstory memories I hadn't had for a while — something about going for walks in the park when I was small. It was dark, too, and I felt a pain in my chest. I didn't know what it was until, with a sound like a tornado, a hot gush of foul air erupted from within me and blew out of my mouth. Before I could recover from this shock, I spontaneously did the opposite and drew in an equally fast gush of air that cooled my teeth and tasted of pine needles.

"It's called breathing," came a voice close at hand. "It's very simple, and everyone does it. Just relax and go with the flow."

"I used to 'take a breath' and 'exhale uneasily' at home," I managed to say, "but this is quite different."

"Those were merely descriptive terms intended to suggest a mood," came the voice again, which sounded how I imagined a cheese straw might sound. "Here you are doing it to stay alive. Can you hear a thumping and a gushing noise, and a few rumbles, grunts, squeaks and growls?"

"Yes."

"It's your body. The thumping is your heart. It's all new to you, so it will fit oddly, like a new pair of shoes, but you'll get used to it. Feel your wrist."

I did so and was surprised to note that my skin was warm, soft and ever so slightly tacky. It was also thumping. It was my pulse, and I was sweating. Not for any descriptive reasons but because I was *alive*. After a few minutes of doing nothing but breathing, I spoke again.

"What's that random sensation of memories I keep getting?"

"It's smells. They have a way of firing off recollections. No one knows why."

I didn't understand and moved rapidly on. "Why can't I see anything?"

"You need to open your eyes."

So I did. I sat and blinked for some minutes. The view was quite astonishing, not only in range but in *detail.* I had been used to seeing only what was relevant within a scene. Back home, anything extra would have been unnecessary and was a pasty shade of magnolia with the texture of uncooked dough. Here there was *everything,* in all directions, in full color and in full detail. Several books' worth of description was just sitting there, with no one except me to revel in its glorious detail. The trees swayed ever so gently in the breeze, and the clouds moved slowly across the heavens. It was summer, and the flower beds had erupted in a sumptuous palette of color, while on the air were delicate tastes of cooking and garbage and rain and earth. I could hear stuff, too, except not one thing at a time, but all things at all times. The delicate symphony of sounds that reached my ears so heaped together that it was difficult to separate anything out at all, and I sat there quite numbed by the overload of sensations.

"How do they filter it out?" I asked.

"Humans filter well," said the voice. "In fact, they can filter out almost anything. Sound, vision, smells, love, anger, passion, reason. Everything except hunger and thirst, cold and hot. No need to hurry. Take your time."

I sat there for an hour, attempting to make sense of the world, and I did reasonably well, all things considered. In that time I managed to figure out I was sitting on a bench in a small and well-kept park hemmed in by redbrick houses on every side. There was a children's play area, a pond, a flower bed and two trees, both silver birch. A main road was to one side, and on a building opposite were two billboards. One was advertising the Goliath Corporation's supposed good work on behalf of the community, and the other promoted "Daphne Farquitt Day" on Friday, which began with a celebration of her works and ended with a Farquitt Readathon. It was a name I recognized, or course. The popularity of the romance author dictated that she had a genre all her own.

"It's beautiful!" I said at last. "I could stay here and watch the clouds for the whole twelve hours alone!"

"Many do," came the voice again.

I looked around. Aside from an impertinent squirrel foraging on the grass, I was entirely alone.

"Who are you?" I asked. "And why can't I see you?"

"Bradshaw asked me to keep an eye on you," came the voice. "The name's Square — Agent Square. If you want to know why you can't see me, it's because I'm from *Flatland* and bounded in only two dimensions. At the moment I'm presenting my edge to you. Since I have no thickness, I am effectively invisible. Watch."

A line a half inch thick and two feet long appeared in the air quite near me. The line separated and opened out into a thin rectangle, which broadened until it was a square, hanging in the air.

"How do you do?" I said.

"Oh, can't complain," said Square. "A spot of trapezoidism in this chill weather, but hey-ho. I worked with the real Thursday several times. Do you really look like her?"

"You can't see, then?"

"Since I am only two-dimensional," said Agent Square, "I can see the world only as a series of infinitely thin slices, like a ham. May I approach and have a look?"

Square moved closer. Out of curiosity I put my hand inside the area bounded by his vertices, and a soft bluish light gave me four rings around my fingers.

"Four disks is all I can see," said Square. "Viewing one dimension up is always a bit confusing. Mind you, for you people bounded in three dimensions, it's no different."

"I don't understand."

"Time," said Square, "is your next dimension, so to anyone in the RealWorld it appears as your third spatial dimension does to me — a thin slice in plain view but with the abstract notions of 'forward' and 'beyond' unseeable. May I?"

Square approached me and then tilted to a narrow rectangle, again became a line, vanished and then reappeared again. It was as though he were tilting in front of me in order, I assumed, to allow his two-dimensional frame of reference to scan my features. Once satisfied, Square withdrew.

"Spooky!" he said. "You *do* look just like her. What's the mission?"

"To find Thursday."

"Nothing hard, then."

I moved to stand up, but everything felt funny, so I sat down again.

"Why does my face feel all draggy?" I

asked. "The underneath of my arms, too, and my boobs — everything feels all . . . well, *weighted down.*"

"That'll be gravity," said Square with a sigh.

"We have gravity in the BookWorld," I said. "It's not like this."

"No, we just talk as though gravity existed. There's a huge difference. In the BookWorld, gravity is simply useful. Here it is the effect of mass upon space-time. It would be manageable if it were constant, but it isn't. Acceleration forces can give one a localized gravitational effect that is quite disconcerting. If you're here for only twelve hours, I'd stay well clear of trains, elevators, airplanes and cars. Very odd, I'm told, although I don't notice it myself. By the way, do you have a timer on your watch? You're here for just twelve hours, remember."

I looked at my watch, which had nothing but hands and a face. "No."

"You'll get used to that, too. If this were the BookWorld, you'd have one of those watches that counts down from twelve hours to add some suspense. Believe me, the plot in this world takes a bit of getting used to. I've not done anything for Bradshaw for six months. That's nothing in the

BookWorld, barely half a dozen words. Out here it really *is* six months. Hell's teeth! The boredom. There's a limit to how much reality TV one can watch, although it's become a lot easier for me since they brought in flat-screens. Now, what do you want to know first?"

"Walking would be a good start."

Agent Square was a good teacher, and within the space of twenty minutes I had mastered the concept of mass and the ticklish practical considerations of coping with momentum. Though easy to someone who'd been doing it for years, being able to lean back when negotiating a sharp stop to avoid falling over was an acquired skill.

"Bipedal movement is the skill of controlled falling," said Square. "If it weren't so commonplace, it would seem miraculous — like much out here, to be truthful."

I found the "walking straight" part fairly easy to master, but learning to conserve momentum while doing a right-hander at speed was a lot harder, and I was flailing my arms for balance until Square patiently taught me how angular velocity, centripetal forces and shoe/ground friction coefficients all worked together.

"Outlanders must be very good at math," I said, struggling with the vast quantity of complex equations necessary to recover after a stumble.

"So good they do it without thinking," he said. "Wait until you see someone riding a unicycle — it's math to die for."

The physical walking I soon got the hang of, but the rapidly moving pavement beneath me I found disconcerting — not to mention the highly constricting pull and drag of my clothes. Square told me to keep my eyes on the horizon and not look down, and after ten or so laps around the small park I was ready to venture farther.

We walked out of the park and down the street, and I stared at the intricate detail with which the RealWorld was imbued. The stains, the corrosion, the reflections — none of it could be adequately explained or described, and I became fascinated by every facet.

"What's that?"

"A spider."

"And that?"

"A dog turd."

"So *that's* what they look like. Who's that person over there?"

"Which one?" asked Square, tilting his body so his infinitely thin frame of reference sliced in the direction I was pointing. "I don't see anything."

But there *was* something there — a wispy humanlike form, through which I could see the wall and hedge beyond. I had met Marley's Ghost once when he was doing one of those tedious grammasite-awareness talks, and it was like him — transparent. I'd queued up for autographs afterwards, but when I'd asked him for a personalization, his agent told me to sod off. He wouldn't sign memorabilia either.

"What did you expect?" Marley's Ghost had said when I protested. "Albert Schweitzer?"

"Ghosts?" said Square when I explained what I could see. "Perhaps. There is much unexplained in the world. It behooves one to be wary at all times. Just when you think you've got the hang of it, along comes string theory, collateralized debt obligations or Björk's new album, and bam! You're as confused as you were when you first started."

We arrived at the Clary-LaMarr Travelport soon after. As in fiction, this was the main transportation hub in Swindon, where the Skyrail and mainline bullet services met. From here you could travel off to the west and Bristol and the steamer ports or east to London and the Gravitube. This was the business district, and the impressively high glassy towers disgorged a constant stream of people, all working together to make Swindon the powerhouse it was, deservedly known as "the Jewel of the M4." My Swindon was pretty similar, even if it lagged behind by eight years, the time that had elapsed since my series was written.

"What's that?" I asked, pointing towards a steel latticework tower that was being built on a hill to the south of the city. It was only half built but looked large enough to dwarf the skyscrapers when complete.

"It's part of the Anti-Smite Strategic Defense Shield that will one day protect a sinful citizenry from God's wrath — a series of force fields supported by steel pylons. Not even the most powerful smiting by the angriest or most vengeful God will make it through — or so it is claimed."

"That sounds pretty daft."

"That's the whole point," he said. "It's *meant* to be daft. The Commonsense Party's unswervingly sensible management of the country has left the nation with a woefully high stupidity surplus that needs to be safely discharged. It's hoped that the extraordinarily pointless and ridiculously expensive defense shield will be enough to deplete the stupidity quickly enough to allow time to more sensibly deal with a bigger problem that's coming up."

"What could be a bigger problem than God's wrath upon his creations and a cleansing fire falling from the heavens?"

"I'm not sure. Something to do with polar bears."

I sighed. "It's been a while since I had any concept of current affairs," I said. "All of this was barely thought of when I was penned."

"I keep abreast of things," said Square. "It's the closest thing to STORY they have out here. Makes me feel less homesick. You've been here an hour and you can walk pretty well, so you're doing okay. The next thing you need to learn is *interaction* and how humans all manage to live together without descending into chaos. The best place for appreciating this is crowds."

"Crowds?"

"Right. Humans are more or less identical except for a few peculiar habits generally delineated by geographic circumstances and historical precedent. But essentially they're all the same and reading from the same rule book. To get along you have to appreciate the rules but also know that other people know the rules — and that *they* know that *you* know the rules. Get it?"

"No."

"You will. Observe the crowds for a moment."

I watched as the thousand or so individuals milled around the Skyrail port, all of them heading in one of six directions and moving on their own yet as one. Astonishingly, *without* bumping into one another and falling over. It was a most remarkable sight. The wispy Marley-like ones had it even easier, since they could go *through* the pedestrians just as easily as around them.

"I'm still seeing the transparent humans."

"How insubstantial are they?"

"Pretty smoky. And they all look so *sad.*"

This was true. They all wandered about looking very dejected, as if the world were pressing heavily on their shoulders. I had tried to catch the eye of one or two, but they'd steadfastly ignore me and, it seemed, everyone else. I knew about "ghosts" but always thought they were a fictional construct, like some of the odder facets of Japanese culture. However, Square was uninterested in my transparent people and wanted to carry on with my education.

"If you can manage crowd work, you can handle almost anything," said Square. "You know about flocks of starlings and schools of fish, how they all seem to move at the same time?"

I told him that I had heard of this but not witnessed it.

"Humans are exactly the same when they get into crowds. By using subtle sensory cues and working to a set of basic rules, you can enter a crowd full of people all heading in different directions and come out the other side without touching anyone or causing an accident."

"How?" I said, looking suspiciously at the swirling mass of humanity.

"Think of it as a subtle dance, where you have to avoid touching anyone. You have to jog and dodge your way around but also have to know when people are going to dodge and jink round *you.* Give it a whirl."

I stepped into the crowd, and almost immediately a woman stopped dead in front of me.

"Sorry," I said, and walked on. I could sense I was disrupting the smooth liquidity of the crowd, and based on the noises people were making, it wasn't appreciated. I got to the other side of the street without bumping into anyone, but only just.

"Not so easy, is it?" said Square, and I had to admit he was right. I had thought being in the RealWorld would be simple, or at least a lot like home, but it wasn't. Nothing here was assumed; everything had to be actually *done,* and witnessed. Weirder still, once something *was* done, it was gone, and the knowledge of it faded almost immediately into memory. Once or twice I found myself attempting to move backwards or forwards in time before realizing that that's not how it worked. If I wanted to be five minutes in the future, I had to laboriously *run* the five minutes in real time, and if I wanted to go back, I couldn't. It was how I imagined the narrator in *À la Recherche du Temps Perdu* spent most of his life — trapped in a noisy, brightly colored cage barely two or three seconds wide.

After twenty minutes I could walk through the crowd without too much difficulty, but once or twice I found myself in the situation where the people I was trying to avoid met me head-on, and I moved left, and they did, so I moved right, and they did, too, and so on, for up to five times, which elicited nothing more than a chuckle from my dancing partner.

"The old 'back and forth' happens a lot when real and fictional people meet," said Square when I'd returned to where he was waiting for me. "If the Outlanders had any idea we were amongst them, it would be the surest way to tell. That and a certain confusion when it comes to everyday tasks. If you see someone unable to boil a kettle, open a sash window or understand he has an appalling haircut, it probably means he's fictional."

"Hmm," I said, "why is that woman in the annoyingly flamboyant clothes staring at me?"

"Probably because she recognizes you."

"Don't I have to know who she is before she can recognize me?"

"It doesn't work that way."

"Thursday?" said the woman, bounding up to me with a huge grin and a clatter of beads. "Is that really you? Where have you been hiding these past few months?"

I recognized her from the vague approximation that had made it through to my series. It was Cordelia Flakk, ex–SpecOps publicity guru and now . . . well, I had no idea what she did.

"Hello, Cordelia."

"How are Landen and the kids?"

"Apparently they're very well."

"Did you hear about Hermione? Went to the slammer for trying to fiddle her taxes and then tried to escape. She was caught between the wire with two saber-toothed tigers. They didn't know what had happened to her until a bangle and parts of her synthetic kidney turned up in one of the sabers' . . . well, I don't want the story to get too gruesome."

"Too late."

"You old wag, you! Will you be coming to Penelope's for the Daphne Farquitt reading party Friday afternoon? She wants us all to come round to her place for the readathon, and she's dying to show off her new man." She leaned closer. "A *neanderthal,* you know. Frightfully polite, of course, but likes to sleep in the garden shed. She has a few stories about matters south, I should warrant — a few glasses and she'll spill the beans, if you know what I mean."

The woman laughed.

"Goodness, is that the time? How I prattle so!" She suddenly lowered her voice. "By the way, are you still dealing in cheese?"

"Not really —"

"A pound of Limburger would set us straight. Just a taster, then — anything, in fact. I mean, it's not like we're asking for any X-14. Oh. Sorry, is that still a sore point? Why not bring a taster of cheese to Penelope's do on Friday? We can enhance them with some pineapple chunks. Cheese and Farquitt! Naughty us! Ta-ra!"

And she tossed her head and moved off.

"Did you understand any of that?" asked Square.

"About one word in eight."

"That many?"

I stood there, stunned by the fact that I had no idea what Thursday actually *did* in the RealWorld, nor what had happened and what hadn't. The recent exchange told me that she *had* been involved in the illegal cheese market, and we had walked past the abandoned Special Operations Division headquarters earlier, so I knew that at least some of her SpecOps adventures had been real. But what else had happened in her life I had no idea. If anyone asked me anything specific, I was going to have to wing it, or simply grin stupidly. Best of all, stay well away from anyone who might know me.

"Was that meeting at all relevant?" I asked Square. "In the grand scheme of things, I mean?"

"Probably not," replied Square. "Just a chance meeting that means nothing. If this were a book, Cordelia wouldn't have survived the first draft."

I spent the next two hours walking around trying to figure out how the world worked. It was confusing and tiring, and it seemed that much energy was expended for very little outcome. I had my first real pee, which was pretty bizarre, then ate some chocolate, which was hugely enjoyable. Mostly I listened in on conversations and was dismayed to note that Professor Plum had been correct. A lot of what was said was superficially very banal. Less of a sense of communication and more to do with being comfortable and secure amongst members of one's own species — the modern equivalent of being huddled together in the dark.

"There seems to be a tremendous fear of being alone," I said once we had stopped for a break in the graveyard of the Blessed Lady of the Lobster.

"My theory is that it's all misdirection."

"From what?"

"The depressing certainty that one day all of us will die."

"Speak for yourself. What's your story, Square?"

"I used to work in *Flatland* but was fired after 'artistic differences' with Circle. After that I was recruited by Bradshaw for deep-cover operations in the Outland. I was here on assignment when the RealWorld travel ban came down, so I took Blue Fairy, became real and volunteered to stay."

He sighed deeply, in a thin, two-dimensional sort of way. "Blue Fairy" was the term used to describe the only way in which fictional people could become real, and unsurprisingly, the Blue Fairy from *Pi-*

nocchio was the only person who could do it. She used to do it for free if you asked nicely and had a chit from the CofG, but now she is not permitted to conduct any realizations at all and is paid handsomely by the council for the honor of doing nothing. Nice work if you can get it.

"When do you get to go home?" I asked.

"I don't get to return home. The only good thing about this place is that it's fantastically roomy. Are you ready?"

I said I was, and we walked the three blocks to Landen and Thursday's house, situated in a quiet part of the Old Town. I asked Square to keep a low profile, took a deep breath, walked up the garden path and stared at the front door, heart beating furiously. This time for real.

21.
Landen Parke-Laine

The manufacture of robots, automatons and assorted mechanical people is undertaken by the Duplex Corporation, situated on the border of Sci-Fi and Fantasy. Most automata are energy cell powered these days, but the factory still produces a "Classic" line of clockwork men to satisfy clients who require something more retro. Despite problems with emotion, adverse wear and the continual windings, the Duplex range of robots (currently in its fifth incarnation) remains popular. Tours of the factory by arrangement.

Bradshaw's BookWorld Companion
(6th edition)

I knocked twice. There was the sound of noises from within, and the door opened. It was Landen, and we stared at each other for a few seconds.

"Hello," I said.

"Hello," said Landen.

"Hello," I said again.

"Are you her?" he asked.

"No, not really."

"Then you'd better come in."

He moved aside, and I stepped into the hallway that was familiar to mine, but only in layout. Thursday's real house was more real, more worn, more lived in. The banisters were chipped, the newel post was draped with discarded clothes, and a tide mark of children's fingerprints ran along the wall and up the staircase. Pictures hung askew, and there was a small cobweb around the lampshade. Landen led me through to the kitchen, which was a big extension at the back of the house, partly consuming the garden and covered with a large glazed roof above the junk-strewn kitchen table. It was packed with the chaotic assortment of the minutiae of life being lived — not the sanitized shorthand we get in the Book-World, even with the Reader Feedback Loop set to max. Life seemed to be a lot messier than people wanted fiction to be. Feedback reflected hopes, not realities. I looked around carefully and sat in the seat he had indicated.

"Tea?" he asked.

"Do I drink it?"

"Gallons of it, usually."

"At a single sitting?"

"No, generally one cup at a time."

"Then I'd love some, thank you."

He went to put the kettle on.

"You look a lot like Thursday," he said.

"I'm often mistaken for her," I replied, feeling less nervous around familiar questions. "In fact, I'm surprised you needed so little convincing I wasn't the real Thursday."

"I don't know that for certain," he replied. "Not yet anyway. I'd like you to be her, naturally, but there have been others who looked a lot like her. Not quite as much as you do, but pretty similar. Goliath is keen to know what Thursday gets up to when she's not at home, and they've sent one or two to try to trick me into giving information. The first was just a voice on the phone, then one who could be seen only from a distance. The last one almost took me in, but up close she didn't pass muster. Her texture was all wrong, the smell was different, the smile lopsided and the ears too high. I don't know why they keep sending them, to be honest — nor where they end up. After I booted the last one out the door, someone from Goliath's Synthetic Human Division came round demanding to know what I'd done with it. Then, after I asked about the legality of such a device, he denied there had been any, or even that he was from the Synthetic Human Division. He then asked to read the meter."

"So how can they lose two synthetic Thursdays?"

"They lost three. There was *another* that I hadn't even seen. They said it was the best yet. They dropped it off two weeks ago near Clary-LaMarr and haven't heard anything since. Are you that one?"

"No."

"Are you sure?"

"Yes," I replied, vaguely indignant. "I'm not a Goliath robot."

"Not a robot — a *synthetic.* Human in everything but name."

I took a deep breath. I had to lay my cards on the table. "She's missing, isn't she?"

There was a flicker of consternation on Landen's face. "Not at all. Her absences are quite long, admittedly, but we're always in constant communication."

"From the BookWorld?"

He laughed. "That old chestnut! It was never *proved* she could move across at will. I think you've perhaps spent a little too much time listening to deranged theories."

It sounded like a cover story to keep the real nature of the BookWorld secret. I didn't expect him to tell me anything. He didn't know who or what I was, after all. But he had to know.

"I'm the *written* her," I told him. "She may have spoken to you about me. I was the tree-hugging version in the Great Samuel Pepys Fiasco, who then took over from the evil Thursday who was deleted with Pepys. I run books one to five now — less along the lines of the old Thursday, but more how the real Thursday wanted them to be. Less sex and violence. It explains why we're out of print."

If I thought he would be surprised or shocked, however, I was mistaken. I guess when you're married to Thursday, the nature of weird becomes somewhat relative. Landen smiled.

"That's a novel approach. Mind you, there's nothing you've told me that I couldn't find out by rereading *First Among Sequels.* Goliath has access to that book, too, so if you *were* one of the synthetic Thursdays, I'd expect you to come up with something like that."

"Commander Bradshaw of Jurisfiction sent me."

He stared at me. The relevance wasn't lost on him. Jurisfiction and Bradshaw were never mentioned in the books.

"I'm not yet convinced," he said, giving nothing away, "but let's suppose Thursday *is* missing — you want my help to find her?"

"If she's missing, then you and I can help each other. I'll be going home in less than twelve hours. Any information learned out here might be helpful."

He took a deep breath. "She's been gone four weeks, that much is common knowledge. Everyone wants to find her. It's a national obsession. *The Mole, The Toad,* Goliath, SO-5, the police, the Cheese Squad, the government, the NSA — and now you claim the BookWorld, too."

"Do you have any idea where she is?"

He poured the boiling water into the teapot.

"No. And the thing is," he added, looking at the clock, "we need to resolve this one way or another pretty soon."

"Because of the police and the NSA and whatnot?"

Landen laughed. "No, not *them.* The kids. Friday won't get away from his shift at B&Q until six, but Tuesday will be home in two hours, and although my mind has been rendered as supple as custard when it comes to things Thursday, the kids are still at an impressionable age — besides, I don't think the doors in the house will take much more slamming."

And he smiled again, but it was sadder, and more uncertain.

"I understand."

"Do you? *Can* you?"

"I think so."

"Hmm," he said, pondering carefully, "does anyone else know you're here?"

"Cordelia Flakk's the only one we need to worry about."

"That's bad," he murmured. "Flakk's the worst gossip in the city. I've a feeling you've less than forty minutes before the press starts to knock at the door, two hours before the police arrive with an arrest warrant and three hours before President van de Poste demands you hand over the plans."

"What plans?"

"The *secret* plans."

"I don't have any secret plans."

"I'd keep that to yourself."

He poured out the tea and placed it in front of me. He was standing close to me, and I felt myself shiver within his proximity. I wanted to take him in my arms and hug him tightly and breathe in great lungfuls of Landen with my face buried in his collar. I'd dreamed of the moment for years. Instead I did nothing and cursed my restraint.

"Does Thursday know the president?"

"He often seeks her counsel. Thursday?"

"Yes?"

"How like her are you?"

I rolled up my sleeve to reveal a long scar on my forearm. "I don't know how I got that one."

"That was Tiger."

"Was Tiger a tiger?"

"No, Tiger was a leopard. Your mother's. Only Mrs. Next would name a leopard Tiger. May I?"

"Please do."

He looked at my scalp where there was another scar, just above my hairline.

"That was Norman Johnson at the close of the 1989 Super-Hoop," I said. "*Something Rotten,* page 351."

He went and sat at the other end of the table and stared at me for a while.

"You even smell like her," he said, "and rub your forehead in the same way when you're thinking. I have a lot of respect for Goliath, but they never got synthetics this good."

"So you believe I'm the written one?"

"There's another possible explanation."

"Who would I be if not Goliath or the written one?"

He looked at me for a long time, an

expression of concern on his face. I understood what he was trying to say.

"You think I might *be* Thursday, but suffering some sort of weird delusion?"

"Stranger things have happened."

"I've spent my entire life in books," I explained. "I'm really only five years old. I can remember popping out of the character press as plain old D8-V-67987, and my first day at St. Tabularasa's. I did well, so I was streamed into the First-Person fast-track program. Long story short, I look after the Thursday books one to five but also work for JAID — that's the Jurisfiction Accident Investigation Department. I can tell you about Sprockett and Carmine, and how Lorina/Pickwick doesn't approve of her bringing goblins home and likes to bore us stupid by quoting Latin mottos, and the new book that arrived in the neighborhood. And there's Bradshaw, and the metaphor shortage, and Jobsworth wanting me to go up-country to help deal with Speedy Muffler in the peace talks on Friday. That's me. I'm *not* Thursday. I'm nothing like her. Show me a frightening situation and I'll run a mile. Square will vouch for me."

And I called his name, but there was no answer.

"Right," I said, wondering where he'd

gone. "That makes me look stupid."

We both fell silent, and Landen stared at me for a long time once more. I saw his eyes moisten, and mine spontaneously did the same.

"I so want to be her," I sniffed as my eyes blurred with tears. "But I'm not."

Before I knew it, I had discovered what crying actually means when you do it for real. He gave me his handkerchief and hugged me, and I responded by wrapping my arms around his neck. It felt *wonderful.* Natural — like two parts in a jigsaw. When I had calmed down, he gently took my hands from around him and held them in his, gazing into my eyes.

"Here's the thing," he said at last. "If you're *not* the real Thursday, we must come clean to the kids and explain that you're not. I can't have them being disappointed again. But if you *are* the real Thursday, you must stay so we can look after you. It's possible that you just *think* you're not Thursday. All that stuff about the BookWorld — it could be Aornis up to her tricks again."

"Aornis, sister of Acheron?"

He raised an eyebrow. "How many children do Thursday and I have?" he asked.

"Two."

"That's in your favor as the written Thursday. Aornis gave the *real* Thursday a mind-worm so she thought she had a third child — another daughter — and Thursday was always worrying about her. We helped her by pretending there was, and occasionally, in lucid moments, she would realize what was going on. Then she'd forget and was worrying about her missing daughter again."

I tried to imagine what it might be like having a child who was a figment but could not. If Aornis was anything like the written Acheron, she was pretty unpleasant. Still, I was kind of glad I didn't know about the extra daughter. I had an idea.

"T minus pumpkin in ten hours," I said, consulting my watch. "If you see me vanish in front of your eyes will you believe I'm from the BookWorld?"

"Yes," he said, "I'll believe you. But if you don't vanish, will you believe that you *might* be Thursday except . . . well, nuts?"

"I could be the missing Goliath *synthetic* Thursday," I said, "with a well-researched cover story."

Landen smiled. "Being married to you has never been boring."

I was pondering over the consequences of being either mad or synthetic when Thursday's mother arrived.

"Thursday!" she squealed, having let

herself in. "You naughty girl! Where have you been?"

The real version of my mother was quite different from the written one. The real one was a lot older — at least seventy, by my guess, but didn't seem to have lost any of her youthful vigor. She was a little gray, a little hunched and a little odd.

"Here for long?" she asked.

"Only until midnight," I managed to mutter.

"Shame!" she said, then turned to Landen. "Is this one of the synthetics?"

"The jury's still out."

Mrs. Next walked up close and peered at me through her spectacles, as one might regard a stubborn stain on the carpet.

"It's very lifelike. Does she have the scars?"

Landen nodded.

"I know how to check," she said, and cut me a slice of Battenberg cake. "Here," she said, and handed it over. "Your favorite."

I took a large bite, and even though it had some paste inside that was almost indescribably nasty, I smiled politely and tried to eat it as quickly as I could.

"Very nice," I managed to say.

"Hmm," said Mrs. Next, "that doesn't

sound like her at all. Thursday *hates* marzipan."

"Is that what it was?" I said, running to the sink to spit it out. I knew I didn't like it, I just didn't know what it was. I had thought Marzipan was the name of a boy band.

"Hmm," said my mother, "this doesn't really help. Hating it *does* make her Thursday, but pretending to like it to spare my feelings definitely does *not* make her Thursday."

"It's a tricky one," agreed Landen.

They eyed me for a long time as they tried to figure out what to do and how best to tell if I was the real one or the written one. Nothing I could say would convince them of either alternative, and the only way to truly know — if I vanished at pumpkin hour — was a bit pointless, since by then I would no longer be around for them to answer any questions I might have, which was a bit like devising a 100 percent destructive test for counterfeit tenners.

The doorbell rang.

"That will be the first of your fan club," said Landen, and he went off to answer it.

"So," said Mrs. Next, "loopy, fictional or synthetic. Which would you prefer?"

"Loopy, I guess," I said sadly.

"Me, too. But the shitstorm that will be

unleashed when you get back is not something I'd like anyone to face. President van de Poste won't be able to make his Antismite Shield without you and the secret plans, and as a key witness in the Stiltonista cheese-smuggling trial, you'll need round-the-clock protection. And that's before we get into the fun Goliath has in store for you."

"She made a few enemies, right?"

"Only a few thousand. Start causing trouble amongst the criminal fraternity and no end of unfair retribution starts coming your way. Would you excuse me? I must avail myself of the facilities. The bad plumbing needs to meet the bad plumbing, so to speak."

And she tottered off in the direction of the downstairs loo.

I sat there for a moment unsure of what to think or do. I called out to Square but to no avail, then heard a noise. I looked up and noticed that the broom-cupboard door was ajar. Looking at me through the crack were two bright eyes. The door opened a little farther, and a small girl aged about eight stepped out. She was like the spirits I had seen around the place — that is to say, mildly transparent. I could see the bottle of Brasso on the shelf directly behind her.

"You're the last person I want to see," I said as my heart fell.

"That's not a very nice thing to say," said the girl.

"Let me guess," I said. "You're the mind-worm."

"I prefer Jenny," said Jenny indignantly. "Who are you?"

"If I can see you, I guess I'm the real Thursday — just insane. Still, at least this way I don't have to worry about Carmine and the goblin anymore."

"You're not insane," said Jenny, "and you're not Thursday either."

"I could be making you up," I remarked, "and making up your denial, too."

She shook her head.

"Creating figments like me takes a serious amount of effort, and you're not that good."

"Thanks. Insulted by someone's else's delusion."

"Jenny."

"Jenny, then. So how can I see you?"

"You're not seeing just *me,* are you?"

"No," I said, "there are others. Lots of them."

"Then you see what I mean. What does Landen think you are?"

I shrugged. "The real Thursday mad, I think."

"Don't upset him," said Jenny. "Thursday wouldn't like it."

"Thursday could be dead."

"I know for a fact that she isn't."

"How?"

But at that moment Landen came pacing down the corridor, and Jenny jumped back into the broom cupboard.

"That was your old buddy Lydia Startright, wanting to get an exclusive before the network vans turn up. I told her you weren't here and I had no idea where you were."

"Did she believe you?"

"She's an excellent journalist — of course not."

We sat in silence for some moments. I didn't think I would tell him I'd just seen Jenny, but the seeds of doubt had been sown. I *could* be the real Thursday. And even though the ramifications of being someone suffering bizarre delusions were *not* good news, the possibility that I would be with the man I loved was some consolation.

"Ask me some questions," I said finally. "I want to convince myself I'm not her."

"What's my middle name?" he asked.

"Is it . . . Whitby?"

"Not even close. Where was our first date?"

"At the Alhambra. The Richard III thing."

"No, that was later. Where did I lose my leg?"

"You've lost a leg?"

Mrs. Next came back into the room. "You never told me you'd bought a gold-plated toilet."

Landen frowned. "We don't have a gold-plated toilet."

"Oh, dear," said Mrs. Next. "I think I've just peed in your tuba."

She then muttered something about "the shocking price of dodo feed" and went out without saying good-bye to either of us.

"Daft as a brush," said Landen, "and just a teeny-weeny bit repulsive."

"Plock."

I turned. A dodo stood at the open door. It was nothing like the Pickwick/Lorina back home. This dodo was *old.* Her beak was worn and scaly, she had no feathers, and her left foot had a tremor. She was dressed in an all-over body warmer made of fleecy material and was regarding me curiously.

"Pickwick?"

"Plock?" said the dodo, cocking her head to one side. She walked unsteadily up to me and looked very closely at me for a long time.

"Plock, plock," she said, and rubbed her

beak affectionately on my trouser leg before walking over to her water dish.

"Pickwick thinks you're real."

"Pickwick has a brain the size of a *petit pois.*"

"True."

The doorbell went again.

"That will be the Toad News Network."

As soon as he had gone, the broom-cupboard door opened again.

"Has he gone?" asked Jenny.

I nodded.

"Right, then. I'll show you what I mean about Thursday not being dead. Come with me."

22.
Jenny

Places to Eat #15: Bar Humbug, 68 *Christmas Carol.* Very cheap food served in an authentically austere and utterly miserable Dickensian atmosphere. Waifs wait at tables, and portions are notoriously small. People with silly names particularly welcome, and those with an archaic job title (beadle, proctor, sexton, etc.) can eat for free.

Bradshaw's BookWorld Companion
(5th edition)

Jenny opened the back door and checked to make sure the coast was clear.

"Why do you do that?" I asked. "Check that no one's coming? Only I can see you, right?"

Jenny looked at me and raised an eyebrow. "When you're illusory like me," she said, with great clarity, "it pays to keep an eye out for imaginary foes."

She checked again and beckoned me out. I followed her down to the end of the garden and opened the door that led into the garage behind. I knew that my car would be kept here, but Thursday's figment had no time to waste and hurriedly led me down the rear access road until we came back out onto the same street. Landen had been correct. Parked outside the house was a large Toad News Network van, complete with transmitter dish ready for bouncing a live feed to a handy airship.

"Landen will be surprised to find me not there."

"Nothing could surprise Landen. This way."

"Miss Next?" asked a man who had just gotten out of a car opposite. "May I have a word?"

I looked around, but Jenny seemed to have vanished. "I suppose so."

"I just heard about your return. I'm a *huge* fan of your work. Adrian Vole of the Wapcaplit and Vole Advertising Agency. We understand you travel in Fiction, and we were wondering if you wanted to do a bit of product placement around the written world."

"I hardly think that's appropriate, do you?" I said, adding quickly, "Even if there is a BookWorld, which is by no means proven."

"Thirty grand to plug the Toast Marketing Board in the Thursday Next series. You can introduce it how you want."

"I've never even *heard* of the Toast Marketing Board."

"You wouldn't. It's new. What do you say?"

"What do you think I'm going to say?"

"Yes," said Vole unhappily, "we thought you'd tell us to stick it in our ear. Here's a check. If you cash it, we know you're on board."

I took the check and moved on. Oddly enough, as soon as Vole turned away, Jenny was back.

"What's going on?" asked Square, who had suddenly reappeared. "It's not like the BookWorld, where I can be five or six places at once."

"Landen thinks I might actually *be* Thursday," I said, "and if I can see Jenny, then he might be right."

"Who's Jenny? I don't see anyone."

"She's one of the wraiths I've been seeing. And if I *am* Thursday, then I'm simply imagining you."

"Who are you talking to?" asked the figment Jenny, which seemed a bit impertinent given her less-than-definite existence.

"Agent Square," I said, "in Jurisfiction deep cover."

"Who are you talking to?" asked Square.

I sighed. This was getting more and more complex, but in a way I was heartened that they couldn't see or hear each other. If they were *both* in my head, they should be able to converse — unless I was more insane than I thought possible.

"I'll tell you about it later," I said as we crossed another road, walked through the graveyard of the Blessed Lady of the Lobster, took a right down the hill and then an immediate left, where we found a small apartment building. Jenny led us into the lobby, and we paused while she consulted the names on the mailboxes.

"Fifth floor."

We took the stairs, as neither I nor Square wanted to get into the elevator, and arrived at the upstairs corridor, from which four apartments could be accessed. As I walked along the corridor, one of the doors opened and a nurse walked out, glanced at me and moved off towards the elevators. As the door closed on the apartment, I could see that other medics were in attendance, clustered around a bed.

"You brought me here to see a guy dying?"

"Sort of," replied Jenny, "but not him in there — him out here."

She pointed. At the far end of the corridor were five more of the wraithlike figures I had seen earlier. They all stood around looking solemn, trying to comfort one of their number, who flickered in and out like a badly tuned TV set. They all spoke in a low growl that I couldn't really understand, and as I walked closer, I noticed that they were dressed rather oddly.

"You brought me here to see some spooks?"

"They're not spooks," said Jenny. "They're like me and you, Thursday — made up. Figments, inventions. Created in the white-hot heat of a child's imagination, they linger on even when redundancy renders them invisible to their creators. Sometimes people catch a glimpse of them, but for the most part they're invisible. You can see them because you're fictional. So can I. You, them, me — we're all one and the same. A living fiction that needs no book."

I looked closer at the figures. They were partially dressed as clowns, had bold, large features and spoke in a simple dialect of basic verbs and a limited number of nouns.

"They're . . . imaginary childhood friends, aren't they?"

Jenny smiled. "Bravo, Thursday — a chip off the old block. They follow their creators about, an echo of a vibrant childhood imagination."

She indicated the one who was flickering.

"Pookles here is about to leave — they can have no independent existence without their creator."

As we watched, the flickering imaginary friend started shaking hands with the others, hugging them and thanking them, and then, with a final bright burst, it vanished. Almost immediately we heard a cry of grief from the bedroom behind us, and one by one the ethereal figures took their leave, walking through us and along the corridor, leaning on one another for support and shaking their heads sadly.

"So where does Thursday come into all this?"

"This is how I know she's still alive. *I'm still here.* Unlike you, who are the figment of a ghostwriter and are now carved into a textual matrix, a part of Thursday is all I am. If she were dead, I wouldn't be around to be thought of. I'm bound to her, like a dog on a leash."

"Right," I said, "I get that. But it doesn't

tell us where she is. Any ideas? The Dark Reading Matter, for instance?"

"That was one of her interests, certainly, but the whole Racy Novel stuff had taken over her life. The last time we spoke, she said something about Lyell being boring."

"Lyell? Boring?"

"Yes. I don't know who Lyell was or why he should be boring, but boring he was — and Thursday didn't like it. Not one little bit." Jenny shook her head and took me by the hand. "I miss her, Thursday. It's lonely not being directly imagined on a day-to-day basis."

We walked back towards Landen's house.

"I'm confused," said Square. "What, precisely, is going on?"

"I'm not really sure. I feel like I'm following in Thursday's footsteps, only several hundred yards behind, and — hello, that's odd."

I looked around. Jenny, who'd been with us just a second ago, was nowhere to be seen. I twisted this way and that to see where she'd gone, and as I was doing so, a black van screeched to a halt in front of me. Within a few moments, the sliding door had opened and I'd been bundled inside in a less-than-polite manner, a sack put over my head. With another screech of tires, the van set off, and to make matters worse, I was then immediately sat upon by someone who smelled strongly of Gorgonzola.

23.
THE STILTONISTA

> The most cost-effective way to tour the BookWorld is by bus. A BookWorld Rover is the preferred method, giving you unlimited travel for a month. Delays might be expected at the borders between islands, but for the discerning tourist eager to see the BookWorld at a leisurely pace, the Rover ticket is ideal. Next page: working your passage on a scrawl trawler. Not for the fainthearted.
>
> *Bradshaw's BookWorld Companion*
> (5th edition)

Any attempt to describe the journey would have been futile, as the varying degrees of gravitational flux that I encountered during the trip were unpleasantly distracting. Suffice it to say that all the lurches, bumps, swerves and twists made me feel quite peculiar, and I wondered how anyone could undertake journeys on a regular basis and not only become ambivalent but actually enjoy them. Fortunately, this journey ended after not too long, and once the van came to a stop and I was rather impolitely hauled from the back and placed on a chair, the sack was pulled off.

I was in a deserted warehouse. There were puddles of water on the floor and holes in the ceiling — which probably accounted for the puddles on the floor. The windows were broken, and green streaks of algae had formed on the walls. In several places brambles had started to grow, and the odd pile of rubble and twisted metal sat in heaps. I wasn't alone. Aside from the four men who had brought me in the van, there was a Rolls-Royce motorcar and three other men. Two of them seemed to be bodyguards, and the third was undoubtedly the leader. He was dressed in a mohair suit and greatcoat, and his features were drawn and sunken — he looked like a skull that someone had thrown some skin at.

"I am Keitel Potblack," he said in the tone of someone who felt I should know who he was and not fail to be impressed, "head of the Wiltshire Stiltonista. Your failure to remain properly dead is becoming something of an inconvenience."

I laughed at the ridiculousness of the situation. This guy dealt in cheese, and he was acting as though he were a Bond villain.

"You're kidding, right?"

"I don't kid," said Mr. Potblack.

"Oh," I said, "right."

I looked at him, then at the men standing next to him, one of whom was carrying a spade. "Going gardening?"

They exchanged glances, as though this were the sort of comment they expected.

"It's up to you. Now, are you the real Thursday or just another copy?"

"I'm not her," I said, "so if you can take me home, I'd be really grateful."

"If you're not her," said Potblack, "I have no further need of you."

"Good. If you could tell your driver to go easy a bit on the way back, that would be —"

"Mr. Blue? Would you do the honors?"

The man with the spade walked towards me, and all of a sudden I realized that if he was digging anything over today, it would be me.

"You want to talk?" I said, the ease with which I stayed calm surprising even me. "Then let's talk."

"So you are Thursday?"

"Yes," I replied, which was no lie — I was *a* Thursday.

The man with the spade walked back to his position to the left of his boss. I noticed as he did that one edge of the spade had been sharpened.

"Okay," said Potblack, who seemed annoyed that I wasn't more frightened than I was. Perhaps if I'd known who he was, I would have been. But this was Thursday's life, not mine.

"In the past," began Potblack in a slow, deliberate speech, "we may have had an 'understanding' over who deals what cheese where. Perhaps you think I was being too harsh when I started dealing in really strong cheeses, but I am a businessman. The stronger the cheese, the more people will pay. Business is good, and we want to keep it that way. If the government lifts the cheese ban as threatened, then it could be very bad business for all of us. The last thing we want is legal cheese."

I vaguely knew what he was talking about, but not the details. I'd heard that cheese in the Outland was subject to a swingingly large amount of duty, but it seemed the government, in an attempt to control the burgeoning illegal-cheese market, had tried cheese prohibition. Judging from Potblack's jewelry, car and ability to supply, the ban didn't seem to be working.

"So what do you want me to do?" I asked. "It's not like I have the ear of the president, now, is it?"

The Stiltonista looked at his henchman with the spade, who picked it up again. I was wrong — I *did* have the ear of the president. Landen had said so earlier.

"Anymore. I don't have his ear *anymore.* But I'm sure I could give him a call and advise him to keep the prohibition in place."

Potblack stared at me and narrowed his eyes. "You're being uncharacteristically compliant."

"But characteristically *realistic,*" I said cheerfully. "You're the one with the sharpened spade."

"Hmm," said the Stiltonista, "very well. But I want to offer an incentive to make sure that once released you don't 'forget' your part of the bargain."

"Bargain?" I echoed. "You mean *I* get something from this?"

"You do. You get to keep your life, your husband gets to keep his, and your children get to keep their fingers."

The man with the spade tapped it on the ground as if to emphasize the point, and the steel rang out with a threatening *ting-ting-ting-ting* sound. I stared at the Stiltonista for a moment, and when I spoke, I tried to convey as much menace as I could — surprisingly easy, for I *was* angry — and it wasn't the sort of anger I get when I fluff my lines or my father misses a cue and comes in late. Or even the sort of anger I felt when Horace the goblin nicked all my stuff or Carmine went AWOL. This was *real* anger. The sort of "don't shit with me" stuff that mothers feel when you threaten their children.

"Dear, oh, dear," I said, sadly shaking my head, "and we were getting on so well. I said I'd help you out, and you respond by threatening my kids. That's not only insulting, it's impolite. There's a new deal: You let me go right now and promise never to even *look* at my husband or children, and I will let you live to see tomorrow's dawn."

The Stiltonista bit his lip ever so subtly. It was clear that I had a reputation, and it moved in front of me like a bulldozer. Despite the fact that I was outnumbered six to one, the Stiltonista obviously considered that at the very least I should not be underrated. Thursday, it seemed, was a formidable foe — and highly dangerous if you got on the wrong side of her.

"You're not in any position to be doing deals."

"I don't want anyone to think me unfair,"

I said. “I’ll give you until the count of three. One.”

There was the sound of safety catches being released from the men behind me. They were quite obviously armed and, from the sound of it, heavily.

“I’m sorry we couldn’t do any sort of deal, Miss Next,” said Potblack with renewed confidence. “Perhaps you would like to reconsider. My men will finish you before you get to three, and you’ll end up with all the others — six feet under the Savernake Forest, a feast for the worms. I apologize if I have been impolite, but as you understand, a lot rides on a lifted prohibition, and I speak not only for myself but for many cheese suppliers up and down the country. We can make this work to the best advantage for all of us, I’m sure — and perhaps even offer up some sort of compensatory payment.”

“Two.”

“You really don’t understand, do you?” said the Stiltonista in a voice that now carried an echo of uncertainty. “It doesn’t have to end for you like this.”

I didn’t have a plan of action, but that didn’t seem to be a problem, for the plan of action had *me,* and before I knew what had happened, I had the barrel of my pistol pressed hard against the Stiltonista's throat and the man with the spade was flat on his back unconscious. The goon next to me had managed to get his hand to the butt of his automatic, but no farther. The rest were just blinking stupidly. Oddly, I didn't feel nervous in the least. It felt like I was someone else. Someone else *inside* me.

"You see what happens when you're impolite?" I said. "And don't struggle. This an armor piercer. Once it's gone through, only Exxon will be able to retrieve it — or you."

He stopped struggling.

"Tell them to drop their weapons."

He did, and they did.

"Right," I said, unsure what to do next. "This is the plan. . . ."

If there was a plan, I never found out what it was, for a voice rang out from one corner of the warehouse.

"*Armed police!* You are surrounded. Do *exactly* as we tell you. Carefully and slowly, put your hands behind your heads."

The Stiltonista's goons did as the voice asked and seemed to know the drill, as they also lay flat on their faces without being asked.

"And you, Next."

I set my pistol on the floor, kicked it away and then obediently placed my hands on the back of my head and lay on the ground quite close to where Potblack now lay.

"I'll get you for this if it's the last thing I do, Next."

He said it without looking at me, his voice a low growl.

"Really?" I replied evenly. "Try to get me or my family and I'll happily ensure that it is."

He grumbled and faced the other way.

I heard the patter of feet, and within a few seconds I felt my arms pulled behind me and bound with a plastic tie. They weren't rough, though — they were almost gentle.

"Got a weapon here," said a voice, quickly followed by, "Got several weapons here."

"Thursday, Thursday," came the voice that had been behind the bullhorn. It was deep and earthy and was exactly how I expected Spike to sound. He was one of Thursday's SpecOps pals — someone who had been more than happy to feature in the series. It was the only recognition he'd ever got.

"Spike?"

"Hello, old friend," he said. "What have you got for us?"

"Keitel Potblack, head of the Swindon Stiltonistas," I said, "threatened to kill me, wanted to bribe me to block the repeal of prohibition and is also guilty of putting three of Goliath's synthetic Thursdays under the Savernake Forest."

"You've nothing to connect me with the Stiltonistas," said Mr. Potblack. "I happened to be here pursuing a potential property development when I was set upon by this madwoman."

"We've got a trunkful of Gorgonzola here," said one of the armed officers. "At least fifty kilos."

"For personal use," said Potblack in an unconvincing tone of voice.

"And your armed associates?"

"I employed them as decorators this morning. I am shocked, *shocked* to discover they are armed."

Spike helped me to my feet and walked me across to the front of the Rolls-Royce.

"It's good to see you again, Thursday. The Cheese Squad will have a field day with this lot. How in heaven's name did you nail Potblack of all people? We've been after him for years."

"Let's just say I have a magnetic personality."

Spike laughed. "Still the same. Tell me, do you want to do some moonlighting? The undead are about to be culled again, and there aren't many with Class IV zombie hunters' licenses about — or at least none who don't drool a lot and mumble."

I thought carefully. "If I'm around tomorrow, I'm totally up for it."

It was quite fun being her. I had a sudden thought.

"Spike, if you weren't here to arrest Potblack, what were you here for?"

"We've been trailing you for the past hour, Thursday."

"Why?"

"Because if *we* know you're here, so will *they.*"

" 'They' being . . . ?"

"Who else? Goliath."

"I can handle them."

"I don't think so," said Spike. "You've been gone a month, right?"

"In a manner of speaking."

"Three weeks ago SpecOps announced it had been privatized. The Goliath Corporation now runs not only SpecOps but the police as well. Almost the first thing Goliath did was charge you with crimes against humanity, murder, theft, illegal possession of a firearm, the discharge of a weapon in a public place, murder, impersonating a SpecOps officer, cheese smuggling, assorted motoring offenses and murder. It's quite a list. They must *really* hate you to dream up so many spurious charges."

"I think the feeling's pretty much mutual. Does that mean I'm under arrest?"

"We tried to, but you escaped." He smiled and removed the plastic cuffs with a flick knife. "Now go before Flanker gets here."

It was too late. A group of blue-suited individuals had arrived, brandishing Goliath IDs and a lot of attitude. Their leader I recognized from the description I had in the series — Commander Flanker, once head of SO-1, the police who police the police, now presumably answering to Goliath.

"Thank you, Officer Stoker," said Flanker, "for securing our prisoner."

"You can have her once we're done," said Spike, pulling himself up to his full height — he was well over six feet six. "Miss Next is charged with the illegal possession of a firearm, and I need to process her."

"The charge of crimes against humanity has precedence, Stoker."

"Your bullshit charge is bigger than my bullshit charge?"

"We could argue this all night, but the outcome remains the same. She is coming with me to be interrogated at Goliathopolis."

"Over my dead body," said Spike.

"I'm sure that can be arranged."

They growled at each other, but there was little, it seemed, that Spike could do. Within a half hour, I was in the back of a large automobile being driven to the Clary-LaMarr Travelport to be put on a private bullet train to Goliathopolis.

I took a deep breath. Being Thursday was exciting and was certainly distracting. I'd hardly thought about Whitby at all.

24.
Goliath

Perils for the Unwary #16: Big Martin. A large catlike beast who is never seen but always leaves a trail of damage and mayhem in its wake. A Big Martin event can always be avoided, due to the ample warning given by a series of cats that gradually increase in size. The universal Rule of Three should be adopted: Simply put, the third Big Martin warning should be considered the last, and it is time to leave.

Bradshaw's BookWorld Companion (2nd edition)

"Well," said Flanker as we sat in the plush interior of the bullet train, "we'll be at Goliathopolis in an hour, and your debrief can begin."

"Mr. Flanker, sir," said one of the accompanying heavies, a small man with a rounded face and a crew cut like a tennis ball, "have you checked she's not one of ours?"

"Good point," said Flanker. "Would you be so kind?"

The two heavies needed no extra encouragement, and while one held me down, the other clasped my upper eyelid and peered underneath. It wasn't painful, but it *was* undignified. Plus, the agent looking at my eye had been eating an onion sandwich not long before, and his breath was pretty unpleasant.

"She's not one of our Thursdays," said the agent, and they released me.

"I'm delighted to hear it," I said — and I was. There were now only two possibilities for who I was: me or Thursday. "Pot black killed them all," I added, "and had them buried in the Savernake."

"I don't know what you're talking about," replied Flanker airily. "Goliath no longer conducts experiments into synthetics. It's against the law. Oh," he added, "I forgot. We *are* the law. Shall I come straight to the point? We've been contracted to complete Phase One of the Anti-Smite Strategic Defense Shield by the end of the year, and the penalties are severe for noncompliance. We're not in the business of paying out severe penalties, so tell us where the secret plans are and we can release you and drop all the charges."

It felt like covering for a character in a book without being told what the book was about, who was in it or even what your character had been doing up until then. I'd done it twice in the BookWorld, so I had some experience in these matters. But at least I was beginning to understand what was going on.

"The plans are in a safe place," I replied, assuming they were, "but if you think you can simply ask questions and I'll simply answer them, you've got another think coming."

"Oh, this is just the preamble," said Flanker in an unpleasant tone, "so I can tell the board that I did ask you and you refused. We can cut the information out of you, but it's a very messy business. Now, where are the plans?"

"And I said somewhere safe."

Flanker was quiet for a moment. "Do you have any idea how much trouble you have caused Goliath?"

"I'm hoping it's a lot."

"You'd be right. Just getting you off the streets is a small triumph, but we have other plans. The Goliath Advanced Weapons Division has been wanting to get hold of you for a long time."

"I won't help you make any weapons, Flanker."

"It's simpler than that, Thursday. Since you have been so devastatingly destructive to us over the years, we have decided that *you* would make the ideal weapon. We can create excellent visual copies, but none of them have the unique skills that make you the dangerous person you are. Now that we have you and that precious brain of yours, with a couple of modifications in your moral compass our Thursday Mark V will be the ultimate killing machine. Of course, the host rarely survives the procedure, but we can replace you with another copy. I'm sure Landen won't notice. In fact, with a couple of modifications we can improve you for him — make the new Thursday more . . . compliant to his wishes."

"What makes you think that I'm not already? If he were only a quarter of the man he is, he'd still be ten times more of a man than you."

Flanker ignored me, and the bullet train moved off. We were soon zipping through the countryside, humming along thirty feet above the induction rail. When another bullet train passed in the opposite direction, we gently moved to the left of the induction wave, and the opposite train shot past us in a blur.

I stared at Flanker, who was sitting there grinning at me. If he could have started to laugh maniacally, he would have. But the thing was, this didn't sound like the Flanker in my books. Pain in the ass he might have been, but Goliath lackey he most certainly wasn't. His life was SpecOps, and although a strict rules man, that's all he was. I had an idea.

"When did they replace you, Flanker?"

"What do you mean?"

"This isn't you. Shit you might have been, evil-toady Goliath-lackey shit you most definitely weren't. Ever had a look at your own eyelid? Just to make sure?"

He laughed uneasily but then excused himself to the bathroom. When he came back, he looked somewhat pale and sat down in silence.

"When was I replaced?" he asked one of the heavies.

I'd not really given them much thought, but now that I looked at them, they also seemed to be vaguely familiar, as though they'd been described to me long ago. There were plenty of Goliath personalities in my book, but the litigious multinational had always insisted that no actual names could be used, nor realistic descriptions — they went further by denying that anything in the Thursday Next books ever took place, something that Thursday told me was anything but the truth.

"This morning," said one of the heavies in a matter-of-fact tone, "and you're due for retirement this evening. You're what we call a day player."

Flanker put on a good face of being unperturbed and picked up the phone that connected him to the central command for the bullet train. Before he could speak, the other heavy leaned forward and placed his finger on the "disconnect" button.

"Even if I am only a day player," said Flanker, "I still outrank you."

"You're not the ranking officer here," said the other heavy. "You're just the friendly face of Goliath — and I say that without any sense of irony."

Flanker looked at me, then at the heavies, then out the window. He said nothing for perhaps thirty seconds, but I knew he was going to make a move. The trouble was, so did the heavies. Flanker reached for his gun, but no sooner had he grasped the butt than he suddenly stopped, his eyes rolled upwards into his head, and he collapsed without a noise. It was as though he'd been switched off. The Goliath heavy showed me a small remote with a single button on it.

"Useful little gadget," he said. "All our enemies should have one. Boris? Get rid of him and then fetch Miss Next a cup of tea."

The synthetic Flanker was unceremoniously dragged from the compartment by Boris, and the first heavy came to sit in Flanker's old place.

"An excellent move," he said with the air of authority, "to pit one of your foes against another. Worthy of the real Thursday. Now, where is she?"

"I'm her," I said, suddenly realizing that while this whole Goliath adventure was kind of amusing, it wasn't helping me find out where Thursday had actually gone. The sum total of my knowledge was that she'd been gone a month, was not dead, and had said that Lyell was boring. Goliath didn't have her, so I was wasting my time here. I needed to get back to Swindon.

"Are you a day player as well?" I asked.

"No," said the man, "I'm real. I check every morning. I know better than most that Goliath can't be trusted. Now, where are you from and where's Thursday?"

"I'm her. You don't need to look any further."

"You're not her," he said, "because you

don't recognize me. It surprised me at first, which was why I had to make sure you weren't one of ours gone rogue. They do that sometimes. Despite our best attempts to create synthetics with little or no emotions, empathy tends to invade the mind like a virus. It's most troublesome. Flanker would have killed you this morning if I'd told him to, and by the afternoon he dies trying to protect you. It's just too bad. Now, where's Thursday?"

Finally I figured it out. The one person at Goliath who had more reason to hate me than any other.

"You're Jack Schitt, aren't you?"

He stared at me for a moment, and smiled.

"By all that's great and greedy," he said, staring at me in wonder, "what a coup. You're the written one, aren't you?"

"No."

But he knew I was lying. Unwittingly, I had revealed everything. Jack Schitt wasn't his real name — *it was his name in the series.* I didn't know what his real name was, but he would certainly have known his fictional counterpart. He pulled the phone off the hook and punched a few buttons.

"It's me. Listen carefully: It's not Thursday, it's the *written* Thursday. . . . Yes, I'm positive. She could melt back any second, so we need to get her Blue Fairyed the second we're on Goliath soil. . . . I don't care what it takes. If she's not real by teatime, heads will roll. And no, I'm not talking figuratively."

He hung up the phone and stared at me with a soft, triumphal grin. "When are you due back?"

I stared at him, a feeling of genuine fear starting to fill me. My actions so far had been based on the certainty that I would return. The idea of staying here forever was not in the game plan.

"What happened to the Austen Rover, Next?"

"The what?"

"The Austen Rover. Our experimental transfictional tour bus. The real Thursday traveled with it on its inaugural flight and never returned. Where is it?"

"I don't know what you're talking about, and besides, the Blue Fairy is fictional and lives inside *Pinocchio.* She doesn't do any actualizing these days. The Council of Genres forbade it."

"Better and better," he said, waving away the second heavy, who had returned with my tea, and closing the compartment door. "So you *are* from the BookWorld. And I was bluffing — we don't have a Blue Fairy. But we have the next best thing: a *green* fairy."

"I've never heard of the Green Fairy."

"It's a concoction of our own. It's not so much a fairy — more like a magnetic containment facility designed to keep fictional characters from crossing back. I understand that the first few hours can be *excruciatingly* painful, and it gets worse from there. You'll talk — they always do. How do you suppose we managed to get the inside information necessary to even begin research into the Book Project? Perhaps we can't make you real, but we can keep you here indefinitely — or at least until such time as you can't bear it any longer and agree to help us. Make it easy for yourself, Thursday: Where is the Austen Rover?"

"I have no idea."

"You'll tell us eventually. A few hours of Green Fairy will loosen your tongue."

"Goliath wouldn't last twenty minutes inside fiction," I said, but I wasn't convinced. If this "Jack Schitt" was even half as devious as the one written about, we were in big trouble. Thursday had spent a great deal of time and effort ensuring that the Goliath Corporation didn't get into fiction, either to dump toxic waste, use the people within it as unpaid labor or even just to find another market to dominate and exploit.

I said nothing, which probably was all he wanted to know. It was rotten luck that he'd been the one to figure me out. The real Thursday had once imprisoned the so-called Jack Schitt within Poe's "The Raven," so here was a man with some experience of being in the BookWorld.

"What's your name, then?" I asked. "If not Jack Schitt?"

"It was a ridiculous name, not to mention insulting," he snorted. "I'm Dorset. Adrian Dorset."

25.
An Intervention

Places to Eat #28: Inn Uendo, 3578 Comedy Boulevard. Made famous as the meeting place of the Toilet-Humor Appreciation Society, most of whose motions are passed while members are seated at the bar. The Double Entendre Bar and Grill is also highly recommended, and if you require satiating, the friendly waitstaff will be able to offer relief at the table.

Bradshaw's BookWorld Companion (5th edition)

"Adrian Dorset?" I said. "Are you sure?"

"No, I'm not sure at all."

"What's your name, then?"

"You're not as smart as her, are you? Of *course* it's Dorset. I think I know my own name."

"The Adrian Dorset who wrote *The Murders on the Hareng Rouge*?"

He looked surprised for a moment. "The

worthless scribblings of a man who was fooling himself that he could write. It was following the death of Anne, but I don't expect you'd know anything about that, do you?"

I shook my head.

"Anne was my wife," he said. "Head of the Book Project. She was on board the Austen Rover's inaugural journey. Thursday told me what had happened to her and what she'd done before she died. I don't blame Thursday. Not anymore. Revenge is for losers, cash is the winning currency. I burned the book a month ago. I didn't need it anymore. I'm over her."

He looked down at his feet, and I suddenly felt sorry for him.

"I'm sorry for your loss."

"Thank you."

He said very little for the rest of the journey, and I watched out the window as the English countryside zipped beneath us at breathtaking speed; we had nothing as fast as this in the BookWorld — not even in Sci-Fi, where they were a lot more conservative than they made out. As we approached Liverpool and the Tarbuck International Travelport, the traffic became more intense as other bullet gondolas joined the induction rail and clumped around for a while before moving off in separate directions. At all times the small, bullet-shaped craft, each no bigger than a bus, kept well spaced from one another, moving apart and together as congestion dictated.

The intercom buzzed, and Dorset picked it up, looked at me, then said, "Security override seventeen," before listening for a while and then saying, "*Bastards.* Very well."

"Problems?"

"Nothing to worry your sweet fictional head about."

We glided to a halt on Platform 24 at Tarbuck International. The doors hissed open, but we didn't move, and a few minutes later a small, meek-looking man arrived. He was wearing a dark suit and a bowler hat, and he was carrying a small briefcase. When he spoke, his voice was thin and reedy, and his nose was red from a recent cold.

"Good afternoon, Mr. Meakle," said my captor, without getting up.

"Good afternoon," said Meakle, who looked strikingly similar to someone who had played a bit part early on in my series. "You will release Miss Next to the custody of a federal marshal."

He indicated several marshals who were all standing on the platform outside the bullet.

"I'm afraid not, old chap," said Dorset or Schitt or whoever he was. "Miss Next is under arrest for crimes against humanity, which effectively trumps anything you might have in store for her."

"You're right *and* wrong," said Mr. Meakle. "She is under arrest, but *house* arrest, and will remain there until the government decides the best course of action. National heroes are not treated as common prisoners, Mr. Dorset."

"I have the authority of the police and SpecOps," replied Dorset coolly, "an authority given to us under mandate from the minister of justice."

The bureaucrat opened his case and took out a sheet of paper. "I repeat, Miss Next is to be taken into custody by a federal marshal. Here is an executive order signed personally by President Redmond van de Poste. Need I say more?"

Dorset took the document and stared at it minutely. I could tell from his expression that all was very much in order. He handed it back, looked at me and told me the game "was far from over."

I was taken across the concourse to where Meakle had his own private bullet with the presidential seal painted upon it, and within a few moments we were skimming back south across the countryside.

"Thank you."

Mr. Meakle seemed distracted, as though this were just one of many jobs he had to do in a single day. It looked, in fact, as though he worked from the bullet.

"My pleasure," said Mr. Meakle. "Where can we drop you?"

I asked for Swindon, and he relayed the instructions through the phone.

"I know I speak for the president when we say how fortunate it is to see you back," he added. "NSA officials and SO-5 will be briefed to protect you from Goliath. Can I schedule a meeting with the president anytime soon? We are eager to receive the secret plans as soon as we can, and we hope that the security arrangements are to your satisfaction."

I told him I'd meet with them tomorrow. Meakle nodded solemnly and returned to his work.

I sat back in my seat and ran the events of the afternoon through my head. I had just gotten to the bit where Spike had rescued me from the Stiltonista when I began to feel very peculiar. I started to have odd thoughts, then couldn't figure out why I'd thought of them. The world would soften around the edges, and I could feel myself almost lose consciousness. I thought for a moment I might be dying, as I could feel my conscious mind nearly close down. Before I knew it, I had closed my eyes and an overwhelming darkness stole over me. I might indeed have died, but I didn't, and I slept quite soundly until Mr. Meakle woke me when we arrived back at Clary-LaMarr.

26.
FAMILY

Places to Visit #7: Poetry Island. Although this is at first glance a wild and powerful place, by turns beautiful, wayward, passionate and thought provoking, any visit longer than a few hours will start to have an *exaggerating* effect on the senses. Upbeat poems will tend to have you laughing uncontrollably, while somber poems will have you questioning your own worth in a most hideously self-obsessed manner. Early explorers of Poetry spent weeks acclimatizing in Walter de la Mare and Longfellow before daring to explore the Romantics.

Bradshaw's BookWorld Companion
(12th edition)

"Where did you get to?" asked Landen as soon as I tapped on the back door to be let in. "I was thinking you'd gone missing again."

"I brought down the Stiltonista, was arrested for crimes against humanity, found out where the other Thursdays are buried, was almost kidnapped by Goliath and was then rescued by the attorney general."

"Is that all?"

"No. I found out what ghosts are. They're childhood memories. Oh, and the president wants to see me tomorrow to discuss the Anti-Smite Strategic Defense Shield — I think it's what the whole 'secret plans' deal is all about."

"Are you sure you're not Thursday?"

"Positive. Hey, listen: Jack Schitt's real name is Adrian Dorset. How weird is that?"

"Not weird at all. You and I have known for years. Jack Schitt is a daft pseudonym — not to mention actionable."

"Perhaps so — but he wrote *The Murders on the Hareng Rouge,* the book I was asking you about."

"And the significance of this is . . . ?"

"I don't know, but the RealWorld's kind of wild with all this strange stuff going on, although it's a good thing this isn't Fiction — it wouldn't really make *any* sense."

I was becoming quite animated by now — randomness has an intoxicating effect on the preordained.

"By the way," I added, "do you want thirty grand?"

Landen raised an eyebrow in surprise. "You earned thirty thousand pounds this afternoon . . . *as well?*"

"From a Vole."

"What the . . . ? No, I don't want to know. But yes, we could do with the cash, so long as it's not illegally earned."

"Here you go," I said, handing him the crumpled check.

I'd have to make good on my side of the bargain, but I felt sure I could drop some Toast Marketing Board references into the series without much problem.

"Oh, and if you see anyone who looks like NSA or SpecOps watching the house, don't be alarmed. The president is protecting us — I don't think Goliath is too keen on me right now."

"Were they ever?"

"Not really. But I know what they're up to, and it's particularly unpleasant. In fact, I shouldn't really hang around. I'll only make things dangerous for you."

"Until we prove you're not my wife," he said, "you're staying."

It seemed like a generous sentiment, so I accepted gracefully.

"Listen," he said, "just in case I'm wrong

and you really *are* written, you should know something."

"Yes?"

"You know I said I didn't know where she was?"

I nodded.

"That's not *strictly* true. I didn't know whether I could trust you. You see, when Thursday went to the BookWorld, she *always* came and went via her office at Acme Carpets. Bowden is the manager over there, and when she went missing, I asked him to go and look for her."

"She wasn't in her office?"

"No — *and the door was locked from the inside.*"

He let this information sink in. She had gone to the BookWorld four weeks ago — and not returned.

"So," he said, "if you're *not* her, it's where you need to be looking. If you *are* her, it's where you need to go to find out what has happened to you."

I stared at him and bit my lip. Thursday was definitely somewhere in the BookWorld. Lost, alone, perhaps hurt — who knows? But at least I had somewhere to start. My mission, such as it was, was at least a partial success.

"Well, then," said Landen, clapping his

hands together, "you'd better meet Tuesday."

So I sat down at the kitchen table and felt all goose-bumpy and hot. I'd been less nervous facing down Potblack, but this was different. Landen and the children were everything I'd ever wanted. Potblack was just a jumped-up cheesemonger.

Tuesday wandered shyly into the room and stared at me intently.

"Hello," I said. "I'm not your mother."

"You look like her. Dad says that you might be Mum but you don't know it."

"That's possible, too," I said, "and I'd like to be."

"Could she be?" asked Tuesday of Landen.

"It's possible, but we won't know until later."

"Oh, well," said Tuesday, sitting next to me at the kitchen table. "Do you want to see what I'm working on?"

"Sure."

So she opened her exercise book and showed me a sketch of an idea she'd been having.

"This is a sundial that works in the overcast — or even indoors. This is a method of sending power wirelessly using music, and what do you make of this?" She showed me several pages of complex mathematical notation.

"Looks important."

"It's an algorithm that can predict the movement of cats with ninety-seven percent accuracy," she explained with a smile. "I'm presenting it to Nuffield College the day after tomorrow. Do you want to come?"

Over the next few minutes, she explained her work, which was far-ranging in its originality and depth. My inventor uncle Mycroft was dead now, and his intellect had crossed to Tuesday. If at age twelve she was working out the complex mathematics required to accurately predict random events, her work when she was an adult would be awe inspiring. She spoke to me of her latest project: a plausible method to crack one of the most intractable problems in modern physics, that of attempting to instill a sense of urgency in teenagers. After that she explained how she was designing daylight fireworks, which would sparkle darkness in the light, and then finally mentioned the possibility of using beamed electron fields as a kind of impermeable barrier with such diverse applications as enabling people to go underwater without need for an Aqua Lung or to protect one from rockfalls or even for use as an umbrella. "Especially useful" remarked Tuesday, "for an electron-field umbrella wouldn't poke anyone in the eye and never needs shaking."

After Tuesday had gone off to fetch a photograph album, I turned to Landen. "*She's* the secret plans, isn't she?"

He looked at me but said nothing, which I took to mean she was. Tuesday's intellect would be the driving force behind the government's Anti-Smite Strategic Defense Shield.

"I guess we're just about to find out if you're the Goliath Thursday," said Landen. "If you are, you'll be contacting them straightaway."

I wouldn't, of course. "How long do you think before they figure it out?"

"I don't know," replied Landen, scraping the carrots he'd been chopping into a saucepan, "but know this: I'll die to protect my daughter."

"Me, too."

Landen smiled. "Are you sure you're not her?"

"I'm sure."

Tuesday came back with the photograph album, and I joined her as she leafed through the family holidays of which I had no knowledge. I stared at the Thursday in the pictures and tried to figure her out. She never looked totally relaxed — not as much as Landen and the kids anyway, but clearly loved them all, even if she seemed to be glancing around her as though on the lookout for anyone wishing to do them or her harm. There were very few pictures in which she was smiling. She took life seriously, but her family kept her anchored, and probably as sane as she could ever hope to be. Tuesday reached for my hand and held it tightly without really thinking, and as we chatted, it crossed my mind that I could *become* Thursday, if the real one never showed up. I could go Blue Fairy, and all this would be mine. For a fleeting moment, it seemed like a good, worthy and attainable idea, but reality quickly returned. I was fooling myself. The longer I listened to Tuesday, the more I realized just how much she needed her mother. Not any mother, but *her* mother. I would never be anything more than a pale reflection.

"Landen," I said when Tuesday had gone off to watch *Bonzo the Wonder Hound, Series Twelve,* "I shouldn't have come."

"Nonsense."

"No, really. It was a huge mistake. I can't be her, no matter how much I want to."

"You sell yourself short — I'm more

convinced by the minute. The way you sat with Tuesday."

"Yes?"

"That's how Thursday used to do it. Proud, loving — but not understanding a single word she said."

"Land, I'm not her. I've got no idea what's going on, I didn't recognize Adrian Dorset, I didn't know that you'd lost a leg and, and, and . . . I can't see Jenny. I should just go and hide in a large cupboard somewhere until I'm whisked back into Fiction."

He stared at me for a moment. "I never said her name was Jenny."

"Damn."

He took a step closer and held my hand. "You saw her?"

I nodded. "Jenny mentioned Thursday saying 'Lyell was boring.' Does that make any sense to you?"

"Thursday didn't discuss her BookWorld work with me. She pretended it was a secret, and I pretended I didn't know about it. Same as the SpecOps work. But I don't know anyone called Lyell, and she *hated* boring people. Except me."

"You're not boring."

"I am, but I'm okay with it. I'm the anchor. The shoulder."

"And you're all right with the support role?"

He laughed. "Of course! It's my *function.* Besides, I love her. More than anything on the planet — with the possible exception of Tuesday and Friday. And I'm actually quite fond of Jenny, too, even though she doesn't exist."

"You're a good man."

He smiled. "No, I'm an average man . . . with a truly extraordinary wife."

I rubbed my temples with the frustration of it. I so wanted to be her and have all this — Landen, the kids. There was a dull throb in my head, and I felt hot and prickly. It was a lot easier being fictional — always assuming that I was, of course.

"That's another reason I should leave," I said in a harsher tone than I might have wished. "This morning I knew who I was and what I was doing. Now? I've got no idea."

And I started to sob.

"Hey, hey," he said, resting a hand on mine, "don't cry. There's four hours to go before you vanish or not, and I'm not sure I can wait that long. I'm pretty confident you're her. You called me 'Land,' you saw Jenny, you're a bit odd, you love the kids.

But there's one simple way I'll be able to tell."

"And what's that?"

"Kiss me."

I felt myself shiver with anticipation, and my heart — my real heart, that is, not the descriptive one — suddenly thumped faster. I placed my hand on his cheek, which was warm to the touch, and leaned forward. I felt his breath on my face, and our lips were just about to touch when suddenly I once more felt the hot needles and Klein-Blue Wagnerian treacle, and I was back in the arrivals lounge at JurisTech. As Plum had promised, there was a glass of water and some cookies waiting for me. I picked up the water glass and threw it at the wall.

27.
Back Early

Plot 9 (Human Drama) revolved around a protagonist returning to a dying parent to seek reconciliation for past strife and then finding new meaning to his or her life. If you lived anywhere but HumDram, "go do a Plot 9" was considered a serious insult, the Outlander equivalent of being told to "go screw yourself."

Bradshaw's BookWorld Companion
(3rd edition)

I found Professor Plum working on his Large Metaphor Collider. As soon as he saw me, he pressed a couple of buttons on his mobilefootnoterphone, uttered a few words and smiled at me.

"Oh!" he said in some surprise. "You're back."

"What happened? I wasn't meant to come back for another four hours!"

"Transfictional travel isn't an exact science," he replied with a shrug. "Sometimes you'll pop back early for no adequately explained reason."

"Can you send me out there again? I was right in the middle of something important."

"If Bradshaw allows it, I'll be more than happy to."

"Please?"

"There are safety issues," he explained. "The more you stay out there, the less time you can spend there. Bradshaw used to travel across quite often, but these days he can barely stay out for ten minutes before popping back."

I thought about the excitement I'd felt just as I was about to kiss Landen and the potential chain of events that might have occurred from there on in.

"I *really* need to get back, Professor. Lives . . . um, depend on it."

"Whose lives?"

Commander Bradshaw had appeared in the laboratory. But he didn't walk in, he had *bookjumped* in. I hadn't seen that for a while; it was considered very common and was actively discouraged. The Ungenred Zone and Racy Novel, to name but two, even had antijump sieves set up on their borders — large sails of a fine mesh that snagged the punctuation in one's description and brought one down to earth with a thump.

"I'm very busy," he said, glancing at his watch. "Walk with me."

So I walked with Bradshaw out of the labs, past the frog-footman, who followed at a discrete distance and up the stairs.

"So," said Bradshaw, "how did you get on?"

"Not very well. *Lots* happened, but I've got no way of knowing which of the facts were significant and which weren't."

"The RealWorld is like that. It's possible that nothing was significant or that everything was. It scares the bejesus out of me, I can tell you — and I don't scare easily. Anything on Thursday's whereabouts?"

I told him about the locked room at Acme.

"Hmm," he said, "*definitely* in here somewhere. I'll ask Professor Plum to attempt another Textual Sieve triangulation." He thought for a moment. "How were Landen and the kids?"

"As good as might be expected. Permission to speak honestly, sir?"

"I welcome nothing else."

"Is it possible that Thursday is alive and well but just suffering some bizarre mental aberration?"

He stared at me. "You think you might be

Thursday?"

I shrugged. "Landen seems to think so. I saw Jenny, and I could do things — fight, think on my feet and disarm a man in under a second. Things I never knew I could do."

He smiled and patted my arm. "It's not uncommon to have feelings of elevated status after visiting the RealWorld. It'll soon pass."

"But *could* I tell if I were real? Could anyone tell?"

"There are lots of signs," said Bradshaw, "but here's the easiest: What am I doing now?"

"I don't know."

"How about now?"

"As far as I can tell, you're not doing anything at all."

Bradshaw took his finger off my nose and smiled. "I suppressed my action line. The real Thursday could have seen what I was doing, but you had to rely on the description. You're fictional, my dear, through and through."

"But I could be just *thinking* you did that — the same as I *thought* I saw Jenny, and all my backstory about being the written Thursday. I could be . . . delusional."

"And part of this delusion is you *thinking* you might be delusional? And me here right now talking to you?"

"I suppose so."

"Pull yourself together, girl," he snapped, "and don't be such a bloody fool. If you *were* Thursday, you'd be saving the BookWorld, not blundering around the Outland like a petulant bull in a china shop. This is Fiction, not Psychology."

"I'm sorry, sir."

"That's okay. Now, is there anything else to report?"

I told him about Jenny, the comment about Lyell and how Goliath had developed a Green Fairy and wanted to know where the Austen Rover had ended up.

"Goliath is an ongoing thorn," said Bradshaw grimly, "but we're dealing with the problem. Anything else?"

I thought for a moment. If I couldn't trust Bradshaw, I couldn't trust anyone.

"This morning Jobsworth and Red Herring asked me to pretend to be Thursday and go to the peace talks on Friday."

"We thought they might."

"Should I go?"

"It would be my advice that you shouldn't. Don't be insulted by this, but civilians are ill equipped to deal with anything beyond that which is normally expected of them. The BookWorld is fraught with dangers, and your time is best served bringing as many readers as you can to your series, then keeping them."

"Can I go back to the RealWorld?"

"No."

"I have unfinished business. I did go on a somewhat risky mission for you — I could have ended up erased or dead — or both."

"You have the gratitude of the head of Jurisfiction," he said. "That should be enough. He's not *your* husband, Thursday. He's Thursday's. Go back to your book and just forget about everything that's happened. You're not her and never can be. Understand?"

"Yes, sir."

"Excellent. Appreciate a girl who knows when to call it a day. The frog guy will see you out. Good day."

And so saying, he turned on his heel and walked into the ballroom. The door closed behind him, leaving me confused, drained and missing Landen. I thought of going to find Whitby to cry on his shoulder, but then I remembered about the nuns.

"Damn," I said, to no one in particular.

The frog-footman saw me to the front door, then handed me the Rubik's Cube I'd lent him.

"Here," he said. "It's got me flummoxed,

I can tell you."

Despite his working on the puzzle during my absence the cube had remained resolutely unsolved — all six sides were still the same unbroken colors.

28.
Home Again

There are multiple BookWorlds, all coexisting in parallel planes and each unique to its own language. Naturally, varying tastes around the Outland make for varying popularity of genres, so no two BookWorlds are ever the same. Generally, they keep themselves to themselves, except for the annual BookWorld Conference, where the equivalent characters get together to discuss translation issues. It invariably ends in arguments and recriminations.

Bradshaw's BookWorld Companion
(2nd edition)

I climbed out of the Porsche, slammed the door and leaned against the stone wall. We'd just done the "bad time" section within *The Eyre Affair,* which was always tiring and a bit spacey. Despite our best endeavors, our sole reader had simply given up and left us dangling less than a page before the end of that chapter — the Outlander equivalent of letting someone reach the punch line before announcing you'd heard the joke before.

Bowden climbed out to join me. I got on better with him than I did with the character who played my father, but that wasn't saying much. It was like saying sparrows got on better with cats than robins. Bowden had a thing going on with the previous written Thursday, and when he tried to hit on me at the Christmas party, I'd tipped an entire quiche in his lap. Our relationship on and off book had been strained ever since.

"That was just plain *embarrassing,*" said Bowden. "You were barely even trying."

I'd taken over from Carmine the second I got home, so I couldn't blame her. I should have let her just carry on — she was doing fine, after all, but . . . well, I needed the distraction.

"So we had a bit of wastage," I said. "It happens."

Reader "wastage" was something one had to get used to but never did. Most of the time it was simply that our book wasn't the reader's thing, which was borne with a philosophical shrug. We'd lost six readers at one hit once when my brother Joffy went AWOL and missed an entire chapter. It had never been more tempting to hit the Snooze Button. Mind you, in the annals of reader wastage, our six readers were peanuts. *Stig of the Dump* once lost seven hundred readers in the early seventies when Stig was kidnapped by *Homo erectus* fundamentalists, eager to push a promegalith agenda. Unusually, terms were agreed on with the kidnappers and a new megalith section was inserted into the book. It messed slightly with the whole dream/reality issue but never dented the popularity of the novel. On that occasion the Snooze Button *was* pressed, which accounts for the lack of a sequel. Kitten death — even *written* kitten death — carries a lot of stigma. Barney eventually handed over the reins to a replacement and works these days at Text Grand Central; Stig is now much in demand as an after-dinner nonspeaker.

"So what's up?" asked Bowden. "I've seen more dynamic performances in *Mystery on the Island.*"

I shrugged. "Things aren't going that well for me at the moment."

"Man trouble?"

"Of a sort."

"Do you want some advice?"

"Thank you, Bowden, I would."

"Get your ass into gear and act like a

mature character. You're making us the laughingstock of Speculative Fantasy. Our readership is in free fall. Want to go the way of *Raphael's Walrus*?"

It wasn't the sort of advice I was expecting.

"So you'd prefer the old Thursday, would you?" I replied indignantly. "The gratuitous sex and violence?"

"At least it got us read."

"Yes," I replied, "but by whom? We want the *quality* readers, not the prurient ones who —"

"You're a terrible snob, you know that?"

"I am not."

"You should value *all* readers. If you want to mix in the rarefied heights of 'quality readership,' then why don't you sod off to HumDram and do a Plot 9?"

"Because," I said, "I'm trying to do what the real Thursday wants."

"And where is she?" he asked with a sneer. "Not been down this way for ages. You keep on banging on about the greater glory of your illustrious namesake, but if she *really* cared for us, she'd drop in from time to time."

I fell silent. There was some truth in this. It had been six months since she'd visited, and then only because she wanted to borrow Mrs. Malaprop to put up some shelves.

"Listen," said Bowden, "you're nice enough in a scatty kind of way, but if you try to add any new scenarios, you'll just make trouble for us. If you're going to change anything, revert to the previous Thursday. It's within the purview of 'character interpretation.' And since she was once that way, there's a precedent. More readers and no risk. Who the hell is the Toast Marketing Board anyway?"

"It's a *secret* plan," I remarked defensively, "to improve readership. You're going to have to trust me. And while I'm in charge, we'll do it my way, thank you very much. I may even decide," I added daringly, "to add some more about the BookWorld in the stories. It would make it more realistic, and readers might find it amusing."

It was a bold statement. The CofG went to great expense to ensure that readers didn't find out about the inner workings of the BookWorld. I left Bowden looking shocked and opened a door in the Yorkshire Dales setting, then took a shortcut through the SpecOps Building to find myself back home. Carmine and Sprockett were waiting in the kitchen and sensed that something was wrong.

"I met Mr. and Mrs. Goblin," said Carmine, "and they seem very —"

"I'm really not that bothered, Carmine. You're taking over. I've added something about the Toast Marketing Board. It'll require line changes on these pages here and an extra scene."

I handed her the additional pages, and she looked at me with a quizzical expression. Making up scenes was utterly forbidden, and we both knew it.

"I'll take responsibility. Now, get on with it or I'll have Mrs. Malaprop stand in for me — she'd kill for some first-person time in her logbook."

Carmine said no more and hurried from the kitchen.

"I'm hungry," said Pickwick, waddling in from the living room.

"You know where the cupboard is."

"*What* did you say?"

"I said you know where the cupboard is."

Pickwick opened her eyes wide in shock. She wasn't used to being talked to that way. "Don't use that tone of voice with me, Miss Next!"

"Or else what?"

Pickwick waddled up and pecked me as hard as she could on the knee. It wasn't remotely painful, as a dodo's beak is quite blunt. If she'd been a woodpecker, I might have had more reason to complain. I held her beak shut with my finger and thumb and then leaned down so close that she went cross-eyed trying to look up at me.

"Listen here," I said, "try to peck me again and I'll lock you in the toolshed overnight. Understand?"

Pickwick nodded her beak, and I let go, and she very quietly sidled from the room. There was a mechanical cough from behind me. It was Sprockett, and his eyebrow pointer was indicating "Puzzled."

"How did the trip to the RealWorld go?" he asked.

"Not great."

"So I observe, ma'am."

I sat down at the kitchen table and ran my fingers through my hair.

"Perhaps if ma'am would like to change out of her work costume? I could run a bath — perhaps a long soak might help."

I looked down at the clothes I was wearing. It was classic Thursday: Levi's, boots and a shirt, faded leather jacket and a pistol in a shoulder holster. I felt more at home in these now than I felt in my Gypsy skirts and tie-dye top. In fact, I would be happy never to see a sandal again, much less wear one.

"You know," I said as Sprockett brought

me a cup of tea, "I thought it was odd in the BookWorld. Out in the RealWorld it's positively *insane.*"

"How was Landen?"

"Dangerously perfect."

I told him all that had happened. Of Jack Schitt being Adrian Dorset, of Goliath, the Toast Marketing Board and the contention from Jenny that Thursday couldn't be dead. I also told him my suspicions that I might actually be her, despite what Bradshaw had said and much evidence to the contrary.

"And then I lost a reader and got pissed off with Bowden, Carmine and Pickwick," I added.

"Any clues as to Miss Next's whereabouts?" asked Sprockett as he attempted to keep me on the task at hand.

"Only that Lyell is boring. How many Lyells are there in the BookWorld?"

Sprockett buzzed for a moment. "Seven thousand, give or take. None of them particularly boring — that's a trait generally attached to Geralds, Brians and Keiths — or at least, here in the BookWorld it is."

"Interviewing every Lyell would take too long. Friday and the peace talks are not getting any further away."

"Did you speak to the Jack Schitt here in the series?"

"First thing when I got back."

"And . . . ?"

"He knew nothing about Adrian Dorset or *Murders*. Didn't even know that Jack wasn't his real name."

"But it's a bit of a stretch, isn't it?" said Sprockett, his eyebrow pointer clicking down to "Thinking." "I mean, it can't be a coincidence. Jack Schitt's book being the accident book?"

"In the Outland there *are* coincidences. It's only in the BookWorld they're considered relevant. What about you? Come up with anything?"

"I went and spoke to TransGenre Taxis. To see if they were missing anyone."

"And?"

"They wouldn't give me any information. I think it was a mixture of corporate policy, laziness and overt coggism."

"Really?" I replied. "We'll see about that."

I went into the study, fetched a chair and pulled Thursday's shield from where it was still embedded in the ceiling. I turned the shiny badge over in my hand. It was encased in a soft leather wallet and was well worn with use. It could get me almost anywhere in the BookWorld, no questions asked.

"Why would the red-haired gentleman have given this to me?"

"Maybe he was asked to," said Sprockett. "Thursday has many friends, but there is only one person she knows she can truly trust."

"And who's that?"

"Herself."

"That's what the red-haired man told me," I said, suddenly realizing that recent events might have had some greater purpose behind them. "Something happened. Thursday must have left instructions for him to get out of his story, find me and ask me to help."

"Why didn't he say so directly?" asked Sprockett, not unreasonably.

"This is Fiction," I explained. "The exigency of drama requires events to be clouded in ambiguity." I placed Thursday's badge in my pocket.

"Is using the shield wise?" asked Sprockett. "The last time you used it, the Men in Plaid were onto us within the hour."

"It opens doors. And what's more, I don't *care* if the Men in Plaid arrive. We'll do as Thursday would do."

"And what would that be, ma'am?"

I opened the bureau drawer, retrieved my second-best pistol and emptied all the ammunition I had into my jacket pocket.

"We kick some butt, Sprockett."
"Very good, ma'am."

29.
TransGenre Taxis

The TransGenre Taxi service has been going for almost as long as the BookWorld has been self-aware, and has adapted to the remaking with barely a murmur. TGTs are clean, the drivers have an encyclopedic knowledge of the BookWorld that would put a librarian to shame, and they can be relied upon to bend the rules when required — for a fee. Traditionally, they rarely have change for a twenty.

Bradshaw's BookWorld Companion
(2nd edition)

The TransGenre Taxi head office was housed over in Nonfiction within the pages of the less-than-thrilling *World Taxi Review,* published bimonthly. But traveling all the way to Nonfiction would take a needlessly long time and would alert the Men in Plaid before we'd even gotten as far as Zoology. Luckily for us, there was a regional office located within *The First Men in the Moon,* located over in Sci-Fi/Classic. It was rumored that the propulsion system used by the taxis was based upon a modified Cavorite design, but this was pooh-poohed by Sci-Fi purists as "unworkable." Mind you, so was the "interior of a sphere" BookWorld, but that seemed to work fine, too.

The dispatch clerk was a small, deeply harassed individual with the look of someone who had unwisely conditioned his hair and then slept on it wet.

"No refunds!" he said as soon as we entered.

"I'm not after a refund."

"You wouldn't get one if you were. What can I do for you?"

"We're looking for a missing taxi. Took a fare from Vanity early yesterday morning."

The dispatch clerk was unfazed. "I'm afraid to say that company policy is quite strict on this matter, madam. You'll need a Jurisfiction warrant —"

"How's this?" I asked, slapping Thursday's shield on the counter.

The dispatch clerk stared at the badge for a moment, then picked up a clipboard from under the counter and started to flick through the pages. There were a lot of them.

"You're fortunate we still have them," he

said. "We file with Captain Phantastic in an hour."

He searched though them, chatting as he did so.

"We lose a couple of taxis every day to erasure, wastage, accidental reabsorption or simply to being used in books. For obvious reasons we're keen to hide the actual number of accidents for fear of frightening people from our cabs."

"Most thoughtful of you."

"You're in luck," he said, staring at his notes. "The only taxi missing that morning was Car 1517. Its last-known fare was a pickup from Sargasso Plaza, opposite the entrance to Fan Fiction."

"On Vanity Island?"

"Right. The driver departed Sargasso Plaza bound for the Ungenred Zone at 0823, and that was the last we heard."

"You didn't think about reporting it?"

"We usually wait a week. Besides, search parties are expensive."

"Do we have a passenger name?"

"Tuesday Laste."

Sprockett and I looked at each other. We seemed finally to be getting somewhere.

"And the name of the driver?"

"Gatsby."

"The Great Gatsby drives taxis in his

spare time?"

"No, his younger and less handsome and intelligent brother — the Mediocre Gatsby. He lives in Parody Valley over in Vanity. Here's his address."

We thanked him and left the office.

"Tuesday Laste?" repeated Sprockett as we hailed a cab.

"Almost certainly Thursday."

Sprockett's eyebrow pointer switched from "Puzzled" to "Bingo," paused for a moment and then switched to "Worried."

"Problems?" I asked as we climbed into the cab.

"In the shape of a Buick," replied Sprockett, indicating a Roadmaster that had just pulled up outside the TransGenre Taxi office. It was the Men in Plaid, and they were following the same trail we were. I leaned forward.

"Vanity Island," I said to the driver, "and step on it."

Vanity wasn't a place that conventionally published people liked to visit, as it was a bizarre mixture of the best and worst prose, where iambic pentameters of exceptional beauty rubbed shoulders with dialogue so spectacularly poor it could make one's ears bleed. We skimmed low across the narrow straits that separated Vanity from the mainland and circled the craggy island, past sprawling shantytowns of abandoned novellas, half-described castles and ragged descriptions of variable quality before coming to land in a small square just outside Parody Valley.

"You can wait for us," I said to the cabbie, who gave me a sarcastic, "Yeah, right," and left almost immediately, which made me regret I'd paid up front and tipped him.

We took a left turn into Cold Comfort Boulevard and made our way past unpublished pastiches and parodies of famous novels that were only on Vanity at all due to their being just within the law. If they had used the same character names from the parodied novel, they were removed to the copyright-tolerance haven of Fan Fiction. This was situated on a smaller island close by and joined to Vanity by a stone arched bridge a half mile long, and guarded by a game show host.

"How long before the Men in Plaid follow us here?" asked Sprockett.

"Five or ten minutes," I replied, and we quickened our pace.

Given that parodies — even unpublished ones — have a shelf life governed by the currency of the novel that is being parodied, the small subgenre was dominated by that year's favorites. We walked on, and once past the still-popular Tolkien pastiches we were in the unread Parody hinterland, based on books either out of print themselves or so far off the zeitgeist radar that they had little or no meaning. We took a left turn by *When Nine Bells Toll; Hello, My Lovely* and *I, Robert* before finding the book we were looking for: an outrageously unfunny Fitzgerald parody entitled *The Diamond as Big as the South Mimms Travelodge.*

Mediocre's apartment was above a set of garages. There was a brand-new taxi parked in an empty bay beneath, and we carefully climbed the rickety stairs. I knocked on the screen door, and after a few moments a woman of slovenly demeanor stood on the threshold gnawing a chicken drumstick. She wore heavy eyeliner that had run, and she looked as though she'd just had a fight with a hairbrush — and lost.

"Yes?" she asked in a lazy manner. "Can I help?"

I flashed Thursday's badge. "Thursday Next," I announced, "and this is my butler, Sprockett. Your name is . . . ?"

"Gatsby."

This was unexpected.

"The Mediocre Gatsby?"

"No, the *Loser* Gatsby, the youngest of

the three Gatsbys. I haven't seen Great for a while. How did it turn out with crazy Daisy? She looked like trouble to me."

"Not . . . *terrific,* as I recall."

"Did they let Mia Farrow play her in the movie?"

"I'm not sure. Is Mediocre here?"

"I've not seen the miserable fart for three days," she sniffed, picking her nose. "How did you know he was missing? I didn't call you."

"May we come in?"

"I guess," said Loser Gatsby with a shrug, and we walked into the apartment. Sprawled in the front room were a half dozen men and women who looked as though life had not been kind to them. One of the women had been crying recently, and two of the men still were.

"This is our Siblings of More Famous BookWorld Personalities self-help group," explained Loser. "That's Sharon Eyre, the younger and wholly disreputable sister of Jane; Roger Yossarian, the draft dodger and coward; Brian Heep, who despite admonishments from his family continues to wash daily; Rupert Bond, still a virgin and can't keep a secret; Tracy Capulet, who has slept her way round Verona twice; and Nancy Potter, who is . . . well, let's just say she's a term that is subject to several international trademark agreements."

"She's a Muggle?"

"Pretty much."

They all nodded a greeting.

"We meet twice daily to try to iron out the feelings of low self-worth we experience, given our more famous family members. It's quite hard, I assure you, being a nobody when an elder sister or brother is iconic for all time. Tracy Capulet was telling us what it was like living in Verona."

"It's 'Juliet this, Juliet that' all day long," said Tracy petulantly. "Juliet's on the balcony, Juliet's shagging a Montague, Juliet's pretending to be dead — blah, blah, blah. I tell you, I'm totally sick of it."

Sprockett moved to the window and peered out. The Men in Plaid would be here soon.

"This is a matter of some urgency," I said. "Does Mediocre have a room?"

Loser pointed to a door, and before she could explain that it was locked, Sprockett had wrenched it off its hinges.

The room was grubby and the floor scattered with discarded pizza containers and empty hyphen cans. The TV was still on and was tuned to a shopping channel, and his record collection contained *Hooked on Clas-*

sics and *Footloose.* Mediocre lived up to his name.

"What do you make of this?" asked Sprockett, who had come across a large model of the Forth Rail Bridge. It had large spans that in reality would have thrust boldly across the Forth Estuary, not just to connect two landmasses separated by a barrier that was also an arterial trade route but to demonstrate man's technological prowess in the face of natural obstacles.

"It's not a bridge," I whispered, "it's *metaphor.*"

We started opening boxes and found three more bridges, two rivers and a distant mountain range, swathed in mist with a road leading to unknown valleys beyond. Loser Gatsby was at the door, mouth open.

"Tell me," I said, "where did your brother get all this?"

"I don't know."

"Truthfully?"

"I'm a loser," she said. "If I'd known about this little lot, I would have sold it all, gone on a bender and had a dolphin tattooed on my left boob."

Her logic was impeccable. I questioned her further, but she knew nothing.

"In two minutes the Men in Plaid will be coming through that door," I told her.

"Believe me, you don't want to be here when they do."

I didn't need to say it twice, and she and the rest of the loser literary siblings made a hasty exit down the stairs.

"So," said Sprockett, staring at all the metaphor, "stolen?"

"Not if Mediocre was as his name suggests," I replied. "How much do you think this is all worth?"

"Twenty grand," said Sprockett. "People will pay good money to get hold of raw metaphor. There's enough here to keep a man comfortable for a long time."

"Or even enroll at character college," I said holding up a prospectus from St. Tabularasa's. "Looks like Mediocre was trying to better himself and shed his epithet. A cabbie couldn't earn this much in a decade of Octobers." I added, "I reckon we're looking at a bribe."

"To do what?"

"I don't know."

I picked up Mediocre's account book. It outlined all the trips he had done and which needed to be billed. The last day was not there, of course, but the previous day *was.*

"Well, well," I said, "looks like Thursday went on a trip to Biography the day before she vanished. And that's not all," I added.

"Every single fare Mediocre accepted was picked up from the same place — Sargasso Plaza, just outside the entrance to Fan Fiction. Coincidence?"

"We have company," murmured Sprockett, who'd been standing at the window.

I joined him and noted that a 1949 Buick Roadmaster had pulled up outside the building. Two Men in Plaid got out and looked around.

"Time we weren't here."

We crossed to the other side of the room and exited though the French windows, which opened onto a veranda. From there we climbed down onto the roof of a garden shed, then let ourselves out into an alley beyond. We walked back around the house and watched as the Plaids went into the building.

"What now, ma'am?"

I handed him a set of keys I'd found in Mediocre's room and nodded towards the brand-new taxi parked outside. "Can you drive one of those?"

"If it has wheels, I can drive it, ma'am. Are we heading for Biography?"

"We are."

"And what will we do when we get there?"

"Find out if Lyell is as boring as Thursday said he was."

30.
High Orbit

Sooner or later a resident of the Book-World will start to question what is *beyond* the internal sphere that we call home. Stated simply, what would happen if one burrowed directly downwards? In pursuit of an answer, noted explorer Arne Saknussemm entered a disused metaphor mine to see if a way through could be found. As this edition went to press, he has not yet returned.

Bradshaw's BookWorld Companion (3rd edition)

Sprockett reversed the cab out of the garage, engaged the Technobabble™ Swivelmatic vectored-ion plasma drive and powered vertically upwards from Parody Valley and Vanity. I was pressed back into my seat by the acceleration and the ascent angle, and I might have been frightened had my mind not been tumbling with what we'd discovered so far — or even with what we had still yet to find out. Within a few minutes, we were hanging in the heavens a couple of thousand feet from the surface, right at the cruising altitude of local books that were being moved around Fiction. Below us the islands that made up the Fiction Archipelago were laid out in precise detail.

"Would it be impertinent to point out that visiting another island in the BookWorld without transit papers is strictly forbidden?"

"What does Thursday Next care for transit papers?"

"I would politely point out that you're not her, ma'am."

"I might as well be. I have a shield and I look like her. Who can say I'm not?"

"Who indeed, ma'am?"

I looked behind us and out to sea. Biography was situated beyond Artistic Criticism, and it was unlikely that any books would be going that way at this lower level. I wound down the window, poked my head out and looked up. Several miles above us, I could see the high-level books crisscrossing the sky, their journey made less arduous by traveling at the precise altitude where the force of gravity from below cancels the force of gravity from above — the gravopause. At that height you could usually find someone going your way — so long as you could get up there. The Technobabble™ drive on the cab would get us to local traffic height, but after that we were on our own.

We had to wait a nail-biting two and three-quarters minutes, every second worrying that the Plaids would spot us.

"Buckle up, ma'am," said Sprockett. "Looks like someone's been discovered."

As we watched, an entire section of Vanity Island seemed to fall away. A book had been accepted into the mainstream and was rising from the flanks of Mount Sleeper, trailing the debris of a ramshackle group of shameless Zadie Smith rip-offs that had been unwisely built on top of it.

The settings — mostly of a winter scene in London, it appeared — rotated slowly about its axis as it rose vertically to meet us, and just as it transitioned into forward flight, Sprockett stepped on the throttle and accelerated to meet the book, which loomed as large as eight cathedrals in the windscreen. As soon as we were close enough, Sprockett slewed the vehicle to a stop on the side of a dream sequence — a picnic the family had once spent on a grassy hill in spring, where a silver pond alive with bulrushes lay within the dappled glade of beech trees.

"Congratulations on the publication," I said to a small boy who was playing with a tin train, and he waved shyly in return. We weren't there for long. Piggybacking around the BookWorld was a dark art that needed calm nerves and good timing; within a few minutes, Sprockett lifted off again and made the short hop to a historical novel that was moving up to join the High Stream in order to make its way to History for fact-checking. They looked less friendly in this book, so Sprockett simply fired one of the vehicle's two grapnels into the soft intratextual matrix to which the book's settings were bolted, and we began the tow into the high orbit dangling on the end of a slender length of steel cable.

"Okay," I said as we moved steadily upwards, the cab's altimeter winding around like a top, "how's this for a scenario? Thursday is investigating something that requires her to stay out of sight. She hides out in Vanity, somewhere near Sargasso Plaza. The Mediocre Gatsby always hangs out there, waiting for fares. He takes her to Biography and the following day picks her up to go to the Council of Genres. He piggybacks *The Murders on the Hareng Rouge,* which is heading — ISBN already scrubbed — towards the Ungenred Zone to be scrapped. Somewhere above Aviation the rhetorical device is activated. The book explodes into a zillion fragments within a fraction of a second, taking with it Thursday, Mediocre, and the TransGenre Taxi. It's just another book coming to grief that would be swiftly investigated, and then as swiftly dismissed as an accident."

"Barmouth Blaster?" asked Sprockett, offering me a cocktail.

"Thank you."

"So we were right — it wasn't an attack on the book at all," murmured Sprockett, adding the ice and lemon to the cocktail shaker along with half a can of Red Bull, a Mucinex and two onions. "It was a hit on the taxi — with Thursday Next inside. Which means that Mediocre must have been bribed to take the particular book —"

"But knew nothing of the reason. He was tricked into attending his own execution, as well as Thursday's."

We sat in silence for some minutes as we were towed ever upwards, thinking about what we had just uncovered. In the Real-World such a convoluted method of murder would be faintly ridiculous, but in the Book-World all murders happened this way.

"Your Barmouth Blaster, ma'am."

"Thank you."

"Ma'am?"

"Yes?"

"Why was Ms. Next murdered?"

There were at least seventy-two people who had tried to kill her over the years, and narrowing it down was going to be tricky. I decided to head for the most obvious.

"Without Thursday the Racy Novel peace talks might well fail. Who would benefit most from a genre war in the north of the island?"

"Men in Plaid," said Sprockett.

"Hardly likely," I replied. "They're probably mopping up for someone else — or simply want to find Thursday — or are just being wicked for the hell of it."

"You misunderstand me, madam," he said politely. "I mean Men in Plaid — *behind us!*"

I turned and looked out the cab's rear window. Sprockett was right. Far below was not one Buick Roadmaster but three. They would also have Technobabble™ Scramjamcious Gravitational Flux Throb-O-Tron Torque Converter drive systems and, knowing the Men in Plaid, ones considerably more advanced than ours and twice as nonsensical.

"How far to the gravopause?" I asked.

"We're almost there."

Despite the gravopause's usefulness for getting about, one had to be careful. If you had the misfortune to move *above* this altitude and had insufficient thrust to escape, you could be caught in the dead center of the sphere forever. There was a small moon in the gravitational dead spot made from accreted book traffic that had accidentally fallen in and been unable to escape. From the dizzying heights we had now reached, I could actually see the moon above us, no bigger than a pea.

Within a half minute more, we had reached the gravopause. Sprockett cast off the towline, and we drifted onwards, safely in orbit. All that was required now was to coast along until we were above Biography and then dip the cab into a downwards trajectory and let gravity take over.

"Ma'am, would you wind me up?" said Sprockett. "I can see fun and games ahead, and I wouldn't want to risk spring depletion at an inopportune moment."

I leaned forward and wound him until his indicator was just below the red line. I felt his bronze outer casing flex with the increased tension.

"The Men in Plaid are gaining," I said, looking behind us.

The three Roadmasters were in V formation about a half mile away and had just reached the gravopause. At the rate they were going, they would be upon us in under five minutes.

"I'm going to head for that cluster of book traffic," announced Sprockett, opening the throttle and accelerating towards a loose gaggle of several hundred books that all appeared to be heading in the same direction. As we drew closer, I could see that they were mostly nonfiction and of considerable size. It was the renegade Oversize Books section, on their way to their new home.

They grew dramatically in size as we approached, and as we passed between *John Deere Tractors* and *Clarice Cliff Tableware,* they towered over us like skyscrapers.

"Hold tight," said Sprockett, and he pulled the cab hard over and darted behind *Lighthouses of Maine.*

"They're still behind us!" I barked, peering out the rear windshield as the Monhegan Island Light Station flashed past on our left-hand side, foghorn blaring. "Or at least one is."

"They only attack one at a time," replied Sprockett, his eyebrow flicking past "Indignant" to "Peeved," "and in that respect they're very like baddies in seventies martial-arts movies. Hold tight."

Sprockett skimmed past *Best of National Geographic* so close I could taste the hot dust of the Serengeti, then pulled up sharply in front of *Chronicle of Britain.* I felt myself pressed hard into my seat. My vision grew gray, then faded out entirely. My arms and head felt intolerably heavy, and a second later I was unconscious as Sprockett — his body designed to tolerate up to 17.6 Gs — pulled the cab into an almost vertical climb. I came around again as soon as he reached the top of the book, and he immediately plunged the cab into a near-vertical dive.

"Still behind us?"

They were. I could see the emotionless features of the Plaids as they edged closer. Sprockett corkscrewed around *Knitting Toy Animals for Pleasure and Profit* as the passenger in the Roadmaster leaned out the window and fired a shot, which flew wide to blow a ragged hole in *Knitting Toy Animals* as we sped on, and a blue knitted giraffe named Natalie began a long, slow fall to the Text Sea, sixteen miles below.

"These Men in Plaid are made of stern stuff," said Sprockett, his eyebrow pointer clicking from "Peeved" to "Puzzled" to "Indignant," then almost to "Severely Peeved" before settling on "Peeved" again. "Hold tight."

The Oversized Books were now moving in a more random fashion as they tried to avoid us, and Sprockett dived to get more speed, then pulled up and headed towards where *What Do People Do All Day?* and *ABC with Dewin the Dog* were about to collide, cover to cover. There was barely a ten-foot gap on either side as we flew between them, and the gap narrowed as we moved on. I barely had a chance to wave a cheery hello to a worried-looking Lowly Worm as the covers closed together a split second before we shot out the other side. The Roadmaster was less fortunate, and there was a tremendous detonation as the car was crushed between the two books, the worried shouts of Scarry's folk mixing with Dewin the Dog's furious barking.

"Do you see the others, ma'am?" asked Sprockett as he swerved hard to miss the Greatest Oversize Book of All Time but the abrupt sideways movement caused a ventral compressor stall on the Technobabble™ drive, and we went spiraling downwards out of control until Sprockett achieved an emergency relight.

"On the left!" I yelled as the second Roadmaster swept past, a shot from an eraserhead removing half the rear bumper and a fender. Sprockett jinked hard, spiraled up

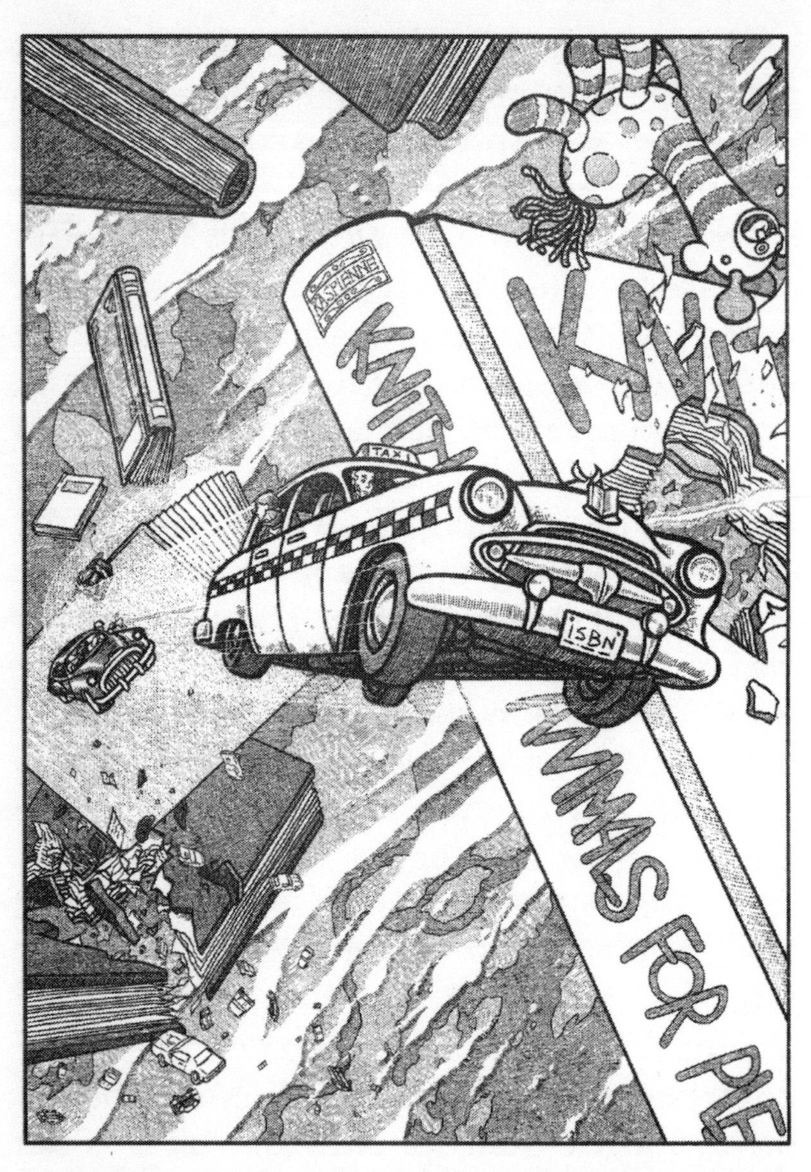

. . . the passenger in the Roadmaster fired a shot, which flew wide to blow a ragged hole in Knitting Toy Animals, and a blue knitted giraffe named Natalie began a long, slow fall to the Text Sea, sixteen miles below.

for a second, then shot past *Cooking for Fusspots* and *Helmut Newton Nudes.*

"Rewind me again, ma'am, if you please," said Sprockett, hauling sideways on the wheel to avoid the *Times Atlas.* The exertions on his frame had depleted his spring at a furious rate — I'd have to remain conscious, if only to rewind him.

"Watch out!"

It was too late. We had taken a hard left at *The Titanic Revisited* and were met by a group of Oversize Books that had bunched together tightly for self-protection. There was no time to avoid them and all we could see was a saber jet fragmenting in front of us as we loomed ever closer to *Lichtenstein Prints.* But just when I thought we were dead for sure, Sprocket pulled the wheel hard over and we entered *The Works of Thomas Gainsborough* through a small thermal-exhaust port near the preface.

I stared wide-eyed as Sprockett drove the cab through the paintings of Gainsborough at over a hundred miles per hour. We shot through early landscapes, dodged past *Cornard Wood* and then burst into portraiture at *John Plampin,* then twisted and turned past a dozen or so well-dressed dignitaries, who for their part looked as startled and horrified as we did. We went between the knees of Mr. Byam and at one point nearly knocked the hat off Mrs. Siddons. But still the Roadmaster stuck to us like glue, not able to fire at us with the constant movement but awaiting the opportunity with a certain calm detachment. We doubled back around *The Blue Boy* as Sprockett searched for the exit.

"Can you see a way out, ma'am?"

"There!" I said, having heard a lowing in the distance, "behind the third cow from the left in *The Watering Place.*"

We passed *The Harvest Wagon* for a second time as Sprockett lowered the nose and accelerated across the painted landscape, the Roadmaster still close behind. We turned sharp left as the Duchess of Devonshire loomed up in front of us, and there was a thump as we collided with something. The Roadmaster behind us had misjudged the turn and struck the duchess on the shins, the resulting explosion scattering metal fragments that hit the back of the cab with a metallic rattle.

In another second we were clear, none the worse for our rapid traverse aside from a brace of partridge that had jammed in the wipers and cracked the screen.

"What did they hit?" asked Sprockett.

"The Duchess of Devonshire — took off both legs."

"She'll be a half portrait from now on. Whoops."

The third Roadmaster had appeared in front of us, and another eraserhead had taken the "taxi" light off the roof and blasted a hole into *Classic Bedford Single-Deckers,* releasing several Plaxton-bodied coaches to tumble out into the void.

"We're causing too much damage," I said, catching sight of the now-chaotic movement of the Oversize Books, some of them on fire, others locked in collision and one, *Detroit's Muscle Cars,* falling to earth in a slow death spiral, the huge forces breaking apart the book and spilling 1972 Dodge Chargers across the BookWorld. "We need to leave the Oversize Books section."

"Logically, it places us in grave danger, ma'am."

"But we are endangering *others,* Sprockett."

"I place our chances of survival in open orbit at less than 1.7 percent, ma'am."

"Nevertheless," I said, "we are causing more destruction and death than we are worth."

His eyebrow pointer clicked to "Puzzled." "I do not understand."

"It's the right thing to do, Sprockett. Not for us but for *them.*"

"Is this *compassion,* ma'am? The following of the correct course irrespective of the outcome?"

The Duplex-5s were never great at this sort of stuff.

"You should always place others before yourself."

"Even if it means certain destruction?"

"Yes, Sprockett, that's *exactly* what it means."

He buzzed to himself for a moment in deep thought.

"Thank you for explaining it to me, ma'am," he replied. "I think I understand now."

He peeled away from the Oversize Books and headed off into clear air. The last Buick Roadmaster was close on our tail, and with no books to take cover behind, the end didn't seem far off. I pulled out my pistol and attempted to load it, but all the cartridges had spilled out of my pockets and into the foot well, and with Sprockett's constant bobbing and weaving they were proving almost impossible to pick up.

But just then the car stopped moving about and all was calm. I seized the opportunity to grab an armor-piercing round and flick it into my pistol.

"Sprockett?"

He wasn't moving. I thought at first he might have run down or been hit, but then I noticed that his eyebrow pointer was stuck firmly on "Thinking." He had committed his entire mainspring to his thought processes and had shut down all motor functions to enable him to think faster. When I looked at his spring-tension indicator, I could see it visibly moving — Sprockett was thinking, and thinking *hard.*

The Buick Roadmaster gained ground until it was no more than ten yards away. The Man in Plaid in the passenger seat leaned out the window, took careful aim and fired.

The eraserhead is one of a series of special-function cartridges that can be chambered within the large-caliber pistol common among BookWorld law enforcers. A long history of implausibly survivable bullet wounds in Thriller and Crime had rendered characters in the BookWorld invulnerable to small-caliber weapons, so the Textual Disrupter was designed to instantly break the bonds that hold graphemes together. A well-placed eraserhead can reduce anything in the BookWorld to nothing more than text — titanium, diamond,

Mrs. Malaprop's sponge cake — anything. The effective range in the pistol was limited to less than forty feet, but the shoulder-mounted, rocket-propelled eraserhead was effective up to a hundred yards, though highly inaccurate.

The eraserhead struck the back of the cab, and the entire trunk section, spare tire, bumper, jack and wheel brace burst into a cloud of individual letters, leaving only the rear part of the chassis and the back axle. One more shot and they would erase me and half of the cab. Two more shots and we would be nothing but a few thousand scrap letters, orbiting at the gravopause until nudged up to the moon or down to the BookWorld.

I fired my own pistol in reply, but the armor-piercing round simply passed through the Roadmaster's windshield and left-side rear door pillar, doing no lasting damage at all. I watched with detached fascination as the passenger reloaded, took aim and fired.

The cab dodged sideways, and the eraser-head flew wide.

"Sprockett?"

"I was thinking, ma'am. I was *calculating.*"

I noticed then with a sense of horror that we were climbing. We were moving *above* the gravopause.

"Sprockett," I said nervously, "if we get too high, we'll be pulled into the gravitational dead spot. We'll *never* get out."

"As I said, ma'am, I was calculating. Do as I instruct and there is an 18 percent probability that we will survive."

"Those aren't good odds."

"On the contrary, ma'am. Next to the 98.3 percent possibility of being erased, they're staggeringly good."

"They may not follow," I said, looking around.

"They're Men in Plaid," replied Sprockett, "and painfully dogged. They'll follow."

I watched the Roadmaster, and after pausing momentarily it was soon following our slow fall towards the moon. Although not gaining, it was certainly keeping pace.

"Do you have any armor-piercing rounds left, ma'am?"

I said that I did.

"Have them at hand, and use them only when I say."

The long fall towards the moon was conducted at a greatly increased velocity. I peered over Sprockett's shoulder and noted that the speedometer went only as fast as .5 Absurd, and we exceeded that speed within half a minute. The glass on the instrument shattered. The moon went from the size of a pea to an orange and to a soccer ball, and as we moved ever closer, I could see that the small moon was about a quarter of a mile in diameter and was indeed made of accreted junk — bits of books that had been nudged from the gravopause and lost. Pretty soon the moon was the biggest object in the sky, and just when we were less than five hundred feet from the surface, Sprockett rolled inverted and pulled the cab into a tight orbit. I felt a lurch as we accelerated rapidly, had time to see several people on the surface waving at us desperately, and then we were off and around and away again, flung out back towards the gravopause in a slingshot maneuver.

"Now we will see if my calculations are correct," murmured Sprockett, his eyebrow pointer clicking to "Doubtful", then "Apologetic," then back to "Doubtful" again before settling on "Worried."

I looked around. The Roadmaster was gaining, perhaps as a result of its greater mass, but we were still out of range of the eraserhead. We cannoned on, still at speeds in excess of Absurd, but all the while slowly decelerating. Sprockett had hoped we would be able to reach the gravopause again, but if he had miscalculated and we fell short by even a few feet, we would fall inexorably back towards the moon and end our days playing cribbage and I Spy with the unfortunate souls who were already there.

"Fire at the Roadmaster, ma'am."

"They're out of range."

"It doesn't matter."

So I did, and the shot missed by a mile, and Sprockett nodded and pointed towards a lone copy of *World Hotel Review* that was orbiting at the gravopause and thereby offering us a convenient yardstick of where safety lay.

I could feel ourselves slow down, and the needle from the shattered speedometer was now reading .25 Absurd and slowing by the second. *World Hotel Review* was less than half a mile away, and it seemed doubtful we would make it.

"Fire at them again."

So I reloaded and did as he asked, and at his insistence I continued to fire.

"Is there a point to this?" I asked after firing five times and managing only to clip a wing mirror.

"If we can make them angry and act irrationally, there is every point to it, ma'am. The cab has no power remaining. I am relying on our momentum to reach the gravopause."

I realized then what his calculations had been for, although I failed to see what we had gained, aside from twenty extra minutes, and a never-before-seen view of the moon. The Men in Plaid would simply wait until we were once more within range and then finish us off.

The gravopause was barely one hundred yards distant when they fired again. We were now moving at less than a fast walking pace and had drifted sideways. The last armor piercer I'd fired had sent us in a gentle end-over-end spinning motion, which, while not unpleasant, was certainly disconcerting.

The first eraserhead took away the front left side of the car and the second the back axle. I returned fire at Sprockett's request, and an odd sight we must have seemed, two helplessly drifting cars less than thirty feet apart, trading shots.

"I hope this was part of your plan, Sprockett. That was my last round, and I missed them again. I think my poor marksmanship has squandered our chances."

"*Au contraire,* ma'am. Every shot you fire pushes us farther towards the gravopause — and every shot they fire stops them from reaching it."

I frowned and stared out the window. The passenger in the Roadmaster pointed his weapon and fired straight at us, but the disrupting power of the eraserhead evaporated a few feet short of the battered cab in a sparkle of light. The Men in Plaid had acted irrationally, and as we drifted behind *World Hotel Review* and safety, the Roadmaster hung in space for a moment and then started to fall away in a slow trajectory that would eventually find it, a few weeks hence, adding permanently to the moon's mass.

I breathed a sigh of relief, rewound Sprockett — who had redlined without my realizing it — and sat back in my seat.

"Well done," I said. "You've just earned yourself an extra week's paid holiday."

"I seek only to serve," said Sprockett, his eyebrow clicking from "Nervous" to "Contented."

He fired the last remaining grapnel into the back of *World Hotel Review,* then hailed a distress signal, and we were taken on board.

"The name's Thursday Next," I said to the duty book officer, a frightfully dapper individual who was also manager of the Hotel Ukraina in Moscow, a place that we soon learned "offers a wide range of modern conveniences to suit both the business and leisure traveler."

"I'd like to use your book-to-Fiction footnoterphone link," I added, flashing Thursday's badge. "And after that I'll need to requisition a small family-run guesthouse in Ghent to take me all the way to Biography."

"Certainly," said the manager, eager to help someone he thought was a Jurisfiction agent in distress. "How about the Hotel Verhaegen? It provides elegant guest rooms in the heart of historic Ghent and offers contemporary style in an authentic eighteenth-century residence."

"It sounds perfect."

"This way."

As we made our way to the Belgium section of the book, we caught a glimpse of the Roadmaster, now a tiny speck in the distance.

31.
Biography

Although Outlander authors kill, maim, disfigure and eviscerate bookpeople on a regular basis, no author has ever been held to account, although lawyers are working on a test case to deal with serial offenders. The mechanism for transfictional jurisdiction has yet to be finalized, but when it is, some authors may have cause to regret their worst excesses.

Bradshaw's BookWorld Companion
(16th edition)

The Hotel Verhaegen landed on the lawn outside one of the biographical tenements. I sat for several moments in silence in the lobby. For some odd reason, my left leg wouldn't stop shaking, and when I tried to speak, it sounded like I was hyphenated. I'd been fine on the trip down, but as soon as I started to think about the Men in Plaid who'd tried so hard to kill us, I suddenly felt all hot and fearful. I thought for a moment it might have been a virus I'd picked up from the RealWorld until I realized I was in mild shock.

I rested for ten minutes, and after downing one of Sprockett's restoratives and writing *"Very nice"* in the guest book, I stepped from the Verhaegen, which lifted off behind us. The manager wasn't going to hang around — the Pay and Display fees in Biography were ridiculous.

"Sp-Sprockett," I said as we walked across the car park, "where d-d-did you learn to d-drive like that?"

"My cousin Malcolm, ma'am."

"He's a r-racing driver?"

"He's a racing *car.* Is madam all right?"

"Madam is surprised she didn't scream, vomit and then pass out. I owe you my life, Sprockett."

"A good butler," intoned Sprockett airily, "should save his employer's life at least once a day, if not more than once."

Luckily for us, the island of Biography had elected to maintain parts of the Great Library model during the remaking, so while the Geographic model gave it the appearance of a low-lying island mostly covered with well-kept gardens, exciting statuary and dignified pavilions of learning, the biographical subjects themselves lived in twenty-six large tower blocks, each designated by a single letter painted conveniently on the front. The lobby of the apartment building was roomy and bright and was connected to a game room, where D. H. Lawrence was playing H. P. Lovecraft at Ping-Pong, and also a cafeteria, where we could see Abraham Lincoln and Martin Luther discussing the struggles of faith over conscience. In the lobby were eight different Lindsay Lohans, all arguing over which biographical study had been the least correct.

Even before I'd reached the front desk, I knew we were in luck. The receptionist recognized me.

"Hello again, Miss Next," he said cheerfully. "How did the peace talks go?"

"They're not until Friday."

"How silly of me. You can go straight up. I'll ring ahead to announce you."

"Most kind," I replied, still unsure whom Thursday had seen. "Remind me again the floor?"

"Fourth," said the receptionist, and he turned to the telephone switchboard.

We took the brass-and-cast-iron elevator, which was of the same design as the one in the Great Library — the two buildings shared similar BookWorld architecture. Even the paint was peeling in the same places.

"How long do you think before the Men in Plaid catch up with us?" asked Sprockett as the elevator moved upwards.

"I have no idea," I replied, opening my pistol and chambering my last cartridge, a disrupter that was nicknamed "the Cherry Fondue," as it was always the last one in the box, and extremely nasty, "but the Hotel Verhaegen won't give them any clues — you signed the register as 'Mr. and Mrs. Dueffer,' yes?"

"Y-e-es," said Sprockett, his eyebrow pointer clicking to "Apologetic."

"Problems?"

"Indeed, ma'am. In an unthinking moment, I may have written 'choice of oils open to improvement' in the comments section of the visitor's book."

"We'll just have to hope they're not curious."

I replaced the weapon in my shoulder holster, and the lift doors opened on the fourth floor. We walked out and padded noiselessly down the corridor. We walked past Lysander, Lyons, Lyndsay, Lynch and Lynam before we got to the Lyells.

"Charles Lyell, Botanist," read the name

on the first door.

"Is botany boring?" Thursday asked.

"I suspect that it isn't, ma'am, given there is an entire island committed to little else."

The next door was for "Sir James Lyell, Politician."

"Boring, ma'am?" inquired Sprockett.

"Politicians' lives are never boring," I assured him, and we moved to the next.

" 'Sir Charles Lyell, Geologist,' " I read. "Is geology more or less boring than politics or botany?"

Sprockett's pointer flicked to "Bingo."

"I believe, ma'am, that as regards boring, geology is less to do with tediousness and more to do with . . . drilling."

"Genius," I remarked, mildly annoyed that I hadn't thought of it myself. Sir Charles Lyell was the father of modern geology. If Thursday had come to him, she was after the finest geological advice available in the BookWorld. I knocked on the door in a state of some excitement, and when I heard a shrill "Enter," we walked in.

The room was a spacious paneled study, the walls covered with bookcases and a large walnut desk in the center. It was not tidy; papers were strewn everywhere, and a chair was overturned. The pictures were crooked, and a plant pot lay on its side. The wall safe, usually hidden behind a painting of a rock, was open and empty.

A man of considerable presence was standing in the middle of the chaos. He had a high-domed head, white sideburns and somewhat small eyes that seemed to glisten slightly with inner thoughts of a distracting nature.

"Thursday?" he said when he saw me. "I have to confess I am not pleased."

"Oh?"

"Yes. You told me that my assignment with you would be of the utmost secrecy. Look at my study — ransacked!"

"Ah," I said, glancing around, "I am most dreadfully sorry, Sir Charles. This was done after we came back from . . . ?"

"An afterlifetime's work *ruined,*" he said in a much-aggrieved tone. "I am most displeased. Good Lord. Who is that mechanical man with the curiously emotive eyebrow?"

"My butler, Sir Charles. You have no objection?"

He stared at Sprockett curiously. "When I was alive, I pursued the advancement of scientific truth with all passion — I am afraid to say that I am at odds to explain Fiction, which often seems to have no basis in logic at all."

"Some enjoy it precisely for that reason."
"You may be right. Can he tidy?"
"We can both tidy, Sir Charles."
And we started to pick up the papers.
"It is most unfortunate," remarked Sir Charles, "after we had done all that work together. *Most* unfortunate."
I suddenly felt worried. "Our work together?"
"The report!" he muttered. "All the maps, notes, core samples, graphs, analysis — stolen!"
"Sir Charles," I said, "this might seem an odd request, but can you go over what was in the report?"
"Again?"
"Again."
He blinked owlishly at me. "Over tea, Miss Next. First we must . . . tidy."
"Sir Charles," I said in a more emphatic tone, "you must tell me what was in the report, and *now!*"
He frowned at me. "As you wish. All that metaphor —"
He didn't have time to finish his sentence. With a tremendous crash, the door was pushed off its hinges, and two Men in Plaid entered. From door to death was scarcely less than fifteen seconds, and much happened. Sprockett was between us and the

MiP, and he valiantly made a lunge for the intruders. The first Plaid was quicker and before we knew it had popped Sprockett's inspection panel and pressed his emergency spring release. In an instant the butler fell lifeless. Before Sprockett hit the floor, the Plaid had advanced, knocked my pistol from my grasp and pushed me sideways. As I lay sprawling, the second Man in Plaid picked up Sir Charles and threw him bodily out the window, while the first Plaid moved towards me, his expressionless eyes boring into mine like a pair of gimlets. We'd just killed six of their compatriots; I didn't think there was much room for negotiation.

I quickly scrambled across the floor and was grabbed by my foot. I wriggled out of my boot, and it was this, I think, that saved us. The Man in Plaid was put off balance and gave me the split second I needed to find my pistol. Without hesitation I turned and fired. There was a *whompa* noise, and the air wobbled as the Cherry Fondue hit home. With an agonizing scream of pain, the Man in Plaid exploded into not graphemes but the infinitely more painful *words,* many of which embedded themselves into the woodwork like shards of glass. The blast caught the second Man in Plaid and cut him in two. He fell to the floor with a heavy thump, the lower half of him spilling cogs, springs and brass actuating rods onto the floor.

"You're robotic?" I said, moving closer. The Man in Plaid was moving his arms in a feeble manner, and his eyes followed me as I approached. He was still functioning, but it was clear he was damaged well beyond economic repair. He looked as though he was out of warranty, too.

"You are impressive, Miss Next," he managed to say. "A worthy adversary."

"Who sent you?"

"I don't answer questions. I ask them."

I noticed I was shaking. I retrieved my boot and walked to the broken window. Lying on the grass four stories below was Sir Charles. The heavy impact had caused the binding matrix of his body to become fused to the ground, and he was beginning to merge with the lawn. I could see several people staring up and pointing, first at me and then at the remains of Sir Charles. We didn't have long before someone called Jurisfaction. Lyell could be rewritten, but these things take time and money, and Biography's budget was tighter than ours.

Sprockett was lying flat on his face in an undignified manner, and I quickly rewound him. As soon as his gyros, thought cogs and speech diaphragm were back to speed, he sat up.

"I've had the most peculiar dream," he told me, his eyebrow clicking through each emotion in turn and then back again, "about being caught by my mother oiling a Mark III Ford Capri in an 'inappropriate' manner."

"I didn't know you had a mother."

"I don't — that's what was so peculiar."

"See what you can get out of him," I said, pointing to the damaged Man in Plaid. "I'm going to have a look around."

I didn't waste any time and hunted through the remains of Lyell's study to see what — if anything — had been left behind. The short answer was not much, until I went through the wastepaper basket and came across a pencil sketch of Racy Novel with WomFic on one side and Dogma on the other. A rough outline of the geology had been sketched in, and for the most part the strata were more or less identical beneath all the genres, except for a shaded patch the shape of a tailless salmon that seemed to be mostly beneath Racy Novel. I returned to where Sprockett had been talking with the badly damaged Plaid.

"He's a Duplex-6," said Sprockett with a sense of deep respect. "I was wondering why they managed to stay on our tail so easily during the Oversize Books section."

"Who is he working for?"

"He won't tell us, but it's of no matter — the Duplex automaton's memories are recorded on punched tape. We can have it read."

"So remove his tape and let's get out of here."

In reply the Duplex-6 took a large brass key from his jacket pocket and inserted it into the socket in the base of his neck. We could see he was almost run down, and before we could stop him, he had started to turn the key.

"Good Lord," said Sprockett. "The Duplex-6 has a self-wind capability."

Sprockett tried to stop the damaged Man in Plaid from winding himself up, but the 6's superior strength was too much, and we watched with increased hopelessness as the Plaid's tension indicator neared the red line.

"We're leaving," said Sprockett, and without waiting for a reply he took me by the hand and we ran to the bathroom window and out the fire escape at the back of the building.

We were two flights down when the Duplex-6's mainspring finally ruptured in an almighty outburst of stored mechanical energy. There was a loud *twuuung* noise, and the shattered remains of the Man in Plaid erupted out the windows of Lyell's apartment. We were showered with minute cogs, sprockets, bevel gears, and dogs, chains, pushrods and actuators.

"A self-winding capability," said Sprockett, who was obviously deeply impressed. "I wonder if they would retrofit that feature for us Duplex-5s?"

32.
Homecoming

Islands to Visit #124: Photography. This beautifully expressive and lyrical island has been divided between Black-and-White and Color for many years, and the two factions are almost constantly at war, an event that is itself documented by resident war photographers. The recording of the war recording is also recorded, with Martin Parr photographing the ears and neckties of those who are recording the people who are recording the people recording the events.

Bradshaw's BookWorld Companion
(5th edition)

We dodged Jurisfaction officers for two hours and eventually negotiated a ride home aboard a copy of the recently discredited *President Formby War Diaries,* which was on a one-way trip to Historical Counterfactuals.

"May I be so bold," said Sprockett once we had landed and were on the train heading back towards Fantasy and home, "as to inquire about our next move?"

"Placating an angry Carmine, I should imagine — I've been away a lot these past few days. After that we'll have to recover anything Horace has stolen again, put up with petulant huffing and tutting from Pickwick — and my dopey father will be complaining about something, I shouldn't wonder."

"I was referring to Racy Novel, ma'am. Should you call Commander Bradshaw again?"

I'd asked myself the same question on the way back from Biography. I'd spoken to him briefly while on board the *World Hotel Review.* He had expressed surprise and alarm about the Men in Plaid and had also checked out Mediocre's address and reported back to us no sign of metaphor — in bridges or otherwise. Unwisely, I had told him we were going on to Biography, and now I didn't know if I could trust him or not.

"He might have tipped off the Men in Plaid," I said after airing my thoughts, "or he simply might be having his footnoterphone messages read in transit."

It wasn't hard, apparently. All you needed do was to sit in the footnoterphone ducts and read the messages as they flitted past.

"Even if he is on the level," I added, "it's not like we have any answers or evidence — just a geologist out to grass and a rough sketch of the strata beneath the northern part of Fiction."

Sprockett nodded agreement.

"But," I added, "we know that Thursday would have been working to avert war at the peace talks. If she *was* silenced, the attacks by the Men in Plaid would seem to implicate the Council of Genres, but the CofG want to avoid a war, not start one. It was Senator Jobsworth *himself* who wanted me to go to the peace talks tomorrow. The only person we know who seems to actually welcome war is Speedy Muffler."

"Would he have access to Duplex-6 automatons that could be made to look like Men in Plaid?" asked Sprockett.

"Duplex will sell to anyone with the cash, but the Council's strict sales embargoes are hard to circumvent. Not impossible, but hard."

"What about Red Herring, ma'am?"

"I'm not sure. Is Red Herring a red herring? Or is it the fact that we're meant to *think* Red Herring is a red herring that is actually the red herring?"

"Or perhaps the fact you're meant to think Red Herring *isn't* a red herring is what makes Red Herring a red herring after all."

"We're talking serious metaherrings here. Oh, crap, I'm lost again. Who's talking now?"

"It's you," said Sprockett.

"Right."

"Whatever is going on," I said, "it's big. *Really* big. If it's big enough to risk killing Thursday Next, destroying a book and subverting the Men in Plaid from their usual duties of frightening the citizenry to the more specific duty of frightening *individual* citizens, then there is no limit to what they might do. We need to keep our eyes open at all times."

We took a cab from Le Guin Central and, deep in thought, walked up to the house. I had my hand on the butt of my pistol, just in case. I needn't have worried. Men in Plaid were never seen without their Buick Roadmasters, and the driveway was empty. I opened the front door and found a dozen members of the cast sitting around the kitchen table.

"Hello," I said, somewhat surprised. "Have we got a cast meeting scheduled for this evening?"

"We have now," replied Carmine.

My eyes flicked from face to face, and they seemed very serious. Most of the major players were there — my father, Bowden, Hades, Jack Schitt, Braxton, Rochester, Paige Turner, Joffy, Stig, Victor Analogy, my mother and even Bertha Rochester, although she had been put in a straitjacket in the event she tried to bite anyone.

"What's going on?"

"You've been acting a bit irresponsibly recently," said Carmine, "running around the BookWorld, pretending to be her. You've been neglecting your duties. I've been covering for you far more than is written in my contract, and only yesterday you were shouting at us all."

"I've had things on my mind," I replied by way of excuse, "*important* things."

"So *you* say. To the casual outside observer, you're simply getting delusions of adequacy. Play a strong character for too long and it tends to have an unhinging effect."

"And today," said Bowden in an annoying "I told you so" sort of voice, "you were threatening to tell the Outland all about the BookWorld. There's a good reason the real Thursday never put that part of the story in her books, you know."

"I admit I might have gone too far on that point," I conceded, but I could see they didn't believe me.

"None of us are happy," said my father, "and we feel you might be leading the series into disrepute. If the book gets punished for your transgressions, then every one of us has to suffer. Punish one, punish all. You know how it works."

I did, far too well. To keep books in line, the entire cast is often disciplined for the misdeeds of one. It generated a certain degree of conformity within the cast — and a lot of ill feeling.

"So what are you saying?" I asked.

My father nudged Bowden, who nudged Victor, who nudged Acheron Hades.

"We're saying," said Hades slowly, "that we might need to make some . . . *changes.*"

"Changes? What sorts of changes?"

"Changes in leadership."

"You want to have me fired? You can't do that."

"In point of fact," piped up Pickwick, "we can. Article 218 of the Textual Code states, 'If the nominated leader of a book acts in an unlawful or reckless manner that might affect the smooth operation of a book, he or she can be removed by a simple show of hands.' "

There was a deathly hush as they waited to see what I would say.

"The series is operating smoothly. It will be hard to prove recklessness on my part."

"We don't need to," replied Carmine. "We need only prove unlawfulness."

"And how would you do that?"

"The Toast Marketing Board subplot. *Totally* illegal. You wrote out the new pages in your own handwriting."

"Listen," I said, changing my tone to one of conciliation, "we have an average weekly ReadRate of 3.7 at present — remaindered, out of print and, technically speaking, unread. You need my leadership to try to turn this series around. If you want to negotiate, we can negotiate — everything's on the table. So let's talk. Who's for tea?"

They all stared at me in a stony-faced manner, and I suddenly felt that things were a lot worse than I'd thought. There had been grumblings before, but nothing like this.

"Well, then," I said, my temper rising, "who's going to lead the book? Carmine?"

"I can handle it."

"You can handle it *now.* What if the ReadRate goes above forty? How screwed will you be then?"

"There is no need to be unkind," said my father. "With our support she'll manage. At least she doesn't spend her days gallivanting around the BookWorld on arguably pointless quests for a namesake who doesn't even like her."

That hurt.

"Well," I replied in a sarcastic tone, "how does consorting with a goblin fare on the 'bringing the book into disrepute' stakes?"

"You can talk," retorted Carmine. "*Your* intended boyfriend set fire to a busload of nuns."

"And puppies," said Pickwick.

"*Orphaned* puppies," added Rochester, dabbing his eyes with a handkerchief.

"Besides," said Carmine, "Horace and I have agreed to a trial separation."

"I think we've all said quite enough," announced Bowden haughtily. "All in favor of replacing Thursday with Carmine, raise a hand."

They all raised a hand except Stig, who I know liked me, Bertha Rochester who was in a straitjacket, and Pickwick.

"Thank you, Pickwick," I said. "Nice to know some friends haven't abandoned me."

"Are we voting now?" asked Pickwick, waking with a start. "I'm in."

And she put a wing in the air.

"All right, you bunch of disloyal ingrates," I said, taking the Snooze Button's access codes and the key to the core containment from around my neck, "have the job. Who cajoled you all when you thought you were rubbish? Who made sure we rehearsed the whole way through the six weeks we were unread last winter?"

Victor looked at the ceiling, and Pickwick stared at her foot. They all knew I'd been holding things together for a while. The previous written Thursday had left the series in a terrible state. Everyone arguing with everyone else, and with a humor deficit that I had only just managed to plug.

"And a fat lot of good it did us," replied Carmine angrily. "We're the laughingstock of Speculative Fantasy."

"We're still being read. Do you know what to do if there is a flameout on the e-book throughput intensifiers?"

Carmine's blank look told me she didn't.

"Or if the metaphor depletes midscene? What about the irony injectors? How often should they be cleaned? Do you even *know* what an adjectivore looks like or what happens if you get Martha Stewarts behind the wainscoting?"

"Hey," said Horace, who had been sitting unnoticed on the top of the bureau, "why don't you go do a Plot 9 on yourself? We can muddle through. With less than twenty active readers, we've certainly got enough time."

"We?" I demanded. "Since when were you anything to do with this series?"

"Since Carmine asked me."

"He has some very good ideas," said Carmine. "Even Pickwick thinks they're quite good. Isn't that so, Pickers?"

"Sort of," said Pickwick, looking the other way huffily.

"We'd better get on," said Hades in a pointed fashion. "We've got some readings to attend to."

"Right," I said, lips pursed as I tried to control my temper, "I'll let you get on with it."

And without another word, I strode out of the house with as much dignity as I could muster. As soon as I was outside, I sat on the garden wall, my heart beating fast, taking short gasps of air. I looked back at the series. It was a jagged collection of settings — the towers of Thornfield Hall set among the floodlights of the Swindon croquet field and the Penderyn Hotel. There were a few airships, too, but only one-tenth scale. It was all I'd ever known. It had seemed like *home.*

"You should look on the bright side, ma'am," said Sprockett, handing me a Chicago Fizz he had conjured up seemingly from nowhere.

"There *is* a bright side? No book, no home, no one to believe in me and no real idea what became of Thursday — or what the hell's going on. And in addition I'd *really* like to punch Horace."

"Punching goblins," replied Sprockett soothingly, "while offering short-term relief, has no long-term beneficial value."

I sighed. "You're right."

"By referring to the 'bright side,' ma'am, I merely meant that the recent upset simply frees your schedule for more pressing matters. You have larger fish to fry over the next couple of days."

I stood up. Sprockett was right. To hell with the series — for the moment at least.

"So where do you suggest we go now?"

"Back to Vanity."

33.
The League of Cogmen

There are two languages peculiar to the BookWorld of which a vague understanding will help the enthusiastic tourist. **Courier Bold** is the traditional language of those in the support industries, such as within the Well of Lost Plots, and Lorem Ipsum is the gutter slang of the underworld — useful to have a few phrases in case you get into trouble in Horror or Noir.

Bradshaw's BookWorld Companion
(1st edition)

Sprockett, I learned, lived in the Fantasy section of Vanity, not far from Parody Valley. I was more at leisure to look about upon this, my second visit, and I noticed that whereas in Fiction the landscape was well maintained, relatively open and with good infrastructure, years of self-publishing into the same geographic area meant that Vanity was untidy, chaotic and overcrowded.

The resident novels with their settings, props and characters now occupied every spare corner of the island and had accreted on top of one another like alluvial deposits. Grand towers of imaginative speculation had arisen from the bare rock, and the island was honeycombed with passageways, tunnels and shafts to provide access to the scenes and settings now buried far below the surface. In some places the books were so close that boundaries became blurred — a tiger hunt in 1920s Bengal merged seamlessly with the TT races on the Isle of Man, a western with the 1983 Tour de France. Space in Vanity was limited.

"Don't let on you're published," remarked Sprockett as we arrived at his book, a badly worn tome cemented into a cliff face of similar books and supported on slender stilts that were anchored to the rock below. He needn't have — I knew the score. Vanity's beef with the rest of Fiction was long-lived and not without some degree of justification.

I wiped my feet on the doormat as we entered and noted that the novel was set mostly in the manor house that belonged to Professor Winterhope, Sprockett's creator, and was populated by a large and mildly eccentric family of mechanical men, none of whom looked as though they had been serviced for years.

"Welcome to *The League of Cogmen,*" said Mrs. Winterhope once the professor had taken Sprockett off for an oil change and general service. "Would you like some tea?"

I told her I would, and we walked into the front room, which was like my kitchen back home, a command center and meeting place all in one. Mrs. Winterhope introduced me to the Cogmen, who had been wound sufficiently to converse but were under strict orders not to move, so as not to wear themselves out — quite literally, as they had a limited stock of spare parts. Despite these obvious drawbacks, they still expressed the languorous attitude of the long-unread. It didn't look as though they rehearsed much either, which was a lamentable lapse in professionalism, although I wasn't going to say so.

"We must thank you for rescuing Sprocky from that rabble in Conspiracy," said Mrs. Winterhope, putting an empty kettle onto a cold stove. "And we were delighted to hear he was employed by Thursday Next — even if not the real one."

"You're very kind."

"Has our Sprockett been serving you well?"

"He has been beyond exemplary," I told her. "A gentleman's gentleman."

"Excellent," she replied. "I can count on you to give good references?"

"I cannot see a scenario where I would let him go," I said with a smile. "He is utterly admirable in every respect."

But Mrs. Winterhope wasn't smiling.

"I understand," she said slowly, "that you have recently found yourself in diminished circumstances?"

This was true, of course. I had almost nothing except Sprockett and the clothes I was wearing.

"At present yes, that is true," I admitted somewhat sheepishly.

Mrs. Winterhope poured the contents of the empty kettle into a teapot that I noted contained no tea.

"Sprockett is the most advanced automaton we possess," she continued, "and whilst not wishing to be indelicate in these matters, I cannot help thinking that his career may not be well serviced by someone who finds herself — I'm sorry to be blunt — in a position of . . . *unreadness.*"

She stared at me with a kind yet desperate expression and handed me an empty cup.

"Would you like no milk?"

"Yes thank you," I said, not wishing to

embarrass her. Not a single reader in over seventeen years had graced the Winter-hopes' pages, so the reader stipend was unavailable to them, and they had, quite literally, nothing. The only possible avenue to a better life was through the one character who might conceivably find a placement in the world of wider readership. Four days ago I'd been a potential help; now I was a millstone. I knew what I had to do.

"Yes," I said to Mrs. Winterhope, "I understand."

She nodded politely and patted me on the arm. "Will you stay with us tonight?" she asked. "We have absolutely nothing, but we would be happy to share it with you."

I told her I would be honored to share in their nothing, then excused myself to go for a walk.

I left the novel and wandered down through the narrow streets to where the Tennyson Boardwalk ran alongside the beach. The walk was full of evening strollers and traders, mostly selling book-clearance salvage from those novels that had been recently scrapped. I stopped to lean on the decorative cast-iron railings and absently watched the Text Sea lap against the foreshore, the jumbled collection of letters heaving and mixing in the swell. Every now and then, a chance encounter would construct a word, and the constituent parts glowed with the joyous harmony of word construction. Farther down, some kids were fishing these new words from the sea with hooked sticks. Three-letter constructions were thrown back to potentially grow larger, but longer ones were pulled ashore for possible sale. While I stood there watching, they caught a "theodolite," a "linoleum" and a "pumpkin," although truth to tell the "pumpkin" was actually a "pump" and a "kin" that were tickled together after being pulled from the Text Sea.

I couldn't help feeling a bit sorry for myself. I had no job, no book, no friends and no immediate prospects. The man I loved was real and wholly unavailable, the deputy man I loved was a mass murderer. More important, I was no nearer to who had killed Thursday, nor to what Sir Charles Lyell had discovered about Racy Novel that was so potentially devastating that it was worth murdering him, Thursday and Mediocre for. The truth was this: I wasn't up to scratch. I'd been trying too hard to be her, and I had failed.

I thought of Whitby, then of Landen, and what he had said about my actually *being*

Thursday and not knowing it. I wasn't in agreement with him over that one, and when I'd vanished in front of his eyes, he would have known that, too. I thought for a minute as I considered putting myself in Landen's shoes. He might try to get in touch with me — after all, we both wanted Thursday back. The question was this: If I wanted to contact someone in the Book-World, how would I go about it?

The Mediocre Gatsby had picked Thursday up in Sargasso Plaza, a stone's throw from where I was now, right on the south-east tip of Vanity. She was likely to have been hiding close by, somewhere she would have been off the Council of Genres' radar — somewhere even the Men in Plaid would fear to tread. And there it was, staring at me across the the bay — Fan Fiction. Where better to hide a Thursday than in a bunch of that? The small island was lit up by thousands of lightbulbs strung from trees and lampposts. It was a busy place, that much I knew, and given that Vanity had been unfairly shunned by the rest of Fiction, the fact that Fan Fiction was isolated still further gave one an idea how poorly it was regarded.

I walked to the entrance of the narrow causeway and approached the two game-show hosts who were guarding the entrance. One was sitting on a high stool and dressed in a gold lamé suit, while the other was holding a hunting rifle.

"Hello, Thursday!" said the first host, beaming happily at me with a set of teeth so perfectly white that I had to blink in the glare. "Back to win further prizes?"

It was Julian Sparkle of *Puzzlemania.* We had met a few years back when the real Thursday was attempting to train me up for Jurisfiction. He was what we called an "anecdotal," someone who lived in the oral tradition, ready to leap to the Outland when puzzles and brain teasers were related — usually during boring car journeys or in pubs. The last time we'd met, I would almost certainly have been eaten by a tiger if not for Thursday's brilliant intervention.

"I was actually thinking of visiting Fan Fiction," I replied.

"No problem," said Julian in his singsong voice. "Anyone can go in — but no one can come out."

As if to bring home the point, the second game-show host showed me the hunting rifle.

"Unless," said Julian Sparkle, "you want to play *Puzzlemania*?"

"What do I win?"

"A set of steak knives."

"And if I lose?"

"We destroy you with a high-powered eraserhead."

"Fair enough," I replied. "I'm in."

Sparkle smiled warmly, and I stepped to a mark on the floor that he indicated. As I did so, the lights seemed to dim, except for a bright spotlight on the two of us. There was a short blast of applause, seemingly from nowhere.

"So, Thursday Next, today we're going to play . . . 'Escape Across the Bridge.' "

He indicated the long, narrow causeway.

"It's very simple. We erase anyone we see walking towards us across the causeway. There is no way to go round the causeway, and you'll be dissolved in the Text Sea if you try to swim."

"And?"

"That's it. We check the bridge every half minute, and it takes four minutes to run across."

As if to accentuate the point, the second host noticed someone trying to sneak across as we were talking. He shouldered the rifle and fired. The unfortunate escapee exploded in a chrysanthemum of text, which was quickly snapped up by the gulls.

"Ha-ha!" said the host, reloading the rifle.

"Bagged another Baggins."

And he made a mark on his tally board, which contained several hundred other Bagginses, three dozen Gandalfs, a plethora of Pratchett characters and sixty-seven Harry Potters.

"Right, then," said Sparkle, "off you toddle."

"Don't you want the answer?"

He smiled in an oddly unpleasant way. "You can figure it out for the return journey."

I walked across the causeway with a curiously heavy heart, as I had no idea how to get back, but once I arrived on the other side, it seemed a party was in full swing. Everyone was chatting to everyone else, and the mildly depressed feeling I had felt over in Vanity seemed to vanish completely.

"What's the party about?" I asked a Hobbit who had thrust a drink into my hand.

"Where *have* you been?" she said with a smile. "Fan Fiction isn't copying — it's a *celebration.* One long party, from the first capital letter to the last period!"

"I never thought of that."

"Few do — especially the authors who should really accept the praise with better grace. They're a bunch of pompous fatheads, really — no slur intended. Nice clothes, by the way."

"Thank you."

And she wandered off.

"Thursday?"

I turned to find myself staring at . . . well, *myself.* I knew she wasn't me or the real Thursday because she seemed somewhat narrow. In fact, now that I looked around, most people here were similar to real characters but of varying thickness. Some were barely flatter than normal, while others were so lacking in depth that they appeared only as an animated sheet of cardboard.

"Why is everyone so flat?" I asked.

"It's a natural consequence of being borrowed from somewhere else," explained the Thursday, who was, I noted, less than half an inch thick but apparently normal in every other way. "It doesn't make us any less real or lacking in quality. But being written by someone who might not *quite* understand the subconscious nuance of the character leaves us in varying degrees of flatness."

This made sense. I'd never really thought about it before, but it explained why the Edward Rochester and indeed *all* the borrowed characters in my series were of varying degrees of depth. Some weren't that bad, but others, like Jane Eyre herself, were thin enough to be slipped under the door and could sleep rolled up and slipped into a drainpipe.

"How's all that cloak-and-dagger stuff going?" asked Flat Thursday.

It seemed she thought I was the real one, and I wasn't going to deny it.

"It's going so-so," I said. "How much did I tell you?"

She laughed. "You never tell us anything. Landen sent another message, by the way."

"That's good," I replied, attempting to hide my enthusiasm. "Lead on."

Thursday turned, and as she did so, she almost vanished as I saw her edge on. I wondered whether perhaps Agent Square might *not* be a Flatlander as he claimed, but a hyperfiction cube or something.

"We all think Landen's totally Mr. Dreamcake," said Flat Thursday as we walked past a reinterpretation of Middle Earth that was every bit as good as the real one, only flatter, "but he won't speak to anyone except the real one."

We walked down Thursday Street, and everything started to look vaguely familiar. The characters and settings were sort of similar, but the situations were not. The combinations were unusual, too, and although I had not personally supposed that Thursday might battle the Daleks with Dr.

Who in a literary landscape, in here it was very much business as usual.

"He's in there," said Thursday, and she ushered me into a large, square room with a stripped pine floor, a thin skirting board and empty walls painted in magnolia. In the middle of the room was Landen, and he smiled as I walked in. But it wasn't actually him; it was just a *feeling* of him.

"Hello, Landen."

"Hello, Thursday. I needed to speak to you."

"What about?"

"I'm sorry," he said apologetically, "my answers are limited."

I stared at him for a moment. Flat Thursday had said this was *another* message, so he must be communicating on a one-way basis by writing a short story — possibly with himself and his wife in conversation.

"Which Thursday do you want to talk to?" I asked.

"The written Thursday."

So far, so good. "Do you *now* believe I'm from the BookWorld?"

"You vanished as I was about to kiss you. Thursday never did that. I'm sorry I doubted you."

"Do you know what the real Thursday was doing with Sir Charles Lyell?"

"I'm sorry," he said, "my answers are limited."

"Do you know who was trying to kill Thursday?"

"The Men in Plaid have tried to murder her on numerous occasions. At the last count, she had killed six of them. She doesn't know who orders them to do it, or why."

This was good news. Between Thursday and Sprockett and me, we'd taken out fourteen Plaids.

"Where is she now? Do you know?"

"I'm sorry," he said, "my answers are limited."

"Why did she ask the red-headed man to give me her badge?"

"She didn't — *I did.* As soon as she was out of touch for over five days, I contacted Kiki."

"Why did she ask *me* to help her?"

"She'd hoped you had evolved into something more closely resembling her. The only person she knew she could truly trust was . . . herself."

This sounded encouraging. "Can I trust Bradshaw?"

"I'm sorry," he said, "my answers are limited."

"Is there anything else I should know?"

"She told me that she would try to contact you. She said the circumstances of your confusion will be your path to enlightenment."

"What did she mean by that?"

"I'm sorry," he said, "I have no more answers for you. I won't know if you even got these. Good luck, Thursday."

He stopped talking and just stood there blinking, awaiting any possible response from me.

"Listen," I said, lowering my voice and looking around to make sure that Flat Thursday wasn't listening, "did you write in a kiss, just to make up for the one I missed earlier?"

"Good luck, Thursday," he said again. "I'm in a hurry, as I told your mother I'd help her with the Daphne Farquitt Readathon. Remember: *The circumstances of your confusion will be your path to enlightenment.* Four pounds of carrots, one medium cabbage, four-pack tin of beans, Moggilicious for Pickwick, pick up dry cleaning, toilet paper."

I was confused until I realized that he had probably written the short story on the back of a shopping list. I watched and listened while he went through "Tonic water, snacks and the latest Wayne Skunk album, *Lick the*

Toad" before he stopped, smiled again and then just stood there blinking in a state of rest.

I walked back outside to where many Thursdays of varying thicknesses were waiting to be told a story and given a few tips. It felt like I was doing a Thursday master class in a hall of mirrors, but I think they appreciated it. By the time I left two hours later, some of the thinner Thursdays were a little bit thicker.

"Might I inquire where madam has been?" asked Sprockett once I had returned to *The League of Cogmen*. "*Vanity* can be a dangerous place for those published. Brigands, scoundrels, verb artists and the Unread lurk in doorways, ready to steal the Essence of Read from the unwary."

"I was in Fan Fiction."

Sprockett's eyebrow shot to "Worried" in alarm.

"How did you get back across the causeway?"

"Quite easily. They shoot anyone trying to escape, and they check the causeway every half minute to make sure. You can't possibly run the distance in less than four minutes, so the answer seemed quite obvious."

He diverted his mainspring to his thought

cogs and whirred and clicked noisily for a full minute before giving up, and I had to tell him.

"That's quite clever."

"Elementary, my dear Sprockett. Julian Sparkle was a bit annoyed. He said that he'd have to change the puzzle. I won these steak knives. Perhaps Mrs. Winterhope would like them?"

"I think she should be delighted. May I ask a question, ma'am?"

"Of course."

"What are we going to do now?"

"I'm going to accept Senator Jobsworth's invitation to go to the peace talks tomorrow masquerading as the real Thursday Next. The paddle steamer leaves at seven A.M. Everything that has happened is to do with Racy Novel and Speedy Muffler, and unless I start getting to the heart of the problem, I'm not going to get anywhere. The Men in Plaid will think twice before doing anything while I'm in plain view, and Landen told me that this was the way to find Thursday: 'The circumstances of your confusion will be your path to enlightenment.' I don't understand that, but I *can* become more confused — going upriver with Jobsworth will *definitely* provide the extra confusion I need."

Sprockett stared at me for a moment, and I could tell by the way his eyebrow was quivering between "Thinking" and "Worried" that he knew something was up.

"Don't you mean 'we,' ma'am?"

I pulled a letter from my pocket that I'd prepared while seated at a You for Coffee? franchise just off Sargasso Plaza.

"These are glowing references, Sprockett. They should allow you to find a position in Fiction without any problem. You have been a steadfast and loyal companion whom I am happy to have known as a friend. Thank you."

I blinked as my eyes started to mist, and Sprockett stared back at me with his blank porcelain features. His eyebrow pointed in turn at all the possible emotions engraved on his forehead. There was nothing for "Sad," so it sprang backwards and forwards between "Doubtful" and "Worried."

"I must protest, ma'am. I do not —"

"My mind is made up, Sprockett. I have nothing to offer. You have a bright future. It will please me greatly if you find onward employment that I can be proud of."

Sprockett buzzed quietly to himself for a moment. "This is compassion, isn't it?"

"Yes."

"I can *recognize* it," he said, "but I am at

odds to understand it. Shall we go indoors?"

We had boiled cabbage for dinner, which might have been improved had there been any cabbage to go in it. But the Winterhopes were more than friendly, and after several rounds of bezique that might have been more enjoyable had there been cards, Sprockett played the piano accordion without actually having a piano accordion, and the empty unread book didn't ring to the tune of the "Beer Barrel Polka" until the small hours.

34.
THE METAPHORIC QUEEN

Journeys up the Metaphoric River are hugely enjoyable and highly recommended. Since every genre is nourished by its heady waters, a paddle steamer can take even the most walk-shy tourists to their chosen destination. As a bonus there is traditionally at least one murder on board each trip — a "consideration" to the head steward will ensure that it is not you.

Bradshaw's BookWorld Companion
(1st edition)

The steamer was called the *Metaphoric Queen,* and when I arrived, it was lying at the dockside just above the lock gates that separated the river from the Text Sea. The *Queen* was built of a wooden superstructure on a steel hull, measured almost three hundred feet from stem to stern and was the very latest in luxury river travel. A covered walkway ran around the upper deck, and behind the wheelhouse on the top deck was a single central stack that breathed out small puffs of smoke. As I approached, I could see the crew making ready. They loaded and unloaded freight, polished the brasswork, checked the paddle for broken vanes and oiled the traction arm that turned the massive sternwheel.

The *Queen* had docked only an hour before, and the cargo was being offloaded when I arrived: crude metaphor, sealed into twenty-gallon wooden casks, each stenciled PRODUCT OF RACY NOVEL. I watched as the casks were taken under guard and moved towards the Great Library, where they would be distilled into their component parts for onward trade.

"Welcome aboard!" said the captain as I walked up the gangplank. "The senator will be joining us shortly. The staterooms are the first door on the left — tea will be served in ten minutes."

I thanked him and moved aft to the rear deck, which afforded a good view of the docks and the river. The other passengers were already on board and were exactly the sort of people one would expect to see on a voyage of this type. There was a missionary, a businessman, a family of settlers eager to make a new home for themselves, two ladies of negotiable affection and, strangely enough, *several* odd foreigners who wore rumpled linen suits and looked a bit mad.

"I think someone made a mistake on the manifest," came a voice close at hand.

I turned to find an adventurer standing next to me. He looked as though he had argued with a rake at some point as a teenager and come off worse; three deep scars showed livid on his cheek and jaw. He was quite handsome in an understated sort of way, with a plain shirt, grubby chinos and a revolver on his belt. He was wearing a battered trilby with a dark sweat stain on the band, and he looked as though he hadn't shaved — or slept — for days.

"A mistake on the manifest?"

"Three eccentric foreigners on a trip like this rather than the mandatory one. Mind you, it could be worse. I was on a similar jaunt last year, and instead of a single insultingly stereotypical Italian, all fast talking and gesticulating — we had six. Hell on earth, it was."

As if in answer to this, the three eccentric foreigners started to jostle one another in an infantile manner.

"It's Thursday Next, isn't it?"

I looked at him, trying to remember where I'd seen him before. I stared for a little too long at the scars on his face, and he touched the pink marks thoughtfully.

"I don't know how I got them," he confessed, "but they're supposed to make me look like I'm a man with an adventurous past."

"Aren't you?"

"I'm really not sure. I was given the scars but no backstory to go with them. Perhaps it will be revealed to me later. It's an honor to meet you, I must say. My name's Foden. Drake Foden."

We shook hands. I didn't want to deny I was Thursday, given my reason for being here, so I decided to hit him with some pseudo-erudition I had picked up in Hum-Dram.

"You're kind," I replied, "but last Thursday and next Thursday are still a week apart."

"Deep," he said with a smile. "Where are you headed?"

"Upriver a bit," I said, giving little away. "You?"

"Beyond Racy Novel," he said, "and into the Dismal Woods."

"Hoping to find the source of the Metaphoric?"

"Is there one?" He laughed.

Most people these days agreed that the

river couldn't actually have a source, since it flowed in several directions at once. Instead of starting in one place and ending in another using the traditionally mundane "downhill" plan, it would pretty much go as the mood took it. Indeed, the Metaphoric had been known to bunch up in Horror while Thriller suffered a drought, and then, when all was considered lost, the river would suddenly release and cause a flood throughout Comedy and HumDram. Not quite so devastating as one might imagine, for the Metaphoric brought with it the rhetorical nutrients necessary for good prose — the river was the lifeblood of Fiction, and nothing could exist without it.

The puzzle, therefore, was how the river replenished itself. It had long been known that the river flowed up into the Dismal Woods a tired and stagnant backwater and emerged four hundred miles to the west reinvigorated and fizzing with a heady broth of creative alternatives. Quite what mechanism existed to make this happen was a matter of some conjecture. Many adventurers had been lost trying to find out. Some said the secret was guarded by a Mysteriously Vanished subplot that would devour all comers, while others maintained there existed a Fountain of Bestsellerdom that could grant eternal life, and no one troubled to expend a further word in consequence.

"No," said the adventurer, "better men than me have been lost searching for the source of the Metaphoric. That's next year. *This* year I'm in training: I'm going to attempt to uncover the legendary Euphemasauri graveyard."

"Good luck," I said, knowing full well that he would doubtless be dead in a week — the Euphemasaurus was a fearsome beast and not conducive to being tracked. It would perhaps be a safer, easier and more productive quest to look for his own refrigerator.

"Who is that?" I asked as a man with his face obscured by a large pair of dark glasses hurried past and went belowdecks, followed by a porter carrying his suitcases.

"He's the mandatory MP-C12: Mysterious Passenger in Cabin Twelve. All sweaty journeys upriver have to carry the full complement of odd characters. It's a union thing."

"Hence the foreigners?"

"Hence the foreigners. Mark my words, there'll be a mixed-race cook with a violent streak who speaks only Creole, a cardsharp and a man from the company."

"Which company?"

"A company with commercial interests upriver. It doesn't really matter what."

"You must have done this many times."

"Actually, it's my first. I graduated from St. Tabularasa's only this morning."

"You must be nervous."

The adventurer smiled confidently. "I'm running around inside screaming."

I excused myself, as Red Herring, Colonel Barksdale and Senator Jobsworth had just arrived. They were accompanied by an entourage of perhaps a dozen staff, most of whom were simply faceless bureaucrats: D-grade Generics who did nothing but add background and tone to the general proceedings. Try to engage them in conversation and they would just blink stupidly and then stare at their feet.

"Good morning, Miss Next," said Herring affably. "A moment of your time, if you would?"

He was dressed in a light cotton suit and was overseeing the arrival of a riveted steel box that had been placed on the foredeck by four burly rivermen and was now being lashed in place.

"Gifts for Speedy Muffler?"

"Two dozen plot lines and some A-grade characterization to show willingness," replied Herring, tipping the rivermen and checking the cords. "Racy Novel doesn't have much of either, so it should go down well."

I thought of saying that this was because of Council of Genres sanctions but thought better of it.

"So," he said, mopping his brow with a handkerchief, "good to see you could make it."

"All BookWorldians have a duty to avert war whenever it presents itself," I said pointedly.

"Goes without saying. Your series is in good health, I trust?"

"Nothing a reissue in the Outland wouldn't fix."

He steered me to the rail and lowered his voice.

"Have the Men in Plaid been bothering you?"

"Why do you ask, sir?"

"Speedy Muffler has . . . *friends* within government. Some people are sympathetic to his cause. They feel that he has been unfairly treated and may try to work against the peace."

I didn't know whom to trust on this boat, so I decided to trust no one.

"I have seen a few Roadmasters following me over the past few days," I replied cagily.

"Not that unusual," said Herring. "Fantasy is a hotbed of Imaginative Fundamentalism; if we didn't keep a Plaid presence on the streets to rein in Fantasy's worst excesses, we'd be in cross-genre anarchy before we knew it. We'd regulate it more than we do if it weren't so damn readable."

Herring was nothing if not conservative in his opinions, but that only reflected the dominant politics of Fiction. The opposition called for more deregulation and even the banning of genres themselves, dubbing them "an affront to experimentation" and "the measles of the BookWorld," while others called for greater formulaicism — if for nothing better than to appease publishers. A noise made me turn.

"Miss Next," said Senator Jobsworth. "I am most grateful for your attendance. Will you join me in the captain's cabin in twenty minutes?"

I told him I would, and he disappeared off towards his private rooms with his entourage. Red Herring looked at his watch nervously.

"Are we late leaving?" I asked.

"We're waiting for the official Jurisfiction delegate."

We were kept waiting another ten minutes until a sleek spaceship that seemed to have been carved from a single block of obsidian approached from the south, circled twice, lowered its landing gear and, with a rolling blast from its swiveling thrusters, landed on the dockside. The entrance ramp descended, and two imperial guards hurried down it while one blue-skinned valet spread rose petals on the ground and two more played a brief alarum on trumpets. After a dramatic pause, a tall figure swathed in a high-collared black cloak strode menacingly down the ramp. He had a pale complexion, high cheekbones and a small and very precise goatee. This was His Mercilessness the Emperor Zhark, tyrannical ruler of a thousand solar systems and undisputed star of the Emperor Zhark novels. He was also a senior Jurisfiction agent and by all accounts quite a sweetie — if you didn't consider his habit for enslaving entire planets to be worked to death in his spice mines.

"Good morning, Your Mercilessness," said Red Herring, stepping forward to greet him. "No entourage today?"

"Hello, Herring old chap. Where's my cabin? I've a splitting headache. I was up all night dealing with Star Corps — bloody nuisance, they are. What am I doing here again?"

"You're the Jurisfiction delegate to the

Racy Novel peace talks."

"Who are we fighting?"

"No one yet — that's why we call them 'peace talks.' "

"Couldn't we just lay waste to the entire region and put everyone to the sword? It would save a lot of boring chat, and I can go back to bed."

"I'm afraid not, Your Mercilessness."

"Very well," he said with a sigh, "just don't expect me to bunk in with the cook again. He frightens me."

"You have your own cabin this time, Emperor. We are already behind schedule. Steward?"

A steward stepped forward to take the emperor's bag, which I noticed was made out of the skin of the uncle he had murdered in order to seize the Zharkian throne. Despite appearances, Zhark was a skilled negotiator; it was he and he alone who had brought Forensic Procedural to the table and averted a potential fracturing of the Crime genre.

"Good Lord," said Zhark when he saw me. "Thursday?"

"The written one, Your Mercilessness," I said, bowing low. "We last met six months ago at the Paragon Tea Rooms."

He stared at me for a moment. Sometimes

he was slow on the uptake. "You're the written one?"

"Yes, sir."

He moved closer, looked to left and right and lowered his voice.

"Do you remember that waitress at the Paragon? The perky one who answered back a lot and was wholly disrespectful?"

"I think so."

"You didn't get her number, did you?"

"I'm afraid not."

"Never mind. Written Thursday, eh? Know where the real one is?"

"No, sir."

"Bummer," he said, and walked off towards his cabin.

35.
We Go Upriver

> For those with adventure on their minds, a trip watching the never-seen Euphemasaurus might be considered. For a fee, intrepid holiday makers will be taken into the Dismal Woods in the far north of the island where they will spend a pestilential four days being eaten alive by insects and bled white by leeches. Recovery is said to be three to six months, but the blurry pictures of "something in the distance" can be treasured forever.
>
> *Bradshaw's BookWorld Companion* (7th edition)

Within a few minutes, the captain ordered the mooring ropes cast off, and with a blast of the whistle, a shudder from the deck and the venting of steam from the pistons, the sternwheel began to rotate and the boat pulled slowly away from the dock.

For a moment I watched the Great Library

recede, and I suddenly realized that I was very much here on false pretenses. I wasn't Thursday, and I was here on the coattails of a mystery that I had singularly failed to uncover. It was frustrating because, this being Fiction, most of the relevant facts would already have been demonstrated to me but safely peppered with enough red herrings to ensure I couldn't see the true picture. Thursday would have spotted it all and indeed, given her "absent" status, had done so long ago. I still had no clear idea as to what was going on, but I was fortified by the simple fact that I was here, not cowering in a cupboard back home being bullied by Pickwick. Luckily, my thoughts were interrupted by the adventurer, who asked me to meet him in the bar in an hour, and after that I went to find my cabin — a cozy wood-lined cubbyhole with the sink bolted to the ceiling to save room. There was no electricity, but a single porthole gave ample light. I unpacked the small case I had brought with me, and after freshening up I stepped outside, then stopped. I was next door to Cabin 12, where the mysterious passenger was staying. I heard raised voices from within.

". . . but I won't take your place at the talks," came the voice. I leaned closer, but the

conversation was muted and indistinct from then on, and I hurried off towards the captain's quarters, which were situated just behind the wheelhouse, two decks up.

The senator was already there and had ensconced himself in a large and very worn wicker chair, from which spot he contemplated the river traffic that floated past as we made our way out of the Ungenred Zone and into Comedy. The captain and the helmsman were also present, and they expertly steered a path around the many underwater obstructions, islands and sandbars. I decided to try to act as much like the real Thursday as I could.

"Do you expect a clear run up the river, Captain?" I asked.

The captain chuckled.

"It's always eventful, Miss Next. Someone will doubtless be murdered, there will be romantic intrigue, and after that we'll pass a deserted village with a lone survivor who will ramble incoherently about something that we don't understand but has relevance later on. Did you meet the adventurer? Youngish chap. Handsome. He's probably met you before."

I said that I had, and both he and the senator laughed.

"What's the joke?"

"He's the fodder. There's always at least one on a trip like this. Someone for you to get attached to, probably sleep with, but who then dies on the journey, probably saving your life. You won't tell him, will you? It'll ruin his day."

"I'll try to keep it under my hat."

"Do you have the route all planned, Captain?" asked Jobsworth, who was sipping on a pink gin handed to him by a steward dressed in starched whites.

"We'll stay on the Metaphoric until we've entered Comedy and moved past Sitcoms," replied the captain, pointing to a map of the river, "and after that we follow a tributary past Mother-in-Law Jokes and then to Edgy Rapids before cruising the flat plain of Bob Hope and Vaudeville. At the foothills of the Scatological Mountains, we'll enter the subgenres of Bedroom Farce and Bawdy Romp. Twenty minutes after that, we stop at Middle Station, which marks the border into Racy Novel."

"Emissaries from Speedy Muffler will meet us at Fanny Hill," added Senator Jobsworth, "and they will accompany us to Pornucopia, the capital."

The conversation fell off after that, and once I'd mustered some courage, I spoke.

"Did you want to speak to me, Senator?" I asked.

"Yes," he replied. "I want you to understand that you are here simply as a face — nothing more. As already explained, we have been putting around the story that you have irritable-vowel syndrome and are mute. You will not be party to talks, or to preparations for talks. You will not express an opinion by gesticulating or written notes unless we decide and are fully briefed. You'll be told where to appear and when. Is that clear?"

"As a bell, sir."

"Good. Off you toddle, then. Ah!" he added, much relieved, "Come in, gentlemen."

Red Herring, Colonel Barksdale and Zhark had just appeared at the doorway. I was no longer needed. I thought for a moment of voicing my concerns over what Thursday might have been up to, but I didn't know for certain what she *had* been up to, so I said nothing, bowed and withdrew politely from the cabin.

I walked down the companionway to the main deck and found my way to the bar. I wasn't particularly bothered by the senator's attitude. It was what I was expecting — a friendly welcome, then being put firmly in my place.

The bar was elegantly paneled in light wood with inlaid etched mirrors to give the the illusion of greater space. The furniture was of leather but had worn badly, and the horsehair stuffing was beginning to sprout at the seams. One of the mad-looking foreigners was asleep in an armchair, and at the bar was the adventurer. He looked handsomer than he had earlier, and his hat was placed on the bar next to him.

"Enjoying the trip?" I asked as I sat down.

"I thought it would be funnier steaming through Comedy."

"It's less funny the closer you get."

"Hmm. Would you permit me to buy you a drink?"

"I buy my own drinks," I told him, doing as Thursday would. It wasn't like it was a real drink anyway. Alcohol doesn't do anything in the BookWorld, except act as narrative furniture in scenes such as these. If you wanted to get off your head, you'd hit the hyphens, but I needed my wits about me.

"A beer for me," I said. "Drake?"

"Scotch."

The barman placed our drinks on the counter, and I took a sip. The beer was a light, amber-colored liquid, but it tasted like warm tea. This wasn't unusual, since everything in the BookWorld tasted like warm tea — except warm tea itself, which tasted of dishwater. But since dishwater tasted of warm tea, warm tea actually might have tasted like warm tea after all.

"Are you part of the diplomatic mission?" asked Drake.

I told him that I was, and he grunted noncommittally. Since the senator said he was fodder and unlikely to last the next few hours, I though it a safe bet to trust him.

"I overheard something odd outside the mysterious passenger's cabin."

"That's entirely normal. You'll probably hear odd noises in the night, too, and if we've got time, someone will be found shot dead with a cryptic note close by."

"Do you want to know what I overheard?"

"Not really. There'll be an impostor on the boat, too — and a shape-changer."

"What, of the alien variety?" I asked, looking nervously about.

"No," he replied, smiling at my naïveté. "Someone or something who is not what it seems."

"Isn't that the impostor?"

"There's a subtle difference." Drake mused for a moment, staring at the ceiling. "But I'm not sure *precisely* what it is. I was born yesterday, you know."

"My name is Florent," announced a new bar steward who had just come on duty. "May I mix you a Tahiti Tingle?"

I frowned, then turned. It was Sprockett, dressed as a bar steward and sporting a ridiculous false mustache on his porcelain features. Since he didn't greet me, I assumed he wanted to remain incognito, so I merely said I already had a drink and resumed my conversation with Drake.

"Are journeys upriver usually like this?" I asked.

"Apparently so. How do they think they're going to stop Speedy Muffler anyway?"

"By telling him that massed armies on the borders of WomFic and Dogma are waiting to invade if he so much as hiccups."

"What makes you think Speedy Muffler is doing anything but rattling his saber? The only people who stand to gain by a war are the neighboring genres who get to divvy up the spoils."

"I knew Speedy Muffler in the old days," said one of the foreigners who had joined us, "long before the BookWorld was remade — even before Herring and Barksdale and that idiot Jobsworth were about."

"What do you know about Speedy Muffler?"

"That he wasn't always the leader of Racy

Novel. He was once a minor character in Porn with delusions of grandeur. Muffler was up here in the days before Racy Novel, when the Frowned-Upon Genres were clustered in the north beyond Comedy. His name came to prominence when he quite suddenly started sending large quantities of metaphor downriver. He wasn't licensed to do so, but because his supplies were consistent, the rules were relaxed. Pretty soon he was taking more and more territory for himself, but he kept on sending down the metaphor, and the CofG kept on turning a blind eye until he publicly proclaimed the area as Racy Novel, which was when the CofG started to take notice."

"By then it was too late," added Drake. "Speedy Muffler's power was established, his genre large enough to demand a chair at the Council of Genres."

"I guess WomFic/Feminism were none too happy?"

"Not overawed, no. Especially when he used to turn up at high-level summits with his shirt open and declaring that feminists needed to 'loosen up' and should groove with his love machine."

"Is he still shipping metaphor downriver?" I asked.

"Not as much as before," said Drake, "but

still more than WomFic and Dogma. The area is rich in metaphor, and whoever can send the most downriver is the wealthiest. Put simply: Whoever controls the Northern Genres controls the metaphor supply, and whoever controls the supply of metaphor controls Fiction. It's not by chance that WomFic and Crime have forty-three percent of the Outland readership. If Squid Procedural had been positioned up here, everyone would be reading about Decapod Gumshoes, and loving it."

"So why isn't Racy Novel read more than Women's Fiction? If he sends more metaphor downriver, I mean?"

"Because of *sanctions,*" said Drake, looking at me oddly, "imposed by WomFic and Dogma — and pretty much everyone else. Like it or not, Racy Novel isn't very highly thought of."

"Is that fair?"

"You're asking a lot of *basic* questions," said Drake. "I thought Thursday Next would be well up on all this — especially if she's here for the peace talks."

"I need to gauge local opinion," I said quickly. "This is Fiction, after all — interpretation trumps fact every time."

"Oh," said Drake, "I see."

I excused myself, as Sprockett had just

left the bar, and I caught up with him farther down the steamer, just outside the storeroom.

"Good afternoon, ma'am," he whispered. "How is it going?"

"What are you doing here?"

"I'm the bar steward."

"I can see that."

"I knew you couldn't *actually* let me go," he said. "I'm too good a butler for that. So I simply assumed you were being compassionate and thought this trip too dangerous for you to take staff. So I came anyway. What do you want me to do?"

I took a deep breath. It seemed as though butlers were like flat feet, dimples and troublesome aunts — you've got them for life.

"There's a mysterious passenger in Cabin Twelve. I want you to find out what he's doing here."

"He doesn't *do* anything — he's simply the MP-C12. Have you figured out who the fodder is yet?"

"It's Drake."

"Ooh. Will he be eaten by a crocodile? A poison dart in the eye?"

"Just find out what you can about the mysterious passenger, would you? I overheard him say, 'I won't take your place at

the talks,' and it might be significant."
"Very good, ma'am. I'll make inquiries."

36.
Middle Station

For those of you who have tired of the glitzy world of shopping and inappropriate boyfriends in Chick Lit, a trip to Dubious Lifestyle Advice might be the next step. An hour in the hallowed halls of invented ills will leave you with at least ten problems you never knew you had, or even knew existed.

Bradshaw's BookWorld Companion
(7th edition)

It took us an hour to steam through Comedy, and whilst mostly light and airy and heard-it-beforeish, the atmosphere became more strained and intimidating as we chugged slowly through Mother-in-Law Jokes and Sexist Banter. Despite being advised to remain out of sight, I elected to stay on deck and brazen out the worst abuses that came shouted unseen from the thick trees that covered the riverbank. The two ladies of negotiable affection had no difficulty with the comments, having heard much worse before, and simply retorted with aplomb — delicately countering the more vulgar insinuations with amusing attacks on the male psyche and various aspersions on their manhood or ability.

We came across the Middle Station at noon. The small trading town was right on the point where the Double Entendre River becomes the Innuendo, and although we had been traveling through the buffer genre of Bawdy Romp, replete with amusing sketches of people running in and out of each other's bedrooms in a retro-amusing manner, we were now very much within the influence of Racy Novel, and we all knew it. The first part of the journey had been a pleasing chug up the river, but now we were here for business, and a sense of brooding introspection had fallen upon the boat.

The arrival of the paddle steamer at the Middle Station was welcomed not by sound but by silence. The constant *tramp-tramp-tramp* of the engines, for five hours a constant background chorus, made things seem deafeningly quiet when the engines were stopped. I stood on the foredeck as the steamer drifted towards the jetty. The Middle Station, usually a throbbing hub of activity, seemed deserted. Drake stood next to me, his hand on the butt of his revolver.

"I'm going ashore to check this out," I said, "and I think it would be better if you stayed here."

"*Au contraire,* Miss Next. It is *you* who will be staying here."

There seemed no easy way to say this, so I came right out with it.

"Drake," I said in a quiet voice, "you're the fodder, due for a tragic yet potentially heroic end."

He looked at me for a moment. "It's very good of you to warn me, but that's not how I see it."

"You think it's someone else?"

"I think the fodder is *you,* Thursday."

"No it's not."

"What are you if you're not the fodder?"

"I'm the impostor."

"You . . . could be the impostor *and* the fodder."

"The unions would never allow it."

"They might."

"Look," I said, "we could argue this all day, but here's the thing: You graduated only this morning with a minimal back-story. I've been working the BookWorld for over three years — who's most likely to cop it in the next few hours?"

"You might just *think* you've been working the BookWorld for three years. It could be *your* backstory."

"Okay," I said, beginning to get angry, "we'll both go out there and see who gets eaten by a crocodile or gets a poison dart in the eye. *Then* we'll know."

"Deal."

The rest of the peace delegation had joined us on deck, and they were staring silently towards the Middle Station. As we drew closer, we could see that the houses had been recently burned, for wisps of smoke hung in the air with the faint smell of scorched custard. We waited for the steamer to drift towards the jetty, until it touched with a faint bump. The crew made the steamer fast before jumping back onto the boat, and we watched and waited as the steamer slowly swung around in the current. There was not a single sign of life anywhere in the station.

"Well," said Colonel Barksdale after a few minutes, "I've seen enough — doubtless skirmishers from Racy Novel causing trouble. Let's steam on deeper into the genre and start getting some face time with this lunatic."

"We're not going anywhere until we load some coal," said the captain.

I stepped off the steamer and onto the rickety old jetty, Drake at my side. We walked slowly into the town. Drake looked about anxiously, but not, I realized, about the deserted Middle Station.

"You'll keep an eye out for crocodiles, won't you?" I asked.

"As long as you watch my back for poison darts."

We came across the first body near the mailbox on the corner. There was an ugly wound in the middle of his chest, and the small letters and words that made up his existence had been caught by the breeze and blown into the fishing nets set up to dry. We looked around and noticed more bodies and the detritus of conflict: discarded rubber chickens, feather dusters, strings of silk flags, spinning bow ties and custard-pie shrapnel that somehow seemed sadder and less funny than usual.

"Is this a garrison town?" I asked.

"No," replied the adventurer.

"Then what's a lance corporal of the Fourteenth Motorized Clown doing up here?"

The corpse was indeed a member of Comedy's frontline troops. He had orange hair, a bulbous red nose, and he was wearing camouflage battle dress, along with a pair of size-twenty-eight shoes. Not much good for marching and a hangover from their days as an Alpine regiment.

Drake placed his hand on the clown's bright red nose.

"Still warm," he said, "probably been dead less than an hour. Any thoughts?"

"I don't know," I said, picking up a nurse's hat from the ground. A little farther on, a stethoscope was lying broken in the dust. "But it wasn't just clowns who died here today."

We walked some more and came across a dozen or so other bodies. All clowns, all dead and none meant to be here. Bawdy Romp was within Racy Novel's control and officially a demilitarized zone.

"This doesn't make sense," said Drake. "Comedy never had any beef with Racy Novel. Quite the reverse — they actually got on very well. Without Racy Novel, Comedy would be very poor indeed — especially for the stand-ups."

"Let's not hang around. Where did the captain say the coal was?"

We walked deeper into the station and saw more evidence of a pitched battle having taken place not long before. We found the remains of several burned-out clown cars; despite their being able to drive in either direction and having a device for shedding all the body work in order to lighten the vehicle for a speedy getaway, it hadn't done any good. There was evidence of atrocities, too. Medical staff had been killed. I noted several pretty nurses and a handsome doctor lying in a doorway, and several crash carts were strewn about. There were a few dead rustic serving wenches, too, a ripped bodice and a couple of horses with ruggedly handsome and now very dead riders lying in the road amidst scorched brickwork and smoking rubble. We came across more dead clowns; it seemed as though an entire company had been wiped out.

"Looks like someone was making sure Comedy couldn't come to Racy Novel's aid," observed Drake.

"It makes me wonder why we're bothering with peace talks. Crocodile."

"What?"

"Behind you."

Drake jumped out of the way as the crocodile's jaws snapped shut. "Thank you."

"Now do you believe you might be the fodder?" I asked.

Drake thought for a moment. "He could have been trying to eat his way through me to get to you."

"Sure," I said with a smile, "and while

we're on the subject: If I were the fodder, why didn't you warn me? I warned you."

"Because I . . . didn't want to ruin your day?"

"How very generous of you."

We found the coal heap amidst a few more civilians — this time pretty secretaries who had died in the arms of their bosses. We filled a couple of wheelbarrows with coal before returning to the steamer. As soon as we were aboard, the crew slipped the moorings and the captain ordered, "Astern slow," and swung the bows into the limpid river. We took the left branch up the tributary known as the Innuendo, and pretty soon the steamer was at full speed once more. Despite others' misgivings, Jobsworth seemed adamant that the peace talks should go ahead.

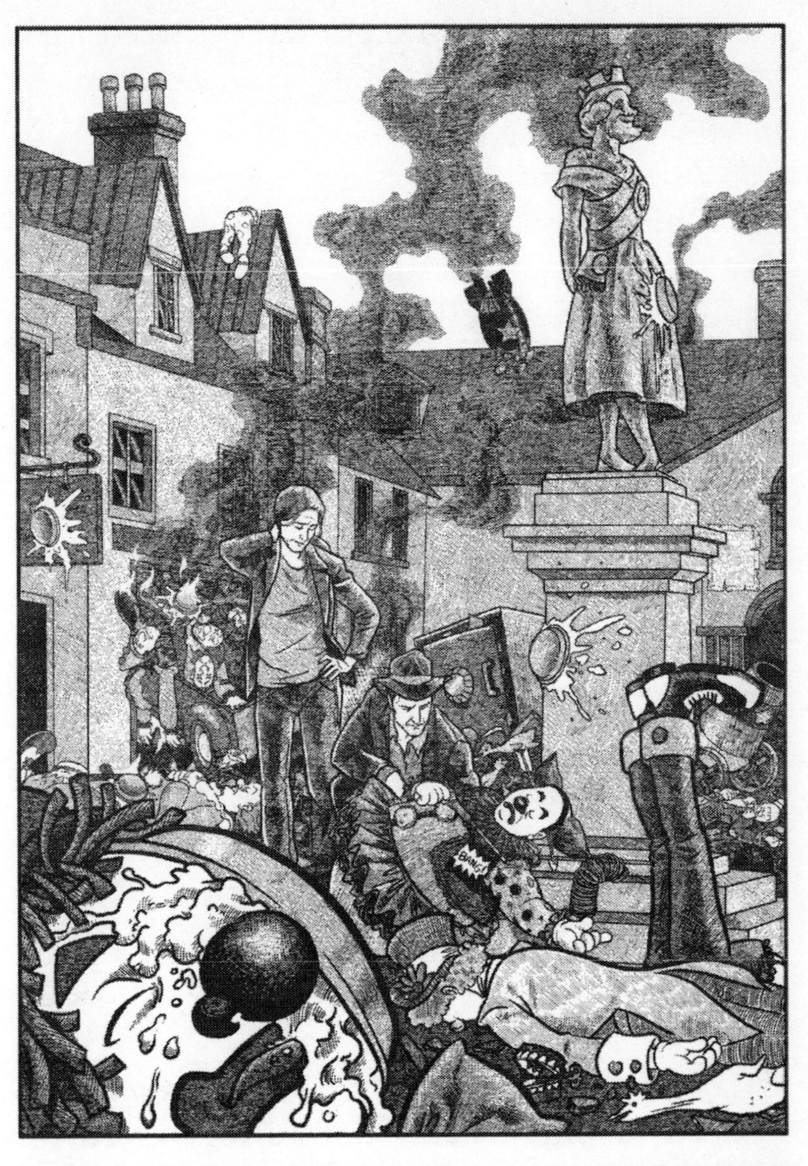

It seemed as though an entire company had been wiped out.

37.
Revision

Amongst all the genres on Fiction Island, Comedy is the only one that still demands compulsory military service and a bucket of water down the trousers for every citizen. Conscripts are trained in the clown martial art of slapstick and do not graduate from military academy until they can kill silently with a frying pan and achieve fatal accuracy with a custard pie at forty yards. It's a bit like Sparta, only with jokes.

Bradshaw's BookWorld Companion
(7th edition)

We convened in the bar soon afterwards and related everything we had seen at the Middle Station. Colonel Barksdale, Herring, Zhark and Senator Jobsworth listened carefully to all we had to say but didn't seem to have any better idea of what was going on than we did.

"There is no reason for the Fourteenth

Motorized Clown to be this far north," declared Colonel Barksdale angrily. "It is a flagrant breach of numerous peace agreements and specifically the 1996 Clown Army Proliferation Treaty."

"Shouldn't you have known about it?" asked Emperor Zhark, who knew better than most the value of intelligence.

"The Textual Sieve network is patchy up here," replied Barksdale in a sulky tone. "We can't know everything. I can only think the Fourteenth Clown must have been massing in the demilitarized zone as the potential allies of Racy Novel."

"Then who killed them and all the civilians?" asked the adventurer, to which question there didn't seem to be much of an answer. They all fell silent for a moment.

"When do we meet with the other delegates?" asked Jobsworth.

"In an hour," replied Herring. "Aunt Augusta of WomFic and Cardinal Fang of Outdated Religious Dogma are meeting us at Fanny Hill. Would you excuse me? We're out of footnoterphone range, and I'm going to have to send a message to the council via the shortwave colophone."

Drake and I were dismissed, as Jobsworth, Barksdale and Zhark had decided to discuss the finer points of the peace talks, something to which we could not be privy.

"I'm going to freshen up before we get there," said Drake, "and maybe rub on some crocodile repellent."

I laughed, saw he was serious, turned the laugh into a cough and said, "Good idea."

We were now well within Racy Novel, and the rustling of bushes, the groans and squeaks of delight echoed in from the riverbanks, where large privet hedges were grown to afford some sort of privacy for the residents. Every now and then, a slip in the riverbank allowed us a brief glimpse of what went on, which was generally several scantily dressed people running around in a gleeful manner — usually in a bedroom somewhere, but occasionally in the outdoors and once on the top deck of a London bus.

I made my way forward, where I was met by Sprockett, who beckoned me into a laundry cupboard.

"I took the opportunity to go through the mysterious passenger's belongings, ma'am."

"And?"

"I came across some shoulder pads, knee pads, a chest protector and a gallon of fire retardant."

"What?"

"Shoulder pads —"

"I heard. It just doesn't make any sense."

"What doesn't?"

"All of it. From beginning to end. We reach Fanny Hill in half an hour, and the peace talks begin as soon as we are escorted to Pornucopia. It's time to go over what we've found. I feel the answer is staring me in the face."

"Shouldn't we gather all the suspects in the bar?" asked Sprockett, who was fast becoming infected by the *Metaphoric Queen*'s capacity for narrative formulaicism.

"No. And another thing —"

I was interrupted by a cry from outside, and the engine went to slow ahead. We stepped out of the laundry cupboard to see several crewmen run past, and we followed them to the upper rear deck, from where we could see across the top of the sternwheel. Behind us in midstream was a figure in one of the riverboat's four-man tenders. The man was rowing in a measured pace away from the boat, and given our forward speed, the distance between the two craft was rapidly increasing.

"Who is it?" asked Herring.

"It looks like the mysterious passenger from Cabin Twelve," replied Drake, who had a small telescope, as befits an adventurer. "He's even taken his luggage with him."

"What's the meaning of this?" asked Jobsworth, who had just arrived.

Herring explained, and Jobsworth looked at us all in turn. "Let me see."

He peered through the telescope for a moment. "He's taken his luggage with him."

"That's what I said," remarked Drake.

"Mr. Herring," said Jobsworth, "what's going on here?"

"I've no idea, Senator."

"Advice?"

"Um . . . carry on?"

"Sounds good to me. Captain?"

"Sir?"

"Carry on."

But the captain, long a riverman, knew more of the perils that can be found on the Metaphoric.

"We can't leave him out here, sir. The forests are full of Sirens eager to . . . well, how can I put it? He'll be captured and made to . . . Listen, he'll be killed."

"Will it be quick?"

"No — it will be long and very drawn out. He might enjoy it to begin with, but he will eventually be discarded, a shriveled husk of a man devoid of any clothes, humanity or moisture."

But the senator was made of sterner stuff.

"This mission is too important to delay,

Captain. The mysterious passenger formerly of Cabin Twelve will have to remain exactly that. In every campaign there are always casualties. Full ahead."

"Yes, sir."

And they all walked away. The engines ran up to full speed again, and after a few more minutes the small boat was lost to view behind an overhanging tree on a bend in the river.

"I guess that's what mysterious passengers do," said Drake with a shrug. "Be mysterious. Drink?"

"I'll see you down there," I replied. "I must admonish this bar steward for the lamentable lack of quality in his Tahiti Tingle."

Drake nodded and moved off, and Sprockett and I sat on the curved bench on the upper rear deck to discuss recent events. From the epizeuxis to the mimefield to the Men in Plaid to Sir Charles Lyell and the bed-sitting room.

"What had Thursday discovered that was so devastating to the peace process?" asked Sprockett.

"I don't know. I wish to Panjandrum I were more like her."

I took the sketch I had found in Sir Charles's office out of my pocket. It was a map of Racy Novel with WomFic to one side and Dogma on the other. There was a shaded patch the shape of a tailless salmon that was mostly beneath Racy Novel.

As I stared at the picture, I felt a sudden flush of new intelligence, as though a jigsaw had been thrown into the air and landed fully completed. Everything that had happened to me over the past few days had been inexorably pointing me in one direction. But up until now I'd been too slow or stupid to be able to sift the relevant facts from the herrings.

"By all the spell checkers of Isugfsf," I said, pointing at Lyell's sketch. "It's *metaphor.* A trillion tons of the stuff waiting to be mined, lying beneath our feet!"

"Yes?" said Sprockett, his eyebrow pointing at "Doubtful."

"That's what Lyell and Thursday had discovered," I said excitedly. "It's as Drake said: 'Whoever controls the supply of metaphor controls Fiction.' "

"If so," said Sprockett carefully, "Racy Novel would be sending more metaphor downriver than anyone else. And they're not."

I thought about this for a moment. "Maybe Speedy Muffler isn't bad at all. Perhaps he's defending the metaphor against greedy genres intent on mining it to exhaustion. Metaphor should be controlled — a glut on the market would make Fiction overtly highbrow, painfully ambiguous and potentially unreadable. The new star on the horizon would be the elephant in the room that might lead the BookWorld into a long winter's night."

"That would be frightful," replied Sprockett, recoiling in terror as the overmetaphorication hit him like a hammer. "But how does that explain the Fourteenth Clown's destruction? Or even who's responsible for all this?"

"I don't know," I said, "but Senator Jobsworth needs to hear about it."

I jumped up and ran down the companionway to the captain's cabin, nearly colliding with Red Herring on the way.

"Sorry," he said, "I'm just going to find a doughnut — do you want one?"

"No thank you, sir."

I found Senator Jobsworth discussing the talks with Emperor Zhark and Colonel Barksdale.

"Have you seen Herring?" asked Jobsworth. "He should really be going through the final details with us."

"He went to get a doughnut."

"He did? Leave us now. We're very busy."

"I have important information. I think I know why Thursday was assassinated."

Jobsworth stared at me. "Thursday's dead?"

"Well, no, because her imagination is still alive. It was an assassination *attempt* — in a crummy book written by Adrian Dorset."

"Adrian Dorset?"

"Jack Schitt, if you must. It was the epizeuxis that got her.

And Mediocre."

"Who's Mediocre?"

"Gatsby."

"He's anything but mediocre, my girl."

And both he and Zhark laughed in a patronizing sort of way.

"Seriously," I said hotly, "Thursday was attacked, and the reason —"

"Whatever it is, I'm sure it's *fascinating,*" said Jobsworth, "but it's going to have to wait. We enter the subgenre Racy Classics in five minutes and meet with the other delegates in forty-five. We have much work to do. If you really want to be helpful, make me a cup of tea or go find Herring."

"But —"

"GO!"

I mumbled an apology and backed out the door, cursing my own weakness.

"That could have gone better," said

Sprockett. "I'll try to find Herring for you."

And with a mild buzz, he disappeared. I walked down to the lower deck feeling hot and frustrated. I didn't like to be talked to that way, but this could indeed wait. I'd leave it until Jobsworth had a quieter moment and then tell him — or perhaps speak to Speedy Muffler's people in private and see if my suspicions were correct. Perhaps it was better *not* to talk to Jobsworth.

I went down to my cabin to wash my face but stopped at Cabin 12, next door to mine. The mysterious passenger's escape from the steamer still made no sense, so I pushed open the door and went in.

The bed was made up, as I might have suspected — we weren't due to return until tomorrow. I searched through the missing passenger's baggage and found none of the shoulder or knee pads that Sprockett had described, although the fire retardant was still there, unopened. There was a change of clothes and nothing else. I was about to close the door when I remembered — *the mysterious passenger had his luggage with him when we saw him rowing away.*

A flurry of unpleasant thoughts went through my head, and I suddenly realized not only why the mysterious passenger would have knee pads, but who had attacked the Fourteenth Clown and what was going on in the Outland that made the whole thing possible. This was a complex plot of considerable dimension, and I was now certain who was behind it all. My first thought was to go and tell Jobsworth exactly what was happening, but I stopped as a far worse realization dawned upon me. The plan would work only if everyone on board the *Metaphoric Queen* were to be assassinated.

I grabbed a fire ax and ran up the companionway to the deck.

38.
Answers

> Off the coast lies Vanity Island, and off Vanity lies Fan Fiction. Beyond Fan Fiction is School Essays and beyond that Excuses for Not Doing School Essays. The latter is often the most eloquent, constructed as it is in the white-hot heat of panic, necessity and the desire not to get a detention.
>
> *Bradshaw's BookWorld Companion* (2nd edition)

One of Jobsworth's D-3 minions had been given the task of keeping an eye on the riveted box that contained the valuable plotline gifts for Speedy Muffler, and he noticed me only when I was halfway across the foredeck, my intention already clear to those present. He dropped his copy of *The Word* and took a pace towards me. I caught him on the solar plexus with the ball of my hand, and he reeled over backwards. The foredeck would have been in plain view from the wheelhouse, and the captain pulled on the steam whistle and sent a deafening blast echoing across Racy Novel, temporarily quenching the sounds of the enthusiastic moans that echoed over the water.

The whistle also drowned out the sound of the padlock being smashed off, and I had the lid open and was looking at the contents when Zhark and Jobsworth arrived beside me. They stopped, too, and stared inside the box.

"Those aren't plot lines," said Jobsworth.

"No," I replied, looking up the river to where I could just see *Lady Chatterley's Lover* appear around the next bend, less than five hundred yards away, "and you need to stop the boat before we get to Racy Classics."

"Captain!" yelled Jobsworth, who knew how to act properly when evidence presented itself. The captain opened the wheelhouse window and leaned out, cupping a hand to his ear.

"Turn the *Queen* about and get us downstream. If we go up, I want to be taking only Racy Pulp with us!"

The captain needed no further bidding, and he ordered the helm hard over to turn midriver.

I leaned in and examined the contents of the box. It was a classy job. There was a single glass jar that contained, as far as I could see, a lot of foam. This was attached to a funnel and a time switch, and wrapped around all this was a series of embarrassingly bad descriptions of sexual congress. Emperor Zhark moved closer and put on his glasses.

"By the seven-headed Zook of Zargon," he breathed. "It's full of antikern."

"It's full of what?"

"Kerning is the adjustment of the white spaces between the letters," he explained, "in order to make the letters seem proportionally spaced. What this does is remove the white spaces entirely — within an instant this entire boat and everyone in it will implode into nothing more than an oily puddle of ink floating on the river."

I pointed to the poorly written descriptions of sexual congress wrapped around the device.

"With a few telltale descriptions of a sexual nature to point the finger toward Speedy Muffler."

"So it would appear. *Blast!*"

Emperor Zhark had been examining the device carefully.

"What's up?" I asked.

"No blue wire. There's usually a choice of wires to cut, and by long convention it's always the blue one. Without that there's no way we can know how to defuse it."

I glanced at the timing device, which also by long convention was prominently featured — and had two and a half minutes to go.

"Can we throw it overboard?" asked Jobsworth.

"Not unless you want to see the entire Metaphoric River vanish in under a second."

"We could abandon the steamer."

"It'll be a tight fit in the one tender remaining — and those high privet hedges along the riverbank won't make for an easy escape."

"I'll take it in a boat with me."

It was Drake Foden, adventurer.

"I don't want any arguments," he said. "This is my function. I'm the fodder."

"I told you he was," said Barksdale, jabbing Jobsworth on the shoulder with his index finger.

There was no time to do anything else, and at a single word from the captain the second tender was lowered over the side and the riveted box placed inside. Drake turned to me and took my hands in his.

"Good-bye, Thursday. I'm sorry we didn't get to sleep together and perhaps have a few jokes and get into a couple of scrapes and thus make this farewell more poignant and mournful, which it isn't."

"Yes," I replied. "I'll always regret not knowing you at all or even liking you very much. Perhaps next time."

"There won't be a next time."

"I know that. Drake?"

"Yes?"

"You have something stuck in your teeth."

"Here?"

"Other side."

"Thanks."

And without another word, Drake clambered aboard, cast off the mooring and began to row quickly away from the steamer.

"Hey!" I yelled across the water. "Aren't you glad it wasn't a poison dart in your —"

But I didn't get a chance to say any more. Drake, the tender and the iron box suddenly imploded with a sound like a cough going backwards, accompanied by a swift rush of air that sucked in to fill the void and made our ears pop. I'd never seen text destroyed so rapidly — even an eraserhead takes a half second to work.

"Slow ahead," ordered Jobsworth, "and wire the delegation that we have been 'unavoidably delayed.' "

He turned to me.

"Just what in Wheatley's name is going on here, Next?"

My mind was still racing. There was the fate of the Fourteenth Clown to think of, and the broader implications of regional stability, pretty nurses, handsome doctors and fire retardant.

"Time is of the essence. Senator, I need you to do something without question."

"And that is?"

"Shut down every single Feedback Loop north of *Three Men in a Boat.*"

"Are you mad?" he said. "That's almost three hundred million books!"

"Mad? Perhaps. But if you don't do what I ask, you'll have a genre war on your hands so devastating it will turn your blood to ice."

"My blood is already ice, Miss Next."

The senator paused, then looked at Zhark, who nodded his agreement.

"Very well."

Jobsworth instructed Barnes to get the message to Text Grand Central in any way he could — and to expedite, code puce.

"And you," said Jobsworth, pointing a finger at me, "have some serious explaining to do."

We convened in the bar almost immediately. Jobsworth was there with Herring, Barksdale, the captain and Emperor Zhark — as well as all of Jobsworth's D-3s and Sprockett, who had divested himself of his bar-steward disguise and was once more in full butler regalia.

"Where would you like me to start?" I asked.

"At the beginning," said Jobsworth, "and don't stop until you get to the end."

I took a deep breath and showed them the map Lyell had drawn.

"We won't find out exactly *how* she knew until we find her, but the real Thursday Next became aware that there might exist a huge quantity of raw metaphor under the Northern Genres. Such a state of affairs would throw the entire power balance of Fiction on its head, so she needed to make sure. She took leading geologist Sir Charles Lyell up-country to conduct some test drilling, and it seems she was right. Buried beneath Racy Novel are the largest reserves of untapped metaphor the BookWorld has ever seen."

I had everyone's attention by now — you could have heard a pin drop.

"It was potentially explosive news, and Thursday knew that she would be in severe danger if this got out — so she hid among the flat Thursdays out in Fan Fiction. Despite her precautions, her activities were being scrutinized without her knowledge, and Thursday — reliably touted as 'the second-hardest person to kill in the BookWorld' — had to be gotten rid of. A cabbie named the Mediocre Gatsby was bribed to hang around Fan Fiction on the off chance she would want picking up. A previously scrapped book called *The Murders on the Hareng Rouge* was being kept in Vanity and as soon as she was in the cab, the book was dispatched to the Council of Genres. Mediocre piggybacked the book for the trip as instructed, and a second later a rhetorical device was detonated, leaving the book, the cabbie and, it was hoped, Thursday herself little more then textual confetti — a million graphemes littered all over Fiction."

There was silence, so I carried on. "That might have been the end of it. Most of the book was just small, tattered remnants not dissimilar to the usual detritus that flutters occasionally from the heavens and is absorbed into the ground, except that for some reason, Adrian Dorset described a bed-sitting room so well that it survived the sabotage intact and came to rest in Conspiracy, and JAID had to be alerted. This was tricky, because a diligent investigator might start to ask awkward questions, so Lockheed was ordered to employ his most useless investigator to look into it. Me. And that's not a coincidence. Why would that be, Sprockett?"

"There are *no* coincidences in the Book-World — so long as you don't count the last chapters in some of Charles Dickens's books."

"Exactly. But we *do* find problems — the fact that someone scrubbed off the ISBN to avoid discovery, and the epizeuxis device. And as we look, we find ourselves one step behind the Men in Plaid, who are silencing anyone who had anything to do with the attempted hit on Thursday Next."

"Rogue Men in Plaid?" said Emperor Zhark in an accusatory tone, staring at Jobsworth and Herring — the two who were responsible for them.

"Scrubbed ISBN?" demanded Jobsworth. "Dead geologists? Epizeuxis devices? Who is responsible for this outrage?"

"One of us present here."

They all looked at one another.

"It was little things to begin with — things that didn't click until later. I learned from Adrian Dorset that he destroyed *The Murders on the Hareng Rouge* a month back, yet it was still floating around Vanity waiting to intercept Thursday. The rules state that it has to be scrapped immediately — on Red Herring's signature."

They all looked at Herring, who had started to go pale.

"He controls the Book Transit Authority, and also the Men in Plaid. He's the second-in-command to the BookWorld, but he wanted more. He was after the top job and, what's more, control of the vast stores of metaphor that are lying under Racy Novel. He knew that whoever controlled the metaphor would control Fiction."

"But how could he control Speedy Muffler and Racy Novel?" asked Zhark.

"That's the clever bit. He planned to invade — using an army mustered from one of the most powerful genres on the island."

"Women's Fiction?" said Colonel Barksdale with a smirk. "Not possible. They have neither the manpower nor the inclination."

Emperor Zhark and Jobsworth nodded their heads vigorously; WomFic was wholly against any sort of warfare and had agreed to sanctions only as a last resort.

"Not WomFic," I said. "A smaller sub-genre with enough shock troops to take on the Fourteenth Clown and win. A genre that has for many years been the buffer zone between WomFic and Racy Novel. A genre that has successfully blended raciness and euphemism to create an empire that sells books by the billion — Daphne Farquitt. More readers than almost any other writer, and eighteen percent of total global readership."

"They don't have any troops," scoffed Barksdale. "You're mistaken."

I chose my words carefully. Despite recent events, I'd be pushing my luck if I admitted I'd been in the RealWorld.

"Today is Daphne Farquitt Day in the Outland. As we speak, a massive readathon is in progress. At even conservative estimates, there must be upwards of two hundred million readers making their way through Farquitt's three hundred seventy-two novels. There will be speed-reading events, trivia quizzes and read-ins. The power of the Feedback Loop will be astronomical — and easy enough to create an unstoppable army of ditzy romantic heroines and their lantern-jawed potential husband/lovers."

"The nurses, secretaries and medical equipment you saw at Middle Station?"

"Exactly," I replied. "Not civilians at all — but the romantically involved honored dead. The Farquitt Army was working against

Racy Novel by taking a preemptive strike and eradicating any possible threat from Speedy Muffler's allies in Comedy. With members of the peace envoy all assassinated in an apparent Muffler attack, there would be no opposition to the total and complete invasion of Racy Novel by the Farquitt Army and, with it, control of the vast stocks of metaphor beneath our feet."

There was silence in the room. They all looked stunned. Barksdale was the first to speak.

"That explanation," he said in admiration, "was of a complexity that would gather plaudits from even the most intractable of political thrillers. With all of us dead in an attack that could be blamed on Speedy Muffler, Red Herring would step into the top slot, direct his allies to annex Racy Novel, secure the metaphor and set himself up as supreme dictator of Fiction."

"It's a brilliant scheme," murmured Zhark in admiration. "I'll *definitely* be using it on the Rambosians next week. The little devils. They love a good subjugation. Senator?"

"A plan of titanic proportions. If he weren't going to be erased for treason, I'd offer him a job."

Red Herring was starting to shake when he heard this. He tried to speak, but only a strangled squeak came out.

"Might I make an observation?" asked Sprockett.

"Go ahead," replied Jobsworth, who was now in a generous mood.

"Mr. Herring is here with us now — how could he seize power if he was assassinated along with the rest of us?"

Barksdale's and Zhark's faces fell, and even Jobsworth's smile dropped from his face. They looked at me.

"Simple," I said, placing my hand on Herring's shoulder. "This *isn't* Red Herring. Figuring that out was the key to the whole thing."

"That's absurd," remarked Jobsworth. "We were discussing the minutiae of the peace talks on the way in. He can't be anything but."

"I assure you," said Faux Herring, who had finally managed to find his voice. "I'm *not* Red Herring."

"He's right," I said. "This is Herring's stunt double, Fallon Hairbag. He took Herring's place when Red Herring made his escape in the boat's tender."

"You're the mysterious passenger?" asked Zhark, and the Herring-that-wasn't nodded unhappily.

"Mr. Herring promised me the pick of all

the stunt work in the BookWorld if I did this for him. He said it was for a prank. That it would be funny."

"I overheard Herring and his stunt double talking in the cabin — about 'not doing the talks' — and my butler discovered knee and elbow pads as well as a gallon of fire retardant."

"Whatever for?" asked Barksdale.

"Just in case I had to set myself on fire and leap out a window waving my arms," replied Fallon wistfully. "It always pays to be prepared."

"The switch was subtly done," I said, "but when I met the replaced Herring later on, he was polite and asked me if I wanted a doughnut — the real Herring would never have been so accommodating."

"I've heard enough," announced Senator Jobsworth, rising to his feet. "Send word that the peace talks are postponed. I want an emergency meeting of everyone in the debating chamber this evening, a press conference at five and the WomFic and Farquitt senators in my office the minute we get back. Barnes?"

"Yes, sir?"

"Implement Emergency Snooze Protocol 7B on the whole Farquitt canon *immediately*. I want every Farquitt reader yawning and nodding off in under ten minutes. We need to not only close down their feedback but send Daphne Farquitt a clear message that we will not be trifled with."

"What about the kittens?" asked Zhark in a shocked tone.

"It's a feline-compliant executive order," replied Jobsworth grandly. "No kittens will be harmed in the great Farquitt Snoozathon."

While Barnes and the rest of the D-3s scurried off to do Jobsworth's bidding, the senator and the others put their heads together. I told Fallon to go hide in his cabin until we got in, by which time he would doubtless be forgotten. He thanked me and gave me his card in case I needed someone to attempt to leap fourteen motorcycles in a double-decker bus or something, and Sprockett and I went and sat on the foredeck to watch the riverbank drift slowly past. Despite keeping a careful eye out for Herring, we saw only the upturned tender he had escaped in and figured that he was either making his escape to Farquitt or had been eaten by a crocodile who had mistaken him for fodder.

"Well," said Sprockett, "that denouement went very well. Your first?"

"Did it show?"

"Not at all."

I was glad of this. "I think Thursday might have been proud."

"Yes," agreed Sprockett, "I think she might."

39.
Story-Ending Options

To finish off your Character Exchange Program break, Thomas Cook (Book-World) Limited is offering tourists the option to choose how they would like to end their holidays. The "Chase" or "Scooby-Doo" endings remain popular, as do the "Death Scene" and "Reconciliation with Sworn Enemy." Traditionalists may be disappointed, though. The ever-popular "Riding Off into the Sunset" option has recently had to be withdrawn owing to irreconcilable cliché issues.

Bradshaw's BookWorld Companion
(15th edition)

The trip back downriver was uneventful and over in only twelve words. By the time the *Metaphoric Queen* had docked, the senator for Farquitt had already denied that her genre had anything to do with Herring's plan and expressed "great surprise" and "total outrage" that someone had "faked Romantic Troops" in order to attack the Fourteenth Clown. For its part, Comedy had mobilized its Second and Sixth Clown divisions to its borders and was demanding reparations from Farquitt, at the same time bringing pressure to bear on WomFic by threatening to withdraw all humor. Not to be outdone, Speedy Muffler had declared that the "presence of untapped metaphor" within his territory was "unproven and absurd," and he had so far refused all offers of commercial extraction contracts, further commenting that individual senators were welcome to see him personally in his "love train."

"Looks like it's business as usual," I said to Commander Bradshaw.

We were in the Jurisfiction offices at Norland Park, and I was having a lengthy debrief that same afternoon. I had entered the offices not as a bit player nor an apprentice but on my own merit. Emperor Zhark had awarded me a gift of some valuable jewelry that he said had been buried with his grandfather, Mr. Fainset doffed his cap in an agreeable manner, and Mrs. Tiggywinkle had kindly offered to do my laundry. It felt like I was part of the family.

"So what are you going to do now?" asked

Bradshaw, leaning back in his chair.

"I had a small mutiny in my series," I explained. "My own fault, really — I was thinking of Thursday and not my books. It'll need a lot of tact and diplomacy to win it back."

Bradshaw smiled and thought for a minute. "The BookWorld is falling apart at the seams," he said, waving his hand at the huge pile of paperwork in his in-tray. "We've got a major problem with e-books that we'd never envisioned. The Racy Novel–Farquitt affair will rumble on for years, and I'm sure we haven't heard the last of Red Herring. Ten Duplex-6s have gone missing, and everyone has escaped from *The Great Escape.*"

"How is that possible?"

"There was a fourth tunnel we didn't know about — Tom, Dick, Harry and *Keith.* There's a serial killer still at large, not to mention several character assassins — and that pink gorilla running around inside *A Tale of Two Cities* is really beginning to piss me off."

He took a sip of coffee and stared at me.

"I'm down to only seven agents. You've proved your capacity for this sort of work. I want you to join us here at Jurisfiction."

"No, no," I said quickly, "I've had quite

enough, thank you. The idea that people actually do this because *they like it* strikes me as double insanity with added insanity. Besides, you've already got a Thursday — you just have to find her. That reminds me." I dug Thursday's shield from my pocket and pushed it across the desk.

Bradshaw picked it up and rubbed his thumb against the smooth metal. "Where did you get this?"

"The red-haired man. I think Thursday knew she was compromised before she set off on her last trip and wanted me to carry on her work."

"So that's why he was out of his book," muttered Bradshaw. "I'll see him pardoned at the earliest opportunity."

Bradshaw looked at the badge, then at me. "So how do you think this story's going to end?"

"I don't know, sir."

"Are you sure you're not her?"

"It's a tricky one," I replied after giving the matter some thought, "and there's evidence to suppose that I am. I can do things only she can do, I can see some things that only she can see. Landen thought I was her, and although he now thinks I'm the written one, that might be part of a fevered delusion. His or mine, I'm not sure.

It's even possible I've been Owlcreeked."

Bradshaw knew what I was talking about. "Owlcreeking" was a Biercian device in which a character could spend the last few seconds of his life in a long-drawn-out digression of what might have happened had he lived. I might be at this very moment spiraling out of control in Mediocre's cab, Herring's coup still ahead of me and perfect in its unrevealed complexity.

"Carmine might actually be the Thursday I think I am," I added. "It's even possible I'm suffering the hallucinatory aftershock of a recent rewriting. And while we're pushing the plausibility envelope, the BookWorld might not be real at all, and maybe I'm simply an Acme carpet fitter with a vibrant imagination."

I shuddered with the possibility that none of this might be happening at all.

"This is Fiction," said Bradshaw in a calm voice, "and the truth is whatever you make it. You can interpret the situation in any way you want, and all versions could be real — and what's more, depending on how you act now, any one of those scenarios could *become* real."

I frowned. "I can be Thursday just by thinking I am?"

"More or less. We may require you to

undergo a short narrative procedure known as a 'Bobby Ewing,' where you wake up in the next chapter and it's all been a dream, but it's pretty painless so long as you don't mind any potential readers throwing up their hands in disgust."

"I can be Thursday?" I said again.

He nodded. "All you have to do is *know* you are. And don't deny that you've had some doubts over the past few days."

It was tempting. I could be her and do Thursday things and never have to worry about falling ReadRates, keeping Bowden in line or dealing with Pickwick. I could even have Landen and the kids. I looked around at the Jurisfiction office. The Red Queen was hopping mad as usual, Mr. Fainset was attempting to figure out why Tracy Capulet had locked her sister in a cupboard, Lady Cavendish was drafting an indictment against Red Herring for "impersonating a red herring when you're not one," and Emperor Zhark was putting together an interim peace deal for the Northern Genres. It looked enjoyable, relevant and a good use of anyone's time.

Commander Bradshaw smiled and pushed Thursday's shield back across the table, where I stared at it. "What do you say?"

"I can be Thursday," I said slowly. "I can

work at Jurisfiction. But at a *fictional* Jurisfiction. I want to depict the real Thursday doing everything she really did. I want her series to feature the BookWorld and you and Miss Havisham and Zhark and all the rest of them. *That's* where I'd like to be Thursday. That's the Thursday I can be. A *fictional* one. I'd like to help you out, but I can't."

Bradshaw looked at me for a long time.

"I *reluctantly* respect your decision to stay with your books," he said at last, "and I understand your wanting to tell it like it is. Naturally we're very grateful for everything you've done, but even if Jobsworth and I sign off on a Textual Flexation Certificate to change your series, I must point out that you can't truly be Thursday without Landen, and even if you get his permission, you still have to get Thursday's approval before you even begin to *think* about trying to change your series. And as far as we know, she may already be . . . dead."

He had trouble saying the final word and had to almost roll it around in his mouth before he could spit it out.

"She's not dead," I said firmly.

"I hope not, too. But without any leads — and we have none — it's going to be an onerous task to find her. Here in Fiction we have over a quarter of a billion titles. That's just one island in a BookWorld of two hundred and twenty-eight different and very distinct literary groupings. Most of those islands have fewer titles but some — like Nonfiction — have more. And then there are the foreign-language BookWorlds. Even if you are right — and I hope you are — Thursday could be anywhere from the Urdu translation of *Wuthering Heights* to the guarantee card on a 1965 Sunbeam Mixmaster."

"But you're still looking, right?"

"Of course. We rely on telemetry from our many unmanned probes that move throughout the BookWorld, all Textual Sieves have been set to pick her up if she makes a move, and Text Grand Central is keeping the waste gates on the imaginotransference engines on alert for a 'Thursday Next' word string. There's always hope, but there's a big BookWorld out there."

"If she's alive," I said in a resolute tone, "I can find her."

"If you do," said Bradshaw with a smile, "you can change whatever you want in your book — even introduce the Toast Marketing Board."

I started. "You heard about that?"

He smiled. "We hear about *everything.*

Take the shield. Use her rights and privileges. You might need them. And if you change your mind and want to be her, call me."

I picked up the badge from the table and put it in my pocket.

"Commander?" said the Red Queen, who had been hovering and stepped in when she saw that our conversation was at an end. "Text Grand Central has reported a major narrative flexation over in Shakespeare. It seems Othello has murdered his wife."

"Again? I do wish that trollop Desdemona would be more careful when she's fooling around. What is it this time? Incriminating love letters?"

The Red Queen looked at her notes. "No, it seems there was this handkerchief —"

"Hell's teeth!" yelled Bradshaw in frustration. "Do I have to do everything around here? I want Iago in my office in ten minutes."

"He's doing that spinoff with Hamlet," said Mr. Fainset from across the room.

"*Iago v. Hamlet*? They got the green light for that?"

"Shylock bankrolled their appeal and got Portia to represent them. They were seriously pissed off about the mandatory European directive of 'give me my .453 kilo of flesh' — hence the anti-European subplot in *Iago v. Hamlet.*"

"Get him to see me as soon as he can. What is it, Mr. Fainset?"

"The Unread, sir."

"Causing trouble again?"

"They're all over Horror like cheap perfume."

I moved off, as tales of the Unread gave me the spooks. Most characters who were long unread either made themselves useful like Bradshaw or went into a downward spiral of increased torpidity. Others, for some unknown reason, went bad and became the Unread. They festered in dark alleys, in holes in the ground, the crevices between paragraphs — anywhere they could leap out and ensnare characters and suck the reading light out of them. Even grammasites, goblins and the Danvers avoided them.

I moved away. Bradshaw was busy, and my debrief was over. Thursday was missed, but Jurisfiction's work couldn't stop just so it could utilize its full resources to find her. It would be the same for any one of them, and they all knew it.

I walked across to Thursday's desk and rested my fingertips on the smooth oak surface. The desk was clean and, aside from a SpecOps mug, a picture of Landen, a stack of messages and a goodly caseload in the in-basket, fairly tidy. I looked at the worn chair but didn't sit down. This wasn't my desk. I opened the drawers but could find little of relevance, which wasn't hard — I didn't know what would *be* relevant.

I stepped outside the Jurisfiction offices and found the frog-footman dozing on a chair in the lobby.

"Wesley?"

He started at hearing his name called and almost fell off the chair in surprise. "Miss Next?"

"Where do I requisition a vehicle?"

His eyes lit up. "We have a large choice. What would you like?"

"A hover car," I said, having always wanted to ride in one. "A convertible."

I picked up Sprockett, who had been waiting outside, and soon we were heading west out of HumDram/Classics in a Zharkian Bubble-Drive Hovermatic. We arrived over Thriller within a few minutes and flew slowly over the area in which *The Murders on the Hareng Rouge* had come down almost a week ago. If Thursday had survived the sabotage, she would have landed somewhere within the half million or so novels along the debris trail.

If Thursday had survived, I reasoned, the cab had come down more or less intact. No one had reported the remains of a taxi falling to earth, and I wanted to know why. We flew up and down the area of the debris trail for a while, searching for even the merest clue of what might have happened but seeing nothing except an endless landscape of novels. We were yelled at several times by cabbies annoyed that we were "hovering about like a bunch of numpties," and on one occasion we were pulled over by a Thriller border guard and made to explain why we were loitering. I flashed Thursday's badge, and he apologized and moved on.

"What are we looking for, ma'am?"

"I wish I knew."

I had a thought and took out my notebook to remind me what Landen had told me when I spoke to him in Fan Fiction.

He had stated that in an emergency, Thursday would try to contact me. As far as I knew, she hadn't. She had also said, *The circumstances of your confusion will be your path to enlightenment.*

I stared at the sentence for a long time, then took my *Bradshaw's BookWorld Companion* from my bag and flicked to the map section at the back. And then all was light.

She *had* been contacting me, and my confusion was indeed the answer.

"Bingo," I said softly.

40.
Thursday Next

A trip to Text Grand Central is a must for the technophile, and a day spent on one of the main imaginotransference-engine floors is not to be missed. A visit will dispel forever the notion that those at TGC do little to smooth out the throughputting of the story to the reader's imagination. Tours around the Reader Feedback Loop are available on Tuesday afternoons, but owing to the sometimes hazardous nature of feedback, exposure is limited to eighteen seconds.

Bradshaw's BookWorld Companion
(15th edition)

It took nearly an hour to find what we were looking for. Sandwiched between Political Thriller and Spy Thriller and well within the condemned book's debris trail was Psychological Thriller. The whole "Am I really Thursday?" stuff I'd been laboring through over the past few days had all the hallmarks of a PsychoThriller plot device and made total sense of Thursday's obscure "confusion enlightenment" sentence.

Finding the genre, however, was harder. It was difficult to spot from the air, as a sense of ambiguity blurred the edges of the small genre, and with good reason. Psychological was another "rogue genre" where nothing could be taken at face value, trusted or even believed, a genre whose very raison d'être was to confuse and obfuscate. Often accused of harboring known felons and offering safe haven to deposed leaders of other rogue genres, PsychoThriller could never be directly indicted, as nothing was ever quite what it seemed — a trait it shared with others that also had a tenuous hold on reality, such as Creative Accounting and Lies to Tell Your Partner When S/He Finds Underwear in the Glove Box.

We found it by using our small onboard Textual Sieve to home in on a trail of confused reader feedback, and Sprockett expertly brought us in for a landing at the corner of Forsyth and Ludlum. We walked across a vacant lot to the unfenced border of Psychological Thriller. The weather, naturally, was atmospheric. On the Thriller side of the border, the skies were clear, but across into Psychological there seemed to be an impenetrable wall of rain-soaked air. Jurisfiction had considerately posted signs along the border at regular intervals, warning trespassers to stay away or potentially suffer "lethal levels of bewilderment." Only fools or the very brave ventured into Psychological Thriller alone.

"Ma'am?" said Sprockett, his eyebrow flickering "Alarm."

"Problems?"

"You find me hugely embarrassed."

"What is it? You need winding?"

"No, ma'am. It's the damp. Humans might fear viruses and old age, two things with which cog-based life-forms have very little issue. But when it comes to corrosion, honey, magnets and damp, I'm afraid to say I must warn you that a rebuild might be necessary, and spare parts are becoming scandalously expensive."

"It's all right," I said. "Just wait for me here."

I stepped across. Inside Psychological Thriller it was raining, and night. The cold wind lashed my face and drove the rain into every crevice of my clothes, until within a very short period I was soaked through. The tops of the trees swayed dangerously in the wind, and every now and then there was a flash of lightning followed by a splintering crack and the sound of a tree falling with a muffled crash somewhere in the dark.

I moved on, occasionally sinking ankle-deep in the marshy ground. After a few hundred yards, I came to a small clearing of tussock grass, pools of brackish water and a scattering of broken branches. On the far side, partially immersed in ooze, were the remains of a TransGenre Taxi. The front had been staved in, the engine torn out and the bodywork rippled and bent. Scraps of tree had been caught in the side mirrors as the taxi tore through the foliage on its way down. While I stared at the mangled wreck, the lightning flashed, and on the side was painted NO TIPS and, farther along, 1517. It was Thursday's cab.

I hurried round to see if anyone had survived. I was perhaps in too much haste and swiftly sank up to my thighs in the fetid waters. I extricated myself with a considerable amount of grunting and swearing and finally made my way to the taxi and peered in. The rear door was open and the empty backseat scattered with papers, mostly about the geology under Racy Novel. The Mediocre Gatsby was still sitting in the front seat, impaled on the steering column. He had been killed by a bad case of selective nostalgia. For some peculiar reason, all TransGenre Taxis were modeled on the 1950s yellow Checker Cab design, at a time when safety standards were nonexistent and fatal accidents embraced by Detroit with an alarming level of indifference. The "hose down the dash and sell it to the next man" attitude pervaded all the way into the BookWorld, and not without good reason. In here there was always a battle between nostalgia and safety, and nostalgia usually won.

I stood up, pushed the wet hair out of my eyes and tried to think what might have happened. As I stared in turn at the taxi, the empty backseat and the remains of Mediocre Gatsby, I suddenly had a thought: The rear door had been open when I got here. I looked around to see where I might have gone if I'd found myself unceremoniously dumped in the middle of a rainy swamp at night, possibly injured and very alone. I took the most obvious way out of the marsh and managed to find a path to higher ground. I followed the trail as best as I could, and after stumbling through the forest for a few hundred yards in a generally uphill direction I came across a doorway in a high brick wall, upon the top of which were the remains of a corroded electrified fence. Attached to the brick wall was a weathered wooden board telling me to keep away from THE WILFRED D. AKRON HOME FOR THE CRIMINALLY INSANE.

If I had been real, I would doubtless have been more nervous than I was, but this was Psychological Thriller, and secure hospitals for the criminally insane were pretty much a dime a dozen, and rarely secure. I found myself in a small and very overgrown graveyard, the lichen-encrusted stones leaning with a frightening level of apparent randomness. I moved through the graveyard towards a mausoleum built of brick and stone but in an advanced state of decay. If I had crash-landed here in the taxi, this is where I would have sought shelter.

The double doors were bronze, heavy and streaked green with age. There was a hole about three feet wide in the middle, so both doors looked as though they had a semicircle cut from each. My foot knocked against something. It was Thursday's well-worn pistol, her name engraved on the barrel — the hole in the locked doors had been blasted out for access. I was getting close. I carefully climbed through the hole and pushed my rain-soaked hair from my face. It was light enough to see, and below the broken skylight was a table that had once held flowers but was now a collection of dirty vases. There were a few personal items scattered about — a picture of Landen and the kids, a five-pound note, an Acme Carpets ID.

"It's difficult to know sometimes who you are, isn't it?"

I turned to see the small figure of a girl aged no more than eight standing in a shaft of light that seemed to descend vertically from the roof.

"Hello, Jenny," I said.

"Did anyone figure you out?" she asked. "Hiding in plain sight as the written version of you. How did the written Thursday feel about taking a backseat for a while? And where is she, by the way?"

"I'm really Thursday?" I asked.

"Oh, yes," replied Jenny with a chuckle. "Doesn't it all seem so obvious now?"

Two days ago I might have believed her.

"No," I replied. "You see, I spoke to Landen, and he told me I vanished from the RealWorld as a good bookperson might do, so don't give me any of your Psychological Thriller bullshit."

"O-o-o-kay," said Jenny, thinking quickly, "how about this: You're actually just witnessing —"

"Don't even *think* to try Owlcreeking me. And while we're at it, you're not Jenny."

"Is she giving you any trouble?" said another voice I recognized.

"A little," said Jenny, and Sprockett — or a reasonable facsimile of him — appeared from out of the shadows. I sighed. My mother would be appearing next, and then probably myself. It was all becoming a little tedious.

"Did you try her on the *You really are Thursday* twist ending?" asked Sprockett.

"She didn't buy it. I tried the *It's all in your last moment before dying* gambit, too."

Ersatz Sprockett thought for a moment. "What about the *You're actually a patient in a mental hospital and we've been enacting all this to try to find out if you killed Thursday*? That usually works."

"Goodness," said Faux Jenny, "I'd clean forgotten about that one."

"And now that you've told me," I said, "I'm hardly likely to go for it, am I?"

"Well done, Einstein," said Faux Jenny to her partner in a sarcastic tone. "Any other bright ideas?"

Ersatz Sprockett looked at me, then at Faux Jenny, then tried to telegraph an idea across to her in a very lame portrayal of someone being in a shower.

"Oh!" said Faux Jenny as she twigged to what he was talking about. "Good idea."

But I had figured it out, too.

"You wouldn't be thinking about pulling a Bobby Ewing on me, would you?"

And they both swore under their breath.

"Well," grumbled Ersatz Sprockett with a shrug, "that's me, clean out of ideas."

And as I watched, they reverted to the strangely misshapen shape-changers who skulked around Psychological Thriller, hoping to trap unwary travelers into thinking they had once been homicidal maniacs but now had amnesia and all their previous visions depicted in horrific nightmares were actually recovered memories. In a word, they were a pair of utter *nuisances.*

"Thank heavens for that," I said. "Let's get down to business. Where is Thursday, and why didn't you report her presence here to Jurisfiction?"

"We send so many conflicting and utterly bizarre plot lines out of the genre that everyone ignores us," said Shifter Once Jenny sadly. "I think Jurisfiction set our messages to 'auto-ignore.' "

"For good reason," I replied. "You're only marginally less troublesome than Conspiracy."

"That's why Thursday asked us to transmit all those ambiguities direct to you. We were hoping you'd get here sooner than this.

We peppered you with as much confusion as we could, but you didn't pick it up."

If I'd been Thursday, I would have. Being confused over identity had been a mainstay of Psychological Thriller for years. I had a lot to learn.

"I'm new to this."

"You'll get the hang of it."

"I hope not. Where is she?"

"In that antechamber."

I turned and followed a short corridor to where there was a small room off the main mausoleum. It was obviously where the shape-changers usually lived, as there were posters of Faceache on the wall. They had given over the one bed to Thursday, who was lying on her back. The room was lit by a gas lantern, and by its flickering jet I could see that she was in a bad state. There was an ugly bruise on her face, and one eye was red with blood. She moved her head to look at me, and I saw her eyes glisten.

"Hey," I said.

"Hey," said Thursday in a weak voice.

I placed my hand on her forehead. It was hot.

"How are you feeling?" I asked.

She gave a faint smile and shrugged, but she winced when she did it.

"Landen?" she whispered.

"He's fine. Kids, too."

"Tell them —"

"Tell them yourself."

I stood up. I had to get her to *Gray's Anatomy* as soon as possible. There was an umbrella in a stand at the door, and I picked it up.

"Thursday? I'm going to fetch someone who can carry you out of here. My butler. I'll be ten minutes."

"You have a butler?" she managed.

"Yes," I replied in a chirpy voice in order to hide my concern. "*Everyone* needs a butler."

41.
The End of the Book

About the author: Commander Bradshaw has been one of the stalwarts of Jurisfiction for over fifty years and has been the Bellman an unprecedented eight times. Hailing from a long-unread branch of British imperialist fiction, he now divides his time between Jurisfiction duties, his lovely wife, Melanie, and continually updating the *BookWorld Companion,* which remains the definitive work on the BookWorld and everything in it.

Bradshaw's BookWorld Companion
(17th edition)

I flew the Hovermatic home from *Gray's Anatomy* two hours later, but Sprockett and I said nothing on the trip. I was quiet because I was thinking about Thursday, and what a close call it had been. She had a fractured skull, a broken femur and eight breaks to her left arm and hand. There were multiple lacerations, a loss of blood, fever and a concussion. Henry Gray himself took charge and whisked her into surgery almost the moment I arrived. Within ten minutes the waiting room was full of concerned well-wishers, Bradshaw and Zhark amongst them. I knew she was in good hands, so I'd quietly slipped away as soon as I heard she was out of danger.

I was quiet also because I had averted a war and saved many lives today, and that's a peculiar feeling that's difficult to describe. Sprockett was quiet, too — but only because I had inadvertently allowed his spring to run down, and he had shut off all functions except thought, and he was thinking mildly erotic thoughts about bevel gears and how nice it might be to have a flywheel fitted in order to give him a little more oomph in the mornings.

The first thing I saw when I got back to my house was Bowden, dressed up as me.

"This isn't how it appears," he said in the same tone of voice he'd used when I found him looking through my underwear drawer the year before. He told me then that he'd "heard a mouse," but I didn't believe him.

"How *should* it appear if you're dressed up in my clothes?"

"Carmine's goblin ran off with a

goblinette, and she locked herself in the bathroom again. I'm standing in for her. *You.* I've just done a scene with myself. It was most odd."

"How many readers we got?" I asked.

"Six."

"You can handle it."

"Oh!" said Bowden, in the manner of one who is pretending to be disappointed but is actually delighted. "If I must. But who will play me?"

"I will," came a voice from the door. I turned to find Whitby Jett standing there.

"Whitby?"

"How's my little Thursday?"

"She's good. But . . . what about the nuns?"

"A misunderstanding," he said. "I hadn't set fire to any of them, as it turned out."

I stepped forward and touched his chest. I could feel that the guilt had lifted. He'd managed to move the damaging back-story on.

"I'm going to mix some cocktails," announced Sprockett, and he buzzed from the room.

"Make mine a Sidcup Sling, Sprocky old boy," said Jett. "Bowden — where are my lines?"

"Here!" said Bowden, passing him a well-thumbed script.

"Whitby?"

"Yes, muffin?"

"Are you busy right now?"

"Only selling useless rubbish for EZ-Read. Why?"

"Nothing." I smiled, but there *was* something. Whitby could play Landen beautifully.

He and Bowden both went off to play a scene in the SpecOps Building, leaving me to sit at the kitchen table trying to figure out if I could have found Thursday earlier. If I'd had more experience, probably.

Pickwick stuck her head around the door and looked relieved when she saw me.

"Thank goodness!" she said. "I can't tell you what a disaster it's been. They threatened to tape my beak shut if I didn't join them. Your father was the ringleader — along with Carmine, of course. She'll come to a sticky end, I can tell you."

"She'll be fine," I said, feeling magnanimous. Carmine had problems, but so did we all. "Make the tea, will you?"

"Isn't that why we have a butler?"

I stared at her and raised an eyebrow.

"So . . . milk and one sugar, right?"

And she waddled into the kitchen to try to figure out which object was the kettle.

"May I come in?"

It was the character who played my father. He was quite unlike his usual abrasive self and seemed almost painfully eager to be friendly.

"Hello, Thursday," he said. "Is . . . that chair comfortable?"

"Don't sweat it," I said, almost embarrassed to see him like this. "I'm going to make some radical changes to your character. It's very simple: Do the new scenes or you can have a transfer. Take it or leave it."

He thought about it for a moment, mumbled something about how he would "look forward to seeing his new lines" and made some excuse before departing.

Pickwick came back in. "The tea is in the jar marked 'tea,' right?"

"Right."

The doorbell rang. It was Emperor Zhark.

"Good evening, Your Mercilessness," I said, opening the door wide. "Come on in and have a cocktail. My man does a Gooseberry Flip so strong it will make your toes swell."

"That's a figure of speech, right?"

"Not at all. Your toes really do swell — to the size of apples."

"I won't, thank you. I'm actually here on business. Do you have an automaton living here, name of Sprockett?"

I think my heart might almost have stopped.

"What is it?" I asked. "What's going on?"

"I am ready, sir."

It was Sprockett. He had his overcoat on and had packed his oils and a spare knee joint, just in case.

"Wait a minute," I said, "you can't take him away. He has a job with me. I'll sign any papers you want."

"Ma'am," said Sprockett, "I am no longer in your employ. If you recall, you gave me glowing references and relieved me of my duties. Emperor, may we go?"

The emperor moved to the door, but I wasn't done.

"Emperor," I said, "I don't wish to appear above my station, but I do feel that a simple work-permit violation could be overlooked on this occasion."

Zhark told Sprockett to get into his car and turned back to me.

"Miss Next," he said in a firm voice, "your butler might be the perfect Thursday's Friday, but he is far too dangerous to allow to remain at liberty. All those laws of robotics you've heard of are pretty much baloney. Good evening, Miss Next, and I'm sorry."

And he turned in a sweep of black velvet

and strode up to his waiting limousine, leaving me shaking with frustration until I had a thought.

"Wait!"

I ran up to the limousine's window.

"This crime," I said, "did it have anything to do with nuns?"

"And puppies," said Zhark with a shudder. "Frightful business."

"You stay right here. Don't move. Understand?"

I think Emperor Zhark started to respect me just then. Not just as a Thursday but as a person. Either that or he was used to taking orders from angry women.

Whitby and Bowden were in the SpecOps office, talking about Hades. I'd found Carmine looking in the fridge for something to eat, and she did a mid-read changeover with Whitby. I took him by the hand and pushed him into an adjoining room. I'll admit it. I was angry.

"What the hell do you think you're doing?" I demanded.

"A scene with Bowden. You told me to."

"Not *that*. I'm talking about Sprockett and the incident with the nuns. What were you doing?"

He shrugged. "Listen, muffin, he approached *me*. Said he'd take on my backstory so you'd be happy. What am I going to do? Turn him down? I want you and me to be happy, pumpkin, and we'll always be thankful to it for such a selfless act."

"Not 'it' — *him*."

I stared at him and shook my head, and he knew then that however much I liked him, I couldn't let it happen this way, and neither could he. He leaned forward and kissed me on the cheek, and I could feel my eyes fill with tears.

"Listen, Whitby, you'll find a way of getting rid of it."

"Yes," he said, "and when I do —"

"You'll know where to find me."

He smiled a wan smile and walked out the door. I wiped my eyes and went and sat down in the kitchen to stare at the wall.

"Here," said Pickwick, panting with the exertion, "your tea."

She pushed it across the table with her beak, and I picked it up.

"Oh," I said, "it's gone cold."

"It was supposed to be hot?"

"No, actually, this is good. Thank you, Pickers."

"That's a relief. What's for dinner? I'm starving after all that tea making. It really takes it out of you."

"Mrs. Malaprop suggested a macarena

cheese," came a voice from the doorway. I turned to see Sprockett standing tall and as straight as a poker, every bit the perfect butler.

I ran across and gave him a hug. He was hard and cold, and although he was outwardly emotionless, deep within him I could hear his cogs speed up as I squeezed.

"Madam, *please,*" he said, faintly embarrassed.

"Thank you, Sprockett," I said. "For everything."

The automaton inclined his head politely, but my eyes were fixed on his eyebrow to see what it would do. I wanted to see what loyal friendship meant to him — whether a man of cogs, dials, chains and sprockets could *really* feel as humans feel.

But I was to be disappointed. He pressed a white-gloved finger to his eyebrow, blocking any movement. All I could see in his face was blank molded porcelain, two lenses for eyes and a slot through which he spoke.

"May I ask a question, ma'am?"

"Of course."

"Was it a compassionate act to take over Whitby's backstory to enable you to be together?"

"Yes."

"I believe I have learned something of

value here today, ma'am. But what made Whitby retake the backstory?"

"He knew it was the right thing to do."

Sprockett buzzed briefly to himself. "Does that sort of thing happen out there in the RealWorld, or is it just in books?"

I thought for a moment. Of the untidy chaos I had seen in the RealWorld; of not knowing what was going to happen; of not knowing what, if anything, had relevance. The RealWorld was a sprawling mess of a book in need of a good editor. I thought then of the narrative order here in the BookWorld, our resolved plot lines and the observance of natural justice we took for granted.

"Literature is claimed to be a mirror of the world," I said, "but the Outlanders are fooling themselves. The BookWorld is as orderly as people in the RealWorld *hope* their own world to be — it isn't a mirror, it's an aspiration."

"Humans," said Sprockett, "are the most gloriously bizarre creatures."

"Yes," I said with a smile. "They certainly are."

ACKNOWLEDGMENTS

First, my thanks to Carolyn Mays and Josh Kendall and all the team at Hodder and Viking for their steadfast support and understanding during the final stages of the book, where events of a daughtering nature conspired to render the manuscript past the ideal delivery time.

My thanks to Dr. John Wooten for his valuable contributions to the understanding of Nextian Physics, and for being at the end of an e-mail if I had a query with regard to the best way to mangle physics while still looking vaguely correct.

The illustrations were drawn by Bill Mudron and Dylan Meconis of Portland, Oregon, and they have, as usual, surpassed themselves in their depiction of the Nextian Universe. Bill can be found at www.excelsiorstudios.net and Dylan at www.dylanmeconis.com.

My apologies to the many, many authors

who have used the "hollow earth" notion as the setting for a book. It *must* have been done before, and I would expect the mechanics of how it functions would be universal, as the concept has a tendency to write itself. In case of unavoidable parallels, my apologies.

BookWorld cartographers. My thanks to the following for submitting wonderful ideas to me about the possible shape and layout of Fiction Island: Alex Maunders, Robert Persson, Laura, Catherine Fitzsimons, Geoffrey Elliot-Howell, Michael O'Connor, Ellie Randall, Steve James, Elizabeth Walter, Derek Walter, Theresa Porst, Sarah Porter, Dhana Sabanathan, Alex Clark, Loraine Weston, Elisabeth Parsons, Jane Ren, Birgit Prihodko and Helen Griin-Looveer.

I am also indebted to my new agents, Will Francis and Claire Paterson, who have filled Tif's recently vacated shoes with an aplomb and unswerving professionalism of which I know she would approve.

No thanks would be complete without special mention of Mari, whose constant and overwhelming support allows me to function as a vaguely sentient creature rather than a mass of quivering jelly. I would also like to thank Ingrid and Ian for much support when we needed it, and finally thanks to my in-laws, Maggy and Stewart, for help and assistance on occasions too numerous to mention.

This book took 108 days to write between December 22, 2009, and September 3, 2010. It was written on a Mac Pro using Pages software. I've been Mac since 1995, when it was OS 7.9.2, and I have used Apple writing software on all my projects. During the writing I consumed thirty-two gallons of coffee, eighteen gallons of tea, and I walked 192 miles. The filing backed up to a depth of seven and a half inches, and I received 1,672 e-mails and sent 380. The average daytime temperature was 9.2 degrees Celsius and I burned 1.2 tons of logs in my wood burner. In that time I lost a faithful hound but gained a fourth daughter.

Jasper Fforde
September 2010

We hope you have enjoyed this Large Print book. Other Thorndike, Wheeler, and Chivers Press Large Print books are available at your library or directly from the publishers.

For information about current and upcoming titles, please call or write, without obligation, to:

Publisher
Thorndike Press
295 Kennedy Memorial Drive
Waterville, ME 04901
Tel. (800) 223-1244

or visit our Web site at:

http://gale.cengage.com/thorndike

OR

Chivers Large Print
published by BBC Audiobooks Ltd
St James House, The Square
Lower Bristol Road
Bath BA2 3SB
England
Tel. +44(0) 800 136919
email: bbcaudiobooks@bbc.co.uk
www.bbcaudiobooks.co.uk

All our Large Print titles are designed for easy reading, and all our books are made to last.

GOWER PENINSULA

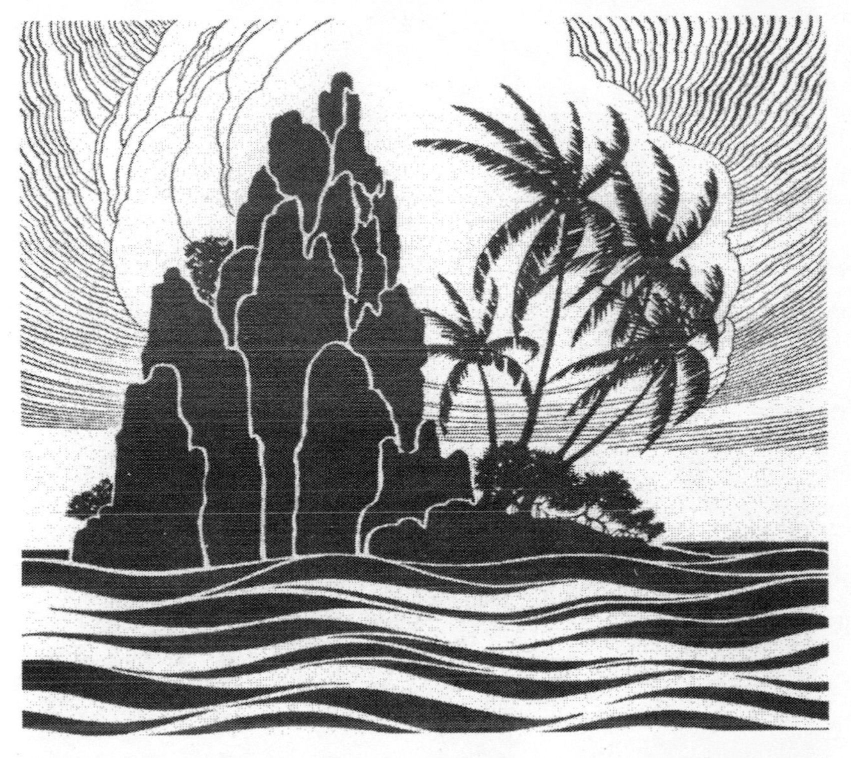

Socialist Republic of Wales

Not *always* raining.

See your local tourist office for details.

Advertisement in *The Word*, August 1915

Congratulations!

Jurisfiction offers its heartfelt thanks and admiration to Mr. Buñuel and the engineers and designers at the Book-World Maintenance Facility for the successful completion of the main footnoterphone trans-genre trunk line between *Human Drama* and *Crime*. August 23, 1915.

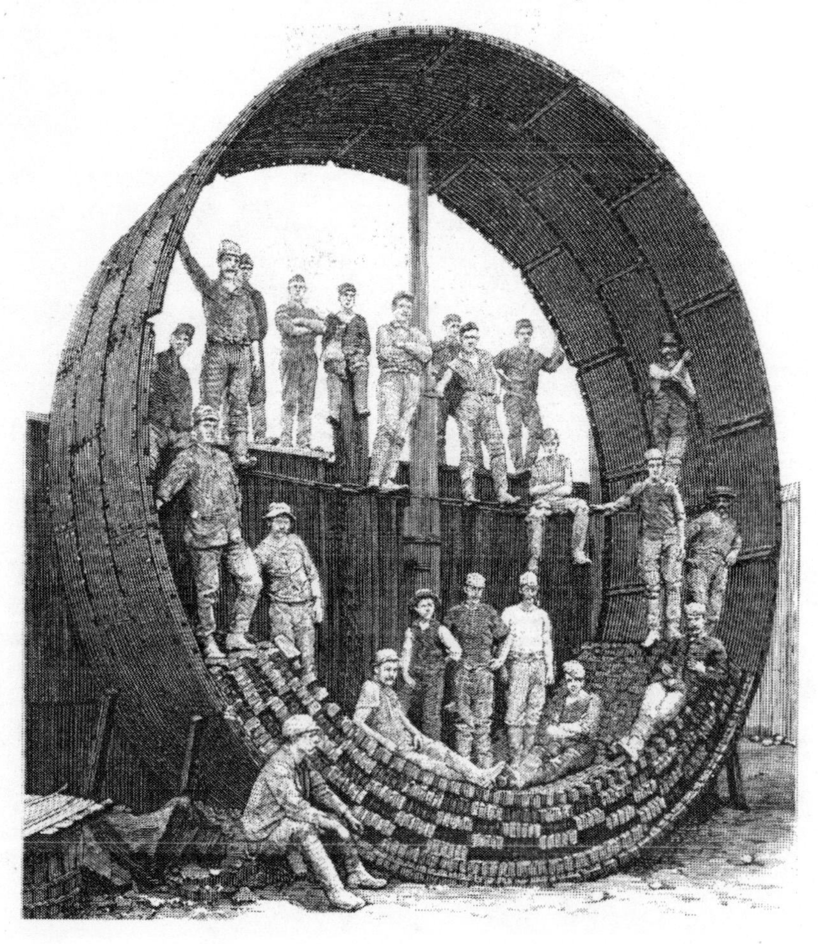

Workers relax on a prefabricated section of footnoterphone conduit.

The Textbook of Children's and Young People's Nursing

Second Edition

Tina Moules
Head of Department of Advanced Practice and Research
Faculty of Health and Social Care
Anglia Ruskin University
UK

and

Joan Ramsay
Associate Director of Nursing
Women and Children's Division
Musgrove Park Hospital
Somerset
UK

with contributions from

Judith Hendrick
Law Department
Oxford Brookes University
Headington
Oxford
UK

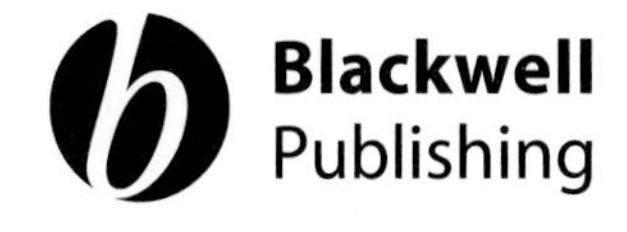

Blackwell Publishing editorial offices:
Blackwell Publishing Ltd, 9600 Garsington Road, Oxford OX4 2DQ, UK
Tel: +44 (0)1865 776868
Blackwell Publishing Inc., 350 Main Street, Malden, MA 02148-5020, USA
Tel: +1 781 388 8250
Blackwell Publishing Asia Pty Ltd, 550 Swanston Street, Carlton, Victoria 3053, Australia
Tel: +61 (0)3 8359 1011

First published 1998 by Nelson Thornes Ltd
Second edition published 2008 by Blackwell Publishing Ltd

ISBN: 978-1-4051-7093-2

Library of Congress Cataloging-in-Publication Data

Moules, Tina.
The textbook of children's and young people's nursing / Tina Moules and Joan Ramsay. – 2nd ed.
p. ; cm.
Rev. ed. of: The textbook of children's nursing / Tina Moules and Joan Ramsay. 1998.
Includes bibliographical *References* and index.
ISBN: 978-1-4051-7093-2 (pbk. : alk. paper)
1. Pediatric nursing–Textbooks. I. Ramsay, Joan, RGN. II. Moules, Tina. Textbook of children's nursing. III. Title.
[DNLM: 1. Pediatric Nursing. WY 159 M926t 2007]
RJ245.M683 2007
618.92′00231–dc22

2007013108

A catalogue record for this title is available from the British Library

Set in 9.5/11.5pt Sabon by Graphicraft Limited, Hong Kong
Printed and bound in Singapore by Fabulous Printers Pte Ltd

The publisher's policy is to use permanent paper from mills that operate a sustainable forestry policy, and which has been manufactured from pulp processed using acid-free and elementary chlorine-free practices. Furthermore, the publisher ensures that the text paper and cover board used have met acceptable environmental accreditation standards.

For further information on Blackwell Publishing, visit our website: www.blackwellnursing.com

Contents

Preface to Second Edition

This second edition has been written not only to meet the interest in and demand for the first edition but also to reflect the vast changes in health care, which have affected children's nursing since the late 1990s. The government has emphasised the quality of patients' experience of health care, involving them much more in the development of local healthcare services and providing them with clear information about the choices of treatment that are available and the location of treatment. They have also emphasised the needs of children as important individuals and not merely small adults. The National Service Framework for Children set standards for children's health and social care for the first time, which promote quality child-centred care that meets the needs of children, parents and families. 'Every Child Matters' is a series of documents that set out the government's commitment to improving outcomes for all children and young people, including the most disadvantaged, in all aspects of children's lives – health, education, social care and the criminal justice system. The Children Act 2004 broadened the remit of child-protection processes and introduced the concept of safeguarding children. This second edition of *The Textbook of Children's and Young People's Nursing* has included these changes throughout the text so the reader can appreciate how government policy affects practice.

Changes in the authors' professional lives have also influenced the second edition. Tina has completed her doctoral study in which she undertook participatory research with young people as co-researchers. Together they explored the role of children and young people in monitoring the quality of care in hospital. Tina has been able to use the experiences and findings from her research in the text to stimulate you to use children's views to help you develop your own areas of children's nursing.

Joan now has a wider management role, which encompasses women's services as well as those for children. This has prompted her to include a new chapter on sexuality problems of adolescence as the increase in teenage sexually transmitted infections and pregnancies relates so closely to children's nursing. This new content aims to promote your interest in this area to enable closer links with maternity and genito-urinary services. Joan also now has a lead role in risk management in her division. This is becoming increasingly important in health care and the new content on risk management should enable you to appreciate the importance of preventing risks and learning from incidents.

Preface to First Edition

> Give a man a fish and you feed him for a day
> Teach a man to fish and you feed him for life
>
> Old Chinese Proverb

This book does not merely give you facts about children's nursing because it aims to teach you how to nurse children in a way that you can remember and apply to any child in your care. It has been written to enable you to explore many different aspects of children's nursing and to actually participate in the learning process by undertaking various activities within the text. We encourage you to add your own notes, either within the text or, if you prefer, in a separate notebook. This idea is based on the philosophy that learning is an active process and occurs more effectively if the learner is actively involved. Because learning is a life-long process, you are encouraged to review the content at a later stage and explore how it has changed. By adding your own thoughts about these changes you will prolong the life of the content and build up a valuable resource of past and current issues.

The book does not profess to give you all the answers. In fact it should stimulate you to ask more questions and to reflect upon your experiences, past and present. The content is structured on a modular format and will provide you with a wealth of literature and a number of learning outcomes, and is divided into parts which can be studied separately, thus allowing you to study at your own pace. You can also choose to use the book as part of a course of study, in which case the modular format could be used to structure your learning.

The book has a strong emphasis on the differing roles of the children's nurse and in particular the role as a health promoter. This is an important role of the children's nurse so that children can be helped to achieve their full potential. The caring role of the children's nurse is complex requiring you to use your skills to make reasonable judgements and decisions about the needs of children of varying ages and levels of development. The book aims to help you in this problem-solving process by encouraging reflection, critical analysis and exploration.

Acknowledgements

The idea for the first edition of this book was conceived on a beach near Herstmonceux in East Sussex many years ago and signed and sealed over a bottle of good red wine. It came to fruition through the dedication of our dear friend and editor Rosemary Morris. Rosemary supported us with her patience, persistence, sense of humour and her continued belief in us. She continued to give us encouragement even through her own difficult times. Rosemary – we continue to be grateful for the support you gave us then. And now we thank Lisa Fraley for initiating this second edition, for her continued faith in our ability to meet her very tight deadlines, and her patience and support in helping us to do so.

We also need to thank Judith Hendrick once again for updating the section on legal and ethical issues. Judith's knowledge and expertise (and her ability to keep to our deadlines) continues to be invaluable.

Several other colleagues have helped us bring this second edition to fruition and we would like to acknowledge their contributions:

Debbie Steele undertook to update Module 3 in a very short space of time. Tanya McFerran, Senior Lecturer in Child, Youth and Family Studies at Anglia Ruskin, updated much of Module 2. Jon Wheater helped to update Chapters 37, 38, 42, 43 and 44 of Module 6. Jon is a Senior Lecturer in Child, Youth and Family Studies at Anglia Ruskin University. Sue Skinner updated Chapter 49 of Module 6. Sue is a Senior Lecturer at Anglia Ruskin University and is Pathway Leader Special and Intensive Care of the Newborn.

Thank you to all of you for your hard work and support.

I would especially like to thank my husband Eddy for his continued support. He has been very tolerant particularly because, after the first edition, I spent the next 6 years doing my doctorate. He has never ceased to have faith in me and he provides me with the motivation to get things done. When I started to write the first edition my children (Tom and Kate) were 7 and 4, respectively. Now Tom is 17 and Kate is 14 and I am faced with the challenges of keeping a cool head in the face of teenage trials and tribulations! Thank you, both of you, for your love and support. The safe delivery of two step-grandchildren (aged 3 and 7), nieces to Tom and Kate, since the first edition has provided me, like Joan, with a different perspective. Finally I thank all my colleagues at Anglia Ruskin University for their support.

Thank you all
Tina

I would like to thank my husband Alex for his continued support by giving up his evenings with the computer to allow me time to type, by tolerating the piles of paper in the study as I collected more and more reference material, and for accepting my refusals to go out at weekends until I had completed my typing! When I wrote the first edition my daughter Helen provided inspiration for problems of adolescence! Now she is married with a daughter of her own. I would like to thank her and her husband for producing my much-loved granddaughter, Nicole. As new parents with a healthy young child they have provided a different source of inspiration for this new edition. Finally I would like to thank all my colleagues at Musgrove Park Hospital for providing me with ideas and support.

Thank you all
Joan

Part 1

Health in Childhood

Module 1
Understanding Families

Tina Moules

Learning Outcomes

The material contained within this module and the further reading/references should enable you to:

- explore the nature of the family with special reference to the changes that have occurred in its structure
- analyse the nature of relationships and roles within families and the factors that influence family life
- consider critically the role of the family in the development of children
- analyse different child-rearing patterns

Introduction

'For most people the family is by far the most significant institution in terms of the impact it has on the quality of their daily life and experience' (White and Woollett, 1992).

Many different types of family structure exist in the UK today, influenced by cultural and social factors. Children are born into and grow up in these units and, as such, develop within the context of the family and have an impact on the family themselves. Debates about the state of the family have been numerous in recent years as changing social constructs have led to changes in family structures and the social 'norm'. Thus children's worlds change as they adapt to cope with, for example, divorce, parents who work, reconstituted families and lone-parent families. It is vital that children's nurses have an understanding of the nature of the family and its role in the development and lives of children, so that they can provide real family-centred care.

This module will begin by examining the nature of the family, the changes in structure that have occurred and the effect of family break-up on children. Families consist of individual members, each with a variety of roles. The way in which these roles and the relationships associated with them interact and influence family members will be explored. One of the main functions of the family is the socialisation of children. It is within the family that most infants develop the first basic social relationships and learn primary social skills. This function and the contribution that the family makes to child development will be discussed. Finally, the module will consider different styles of child rearing. Throughout the module you will be urged to consider the implications of issues for your practice.

Chapter 1

The Family

Introduction

'The family' is considered by many people to be the smallest and most personal of all social institutions and one that is a universal phenomenon, varying from culture to culture. The structure of the family in the UK has changed since the mid-1950s and continues to do so. It is not a static concept, but one that alters and adapts to the needs of a changing society. Before exploring the ways in which the nature of the family has changed it is worth considering some definitions of the family.

According to various authors the family is:

- a group of people tied by relationships of blood, marriage or adoption (Jorgensen, 1995)
- a group of people living with or near each other, who are closely related by marriage or blood (Moore, 2001)
- two or more persons who share resources and responsibilities for decisions, values and goals, and have a commitment to each other over time (Davidson and Moore, 1996)
- a married or cohabiting couple with or without children or a lone parent with children (CSO, 1995)
- a social group, characterised by common residence, economic cooperation and reproduction; it includes adults of both sexes, at least two of whom maintain a socially approved sexual relationship, and one or more children, own or adopted, of the sexually cohabiting adult (Murdock, 1949)
- two generations of people: at least one dependent child and at least one adult who is responsible for the child (Barnes *et al.*, 2005)

Study activity

Consider and analyse each of the definitions above. What does each really say? Do they reflect the concept of the family as you perceive it? Using the definitions try to write one that you feel reflects society today.

The concept of what constitutes a conventional family seems to have changed, so any definition of the family must allow for all possibilities. Narrow definitions based on the conventional family may increase the social pressures on individuals to conform. When caring for children and their families it is important to recognise the value of all forms of family unit and acknowledge the importance placed on individuality. What is considered to be the conventional family? According to White and Woollett (1992), conventional families:

- are headed by a married heterosexual couple
- consist of two to three children genetically and biologically linked with their parents
- consist of children born to mothers between the ages of 20 and 35
- live together in a nuclear household unit
- have fathers who are breadwinners and mothers who are full-time housewives

Study activity

To what extent do you believe that this type of family exists today? Draw up a plan of your family. Is it conventional? If not, how does it differ from the ideas above? If possible share your ideas with a colleague.

Family Structures

You may have identified many ways in which your family differs from the idea of the 'norm' or the 'conventional family'. In this section we will examine the various ways in which the structure of the family has changed over recent years in relation to the characteristics of the conventional family.

The conventional family is headed by married, heterosexual couples

Statistics show that, in 1991, 71% of children lived in married-couple families with both parents. However, there has been a decrease in the proportion of households comprising the traditional family unit – couple families with dependent children – from just over half in 1997 to just over one-fifth in 2004 (ONS, 2005a). It may be argued that the family is in decline but the majority of children still experience this type of family at some stage of their lives.

Marriage rates (see Table 1.1) have declined overall, with a drop of 24% between 1979 and 1991 to 340 000, a slight rise in 1992 to 347 000 but then a fall to 306 000 in 2003 (ONS, 2005a). However, marriage is still the most common form of partnership. In 2003, half the UK's population was married. In 2003 there were just over 123 000 remarriages, accounting for two-fifths of all marriages.

Table 1.1 Marriage rates: 1981, 1992 and 2001 EC Comparison (rates per 1000 population) (adapted from OPCS, 1992; ONS, 2005a)

Country	1981	1992	2001
UK	7.10	5.40	5.10
Belgium	6.50	5.80	4.20
Denmark	5.00	6.20	6.60
France	5.80	4.70	5.10
Greece	7.30	4.70	5.40
Irish Republic	6.00	4.50	5.10
Italy	5.60	5.30	4.90
Luxembourg	5.50	6.40	4.50
Netherlands	6.00	6.20	5.10
Portugal	7.70	7.10	5.70
Spain	5.40	5.50	5.20

Study activity

Using the material in Table 1.1, compare marriage rates in the various EU countries. What factors might be responsible for the differences?

It is interesting to note that the age at which people marry is increasing. In 1971 the average age was 25 for men and 23 for women. By 2003 this had risen to 31 for men and 29 for women. This might be explained partly by the increase in cohabitation. The increase can be deduced partly by the number of births registered outside marriage, which has risen steeply from 12% in 1980 to 31% in 1992 and to 41% in 2003 (ONS, 2005a). Nearly 80% of all jointly registered births outside marriage in 1998 were to parents living at the same address. This might indicate that more cohabiting couples are providing a stable environment for children. In 1991, 7% of children aged 0–4 were living with their natural cohabiting parents. Cohabitation is increasingly favoured by couples where one or both partners is separated or divorced with children (Utting, 1995). Although cohabitation is more popular for a variety of possible reasons, it has been suggested that cohabiting relationships are less stable than marriages. Buck *et al.* (1994) suggest that cohabiting couples are four times as likely to separate as married couples. About 65% of cohabiting unions into which a child is born dissolve, compared with 40% of childless unions. In other words, only 35% of children born into a cohabiting union will live with both parents throughout their childhood (to their sixteenth birthday), compared with 70% of children born within marriage (Ermisch, 2001).

Alongside the fall in marriage rates there continues to be a large number of divorces (Table 1.2). The UK had one of the highest divorce rates in the EC in 1992 with 173 000 decrees registered. In 2000 this figure had fallen to 155 000 but by 2003 it was back up again to 167 000. In 2004 149 275 children aged 0–16 experienced the divorce of their parents (ONS, 2005b).

Factors leading to rise in cohabitation

- Changes in social attitudes
- Less importance placed on the institution of marriage
- Economic factors – cost of weddings
- Declining influence of religion
- Rising divorce rates

Table 1.2 Divorce – worldwide comparison (per 1000) (source: Jorgensen, 1995; www.divorceform.org)

Country	1995	2002
Australia	2.50	2.60
Austria	2.00	2.40
Belgium	2.00	2.60
Canada	2.40	2.28
Denmark	2.80	2.70
Finland	2.00	2.70
France	2.00	2.00
Germany	2.10	2.30
Greece	0.90	0.90
Iceland	2.20	1.90
Ireland	—	—
Italy	0.50	0.60
Japan	1.30	1.92
Luxembourg	2.00	2.30
Netherlands	1.90	2.10
New Zealand	2.50	2.65
Norway	1.90	2.20
Portugal	0.90	1.90
Spain	0.50	0.90
Sweden	2.30	2.40
Switzerland	1.80	2.80
Turkey	0.40	0.50
UK	2.90	2.60
USA	4.80	4.10

Several factors contribute to the large number of divorces:

- changed attitudes – there is less stigma attached to divorce
- changes in legislation – changes in the law have made it easier for couples to divorce
- changing roles of women – more than 75% of petitions for divorce are made by women
- changing expectations of marriage – today the emphasis appears to be on equality and partnership between husbands and wives, perhaps putting more stress on relationships
- family experience of divorce – it is suggested that individuals are more likely to divorce if they have experienced the divorce of their parents

Study activity

Consider each of these possible factors. Using your life experiences and reference to literature, how does each reflect the reality of life?

In the United Kingdom, there has been an increase in the proportion of dependent children living in lone-parent families, with 23% of dependent children living in a lone-parent family in 2001 compared with 18% in 1991. The number of dependent children living in one-parent families

Factors leading to rise in lone-parent families

- Rapid rise in divorce
- Demands placed on partners in marriage make single parenthood preferred option
- Women less dependent on men
- Rise in unmarried mothers with increasing sexual activity among the young
- Greater unpredictability during the lives of many people
- Effects of media increasing the acceptability of lone parenthood

rose from 1 million in 1971 to 2.3 million in 1991 and to over 3 million in 2004 (ONS, 2005c). Children in lone-parent families are more likely to live with their mother than with their father. In 2004 nearly 9 out of 10 lone parents were lone mothers. Lone-parent families can occur as a result of divorce, separation (from marriage or cohabitation), death, through choice (the woman who deliberately chooses to have a child outside of a stable relationship) or through unplanned pregnancy. Lone-parent families are more frequent among black communities than among other ethnic groups, and are least likely to be found among the Asian and Chinese community. The circumstances in which lone-parent families live can vary tremendously and it is impossible to generalise. However, statistics show that the majority of lone-parent families experience significantly more hardship than families consisting of couples. In 1990, 53% of lone-parent families had a weekly income of £100 or less, compared with 4% of married or cohabiting families (OPCS, 1993). In 2002/3 lone-parent families were twice as likely as the population as a whole to be living in low-income households (ONS, 2005a).

Study activity

Consider the implications of lone-parent families for your practice.

Further reading on gay and lesbian families

Patterson, C. J. Gay and lesbian parenting – research findings. http://www.apa.org/pi/parent.html

American Pyschiatric Association – Gay and Lesbian Issue. http://healthyminds.org/glbissues.cfm

Not all families are headed by a heterosexual couple. Although figures are not available, more families may be headed by gay or lesbian couples. A developing freedom allowing gay couples to live openly together has resulted in the controversial issue of children in gay families. Gay families usually occur through one partner having been divorced and being given custody of the children from a heterosexual relationship. Recently, increasing numbers of gay parents have conceived children and raised them from birth either as single parents or in committed relationships. This is often done through alternative insemination or through foster parenting. There has never been a law preventing lesbian, gay or bisexual individuals from adopting children. The Adoption and Children Act 2002 now allows same-sex couples to apply for adoption jointly in England and Wales. This change in behaviour requires us to reconsider our views on relationships and the raising of children. Many assumptions about children in gay relationships are based on the maxim that gay parents equal gay children. However, children do not simply follow in their parents' footsteps – many other factors influence the way in which they grow and develop. According to Wainright *et al.* (2004), teenagers raised by a same-sex couple develop as well as teens raised by opposite-sex parents. These researchers drew from a large US sample of 12–18-year-olds, looking at measures of psychosocial well-being, romantic relationships and behaviour in school. There were no significant differences between the two groups of teens in terms of depression, anxiety, sexual activity, self-esteem and school grades. Previous research compared children of homosexual and heterosexual couples and found no significant difference in their well-being or sexual orientation (Allen and Burrell, 1996). Many gay couples are as committed to a permanent relationship as married couples.

Study activity

Consider your own views on the gay family issue and discuss with colleagues the implications for practice.

The conventional family consists of two or three children genetically and biologically linked with their parents

This may be true for the majority of children but increasing numbers are being raised in families where the genetic links between child and parents have been partially or completely broken.

In 1991 it was suggested that nearly 500 000 *step-families* (reconstituted families) existed in Great Britain, including about 800 000 step-children (most from women's previous relationships) (Haskey, 1994). By 2001 there were 700 000 step-families. Of these 400 000 were married-couple step-families and 300 000 were cohabiting-couple step-families (ONS, 2005c). The data suggest that 30% of children will experience living in step-families during their childhood. Step-families come in many different forms, with children from one (or both) partner's previous relationships. At the same time new partners may have children of their own, which adds to the difficulties that many of these families experience.

step-family
'A step-family is created when two adults form a new household in which one, or both, brings a child/children from a previous relationship'.

(De'Ath, 1996)

A relatively small proportion of families occur through *adoption*. This is a common form of family building for those who are unable to conceive and have children naturally. However, the numbers of children adopted are small. In 1988 approximately 1000 babies and 4000 children were adopted out of the 780 000 children born (Humphrey and Humphrey, 1988). In 2003 the figures remained about the same, with 4800 adoptions in England and Wales and 47% of adopted children between 1 and 4 years old (ONS, 2005a). In these cases there is normally no genetic link between the child and adopted parents.

An even smaller number of children are born with the aid of *reproductive technology*. Approximately 1 in 7 couples have difficulty conceiving naturally; help is now at hand for some with new fertility treatments. One such treatment is artificial insemination by donor (AID). This method helps to overcome infertility in men by inseminating their partners with either fresh or frozen donated sperm. The annual figures for the UK in 2005 show that 8544 children were born by *in vitro* fertilisation (IVF) and a further 818 by donor insemination (Human Fertilisation and Embryology Authority, 2005). Another method leading to disrupted genetic links is *surrogacy*. This increasingly controversial method exists in different forms but usually involves a surrogate mother being artificially inseminated with the father's sperm. In this case the child will have a genetic link with the father but not with the mother. According to COTS (http://www.surrogacy.org.uk/About_Surrogacy.htm, accessed 5 April 2006), there were 500 surrogate births up until 2004.

For a debate on fertility treatment, see http://www.politics.co.uk/issues/fertility-treatment-$2413554.htm (accessed 30 January 2006).

Surrogacy
Four pieces of legislation relate to issues of surrogacy:

- the Warnock Report (1984)
- the Surrogacy Arrangements Act (1985)
- the Human Fertilisation and Embryology Act (1990)
- the Parental Orders (HF&E) Regulations (1994)

There are moral and ethical issues involved with alternative forms of family building. The methods tend to be tightly controlled and limited to those couples considered suitable, as being:

- not too old
- heterosexual
- married
- in long-term, stable relationships

Recent controversy has surrounded applications from gay couples and there is a tendency for single-parent adoption to be shunned. Issues concerned with reproductive technology tend to be centred around the idea that it is wrong to interfere with nature. There are a number of psychological issues that are common to both adoption and reproductive technology, which are worth considering:

- With genetic links partially or completely broken, it is suggested that this can interfere with the sense of continuity and commitment to the future that conventional parents may have.
- In the case of adoption, the mother misses out on the experience of birth, which some say is important in the development of relationships between mother and child (White and Woollett, 1992). The later the adoption occurs, the more the early experience is missed. The same is true for many step-parents who have to accept that the children have had experiences of which they were not a part. It can be quite difficult to adjust to caring for a child who may have been brought up with a different set of ideals.
- With AID, step-parenting, in gay and lesbian families and some forms of surrogacy, the child is clearly genetically linked to only one parent. This may lead to possible conflict within the relationship, especially during stressful times. The child may become 'mine' or 'yours', leading to accusations of blame.
- Parents who have children by alternative methods may choose to keep quiet about their children's origins. For some, the differences are obvious – for example, parents who adopt older children or suddenly bring home a baby with no previous signs of pregnancy. For others, it may be possible to pass the birth off as entirely natural. While there is no right or wrong, keeping secrets has its disadvantages. Issues related to the rights of children to know their origins are central to the debate. Parents have no legal duty to tell children of their origins. Adopted children have the right to obtain information about their birth parents but only if they have been told of the adoption. In January 2004 the government changed the rules for egg and sperm donation, ruling that children conceived through fertility treatment would have the right to know who their biological parents were. Egg and sperm donors would have no obligation to meet with their biological children or to provide them with financial support. The new rules came into effect in April 2005 and are not retroactive, so children conceived before this date would not be able to access details about egg and sperm donors.

Study activity

Consider the implications of alternative methods of family building for your practice.

The conventional family consists of children born to mothers between the ages of 20 and 35

Statistics show that women are choosing to give birth to their first child later in life. In 1971, the mean age at first birth was 24; by 1992 it was approaching 28 (OPCS, 1994). More women are delaying childbirth until their thirties and this applies more to women who have further education qualifications than those who do not (OPCS, 1993). At the same time, growing numbers of women are choosing to remain childless. Projections suggest that this will continue to increase so that about 23% of women born in 1973 will be childless when they reach the age of 45 (ONS, 2000).

'One of the main features of recent British fertility behaviour is the postponement of parenthood'.

(Utting, 1995)

The conventional family lives together in a nuclear household unit

Statistics seem to support the idea that the nuclear family is dominant. However, it does depend on how the statistics are interpreted. Table 1.3 shows us that in 2004 more than a quarter of all households consist of people living alone; one-third are households of adults only (about 40% of whom have grown-up children); 30% of households contain dependent children but one-fifth of these are lone-parent families. The figures have not changed much since 1990/91. If one considers the data as presented, then it would appear that married couples with children are relatively rare occurrences. However, if one takes into account those families who have yet to have children and those with non-dependent children, nearly two-thirds of households conform to the stereotype nuclear family. Most of us are likely to experience life in a nuclear family at some stage (Muncie *et al.*, 1995).

nuclear family

- *Conventional* – husband, wife and their children living in same residence
- *Non-conventional* – two adults and children living in the same residence

The concept of the extended family offers an alternative family structure, which is perhaps more commonly found in its true form among ethnic minorities. Evidence suggests that, although immigrants adapt to their new environments, the fundamental basis of their beliefs about family life remain intact. For example, Asian households are more likely than white British ones to contain extended family members. Although

Table 1.3 Households by type in 1990–91 and 2004, Great Britain (adapted from OPCS, 1992; ONS, 2005a)

Household	Percentage 1990/91	Percentage 2004
Single person:		
pensionable age	15	15
under pensionable age	11	14
Two or more unrelated adults	3	3
Married couple:		
No children	28	29
Dependent children	24	22
Non-dependent children	8	6
Lone parent:		
Dependent children	6	7
Non-dependent children	4	3
Two or more families	1	1

extended family

- *Conventional* – more than two generations living in the same household
- *Modified* – extended family members living in close proximity or maintaining contact though living far apart

British housing makes the formation of three-generation households difficult, the extended family remains an important source of mutual support in Asian life. On the other hand, British Afro-Caribbean households rarely contain an extended family (Ballard and Kalra, 1994). Although very few three-generation households exist in the UK – estimated in 2001 as 1% (ONS, 2002) – there is evidence that the extended family continues to be important in Britain. Willmott (1988) identified the 'dispersed extended family' as being members of a family giving support to each other even though they lived some distance apart. Members of the extended family also play a vital role in child care, thus allowing mothers to work. The results from a national survey in 2001 (ONS, 2001) show that the majority of grandparents looked after grandchildren under the age of 15 years in the daytime (60%) or babysat (54%). They were also likely to give grandchildren money (64%) or have children to stay overnight (52%).

Study activity

To what extent does the existence of an extended family affect your practice?

The conventional family has fathers who are breadwinners and mothers who are full-time housewives

This is no longer necessarily the case. The working pattern of families can be very complex. One or either partner may work part time or full time, from home or outside the home. More mothers are working than ever before and many men are no longer the main or only breadwinners. Employed parents now work at 'atypical times' of day (outside 9 to 5) more than other workers; 53% of mothers, 54% of lone mothers and 79% of fathers frequently work atypical hours (La Valle *et al.*, 2002). Some parents (29% of partnered mothers) have adopted 'shift parenting', where each parent works at times of day that do not overlap with the other, in order to share child care (La Valle *et al.*, 2002). The dominant pattern for UK families at the beginning of the 21st century is to have 1.5 earners, most often a full-time employed father and a part-time employed mother (Dex, 2003).

The female workforce has been on the increase for some years and rose by 3 million between 1971 and 1990. In 2005, 52% of mothers with children under 5 years and 80% with children over 11 years were in work (Equal Opportunities Commission, 2005). Many of these women are in part-time work. Even in dual-earner families, or those where only the mother is in paid work, it is rare for fathers to identify themselves as the main carers. However, it is common for couples to say they take an equal share of being with and looking after their children (Lewis, 2000).

Some fathers remain at home either from choice or through unemployment. In some cases fathers take on role reversal: they stay at home to care for the children while the partner goes out to work. This usually occurs where the woman's earning potential is more than the man's. Whatever the reason, the father is no longer the 'breadwinner'. This may have psychological effects as many men still see it as their role to provide for their families.

Study activity

Reflect on children you have cared for whose parents had diverse employment patterns. What effect did this have on family-centred care?

So the debate is: is the conventional family still the norm? Much of the data examined would seem to support the idea that the conventional family does indeed still exist. Most people in the UK marry and have children; most children are brought up by both birth parents and the nuclear family predominates. It is noticeable that some modifications have occurred in recent years, leading to what some would describe as the 'neoconventional' family. The diverse nature of the family must be taken into account, especially when care for sick children and their families is being planned. Each family will have different needs and will need different kinds of support. At the same time, it is important to recognise that families are not static units: they change and evolve. The conventional family goes through stages (Figure 1.1) beginning with possible cohabitation, then marriage without children, followed by the birth of the first and subsequent children. When the children leave home, the family changes yet again, only to be transformed with the birth of grandchildren. The final stage is one of bereavement, as one or other partner dies. At the same time as one family is changing, others are evolving as children marry.

When one considers the non-conventional family, these stages may well overlap. Some families may reshape themselves several times over within the lifetime of their members.

Study activity

John and Jenny Smythe have recently married. John has two children from his former partner who died. Jenny has one child as a result of an unplanned pregnancy and one child from her previous marriage. John and Jenny have one child of their own. Taking each member of the family, map the various forms of family they may have experienced.

Family Break-up and its Effects on Children

The above discussion has shown that many children will experience family break-up at some time. If one acknowledges the significant role that the family plays in the life of a child, then it is safe to assume that any disruption will have some effect on that child. Family break-up results in:

- new routines and patterns
- financial changes with a tendency towards lower family income
- loss of family identity
- possible environmental changes, such as a new home or new school

Research findings

For research on this issue go to www.jrf.org.uk where you will find a wealth of different projects about families and family life.

Children's views

In 2001 Dunn and Deater-Deckard carried out research to find out how children view their experiences within different kinds of families, including step-father, step-mother and single-parent families. They found that:

- A quarter of the children whose parents had separated said no one talked to them about the separation when it happened. Only 5% said they were given full explanations and the chance to ask questions.
- Most reported that they were confused and distressed by the separation.
- The children rarely confided in fathers and siblings, choosing to talk to grandparents and friends in the weeks following separation.
- Children who felt they had poor relationships with their parents and were more involved in conflict between parents and step-parents tended to have more adjustment problems.
- Children who felt close to their maternal grandparents had fewer adjustment problems.
- More than half the children who lived in two households because of separated parents were positive about their 'divided' lives.
- Those who participated in decisions about living arrangements and those who said they were able to talk to parents about their problems concerning their 'divided' lives were more likely to have positive feelings about moving between households.
- The views of children as young as 5 were similar to the verbal accounts given by older children.

(Dunn, J. and Deater-Deckard, K. (2001) Children's views of their changing families. Available at www.jrf.org.uk)

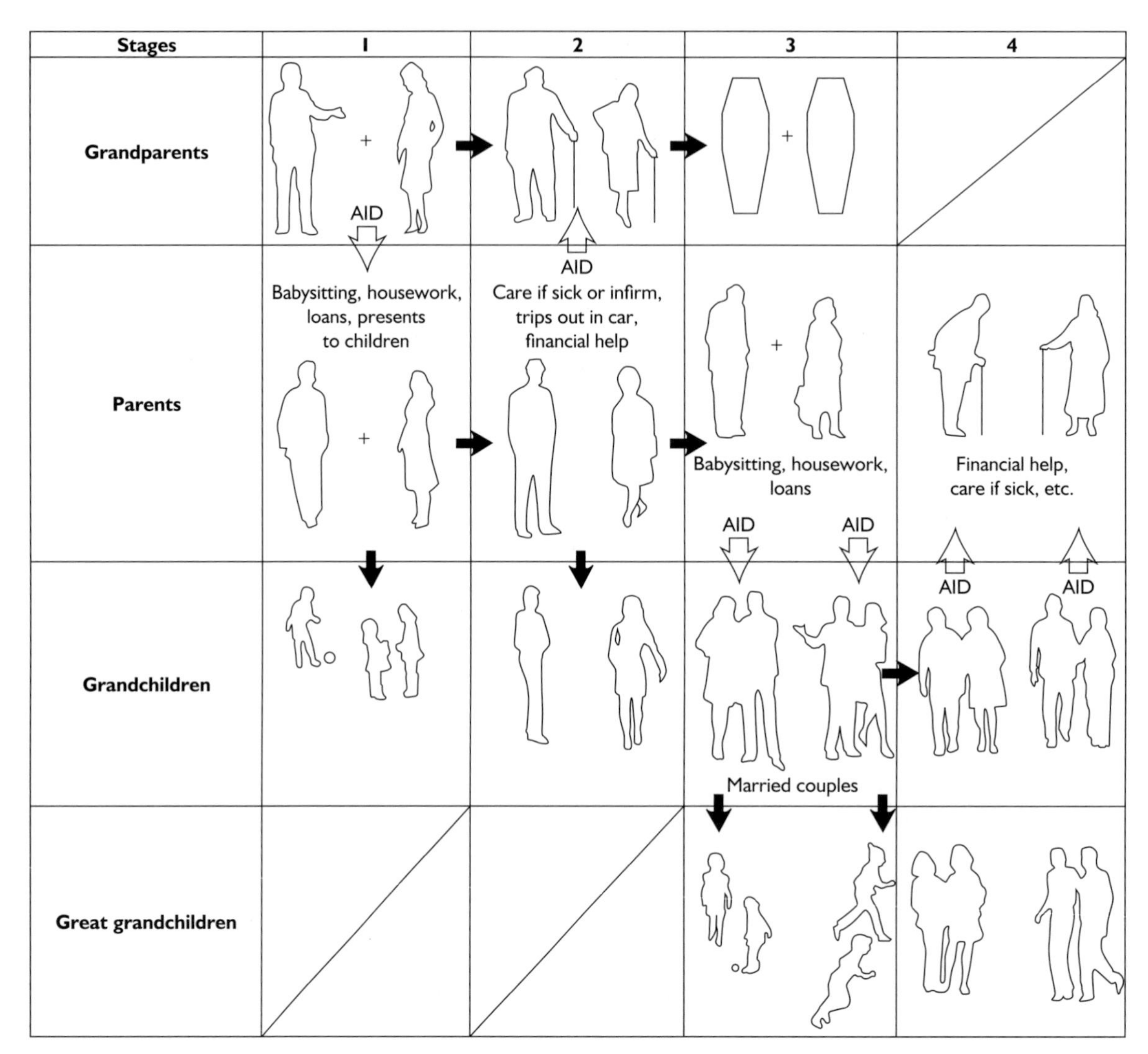

Figure 1.1 The conventional family life cycle (source: Moore, 2001).

The consequences will depend on many factors including:

- circumstances of the break-up
- the existence of family conflict before, during and after the break-up
- gender of children
- age of the child/children
- personalities of those involved
- changes to lifestyle following disruption
- reaction of parents to the break-up
- financial situation
- parental ability to recover from distress of separation
- multiple changes in family structure
- the quality of contact with the non-resident parent

Bearing this in mind, it is useful to develop an understanding of the possible effects on children (*see also* Separation p. 194).

In the early period following family break-up, all family members have to make adjustments and changes. Children are likely, in the short term, to experience unhappiness, low self-esteem and problems with behaviour and friendships. They may become socially withdrawn and inattentive. Young children may regress, become clingy and less likely to cooperate and comply with requests. They may fear being left by the remaining parent. The reactions can be likened to those following bereavement, with an initial expression of denial and guilt. Reactions of children to the break-up will be influenced by the way in which the custodial parent deals with the situation. More than 80% of custodial parents are mothers and for most of them the first year of bringing up children alone will be emotionally and energetically demanding.

The immediate distress surrounding parental separation usually fades with time and most children settle into a pattern of normal development. After the initial period of readjustment, the well-being of all members of the family improves. Routines become re-established as individuals adapt to new circumstances. Nevertheless, studies have found that there is a greater probability of poor outcomes for children from separated families than others – and that these can be observed many years after separation, even in adulthood. Children of separated families tend to grow up in households with lower incomes, poorer housing and greater financial hardship than intact families. They are at an increased risk of developing behavioural problems, including bedwetting, withdrawn behaviour, aggression, delinquency and other antisocial behaviour. They tend to perform less well in school and are more likely to be admitted to hospital following accidents, to have more reported health problems and to visit their family doctor (Kelly, 2003). A review of research has also shown that children who experience the separation of their parents are more likely to leave school and home when young and tend to report more depressive symptoms and higher levels of smoking, drinking and other drug use during adolescence and adulthood (Rodgers and Pryor, 1998). However, the research concludes that there is no simple or direct relationship between parental separation and children's adjustment, and poor outcomes are far from inevitable.

Further reading

Hetherington, E. M. and Kelly, J. B. (2002) *For Better or For Worse: Divorce Reconsidered.* New York: Norton.

Study activity

A 4-year-old boy is admitted to the ward for planned surgery. He has one older brother and a younger sister. On assessing the family you find out that the children's father left home 6 months ago. How might this information influence the care you plan to give this family?

There can be positive results of family break-up. These include:

- reduction in/removal of conflict
- children developing a more mature and sensitive approach and benefiting from additional responsibility
- the relationships between the custodial parent and children becoming very close
- siblings becoming closer

Further reading

Jensen, A. M. and McKee, L. (2003) *Children and the Changing Family.* London: Routledge Falmer.

This book is part of The Future of Childhood Series and it explores how social and family change are impacting on the experience of childhood. It focuses on three main changes: parental employment, family composition and ideology.

Cheal, D. (2002) *Sociology of Family Life.* Basingstoke: Palgrave.

This accessible introductory text provides students who are encountering the sociology of the family for the first time with a systematic way of thinking about the subject, based on a core set of analytical questions. It blends theory with empirical examples drawn from all over the world, thus offering valuable insights into the differences and commonalities between families in quite diverse social and cultural contexts.

Study activity

Carry out some further reading on the effects of family break-up on children. You might look especially at the effects of step-parenting. How do children adjust to this new situation? Perhaps you have experienced family break-up yourself? Reflect on how it affected you and other members of your family.

Summary

This chapter has examined the nature of the family in the UK today. The concept of the 'conventional family' has been explored, examining the changes that have occurred in recent years. Material has been offered to encourage you to reach your own conclusions about the state of the family today and you have been asked to consider the implications of family changes for your practice. Try to take the time to explore some of the further reading and to analyse the current trends that affect families today.

Key Points

1. It is difficult to define the 'family' because of its complex and changing nature.
2. It is important for health professionals to recognise the value of all forms of family units and to acknowledge individuality.
3. The majority of children live in married family couples with both natural parents but an increasing number of children will experience other family forms at some stage during their lives.
4. Most men and women eventually marry but the divorce rate has risen markedly in recent years.
5. Alternative forms of family building bring with them considerable ethical and moral issues.
6. Most of us are likely to experience life in a nuclear family at some stage.

Chapter 2

Roles and Relationships

Introduction

Within each family there is a complex system of relationships and interactions. If we acknowledge diversity of family forms, then these relationships can themselves be diverse. At the same time as belonging to various subsystems, each member of the family fulfils several roles. Understanding how these roles and relationships work may help you to meet the needs of different family members more appropriately.

It is possible to identify subsystems within all families. These will depend on the type of family, but in a conventional nuclear type they will consist of (Figure 2.1):

- mother–child/children
- father–child/children
- child–child
- father–mother

Further reading
Ribbens, J. (1990) *Accounting for our children: different perspectives on 'family life' in middle income households.* PhD thesis, CNAA, South Bank Polytechnic, London.

If one takes into account the extended family, then the relationships may become even more complex and, in fact, too complex to draw. Try it for yourself. It is not surprising that families sometimes argue and find it difficult to reach common ground.

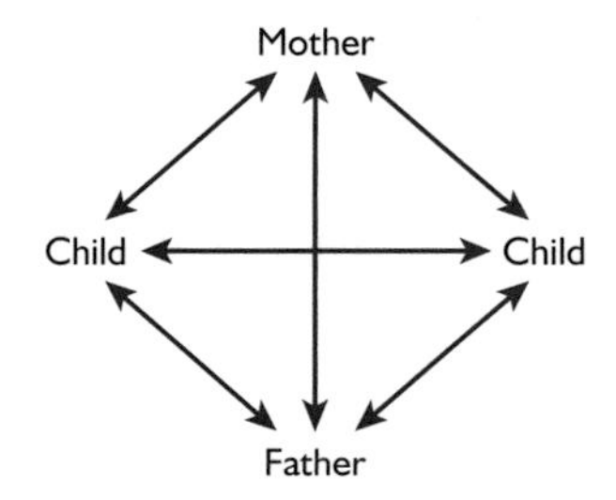

Figure 2.1 Subsystems within the conventional nuclear family.

Study activity

Draw a diagram to reflect the possible subsystems within:

- a step-family
- a lone-parent family
- a step-family with a close extended family
- a gay or lesbian family with children from both partners.

How might an understanding of these subsystems assist your practice?

Many factors will affect relationships and interactions between the different subsystems, including:

- number and age of children
- age gap between children
- age of parents
- the family form
- the presence of twins/triplets
- the roles each individual fulfils

It is important to remember that there is no typical family with typical relationships. We must not generalise about families; rather we should look at the issues surrounding relationships and roles so that we are in a better position to understand. Whatever the type of family structure, research suggests that the physical and psychological well-being of parents and children are shaped primarily by family processes, by the personality of parents and by the relationship between them (McKeown *et al.*, 2003).

Mother–Child Relationship

The relationship between a mother and her child has been described as being more highly charged emotionally than others. Personal experience will probably vouch for this. One minute children baulk at their mother's constraints, shouting and screaming because they cannot do or have what they want. Perhaps the mother, tired and weary after a hard day's work, begins to shout back, frustrated because the child is misbehaving. A vicious circle builds up. Shortly afterwards, both demonstrate almost overwhelming love and affection, cuddling and apologising. Not an everyday occurrence, perhaps, but one that will ring a bell with many mothers. It is worth exploring for a while this emotional relationship as those of us who care for sick children need to understand it (*see also* Parent–child relationship p. 193).

Mothers generally give most care, especially to young children, and consequently develop close and strong emotional bonds with them. The bond often seems to have a special quality which no one can describe accurately. Perhaps it begins with the moment of birth? Perhaps it has something to do with a natural tendency for women to feel a close bond with babies and children? Perhaps it is a social expectation? What would be the argument regarding women who adopt, or women who choose not to have children and have a genuine dislike of them? One could argue for and against each of the suggestions. Whatever the special bond is, it is never more obvious than when a child is ill. Experience has shown that mothers feel intensely about their children's illness, even when the problem may be minor. This can be illustrated by a particular incidence. A very experienced ward sister became frustrated with a mother who was very upset about her son's forthcoming circumcision. The sister declared that she was making a fuss and said 'it's only a circumcision'. Some years later, the same sister was admitted to the ward with her son for the same operation. She was distraught and crying and obviously distressed about the forthcoming operation. Something had changed her – becoming a mother.

The emotional relationships that mothers have with their children is said to be generally warm, responsive and child centred. At the same time, their behaviour towards the child has been categorised into one of four types (Baumrind, 1991; Berk, 2000):

- *Authoritarian* – this type of behaviour is strict and controlling. The mother demands good performance and expects behaviour to be mature. There is no discussion and no reasons given for requests, demonstrating unclear communication. When the child misbehaves, the mother punishes and shows little affection. Firm limits and controls are set.
- *Authoritative* – this mother behaves on the assumption that she has more knowledge and skills than the child. A high degree of compliance is expected and, although she is not intrusive, she is prepared to impose restrictions. Children's demands and reasons are respected.
- *Indulgent* – this type of mother is responsive and highly involved but places few demands on children. She is non-traditional and lenient, does not require mature behaviour, allows considerable self-regulation, and avoids confrontation.
- *Uninvolved* – this mother is low in both responsiveness and demandingness.

Baumrind's work has been criticised by Ribbens (1994) who suggests that the study on which the types were based did not take any account of variable social contexts nor was it expressed in terms that women or parents might use themselves.

Research has shown that most mothers recognise the need to remain in control while allowing the child autonomy (especially after the age of 4 years). This can be difficult to achieve especially when the child is ill as there is a tendency to overindulge the child. The way that a mother behaves with her children will be influenced by a number of factors. Behaviour may change from hour to hour and from day to day, depending on the circumstances. It is possible that many mothers' behaviour is a combination of the above.

Factors affecting type of parenting

- Depth of understanding of child's ability to understand and reason at different ages
- Pressures on the mother – work, housework, number of children
- Mother's expectations of child
- Social circumstances – lone parent, relationship with father, unemployment

Study activity

Reflect on some of the mothers you have met. Which type did they seem to fit into? Did their behaviour vary and, if so, what influenced this?

It is interesting to examine the way in which mothers interact with babies and infants. Relationships and interactions are more intense during this stage. The mother uses the same signals as she does in other relationships but in this case they are more exaggerated – for example facial expressions are exaggerated. Smiles are broader, eyes open wider, the pitch and pace of the voice are extreme. The language that mothers use has been described as 'motherese'. This language is short, simple, highly intelligible, of high frequency and pitch and contains more nouns and fewer verbs. It tends to be bossy in nature, containing many questions and instructions. The main features of motherese are the same in all cultures and are found across various languages such as English, Russian and Swedish. It is important to note that the child's behaviour has an effect on the mother. Positive responses make the mother feel she is being a good mother: the baby cries, is cuddled and fed, and then settles back down. The mother feels complete. The baby who cries and is fed and cuddled but does not settle and continues to cry can make the mother feel inadequate and question her own ability and confidence. Interactions between the mother and child are therefore reciprocal.

Watching motherese

Go to http://www.pbs.org/wnet/brain/episode2/babytalk/ to watch a video clip of motherese and see http://www.personal.psu.edu/users/c/r/crm195/ for more information.

Study activity

Take an opportunity to listen to a mother talking to her baby. Make a note of what she says and then analyse it.

The way that a mother interacts and relates to her child will depend on many factors, including:

- mother's personality and sexual orientation
- confidence
- mother's state of health
- support networks available
- whether the mother works or not
- cultural factors
- the child's gender, age, health, temperament
- experience of motherhood

If we really want to give family-centred care, we ought to make time to attempt to assess the mother's relationship with her child.

Study activity

Next time you carry out an assessment, reflect on how well you were able to assess the mother's relationship with her child.

Father–Child Relationships

Historically, a father's interactions with his children have been limited. Fathers were very much on the periphery, generally responsible for discipline and punishment. Truby King (1938) suggested that the father's role was very much a supervisory one, ensuring that the mother was able to get out for occasional 'wholesome amusement and fresh air'. Memories of childhood remind me of 'wait until your father gets home'. Fathers were unlikely to become involved in child care. Some things may not have changed very much, but fathers are now more likely to have more intimate relationships with their children. It is important to understand father–child relationships because their quality affects the well-being of children directly (Lamb, 1997). Research indicates that children deprived of a positive paternal relationship may be at increased risk of problems such as drug misuse, delinquency and depression (Blankenhorn, 1995; Hetherington and Stanley-Hagan, 1997). In contrast, school-aged children and adolescents show better academic achievement and a more positive self-concept when relationships with fathers are positive (Biller and Kimpton, 1997). Research by Brotherson *et al.* (2003) concludes that it is not the mere presence of fathers that is important but their actual involvement with their children (for example playing together and going on recreational outings).

Fathers' relationships with children, like those of mothers, are influenced by a number of factors. One particular factor is the gender of the child, especially as the child moves into adolescence, when role modelling becomes more important. This does not appear to be as influential for mothers. McQuire (1991) suggests that fathers (and mothers) may not acknowledge gender differences in treatment but that outside observers might pick up on them. Fathers spend much more time with their sons, generally being more involved, particularly as they get older (Pleck, 1997); fathers spend nearly twice as much time with their adolescent sons as compared to their adolescent daughters. Fathers interact more through play than do mothers. Play tends to be boisterous, more so with boys. Throwing children up in the air or 'rough and tumble' are classic games that fathers play. On the other hand, interactions with girls tend to be quieter, involving more cuddling and fewer conversations (Hosley and Montemayor, 1997). It is not clear why fathers should show this preference. Perhaps they feel more comfortable with boys as they know more about males than about females. They have more insight into the needs of boys than girls.

Further reading

Lewis, C. (2000) *A man's place in the home: Fathers and families in the UK.* A study carried out for the Joseph Rowntree Foundation. http://www.jrf.org.uk/knowledge/findings/foundations/440.asp (accessed 29 March 2007).

Lamb, M. E. (1997) *The Role of the Father in Child Development,* 3rd edn. New York: Wiley.

Study activity

Consider the fathers you know. How do they relate to their children? Do they demonstrate a preference for their sons? What implications might this have for your practice?

Another factor that has been shown to influence the relationship between fathers and their children is the state of marital harmony. When marital harmony is high, fathers are shown to be warmer, more positive and happier with their children than when marital harmony is low. Marital stress leads to less interaction and a feeling of anger and contempt towards the children (Cummings and O'Reilly, 1997). The quality of relationships before and around the birth is also likely to influence the way fathers behave and interact with children.

O'Brien and Jones (1996) carried out a survey to study children's perceptions of the role of their fathers and their relationships with them. The results showed that girls were more dissatisfied with the amount of time given to them by their fathers than boys. Fewer girls (23%) than boys (44%) felt that their fathers understood them very well. In a small study by Milligan and Dowie (1998) interviews with children revealed that what they needed from their fathers was:

- a role model
- quality time
- supportive behaviour
- expressions of love
- physical contact

For many children, relationships with their natural fathers will be disrupted by divorce and separation. Researchers have found that as many as a quarter of children will have lost contact with their fathers within 3 years of a divorce (Hetherington and Kelly, 2002). Evidence from the research suggests that father absence may be harmful, not necessarily because of the lack of a sex-role model but because many of the paternal roles – economic, social and emotional – go unfulfilled. The research concludes that it is important to recognise the multiple roles that fathers take in relation to breadwinning, parenting and emotional partnership.

Fathers' relationships with their children are varied and depend on many factors. While it is generally the mother who stays with a child in hospital, there are many times when the father will be present and will even stay in place of the mother. It is therefore important to consider and assess the father's, as well as the mother's, relationship with the child.

Study activity

Identify two fathers that you have known while caring for children. Compare and contrast their relationships with their children.

Sibling Relationships

Relationships between brothers and sisters have often been called life's most influential and longest lasting relationships – lasting longer than ties to parents, spouses or children (Bank and Kahn, 1997). You might encounter a variety of siblings in your practice, including full siblings, half siblings, step-siblings, twin siblings, foster siblings and adoptive siblings. Many children have several different types of sibling. Relationships between siblings vary tremendously, from family to family, from day to day and from minute to minute. You may be familiar with the following scenario: Tom (aged 7) and Kate (aged 4) adore each other: they tell each other 'I love you' frequently. They play together, watch television together and cuddle. However, by the same token they 'hate' each other frequently, especially when one does something to annoy or tease, or takes a special toy. Generally speaking, however, they are buddies, companions, playmates. They depend on each other when the going gets tough (when one is punished for wrongdoing). A typical sibling relationship perhaps?

Study activity

If you have brothers and sisters, what were your relationships like when you were young and what are they like now?

Relationships between siblings tend to be more reciprocal than those with adults. Children share more jokes, games, role play and pretend play than children and adults together. Tom and Kate love to dress up and play weddings, something they would never get their mother to do. Siblings tend to spend more time with each other than with their parents. They understand each other and have a degree of empathy:

- Kate comes running in from the garden – 'Tom's hurt himself, he needs you'
- Kate has been told off and begins to cry. Tom puts his arm around her – 'Don't worry darling, Tom's here'
- Kate has been told off (again) – 'I want Tom!'

Sibling relationships offer children one of the first contexts in which they can show their feelings for others.

Younger children tend to copy older siblings. At this stage there is an obvious imbalance of skills, physical as well as psychological. The older sibling gives physical and verbal aggression, takes control and leads the play. As the children grow older the imbalance of skills becomes less. The younger child takes a more active role and will begin to challenge the older child: this results in fights and arguments. Older siblings, in particular, provide several very useful sources of support for their little brothers and sisters – the younger child is treated to a ready source of companionship, help and learning. The older child gains the chance to develop responsibility, and learns to share and protect others. Both are likely to receive a very intense initiation into the human social world of needs, intentions and feelings.

Dunn (1984) suggests that although sibling relationships are, on the whole, positive, negative emotions are frequently displayed. They tease and mock each other, quarrel and bicker, hit and pinch one another, take each other's toys and generally annoy each other. One study found that siblings typically fight over possessions and each other's behaviour towards one another (and, to a lesser extent, over rivalry regarding parental attention) (McQuire *et al.*, 2000). The conflict, companionship, love and affection tend to continue throughout childhood, forming an ideal ground for searching out social rules and forming ideas about social issues.

Some siblings get on better together than others. Perhaps you know some who have no time for each other, even hate each other. There are several factors that will affect sibling relationships:

- *Gender*. Same-sex siblings show a tendency to get on better. Perhaps this is because they have similar interests or because parents tend to treat boys differently from girls. I remember when I asked if I could stay out late because my brother did. 'He's a boy' was the reply. I hated my brother for that. In all types of families, sisters are more warm and supportive and less antagonistic and conflicted than brothers (Dunn *et al*., 1999). As a whole, same-sex siblings tend to get into more conflict and show more aggression than opposite-sex siblings.
- *Age gap*. A small age gap could mean that there is a greater similarity of interests and perhaps more warmth and closeness. This can be seen in twins. However, at the same time, there is the possibility of greater discord and jealousy. With a large age gap there are few shared interests but there may be fewer arguments as a result. It is also possible that an age gap of 2–4 years can produce more conflict and rivalry because siblings this close have especially similar lives.
- *Parental preferences*. When actual (as opposed to perceived) preferential treatment of one sibling occurs, one sibling is treated with less affection and more coercion and punishment by the parents. Sibling rivalry, sibling aggression and sibling avoidance are more intense (Boer and Dunn, 1992). The way in which a mother treats her children can affect their relationships. If there is disparity in treatment and if the mother tends to interfere frequently in sibling conflicts, sibling relationships tend to be more negative. It tends to be the older child who takes the brunt of this interference. Where a mother involves a young child in preparations for the birth of a new baby, sibling relationships are more likely to be positive (White and Woollett, 1992).
- *Birth order*. The order in which siblings are born is seen as having implications for identity. Firstborns are said to develop dominant, conscientious and conforming personalities and to feel resentment or ambivalence towards their younger siblings; children born later take risks and are creative; middle children act as peacekeepers (Mitchell, 2000; Sulloway, 2001).
- *Middle childhood*. Sibling relationships during this period are often put on hold. The children make more friends outside the home, friends who have the same interests and are dealing with the same experiences.

Children's views on sibling relationships

Findings from a research study: http://www.jrf.org.uk/knowledge/findings/socialpolicy/0245.asp

Study activity

Talk to friends and examine your own brother–sister relationships. What is the age gap? How has this affected relationships? Compare and contrast your findings.

Father–Mother Relationships

No two mother–father relationships are the same. None progress the same or end the same. Relationships are directly related to the roles each

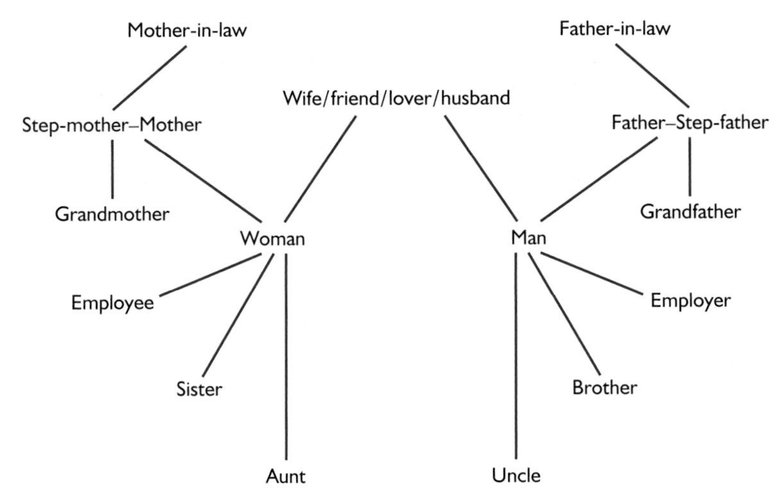

Figure 2.2 The complexity of mother and father roles.

fulfils and so are complex. It is possible that each partner fulfils several roles depending on the structure and form of the family (Figure 2.2).

Each partner will have different relationships within the context of each role, and each relationship will be affected by another. One can therefore never really understand how an individual's relationships are formed and develop. What we can do is look at how mother/father roles and relationships have changed.

Moore (2001) shows how sociologists have divided the changing roles and relationships between mothers and fathers into three phases:

- In *pre-industrial families*, husband and wife tended to work together on the land. They relied heavily on each other and both worked. However, relationships between them were not particularly close.
- In *industrial families*, men were the breadwinners, women took on the role of housewife and withdrew from the workplace. The father was the head of the household and took charge. The men tended to dominate the relationship.
- In *contemporary families* there has been a move to more equality. Women have moved back into the workplace and have found a degree of financial independence. This, in turn, has made them look for more involvement from the fathers in relation to household chores and child care. This new equality led to the term 'symmetrical family' (Young and Willmott, 1975). This equality has been disputed by many sociologists who argue that male dominance still exists and that there is not equality, especially in the area of power and delegation of household chores.

Study activity

Take a look back at your family. Talk to parents, grandparents, great-grandparents. How would they describe the roles and relationships between them? How have they changed over the generations?

The symmetrical family

'Identified by Young and Willmott as a type of family evolving in the late 20th century in which husbands and wives have a more egalitarian relationship in the home; household and childrearing activities are increasingly shared'.

(Jorgensen, 1995)

Further reading

Davidson, J. K. and Moore, N. B. (1996) *Marriage and Family: Change and continuity*. Boston: Allyn and Bacon.

Family Policy Studies Centre. This centre closed in April 2003 but you can still access useful information here: http://www.apsoc.ox.ac.uk/fpsc/ (accessed 29 March 2007).

Relationships between mothers and fathers fluctuate and are affected by many things. They fluctuate from day to day and from one stage of the family life cycle to another.

Study activity

List the factors that affect your relationships with your partner, or the relationships between your parents.

You may have found some of the following:

- *Age gap.* A wide age gap may result in different expectations, interests, even a different approach to life in general.
- *Own parental relationships.* Experience of conflict and fights or conversely warmth and affection.
- *Financial circumstances.* Worries over money can cause conflict and disagreement.
- *Employment or unemployment.* Women going out to work, fathers becoming unemployed.
- *Loss and bereavement.* Loss of a parent, loss of a child.
- *Parenting style.* May differ causing conflict.
- *Sexual relationship.* Different expectations, needs.
- *Birth of a baby.* A transitional stage. Can lead to conflict, stress, less time together, jealousy. More likely to adjust if relationship is stable before birth.
- *Social life.* Friends, hobbies, spending time together.

There may be numerous other factors not mentioned here but this serves to highlight how complex adult relationships can be.

Summary

This chapter has examined some of the issues surrounding roles and relationships within the family. It is clear that these issues are complex and cannot fully be given justice here. It is also clear that in attempting to implement family-centred care, we must try to understand where the family is coming from. We are not able to assess all facets of family life but we need to acknowledge and be mindful of the various factors that can affect relationships within families.

Study activity

Consider a family that you have cared for. Analyse the roles and relationships between various family members. How did this affect the care you were able to give? Reflect on how more knowledge of roles and relationships may have helped you.

Key Points

1. There is a complex system of relationships and interactions within each family.
2. The mother–child relationship has been described as being more highly charged than any other.
3. Fathers are now more likely to have more intimate relationships with their children.
4. Relationships between siblings tend to be more reciprocal than those between adult and child.
5. Relationships between mothers and fathers are directly related to the roles that each fulfils, and so are complex and changing.

Chapter 3

Functions of the Family

Introduction

A variety of views exist about the role of the family in society, ranging from those that are positive and see the family as beneficial to those that are negative and see the family as a damaging social institution. Government policy recognises that parents, carers and families are the most important influence on children and young people's outcomes (DfES, 2003).

The *positive view* is generally that expressed by the functionalist theorists. They believe that the family acts as the link between society and the individual and, as such, benefits both. The functions of the family are seen as being (Parsons, 1959; Fletcher, 1966):

- *The socialisation of children.* This aspect benefits children by preparing them for their role in society. It benefits society by producing individuals who will conform to the rules and regulations of that society. The family teaches its members the roles they will play in society and helps them to accept the rights, duties and obligations accompanying those roles.
- *The stabilisation of the adult personality.* The family serves as a comfortable and secure place within which individuals can deal with the pressures and demands of life outside.
- *The regulation of sexual behaviour and the procreation of children* in a responsible environment.
- *The care of dependent members*, whether young or old.

The *negative view* is held by sociologists who are critical of the functionalist ideas and thus highlight the harmful aspects of family life:

- *Marxist theories* see the family as an instrument of exploitation and oppression, particularly of women.
- *Feminist theories* see the family as a patriarchal structure, which is the cause of the oppression of women. Radical feminists believe that true liberation for women will only result with the abolition of the family and associated patriarchy.

Marxist theorists

- Karl Marx
- Friedrich Engels
- Loius Althusser
- Eli Zaretsky
- Michele Barrett and Mary McIntosh

- *Radical psychiatrists* offer a view that sees the family as the main source of human unhappiness and the root of some psychiatric disorders including schizophrenia. The darker side of family life is emphasised including abuse and violence.

Whichever view one takes of the family, it is clear that one major role must be concerned with the development of children. It has been suggested that it is the combination of parenting characteristics – parental warmth/affection, behavioural control and psychological control, in particular – that is influential in child development (Steinberg, 2001). It is the context in which children grow and become adults. The experiences and relationships within the family in the first years of life are vital if children are to realise their full potential to relate to others – to become social beings.

patriarchy
'A system or an instance of social organisation marked by the supremacy of the father in the clan or family, the legal dependence of wives and children, and the reckoning of descent and inheritance in the male line'.

(*Longman New Universal Dictionary*, 1982)

Further reading
For a more in-depth discussion of different theoretical views on the functions of the family see Chapter 8 Families and Households in Haralambos, M. and Holbourn, M. (2000) *Sociology. Themes and Perspectives*, 5th edn. London: HarperCollins.

Further reading
Tasker, F. L. and Golombok, S. (1998) *Growing Up in a Lesbian Family: Effects on Child Development.* Guildford: Guildford Press.

Explores the similarities and differences among young people brought up by lesbian mothers and a comparable group of young adults who were raised by single heterosexual mothers.

Role of the Family in Child Development

The socialisation of children

Socialisation has been described by Booth (1975) as 'the process by which an individual born with behaviour potentialities of an enormously wide range is led to develop actual behaviour confined within the narrow range of what is customary for him (her) according to the standards of his (her) group'. A simpler definition is given by Sroufe *et al.* (1996): 'the acquisition by the child of the rules, standards and values of society'.

Study activity

Take 2 minutes to reflect on these definitions. Compare and contrast them.

The first definition acknowledges that human behaviour is the result of an interaction between nature (inborn characteristics) and nurture (experiences). Perhaps the latter does not explicitly impart this aspect, rather seeing behaviour as a result of experience alone. Whichever definition we choose to work with, socialisation of children usually begins within the context of the family. During the process of socialisation children internalise societal norms, values and roles. However, whereas socialisation researchers often depicted parents as 'moulding' children to function adequately in the society (Hartup, 1989; Macoby, 1992), contemporary evidence clearly points towards multiple roles for parents that often do not imply the deterministic effect once attributed to them. Socialisation research is guided by an ecological perspective on human development (Bronfenbrenner and Morris, 1998). Families are seen as important influences on children, but the effect can only be understood in light of other simultaneous influences, such as peer groups and schools. These influences occur within broad contexts (for example, neighbourhood, cultural context) that add to, shape and moderate the effect of the family.

All types of expression are found within family relationships – love, hate, anger, companionship, despair, aggression. It is within this context that children gain an idea of the causes of various emotions and of the rules that operate inside and outside the family. Parents facilitate the socialisation process by providing a nurturing environment and social contact. The family helps children to prepare for life in the wider world and it serves to promote the continuation of cultural beliefs from generation to generation (*see also* Attachment pp. 86 and 87).

Study activity

Reflect on your own childhood. What do you consider you learned from your parents about life outside the family?

You may have come up with some or all of the following. Interactions with parents help children to learn about:

- taking turns, sharing, cooperating with others
- rules – how to recognise them, why they exist
- how to interact with others and respond to others' needs
- moral values – the difference between right and wrong
- how to act and behave appropriately within social contexts
- the roles they will play in later life, for example as parent, friend, worker
- cultural beliefs and expectations – the continuity of beliefs

The earlier children meet others, the more effectively they learn to interact and the more they will be accepted as companions. To some extent parents are able to manage children's social lives (especially those of young children) and thus have an impact on peer relationships. Research has shown that the particular peers a young person selects as friends and the extent to which he or she is susceptible to their influence are both affected by parenting (Collins *et al.*, 2000).

As children develop, so other influences contribute to the socialisation process:

- playgroups and schools
- mass media
- play
- friends/peers
- religion and culture (sometimes other than those of the parents)
- legal structures

Socialisation is a lifelong process and children need to learn new norms at each stage of the lifespan. They have to cope with learning new rules at school, when they join new groups, on leaving school, going to university or finding employment. Children also act as socialising agents for their parents, therefore making the process reciprocal.

General Aspects of Development

The family is the context in which other facets of development take place. There is a tendency for development to be considered without reference to the family, assuming that children's development follows certain patterns and stages regardless of their environment. However, it is important that we acknowledge the social network of the family and recognise that the family is also embedded in a social system. Mothers and fathers interact with children in unique and different ways. These roles are not equal or interchangeable, but each makes its own contribution to child development.

The process of family gender socialisation is very complex, but parents influence their child's *development of sexual identity* from birth intentionally and non-intentionally (Witt, 1997), directly and indirectly. The direct influence comes from the way the parents behave and the attitudes they hold, and is affected by their own gender-role attitudes. These attitudes determine their own behaviour and the way in which they treat sons and daughters (Basow, 1992). Indirect influence comes from the way in which parents control aspects of children's lives. Parents treat sons and daughters differently. Before children can express their own preferences, parents begin to create different environments for boys and girls. Bedrooms are decorated with colours and themes and infants are dressed in gender-specific colours – pink for girls and blue for boys. Parents encourage their sons and daughters to participate in sex-typed activities. Girls are encouraged to play with dolls and tea sets and boys are encouraged to play with cars and footballs (Berk, 2000). Early in development, parents provide experiences that encourage assertiveness, exploration and emotional control in boys. In contrast they promote imitation, dependency and emotional sensitivity in girls (Berk, 2000).

Further reading

McHale, S. M., Crouter, A. C. and Whiteman, S. D. (2003) The family contexts of gender development in childhood and adolescence. *Social Development*, **12** (1), 125.

Reviews research on the family's role in gender development during childhood and adolescence.

Study activity

Critically reflect on your own childhood. In what ways do you feel that your parents influenced the development of your gender identity? Take opportunities to observe children and their parents, television programmes and advertisements. Is sex stereotyping going on?

sex stereotyping
Conforming to general pattern of gender.

It is accepted that a complicated mix of heredity and experience shapes *brain development*. The environment has an important effect on early learning and it seems that relationships are the core of it all in early childhood. Good prenatal care, warm and loving attachments between young children and adults and positive stimulation from birth make a difference in children's ability to learn. There is evidence that early experiences can dramatically alter the way genes are expressed in the developing brain (Shonkoff and Phillips, 2000). The features found to encourage intelligence and cognitive development include the use of varied, developmentally appropriate stimulation, and responsiveness to cues. Guided play with objects helps to develop exploratory skills and imagination. Several studies (Bee, 1995; Shonkoff and Phillips, 2000) have suggested that certain features of family interaction seem to make a difference to a child's IQ level:

- the provision of an interesting and complex physical environment
- parents who are emotionally responsive towards and involved with their child

- parents who talk to their child using accurate, rich language
- parents who avoid excessive restrictiveness and who give the child room to explore
- parents who expect their children to do well

The children of parents who are aware of what their child is doing during leisure time and at school are more likely to do well at school and are less likely to have behavioural problems (Crouter *et al.*, 1990). It is important to consider the role of heredity in the development of the brain but the influence that the family can have on a child should not be dismissed.

As regards *language development*, parents do not formally teach their children about language; they do it informally and indirectly. They use language to communicate and by doing so they expose children to language. Infants and children who are talked to, read to and engaged in lots of verbal interaction show more advanced linguistic skills than children who are not as verbally engaged by their caregivers. Parents encourage language development by the use of:

- early interactions with the infant, encouraging the development of vocalisation and communication
- word games, telling stories
- repeating and expanding upon what their child has said (this often includes using more adult forms of speech, thus helping the child to learn)
- explaining and asking questions
- reading stories

The mother plays an important role in her child's language development. It has been shown that mothers and their babies engage in 'proto-conversation' as early as 6 weeks after birth, when mutual smiling games have been observed. The mother and baby are seen to take turns, as in a conversation (Powers, 2001). This type of 'chat' has also been seen to take place between fathers and their babies (Trevarthen, 2004). This is the basis on which further language and communication skills are based. As children begin to talk, so mothers structure their language in order to provide clear, simple and easy-to-understand communications. This type of language has been called 'motherese' and it appears to be used unconsciously (*see also* Language development p. 77).

Further reading

Learning about ourselves, from children: why a growing human brain needs interesting companions, by Colwyn Trevarthen (2004). Read more about this fascinating subject at http://www.perception-in-action.ed.ac.uk/PDF_s/Colwyn2004.pdf (accessed 29 March 2007).

Summary

This chapter has focused on the role of the family in the development of children. It has skimmed the surface of this subject and encourages you to explore some of the ideas raised more fully. When you are working with children it is important to remember that they are part of a family and that their development goes on within that context. You need to bring together ideas about different family structures and investigate the influences that family life can have upon children. Whether nursing a sick child or promoting health, you should assess the child against the family background and take into consideration the different forces acting upon the child. Although the discussion has focused mainly on the role of the parents in child development, other members of the family will play a role in a child's development. These include siblings, grandparents, aunts and uncles, and members of reconstituted families. The family plays a role in all aspects of a child's development, and therefore should be considered in all aspects of a child's care.

'Children are invariably born into a social network, typically a family. The family, too, is embedded in a social system. The family, the primary institution responsible for transforming societal maintenance and perpetuation goals into directives for the new individual, is thus at the core of socialization. Hence the family is society's adaptational unit'.

(Lerner and Spanier, 1978)

Key Points

1. There are two major views regarding the functions of the family – the positive and the negative.
2. Whichever view one takes, it is clear that the family plays a major role in child development.
3. The family is regarded by many as being the primary socialising agent for children, but it is acknowledged that other influences make the role of parents very complex.
4. The part that nature plays in child development is acknowledged, but the role that the family plays should not be dismissed.
5. The importance of assessing the child with the family is stressed.

Areas for further study

- The effect of birth order on a child's development
- The effect of reconstituted family life on children
- The role of heredity in intellectual development

Chapter 4

Child-rearing Practices

Introduction

One of the functions of the family is seen by many to be that of rearing children. The *Longman New Universal Dictionary* gives a definition of rearing: 'to raise upright, to build or to construct'. It is within the context of family life – whatever its structure – that parents undertake the responsibility of 'building the individual', helping to 'construct' a person who will reach his/her optimal potential.

Each family will have its own beliefs about how children should be raised. These beliefs will be based on many factors, including past experiences (especially related to their own upbringing), culture, religion and media influence (programmes and books on 'how to raise children' are plentiful). It is very difficult to make rules about how to bring up children. Each child is an individual and what we do for one child may not work for another.

Patterns of child rearing have changed considerably over the centuries. In the 18th and 19th centuries people had plenty to say about the moral upbringing of children. It was considered important to save them spiritually, given the high death rate among the young. As the infant mortality rate fell, more and more children survived into childhood, and the emphasis was placed on physical upbringing, following fairly rigid rules. This rigid approach survived into the 20th century and in the 1930s authors of child-rearing books gave quite authoritative views on the subject. One writer told mothers 'Never kiss and hug them. If you must, kiss them once on the forehead.' Truby King (1938) suggested 'the establishment of perfect regularity of habits initiated by feeding and sleeping by the clock' as being the ultimate foundation of all-round obedience.

Current trends are not so dictatorial, although they still vary in their approach and, in fact, often go to the other extreme with the concept of non-advice – do what you find suits the child best. Leach (1989) suggests that it is impossible to give a child too much attention or love. She believes that rearing a child by any book or set of rules can only work if the rules happen to fit the baby – a minor misfit can cause misery. What parents actually do is to take advice (from books, professionals, from family) and then try to find what suits them and their children best. There is a wealth of knowledge about child rearing upon which today's parents can base their decisions about parenting.

Study activity

Read:

Holt, K. (2004) Just in the niche of time: in this age of specialization, publishers are targeting ever-more-specific child-rearing issues. *Publishers Weekly*, **251** (8) (23 February 2004), 38.

Then try and find some of the books she mentions and consider their usefulness or otherwise to parents. How might you feel as a parent faced with all this advice?

Study activity

Reflect on your own upbringing. Talk to your parents about how they found their way through the maze of advice on child care. Who influenced them most?

Principles of Child Rearing

The principles of child rearing are based on meeting the child's physical needs (nourishment, safety, sleep and comfort) and psychosocial needs.

Pringle (1980) identified four main psychosocial needs:

- The need for love and security – the child needs to be valued and cherished for his own sake without any expectation of gratitude. The security of predictability and continuity helps the child to come to terms with his developing self.
- The need for new experience – the child must experience new things and situations if he is to grow and mature. He needs the support and safety of a family in which to explore the world around him. At the same time he needs clear boundaries in which to experiment. Discipline is vital for the child to show him the boundaries.
- The need for praise and recognition – often parental expectations are too high and disappointment leads to punishment and recrimination. Children need an incentive, and expectations must be geared to each individual, neither too high nor too low. Each child needs the right to make mistakes and to experience failure without the fear of reprimand.
- The need for responsibility – allowing children to take responsibility for their actions is essential but parents often fear the consequences. Children need to learn to do things for themselves and need to be given increasing responsibility as their age dictates. This part of child rearing would seem to me to be the hardest part. When are children old enough to go to the park on their own? Will they be attacked, abducted? How do they know whom to ask for help? Unfortunately, there are no answers; parents must go with their own convictions.

General objectives for parenting

- Protection from environmental and social dangers
- Development of social skills
- Development of identity
- Development of self-esteem
- Spiritual development
- Cognitive development
- Affection and trust
- Moral guidance
- Economic support
- Self-regulation
- Stability of close relationships
- Adequate nutrition
- Education
- Physical care
- Preparation to be an adult who can contribute to society
- Modelling of socially desirable behaviour
- Development of independent living skills

(Campion, 1995)

Green (2006) takes a sensible, no-nonsense, humorous look at child rearing with particular reference to toddlers. He suggests that 'the important things in child care will always remain the same: love, consistency, example, tension-free homes, sensible expectations and confident parents at the helm'. He believes that childcare is natural and that parents have been doing it well for years.

Campion (1995) suggests that there are universal objectives for parents in the rearing of their children which constitute the job of parenting. She sees these as the same for all cultures, although she acknowledges that the specific nature of each will vary depending on cultural norms.

The *Every Child Matters* Green Paper (DfES, 2003) identified the five outcomes that are most important to children and young people:

- be healthy
- stay safe
- enjoy and achieve
- make a positive contribution
- achieve economic well-being

These five outcomes are universal ambitions for every child and young person, whatever their background or circumstances and the role of parents and carers in achieving these outcomes is clearly important.

Parenting Styles

Many writers have noted that the broad pattern of parenting is important in predicting child well-being. Parents may differ in how they try to control or socialise their children and the extent to which they do so. The overall pattern of interactions shapes a child's behaviour rather than one single act. Parents develop various styles of interacting with their children. Research has identified a typology of four parenting styles: authoritarian, authoritative, permissive and uninvolved, each of which influences how the child develops (Macoby and Martin, 1983; Berk, 2000). The way in which the principles of child rearing are put into practice will depend very much on the style of parenting adopted. Two dimensions are identified as being important in child rearing:

- the level of demand and control
- the level of acceptance or responsiveness

By putting these two dimensions together they came up with four types of parenting style (*see also* Parental behaviour p. 196), each with its own influence on child development:

- *Authoritarian.* Parents tend to exert a high degree of control, are demanding but at the same time display little warmth or responsiveness. They exert power over the child. Children with this type of parent tend to have low self-esteem and may be subdued or out of control and have lower peer affiliation (Jewell and Stark, 2003; Wolfradt *et al.*, 2003).
- *Authoritative.* This type of parent, whilst exerting high levels of control and demand, also shows a high level of warmth and is responsive to the child's needs. These children show a higher self-esteem, are

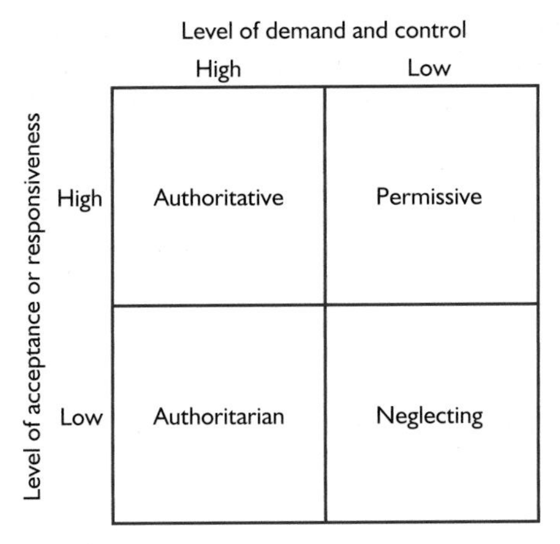

Figure 4.1 Parenting styles.

more compliant, self-confident and more independent. Authoritative parenting was shown to be positively associated with adjustment in children of various ages (Hart *et al.*, 2003).

- *Permissive*. This type of parent is sometimes referred to as indulgent. Although they show warmth and respond to the child's need, these parents exert little control. They make few rules and demands for good behaviour; they do not restrict noise, climbing about on furniture; they allow freedom to play without supervision (Mussen *et al.*, 1994). Children tend to show negative outcomes – aggression, immaturity in relationships with peers. They are more dependent.
- *Neglecting*. Sometimes this type of parent is referred to as uninvolved. These parents show little warmth and responsiveness and at the same time little control. Children may show insecurity and difficulty in forming relationships. They are more likely to be impulsive, behave in an antisocial manner and demonstrate withdrawn behaviour and conduct disorders (Jewell and Stark, 2003; Wolfradt *et al.*, 2003).

Study activity

Reflect on your own parents, parents of friends. What type are they? If you are a parent yourself, reflect on and try to analyse your own style.

Other aspects of child rearing worth exploring

- Toilet training
- Weaning/breastfeeding
- Caring practices – hygiene, dental care

Aspects of Parenting

There are many aspects of parenting, all of which will be influenced by the factors discussed above. For the purposes of this module, two aspects will be examined in more detail: discipline and sleep.

Discipline

Discipline is probably one of the most contentious issues in the area of childcare. Disciplining children is very difficult; it can be emotionally

Cultural perspective

In the Asian culture there is virtually no discipline for the first 3 years. When it does start, total obedience is expected. Discipline tends to be physical and outside interference is not tolerated.

(Mayor, 1984)

discipline
'The use of instruction, control, rewards or punishment as a means of training or correcting, in order to instill self-discipline.'

(Davidson and Moore, 1996)

draining. The problem is that there are no hard-and-fast rules. Different parents have different views on how to discipline their children. Limit-setting is important for children; unrestricted freedom is often a threat to security and safety.

Study activity

Begin by examining your own views about discipline. Do you withdraw privileges, withhold affection, scold, impose unpleasant tasks/penalties?

Discipline is just part of the process of guiding children with the aim of their becoming happy, healthy, fully functioning adults. To try to get it right, Davidson and Moore (1996) suggest that parents need to know why a child misbehaves. Once this is understood, they propose that it is easier to select appropriate methods of discipline.

Reasons for a child's misbehaviour include:

- *Age of the child.* Knowing what type of behaviour is expected of a child is important when deciding on discipline. For example, we all know about 'the terrible twos'. It is not worth punishing a 2-year-old having a temper tantrum. The best way of dealing with this type of behaviour is to tolerate it if you can.
- *Unsatisfied demands.* Very often, bad behaviour occurs when children cannot have what they want (or think they need). First, it is important to decide if the desired demand is legitimate. If it is, then it may be appropriate to acknowledge this but remind the child of how to ask. If the desire is not legitimate, for example if the child wants a new toy, then it is important to be consistent – no means no. It is no good changing one's mind just to avoid confrontation. It is better to try some other tactic. Diversion is a useful one. Children, especially young ones, can usually be diverted quite easily.
- *Lack of social knowledge about appropriate behaviour.* It is unwise to punish children for not knowing how to behave. It is far better simply to show them or tell them what to do. It is preferable to indicate what to do rather that what *not* to do, as the latter is very negative.
- *Inappropriate environment.* It is difficult for children to behave when their environment is not suited to their developmental needs. Children are curious; they love to experiment and try out new things. They need to run about and expend energy. If they are restricted they may resort to bad behaviour. Experience has shown that it is better to let children play outside when they want to, even if it is cold, rather than make them come into the house. The latter choice always ends up in a shouting match when the noise and mess become too much.

Study activity

Consider what actions you might take in the following situation: a 2-year-old child in your care has a tantrum at the top of a flight of stairs in a busy department store. Discuss this situation with colleagues and explore different ways of dealing with it. What other behaviours are age related and should be taken into account when disciplining children?

Table 4.1 Acceptable or unacceptable behaviour in children

Behaviour	Yes/No	Reason
A toddler pokes a pencil into an electric socket		
A 4-year-old will not put his toys away		
A 2-year-old swears at his teddy		
A 4-year-old smacks his sister after he has been scolded		
A 3-year-old boy plays with his penis		
A 4-year-old refuses to eat his dinner and hurls it on the floor		
A 5-year-old says he did not do something when he did		
A 5-year-old keeps making rude noises with his mouth		
A 3-year-old will not let a friend have a turn on his bike		
A toddler bashes another toddler with a toy		
A 4-year-old kicks and bites other preschool children		

Study activity

For each of the behaviours listed in Table 4.1, indicate whether you find it acceptable or unacceptable. If you find the behaviour unacceptable indicate your reason from the list in the box. Discuss your answers with (a) your mother, (b) a friend and (c) a colleague.

Reasons for unacceptable behaviour

You think it is:

- dangerous
- unhygienic
- the cause of distress, a nuisance or inconvenience
- the cause of damage, expense or extra work
- against rules or conventions
- babyish
- bad manners or impolite
- disobedient
- irritating or embarrassing
- bad tempered or emotional
- a lie or dishonest

Research

Simon Anderson and Lorraine Murray (NFO System Three Social Research) and Julie Brownlie (Stirling University). Disciplining children: research with parents in Scotland, available at http://www.scotland.gov.uk/cru/kd01/blue/dcrp-00.asp (accessed 29 March 2007).

Whatever discipline techniques are used, certain principles apply:

- Discipline is best carried out within a warm, responsive caring family.
- To be effective, punishment should either interrupt the undesirable behaviour or take place immediately after it. 'Wait till your father gets home' is of little use as the child will probably have forgotten all about the incident by then.
- The punishment chosen should be worthy of the crime. It should also be feasible. 'We will go out without you if you're not ready in time' is a wasted threat for a 4-year-old.
- Discipline must be consistent between parents and from day to day. Once a rule is set it must be observed.
- Discipline must not be overused as it loses its potency and becomes an entertaining game.

Various techniques are suggested from which parents can choose those most congruent with their beliefs and their behaviour:

- *Positive parenting*. This is recommended by the NSPCC (http://www.nspcc.org.uk/html/home/needadvice/encouragingbetterbehaviour.htm), which says that the techniques work regardless of temperament, background, culture or tradition. They build on a child's natural wish to please you and will ensure a happier child and less stressed parents.
  - Give as much love and warmth as possible.
  - Have clear, simple rules and limits.
  - Set a good example – actions speak louder than words.
  - Praise good behaviour.
  - Ignore behaviour that you do not want repeated.

- Don't criticise your child – criticise the behaviour.
- Reward good behaviour with hugs and kisses.
- Distract children from bad behaviour – redirect them to another activity before the bad behaviour has a chance to take hold.
- Allow children some control – they need choices and joint decision-making.

- *Time out*. This technique can bring a rapid response. The aim is to remove the child from a situation and place him in another room for a short time. He then has time to cool off. It also allows time for the parent to calm down so that the situation does not deteriorate further.
- *Removal of privileges*. This technique works for children over the age of about 6. It is of little use for younger children as they do not think much about the future. Privileges such as playing out, watching television, riding a bike, extra pocket money for good behaviour can be withheld. The child needs to know the standard of behaviour expected and the results of misbehaviour.
- *Behaviour modification therapy*. This technique is based on the premise that behaviour reinforced by rewards will be repeated, and behaviour that is not reinforced will probably disappear. Rewards can be in the form of praise, attention and cuddles, or more tangible items such as stickers, stars or small toys.
- *Smacking*. Article 19 of the UN Convention on the Rights of the Child (1989) states that appropriate measures should be taken to 'protect the child from all forms of physical or mental violence . . . while in the care of parent(s), legal guardian(s), or any other person who has the care of the child'. In some countries, smacking is prohibited (Sweden, Finland, Denmark and Norway). In England and Wales, Section 58 of the Children Act 2004, which allows the common assault of children to continue to be justified as 'reasonable punishment', came into force on 15 January 2005. This new law limits this form of punishment to mild smacking, but any hitting or smacking that results in lasting bruises, cuts, scratches or swellings can now face up to 5 years in jail for child abuse.

UN Convention of Rights

The UN Convention on the Rights of the Child was adopted by the UN General Assembly on 20 November 1989. It provides detailed minimum standards against which to test the treatment of the world's children and young people. It was ratified by the UK Government in 1991 'with some reservations'.

Other relevant articles of UN Convention of Rights

- Article 28 states that 'Parties shall take all appropriate measures to ensure that school discipline is administered in a manner consistent with the child's human dignity'.
- Article 37 states that 'No child shall be subjected to torture or other cruel, inhumane or degrading treatment or punishment'.

Study activity

It is important to continue with discipline even when a child is ill. Consider how you might deal with discipline for a child in hospital.

Study activity

Arrange a debate with colleagues – 'There should be a total ban on smacking children as a form of punishment in the UK'.

Sleep and sleep problems

Sleep is a complex phenomenon that is taken for granted until it is disturbed. It is expected that children should develop 'acceptable' sleeping

Children talk about smacking

It hurts you inside – children talking about smacking, by Carolyne Willow and Tina Hyde (National Children's Bureau, 1998), available at http://www.endcorporalpunishment.org/pages/frame.html (accessed 16 February 2006).

Seventy-six 5- to 7-year-olds talked to researchers about smacking. Here are some of their responses to the question 'What does it feel like to be smacked?'

- 'It feels like someone banged you with a hammer' (5-year-old girl)
- 'It hurts and it's painful inside – it's like breaking your bones' (7-year-old girl)
- 'It's like when you're in the sky and you're falling to the ground and you just hurt yourself' (7-year-old boy)
- '[It feels] like someone's punched you or kicked you or something' (6-year-old boy)
- '[Children feel] grumpy and sad and also really upset inside' (5-year-old girl)
- '[It] hurts your feelings inside' (7-year-old girl)
- 'You feel you don't like your parents any more' (7-year-old girl)

On the web site you will also find children from different countries speak up about smacking.

This can be purchased through:
National Children's Bureau, 8 Wakley Street, London EC1V 7QE
Tel: 020 7843 6000
Website: http://catalog.ncb.org.uk/

patterns – that is, they should go to bed when the parent decides, sleep through the night and wake at a reasonable time in the morning. In reality, this expectation is not always fulfilled, causing anxiety and stress among families.

When looking at the development of sleep patterns in children (Table 4.2), we see that the sleep pattern of newborns is 'polyphasic' with short cycles of sleep and wakefulness occurring throughout the day and night. Total sleep time (about 15–18 hours) is distributed over the 24-hour period. As the central nervous system matures, the pattern changes and the infant spends more time awake in the day and more

Table 4.2 Stages in the sleep cycle with age

Age	Sleep pattern	Length of each sleep cycle (min)	%REM	Total sleep time (h)
Newborn – polyphasic	Wake, REM, non-REM	<45	50	18–20
3 months–1 year – polyphasic	Wake, non-REM, REM	45–50	35	15–18
2–3 years – biphasic	Wake, non-REM, REM	50–60	20–25	12–15
4–10 years – monophasic	As above	60–70	20–25	12 reducing to 7–8
Adult – monophasic	As above	90	20	6–8
Elderly – multiphasic	As above	90	20	Often less than 6

UK measures against physical punishment

- Physical punishment outlawed in all state-supported schools
- Children in various categories of children's homes protected under the Children Act 1989
- Local authority foster carers prevented from using physical punishment under the Children Act 1989
- Children Act 2004 – smacking allowed if justified as reasonable punishment

The case against physical punishment – smacking

- Serves as a model of violence
- Erodes the positive influence of the parent
- Creates a family climate of rejection instead of warmth
- Lowers a child's self-esteem
- Damages parents' self-concept because they lose control of their emotions
- Promotes dependency on external rather than internal control
- For further information contact: EPOCH, 77 Holloway Road, London N7 8JZ

sleep

'The natural periodic suspension of consciousness that is essential for the physical and mental well-being of higher animals' (*Longman Universal Dictionary*, 1982). The English word *sleep* is of Germanic origin and derives from the Gothic word *sleps*.

time asleep at night. Longer periods of behavioural inhibition become possible and a bulk sleep of 8 hours is usually established by about 4 months of age. As the infant grows and develops, so total sleep time decreases and occurs mainly at night. By the age of about 2 years, most children have developed a biphasic sleep pattern with a nap at some stage of the day. A monophasic pattern (the bulk of sleep at night-time) is generally established by about the age of 4 years. The development of the monophasic sleep pattern of adulthood is affected not only by maturation of the brain but also by environmental and cultural factors. In Mediterranean countries it is common for adults to maintain the biphasic pattern of childhood by taking afternoon siestas to avoid the hottest time of the day. Thus it is acceptable practice for children to do the same and so have a later bedtime than would generally be accepted in this country.

Study activity

Consider your own views on what is an acceptable sleep pattern for children. If you have children of your own, how do you manage this aspect of child rearing? If not, explore your parents'/friends' views.

REM

Rapid eyeball movement associated with paradoxical sleep, increased electrical activity of the brain and dreaming.

Cultural issues – sleeping

Read these interesting articles for more information:

McKenna, J. J. (2000) Cultural influences on infant and childhood sleep biology, and the science that studies it: toward a more inclusive paradigm. In Loughlin, J., Carroll, J. and Marcus, C. (eds), *Sleep and Breathing in Children: A Developmental Approach*. London: Marcel Dekker; pp. 199–230.

Jenni, O. G. and O'Connor, B. B. (2005) Children's sleep: an interplay between culture and biology. *Pediatrics*, **115** (1), 204–216.

Sleeping arrangements differ from culture to culture. One of the most interesting features that has been studied is *bed sharing*. It is common practice for Western babies to be placed in their own cots or beds, usually in their own room. It is not generally acceptable to admit to sleeping with babies/children in the marital bed. However, for many cultures there are no special sleeping arrangements for babies. In parts of India and Kenya, babies and small children sleep with their parents for several years. Japanese infants and children usually sleep adjacent to their mothers and, in general, children sleep with someone (fathers or extended family members) through to the age of 15. In the Philippines, infants sleep with their mothers except during weaning when they are moved to another room with aunts or a grandmother. Mayan mothers in Guatemala share their bed with infants during the first year of life and toddlers sleep in the same room (Morelli *et al.*, 1992). In a study of bed sharing in Korean children, Yang and Hahn (2002:155) found that 73.5% of mothers approved of bed sharing with children between 3 and 6 years of age. The main reasons for bed sharing were 'to look after the child while sleeping' and 'the child is too young to sleep alone.'

Many Western child health professionals emphasise the hazards of cosleeping, such as impediment of the development of autonomy and independence, increased dependence on parents, inappropriate sexual arousal, risk of sleep problems and interference with parental sexuality and intimacy. There may also be a concern that sleeping with children may in itself have sexual connotations. Health visitors and other professionals advise us against bed sharing and give parents ideas on how to encourage babies to sleep on their own. The Foundation for the Study of Infant Deaths (FSID, 2006) advises against it, saying that the safest place for a baby to sleep is in a cot in the parents' bedroom for the first 6 months. They go on to state that there is a proven risk of sudden infant death when bed sharing if either partner smokes (even if you never smoke in bed or in your home), has been drinking alcohol, has taken drugs or medication that causes drowsiness, or is very tired.

Study activity

Talk to children and parents with different cultural backgrounds from your own. Find out their views about sleeping arrangements for infants and young children. Make notes in the margin for future reference.

Concerns regarding an infant's sleeping patterns are often expressed. Sleep problems resulting from behavioural disturbances affect 20–25% of children aged 1–5 years (O'Connor and Gregory, 2002). A number of factors, both within the child and the family, have been suggested as contributing to the development of sleep disturbances. At the same time it must be recognised that what constitutes a problem for one family may be considered normal for another. This is especially important when considering cultural differences. Affective factors such as fear of the dark and other anxiety-provoking events (such as moving house or birth of a sibling) may cause reactions that can be reflected in a child's sleeping pattern. Whatever the cause of the problems, the effects on the family can be devastating.

Sleep problems fall into two main categories which are collectively referred to as disorders of initiating and maintaining sleep (DIMS) (Stores, 2001):

- inability to settle or sleep alone, and/or
- repeated night waking, often with disruptive behaviour and early morning arousal.

It might be possible to solve sleep problems with some commonsense advice, with cultural differences taken into account. However, for more serious problems, further professional advice and treatment may be needed.

Behaviour modification has been increasingly advocated as an effective tool for managing sleep problems. The approach requires careful analysis of the individual problem, establishment of goals of treatment and the setting of gradual steps to attain them. Several studies have attempted to examine the effectiveness of this (Owens *et al.*, 1999; Ramchandi *et al.*, 2000). All the studies suggest that the techniques can be an effective therapy for sleep problems, provided that the treatment is carried out by professionals with experience and knowledge of the technique. It must also be acknowledged that it may not be suitable for all children and that parental involvement in goal setting and evaluation is essential, with the programme being individually tailored to suit each child.

Ideas for dealing with minor sleep problems

- Give child plenty of exercise during the day – both mental and physical
- Go through the same routine every night
- Try to make the period just before bed a quiet time to allow child to wind down
- Leave a small night light on – some children like the comfort of a light being left on overnight
- Allow the child to listen to music or a story tape, or allow them to play for a short while – offer quiet toy or a book
- If the child cries or makes a fuss, wait 10 minutes and go back in, resettle and leave. Repeat as necessary *but* be firm

Further reading

Wiggs, L. (2004) Effective services and programs for managing infant/child sleeping disorders and the impact on the social and emotional development of young children (0–5). In Trembly, R. E., Barr, R. G. and Peters, R. deV. (eds), *Encyclopaedia on Early Childhood Development* (online). Montreal, Quebec: Centre of Excellence for Early Childhood Development. Available at http://www.excellence-earlychildhood.ca/documents/WiggsANGxp.pdf (accessed 17 February 2006).

Cultural Perspectives on Child Rearing

Child-rearing practices differ between cultures and ethnic groups, and it is important to remember this when assessing and working with

Cultural aspects

Reynolds, T. (2005) *Caribbean Mothers: Identity and Experience in the UK*. London: Tufnell Press.

This book provides accounts of historical and cultural patterns of mothering and family ideologies in the cross-national context of the Caribbean, USA and UK. It presents an analysis of the relationship between black and white mothers, black men and women, and mother and child, in order to challenge and deconstruct stereotypical (and pathological) images of black mothers, such as the 'babymother', 'welfare queen' and 'superwoman'.

Transcultural healthcare practice with children and their families, Part one: Well-being, health and development across cultures. Section One: Family life and child rearing practices. RCN Online: http://www.rcn.org.uk/resources/transcultural/childhealth/sectionone.php

This is a great site which contains a wealth of information about cultural differences in child rearing and also activities to help your learning.

children and families. It is wrong to make assumptions based on your own values and beliefs. Chinese parenting practices are still significantly influenced by Confucian principles about family and relationships. Parental control, obedience, strict discipline, filial piety, respect for elders, reverence for tradition and maintaining harmony are all attributed to the influence of Confucianism. Furthermore, Confucian principles require that the elders must responsibly teach, discipline and govern their children. According to Chao (1994) the Chinese and other Asian (for example Japanese, Korean) parenting styles are steeped in Confucian tradition and may best be described as 'training'. The socialisation of Indian children is strongly rooted in patriarchy, hierarchical kinship structure and Hindu religious beliefs. Obedience to authority, passivity and interdependence are highly valued. Mothers are typically kind, indulgent and affectionate, whereas fathers are strict decision-makers who maintain considerable distance from care-giving activities (Konantambigi, 1996). Dosnajh and Ghuman (1997) carried out a study to explore the child-rearing practices of two generations of Punjabi parents. The purpose of the research was to show the effect of acculturation on the child-rearing practices of an ethnic minority community resident in the English Midlands. They found that many of the elaborate customs and rituals had disappeared but there was little difference in feeding and sleeping habits. They concluded that, although there are many factors affecting changing practices, there is a tendency for second-generation Punjabi mothers to adopt and adapt some of the customs and practices of white indigenous mothers (*see also* Children's nursing in a multicultural society pp. 660–668).

Study activity

Find out about the child-rearing practices of as many different cultures/ethnic groups as you can. Consider the implications for your practice with sick children in each case.

Summary

Rearing children has been described as being fulfilling, frustrating, difficult, rewarding and much more, all at the same time. There are no simple prescriptions about how to rear children. The task for parents is to choose the system that works for them from a range of alternatives. Campion (1995) suggests that there are three criteria that interact and contribute to whether good parenting can take place:

- *the child* – age, personality (some children are more demanding and difficult), sex, health
- *the parents* – background and upbringing, relationships with each other, employment, income, health, expectations of the child/children
- *physical and social environment* – housing, supportive networks, transport, schools, assistance with childcare, cultural perspectives

Study activity

Take each of the criteria above. For each one, reflect on issues that facilitate and inhibit good parenting. How might this have implications for your practice?

Key Points

1. Each family will have its own beliefs concerning child rearing, influenced by many factors, including past experience, culture, religion, society and the mass media.
2. The general objectives of child rearing are universal to all parts of the world but the specific nature of practices will depend on culture and the needs of the society in which the child lives.
3. The principles of child rearing are based on meeting the physical and psychosocial needs of the child.
4. The style of parenting adopted will influence the way in which the principles and objectives of child rearing are achieved.
5. Limit setting is important for children, as unrestricted freedoms offer a threat to security and safety.
6. There is no correct way to rear children but there are many suggestions as to how it might be done.
7. Child-rearing practices differ between cultures and ethnic groups.

References

Allen, M. and **Burrell, N.** (1996) Comparing the impact of homosexual and heterosexual parents on children: meta-analysis of existing research. *Journal of Homosexuality,* **32** (2), 19–33.

Ballard, R. and **Kalra, V. S.** (1994) *The Ethnic Dimensions of the 1991 Census: A Preliminary Report.* Manchester: University of Manchester.

Bank, S. P. and **Kahn, M. D.** (1997) *The Sibling Bond.* New York: HarperCollins.

Barnes, M., *et al.* (2005) *Family Life in Britain: Findings from The 2003 Families and Children Study (FACS).* Leeds: Department of Work and Pensions.

Basow, S. A. (1992) *Gender Stereotypes and Roles,* 3rd edn. Pacific Grove, CA: Brooks/Cole.

Baumrind, D. (1991) The influence of parenting style on adolescent competence and substance use. *Journal of Early Adolescence,* **11** (1), 56–95.

Bee, H. (1995) *The Developing Child,* 7th edn. New York: HarperCollins.

Berk, L. (2000) *Child Development,* 5th edn. Boston: Allyn & Bacon.

Biller, H. B. and **Kimpton, J. L.** (1997) The father and the school-aged child. In Lamb, M. E. (ed.), *The Role of the Father in Child Development,* 3rd edn. New York: Wiley.

Blankenhorn, D. (1995) *Fatherless America: Confronting our Most Urgent Social Problem.* New York: Basic Books.

Boer, F. and **Dunn, J.** (1992) *Children's Sibling Relationships: Developmental and Clinical Issues.* Hillsdale, NJ: Lawrence Erlbaum.

Booth, T. (1975) Growing up in society. In Herriot, P. (ed.), *Essential Psychology.* London: Methuen.

Bronfenbrenner, U. and **Morris, P. A.** (1998) The ecology of developmental processes. In Damon, W. and Lerner, R. M. (eds), *Handbook of Child Psychology: Theoretical Models of Human Development,* Vol. 1, 5th edn. New York: Wiley.

Brotherson, S., Yamamoto, T. and **Acock, A. C.** (2003) Connection and communication in father–child relationships and adolescent child well-being. *Fathering,* October 2003. http://www.findarticles.com/p/articles/mi_m0PAV/is_3_1/ai_111268930 (accessed 29 March 2007).

Buck, N., *et al.* (1994) *Changing Households: The British Household Panel Survey 1990–1992.* Colchester: ESRC Research Centre on Micro-social Change, University of Essex.

Campion, M. J. (1995) *Who's Fit to be a Parent?* London: Routledge.

Chao, R. (1994) Beyond parental control and authoritarian parenting style: understanding Chinese parenting through the cultural notion of training. *Child Development,* **65**, 1111–1119.
Collins, W. A., *et al.* (2000) Contemporary research on parenting. The case for nature and nuture. *American Psychologist,* **55** (2), 218–232.
Crouter, A. C., *et al.* (1990) Parental monitoring and perceptions of children's school performance and conduct in dual and single-earner families. *Developmental Psychology,* **26**, 649–657.
CSO (1995) *Social Trends.* London: HMSO.
Cummings, E. M. and **O'Reilly, A. W.** (1997) Fathers in family context: effects of marital quality on child adjustment. In Lamb, M. E. (ed.), *The Role of the Father in Child Development,* 3rd edn. New York: Wiley.
Davidson, J. K. and **Moore, N. B.** (1996) *Marriage and Family: Change and Continuity.* Boston: Allyn & Bacon.
De'Ath, E. (1996) Family change: step-families in context. *Children and Nursing,* **10**, 80–82.
Dex, S. (2003) *Families and Work in the Twenty-first Century.* http://www.jrf.org.uk/knowledge/findings/foundations/923.asp (accessed 6 April 2006).
DfES (2003) *Every Child Matters.* London: The Stationery Office.
Dosnajh, J. S. and **Ghuman, P. A. S.** (1997) Child rearing practices of two generations of Punjabi parents. *Children and Society,* **11**, 29–43.
Dunn, J. (1984) *Sisters and Brothers.* London: Fontana.
Dunn, J., *et al.* (1999) Siblings, parents and partners: family relationships within a longitudinal community study. *Journal of Child Psychology and Psychiatry,* **40**, 1025–1037.
Equal Opportunities Commission (2005) *Facts about Women and Men in Great Britain.* http://www.eoc.org.uk/pdf/facts_about_GB_2005.pdf (accessed 7 April 2006).
Ermisch, J. (2001) Births outside marriage: the real story. *The Edge,* **8**. http://www.esrc.ac.uk/ESRCInfoCentre/about/CI/CP/the_edge/issue8/births_1.aspx?ComponentId=2407&SourcePageId=6573 (accessed 6 April 2006).
Fletcher, R. (1966) *The Family and Marriage in Britain.* Harmondsworth: Penguin.
FSID (2006) *Questions and Answers about Cot Death.* http://www.sids.org.uk/fsid/question.htm (accessed 7 April 2006).
Green, C. (2006) *New Toddler Taming: The World's Best Selling Parenting Guide.* London: Vermillion.
Hart, C. H., Newell, L. D. and **Olsen, S. F.** (2003) Parenting skills and social-communicative competence in childhood. In Greene, J. O. and Burleson, B. R. (eds), *Handbook of Communication and Social Interaction Skills.* Mahwah, NJ: Lawrence Erlbaum Associates.
Hartup, W. W. (1989) Social relationships and their developmental significance. *American Psychologist,* **44**, 120–126.
Haskey, J. (1994) *Stepfamilies and Stepchildren in Great Britain.* Population Trends 76. London: HMSO.
Hetherington, E. M. and **Kelly, J. B.** (2002) *For Better or For Worse: Divorce Reconsidered.* New York: Norton.
Hetherington, E. M. and **Stanley-Hagan, M. M.** (1997) The effects of divorce on fathers and their children. In Lamb, M. E. (ed.), *The Role of the Father in Child Development,* 3rd edn. New York: Wiley.
Hosley, C. A. and **Montemayor, R.** (1997) Fathers and adolescents. In Lamb, M. E. (ed.), *The Role of the Father in Child Development,* 3rd edn. New York: Wiley.
Human Fertilisation and Embryology Authority (HFEA) (2005) http://www.hfea.gov.uk/PressOffice/Factsandfigures (accessed 6 April 2006).
Humphrey, M. and **Humphrey, H.** (1988) *Families with a Difference: Varieties of Surrogate Parenthood.* London: Routledge.
Jewell, J. D. and **Stark, K. D.** (2003) Comparing the family environments of adolescents with conduct disorder and depression. *Journal of Child and Family Studies,* **12**, 77–89.
Jorgensen, J. (1995) *Investigating Families and Households.* London: Collins Educational.
Kelly, J. B. (2003) Changing perspectives on children's adjustment following divorce. *Childhood,* **10** (2), 237–254.
King, T. (1938) *Mothercraft.* New York: Meredith Press.
Konantambigi, R. M. (1996) Beliefs about child, childhood, and upbringing: a crucial component of the developmental niche. ERIC Document Reproduction Service No. ED 407 104. http://www.eric.ed.gov/ERICDocs/data/ericdocs2/content_storage_01/0000000b/80/26/2b/0a.pdf (accessed 7 April 2006).
Lamb, M. E. (1997) *The Role of the Father in Child Development,* 3rd edn. New York: Wiley.
La Valle, I., *et al.* (2002) *Happy Families? Atypical Work and its Influence on Family Life.* Bristol: The Policy Press. http://www.jrf.org.uk/knowledge/findings/socialpolicy/982.asp (accessed 7 April 2006).
Leach, P. (1989) *Baby and Child.* London: Penguin.
Lerner, R. M. and **Spanier, G. B.** (1978) *Child Influences on Marital and Family Interaction: a Lifespan Perspective.* New York: Academic Press.
Lewis, C. (2000) *A Man's Place in the Home: Fathers and Families in the UK.* http://www.jrf.org.uk/knowledge/findings/foundations/440.asp (accessed 6 April 2006).
Macoby, E. E. (1992) The role of parents in the socialization of children: an historical overview. *Developmental Psychology,* **28**, 1006–1017.
Macoby, E. E. and **Martin, J. A.** (1983) Socialisation in the context of the family: parent–child interaction. In Mussen, P. H. (ed.), *Handbook of Child Psychology,* Vol. 4, 4th edn. New York: Wiley.

Mayor, V. (1984) Pregnancy, childbirth and child care. *Nursing Times*, 13 June, pp. 57–58.
McKeown, K., Pratschke, J. and **Haase, T.** (2003) *Family Well Being. What Makes a Difference?* http://www.welfare.ie/publications/famwelloct03.pdf (accessed 29 March 2007).
McQuire, J. (1991) Sons and daughters. In Phoenix, A., Woollett, A. and Lloyd, E. (eds), *Motherhood*. London: Sage.
McQuire, S., *et al.* (2000) Children's perceptions of sibling conflict during middle childhood: Issues and sibling (dis)similarity. *Social Development*, **9**, 173–190.
Milligan, C. and **Dowie, A.** (1998) *What do Children Need from their Fathers?* The University of Edinburgh, Centre for Theology and Public Issues.
Mitchell, J. (2000) *Mad Men and Medusas: Reclaiming Hysteria and the Effects of Sibling Relationships on the Human Condition*. London: Penguin Books.
Moore, S. (2001) *Sociology Alive!* Cheltenham: Stanley Thornes.
Morelli, G. A., *et al.* (1992) Cultural variation in infants' sleeping arrangements: questions of independence. *Developmental Psychology*, **28**, 604–613.
Muncie, J., *et al.* (1995) *Understanding the Family*. London: Sage.
Murdock, G. P. (1949) *Social Structure*. New York: Macmillan.
Mussen, P. H., *et al.* (1994) Dimensions of parent behaviour. In Gott, M. and Maloney, B. (eds), *Child Health: A Reader*. Oxford: Radcliffe Medical Press.
O'Brien, M. and **Jones, D.** (1996) Fathers through the eyes of their children. *Family Policy Bulletin*, November, 4–5.
O'Connor, T. G. and **Gregory, A.** (2002) Sleep problems in childhood: a longitudinal study of developmental change and association with behavioural disturbances. *Journal of the American Academy of Child and Adolescent Psychiatry*, **41**, 964–971.
ONS (2000) *Social Trends 30*. Basingstoke: Palgrave Macmillan.
ONS (2001) *Social Trends 33*. Basingstoke: Palgrave Macmillan.
ONS (2002) *Social Trends 32*. Basingstoke: Palgrave Macmillan.
ONS (2005a) *Social Trends 35*. Basingstoke: Palgrave Macmillan.
ONS (2005b) *Population Trends 121*. Basingstoke: Palgrave Macmillan.
ONS (2005c) *Focus on Families*. http://www.statistics.gov.uk/focuson/families/ (accessed 6 April 2006).
OPCS (1992) *Social Trends 22*. London: HMSO.
OPCS (1993) *General Household Survey 1991*. London: HMSO.
OPCS (1994) *General Household Survey 1992*. London: HMSO.
Owens, J. L., France, K. G. and **Wiggs, L.** (1999) Behavioural and cognitive-behavioural interventions for sleep disorders in infants and children: a review. *Sleep Medicine Reviews*, **3** (4), 281–302.
Parsons, T. (1959) The social structure of the family. In Ashen, R. N. (ed.), *The Family, Its Functions and Destiny*. New York: Harper & Row.
Pleck, J. (1997) Paternal involvement: levels, sources, and consequences. In Lamb, M. E. (ed.), *The Role of the Father in Child Development*. New York: John Wiley & Sons.
Powers, N. (2001) Intrinsic musicality: rhythm and prosody in infant-directed voices. In *Annual Report, 1999–2000, No. 23*. Research and Clinical Center for Child Development, Faculty of Education, Hokkaido University, Japan, pp. 1–19.
Pringle, M. (1980) *The Needs of Children: A Personal Perspective*. London: Hutchinson.
Ramchandi, P., *et al.* (2000) A systematic review of treatments for settling problems and night-waking in children. *British Medical Journal*, **320** (7229), 209–213.
Ribbens, J. (1994) *Mothers and their Children: A Feminist Sociology of Childrearing*. London: Sage.
Rodgers, B. and **Pryor, J.** (1998) *Divorce and Separation: the Outcomes for Children*. http://www.jrf.org.uk/knowledge/findings/foundations/spr6108.asp (accessed 6 April 2006).
Shonkoff, J. and **Phillips, D. (eds)** (2000) *From Neurons to Neighborhoods: The Science of Early Childhood Development*. Washington, DC: National Academy Press.
Sroufe, L. A., Cooper, R. G. and **Dewart, G. B.** (1996) *Child Development: Its Nature and Course*, 3rd edn. New York: McGraw-Hill.
Steinberg, L. (2001) We know some things: parent–adolescent relationships in retrospect and prospect. *Journal of Research on Adolescence*, **11**, 1–19.
Stores, G. (2001) *Sleep Disorders in Children and Adolescents*. Cambridge: Cambridge University Press.
Sulloway, J. (2001) *Sibling Order – Effects*. http://www.sulloway.org/Sibling-order-effects(2001).pdf (accessed 6 April 2006).
Trevarthen, C. (2004) Learning about Ourselves, from Children: Why a Growing Human Brain Needs Interesting Companions. http://www.perception-in-action.ed.ac.uk/PDF_s/Colwyn2004.pdf (accessed 29 March 2007).
United Nations (1989) *UN Convention on the Rights of the Child*. New York: United Nations.
Utting, D. (1995) *Family and Parenthood: Supporting Families, Preventing Breakdown*. York: Joseph Rowntree Foundation.
Wainright, J. L., Russell, S. T. and **Patterson, C. J.** (2004) Psychosocial adjustment, school outcomes, and romantic relationships of adolescents with same-sex parents. *Child Development*, **75**, 1886.
White, D. and **Woollett, A.** (1992) *Families: A Context for Development*. London: Falmer Press.
Willmott, P. (1988) Urban kinship past and present. *Social Studies Review*, November.

Witt, S. D. (1997) Parental influence on children's socialization to gender roles. *Adolescence,* **32** (126), 253–259.
Wolfradt, U., Hempel, S. and **Miles, J. N. V.** (2003) Perceived parenting styles, depersonalisation, anxiety and coping behaviour in adolescents. *Personality and Individual Differences,* **34**, 521–532.
Yang, C. K. and **Hahn, H. M.** (2002) Cosleeping in young Korean children. *Journal of Developmental Behaviour Pediatrics,* **23**, 151–157.
Young, M. and **Willmott, P.** (1975) *The Symmetrical Family.* London: Penguin.

Module 2
The Growing Child
Tina Moules

Learning Outcomes

The material in this module and the further reading/references will enable you to:

- explore the nature of childhood and how it has changed over recent years
- investigate the factors that can influence the growth and development of children
- develop an understanding of life before birth and its implications for the care of sick children
- develop a knowledge of the way in which children grow and in which the body systems mature with time
- critically analyse the various theoretical views on cognitive and social development
- examine the role of play and education in child development

Introduction

In China, age is determined not by date of birth but by date of conception. This is an appropriate concept in the study of children because growth and development begin at the moment of conception. Then follows a process that is both fascinating and mysterious to observe.

The growth and development that take place during this period are common to nearly all children but they occur at different rates and with different outcomes. Some aspects of development are universal; the child's environment and experiences affect others. Babies all develop their own personality, intellect and social disposition within the context of a 'family', developing skills, knowledge and attitudes to equip them for the society into which they have been born. The baby changes from the infant 'mewling and puking in the nurse's arms' to the adolescent ready for independence and the challenge of adult life.

Many different psychologists have attempted to unravel the mysteries of child development, exploring the influence of environment on developmental processes and trying to make sense of the child's world. Theories of normal development provide parameters to help make sense of personal lives, showing what is generally expected at different stages of the life cycle and anticipating potential crises. Whatever the answers are (and there are many different answers) it is essential that those of us who work with children understand the changes that take place so that we can give appropriate age-related care. A child is a precious gift and as such deserves to be treated as an individual, nurtured and cared for by responsive,

growth
An increase in size and number of cells, resulting in an increase in size and weight of the whole or any of its parts.

development
An increase in complexity; the emerging of an individual's capacities through learning, growth and maturation.

maturation
An increase in competence and adaptability; a change in the complexity of a structure that makes it possible for that structure to work.

understanding adults. To do this we need to be aware of the ways in which children think about the world and the people around them.

This module is intended to give you an overview of the various aspects of child development and to encourage you to explore further by providing you with ideas for additional reading and by inspiring you with a thirst for more knowledge. It begins by exploring the nature of childhood and the factors that influence growth and development, considering both prenatal and postnatal factors. Some discussion follows on growth and maturation, examining the way in which various systems of the body mature. The module moves on to analyse some of the various theoretical views on development, considering first cognitive development (including language development) and then the social world of the child. To conclude the module we look at the role of play and education in the development of the child, with special reference to children with special needs.

Chapter 5

The Nature of Childhood

Introduction

It would seem from the extensive literature on childhood that the nature of this concept is complex and continuously evolving. There is very little consensus between writers, with some suggesting that childhood was evident as early as the fourth century BC (Watt and Mitchell, 1995) and others that it did not really emerge until the 17th century. Aries (1962) suggested that childhood was invented in the 13th century. This is not to say that children were neglected, abused or unloved, but in medieval times adults were simply unaware that there was a difference between childhood and adulthood and treated children as adults.

The nature of childhood is dependent on, and relative to, the views that adults have about children at any one time. Childhood, for the children of the poor in previous centuries, was always brief. Children born into poverty were a burden to their parents and were put to work as soon as possible. Children as young as 4 years worked in the textile mills, picking up waste cotton from underneath unguarded machinery. Young children worked up to 12 hours a day in coal mines. Infant and child mortality was high but it was not dwelt on too much as other children were soon born to take their place. Children of the more affluent were a different kind of investment, cementing social status through marital alliances (Lester, 1993). There was little, if any, state intervention in the lives of children; they were their parents' possessions. In pre-industrial Britain there were no laws specifically governing the work of young children, and it was only when children began to be seen in greater numbers in workplaces (as a result of the Industrial Revolution) that a series of questions started to be asked about the appropriateness of certain types of work for children. The 1833 Factory Act provided the first intervention in the labour market to protect children and for the first time they were seen as having specific, enshrined rights.

According to Heward (1993) profound changes in the nature of childhood began to take place in the 19th century. This century saw

Important dates in the development of childhood

- Elementary Education Act 1870
- Sandon Act 1876 (made parents responsible for ensuring their children went to school)
- Mundella Act 1880 (established School Attendance Committees)
- United Nations Convention on the Rights of the Child 1989
- The Children Act 1989
- Human Rights Act 1998
- The Children Act 2004

developments that contributed to a change in the way adults viewed their children. One of the most important of these was the introduction and enforcement of compulsory education between the ages of 5 and 10 years, and with it a move towards acceptance of state intervention. In 1880, the enforcement of school attendance (in England) made childhood more standardised, with all children beginning to have a settled period at school. Education served to separate children from adults, giving them their own place in society.

There was a steady decline in child labour, brought about by rising standards of living, technological advances in agriculture and industry, and parents began to realise the benefits of investing in and prolonging their children's education (Nardinelli, 1990). However, children's experiences of schooling remained heavily dependent on their class and gender. Thirdly, as the status of children and the concept of childhood changed, studies of child development began. One of the earliest studies was made by Charles Darwin – of his own son. He believed that by observing children one could reveal the descent of man.

The health of children began to improve. Services specifically designed for children began to emerge in Europe and in the United Kingdom. Children's dispensaries were opened in London (1816), Manchester (1829), Liverpool (1851), followed by the founding of the Hospital for Sick Children, Great Ormond Street, London, in 1852 (Kosky and Lunnon, 1991).

The 20th century and the beginning of the 21st century have seen further changes as smaller families allow deeper relationships between children and their parents. The birth rate has fallen and children have become more 'precious'. There is a general acceptance that children need to be protected and guided. The views of children are being taken more seriously as we deal with issues of children's rights and their role in society. Although gender differences remain, they are becoming less important. Opportunities and education are seen as being just as important for girls as they are for boys. Numerous theorists have pondered the nature of childhood, giving us views on how children become adults. We are more interested in ensuring that all children grow up healthy and that they are given every opportunity to develop to their full potential, and recognise that childhood experience will affect adult lives.

Schaffer (2004) observes that we begin to understand the constructed nature of what childhood is when we start to consider how concepts of childhood had particular importance at certain points in time and in certain cultures. So, how children are viewed depends on many social, political and religious forces that exist at a particular time and place. The answer to the question 'What is childhood?' depends upon the nature of a particular society and its beliefs and customs in which a child is brought up.

Study activity

Talk to your parents and grandparents. What was childhood like for them? Talk to the parents and children of different cultures that you will come across in practice. Compare their stories with that of your own childhood.

Study activity

Key (1909) claimed that the 20th century would be the century of the child, in which children would take their rightful place beside adults as full and equal participants in society. Take time to consider whether we have reached an effective understanding to support this dream for the 21st century.

Factors Influencing Growth and Development

Many of the debates about child development have centred around the nature-versus-nurture controversy. Those that favour the former believe that human behaviour is guided by inborn biological factors. They would argue that individual differences are a result of heredity. Those that favour the concept of nurturing stress the importance of acknowledging the influence of a child's physical and social environment. According to them, individual differences are a result of the various experiences that children have. In truth the reality is probably somewhere in between, with both inherited and environmental factors playing an important role. Development is a complex process and it occurs as a result of an interaction between many variables, the effect of which will be different for each child. No two children are the same, even when they have the same parents and a similar home environment. Many factors have been identified as being influential in the development of children (Figure 5.1) but generally they fall into two categories – inherited and environmental.

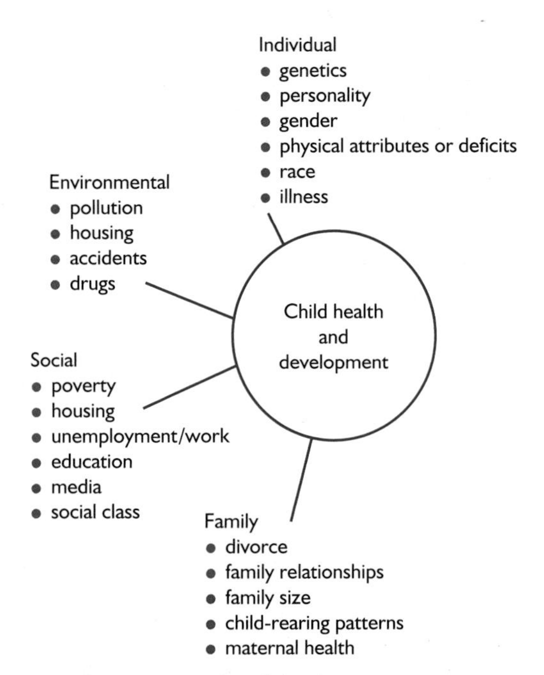

Figure 5.1 Factors influencing growth and development.

Heredity

This refers to the transmission of characteristics from one generation to the next. Many of our characteristics or traits are influenced by our genotype – a unique genetic blueprint that each of us possesses, based on the mix of genes from our parents. There are many ways in which genetic disease can arise through the variation in the number of chromosomes, the sets of chromosomes and their order, and mutations at the level of the gene. At its simplest level, change in a gene could bring about the absence or presence of disease. Identification of many specific genes and their loci on specific chromosomes has progressed rapidly over recent years. As well as knowing the locus of some genes that control characteristics such as hair and eye colour and blood group, researchers now know the loci for those that lead to genetic disorders such as cystic fibrosis. This brings diagnosis and treatment of these conditions ever nearer. Genes are classed as either *dominant* or *recessive* and as such result in various patterns of inheritance (*see also* Genetic factors p. 128).

Dominant inheritance

A dominant gene exerts its influence over the other gene with which it is paired. The gene can be transmitted by either sex. It affects both males and females, and often individuals are affected in more than one generation. For example, parents who have different-coloured eyes will each pass on different genes to their offspring. In this case whichever gene is dominant will exert its influence and will therefore determine eye colour. This principle can also be applied to those diseases passed on through dominant inheritance (Figure 5.2).

Recessive inheritance

A recessive gene needs to be paired up with another carrying exactly the same information for it to influence a characteristic's outcome. For example, the gene for blue eyes is recessive; therefore each parent must himself or herself carry the gene (although they may not have blue eyes) and there must be a successful pairing of these genes in the offspring (Figure 5.3).

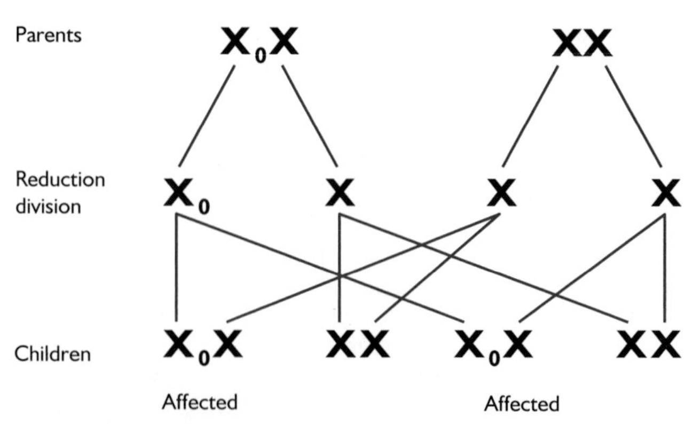

Figure 5.2 Dominant inheritance. Each pregnancy has a 1:2 risk of an affected child of either sex. X_0 = affected gene.

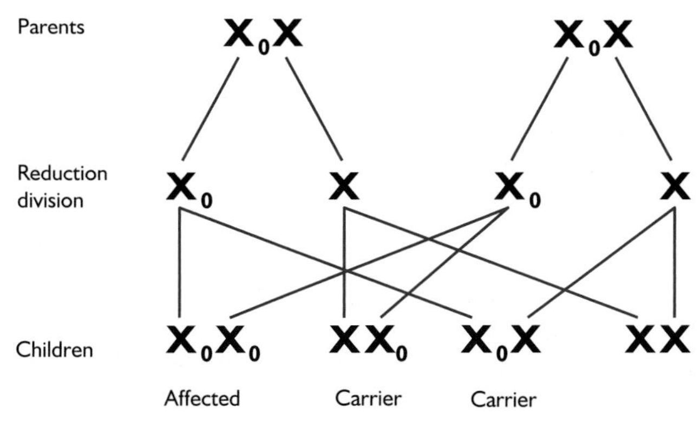

Figure 5.3 Recessive inheritance. There is a 1:4 chance of a child inheriting a recessive genes from both parents, and a 1:2 chance of each child being a carrier. X_0 = affected gene.

The inheritance of some disorders follows the same principles – for example, Tay–Sachs disease, cystic fibrosis and sickle-cell anaemia. It is possible, in this instance, for a characteristic (or disease) to appear 'out of the blue' with no recent family history, or to miss generations.

Sex-linked inheritance

Some characteristics (and diseases) are carried on the female chromosome. Genes on the X chromosome have no counterpart on the Y chromosome, so a characteristic that is determined by a gene on the X chromosome is *always* expressed in the male and so always acts as a dominant gene. If a woman is a carrier of a recessive gene (for example haemophilia) there is a 1:2 chance of her sons having the disease and a 1:2 chance of her daughters being carriers (Figure 5.4). An affected male will only pass on the affected gene to his daughters, meaning that all his daughters will carry the affected gene.

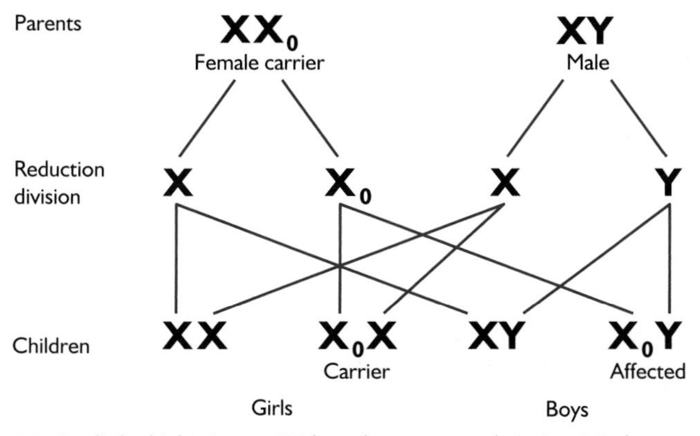

Figure 5.4 Sex-linked inheritance. With each pregnancy there is a 1:2 chance of each girl being a carrier or unaffected, and a 1:2 chance of each boy having the disease or being unaffected.

Chromosomal abnormalities

Sometimes there is a disruption on one or more of the chromosomes when they unite following fertilisation in the ovum. The precise cause of chromosome abnormalities is not known but much of the information suggests a link with maternal age (Glasper and Richardson, 2006). The incidence of Down's syndrome, for example, increases markedly with maternal age regardless of the number of pregnancies. There is also some evidence to suggest that some teratogens may cause defects.

Chromosome defects are mainly caused by:

- Non-disjunction – this is the failure of chromosomes to separate during meiosis or mitosis. Unequal distribution of chromosomes between the two resulting cells follows. Down's syndrome, Turner's syndrome and Klinefelter's syndrome result from non-disjunction.
- Translocation – this occurs when two chromosomes exchange material. These exchanges are usually spontaneous and may result in a spontaneous miscarriage.

Results of these defects can be detected through the use of amniocentesis or chorionic villus sampling (CVS) during the early stages of pregnancy.

The Human Genome Project
This project started in 1990 and was completed in 2003. Its main aim was to identify all the approximately 20 000–25 000 genes in human DNA. Visit the web site to find out more about this project:

http://www.ornl.gov/sci/techresources/Human_Genome/home.shtml

The Human Genome Project

Many disease-causing genes have been identified through scientific endeavours such as the genome project. It is expected that most genetic diseases will be mapped and sequenced before the late 2020s and as such it is possible that many congenital abnormalities of unknown origin will be identified and treatments will be made available. This will have major implications in relation to prenatal care and could lead to the abolition of some genetic abnormalities such as Down's syndrome, cystic fibrosis and some cancers.

The Environment

The extent to which any child's growth and development is influenced by his environment will depend on many complex interactions. Some factors will influence the child both before and after birth. Others will only come into play as the child grows (see Figure 5.1). It is impossible to give due consideration to all factors, so only the major ones will be examined.

Nutrition

This is considered by many to be the most influential factor at any stage of development from the moment of implantation. The fetus receives nutrition from the maternal system and therefore any deficiencies will manifest in fetal development. Chronic intrauterine malnutrition might have a negative effect on complex functions such as social development or intelligence in the absence of early, detectable, severe deficits.

Severe malnutrition in pregnancy has been cited as being responsible for a permanent reduction in the total number of fetal brain cells, thereby influencing the child's later intellectual functioning (Glasper and Richardson, 2006). Grantham-McGregor *et al.* (1994) suggest that infants who are malnourished during pregnancy exhibit tired and restless behaviour, causing their mothers to be less sensitive and stimulating. Thus the babies become even more passive and withdrawn, requiring intervention to enable successful interaction and social engagement. Bee and Boyd (2004) suggest that those who are reared in a stimulating environment have been shown to overcome fetal malnutrition. Other effects of malnutrition in pregnancy include a greater risk of stillbirths, low birthweight babies and infant death during the first year of life.

A link between adult health problems (such as ischaemic heart disease, stroke, hypertension and non-insulin-dependent diabetes) and nutrition in early life has been suggested by various researchers (Fall *et al.*, 1992; Eriksson *et al.*, 2001; Barker *et al.*, 2002). The explanation for these links may lie in the role of nutrition in the programming of organs during development. Nutritional inadequacy may prevent organs developing to their full potential, thus predisposing the infant to chronic disease in later life (Department of Health, 1994).

Teratogens – diseases and drugs

A teratogen is any substance, agent or process that brings about developmental abnormalities in the fetus as a result of exposure. Before birth, the effect of any teratogen will depend on the time at which exposure occurs. Each organ is most vulnerable to disruption when it is developing most rapidly. These periods are known as 'critical' or 'sensitive' periods (Moore and Persaud, 2003) (Table 5.1).

One substance known to cause developmental problems is tobacco. The best known side-effect of smoking during pregnancy is low birth weight. The more a mother smokes, the higher are the chances that her baby will be affected. There are numerous effects, including miscarriage, prematurity, cardiac and respiratory problems, and increased risk of sudden infant death syndrome (SIDS), glue ear and cancer in later childhood. Some women are exposed to the effects of nicotine through passive ingestion of smoke from their partners and co-workers. There are still implications associated with passive smoking, albeit at a lesser level (*see also* Immunisation schedule p. 512 and Incubation/infectious period p. 502).

Table 5.1 Sensitive periods in organ development before birth (adapted from Moore and Persaud, 2003)

Week of gestation	Common sites of damage from disease, drugs, or other outside disturbances
3	Central nervous system and heart
4 + 5	Eyes, heart, limbs
6	Ears, teeth
7	Palate
8	Ears, external genitalia
12	Central nervous system, external genitalia
16	Central nervous system
20–36	Brain

Note: the embryonic period is generally the time of greatest vulnerability

There are many diseases that, if they occur during pregnancy, can cause disruption to one or more of the developing organs:

- *Rubella*. The effects of this infectious disease during pregnancy are becoming rare due to the national immunisation programme. Rubella is a relatively mild infectious disease but one that can have devastating effects on the fetus if contracted within the first 3 months of pregnancy. Damage can include learning disability, genital, urinary and intestinal defects, congenital cataracts, blindness, underdeveloped eyes and, sometimes, congenital deafness. Brown and Susser (2002) have identified that there are links between brain abnormalities as a result of prenatal rubella and subsequent severe mental illness such as schizophrenia.
- *Toxoplasmosis*. This infection is caused by a parasite found in the faeces of infected cats and in infected meat. The mother's infection is not obvious and she may not know she has been in contact with the parasite. However, it can cross the placental barrier and can lead to stillbirth and damage to the developing eyes or brain. Infection in later pregnancy can lead to an enlarged liver or spleen, jaundice or convulsions. Problems can even arise some years after birth. About 80% of children infected during pregnancy with no obvious signs of damage develop learning and visual disabilities in later life.
- *Listeriosis*. This mild, feverish condition in adulthood is caused through a food-borne infection commonly associated with soft cheeses and undercooked chicken. If contracted during pregnancy, it can lead to premature birth, meningoencephalitis, hydrocephalus or intrauterine death.
- *Cytomegalovirus* (CMV) is a virus in the herpes group. It is a common prenatal infection (transmitted through respiratory or sexual contact) for which there is no vaccine or treatment. Very few babies whose mothers have the CMV virus become infected before birth, but those who do have a variety of severe problems, including deafness and damage to the central nervous system leading to retardation. Infected babies are often born prematurely.
- *AIDS*. A proportion of babies born to HIV-positive mothers are themselves seropositive (European Collaborative Study, 1991). Although the incidence of AIDS has declined in industrialised nations, the disease shows a steady increase in developing nations. In South Africa, 25% of all pregnant women are HIV positive and transmit the virus to their unborn child at a rate of 20–30% (Kasmauski and Jaret, 2003). Untreated, these babies will have repeated respiratory infections and weight loss; they are prone to brain damage as a result of the virus and will have delayed motor and cognitive development.

There are a number of drugs that, if taken during pregnancy, can cause abnormal development of the fetus.

Study activity

List the drugs that you know that can cause problems if taken during pregnancy. Make your notes in the margin. Check your list against that given in the box on p. 59.

Sociological Factors

A variety of sociological factors affect a child's development before and after birth. The following can be considered to have a direct or an indirect effect:

- the family, including family structure, the loss or absence of parents, the size of the family and child-rearing styles
- housing, poverty, unemployment
- access to preschool education
- culture and ethnicity
- social inequalities
- relationships
- health

Bronfenbrenner and Morris (1998) see the family as the centre of a network of interdependent relationships, with the behaviours of each family member have an impact on each other (*see also* Family p. 4 and Relationships p. 17).

Study activity

Explore each of the above and critically analyse the effect each may have on child development.

The media

The degree to which the media influence children has been a topic for debate for some time. There are many who believe that the mass media have negative influences on children and there is a growing concern about the effects of violence on television and in the cinema. There is no doubt that all forms of media exert a strong influence on children. The media in all their forms are part and parcel of children's everyday lives. The developments of the computer and the Internet have opened up even more avenues for children to explore a huge range of material. Lindsay (1994) summarises the suggested undesirable influences of the mass media but counters each with positive arguments:

- Mass media take children away from other more fulfilling and interactive occupations. Subrahmanyam *et al.* (2001) found that there was evidence of a concomitant increase in obesity, hand injuries and epileptic seizures as a result of increased computer use, and suggest that children and young people could be using their computers for up to four and a half hours per day. Fishbein (1987) found that other activities, such as reading, suffered as a result of watching television, but Subrahmanyam *et al.* suggest that computers and the Internet are used to support learning, that users may be connecting to other young people in a social context, and that hobbies such as sport, and time with friends did not suffer.
- The mass media promote unrealistic stereotyping, which can lead to undesirable attitudes. However, although this may be true in some instances, it is suggested that television can and is presenting more positive representations of some groups (for example women or

Your list may include some or all of the following:

- aspirin
- antibiotics
- anticonvulsants
- pesticides
- radiation at high doses
- lead
- cocaine
- alcohol

ethnic minority groups), leading children to view both sexes and other minority groups in positive ways (Gunter, 1986).

- The mass media use marketing strategies specifically aimed at children, thereby encouraging consumerism. Woodward (1998) suggested that children will not avoid exposure to consumerist messages and that this may lead to a fall in social standards and to subsequent criminal behaviour; however, his cross-sectional study did not support his initial hypothesis. Children are subjected to marketing in many forms, through programmes featuring media characters such as Thunderbirds and Barbie, and role models, and through advertisements for anything from sweets to clothes and even undesirable commodities such as cigarettes and alcohol. The government has taken steps to prevent the overt advertisement of alcohol and cigarettes within sports fixtures and other situations to which children and young people may be exposed. There may be some positive effects of marketing. If children's consumption of sweets and use of toys is influenced by the media, it might be possible to positively influence their lifestyles. The empowerment of children through the development of effective health promotion, which is seen as the responsibility of the media and healthcare professionals, can only enable the development of autonomy and responsibility.
- The mass media encourage young people to develop antisocial behaviour. Evidence to support this is slim but there is a link between mass media use and risk-taking behaviours in adolescence (Klein *et al.*, 1993). Comstock and Sharrer (2001) concluded that television can provide children with an extensive 'how to' course in aggression, and Anderson and Bushman (2001) suggest that playing violent video and computer games has similar effects. Berk (2005) cites a series of longitudinal studies that have found that time watching TV in childhood and adolescence predicted aggressive behaviour in early adulthood (after accounting for a number of factors such as IQ, parent education and income, and neighbourhood crime). Berk suggests that media violence hardens children to aggression and makes them more tolerant of it. The newer forms of media have not been studied adequately but concern is warranted through the logical extension of earlier research on other media forms and the amount of time the average child spends with increasingly sophisticated media. It is possible that children's access and exposure to these media can be regulated and restricted, but parents need to consider the value of access to multimedia resources in such a way that they can exert a positive influence and encourage pro-social behaviour (*see also* Parental behaviour p. 196).

Study activity

What impact do you think that the media has on children and young people? Is the Internet a useful learning and social aid or does it make children dangerously accessible to those who wish to exert undue pressure on them? Can you think of ways in which children and young people's vulnerability can be protected?

Can you think of positive ways that mass media can be used to bring about changes in health? You might carry out some small-scale research to answer some of the questions posed here.

Summary

There are many factors that impact upon children's growth and development. What is certain is that development occurs within a complex context where factors interact with each other to exert a variety of influences. It is probably impossible to identify some of the influencing factors in a child's life. We must assess each child as an individual and take into account aspects of his or her life and experiences that may impact upon development. The preceding discussions aim to encourage you to be aware of influencing factors when caring for children, and to explore issues raised in more detail.

Study activity

Identify two children you have cared for. Reflect on each child's growth and development and identify factors that may have been influential. Compare and contrast your ideas with the issues covered within this chapter.

Key Points

1. Childhood is a complex and evolving concept – our understanding is based on the views that adults have, and have had, of children at various times throughout history.
2. The growth and development of children is influenced by both genetic and environmental factors.
3. Heredity accounts for some of our physical characteristics, but other inherited features can be influenced by environmental factors and life experience after birth.
4. There are environmental factors that can influence growth and development today, including aspects of family and relationships, lifestyle, disease and sociological issues.
5. The mass media have been accused of exerting a negative influence on development, but there are some who would argue that there could also be positive outcomes.

Chapter 6
Growth and Maturation

Introduction

According to the Chinese, life begins at conception and this is the point from which age is calculated. This belief acknowledges the importance of life before birth and the fact that intrauterine life and neonatal life constitute a continuum. It therefore seems appropriate when exploring child growth and development to start at the moment of conception. Life before birth is usually divided into three phases:

1. *Germinal stage – from day 1 to day 14.* On day 1 fertilisation occurs and the zygote divides into two cells. By day 3 there are several dozen cells, now called a blastocyst, and by day 5 the blastocyst divides. A cavity forms within the ball of cells and the cells divide into an outer layer of cells, which will become the support for the developing embryo, and the inner mass which will become the embryo. Implantation of the blastocyst in the wall of the uterus begins at about 7 days and is complete within the first 2 weeks.
2. *Embryonic stage – 2–8 weeks.* This is a crucial time as the basis of all the major organs develop during this stage. The supportive structures also develop. These consist of the amnion (the sac in which the fetus floats), the placenta (fully developed by about 4 weeks after conception) and the umbilical cord (which connects the embryo's circulatory system to the placenta). The placenta acts as the embryo's lifeline, providing nutrients and oxygen and disposing of waste products. It also acts as a barrier that filters out many harmful substances, such as viruses; however, there are some that can cross the placental barrier, such as drugs, anaesthetics and some diseases. At day 16 the blastocyst differentiates into three layers of cells, called the embryonic plate. Cells of the ectoderm will become the brain, nervous tissue and epidermis; cells of the mesoderm will give rise to connecting tissue, kidneys and genitalia; cells of the endoderm will become other internal organs, including the digestive tract. By 4–5 weeks, folding of the embryonic plate transforms the plate into a tiny

embryo that has a primitive heart, the beginnings of a nervous system, embryonic eyes and ears, and the first suggestion of developing limbs (Figure 6.1). By 8 weeks the embryo is about one and a half inches long and all the basic structures of the organs are formed. No further fundamental changes will take place. The embryo begins to look human and is floating in a fluid-filled cavity.

Study activity

Consider the implications of adverse effects on the embryo during the folding of the neural plate.

Further reading

http://classweb.gmu.edu/awinsler/ordp/prenatal.html

An interesting site with many links to all manner of web pages showing fetal development. Some pages aimed at parents to be, but still of use for you in your exploration of this fascinating area.

http://departments.weber.edu/CHFam/Prenatal/frames1.htm

This web site gives you some really good views of the fetus *in utero*. Interactive too.

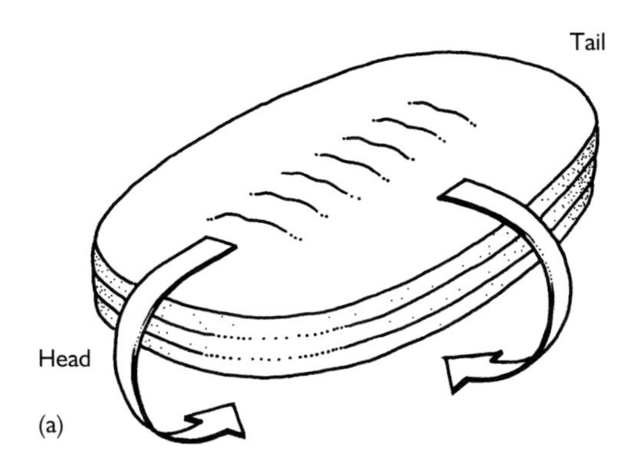

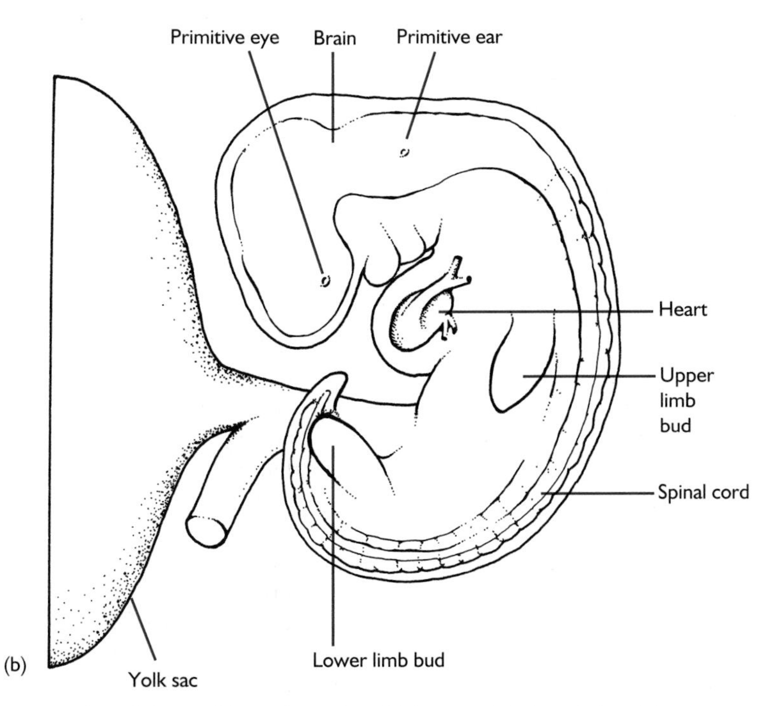

Figure 6.1 (a) Folding of the embryo plate. (b) Embryo at 4–5 weeks' gestation.

Module 2

Study activity

Considering that all the basic structures are present and formed by 8 weeks, what are the implications for the care of pregnant women?

3. *Fetal stage – 9 weeks to birth.* Maturation of the systems continues during this stage. Between 9 and 12 weeks the kidneys begin to produce urine, the bones grow, ossification begins and the genitalia develop. The fetus becomes active as the nervous system begins to mature. Neurons begin to appear at about 12 weeks and are virtually all present by 28 weeks. However, the axons are only very short and there are no dendrites. By the fifth month the fetal ovaries have produced *all* the 5 million ovarian follicles, and a soft downy hair – lanugo – covers the skin. During the final 3 months the fetus grows rapidly and gains most of its birth weight. If the baby continued to grow at such a rapid rate after birth, he would weigh 160 lb (73 kg) on his first birthday. Hair begins to grow on the baby's head and the lanugo is shed. By the seventh month, the testes in a male fetus have reached the scrotum. During the eighth month the fetus develops an insulating layer of fat which helps to keep him warm after birth. It is during this time that antibodies and gamma globulin are passed from the mother across the placenta to the fetus. This gives the baby protection from infections, which will gradually wear off within the first 6 months of life. In the last 2 months the nervous system matures considerably as the axons lengthen and the dendrites grow, giving rise to a vast number of synapses.

The moment of birth

The fetus usually stops growing by day 260, probably because the ageing placenta loses much of its efficiency. Although many suggest that it is the ageing of the placenta that brings about the change in maternal hormone balance, which sets off labour, Nathanielsz (1996) argues that there is evidence to support the idea that the fetus decides when it is time to be born. It is thought that the fetus does this by releasing hormones that convert progesterone to oestrogen, which in turn stimulates the mother to produce oxytocin. Oxytocin stimulates the production of prostaglandin, which enhances the ability of the uterus to contract.

Principles of growth and development

- Development proceeds from the head downward
- Development proceeds from the centre of the body outward
- Development depends on maturation and learning
- Development proceeds from the simple (concrete) to the more complex
- Growth and development is a continuous process
- Growth and development proceed from the general to specific
- There are individual rates of growth and development

(Ruffin, N. J. (2001) Human growth and development – a matter of principles. http://www.ext.vt.edu/pubs/family/350-053/350-053.pdf)

Biological Maturation, Growth and Development after Birth

Universal, predictable patterns of growth are basic to all human beings. However, children differ in the rate at which they grow and in their ultimate size, making each unique. It is important for children's nurses to have an understanding of how children grow and the development of physical abilities, in order that they can recognise the abnormal. At the same time, knowledge of the maturation process of systems of the body assists the nurse in planning appropriate care.

Maturation

All the organs' basic structures are laid down by 8 weeks of intrauterine life, with more maturation occurring prior to birth, but there are still aspects that require further maturation:

- *Bones.* Development of the bones begins early in embryonic life and is usually complete by the late teens or early twenties. During the growth of long bones, a thin strip of cartilage persists between each epiphysis and diaphysis, called the epiphyseal plate. The bones will continue to grow as long as new cartilage develops to maintain this plate. Cessation of bone growth occurs when it becomes ossified and fusion occurs. The growth and development of bone consists of two processes that occur at the same time, namely the creation of new cells and tissues (growth) and the consolidation of these tissues into a permanent form (maturation). An increase in the number of bones occurs in the hands and feet. For example a 1-year-old has three bones in the wrist, an adult has none. Term infants have well-formed skull bones separated by strips of connective tissue, sutures and fontanelles. Mature suture closure occurs by 12 years of age, but completion continues into the third decade of life and beyond. The fontanelles close at different times, the posterior closes at 3–6 months and the anterior at 9–18 months (Kabbani and Raghuveer, 2004).
- *Muscles.* Virtually all muscles are present at birth. After birth they become thicker, longer and less watery until adolescence, when there is a growth spurt in muscles. Finger and toe muscles (used in fine motor dexterity) are the last to develop. A noticeable increase in strength accompanies this growth and is greater in boys than girls.
- *Neurological system.* Most systems grow rapidly after birth but not so the nervous system. The two most rapid periods in the development of the nervous system occur during fetal life. At 9 months of gestation, the brain generally looks quite adult but it has far to go. The average newborn human brain weighs less than 400 g, whereas the typical human adult brain weighs about 1400 g. Much of the weight increase occurs during the first 3 years after birth, but the brain does not reach its maximum weight until about 20 years of age. The cranium continues to expand until about 7 years. Postnatal growth and maturation are mainly related to an increase in communication ability by the advancement of peripheral axons (thereby increasing control over reflexes) and an increase in the amount of cytoplasm around the nuclei. Most of the dendritic growth occurs in the cortex during the early years, aiding the development of imagination and language. Myelination is crucial to the development of the nervous system. Myelin sheaths protect the axons and improve conductivity. Myelination develops in the cephalocaudal direction. The spinal cord and brain stem (which controls vital body functions such as respiration, heart rate and gastro-intestinal function) are essentially fully organised by birth, and myelination of the axons in these regions is quite complete. Shortly after birth, myelination of axons in the cerebellum (concerned with motor coordination) and midbrain begins, and thereafter – by the end of the first year or early in the second year – it begins in various parts of the forebrain, including the cerebral cortex. The last brain structure to mature is the cerebral

cephalocaudal
Head to toe direction.

Question
What are the implications for practice of closure of the fontanelles?

Question
The cranium expands until the age of 7 years – what are the implications for practice?

glomerular filtration rate
The rate at which fluid is filtered by the glomerulus. It is measured by determining the excretion volume and plasma concentration of a substance that is readily filtered through the glomeruli but not secreted or reabsorbed by the renal tubules.

(Watson, 1979)

Question
Infants of 0–4 weeks are nose breathers – what are the implications for practice?

cortex. Myelination is normally complete by about 2 years of age (Dowling, 2004).

- *Renal system.* Most kidney growth occurs during the last 20 weeks of fetal life, with all the nephrons formed by 28 weeks. After birth, kidney size increases in size in proportion to body length, the weight doubling in the first 10 months of life as a result of tubular growth. The glomerular filtration rate (GFR) increases after birth to reach adult values by the age of 2–3 years. In the first few hours after birth there is a high urine volume with low concentration as a result of immaturity of the sodium- and water-regulatory systems. Following a diuresis of water the volume gradually falls and the concentration rises. The newborn infant is able to excrete amino acids and conserve sodium and glucose as well as the adult, but the ability to excrete free water and to concentrate water is immature. Therefore the infant is less able to excrete large water loads and less able to concentrate the urine in response to dehydration. The regulation of acid–base balance is relatively efficient in infancy but the ability to secrete hydrogen ions is relatively immature, leading to a limited renal concentration for metabolic acidosis. Dehydration, hypotension and hypoxaemia all produce a marked fall in GFR, so renal function becomes compromised quickly in a crisis (*see also* Maintaining fluid balance p. 342).
- *Respiratory system.* Every component of the respiratory system is immature at birth. The lungs mature after birth with increased airway dimensions and more alveoli. The airways of the infant are small and easily blocked. By the age of about 10 the increase in alveoli ceases and is followed by an increase in size. By this time there are about nine times as many alveoli as there were at birth. It is also important to recognise that from 0 to 4 weeks the infant breathes through its nose. In the young infant the chest wall is very compliant, gradually becoming more rigid. It is therefore easily distorted, increasing the work of respiration.
- *Gastro-intestinal system.* Most biochemical and physiological functions are established at birth. Secretory cells are functional but depend on a specific relationship, which is gradually acquired with age, therefore efficiency may be reduced. The newborn's glands, reaching full size and function by the age of 2 years, only produce small amounts of saliva. Acidity of the gastric juice is low in infancy, rising to adult levels by about 10 years. The mechanical functions are relatively immature. The oesophageal sphincter is functionally immature during the first 4–6 months of life. Swallowing is an automatic reflex for the first 3 months until the striated muscles in the throat establish cerebral connections. By 6 months the infant is capable of swallowing, holding food in the mouth or spitting it out. The stomach lies horizontally and is round in shape until about 2 years. It then gradually elongates until it assumes the adult position by about 7 years. The capacity of the stomach changes with age (Table 6.1). The immaturity of the digestive system in the infant is shown by the rapidity with which food is propelled through the gastro-intestinal tract. Emptying time in the newborn is 2.5 to 3 hours, in older infants and children it is 3–6 hours. Peristalsis is more rapid in infancy than at any other time and can reverse, resulting in posseting.

Table 6.1 Stomach capacity

Age	Capacity (ml)
Newborn	10–20
1 week	30–90
2–3 weeks	75–100
1 month	90–150
3 months	150–200
1 year	210–360
2 years	500
10 years	750–900
16 years	1500
Adult	2000–3000

- *Body water.* Water is the largest constituent of body tissues – about 70% in the infant and about 60% in the young adult. Water is found in the cells (intracellular) and outside the cells (extracellular). In the adult most water is found inside the cells (67%) but in the infant the larger proportion of water is found outside the cells and there is a higher turnover of water (due to heat production and an inability of the kidneys to conserve water).

Other important points to note related to maturation of the systems include:

- Infants and young children have large surface area/volume ratios
- Infants under 6 months cannot shiver to generate heat – they produce heat through 'non-shivering thermogenesis'
- Children have a higher metabolic rate
- The liver is immature during infancy and less able to metabolise toxic substances
- Infants frequently develop hypoglycaemia during periods of stress because they have high glucose demands and low glycogen stores
- Heart rate is more rapid and stroke volume smaller than in the adult
- The child's circulating blood volume is greater per kilogram than that of an adult, but volume is low. Therefore a small blood loss may affect blood volume significantly

non-shivering thermogenesis

The breakdown of brown fat to create heat. The process requires energy so that the infant's oxygen requirement will increase. The regeneration of brown fat requires good nutrition. A poor calorie intake will mean that brown fat is not replaced and the infant will be less able to maintain body heat in a cool environment.

Further reading

Polin, R. A., Fox, W. W. and Abman, S. H. (2003) *Fetal and Neonatal Physiology*, 3rd edn. Philadelphia: Saunders.

An in-depth compendium of knowledge on the normal and abnormal physiology of the fetus and neonate.

Study activity

Knowledge of the maturation of the body systems can be invaluable when caring for sick children. Using the information given here, and following further reading, explain why an infant is more prone to dehydration than an adult, giving a rationale for your explanation.

Growth

Growth is the result of the interactions of hormones in the body's endocrine system. The rate at which children grow varies from child to child, with periods of rapid growth alternating with periods of slow growth. Research has shown that normal growth (particularly height) may even occur in short (even 24-hour) periods that come between long periods with no growth (Lampl, 1992). Growth is rapid during the first year of life and then slows between 1 and 2 years of age. Average children grow about 5 inches (13 cm) between their first and second birthdays. After 2 years of age, growth continues at a slower but steady rate of 2.5 inches (6 cm) per year until about the age of 11 in girls and 13 in boys, when the growth spurt that accompanies adolescence usually begins. The pubertal growth spurt lasts about 2 years. Normal growth stops when the growing ends of the bones fuse. This usually occurs between the ages of 13 and 15 for girls and between 14 and 17 for boys.

Variations in the rate of growth of different tissues and organs produce significant changes in body proportions. A cephalocaudal trend is evident. During fetal life the head is the fastest growing part of the body. In infancy, growth of the trunk predominates. In childhood it is the legs. In adolescence it is the trunk again and the hands and feet. In infancy and early childhood the face is small in relation to the skull. After the first year the bones grow more rapidly than the brain case. Main growth is in the muscles and in the jaws as they enlarge to accommodate the teeth.

Increase in height and weight with years

- *Height* – at 3 years there is a steady rate of growth of 5–6 cm/year. At about 12 years of age there is a growth spurt lasting about 2 years. During this time girls can grow as much as 16 cm, boys 20 cm
- *Weight* – birth–6 months: 140–200 g/week; 6–12 months: 85–140 g/week; 1 year–adolescence: 2–3 kg/year

Further reading

Sinclair, D. and Dangerfield, P. (1998) *Human Growth after Birth*, 6th edn. London: Oxford University Press.

Looks at the processes of growth in an accessible way; discusses both the biological and environmental factors influencing growth; covers disturbances of growth, and repair; and includes a chapter on old age.

Study activity

Take time to observe children around you. Note their age and their body proportions. Analyse your results.

Growth is usually measured in terms of height and weight. It is interesting to note that at birth babies are one-third of their adult height and by 2 years they are half of their eventual adult height. New growth standards have been developed by the World Health Organization in collaboration with research institutions worldwide. The WHO Multicentre Growth Reference Study (MGRS) was undertaken between 1997 and 2003 to generate new growth curves for assessing the growth and development of infants and young children around the world. The MGRS collected primary growth data and related information from approximately 8500 children from widely different ethnic backgrounds and cultural settings (Brazil, Ghana, India, Norway, Oman and the US). The new growth curves are expected to provide a single international standard that represents the best description of physiological growth for all children from birth to 5 years of age and to establish the breastfed infant as the normative model for growth and development.

Further reading

http://www.who.int/childgrowth/en/

This site provides full details of the WHO Multicentre Growth Reference Study (MGRS) and links to other sites related to growth.

Study activity

Check out the WHO Web site and find out how these new standards impact on your practice.

Physical development

As children grow and mature so their bodies develop and they are able to perform more skilful and complex movements. This is often referred to as motor development and is usually divided into gross motor development and fine motor development. The stages at which children reach different milestones will vary and it is always important to look at the whole child and not just one aspect of development. Knowledge of the milestones helps us to measure the progress that children are making and to identify any deviations from the norm as quickly as possible.

Gross motor skills involve whole body movements: crawling, sitting, walking, running. Fine motor skills involve the manipulative skills associated with hand and eye coordination; finger play, grasping objects, pincer grasp. Nearly all the basic skills of both types are achieved by the age of about 6–7 years. Figure 6.2 gives an overview of the milestones in motor development.

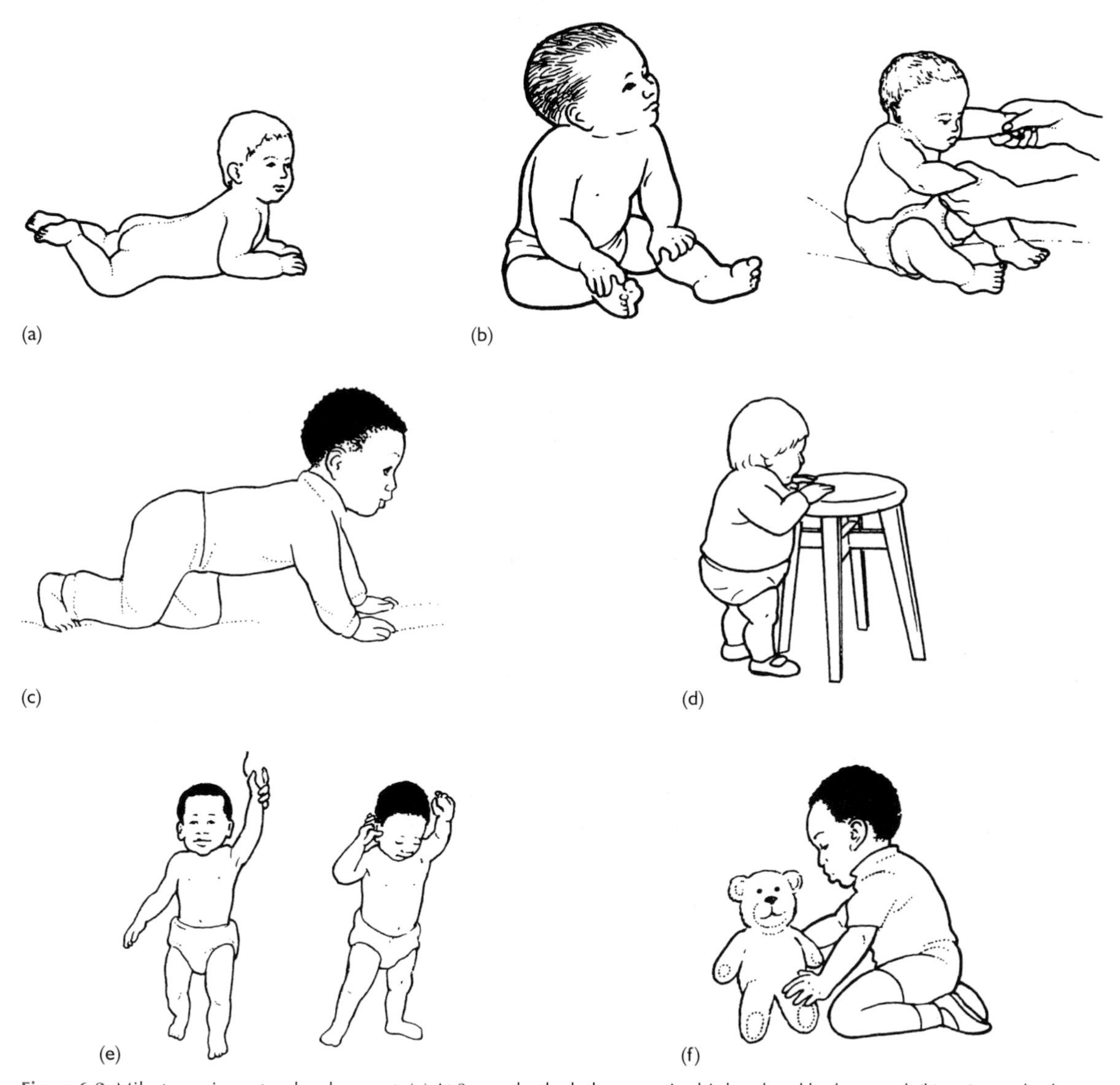

Figure 6.2 Milestones in motor development. (a) At 3 months the baby can raise his head and look around; (b) at 6 months the baby can sit unsupported for a short while; (c) at 9 months the baby can crawl quite well; (d) at 10 months the baby can pull himself up by the furniture; (e) at 12 months the baby is beginning to walk; (f) at 18 months the baby can walk well, bend down, push and pull his toys.

Summary

The development of the individual from conception to maturity is a marvellous, complex process. It is important to acknowledge that life begins at conception and that there are many influences acting upon the developing fetus. The exciting moment of birth is but one stage and signifies the beginning of independence. Infants continue to grow and mature throughout childhood but achieve many of their abilities within the first few years of life. Consider the first year. They are born with little capacity to control their bodies and by 1 year they are nearly ready to walk. It is worth observing children in different settings in an attempt to learn more about the way in which they grow and develop motor skills.

Further reading

More detailed information about motor development:

Sheridan, M., Frost, M. and Sharma, A. (1997) *From Birth to Five Years: Children's Developmental Progress.* London: Routledge.

Gallahue, D. L. and Ozmun, J. C. (2005) *Understanding Motor Development: Infants, Children, Adolescents and Adults,* 6th edn. New Jersey: McGraw-Hill.

http://www.psy.pdx.edu/PsiCafe/Areas/Developmental/PhysDev-Child/index.htm (accessed 2 March 2006).

Provides links to Web sites on (children's) physical development, such as height, weight, and motor skills. A vast majority of the links are to general developmental milestones in childhood, which include physical, social and cognitive development.

Study activity

Find a family with a baby under 6 months (use your own family where possible). You need to be able to have access to the baby at about monthly intervals for about 4–6 months. On each occasion make observations of the infant, noting aspects of growth and physical development. Use charts to plot the infant's progress. On completing the observations compare your findings with those given in Figure 6.2. Where time permits, repeat with another child and compare the two.

Key Points

1. Intrauterine life and neonatal life constitute a continuum – life begins at conception.
2. Life before birth is divided into three stages: germinal (0–2 weeks), embryonic (3–8 weeks) and fetal (9 weeks to birth).
3. Universal predictable patterns of growth and maturation are basic to all human beings.
4. All the organs' basic structures are laid down by week 8 of gestation. The systems continue to mature up until and after birth.
5. A knowledge of the maturation process is vital as it forms a basis on which to rationalise care.
6. The rate at which children grow varies from child to child but follows a predictable pattern.
7. Children have achieved nearly all the basic motor skills by the age of 6–7 years.

Chapter 7

Theoretical Perspectives – Cognitive Development

Introduction

The development of thought and understanding in children is a fascinating and mysterious process. How often have you wondered what children are thinking or asked yourself how they see the world? While all of us have been there, it is unlikely that we can consciously remember how we developed an understanding of our world. In studying cognitive development we can only make assumptions based on what children say, so we are, in fact, relying on adult explanations of children's thinking. Perhaps that is why some of the theories seem difficult to assimilate.

Cognition is the term generally used in developmental theory to refer to thought and understanding. However, there is more to cognition than just these two aspects, as we can see in Figure 7.1. All these aspects interact to enable children to make sense of their world.

For the purposes of this module the discussion will concentrate on three aspects of cognitive development, the development of:

- visual perception
- thinking
- language

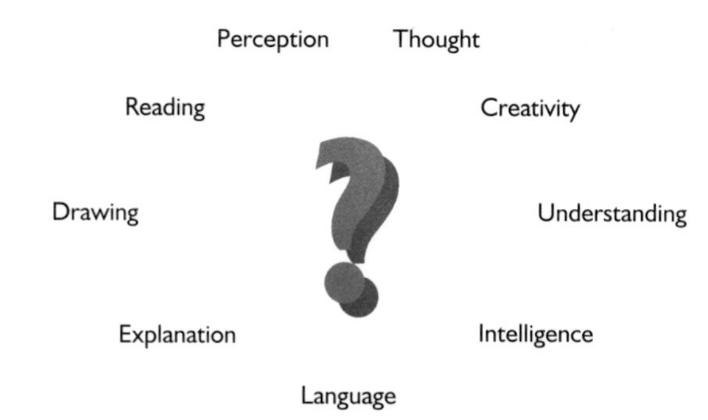

Figure 7.1 What is cognitive development?

Research
See the Web site of the New York University (NYU) Infant Perception lab, where research is conducted on perceptual and cognitive development in infancy and childhood.

http://www.psych.nyu.edu/johnson/infantperceptionlab/learn.html

Visual Perception

Perception refers to the way in which the brain interprets sensory information. According to Gibson and Spelke (1983:2) 'perception is the beginning of knowing and so is an essential part of cognition'. There are two main views on the development of perception in children. The nativists believe that a baby senses the world like an adult from birth and therefore sees things as we do. The empiricists, however, believe that the baby has to learn how to perceive things. The third possible view, and the one that seems to be supported by many psychologists today, is that the development of perceptual skills is a result of both innate and learned experiences.

Visual perception includes a number of abilities such as pattern and depth perception, size and colour constancy. It has been shown that, although babies do not have the same visual acuity as adults, some perceptual abilities exist at birth (for example, basic vision, auditory location and face preference), whereas others (for example, colour, binocular disparity, depth perception and constancy) do not occur in full until later (Eysenck, 2004).

- Bower *et al.* (1970) investigated infants' ability to judge distance and direction. They found that babies could tell the direction of an approaching object and that they became distressed if an object appeared to be heading straight for their face. They concluded that the defensive reaction was innate. Ball and Tronick (1971) reported a similar result and came to the conclusion that this aspect of depth perception was innate.
- Bower (1965) also conducted research to test size constancy. His sample consisted of babies who were only a few weeks old. He found that babies were able to recognise the same object at different distances and concluded that size constancy was innate. Slater *et al.* (1990) came to a similar conclusion.
- In the early 1960s Frantz carried out a number of experiments to test infants' ability to discriminate between patterns and their preference for the human face. He used three pictures (Figure 7.2) and showed them to babies between the age of 4 days and 6 months. He concluded that babies had a preference for the picture of the human face and therefore suggested that there is an unlearned meaning in the

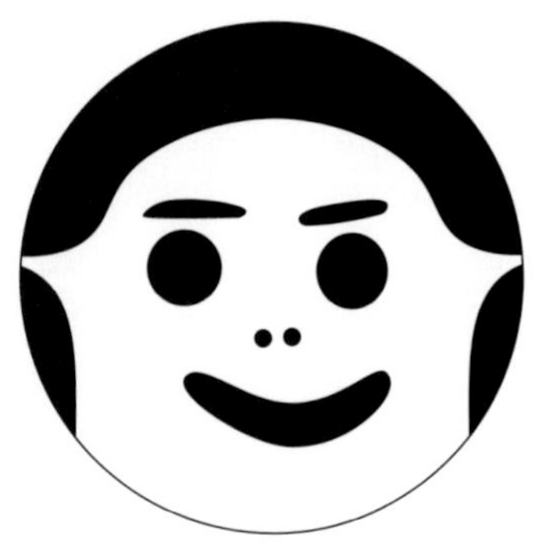

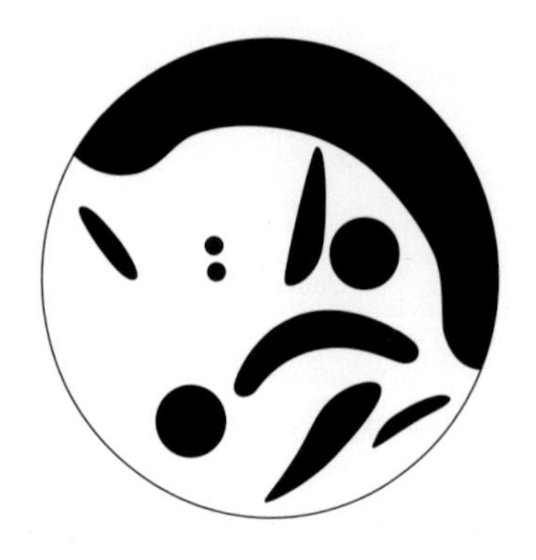

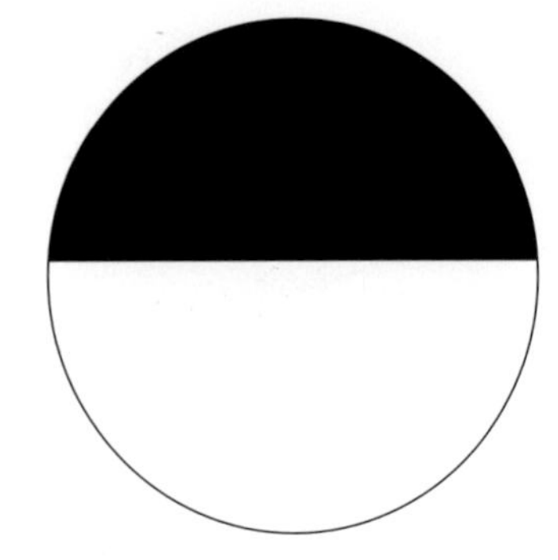

Figure 7.2 Frantz faces.

form perception of infants. There have been many criticisms of Frantz's work, the main one being that a baby looking at one shape more than another does not mean that he prefers that one to the other. In the case of faces, infants develop considerable skill in discriminating different facial expressions over the first 2 years of life and there is reason to suspect that a component of the ability to recognise facial expressions is unlearned (Nelson, 1987). Infants are also very attracted to people's eyes and develop the ability to follow another person's gaze (Butterworth and Jarrett, 1991).

- Walton *et al.* (1992) carried out research that allowed newborn infants to produce the images they wanted on a TV screen by sucking on a pressure-sensitive dummy. When the infant sucked hard an image appeared on the screen. Which image appeared (mother or stranger) depended on the rate of sucking. They concluded that not only did newborns behave in a very competent way, but they were able to distinguish a familiar face from a strange one. More recently, Pascalis *et al.* (1995) replicated this finding but showed that this preference was extinguished when women wore headscarves. The authors suggest that neonates store a representation of their mothers' faces in which the hairline and outer contour play a prominent role.

Question
Ponder this: 'I think it is going to rain'. What might be the basis for your thoughts?

Study activity

Find out more about these experiments and critically review the methodology of each. Make your own criticisms of the research. Search for any more recent research in these areas and compare with that presented here.

Thinking

According to Campbell and Olsen (1990:192), thinking is 'an effortful activity, involving mental "work", in which the organism forsakes its normal outward orientation on the presented world and struggles instead with a world indexed only imperfectly by a shadowy inner structure of mental symbols'. Thinking is also about making meaning out of what goes on around us and understanding concepts. Thinking is something you and I do quite often during our everyday lives. We know what we are thinking about and are able to use symbols and imagery to carry out sometimes complex work in our minds.

Study activity

Think of a number, double it, add three and then take away four. What is your answer? It is quite likely that you carried out this activity without having to use any form of visual aid. Try the same exercise with children of different ages. How do they work it out?

The development of thinking is a mysterious process and one that we can only judge on the basis of adult speculations, for we will never truly

Key terms used by Piaget

- *Schema* – all the ideas and information that a child might have about an object, formed through the child's interaction with the outside world
- *Assimilation* – the way in which a child takes in important elements of any experience
- *Accommodation* – the process of fitting what has been learned into existing schema
- *Adaptation* – the result of interaction between assimilation and accommodation; the child has learned more about the world and can act upon it

Criticisms of Piaget's view of object permanence

Bower (1981) carried out experiments in which he concluded that infants younger than 8 months know that objects exist even when they are occluded. He found that the infants in his study demonstrated this knowledge with their eyes but not with hand or arm movements. This work only suggests that Piaget underestimated the abilities of young infants and does not necessarily negate Piaget's theory.

know what a young child is thinking. Three views on cognitive development are offered for you to consider.

Jean Piaget (1896–1980)

Jean Piaget is perhaps the most well-known psychologist in this area and one who has influenced the care of children through his work. Piaget was a biologist who became interested in children's thinking while carrying out tests on intelligence. He attempted to find explanations for the way in which children come to understand their world and make judgements about it. His studies were based on the qualitative development of children's ability to solve problems and therefore involved clinical interviews that used an open-ended, conversation-like technique for eliciting children's responses. From these studies Piaget concluded that children's thinking develops in stages and that each stage is a prerequisite for the next one. He gave approximate age ranges for each stage. With each stage, thinking becomes more complex until the child reaches maturity. His theory is based on the premise that children learn largely unassisted through interaction with the world around them, using experiences to build on their understanding.

- *Sensori-motor stage: birth to 2 years.* At this stage babies learn through the senses and through movement. At the beginning of this stage Piaget believed that babies have no concept of the difference between self and non-self and have no understanding of the permanent existence of anything other than themselves. It is during this stage that they develop object permanence. Piaget claimed that babies under 8 months of age do not have the concept of permanence: once an object is out of sight they do not understand that it still exists. His explanation for this was that they do not have the necessary ability to conjure up an image of the object in its absence. Between 8 months and 2 years this concept develops, so that by the age of 2 years the child understands that things go on happening and objects have their own independent existence. Piaget concluded that by the end of this stage children are able to make mental predictions about their actions through the use of symbolism.
- *Pre-operational stage: 2–7 years.* The ability to form and use symbols is the main feature of this stage. The symbols Piaget described include language, drawing, music and dance. Through the use of these symbols the child continues to learn about the world and develops the ability to solve problems. However the child's thinking is intuitive and subjective rather than logical and objective. Piaget suggested that children are egocentric at this age and are incapable of seeing things from somebody else's point of view. Linked to this is an inability to understand and apply principles. Piaget reached his conclusions about this stage by setting children tasks and seeing whether they gave correct or incorrect answers. Children under 7 years nearly always gave incorrect answers. One test addressed the concept of conservation. The child watches as two short, wide jars are filled with water to the same level. The content of one of the jars is then poured into a tall narrow jar and placed next to the remaining short wide jar. The level of water in the tall, narrow jar is much higher. Piaget found

that nearly all the children under 7 years said that there was more water in the tall jar than in the short one. Instead of attending to a principle – that no water was added or taken away – the children gave intuitive answers based on what they could see, namely an increased water level. Piaget subdivided the pre-operational stage into two:

- *Pre-conceptual stage – 2–4 years.* Concepts are not fully formed. Children are not able to distinguish the different properties of objects within a different class. Hence all men are 'daddy', including the milkman! This might explain why young children seem capable of believing in Father Christmas. Even when they see a number of Father Christmases in different places and they all look subtly different, they believe that it is the same one.
- *Intuitive stage – 4–7 years.* The ability to classify and organise develops but the children are still unaware of the principles that underlie the concepts.

- *Stage of concrete operations – 7–12 years.* According to Piaget, children in this stage use logical thinking based on principles to solve problems. Children over 7 give the correct answers to the tests of conservation and realise that their view of something is only one of many possible views. However, they cannot deal with abstract or hypothetical dilemmas, they are firmly rooted in the real world and cannot handle a problem that asks them 'just suppose . . .'.
- *Stage of formal operations – 12 years onwards.* Characteristics of this stage include the ability to think logically and to deal with abstract ideas. Problems can be solved on a purely mental level with no visual aids. Problems are approached in a logical, systematic and patterned manner using reasoning based on a clear understanding of the underlying principles. Piaget suggested that not everybody reaches this level of thinking.

Study activity

Try out the water conservation test with children in your family or with children you care for (remember to get permission before you start). Analyse your results. How do they compare with those of Piaget? What other conservation tests did Piaget use? Try them out too.

conservation

'. . . understanding that transformation of appearance need not result in alteration of the underlying reality. The underlying reality remains constant and is therefore conserved'.

(Mitchell, 1992)

Psychologists have attempted to assess the accuracy and appropriateness of Piaget's work. There are many who would argue that his theory should be rejected; others accept that it needs modification. There seems to be a consensus that, if anything, Piaget underestimated the abilities of young children.

Study activity

Find out more about the criticisms of Piaget's work.

Criticism of Piaget's tests

Donaldson (1978) felt that the reason so-called pre-operational children gave the wrong answers was because they misunderstood the questions and not because they did not have any logical abilities. She argues that Piaget's questions did not make sense to the children and that they answered according to how they thought he wanted them to.

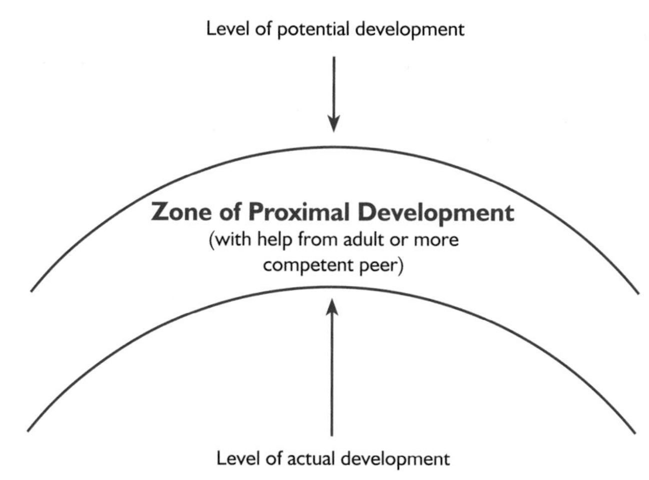

Figure 7.3 Vygotsky's zone of proximal development.

Lev Vygotsky (1896–1934)

Vygotsky provides an alternative view and challenges those of Piaget. While Piaget saw children as being largely unassisted in the development of their thinking, Vygotsky emphasised the role of the social context and, in particular, the role of direct intervention by more knowledgeable others. He believed that it was wrong to judge children merely on what they could do alone, but that what they were capable of doing with help should be taken into account. The central concept of Vygotsky's theory is that of the *zone of proximal development (ZPD)* (Figure 7.3).

The ZPD is the distance between the child's actual cognitive level and his potential level under the guidance of more knowledgeable adults or collaboration with more competent peers. Any intervention that aims to increase a child's existing repertoire of cognitive skills is most effective when it is within the ZPD. That is, it should be at a level beyond the child's existing abilities but not so far above that it is incomprehensible. It would appear from the work of Vygotsky that, if we were to judge children's cognitive level on what they could do with help, then Piaget's description of the ages at which children could do things could be seriously underestimated. The suggestion is that young children have representational powers but can only exercise them with promoting or adult help. A second important concept in Vygotsky's work was the emphasis that he placed on the role of language in the development of thinking and thought. Piaget argued that thinking develops out of action, not language, but Vygotsky thought the opposite. He suggested that by 7 years speech becomes internalised, allowing dialogue with oneself, which in turn helps to guide actions.

Jerome Bruner

Bruner (1966) developed Vygotsky's ideas and identified three stages of cognitive development:

1. *Enactive – 0–2 years.* Children represent the world around themselves by actions.

2. *Iconic – 2–6 years.* Children begin to use images.
3. *Symbolic – 7 years upward.* Children are freed from the present and real world and are able to use symbols. This ability, largely dependent on language, is at the centre of the child's ability to deal with the abstract.

Study activity

Carry out further reading on the ideas of Vygotsky and Bruner. Analyse your findings and compare and contrast their ideas with those of Piaget.

Language

The use of language is the main way in which humans communicate. Language is a complex, organised system of symbols that can be spoken, written or signed (used by people who are deaf and who have no speech). Language acquisition is one of the central topics in cognitive science and children must acquire four main areas of language competence:

- Phonology – the rules of sounds (phonemes). These are the basic sounds that make up a language. Each language has its own phoneme system.
- Syntax (grammar) – this refers to the way in which words are put together to make grammatically correct sentences.
- Semantics – this refers to the meaning of words and sounds.
- Pragmatics – refers to knowledge about how language is used in different contexts. A child will need to be able to adjust and adapt his language according to the situation in which he finds himself.

By the time children reach the age of 5–6 years they have grasped the essentials of their language and are, in fact, highly competent in its use. The acquisition of language appears to proceed with no real effort on behalf of the child and no formal education. Sequential stages in the development of language are identifiable (Table 7.1). It is interesting to note that children learning any language seem to progress through the same stages, in the same order and at approximately the same ages (Slobin, 1973).

Study activity

Tape conversations with children of various ages. Analyse what they say, compare and contrast your findings with the information given in Table 7.1.

Theories of language development

Several psychologists have attempted to explain how children learn a language. As with many areas of development, there are two main views emphasising nature and nurture. The debate is inconclusive, with a consensus gradually emerging that the relevant issue is not nature

Further reading

Harris, M. and Butterworth, G. (2002) *Developmental Psychology.* Hove: Psychology Press.

Eysenck, M. W. and Keane, M. T. (2005) *Cognitive Psychology: A Student's Handbook,* 5th edn. Hove: Psychology Press.

Goswami, U. (ed.) (2004) *Blackwell Handbook of Childhood Cognitive Development.* London: Blackwell.

This book covers all the major topics in research and theory about childhood cognitive development. It synthesises the latest research findings in an accessible manner.

Table 7.1 Age-related development of language

Approximate age	Characteristics of language development
Birth–1 month	Crying – three distinct types identified: basic, usually due to hunger, at first quiet and intermittent but becomes louder angry – same sequence as basic cry but characterised by differences in length of sound and pauses between sounds pain – sudden and loud from the onset – long cry followed by long silence and series of short gasping sounds (Smith *et al.*, 2003)
1–6 months	The infant's repertoire increases and includes laughing and 'cooing'; it uses mainly vowel sounds with a developing variety of pitch. Turn-taking is evident between infant and carer
6–9 months	The infant begins to babble, using a combination of vowels and consonants with no meaning, such as dadadadada, mamama, babababa. There may be identifiable sounds; important for practising sound-producing mechanisms. The infant can understand simple words like 'no'
9–12 months	Babbling continues and begins to reflect intonation of speech. By 12 months the first words appear, usually names of people or objects with which infants are familiar. Respond to simple commands. 0–12 months considered as the pre-linguistic stage in language development
12–24 months	12-month-olds can distinguish between words, mouth sounds and object noises. They have linguistically specific knowledge of the privileged status of language (Hollich *et al.*, 2000). By 18 months vocabulary increased to about 10 words, by 20 months about 50 words and by 24 months to about 300 words – mainly nouns (Mitchell, 1992). Uses holophrases – one-word utterances used to convey many different meanings. For example 'cat' could mean 'there is a cat' or 'where is my cat?'
2–3 years	Sentences become longer but tend to be telegraphic – uses mainly content words and misses out function words such as 'to', 'at', 'of'. Order of words sometimes incorrect. Tends to over-generalise and see all men as 'daddy', all animals as 'dog'
3–4 years	Speech becomes less telegraphic, beginning to acquire the finer points of language. Uses the past tense and three- to four-word sentences. Has a vocabulary of about 1000 words (Smith and Cowie, 1991); enjoys the use of rhyming poems
4–5 years	Using longer sentences with complex constructions; tendency to overregulate, for example assuming that '-ed' is added to all words to make the past tense ('I goed to the park')
5–6 years and upwards	Good grasp of language, although still makes some mistakes with grammar, for example 'it was the bestest'. The average 6-year-old has a vocabulary of about 14 000 words. The child continues to develop and refine language and develops the ability to use embedded sentences and negative forms

versus nurture but rather the process of interaction between the two (Elman *et al.*, 1996). A study of twins (Kovas *et al.*, 2005) suggested that diverse aspects of language, such as expressive and receptive grammar, phonology, articulation and verbal memory, show moderate heritability and moderate influence of environment (*see also* Role of the family in development p. 29).

Nurture

Skinner (1957) believed that language development occurs, like other learning, through reinforcement of appropriate behaviour. When infants make sounds and words they are greeted with a positive response, which acts as reinforcement. Language is then progressively shaped by adults who reward and reinforce correct usage. More recent research appears to give us evidence that the acquisition is far more complex than this. In reality it has been found that mothers rarely correct the grammatical structure of their children's speech, being more interested in the content (Brown *et al.* cited by Smith and Cowie, 1991). However, the role of adults in a child's acquisition of language is clearly important, as has been shown by research into the use of Baby Talk Register by mothers and fathers. The role of siblings in the development of language is also an aspect to be considered. Oshima-Takane *et al.* (1996) suggested that overheard conversations between caregivers and older siblings in addition to child-directed speech are important resources for second-born children learning personal pronouns.

Nature

Noam Chomsky (1986) argued against Skinner's views and suggested that babies are born with an innate ability to acquire language. He claimed that the process of acquiring language was so easy for children because the rudiments of language already exist in their brains in the form of a 'language acquisition device' – LAD. He believes that children learn language on their own and that the environment plays little part. Stromswold (2001) concluded that almost all aspects of language ability, from syntax and semantics to phonology and articulation, are influenced by genetic factors to some extent.

Study activity

Consider how knowledge of language development would help you in your practice.

Summary

This exploration has tried to give you an overview of three important areas in cognitive development. It is important to acknowledge that no one aspect of development occurs in isolation and all are interlinked in some way. Children are an exciting mixture of innocence and maturity. I was often amazed at the degree of understanding that my young children had about the world around them. When my daughter was 4 she had developed an acute awareness of subtle innuendoes and could

Further resources – language development

http://www.childdevelopmentinfo.com/development/language_development.shtml

A good site with a range of different resources and also guidance for parents.

Smith, P. K., Cowie, H. and Blades, M. (2003) *Understanding Children's Development*, 4th edn. Oxford: Blackwell, Chapter 11.

articulate her feelings very clearly. Her thirst for knowledge was sometimes overwhelming. It is fascinating to observe at close quarters the development of a child's thinking, but at the same time one can easily overlook the important developments. If you have children, reflect back on the way they developed – it is likely that you have forgotten much of what happened. Consider your practice and try to focus on what children are thinking and how their cognitive processes are developing. It is important to attempt to see into the child's world in order to plan and implement care appropriately.

Other areas related to cognitive development worth exploring

- Children's drawings
- Children's story telling
- Children's explanations
- Intelligence
- Development of writing and reading

Key Points

1. In the study of cognitive development, we can only make assumptions based on what children say. Therefore, we rely on an adult's explanation of children's developing minds.
2. The term 'cognitive' encompasses language, perception, thinking, creativity, memory, concentration and intelligence.
3. Research has shown that, while babies do not have the same visual acuity as adults, they do have some innate capabilities.
4. We can only speculate as to what children are thinking – but it is better to attempt to understand how they view the world in which they live so that we can give appropriate care.
5. The process of the development of language is unclear: however, stages in language acquisition have been identified and can be related to nearly all children.
6. Each aspect of cognitive development is interlinked – development in one area does not occur in isolation.

Chapter 8

Theoretical Perspectives – The Social World of the Child

Introduction

Becoming a social being is an important process for all children, whatever culture they are born into. There is a wealth of evidence to suggest that the quality of a child's early relationships will affect the development of social competence. Thus it is important to acknowledge the role of the family and others in a child's social development, as the development of a sense of identity is a basic task of childhood. For the purposes of this module the discussions will concentrate on three aspects of social development:

- the development of the concept of self and a child's personality
- the development of social relationships with parents and others
- the development of social cognition (moral development)

(*see also* Roles and relationships p. 17)

The Concept of Self

Study activity

Before reading on, take 2 minutes to consider your answer to the question 'Who am I?' Attempt to give 20 answers. Compare your answers with those of colleagues.

It is likely that you will have identified a range of characteristics that you see as being 'yours'. These could range from physical characteristics to other qualities such as stubbornness, aptitudes, even including ideas about your sex role. These are aspects of your self-concept that shape and influence how we respond to others and how we deal with social relationships. Our ideas about our sex role form a powerful part of our self-concept. During early childhood, the development of new powers and abilities of representation enable children to reflect on themselves. Through language, preschool children are able to vocalise their inner mental states and develop knowledge of their own characteristics and their sense of personal self. Berk (2005) suggests that they develop a self-concept: the set of attributes, abilities, attitudes and values that an individual believes defines who he or she is. Initially, their self-concept is restricted by specific possessions and actions. What could be seen as selfishness and struggles are actually an attempt to clarify boundaries between themselves and others. Self-esteem also contributes to a young child's ability to deal with and master their environment, and its development is highly dependent on social interactions.

Ideas about how self-concept develops have been influenced by Piaget and Freud, who both believed that a baby begins life with no sense of separateness. According to Lewis (1991) babies must first work out that they are separate from others and that this endures over time. The key would seem to be the idea that 'I exist'. Lewis believes that this occurs within the first 2 to 3 months and is achieved through babies learning from experimentation that they can make things happen. For example, smiling at their mother will evoke a response; touching a mobile will make it move. Lewis sees the development of object permanence as being a crucial step and that only when this has occurred, at about 8–9 months, will the real subjective self have emerged. This coincides with Piaget's ideas on object permanence and, although being somewhat controversial, could go some way to explaining the sudden onset of a wariness of strangers that occurs at this age.

Rochat (2004) identifies that the emergence of self-concept is linked to the development of language through self-recognition, as shown by Lewis and Brooks-Gunn's (1979) mirror and rouge test (you can try this out yourself).

This self-recognition is apparent from the age of 18–20 months, suggesting an emerging self-concept. While language and self-concept appear to be connected (because of the timing of their emergence), they are not necessarily reciprocally dependent. Children have a clearly defined perception of others and themselves as communicators, and do not wait until they are symbolically competent to demonstrate some implicit or explicit self-knowledge. From the age of 2–3 months they learn to be effective in relation to objects and subjects, suggesting that they are active participants (and not passive recipients) in their development. However, they expect to be responded to in certain ways (smiling and cooing) and may react with strong negative facial responses and cry if presented with a sudden change of facial expression. Thus Lewis (1991) identifies that, in infancy, the implicit sense of self essentially develops through relationships with others. Between 2 and 6 months, the infant develops a sense of self as a result of interaction with people and can distinguish individuals as separate entities. Rochat (2003) suggests that there are five levels of self-awareness.

Self-concept becomes increasingly differentiated and consistent as children develop. They move from abstract concepts to realistic concepts, as they are able to consider themselves in relation to others. Initially the self-concept is very concrete and linked to visible characteristics such as 'where I live', 'what I look like' or 'what I am good at

The rouge test

Children of various age groups (from 9 to 24 months) were placed in front of a mirror. On being removed, the infant's nose was discreetly rubbed with 'rouge'. Then they were placed in front of the mirror again. The results, which have been replicated several times, show that although all the children smiled at the image, only those aged between 21 and 24 months reached for their own noses. This would suggest that by about this age an infant has a fairly good idea that the reflection in the mirror is a representation of himself.

Five levels of self-awareness (Rochat, 2003)

- Level 0: Confusion shown at birth
- Level 1: Differentiation shown from 2 months
- Level 2: Situation shown from 4 to 6 months
- Level 3: Identification shown from 18 months
- Level 4: Permanence shown from the age of 3
- Level 5: Self-awareness shown from 4 to 5

doing'. Over the school years this gradually changes as children become more abstract in their thinking and focus more on internal qualities, progressing to increasingly sophisticated but realistic self-descriptions. By the age of 6, children become aware of the difference between private thinking and public behaviour and as a result they can start to monitor their experiences and develop self-control. Rochat (2003) suggests that adults vary in the level of self-awareness as do children, but in direct response to their interactions with others.

Adolescence is a period of considerable change, both psychologically and physically. Children's appearance can change so rapidly that they may be left with the feeling that they really are different. It is largely through the writing of Erikson that adolescence has come to be thought of a time of identity crisis, suggesting a temporary period of confusion and low self-esteem. The question of 'Who am I?' takes on a sense of urgency as many adolescents go through a period of redefining themselves, of trying out new aspects of identity. Erikson called this 'crisis identity versus role confusion' and considered it to be normal or a developmental task. Various criticisms have been made of these ideas largely because Erikson's ideas were based on observations and on clinical practice. Since then, attempts have been made to test his ideas using research. The findings seem to suggest that the sense of self changes gradually and not necessarily as a result of adolescence. Berk (2005) notes that for some young people identity development is traumatic but for most it is not, and that we should consider an alternative to the term 'crisis', such as 'exploration'.

Tied in with the development of self-awareness is the concept of self-esteem – the global value of one's worth. We tend to compare ourselves with others and make evaluations about our own worth from that. Harter (1999) suggests that self-esteem is a product of what the child thinks he ought to be and what he thinks he is. When the difference between the two is low, self-esteem is high and vice versa. The level of self-esteem can vary; children's self-esteem can be influenced by their beliefs about their own self-worth, their peers' beliefs about them and the support of others around them. Gender is an important aspect, as many more teenage girls worry about their appearance and their abilities than the same-aged boys. Berk (2005) suggests that authoritative parenting with elements of warmth, approval and supportive problem-solving has a strong correlation with the development of positive self-image.

Study activity

Reflect on your own self-esteem. What factors have influenced the value that you place upon yourself?

Development of Personality

Four approaches related to the development of personality are offered for you to consider.

Further reading

The journal *Social Development*, published by Blackwell, is a major international journal dealing with all aspects of children's social development as seen from a psychological stance. Coverage includes a wide range of topics such as social cognition, peer relationships, social interaction, attachment formation, emotional development and children's theories of mind. An example of one interesting article is:

Steele, M. (2004) Fitting the puzzle pieces together: The complexities of infant–mother interaction and disorganised attachment patterns. *Social Development*, **13**, 479.

Smith, P. K. and Hart, C. (eds) (2004) *Blackwell Handbook of Childhood Social Development.* London: Blackwell.

This handbook provides an up-to-date overview of research and theory about social development in children from preschool age to the onset of adolescence.

personality

It is difficult to find a consensus definition of this term. However, the idea that seems to underlie different theoretical perspectives is that 'each individual has a relatively unique and enduring set of psychological tendencies and reveals them in the course of his or her transactions with various social environments . . .'

(Berryman *et al.*, 2002)

The biological approach

Theorists who support this view have tended to look more closely at temperament – that part of the personality pertaining to mood, activity and general level of energy. Their premise is based on the concept that children are individuals from birth and indications of that individuality can be found in every aspect of behaviour. They propose that:

- Each individual is born with characteristic patterns of responding to the environment and to people.
- These behavioural dispositions are based in variations in fundamental physiological processes and are therefore influenced by the way the brain, nervous system and hormones work. In other words we inherit tendencies to react in particular ways.
- Temperamental dispositions persist through childhood into adulthood and, although subject to change through experience, a bias for certain patterns remains.
- Temperamental characteristics influence the way a child responds to people and vice versa.

Rothbart and Bates (1998) suggest that temperament consists of stable individual differences in the quality and intensity of emotional reaction, activity level, attention and emotional self-regulation. This suggests a genetic foundation for individual differences in personality. Evidence to support this view comes from studies on identical twins, who are more alike in temperament than non-identical twins, even when reared apart. There are consistent ethnic and sex differences in early temperament but the role of heredity lessens as children mature and temperament becomes more stable.

The learning approach

Learning theorists (such as Skinner, Watson and Bandura), although they do not reject the biological basis of behaviour, stress the importance of reinforcement patterns in the environment. It could be said that nature takes a back seat to nurture in this approach. Children also learn from modelling others and therefore develop personality characteristics as a result of this learning. Basic points emphasised by these theorists are:

- Behaviour is strengthened by reinforcements, which can be perceived as positive or negative. Watson saw the developing child as very easily influenced by environmental effects. In an experiment he brought about fear in a child who had previously been content.
- Inconsistent reinforcement is likely to lead to highly persistent behaviour.
- Children learn new behaviour through watching and imitating the behaviour of others, known as modelling. They become increasingly selective about who and what they imitate and they select positive role models for their behaviour.
- As well as learning overt behaviour by modelling, children also acquire ideas, expectations, standards and self-concepts this way.

The learning theory helps to explain why children can be so inconsistent in their behaviour, something that would be hard to explain using biological approaches. A child may be calm, well behaved and do as he is told at school, but be aggressive, wilful and disobedient at home. Learning theorists would explain this as being the result of a variety of reinforcement patterns. There is also room for change within this theory. Many programmes based on reinforcement exist for a variety of behaviour problems, for example sleep, bowel training, language delay and aggressiveness. However, many theorists believe that this approach offers too narrow a view of important environmental influences and does not consider children's contribution to their own development.

The psychoanalytical approach

The basic premise of this approach is that a child's personality is influenced by an interaction between inborn patterns and environmental influences. These theorists suggest a clear developmental pattern as children grow older (Tables 8.1 and 8.2). They propose that:

Table 8.1 Erikson's psychosocial stages in the development of personality

Age (years)	Normative crisis	Tasks and activitites
0–1	Trust versus mistrust	To develop trust in central caregiver(s); an early secure attachment
1–2	Autonomy versus shame and doubt	Physical development leads to more free choice, e.g. walking, grasping; toilet training; more control
3–5	Initiative versus guilt	Become more assertive; Oedipus-like feelings may lead to guilt
6–puberty	Industry versus inferiority	Main social interaction outside home; absorb all basic cultural norms
Adolescence	Identity versus role confusion	Main social interaction with peers; identity crisis; search for new values

NB Erikson proposed three additional stages during adulthood.

Table 8.2 Freud's psychosexual stages of personality development

Stage and approx. age (years)	Erogenous zone	Main characteristics	Tasks to achieve (potential source of conflict)
Oral (0–1)	Mouth	Main source of pleasure is mouth; main concern is with immediate gratification of urges	Satisfactory feeding/weaning
Anal (1–2)	Anus	Controlling bowels and bladder	Toilet training
Phallic (2–6)	Genitals	Playing with genitals; Oedipus and Electra complex	Successful solution to Oedipal and Electra conflicts
Latency (6–11)	None – sexual energy quiescent	Same-sex parent identification	None
Genital (11 on)	Genitals	Increasing concern with adult ways of experiencing sexual pleasure	Mature sexual intimacy

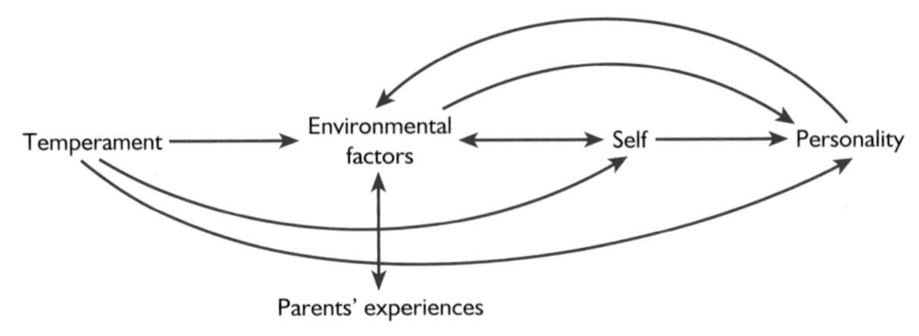

Figure 8.1 A model of personality development (adapted from Bee, 1995).

- Behaviour is governed by unconscious as well and conscious motives. Freud identified three sets of motive – sexual (libido), life preserving and aggressive – which arise out of the three parts of the personality: the id, the ego and the superego. Erikson noted only one – identity. However, Erikson emphasised that normal development must be understood in relation to each culture and that child rearing can only be understood in relation to a particular society or group.
- Personality develops over time as a result of interaction between inborn drives and the responses by key people in the child's life.
- The development of personality occurs in stages, each stage centred on a particular task.
- The specific personality a child develops will depend on the success in dealing with the stages.

Although many psychoanalytic ideas are vague and highly subjective, Erikson captures the concept of personality development and developmental tasks across the lifespan.

The interactive approach

Bee (1995) gives us a model that attempts to integrate the three previous approaches. She suggests that the basis for the development of a child's personality is the inborn temperament. Thereafter a complex interaction of a variety of factors influences personality (Figure 8.1).

Study activity

Take each of the approaches offered above and critically analyse each one. Do the approaches have meaning and relevance in your practice? Attempt to make your own model from the ideas given.

The Development of Social Relationships with Parents and Others

Hartup (1989) describes two types of relationships that he considers vital to the child:

- Vertical – relationships with others who have greater knowledge and power. These could include parents, teachers and older siblings.

These relationships give protection and security and enable the acquisition of knowledge and basic social skills.
- Horizontal – relationships that are egalitarian and reciprocal. These could include same-age peers. These important relationships give children the opportunity to practice social skills that can only be learnt by interaction with equals, for example cooperation, competition and intimacy.

However, relationships do not exist in isolation from other relationships and they tend to occur in networks with implications for interactions.

Vertical relationships

The formation of attachments with caregivers is perhaps one of the most important early social relationships. Others become important as the child grows older. The discussion that follows will concentrate on early attachment relationships.

Attachment is a long-enduring emotional tie to a specific individual. Much of the work on attachment theory has been based on ideas developed by John Bowlby during the 1950s and 1960s. In 1969 Bowlby described four phases in the development of a child's attachment (ages are approximate):

- *The pre-attachment phase – birth to 6 weeks.* Little evidence of attachment. Infants are able to recognise their mother's smell and voice but signal without discriminating between different people. Behaviours include crying, smiling and responding to caregivers, but they are not directed towards anybody in particular.
- *The attachment-in-the-making phase – 6 weeks to 6–8 months.* Infants begin to aim attachment behaviours more narrowly, directing them towards one or more individuals. They begin to rely on the response of their caregiver to their behaviours. They display no special anxiety at being separated from parents or being with strangers.
- *The phase of clear-cut attachment: 6–8 months to 2 years.* The infant uses the mother as a secure base (but it could be another caregiver) from which to explore. If you watch the behaviour of children over the age of 8 months, especially those that can crawl, you might see evidence of attachment behaviours – children crawl away for some distance but occasionally check out the secure base to look for reassurance and protection. They may cry or protest if their mother leaves, but separation anxiety does not always occur. It is at this time that the infant becomes wary of strangers.
- *The formation of a reciprocal relationship – 2–3 years.* Children begin to accommodate the mother's needs. They will be more willing to wait alone if requested until mother returns. However, they still show attachment behaviours such as cuddling. By the age of about 4 years children understand that the relationship exists even when their mother is not there. Attachment behaviours become less noticeable but may occur at times of stress (*see also* Separation anxiety p. 201).

Bowlby suggests that these ties have both an evolutionary and biological basis as they enable protection and survival. He states that the ties are highly selective and focus on specific individuals; they involve an attempt to stay physically close while providing comfort and security, and produce a separation upset when the tie is severed. He also suggests that if children do not develop a secure relationship with their mother they will be unable to form any type of meaningful long-term relationship as adults. Rutter (1981) felt that there was an overemphasis on the role of the mother and that separation is not the crucial factor in emotional disturbance. He suggests that there needs to be a clear distinction between loss of a maternal attachment and the lack of one altogether. He suggests that the very factors that lead to a separation may be those that lead to emotional maladjustment, rather than separation being the only cause of the emotional problems.

Study activity

The next time you have the opportunity, obtain permission to try an experiment with a baby between 3 and 7 months. Separate him from his mother and/or pass him round a few strangers. Observe his reactions. Then try to repeat the test with an older infant (9 to 10 months). Compare and contrast the results.

Ainsworth *et al.* (1978) went on to develop a method for testing the security of attachments – the Strange Situation – and initially identified three main types of attachment. Main and Solomon (1986) identified a fourth disorganised type:

- *Secure attachment.* This type of attachment is evident in about 55% of relationships in industrialised countries (Van Ijzendoorn *et al.*, 1992). Infants show some level of seeking proximity to their mothers but greet them positively on their return from any absences. Infants do not display aggressive behaviour towards them.
- *Avoidant attachment.* Infants are more likely to cry when their mothers leave them but less likely to greet them warmly on their return. After a period of separation infants may avoid or be slow to initiate contact with their mothers. They may react to strangers in the same way that they react to their parents. About 20% of children react in this way.
- *Resistant attachment.* Infants appear to want comfort and attention from their mothers but then react in a hostile fashion. Infants are distressed when their mothers leave but on her return mix clinginess with angry resistant behaviour and cannot be comforted easily. About 10% of children react in this way.
- *Disorganised/disorientated behaviour.* Children show a variety of confused and contradictory behaviours. They may cry but also show flat depressed-type behaviours. About 15% of children react in this way and their response is grounds for great concern.

Cultural perspective

According to Oates (1994) the establishment of either one or a small number of ongoing relationships between baby and carer(s) is a virtually universal feature.

Further reading on attachment

Cassidy, J. (2002) *Handbook of Attachment: Theory, Research, and Clinical Applications.* New York: The Guilford Press.

Smith, P. K., Cowie, H. and Blades, M. (1998) *Understanding Children's Development*, 3rd edn. Oxford: Blackwell.

Rogoff, B. (2003) *The Cultural Nature of Human Development.* Oxford: Oxford University Press.

Study activity

Consider the implications of attachment theory for your practice.

From observing children it is clear that they show differing behaviours demonstrating that the quality of attachment differs. This is perhaps because they have different internal working models of their relationships with their parents. The internal working model comprises the way in which they see the attachment, including the confidence they have in the attachment, expectations of rebuff or affection, and the quality of the secure base. Some theorists have pondered whether the quality of attachment remains stable over time. According to various studies, as many as 70% of children remain in the same attachment group. Attachment is usually secure and stable for middle-class babies. Securely attached babies are more likely to maintain their attachment status than insecure babies, whose relationship with their carers may be fragile and uncertain. There is also stability in insecure attachment behaviours and these behaviours are likely to continue into early childhood. Stability of the environment is important; however, if circumstances change, such as change of caregiver, divorce, abuse, bereavement, then the secure attachment and its quality may also change.

Questions for further consideration:

- What happens when attachment fails?
- What are the effects of long-term deprivation and can they be reversed?
- What can the effects of bereavement be on a child's attachments?
- What are the implications for care outside the home?

Study activity

Reflect critically on some of the children you have cared for. Attempt to identify those who appear have maintained the quality of their attachments and those who have not. Can you identify the reasons?

Horizontal relationships

Peer relationships are important in the development of social behaviour, values and personality. In fact much of what children learn about social behaviour comes from their association with peer groups. The peer group enables a child to learn things that cannot be learned in the same way from parents by sharing problems and feelings. It is usually within this level of relationship that friendships occur. Rutherford (1998) identifies that peer relationships enable social comparison, emotional support, positive stimulation and the provision of attention and, while friendships vary, they are significant in the development of social competence. Same-sex friendships tend to dominate and not only do children choose friends similar to themselves, but they become more similar to each other over time. Peer relationships are important, but most of the benefits of friendships can be achieved by relationships with family members. However, children who have friends are able to learn about perspective taking, cooperation, altruism, social competence and conflict management. Table 8.3 gives an overview of the development of friendships throughout childhood.

Study activity

Take opportunities to observe children in their relationships with their friends. Compare and contrast what you see with the table.

Table 8.3 Age changes in the development of friendships

Age range	Friendship behaviour	References
< 2 years	Clearly interested in other infants of same age. Looks at them, smiles, makes noises, shows toys. Many short overtures to different children. Low level of peer interaction. Playing together is usually around common toys	Brownnell and Brown (1992); Howes (1987)
3–4 years	Prefers to play with peers rather than alone, play is more cooperative. Friendships become clearer and more stable *but* based on proximity and shared interests	Hartup (1992); Hinde *et al.* (1985)
School age	Peers even more important and more perferable than being with older people. Sex segregation appears as a clear pattern in many cultures. Boys play with boys and girls with girls, each sex with own games. Friendships also sex segregated. Boys' relationship tend to be extensive; girls' more intensive	Harkness and Super (1985); Gottman (1986)
Adolescence	Mixed-sex friendships appear, more sharing of feelings. Peer group becomes the vehicle for the transition to adulthood. Conformity to group is essential *but* some research suggests that, in reality, peers have much less influence than we believe them to have	Bernt (1992)

The Development of Moral Reasoning and Social Cognition

Learning the difference between what is right and what is wrong, the rules of good and bad are an important part of becoming a social being. According to Berryman *et al.* (2002) moral awareness consists of at least four interrelated facets:

- resistance to temptation – this enables individuals to resist bad behaviour even when they are not being watched
- guilt – this refers to the emotional discomfort that is felt following wrongdoing
- altruism – prosocial acts such as kindness, helpfulness, service to others
- moral belief and insight – covers all aspects of what people say and do with relation to morality

Several psychologists have investigated this area of development. Kohlberg built on Piaget's ideas, agreeing with him that moral development is one aspect of intellectual development and, as such, occurs in stages. Kohlberg's work (1964–81) concentrates on justice and fairness. He pioneered the practice of assessing moral development by giving children a series of hypothetical dilemmas in story form, each one with a specific moral theme. One of the most famous is the story of Heinz. From his work he identified six stages of moral development extending to adulthood. The six stages are made up from three levels, each with two substages (Table 8.4).

- *Pre-conventional morality* – children are at this level until about 9–10 years of age. The child is concerned with the consequences of an act and judges what is wrong on the basis of what is rewarded or punished. Reasoning is in relation to himself and not based on

The story of Heinz

A woman was near to death from a special kind of cancer. There was one drug that the doctors thought might save her. It was a form of radium that a chemist in the same town had recently discovered. The drug was expensive to make but the chemist was charging ten times what the drug cost him to make. The sick woman's husband, Heinz, went to everybody he knew to borrow the money but he could only get together about £1000, which was half of what it cost. He told the chemist that his wife was dying and asked him to sell it cheaper or let him pay later. But the chemist said 'No; I discovered the drug and I'm going to make money from it'. So Heinz became desperate and considered breaking in to steal it. Should Heinz steal the drug? What are the reasons for your answer?

Table 8.4 Kohlberg's stages of moral development

Level	Stage
Level 1: Pre-conventional morality	Stage 1: Punishment and obedience Stage 2: Rewards
Level 2: Conventional morality	Stage 3: Good intentions Stage 4: Obedience to authority
Level 3: Post-conventional morality	Stage 5: Difference between moral and legal right Stage 6: Individual principles of conscience

societal rules. At stage 1 the child understands that whatever leads to punishment is wrong and tries to be obedient. At stage 2 the child understands that the right way to behave is the way that is rewarded.

- *Conventional morality* – this is the level of moral reasoning that most adults reach. It is concerned with upholding rules, expectations and conventions. Being good is seen as important for its own sake. Judgements about moral issues are based on what most people would think. At stage 3 the child behaves in ways that conform to society's ideas of good behaviour. At stage 4 the importance of doing one's duty is emphasised.
- *Post-conventional morality* – according to Kohlberg this level is reached by a minority of adults who are able to judge issues by an individual set of beliefs based on principles rather than rules. It is concerned with achieving the greatest good for the greatest number. At stage 5 an individual can recognise that rules should be broken on occasion. At stage 6 an individual takes into account the likely views of everyone affected by a moral decision and it becomes a matter of personal conscience.

Cultural perspective

Snarey (1985) reviewed a number of studies related to those of Kohlberg. The studies had been carried out in a variety of different countries including Canada, Turkey, India, Israel, Indonesia and New Guinea. The results all broadly confirmed that the stages of moral development described by Kohlberg occur in other societies.

Critics of Kohlberg's work say that he looks at how children make moral decisions and justify them, but does not look at how they behave in the real world when faced with their own dilemmas. They argue that behaviour may vary depending on the circumstances. Other criticisms are based on the fact that he used only males in his study and that the clinical method of interviewing that he used was very subjective. Turiel (1983) accuses Piaget and Kohlberg of gender bias, on the basis that Piaget considered girls to have a less-developed legal sense than boys. However, Piaget saw girls as being more orientated towards tolerance, innovation with rules and cooperation. Others would ague that he underestimated the ways in which young children see moral issues due to methods that relied on understanding of language and the ability to communicate. Finally, social learning theorists would ague that the development of moral reasoning in a stage-like way is impossible because children learn from other people and thus could vary in their reasoning depending on the circumstances.

Eisenberg (1986) tried to ascertain the type of reasoning used by children in making decisions about right or wrong. The dilemmas she presented to children included the difficult decision of choosing between self-interest and helping others. For example, would a child choose to stop and help someone who had fallen over if it meant missing ice cream and jelly at a birthday party? She identified two types of reasoning:

- *Hedonistic reasoning (preschool).* At this stage the child was more concerned with the self-oriented consequences of his actions.
- *Needs-oriented reasoning.* Children at this stage express concern for other people's needs. They do not use principles to make decisions but respond to needs. Their helping behaviours are related to sociability rather than moral reasoning. This develops further during adolescence into doing things because it is expected of one and then on to internalising the values that guide them.

The work of Eisenberg bears a similarity to that of Selman (1980), who investigated children's ability to adopt a social perspective or viewpoint, that is, their development of social cognition. At first, children have a limited idea of what others might be thinking or feeling, but this evolves to a point where they are able to consider different people's perspectives simultaneously. Social cognition is an area related closely to moral reasoning and is concerned with the child's ability to understand social relationships – empathy, self-control and social problem-solving. Selman proposed five levels of social understanding:

- *Undifferentiated perspective taking: 3–6 years.* Children recognise that they can have different thoughts from their peers but become confused and may not understand that people think or feel differently from themselves.
- *Social informational perspective taking: 4–9 years.* The child is capable of appreciating other people's perspectives because people have access to different information.
- *Self-reflective perspective taking: 7–12 years.* The child is capable of taking a self-reflective and reciprocal perspective.
- *Third-party perspective taking: 10–15 years.* The young person is capable of adopting a third-person, impartial perspective. He is able to stand back and view a relationship as if he were an outsider.
- *Societal perspective taking: 14–adult.* The young person is capable of adopting an in-depth perspective and understands that other people's actions are influenced by a variety of factors (for example social values, personality) and is able to take these into account.

A moral dilemma – Selman's story

Holly is 8 and likes to climb trees. She is the best tree climber in the neighbourhood. One day while climbing down from a tall tree she fell off the bottom branch but did not hurt herself. Her father saw her fall. He was upset and asked her to promise not to climb trees any more. Holly promises. Later that day Holly meets her friend Shawn. Shawn's kitten is caught up a tree and can't get down. Something has to be done or the kitten will fall. Holly is the only one who climbs well enough to reach the kitten but she remembers her promise to her father.

- Does Holly know how Shawn feels about the kitten? Why?
- How will Holly's father feel if he finds out she climbed the tree?
- What do you think Holly should do?

Study activity

Try out Selman's dilemma on children of different ages. What do you find?

It would appear from the last two studies that there is a change in children's social awareness at round about the age of 5 or 6 years, when they begin to entertain ideas about the well-being of others. Work by Piaget also found that pre-operational children could not take account of someone's intentions because they were egocentric. They were more likely to make judgements based on appearances – for example how big a lie has been told or how many things have been broken. Perspective taking varies greatly among children of the same age. These individual differences may be due to cognitive maturity and the way in which adults and peers explain their viewpoints and encourage perspective taking.

Study activity

Here are two stories that Piaget used to test children's moral development. Try them out on pre-operational and post-operational children, recording the children's responses if you can. Analyse the results in light of the theories discussed above.

Story 1: John is in his bedroom when called for dinner. He enters the dining room but does not know that there is a tray with 15 cups on it just behind the door. The door knocks the tray over and all the cups are broken.

Story 2: Henry decides to have some jam one day when his mother is out. He climbs on to a chair to try to reach the jam jar that was in a high cupboard. While stretching up he knocks over a cup, which falls to the floor and breaks.

Questions:

1. Which would you say was the naughtier child?
2. Why?

Both Piaget and Kohlberg agree that there is an association between moral reasoning and moral action and that, as children's moral awareness grows, they are able to make judgements about right and wrong and are able to behave accordingly. However, Kohlberg (1978) makes the point that 'one can reason in terms of one's principles and not live up to them'. In reality moral behaviour is probably the result of many interacting influences and is therefore dependent on the circumstances in which individuals find themselves (Figure 8.2).

Study activity

Reflect on your own childhood, can you recall any times when your moral behaviour was influenced by those given in Figure 8.2 and Table 8.5?

Factors that can facilitate the development of moral and social awareness

- Strong ties of affection between parents and children
- Firm moral demands made by parents on their children
- The consistent use of sanctions
- Psychological techniques of punishment
- The use of reasoning and explanations
- Giving responsibilities to young children
- Encouraging the child to see other people's points of view
- Increasing child's level of moral reasoning by discussion

(Berryman *et al.*, 2002)

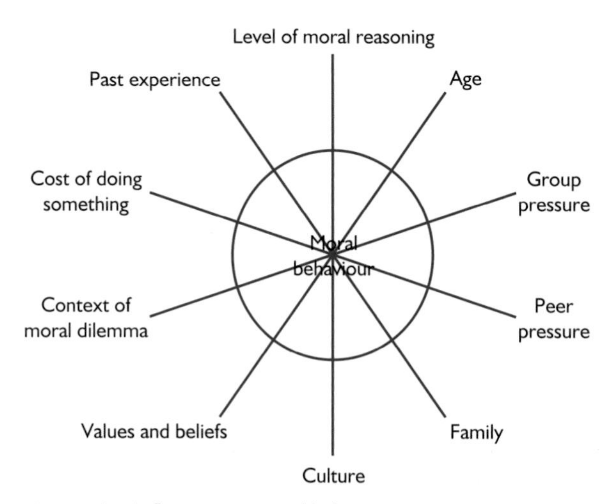

Figure 8.2 Interacting influences on moral behaviour.

Module 2

Table 8.5 An alternative view from Hoffman (1988) on the development of empathy

Stage and approximate age (year)	Type of empathy	Characteristics
Stage 1 (0–1)	Global	Infant may match the emotions of others, e.g. when another baby cries
Stage 2 (1–2)	Egocentric	Child responds to other's distress with some distress of own. May try to help by offering what they know works for self
Stage 3 (2–13)	Empathy for another's feelings	Child notes other's feelings and responds in non-egocentric ways. Over the years, child displays wider and wider range of emotions
Stage 4 (adolescence)	Empathy for another's life conditions	Responds not only to other's feelings, but also to their general situation or plight

Summary

This part of the module has tried to give an insight into a child's social development. Children need to know the expectations of the society into which they were born if they are able to function to their full potential. It is possible that they are born with some inherited, inborn ability to be social. However, it is clear that much social behaviour will depend on the child's environment and cultural background. Children are unique and develop their own self-concepts and personalities. As parents we all hope that they will develop an acceptable moral code of conduct based on the rules and expectations of society. It can be difficult for some children to fit into society, perhaps because they are influenced by adverse circumstances. What happens in the lives of children who lie, cheat, bully and murder? Is this behaviour inborn or is it a result of social forces and influences on young lives? What we do know is that a child's relationships, especially in the early years, are an important basis on which all future relationships and social behaviour are built. However, it is important to acknowledge that other areas of development, such as cognition and language development, will influence social development. It is important to look at the whole child and not just the social being.

Key Points

1. Evidence suggests that the quality of a child's early relationships will affect the development of social competence.
2. Initially, self-concept is very concrete and linked to visible characteristics – this gradually changes as children become more abstract in their thinking and more focused on internal qualities.
3. Although inborn temperament may be the basis for the development of personality, a variety of factors interact thereafter in a complex way to influence it.
4. The formation of both vertical and horizontal attachments is important for a child's social development.
5. As children's moral awareness grows, they can make judgements about what is right and wrong and are able to behave accordingly.

Chapter 9

Play and Education

Play

Time for play is one of the emergent issues of the 21st century and its significance is recognised by a wide range of influential theorists. Children seem to spend a great deal of time 'playing' but the purpose and nature of this activity continues to defy classification. Views on play have changed during the past century. In the early 1900s play was seen as dangerous in that it was thought to present sensual impulses that ought to be guarded against. Other early theories of play suggested that children played so that they could rid themselves of their primitive instincts, restore their lost energy, get rid of surplus energy and practise skills that would be required in later life. In the early 1920s, play was linked directly to children's development, but this behaviourist approach was appropriated by the early educationalists such as Froebel, Montessori, Steiner and Isaacs, who saw play as nature's means of individual education (Moyles, 2005). Play supporters received encouragement from the theories of Piaget, Bruner and Vygotsky, who saw play as the development of a range of exponential and exploratory skills. According to Bruce (2005), play is about the universe and everything – it may have to take place in an environment where it is not supported or enabled, but when it is actively supported it has a major impact on the development of individuals and humanity as a whole. In order to explore the role of play in a child's development we should try to explore the nature of play.

Study activity

What do you understand by the term 'play'? List as many characteristics of play as you can and then try to write your own definition.

Most theorists do not attempt to define play using one sentence. Instead they look at the characteristics of play and try to distinguish between what is play and what is not. Rubin and Fein (1983) identify the following characteristics of play, it:

- is intrinsically motivated
- is characterised by the attention to means rather than the end result
- can be clearly distinguished from exploratory behaviour
- is characterised by symbolism or pretence
- is free from externally applied rules
- is characterised by active participation

They suggest that the more of these characteristics that can be observed in an interaction, the more likely that play is taking place, but the quality of play is not measurable by the number of observed characteristics. Garvey (1990) sees play as a 'non-literal' activity and one that can be contrasted with the 'real' thing. Children recognise when something is the non-real situation but adults can often misinterpret this. For example, children often tease each other and then one begins to 'cry'. The crying appears real and I intervene only to be told 'We're only playing'!

Play can be considered to have an impact on three areas of development: learning, emotion and social understanding. Barnes and Kehily (2003) suggest that children play because they are young and that this immaturity is important as it allows time for the child to learn the intricate skills required for adult maturity. Piaget understood play as an opportunity to practise and consolidate (or assimilate and accommodate) new skills in a safe environment, whereas Vygotsky felt that play is a crucial tool through which children extend their skills, enabling them to explore ways of talking, thinking and behaving. Freud suggested that the inner world of children's thinking is revealed through their play and that they use play to explore situations over which they can exert control. Anna Freud developed his theory of the emotional significance of play into an exploration of therapeutic work that forms the basis for some approaches to play therapy. Anthropologists such as Margaret Mead suggest that imaginary play enables a child to develop a distinct sense of identity through the exploration of different social roles. They are also able to use imaginary play to make sense of their current situation.

Hutt (1971) distinguished play from exploration. She suggested that, although play could lead on from exploration, the two were distinctly different in that exploration is a serious activity and essentially object based, focusing on 'What can this object do?', whereas play is relaxed and diverse and essentially asks 'What can I do with this object?' She found that children's interest in objects waned when the properties of the object did not maintain their attention, i.e. noises and different actions.

Although the nature of play is complex and difficult to define, it is clear from observations that children use different types of play at different ages:

- *From 0 to 2 years.* Play is mainly used to explore the environment and to master skills. Actions are repetitive and are usually those that give the child pleasure: shaking, rattling, building and knocking down, filling and emptying containers. The child explores and manipulates objects by using many of the five senses. As language develops, play with sounds becomes evident. Constructive play becomes apparent in the second year when children build towers, assemble puzzles and mould materials into shapes. Towards the end of the first year pretend play begins to emerge. Initially, the distance between the imaginary prop and the real or physical object is not great, but eventually almost anything can be made to stand in for something else and play becomes increasingly internalised and symbolic. However, Leslie (1988) suggests that although children may substitute symbolic meanings for objects, to do so they have to have a fundamental understanding of the original characteristics of the object. Children who take part in pretend play have better powers of concentration, are varied in their idea production, flexible in their problem solving and show advanced planning skills when organising make-believe activities in the more mature stages of play. Motor development results in the practice of motor skills, running and jumping.

- *From the age of 2.* Towards the end of the first year the development of pretend play begins to emerge. To engage in pretend play children need to be able to distinguish play from reality. Three parallel aspects of this development have been identified. The first is *decentration.* Initially the child's actions are directed towards the self – pretend drinking from an empty cup. Then the same actions begin to be directed towards others – perhaps giving a doll a pretend drink. Finally, by about the age of 2 the child is able to get the doll to pretend to drink from the cup. The second aspect is *decontextualisation.* To begin with the child relies on real objects – the cup. He then moves on to be able to represent the cup with something else – perhaps an empty yoghurt pot or a shell. Finally, by about the age of 3 years he is able to use imaginary objects. It is around this time that imaginary friends appear on the scene. Imaginary play is a means of subjecting things to the child's activities without roles or limitations. The third aspect in the development of pretend play is *integration.* Initially the child uses one action – feeding the doll. By the age of 2 the child is able to use multischeme combinations and immerse himself in mini-stories. This enables him to progress to more complex sociodramatic play, such as mummies and daddies, cowboys and Indians. Some elements of fantasy will occur at various levels within children's play, depending on their maturity. Smilansky and Sheftaya (1990) identify valuable differences between pretend play and fantasy play, which is more concerned with the nature and the role of social interaction. In fantasy play children show a developing awareness of their social surroundings and act out interactions.
- *From 7 years onwards.* The emergence of games with formal rules. Children now understand that play can be governed by rules to which they must conform, particularly if they want to continue playing with others. Prior to this age children find it difficult to understand the properties of rules or their abstract and artificial nature. Although children often have rules in their games, the boundaries frequently change according to the moment, and the rules are particular to a game. Now they are able to take part in games with more formal, public rules with little scope for change, for example football and board games. However, within pretend play, inherent rules can exist that are complex and are only understood by those taking part in the

Criteria for fantasy play

- Imaginative role play
- The substitution of replica objects for real objects
- Verbal make believe
- Persistence (in time) in the role play
- Interaction between at least two members
- Verbal communication

play scenario. They can be highly inclusive and exclusive at the same time.

Although these distinct periods of development exist, the change is gradual and some forms of play will persist into adulthood. There is a degree of overlap between the stages, and some play activities, such as physical play, can be seen to fit into each of the stages. Pretend play does not necessarily stop at 7 years of age; rather, it becomes more complex.

Study activity

Observe children at play – this could be a group of children that you know or in a structured setting such as a playgroup. There needs to be a range of age groups. Observe the children's play activities for a period of time. Make notes as to the activities of each child. Analyse your findings with reference to the suggested stages in the development of play.

Study activity

A hierarchy of play within a social dimension for preschool children has been suggested:

- unoccupied behaviour
- solitary play
- parallel play
- associative play
- cooperative play

Observe a group of preschool children at play and critically comment on their level of social interaction and play.

The way a child plays will be influenced by a number of factors:

- *The role of adults.* Tamburrini (1981) suggested that adult intervention in a child's play will inhibit it. This is based on an assumption that play is universal and spontaneous. Research into the effect of adult tutoring in play has been carried out and seems to indicate that adult participation in play can facilitate and enhance play. Bruce and Meggitt (1996) identified that adult-led structured play can enhance children's level of learning but it has to take place with sensitivity. Play can become undervalued if the children are left to play without any help or guidance. Adults have the opportunity to prolong the play episode and extend its inherent value. Moyles (2005) notes that adults can give inherent messages about the purpose and value of play and caution needs to be advised. Tizard (1977) found that in nurseries where adults adopted a passive role, play was frequently of short duration with limited use of available materials. Sylva *et al.* (1980) in a study conducted in playgroups made suggestions as to how playgroup leaders could enhance the meaning of play for children. They suggested that there should be a balance of structured and unstructured play, with adults being actively engrossed in some play activities.

- *The child's personality*. Singer (1973) identified children as being of 'high fantasy' and 'low fantasy' dispositions. He suggested that those with the former were more creative in some respects than the latter.
- *The child's gender*. Harris and Butterworth (2002) suggest that as preschool children use play to explore familiar roles (such as teacher, cook, train driver, doctor or nurse) they adopt these roles along gender-specific lines, with girls selecting roles usually occupied by females and boys taking the male role. This suggests that symbolic play may contribute and reinforce the acquisition of gender identity. Parents may unwittingly provide play materials that are gender typed. Research has shown that from the age of 2 children select toys and games that fit gender stereotypes. Boys tend to choose more masculine toys such as cars, guns, Action Man, building blocks, Lego. Girls tend to engage in more feminine play such as dressing up, soft toys and dolls, imitating household chores (O'Brien and Houston, 1985; O'Brien, 1992). Rough and tumble play seems to be preferred by boys (Smith and Cowie, 1991). There is much debate about why children show gender differences in play; it may be that their parents treat them differently, but experience suggests that young children can be equally happy playing with toys appropriate for either gender.
- *The environment*. The degree to which a child plays will depend on numerous environmental factors, including cultural contexts, the terrain of the play area, the access to play space, physical and psychological safety. Cross-cultural studies show that children in some cultures may be required to take care of younger siblings, tend crops or help with household chores (Hobsbaum, 1995).

The purpose of play

Various theorists have suggested many different views on the purpose of play. Freud believed that play compensated for the frustrations and anxieties encountered in everyday life. Within play, the child's desire for mastery could be acted out in a safe, secure environment. This idea is the basis of play therapy in which children use play for the release of tension. Piaget believed that play was important in, and linked to, the development of cognitive and intellectual skills. In play, reality is moulded to fit in with the child's own experiences and understanding. Social learning theorists see play as important for learning those social skills needed as adults (*see also* Use of play in hospital p. 271).

Bergen (2002) suggests that there is a growing body of evidence supporting the many connections between cognitive competence and high-quality pretend play:

- high-quality pretend play is an important facilitator of perspective taking and, later, abstract thought
- research has shown some clear links between social and linguistic competence and high-quality pretence; engagement in pretend play with friends may assist children's development in these areas

Some researchers have attempted to find out what children learn through play by comparing the performances of children who have been given play experiences and those who have not. Dansky and Silverman (1973) showed that free play promotes creative thinking, while Sylva

Alternative views on play

- *Froebel (1906)* – 'Play, truly recognised and rightly fostered, unites the germinating life of the child attentively with the ripe life of experiences of the adult and thus fosters the one through the other'.
- *Karl Groos (1900)* – Practice theory of play: 'Play provides exercise and elaboration of the skills needed for survival'.
- *Maria Montessori (1920s and 30s)* – She did not value pretend or sociodramatic play, and thought that this was escape from reality. More emphasis was put on real-life play and the use of constructive play materials.
- *Susan Isaacs (1929)* – She saw play as essential for emotional and cognitive growth of young children.

Cultural perspective

A study by Bornstein *et al.* (1999) found patterns of similarity and difference between Argentine and US cultures. In both cultures boys engaged in more exploratory play than girls, and girls engaged in more symbolic play than boys. US children and their mothers engaged in more exploratory play whereas Argentine children and their mothers engaged in more symbolic play.

Further reading

Landreth, G. L. (2002) *Play Therapy: The Art of the Relationship.* New York: Brunner Routledge.

Provides comprehensive and detailed information for creating therapeutic relationships with children and facilitating the play therapy process.

Kaduson, H. G. and Schaefer, C. E. (2001) *Short-Term Play Therapy for Children.* New York: Guilford Press.

Brings together play therapists to share their expertise on facilitating children's healing in a short time frame. Chapters are filled with lively illustrations and step-by-step guidelines for implementation.

'Play is indeed the child's work and the means whereby he grows and develops'.

(Isaacs, 1929)

Table 9.1 Challenging versus ordinary play (adapted from Sylva *et al.*, 1980)

Challenging play	Ordinary play
A child playing with 'Lego' spreads the bricks out onto the floor. He carefully chooses the bricks the wants and proceeds to build a model. The child is playing in a systematic and purposeful way.	A child playing 'Lego' builds a tower of bricks – does not choose any specific bricks but just uses bricks as they come to hand. He takes the bricks apart and then builds another tower in the same way. Routine, repetitive play with no new elements or ideas.
A child sets up an obstacle course around which he rides his bike. This behaviour is challenging as the child is required to use his skills to steer the bike and not bump into the obstacles.	A child rides his bike up and down the track. He does not try to steer the bike round obstacles but looks as if he is letting off steam.

et al. (1976) found that it improved the problem-solving skills of 3–5-year-olds. They and others have concluded that children learn through play. Most studies show positive benefits of play. However Pellegrini and Smith (1998) urge caution when interpreting the results of research in this field. They conclude that, although certain play activities undoubtedly result in certain types of learning, play is only one way in which children learn and it is important not to over generalise (Table 9.1).

Study activity

Consider ways in which you could research the role of play in development. What are the problems inherent in this type of research?

Education

For most children, school is an important part of the socialisation process, providing social contacts outside the home. At the same time as 'teaching' children different subjects, the school acts as a form of social control, transmitting values through formal and informal (hidden curriculum) control (Moore, 1996) (Figure 9.1).

The history of education

Prior to 1870 there was no organised education system. The rich employed private tutors or sent their children to private schools. Most children had no formal education. The Elementary Education Acts of 1870 and 1880 saw the development of a basic network of state-supported elementary schools with compulsory attendance up to the age of 10 years. Following this, the school-leaving age rose to 14 and then to 15 in 1944. Prior to 1944 attendance at school was based on ability to pay. The 1944 Butler Act attempted to ensure equality of opportunity and introduced grammar schools and secondary modern schools. Children were sent to one or other of these depending on their academic

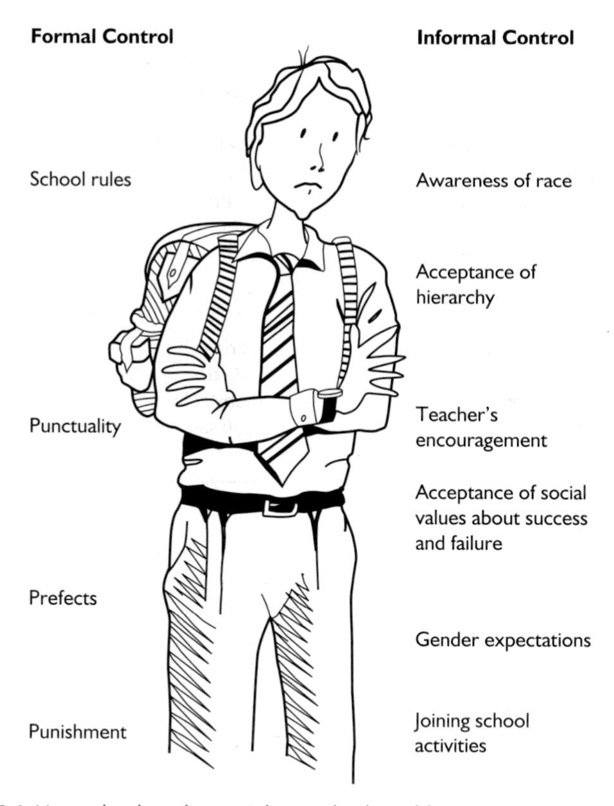

Figure 9.1 How school teaches social control (adapted from Moore, 1996).

ability, as judged by the 11-plus exam. The option of staying on until the age of 17 was offered. A change of government in 1964 brought about the shift towards comprehensive education, which was intended to remove the division between grammar and secondary modern schools, thus enabling all children to have access to equal opportunities. This principle still exists but many areas have retained grammar schools and some have developed their own approaches. The 1988 Education Act introduced some significant reforms, including the establishment of a national curriculum, and the opportunity for schools to opt out from the control of local education authorities to become 'independent state schools'. In November 2001 the White Paper *Schools Achieving Success* proposed:

- allowing successful primary schools to opt out of the National Curriculum and develop curriculum innovations
- more involvement of the private sector in state provision
- 'standards contracts' to enable private, religious and voluntary organisations to support the management of both failing and successful schools
- more 'specialist schools' and 'city academies' attracting private sponsorship
- 'advanced specialist schools' to train teachers
- more vocational education from 14+.

These proposals formed the basis of the Education Act 2002.

The National Curriculum

- *The foundation stage* was introduced in September 2000 as a distinct phase of education for children aged 3–5. Guidance sets out six areas of learning that form the basis of the foundation stage curriculum: personal, social and emotional development; communication, language and literacy; mathematical development; knowledge and understanding of the world; physical development; and creative development.
- *Key Stage 1 (5–7) and Key Stage 2 (7–11).* Consists of three core subjects (English, Maths and Science) and eight foundation subjects (History, Geography, Design and Technology, Information Technology, Art, Music, Physical Education and Religious Education).
- *Key Stage 3 (11–14).* The same subjects with the addition of Citizenship.
- *Key Stage 4 (14–16).* English, Maths, Science, Information and Communication Technology (ICT), Physical Education, Citizenship, Religious Education, Sex Education, Careers Education and Work-related Learning.

Study activity

Education in England differs from the system used elsewhere in the UK. Find out about the systems used in Scotland, Wales and Northern Ireland.

Compulsory education in England begins the year in which a child is 5 years old. Some children start school the term in which they are 5, others start at the beginning of the school year. This means that some children, whose birthdays fall in the summer months, will only just have turned 4 when they begin school. Starting school brings a dramatic change in certain aspects of a child's life. Socialisation to a new culture is one of the most vital aspects of this transition. Children have to learn new rules and routines; they meet many new people, adults and children, and have to find their way round a new environment. Even negotiating the toilets and the dining room can cause alarm and fear in the young child.

Study activity

Reflect, if you can, on your own first day at school. If this proves too distant a memory, reflect on those of your own children or of family and friends. What was it like for them, how did they cope?

Parents play a crucial role in their children's transition from home to school, and the significance of this transition is receiving increasing attention from policy makers and researchers (Bennett *et al.*, 2005). If the transition is not successful, it can impact upon the child's entire education, including grades, retention, anxiety levels and self-esteem (Timperley *et al.*, 2003). In addition, the transition to school will be affected by various other factors:

- age of the child
- siblings already at school
- the child's personality
- preparation for school, including attendance at nursery or play-group, parental views on school
- the philosophy of the school
- expectations of the child, teachers and parents

Once a child has made the transition to school life, many factors will impact upon his education (Figure 9.2) including:

- *Parental attitudes*. The degree to which parents show encouragement and interest in their children's schooling plays an important part in academic success. It may even help to overcome deprivation and poverty (Moore, 1996). A literature review by Desforges and Abouchaar (2003) gives an overview of research in this area.
- *Culture, race, ethnicity*. Black pupils, on average, tend to do less well in the British educational system than white children. The Swann

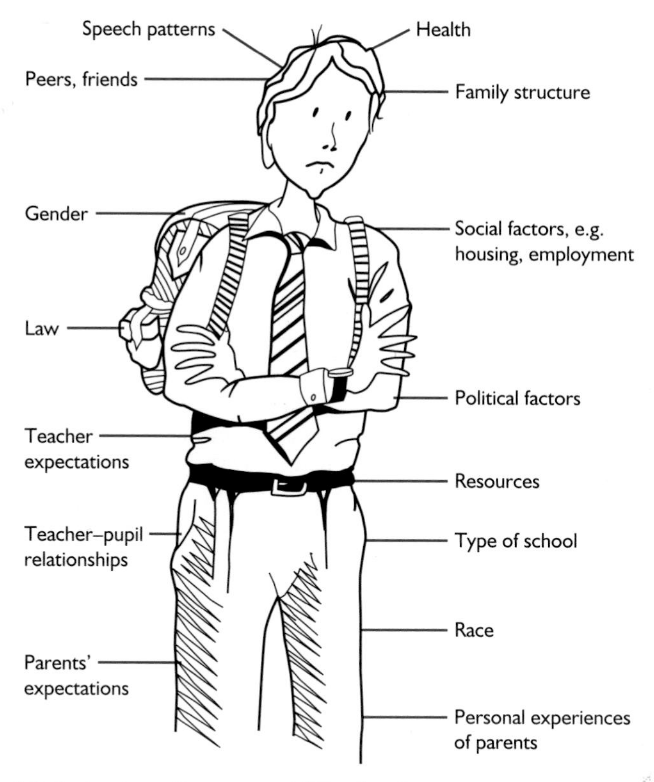

Figure 9.2 Factors impacting upon a child's education.

Report of 1985 (cited by Giddens, 1993) indicated that although 13% of the white population obtained one or more passes at A level in 1981/2, only 5% of West Indian school leavers achieved similar results. In 2002, only 30% of those from black Caribbean backgrounds got five or more good GCSEs. Other studies indicate that racist discrimination exists, leading to inequalities in education success (Craft and Craft, 1985).

- *Gender*. Many studies have been conducted that indicate gender differences in educational attainment. Girls tend to do better than boys during the primary school years and in the early secondary years (Younger and Warrington, 2005).
- *Relationships between teachers and pupils*. Rutter (cited by Giddens, 1993) studied the educational achievement of a group of boys over several years. He concluded that schools have a direct influence on the academic achievement of children. Among the factors that impact upon children are the quality of teacher–pupil interaction, an atmosphere of cooperation and caring between teachers and children, and well-organised preparation. Lacey (1970) found that the attitudes of teachers affected a child's level of achievement. Most of the teachers in his study disliked teaching the lower streams and this showed in their attitudes towards the children.

Further reading

Younger, M. and Warrington, M. (2005) *Raising Boys' Achievement*. Final Report. Research Report No. 363. London: HMSO.

http://www.standards.dfes.gov.uk/genderandachievement/pdf/HomertonReport-final.pdf?version=1 (accessed 7 March 2006).

This very comprehensive report follows a 4-year project looking at issues surrounding 'boys' underachievement'. The authors make the valid point that, although boys' achievements are rising more slowly than those of girls, they should be set against a background of a generally rising trajectory of achievement for both boys and girls. Also, many boys continue to achieve extremely well at school, while, equally, there are some girls whose needs are not recognised within schools and who underachieve.

Study activity

Look for research/articles on any of the other factors identified in Figure 9.2. Make notes here in the margin.

Educational provision for children with special needs

In any given year there are some 100 000 children and young people who require education outside school because of illness or injury. In addition, there is a significant number of children and young people who experience clinically defined mental health problems. The situations of these children and young people will vary widely, but they all run the risk of a reduction in educational achievement. The primary aim of educating children and young people who have medical needs is to minimise, as far as possible, the disruption to normal schooling, by continuing education as normally as the incapacity allows. Enabling children and young people to access education appropriate to their medical condition is important to their future mental and physical development (*see also* Educational needs p. 227 and Living with a disability p. 224).

Section 19 of the Education Act 1996 states that 'each local education authority shall make arrangements for the provision of suitable education at school or otherwise than at school for those children of compulsory school age who, by reason of illness, exclusion from school or otherwise, may not for any period receive suitable education unless such arrangements are made for them'. Local education authorities (LEAs) also have the power to provide suitable education otherwise than at school for young people over compulsory school age but under the age of 19. Suitable education is defined as efficient education suitable to the age, ability and aptitude and to any special educational needs the child (or young person) may have.

Hospital schools are special schools, maintained by LEAs, within the premises of a hospital. They are subject to the procedures laid down in Section 31 and Schedule 6 of the School Standards and Framework Act 1998 in relation to establishment, discontinuance or making prescribed alterations. Education law reflects the special nature and variable circumstances of hospital schools by providing, in some areas of legislation, more flexible arrangements than those applying to other special schools. Hospital schools are not under a legal obligation to offer the National Curriculum. All hospital schools have local management and delegated responsibility for their budgets. Most of the children for whom hospital schools or hospital teaching provide services are hospital inpatients, although a few chronically ill children may attend daily from home.

The responsibilities of LEAs towards pupils who are unable to attend school because of their medical needs include ensuring that:

- pupils are not at home without access to education for more than 15 working days
- pupils who have an illness/diagnosis, which indicates prolonged or recurring periods of absence from school, whether at home or in hospital, have access to education, so far as possible, from day one

- pupils receive an education of similar quality to that available in school, including a broad and balanced curriculum
- pupils educated at home receive a *minimum entitlement* of 5 hours' teaching per week

This is a minimum and should be increased where necessary to enable pupils to keep up with their studies. This is particularly important when a pupil is approaching public examinations. Whether the child or young person is able to access this entitlement will depend on medical advice and, perhaps more importantly, when they feel able to cope with it. The right balance must be struck between encouraging pupils to study and recognising when they are not well enough to benefit from teaching. This must be kept under regular review. Some specialist hospital schools providing for children and young people who require long-term care also make, or help to arrange, provision for well siblings in cases when the whole family has moved to the area temporarily to be close to the pupil who is in hospital. This should happen wherever possible.

Summary

Play and education are a major part of a child's life. They impact upon children's development and serve to enable them to grow up to reach their full potential. There are many aspects of play that provide continuing areas for research. However, it would appear that play is important in children's development and in their learning about life and the world around them. An understanding of how children play serves a vital basis for playing with sick or chronically ill children, or with children who have special needs. As a children's nurse you should be able to appreciate the many facets of play, so that you can enhance play for children in hospital and also use play as therapy to help overcome some of the psychological trauma associated with hospitalisation. All children receive a unique education as the impact of education on each of them will be influenced by many factors. The education of our children provides them with a basis for ongoing education in adulthood and helps to prepare them for a future role in society. The importance of education is recognised in the provision of school for sick children (*see also* Play in hospital p. 263 and 271).

Study activity

Contact a play leader in your hospital and discuss the role of play in therapeutic care.

Study activity

Contact your hospital schoolteacher and discuss school in hospital. Find out about legislation and the organisation of schooling for children who are in hospital. Analyse some of the issues related to school in hospital.

Module 2

Key Points

1. The extent to which play influences development continues to be debated, especially as the nature of play is so complex and unclear.
2. Different types of play are evident at different ages.
3. The way a child plays will be influenced by the role of adults, the child's personality, age and gender, and the environment.
4. The purpose of play has been suggested by various theorists as being important in all aspects of development. However, it is important to note that it is only one way in which children learn.
5. For most children, education is an important part of the socialisation process and is influenced by a variety of factors that are unique to each child.
6. Education for children with special needs is based on assessment of need in partnership with parents and is provided, where possible, alongside peers in mainstream schools.

References

Ainsworth, M. D. S., *et al.* (1978) *Patterns of Attachment: A Psychological Study of the Strange Situation.* New Jersey: Lawrence Erlbaum.

Anderson, C. A. and **Bushman, B. J.** (2001) Effects of violent video games on aggressive behaviour, aggressive cognition, aggressive affect, physiological arousal and prosocial behaviour; a meta-analytic review of the scientific literature. *Psychological Science*, **12**, 353–359.

Aries, P. (1962) *Centuries of Childhood.* London: Penguin.

Ball, W. and **Tronick, E.** (1971) Infant responses to impending collision: optical and real. *Science*, **171**, 818–820.

Barker, D. J. P., *et al.* (2002) Foetal origins of adult disease, strengths of effects and biological basis. *International Journal of Epidemiology*, **31**, 1235–1239.

Barnes, P. and **Kehily, M. J.** (2003) Play and the cultures of childhood. In Kehily, M. J. and Swann, J. (eds), *Children's Cultural Worlds.* Milton Keynes: Open University Press.

Bee, H. (1995) *The Developing Child.* New York: HarperCollins.

Bee, H. and **Boyd, D.** (2004) *The Developing Child.* Boston: Allyn & Bacon.

Bennett, P., Elliot, M. and **Peters, D.** (2005) Classroom and family effects on children's social and behavioural problems. *The Elementary School Journal*, **105** (5), 461.

Bergen, D. (2002) The role of pretend play in children's cognitive development. *Early Childhood Research and Practice*, **4** (1). http://ecrp.uiuc.edu/v4n1/bergen.html (accessed 17 April 2006).

Berk, L. (2005) *Infants and Children*, 5th edn. Boston: Allyn & Bacon.

Bernt, T. J. (1992) The features and effects of friendship in adolescence. *Child Development*, **53**, 1447–1460.

Berryman, J. C., *et al.* (2002) *Developmental Psychology and You*, 2nd edn. Oxford: Blackwell.

Bornstein, M. H., *et al.* (1999) Play in two societies: pervasiveness of process, specificity of structure. *Child Development*, **70** (2), 317–331.

Bower, T. G. R. (1965) Stimulus variables determining space perception in infants. *Science*, **149**, 88–89.

Bower, T. G. R. (1981) Cognitive development. In Roberts, M. and Tamburrini, J. (eds), *Child Development 0–5.* Edinburgh: Holmes McDougall.

Bower, T. G. R., Broughton, J. M. and **Moore, M. K.** (1970) Infant responses to moving objects: an indicator of response to distal variables. *Perception and Psychophysics*, **8**, 51–53.

Bowlby, J. (1969) *Attachment and Loss*, Vol. 1. London: Hogarth Press.

Bronfenbrenner, U. and **Morris, P. A.** (1998) The ecology of the developmental process. In Lerner, R. M. (ed.) *Theoretical Models of Human Development*, Vol. 1, 5th edn. New York: Wiley.

Brown, A. S. and **Susser, E. S.** (2002) In utero infection and adult schizophrenia. *Mental Retardation Developmental Disabilities Research Review Journal*, **8** (1), 51–57.

Brownell, C. A. and **Brown, E.** (1992) Peers and play in infants and toddlers. In Hasselt, V. and Hersen, M. (eds) *Handbook of Social Development: a Lifespan Perspective.* Plenum Press: New York.

Bruce, T. (2005) Play, the universe and everything. In Moyles, J. (ed.), *The Excellence of Play*, 2nd edn. Maidenhead: Open University Press.

Bruce, T. and **Meggitt, C.** (1996) *Childcare and Education.* London: Hodder & Stoughton.
Bruner, J. (1966) On cognitive growth. In Bruner, J. S., Oliver, R. R. and Greenfield, P. M., *Studies in Cognitive Growth.* New York: Wiley.
Butterworth, G. and **Jarrett, N.** (1991) What minds have in common is space: spatial mechanisms serving joint visual attention in infancy. *British Journal of Developmental Psychology*, **9**, 55–72.
Campbell, R. and **Olsen, D.** (1990) Children's thinking. In Grieve, R. and Hughes, M. (eds), *Understanding Children.* Oxford: Basil Blackwell.
Chomsky, N. (1986) *Knowledge of Language: its Nature, Origin and Use.* New York: Praeger.
Comstock, G. A. and **Sharrer, E.** (2001) The use of television and other film related media. In Singer, D. G. and Singer, J. L. (eds), *Handbook of Children and the Media.* Thousand Oaks, CA: Sage.
Craft, M. and **Craft, A.** (1985) The participation of ethnic minority pupils in further and higher education. *Education Research*, **25** (1), 10–19.
Dansky, J. L. and **Silverman, I. W.** (1973) Effects of play on associative fluency in pre-school children. *Developmental Psychology*, **9**, 38–43.
Department of Health (1994) *Weaning and the Weaning Diet.* London: HMSO.
Desforges, C. and **Abouchaar, A.** (2003) *The Impact of Parental Involvement, Parental Support and Family Education on Pupil Achievement and Adjustment: A Literature Review.* Research Report No. 433. London: HMSO.
Donaldson, M. (1978) *Children's Minds.* London: Fontana.
Dowling, J. (2004) *The Great Brain Debate: Nature or Nurture?* Washington: Joseph Henry Press.
Eisenberg, N. (1986) *Altruism Emotion, Cognition and Behavior.* Hillsdale, NJ: Lawrence Erlbaum.
Elman, J. L., *et al.* (1996) *Rethinking Innateness: A Connectionist Perspective on Development.* Cambridge, MA: MIT Press.
Eriksson, J. G., *et al.* (2001) Early growth and coronary heart disease in later life: longitudinal study. *British Medical Journal*, **322**, 949–953.
European Collaborative Study (1991) Children born to women with HIV-1 infection: natural history and risk of transmission. *Lancet*, **337**, 253–260.
Eysenck, M. (2004) *Psychology: An International Perspective.* Hove: Psychology Press.
Fall, C. H. D., *et al.* (1992) Relation of infant feeding to adult serum cholesterol concentration and death from ischemic heart disease. *British Medical Journal*, **304**, 801–805.
Fishbein, H. (1987) Socialisation and television. In Boyd-Barrett, O. and Braham, P. (eds), *Media, Knowledge and Power.* London: Croom Helm.
Garvey, C. (1990) *Play.* London: Fontana/Open Books.
Gibson, E. J. and **Spelke, E.** (1983) The development of perception. In Mussen, P. (ed.), *Handbook of Child Psychology*, Vol. 3. New York: Wiley.
Giddens, A. (1993) *Sociology*, 2nd edn. Oxford: Blackwell.
Glasper, A. and **Richardson, J.** (2006) *A Textbook of Children's and Young People's Nursing.* Edinburgh: Churchill Livingstone.
Gottman, J. M. (1986) The world of co-ordinated play: same and cross-sex friendship in young children. In Gottman, J. M. and Parker, J. G. (eds), *Conversations of Friends: Speculations on Affective Development.* Cambridge: Cambridge University Press.
Grantham-McGregor, S., *et al.* (1994) The long-term follow up of severely malnourished children who participated in an intervention program. *Child Development*, **65**, 428–439.
Gunter, B. (1986) *Television and Sex-role Stereotyping.* London: John Libbey.
Harkness, S. and **Super, C. M.** (1985) The cultural context of gender segregation in children's peer groups. *Child Development*, **56**, 219–224.
Harris, M. and **Butterworth, G.** (2002) *Developmental Psychology.* Hove: Psychology Press.
Harter, S. (1999) *The Construction of Self: A Developmental Perspective.* New York: Guilford.
Hartup, W. W. (1989) Social relationships and their developmental significance. *American Psychologist*, **44**, 120–126.
Hartup, W. W. (1992) Peer relations in early and middle childhood. In Hasselt, V. and Hersen, M. (eds), *Handbook of Social Development: A Lifespan Perspective.* New York: Plenum Press.
Heward, C. (1993) Reconstructing popular childhoods. *Children and Society*, **7** (3), 237–254.
Hinde, R. A., *et al.* (1985) Incidence of friendship and behaviour toward strong associates versus nonassociates in preschoolers. *Child Development*, **56**, 234–245.
Hobsbaum, A. (1995) Children's development. In Carter, B. and Dearman, A. K. (eds), *Child Health Care Nursing.* Oxford: Blackwell Science.
Hoffman, M. L. (1988) Moral development. In Bornstein, M. H. and Lamb, M. E. (eds), *Developmental Psychology: An Advanced Textbook*, 2nd edn. Englewood Cliffs, NJ: Erlbaum.
Hollich, G. J., **Hirsh-Pasek, K.** and **Golinkoff, R. M.** (2000) *Breaking the Language Barrier: An Emergentist Coalition Model for the Origins of Word Learning.* Malden, MA: Blackwell.
Howes, C. (1987) Social competence with peers in young children: developmental sequences. *Developmental Review*, **7**, 252–272.
Hutt, C. (1971) Exploration and play in children. In Herron, R. E. and Sutton-Smith, B. (eds), *Child's Play.* London: Wiley.
Isaacs, S. (1929) *The Nursery Years.* London: Routledge & Kegan Paul.

Kabbani, H. and **Raghuveer, T. S.** (2004) Craniosynostosis. *American Family Physician,* **69** (12), 2863–2870.
Kasmauski, K. and **Jaret, P.** (2003) *Impact: On the Frontlines of Global Health.* Washington DC: National Geographic.
Key, E. (1909) *The Century of the Child.* New York: G. P. Putnam. http://www.socsci.kun.nl/ped/whp/histeduc/ellenkey.
Klein, J. D., *et al.* (1993) Adolescents' risky behaviour and mass media use. *Pediatrics,* **92** (1), 24.
Kohlberg, L. (1978) Revisions in the theory and practice of moral development. *New Directions for Child Development,* **2**, 83–88.
Kosky, J. and **Lunnon, R. J.** (1991) *Great Ormond Street and the Story of Medicine.* London: The Hospitals for Sick Children.
Kovas, Y., *et al.* (2005) Genetic influences in different aspects of language development: the etiology of language skills in 4.5-year-old twins. *Child Development,* **76** (3), 632–651.
Lacey, C. (1970) *Hightown Grammar.* Manchester: Manchester University Press.
Lampl, M. (1992) Saltation and stasis: a model of human growth. *Science,* **258**, 801.
Leslie, A. A. (1988) Some implications of pretence for mechanisms underlying the child's theory of mind. In Astington, J. W., Harris, P. L. and Olson, D. R. (eds), *Developing Theories of Mind.* Cambridge: Cambridge University Press.
Lester, J. (1993) Changing attitudes to children. *Health Visitor,* **66** (5), 162–163.
Lewis, M. (1991) Ways of knowing: objective self-awareness of consciousness. *Developmental Review,* **11**, 231–243.
Lewis, M. and **Brooks-Gunn, J.** (1979) *Social Cognition and the Acquisition of Self.* New York: Plenum Press.
Lindsay, B. (1994) Influencing development: the media. In Lindsay, B. (ed.), *The Child and Family: Contemporary Nursing Issues in Child Health and Care.* London: Bailliere Tindall.
Main, M. and **Solomon, J.** (1986) Discovery of an insecure-disorganised/disorientated attachment pattern. In Brazelton, T. and Yogman, M. (eds), *Affective Development in Infancy.* Norwood: Ablex.
Mitchell, P. (1992) *The Psychology of Childhood.* London: Falmer Press.
Moore, K. L. and **Persaud, T. V. N.** (2003) *Before We Were Born,* 6th edn. Philadelphia: Saunders.
Moore, S. (1996) *Sociology Alive!,* 2nd edn. Cheltenham: Stanley Thornes.
Moyles, J. (ed.) (2005) *The Excellence of Play,* 2nd edn. Maidenhead: Oxford University Press.
Nardinelli, C. (1990) *Child Labour and the Industrial Revolution.* Bloomington: Indiana University Press.
Nathanielsz, P. (1996) *Life before Birth: the Challenges of Foetal Development.* New York: W. H. Freeman.
Nelson, C. A. (1987) The recognition of facial expressions in the first two years of life: mechanisms of development. *Child Development,* **58**, 889–909.
Oates, J. (ed.) (1994) *The Foundations of Child Development.* Milton Keynes: Open University Press.
O'Brien, M. (1992) Gender identity and sex roles. In Hasselt, V. B. V. and Hersen, M. (eds), *Handbook of Social Development: A Lifespan Perspective.* New York: Plenum Press.
O'Brien, M. and **Houston, A. C.** (1985) Development of sex-typed play behaviour in toddlers. *Developmental Psychology,* **21**, 866–871.
Oshima-Takane, Y., Goodz, E. and **Derevensky, J. L.** (1996) Birth order effects on early language development: do second born children learn from overheard speech? *Child Development,* **67** (2), 621–634.
Pascalis, O., *et al.* (1995) Mother's face recognition by neonates: a replication and an extension. *Infant Behavioural Development,* **18**, 79–85.
Pelligrini, D. and **Smith, P. K.** (1998) The development of play during childhood: forms and possible functions. *Child Psychology and Psychiatry Review,* **3** (2), 51–57.
Rochat, P. (2003) Five levels of self-awareness as they unfold early in life. *Consciousness and Cognition,* **12**, 717–731.
Rochat, P. (2004) Origins of self-concept. In Bremner, G. and Fogel, A. (eds), *Blackwell Handbook of Infant Development.* Oxford: Blackwell.
Rothbart, M. K. and **Bates, J. E.** (1998) Temperament. In Eisenberg, N. (ed.), *Handbook of Child Psychology,* Vol. 3. *Social, Emotional and Personality Development,* 5th edn. New York: Wiley.
Rubin, K. H. and **Fein, G. G.** (1983) Play. In Hetherington, E. M. and Mussen, P. H. (eds), *Handbook of Child Psychology.* New York: Wiley.
Rutherford, D. (1998) Children's relationships. In Taylor, J. and Woods, M. (eds), *Early Childhood Studies.* London: Arnold.
Rutter, M. (1981) *Maternal Deprivation Reassessed,* 2nd edn. Harmondsworth: Penguin.
Schaffer, H. R. (2004) *Introducing Child Psychology.* Malden: Blackwell.
Selman, R. L. (1980) *The Growth of Interpersonal Understanding.* New York: Academic Press.
Singer, J. L. (1973) *The Child's World of Make-believe.* New York: Academic Press.
Skinner, B. F. (1957) *Verbal Behaviour.* New York: Appleton-Century-Crofts.
Slater, A., Mattock. A. and **Brown, E.** (1990) Size constancy at birth: new-born infants' responses to retinal and real size. *Journal of Experimental Child Psychology,* **51**, 395–406.
Slobin, D. (1973) Cognitive prerequisites for the development of grammar. In Ferguson, C. A. and Slobin, D. (eds), *Studies in Child Development.* New York: Holt, Reinhart & Winston.
Smilansky, S. and **Sheftaya, L.** (1990) *Facilitating Play: A Medium for Promoting Cognitive, Socio-emotional and Academic Development in Young Children.* Gathersburg, MD: Psychological and Educational Publications.
Smith, P. K. and **Cowie, H.** (1991) *Understanding Children's Development,* 2nd edn. Oxford: Basil Blackwell.
Smith, P. K., Cowie, H. and **Blades, M.** (2003) *Understanding Children's Development,* 4th edn. Oxford: Blackwell.

Snarey, J. R. (1985) Cross-cultural universality of social-moral development: a critical review of Kholbergian research. *Psychological Bulletin,* **97**, 202–232.
Stromswold, K. (2001) The heritability of language: a review and metaanalysis of twin, adoption, and linkage studies. *Language,* **77**, 647–723.
Subrahmanyam, K., *et al.* (2001) New forms of electronic media: the impact of interactive games and the Internet on cognition, socialization and behaviour. In Singer, D. L. and Singer, J. L. (eds), *Handbook of Children and the Media.* Thousand Oaks: Sage Publications.
Sylva, K., Bruner, J. S. and **Genova, P.** (1976) The role of play in the problem-solving of children 3–5 years old. In Bruner, J. S., Jolly, A. and Sylva, K. (eds), *Play: Its Role in Development and Evolution.* Harmondsworth: Penguin.
Sylva, K., Roy, C. and **Painter, M.** (1980) *Childwatching at Playgroup and Nursery Schools.* London: Grant McIntyre.
Tamburrini, J. (1981) What is play? In Roberts, M. and Tamburrini, J. (eds), *Child Development 0–5.* Edinburgh: Holmes McDougall.
Tamir, L. (1984) Language development: new directions. In Lock, A. and Fisher, E. (eds), *Language Development.* London: Routledge.
Timperley, H. *et al.* (2003) Transitioning children from early childhood education to school: teacher beliefs and transition practices. *Australian Journal of Early Childhood,* **28** (2), 32–39.
Tizard, B. (1977) Play – the child's way of learning. In Tizard, B. and Harvey, D. (eds), *The Biology of Play.* London: Heinemann.
Turiel, E. (1983) *The Development of Social Knowledge: Morality and Convention.* Cambridge: Cambridge University Press.
Van Ijzendoorn, M. H., *et al.* (1992) The relative effects of maternal and child problems on the quality of attachment: a meta analysis of attachment in clinical samples. *Child Development,* **63**, 840–858.
Walton, G. E., Bower, N. J. A. and **Bower, T. G. R.** (1992) Recognition of familiar faces by newborns. *Infant Behaviour and Development,* **15**, 265–269.
Watson, J. (1979) *Medical, Surgical Nursing and Related Physiology.* Eastbourne: Saunders.
Watt, S. and **Mitchell, R.** (1995) Historical perspectives. In Carter, B. and Dearmun, A. K. (eds), *Child Health Care Nursing.* Oxford: Blackwell Science.
Woodward, E. H. (1998) *By All Means, Consume! A Multi-method Investigation of the Relationship between Television, Consumerism, and Criminal Behavior.* Philadelphia: University of Pennsylvania – Electronic Dissertations.
Younger, M. and **Warrington, M.** (2005) *Raising Boys' Achievement.* London: Department for Education and Skills.

Module 3

Promoting Child Health

Tina Moules

Learning Outcomes

The material in this module and the further reading/references should enable you to:

- explore the state of health of children in the UK today and investigate changing patterns of illness and disease
- examine the factors and trends that affect children's health
- explore children's beliefs about and concepts of health
- analyse and critically review various models of health promotion/education and consider how theoretical underpinnings can be applied to practice
- investigate the changing role of the nurse in promoting health in children
- consider the strategies and interventions implemented for a range of child health issues
- act as an advocate for children's health and contribute to promoting healthy behaviours among children

Introduction

There has been an upsurge in interest regarding the health of our children in Britain today. It is now well recognised that children's health is important because they are tomorrow's adults. What they take with them from childhood in the way of health or ill health may influence their health for the rest of their lives. Children are the future and, as such, need to be able to reach their full potential to meet the demands that adulthood brings. In recent years a number of key documents and strategies have been produced to ensure that every child has the opportunity to good health and increased life chances. In 2003, the Green Paper *Every Child Matters* (DfES, 2003) set five objectives to help children achieve their full potential:

- being healthy
- staying safe
- enjoying and achieving
- making a positive contribution
- achieving economic well-being

Every Child Matters provided a shift in focus to prevention, early identification and intervention in child protection and children's services, and placed a stronger emphasis on the integration of agencies and professionals around children's services. It set out a number of commitments that were taken forward into the Children Act 2004. The Children Act 2004 builds upon the Children Act 1989 by setting out a new duty for agencies to work together to provide better coordinated and effective support for children. In the National Health Service (NHS) one of the mechanisms for improving the health of children is the *National Service Framework (NSF) for Children, Young People and Maternity Services* (DH, 2004b). This is a 10-year programme developed to deliver sustained improvement in children's health and well-being. The NSF is an integral part of *Every Child Matters: Change for Children* (DfES, 2004), which can only be delivered by a number of organisations working together. The NHS will contribute directly to 'being healthy' and 'staying safe' and indirectly to others. A child who is suffering from ill health or malnutrition will be less likely to 'enjoy and achieve' and may have difficulty 'making a positive contribution'.

The Children Act 2004 and *Every Child Matters* are key to underpinning the reform of children's services but they are only part of a wide programme of change that will require sustained partnerships both locally and nationally. Recognising that patterns of behaviour are often set early in life, the government has strengthened the emphasis on preventative health, through the White Paper *Choosing Health: Making Healthier Choices Easier* (DH, 2004a). The first ever White Paper in public health sets out a number of actions for health services, public and voluntary sectors to promote healthier choices early in life and provide a supportive environment for children, young people and their families or carers.

Nurses will play a central role in an integrated children's service across all sectors, but there is a particular emphasis on the role of health visitors and school nurses who will lead and oversee many new developments. Health visitors and school nurses will work in children's centres, Sure Start programmes, general practice and through links with local voluntary and statutory providers to deliver measurable outcomes to improve the life chances of vulnerable children. The role of the nurse is therefore changing to incorporate an increased concern with health promotion. In order to fulfil this role, nurses must have an understanding of theories and models of health promotion so that they can become effective health promoters.

This module concentrates on issues related to health and its promotion. It begins by examining the health of children in the UK today and discussing the changing patterns of childhood illness. Some of the factors that affect child health are reviewed, with special reference to poverty and its effects on health. Children's beliefs about health and its meaning are explored, and you are encouraged to ascertain children's views regarding their own health behaviours. Different age groups have different views of health and this needs to be recognised when promoting health. An outline of some of the views regarding health promotion and education are given. Several models are put forward for you to consider, helping you to analyse critically health promotion in practice. Issues of child health that were particularly relevant at the time of writing are explored and will give you an insight into how health promotion is put into practice. The role of the nurse in health promotion is discussed, examining the roles of children's nurses and also other nurses who have contact with children. Finally, several aspects of health are considered with the purpose of enabling you to contribute effectively to encouraging children (and carers) to make healthy choices.

Chapter 10

Trends in Child Health

Introduction

The health of children in the UK has improved markedly since the mid-1960s. In the middle of the 19th century many children suffered severe ill health and lived in appalling conditions. One-third of children died before the end of childhood. Childhood was a fragile time and engendered a kind of indifference. Now childhood death and serious infection are becoming rare and, in general, living conditions have improved. Advances in medical technology have improved the life chances of premature infants and children with serious illness. However, detailed analysis of data reveals that although infant mortality rates have decreased, morbidity has increased. Child poverty continues to affect health.

The proportion of children living in low-income households more than doubled between the late 1970s and mid-1990s (HM Treasury, 2004). In 2003, 3.5 million children (28% of all children) were living in poverty. This was an increase from 13% in 1979 (Flaherty *et al.*, 2004). Many children living in poverty have limited opportunities to play safely, often live in overcrowded and inadequate housing, eat less nutritious food, suffer more accidents and ill health and achieve less at school (HM Treasury, 2004). Reading (1997) ascertains that virtually all aspects of health are worse 'among children living in poverty than among children from affluent families'.

This section looks critically at the trends in child health and considers the epidemiology of childhood illness and disease.

Mortality Rates

mortality rate
The number of deaths as a proportion of the population of a given age.

morbidity
All forms of ill health including acute and chronic conditions.

Trends in mortality rates (particularly infant mortality rates) have long been considered to be among the best indicators of children's health. It is suggested that mortality reflects the cumulative interaction of biological and social factors over time. As mortality data have been well documented for many years, trends can be traced and analysed. However, one must recognise that these data are only the tip of the iceberg

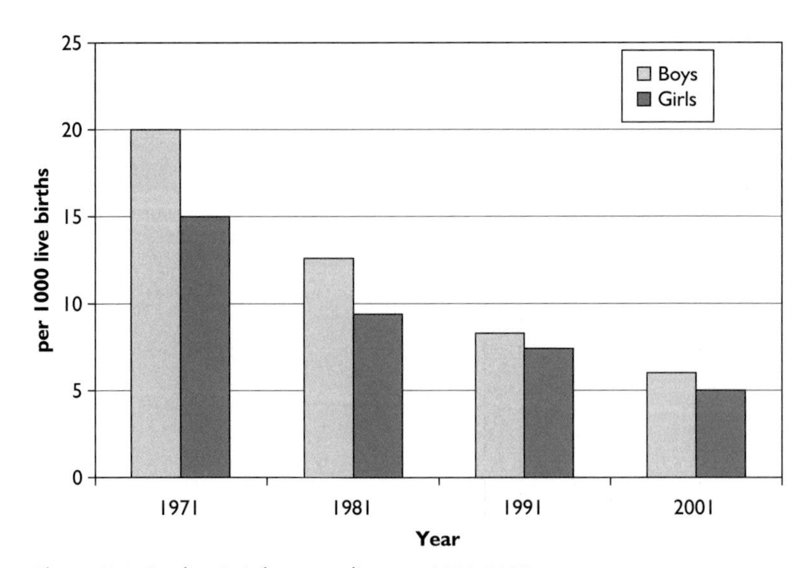

Figure 10.1 Decline in infant mortality rates 1971–2001.

and other factors contribute to the judgements made about child health, including data on morbidity.

Infant mortality rates (deaths under 1 year per 1000 live births)

In England and Wales there has been a steady decline in infant mortality rate (IMR) since the 1940s. In the period 1941–5, the rate was 50 per 1000 live births. By 2001 it had fallen to 5.6 per 1000 live births, the rate being slightly higher for males (6) than females (5) (Figure 10.1).

Although a general decline in the IMR is evident, there are still variations among social groups and regions of the country. Regional variations partly reflect the ethnic and social class make-up of populations. Health districts with higher than average IMRs tend to have above-average proportions of mothers born in Pakistan and the New Commonwealth and an above-average population of fathers in social classes IV and V (Britton, 1989). In 2002, babies of mothers born in Pakistan had the highest infant mortality rate, of 11.4 per 1000 live births, more than twice the overall infant mortality rate (5.3) (Health Statistics Quarterly, 2003). The IMR is lowest (4.4) in the Eastern region and highest (6.9) in the Northern and Yorkshire region and the West Midlands (Figure 10.2). Social class variations in the IMR have existed for many years and data show that inequalities persist.

The infant mortality rate is highest in mothers under 20 years of age (8 per 1000 live births) and mothers over 40 years (7.1 per 1000 live births) (Health Statistics Quarterly, 2003).

stillbirths
Fetal deaths after 24 weeks' gestation.

Study activity

Look critically at the possible factors that lead to regional differences in the infant mortality rate. Try to trace the data to see how the differences compare with previous years.

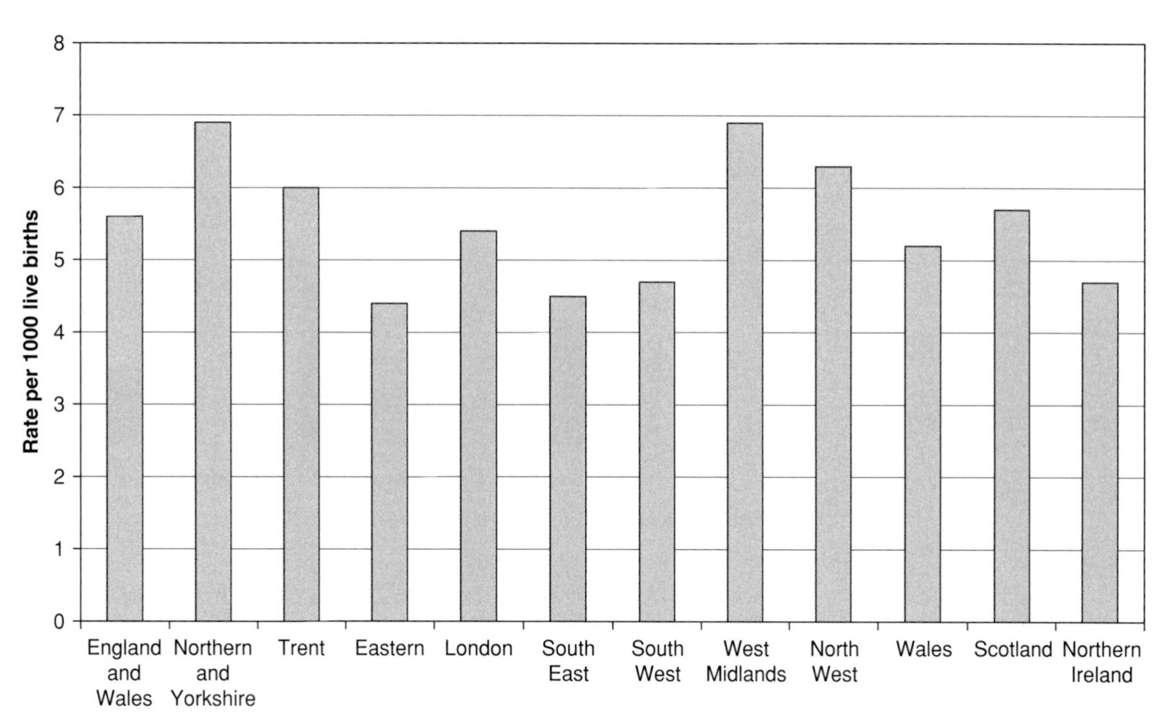

Figure 10.2 Infant mortality rate per region, 2000.

There are large variations in infant mortality rates in the UK by social class. For babies born inside marriage in 2002, with a father in a semi-skilled occupation, the infant mortality rate was two and a half times higher than those whose fathers were in the professional social class (rates of 7.5 and 2.7 per thousand, respectively). For babies born outside of marriage, the mortality rate was 6.9 deaths per thousand live births compared with 5.2 for those born inside marriage. However, there has been a large increase in the proportions of babies born outside marriage across all social classes, reflecting the increase in cohabitation. Although infant mortality rates in each class have decreased over the past decade, there is no evidence that the class differential has decreased over this period (Matheson and Babb, 2002).

Infant mortality is subdivided into:

- perinatal deaths: stillbirths and deaths in the first week of life
- neonatal deaths: deaths within the first 27 days of life
- post-neonatal deaths: deaths at 28 days and over (but under 1 year)

Study activity

Before reading on, take a few minutes to consider what might be the major causes of death in the neonatal period and why there has been a large decline in mortality rate.

Infancy remains the most vulnerable period of a child's life, with the vast majority of deaths in childhood occurring in the first 12 months.

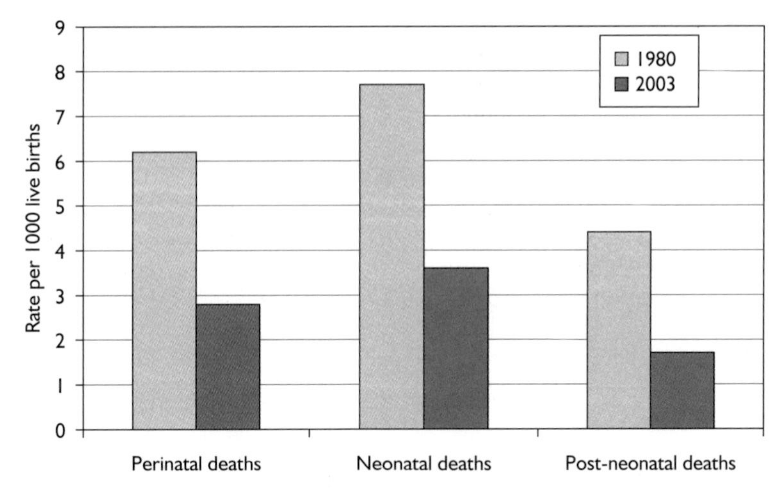

Figure 10.3 Decline in infant mortality rates 1980–2003.

Two in every three infant deaths in 2002 occurred in the first 28 days. The main causes of these deaths were conditions related to premature birth, such as very low birth weight or respiratory difficulties (57%) and congenital anomalies (26%) (Fitzpatrick and Cooper, 2001). However, deaths in the first year of life continue to fall (Figure 10.3).

Although infant mortality rates have dropped significantly since the 1980s, the rate of stillbirths is rising. In 2002 the rate of stillbirths increased from 5.3 per 1000 live births to 5.6, the first rise since the change in definition of stillbirths in 1992. An exploration of the data showed that there was little relationship between birth weight, age of mother, gestation, sex, mother's country of birth and cause of stillbirth. However, the report concluded that factors associated with the increase were: being a single mother (but no increase at all among births outside of marriage registered by both parents), singleton births (there were nine times more singleton stillbirths than multiples) and higher rates of stillbirth in the summer of 2002 (there is usually a drop in the rates of stillbirth in summer months) (Health Statistics Quarterly, 2003). It remains to be seen whether this trend will continue.

Several factors have contributed to the fall in neonatal deaths. Recent advances in the care and management of low birthweight babies has led to an increased survival rate. However, the number of babies born with a congenital defect has risen since the mid-1990s despite improved antenatal screening and the provision of terminations. The highest notification rates for total congenital anomalies were seen among mothers aged 40 years and over, the number of congenital anomalies increased in this age group from 145 per 10 000 births in 1991 to 152 per 10 000 in 2001. The second highest notification rates were among mothers under 20 years (113 per 10 000 births in 1991 compared with 125 per 10 000 births in 2001) (ONS, 2004a). The trend for delayed childbirth, with many mothers delaying starting a family until well into their forties (Harper, 2003), and the high level of teenage pregnancies may be the underlying cause for this rise.

One of the major reasons for the improvement of death rates in this age group is the fall in sudden infant death syndrome (SIDS). A considerable decrease in the number of deaths from SIDS has been evident since a peak in 1988 when the rate was 2.3 per 1000 live births. By 1999 the rate had fallen to 0.39 (ONS, 2002a). The decline has been rapid and has been attributed in part to campaigns to make parents aware of the dangers of the prone position for sleeping babies (*see also* SIDS p. 42 and 576).

For post-neonatal deaths, 34% were related to congenital anomalies and 14% were from SIDS. Rates for all infant deaths show marked class gradients, with rates for neonatal deaths as much as nine times higher for the lowest social class compared to professional social classes (ONS, 2002a).

Childhood mortality (based on the estimated population in the relevant age group)

Childhood mortality figures are generally given within the following age ranges:

- 1–4 years
- 5–9 years
- 10–14 years
- 15–19 years

The death rates for children aged 1–14 are based on small numbers so should be examined with care.

The risk of death in childhood is significantly less than the risk in infancy. In general the rate of decline in childhood mortality has levelled off since the early 1980s. During the period from 1998 to 2000 cancers were the most common cause of death among girls aged 5 to 15, accounting for 23% of deaths in this age group. Accidents were the most common form of death in boys of the same age, accounting for 27% of deaths (ONS, 2002b).

Mortality is twice as high among preschool children and teenagers as among school-age children. Among older children a gender differential is seen, with the death rate in boys (2 in every 10 000 of the population) being double that in girls (1 in every 10 000 of the population) (ONS, 2002b).

Study activity

Take some time to consider the factors that may have contributed to changes in childhood mortality since 1963.

The number of deaths due to accidents has been steadily declining. In 1997, 2.5 million children under 15 years were taken to hospital following an accident, in 2002 the number was 2.01 million. However, in the UK in 2004, 275 children under the age of 15 died as a result of an accident, this is many more than died from cancer or meningitis (CAPT, 2006). Accidental injury is one of the biggest causes of death in children over the age of one in the UK. Accidents are also a major cause of disability and ill health. Many accidents are preventable, meaning that much work is still to be done to make childhood a safer time (*see also* Factors influencing accidents in childhood p. 158).

Class differences are particularly evident in relation to accidents. According to Jarvis *et al.* (1995) accidental injury is the cause of death with the steepest social gradient. Reasons for this are multifactorial but are likely to include lack of safe areas to play and lack of resources to make homes safe. Despite recent initiatives to reduce inequalities, children in lower social classes are one and a half times more likely to die as a result of accidents than children from a higher social class (CAPT, 2006). The sex of a child also seems to be a factor as boys are twice as likely as girls to be involved in accidents (CAPT, 2006).

Morbidity

morbidity
The relative incidence of disease and illness.

Morbidity is the second major indicator used for measuring health. It looks at the prevalence or incidence of disease. Information regarding child morbidity is gained from population surveys (particularly the General Household Survey, GHS), notifications of infectious diseases, registers of children with specific conditions (such as cancer) and hospital admission data.

Study activity

Each of the methods of gaining data on morbidity has strengths and weaknesses. Critically review each of the methods and analyse the role of each in its contribution to knowledge regarding the incidence and prevalence of disease in childhood.

Many of the data presented here are from the GHS, conducted by OPCS. This survey was introduced in the 1970s. It surveys 10 000 private households sampled from the electoral register. Participants in the survey are asked to report any long-standing illness, disability and visits to the GP. Information gathered from the GHS and other sources, including the census, is now collated and stored by the Office for National Statistics (ONS). The information is available online as raw data or is analysed in the form of reports.

According to the GHS (ONS, 2001b) there was a threefold increase in chronic illness in children between 1972 and 2001. Alongside this there has been a rising trend in disability reported in all age groups.

Factors that have influenced childhood morbidity include:

- Improved management and treatment of children with childhood cancers. The survival rates for lymphoblastic leukaemia have improved dramatically since the 1970s. However, at the same time concerns have been raised about possible long-term side-effects of treatment.
- Improved management and treatment of low birthweight infants. Unfortunately this improvement has brought with it increased risks of blindness, deafness and cerebral palsy. For children born in 1984–8, the rate of deafness in survivors to 28 days was 15 times higher in babies who weighed less than 1500 g at birth than it was for all babies (Woodroffe *et al.*, 1993). The incidence of cerebral palsy in

very low birthweight babies (under 1500 g) has increased markedly (Woodroffe *et al.*, 1993).

- Improved survival rates for children with cystic fibrosis. This has contributed to an increase in chronic illness. The median life expectancy for a child born with cystic fibrosis in 2006 is estimated at 30–40 years (Cystic Fibrosis Trust, 2006).
- Improvements in the diagnosis and treatment of respiratory diseases. Respiratory diseases are a major cause of long-term illness and disability in childhood. According to the ONS, in 2000 asthma was the most common condition reported among under-20-year-olds with a longstanding illness or disability, with 42% of total impairments (ONS, 2004a). Asthma, eczema and hay fever are among the most common chronic diseases of childhood. In 1996, 21% of children aged 2–15 years had been diagnosed with asthma in England, 24% with eczema and 9% with hay fever. However, there does seem to be a substantial change in the effect of asthma on children's health and well-being. In England and Wales, hospital admission rates for childhood asthma increased substantially during the 1960s, 1970s and early 1980s, but declined steadily during the 1990s. Between 1990 and 2000, hospital admission rates had decreased by 52% among children under 5 years and by 45% among children aged 5–14 years. The weekly incidence of acute asthma attacks diagnosed by a general practitioner (GP) increased markedly during the 1970s and 1980s, peaked in the early 1990s, and by 2000 declined quite substantially for both age groups (ONS, 2004a). This could be due to better diagnosis, a greater understanding of the disease, improved treatments and greater compliance with drug treatments. (*See also* Treatment of leukaemias p. 578, Cerebral palsy p. 515, Cystic fibrosis p. 513 and Respiratory problems p. 514).

As with mortality, social class differences still exist, although they are not as significant (ONS, 2004a). One of the difficulties in interpreting the data is that parental self-reporting (the major method of data collection in the GHS) can lead to underreporting of children's illness by mothers in the lower social classes (Bornam and Prior, 1999).

Other Indicators of Child Health

Dental health

There has been considerable improvement in the dental health of children since the 1970s, largely due to the fluoridation of toothpaste and drinking water. However, dental caries remains a major health problem. It is preventable and there is no reason why it should not be eradicated in childhood. In the 10 years from 1973 to 1983 improvements were seen in all ages from 5 to 15 and in all regions of England and Wales. The proportion of 5-year-olds with dental caries fell from 73% to 48%. The most recent survey published (ONS, 2004a) shows a continued improvement, with dramatic falls in the prevalence of dental caries. The improvement was particularly strong among 15-year-olds, with the proportion having decay into dentine falling from 42% in 1983 to 30% in 1993 and to 13% in 2003. The proportion of 5- and

The work of George Davey Smith has great implications for child health. To learn more look at:

Davey Smith, G., Hart, C., Blane, D. and Hole, D. (1998) Adverse socioeconomic conditions in childhood and cause specific adult mortality: prospective observational study. *British Medical Journal*, **1316**, 1631–1635.

Davey Smith, G., Hart, C., Upton, M., Hole, D., Gillis, C., Watt, G. and Hawthorne, V. (2000) Height and risk of death among men and women: aetiological implications of associations with cardiorespiratory disease and cancer mortality. *Journal of Epidemiology and Community Health*, **54**, 97–103.

8-year-olds with filled primary teeth has fallen since 1993, with 12% of 5-year-olds and 26% of 8-year-olds having filled primary (or 'milk') teeth. The survey found marked social variations in tooth decay, depending upon whether the school was considered to be deprived or not. Fifty-six per cent of 5-year-olds and 64% of 8-year-old children from deprived schools had dental caries, compared to 37% and 48% in non-deprived schools (*see also* Dental hygiene p. 181).

Growth

Height is taken as a sign of the state of health of a population. Over recent centuries the average height of people in the UK has increased and the trend continues. In general, children's heights are increasing but a class differential has been identified. Work by Professor George Davey Smith has shown that small stature in adults is strongly related to coronary heart disease, stroke, respiratory disease and some cancers. He suggests that a short height in adults is related to socio-economic circumstances and nutritional status during childhood (Davey Smith *et al.*, 2000). This means that a disadvantaged childhood can affect health throughout the lifespan. Davey Smith's work has influenced the child health agenda and underpins much of the focus on child inequalities, such as Sure Start (*see also* Weighing children and babies p. 285).

Mental health

In 2004, around 10% of children in the UK had a clinically recognised mental disorder (ONS, 2004b). Mental health disorder in children varies by some family characteristics. Mental disorders are greater among children in lone-parent families (16%) than among those in two-parent families (8%), and in families with neither parent working (20%) compared with those in which both parents work (8%). Autistic spectrum disorder presents in 1% of children. The majority of these children are boys (82%). However, unlike children with the more common disorders, autistic children tend to have more highly qualified parents than other children: 46% have parents with qualifications above GCSE, compared with 35% of other children. Similarly, autistic children are less likely to live in low-income families: only 9% live in households with a gross weekly income of less than £200 per week compared with 20% of other children (ONS, 2004b). In the UK in 1999 there was a marked variance in the prevalence of mental disorders among children, related to household income (DH, 2004a) (Figure 10.4).

Nutrition and diet

The nutritional status of children is a key indicator of health status. There is mounting evidence to justify a growing concern about children's diets in recent years.

Breastfeeding gives an infant a healthy start in life, protecting against infection and allergy. It also provides the correct amount and balance of nutrients for healthy growth and development. In the early 1970s the incidence of breastfeeding was at its lowest level but it has increased consistently since the mid-1990s. In 2000, 71% of babies were breastfed (DH, 2002). However, there are marked variations in breastfeeding.

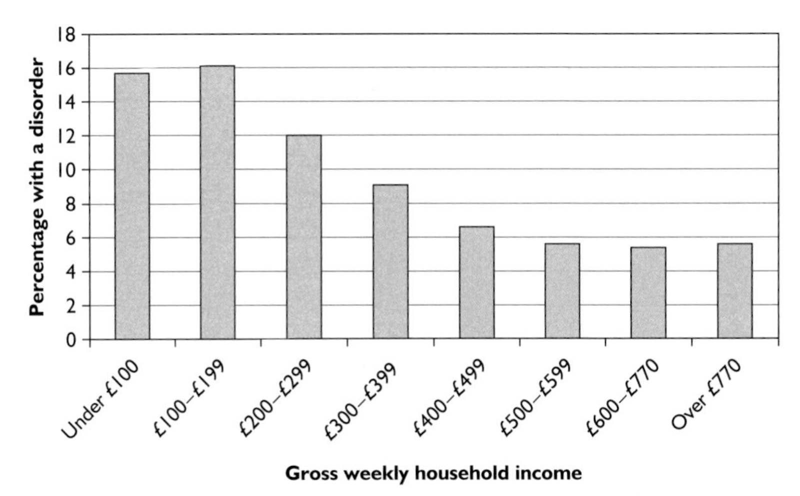

Figure 10.4 Prevalence of mental disorders among children, UK 1999 (adapted from DH, 2004a).

There is a steep social class gradient in breastfeeding initiation in the UK, rising from 57% of mothers in social class V to 91% in social class I. The incidence of breastfeeding varies with age, in the UK 46% of teenage mothers breastfeed compared to 78% of mothers aged 30 years and over. Mothers who left full-time education at 16 or below are less likely to breastfeed (54%) than mothers who were educated to at least 19 (88%) (DH, 2002) (*see also* Nutrition p. 56 and Breastfeeding p. 175).

Breastfeeding and cognitive development

Studies have investigated the role of breast milk in neurological development and suggest that there may be a small advantageous effect of breastfeeding:

Lucas, A. *et al.* (1992) Breastmilk and subsequent intelligent quotient in children born preterm. *Lancet*, **339**, 261–264.

Lanting, C. I. *et al.* (1994) Neurological differences between 9-year-old children fed breastmilk and formula as babies. *Lancet*, **344**, 1319–1322.

Study activity

Which factors may contribute to the social class differences with regard to breastfeeding? How might some of these be overcome?

Obesity

Obesity in childhood is likely to lead to obesity in adulthood. Many diseases are linked to obesity, for example heart disease and stroke. There is growing concern regarding the proportion of young people who are too heavy for their height and the nutritional quality of food that children in the UK consume regularly. Between 1995 and 2000 the proportion of overweight boys in England aged 2–19 years increased by 2% and the proportion of overweight girls in the same age range increased by 3% (Table 10.1). In the same time period, the proportion of obese boys and girls increased by 1%. In 2000, 27% of girls aged 2–19 years were overweight, compared with 20% of boys. In the same year, 7% of girls were obese compared with 5% of boys (ONS, 2004a).

body mass index (BMI)

This summarises the relationship between height and weight:

Obesity = BMI of over 30.

Overweight = BMI of 25–30.

The first major study to highlight the nature of children's diets was commissioned by the Department of Health in 1983. Interestingly, the full report was not published until 1989. This study found that the main sources of dietary energy for British schoolchildren were bread, chips, biscuits, milk, meat, cakes and puddings. Three-quarters of the

Table 10.1 Proportion of overweight and obese children and adolescents aged 2–19 years, by sex, 1995–2000 (source: ONS, 2004a)

England	% Overweight	% Obese
Boys		
1995	18.6	3.7
1996	19.3	4.1
1997	17.7	4.0
1998	21.1	4.2
1999	23.0	5.9
2000	20.3	4.8
Girls		
1995	23.5	5.7
1996	22.7	5.9
1997	22.9	5.8
1998	25.5	7.0
1999	25.2	7.1
2000	26.6	6.8

children in the study had fat intakes above the recommended level. However, the Department of Health deduced that the diets of children were satisfactory.

A study in 1997 looked at a typical week's diet for children aged 4–18 years. It found that the most popular foods, eaten in the highest proportions by four out of five 4- to 18-year-olds, were chips, other potatoes, savoury snacks, white bread, biscuits and chocolate. Three out of five children in this age group had not eaten any leafy green vegetables, although half had eaten cooked carrots; only one in four had eaten citrus fruits and, although the majority had drunk carbonated drinks, less than half had drunk fruit juice. Girls were more likely than boys to have eaten raw or salad vegetables and less likely to have eaten breakfast cereals or sausages (http://www.statistics.gov.uk/cci/nugget.asp?id=718, accessed 22 May 2006).

Child Poverty Action Group
94 White Lion Street, London N1 9PF
Tel: 020 7837 7979; fax: 020 7837 6414; www.cpag.org.uk

Study activity

Arrange to talk to a group of children about their eating habits. Compare different age groups. What are your findings and how do they compare with the above research?

Immunisations

Immunisation is one of the best-documented ways of protecting children's health. Deaths from infectious diseases have reduced markedly since the early part of the century due, in part, to public health reforms in the 19th and early 20th centuries. However, the role of immunisations in the eradication of many diseases and the reduction in incidence of others must not be negated (*see also* Immunisation schedule p. 512 and Immunisation p. 182).

The *diphtheria, tetanus and polio* vaccine was introduced throughout the UK during the 1940s and has continued uninterrupted. The target of

95% coverage set by the World Health Organization (WHO) has been reached since the mid-1990s and has resulted in very few cases of the diseases being reported (ONS, 2004a). This has been a successful immunisation campaign.

Haemophilus influenzae type b was a leading cause of meningitis until a vaccine was introduced in 1992. Uptake has been good and coverage stands at 95% (ONS, 2004a).

Meningococcal meningitis group C has been endemic in the UK for many years. A vaccine was introduced across the UK in 1999. A catch-up dose of this vaccine was offered to all children from 1 to 17 years as part of the initial campaign. A high uptake (85%) has led to an 80% reduction in the incidence of the disease.

Tuberculosis (TB) has re-emerged in the 1990s, not just in the UK, but across many countries, notably Africa. This led WHO to declare TB as a global emergency in 1993 (WHO, 2002). The greatest increase of childhood TB the UK is found in children of black African origin, which quadrupled from 14.6 per 100 000 population in 1988 to 70.6 per 100 000 population in 1998 (ONS, 2004a). The incidence of TB in children of white and Indian subcontinent ethnicity has declined over the same period. Some parts of the country are affected more than others, with London having a particular problem.

A high uptake rate is essential for all children if infectious diseases are to remain a thing of the past. However, with the near elimination of these diseases can come complacency. Parents who have never experienced measles, diphtheria and pertussis may question the need for immunisation. There then comes the danger that uptake rates will fall and epidemics will flare up once more. Evidence of the dangers of complacency can be seen in the cases of pertussis and MMR (measles, mumps and rubella) vaccines, both of which have had controversies that have resulted in poor uptake. Many parents involved had not witnessed an outbreak of the disease; this left them susceptible to suggestions that immunisations were unnecessary or that the immunisation is more harmful than the disease itself.

A *pertussis (whooping cough)* vaccine was introduced across the UK in 1950. The rapid uptake of the vaccine led to a dramatic reduction in the number of reported cases of this virulent disease. However, in 1974 poor publicity and persistent negative media coverage led to a loss of confidence in the vaccine. Coverage dropped to 30% and was followed by a number of epidemics between 1979 and 1983; 200 000 cases of pertussis were reported and 50 deaths from the disease. Eventually public confidence was restored and coverage is now 94%.

Measles, mumps and rubella vaccine was introduced across the UK in October 1988. By 1991 coverage for 2-year-olds was 90% and reported cases of measles had fallen to less than 10 000. In 1994, to boost immunity and forestall a predicted epidemic, an MR (measles and rubella) campaign was conducted for school-age children. Since 1996 a second MMR vaccine has been offered to preschool children to ensure immunity in this age group. Measles became very rare, only 2378 cases were reported in 2001 (ONS, 2004a). Before the introduction of the MMR vaccination, mumps was the biggest cause of meningitis in the UK. The introduction of the vaccine saw a rapid decline in the number of cases. High coverage of the MMR led to a rapid reduction in the number of reported cases of rubella and in the number of pregnancies complicated by rubella (congenital rubella syndrome). In 1995, a paper reported in the *Lancet* by Professor Andrew Morton suggested that the MMR vaccine may be linked to Crohn's disease and autism (Thompson *et al.*, 1995). Despite a number of national and international studies that have rigorously investigated and strongly refuted this claim, the public has lost confidence in this vaccine. In 2001, the coverage for 2-year-olds dropped to 84%, not enough to create herd immunity or to prevent outbreaks. However, Macdonald *et al.* (2004) explored the reasons for low uptake of the MMR vaccine and found that parents declining the vaccine for their children did not do so lightly – in fact they invested a large amount of time researching the subject before making their decision. The study suggested that parents no longer trust the government to provide accurate information and guidance on immunisations but they do trust experts who appear to hold similar views to themselves. It will take a considerable amount of time and effort on behalf of health professionals to restore public confidence; nurses working with children and families will play a pivotal role.

A *pneumococcal vaccination* was introduced in the summer of 2006 (DH, 2006a). Pneumococcal infection is most common in babies, young children and the elderly. Each year there are around 5000 cases in England and Wales. Some 530 of these are in children under 2 years. Around one-third are cases of pneumococcal meningitis. The Department of Health estimates that around 50 children under the age of 2 die each year from invasive pneumococcal disease (DH, 2006a). Approximately two-thirds of deaths are from pneumococcal meningitis. Of the children who survive pneumococcal meningitis, 50% suffer permanent disabilities, including deafness, cerebral palsy or blindness. The immunisation will be routinely offered to children at 2, 4 and 13 months of age. A catch-up programme is planned to ensure that all children up to 2 years of age are offered the vaccine.

Health professionals may have to work harder to convince some parents that immunisations are necessary. Sustained efforts to achieve the national targets and to reduce inequalities in uptake are required.

Study activity

Find out what the uptake figures are for the area in which you work. Compare the figures with the national average. What are your conclusions?

Changing Patterns of Health and Disease

An examination of the data has revealed that the epidemiology of childhood diseases, although changing, remains the same in some respects. The incidence of infectious disease remains fairly low, whereas deaths from accidents remain high. Chronic illness is increasing as medical advances prolong the life of children with congenital disorders and of low birthweight infants. Between the 1970s and 2001 the proportion of children who were reported to have a limiting longstanding illness almost doubled, from 2 to 4% for 0- to 4-year-olds and 5–8% for 5- to

15-year-olds (ONS, 2001b). In 2001, 17% of boys aged 0–4 years and 20% aged 5–15 years had a longstanding illness, compared to 12 and 16% of girls, respectively.

Childhood cancer is one of the major causes of ill health, particularly in 5- to 15-year-olds. In fact cancer was the most common cause of death in girls of this age group (ONS, 2002a). In 2000, there were around 1400 new cases diagnosed in the United Kingdom. However, cancer accounted for around 20% of all deaths in children aged 1–14 years. Around one-third of all childhood cancers are leukaemias. About 80% of all leukaemias are acute lymphoblastic leukaemias (ALL). Childhood cancer is around one-fifth more common among boys than girls. Between 1996 and 2000, there was a peak in the incidence of ALL at ages 2–3 years. In the UK, the incidence of ALL is more prevalent in children from families of higher socio-economic status, particularly in early childhood (ONS, 2004a).

The most recent infectious disease, requiring sensitive handling, is HIV and AIDS. Between 1985 and the end of January 2001, 1101 children aged under 14 years were diagnosed with HIV in the UK. Of all the children diagnosed, 27% are known to have died. Two-thirds of all the children diagnosed acquired their infection from their mother at or around the time of birth, and most of the remainder acquired their infection through blood-factor treatment for haemophilia. In 2002, almost all new infections diagnosed in children were acquired from the mother and no new infections resulting from blood transfusion were identified. In 2001, 4974 new HIV cases were diagnosed. Just under 2% of these were among those aged 16–19 years and 89% of these acquired the infection through sexual transmission. In this age group, 61% of the infections were in females (ONS, 2004a). (*See also* Caring for children with HIV disease p. 507.)

Factors Affecting Child Health

Many factors affect children's health and development today. The purpose of this section is to identify and examine some of these factors and encourage you to explore the issues more fully. Before reading on, try the next activity.

> **Study activity**
>
> List as many factors as you can that you think have an impact on child health and development. Then try to put them into categories. Compare your thoughts with those in Figure 10.5.

Environmental

Concerns have been raised about the impact of many environmental issues in recent years. The threat to children from leaded paint has been known for many years, with cases of lead poisoning reported up until 1982. Various regulations now exist in the UK that limit the lead content of paint applied to surfaces that children might chew or suck. However, the main problem now is from old lead paint that might still

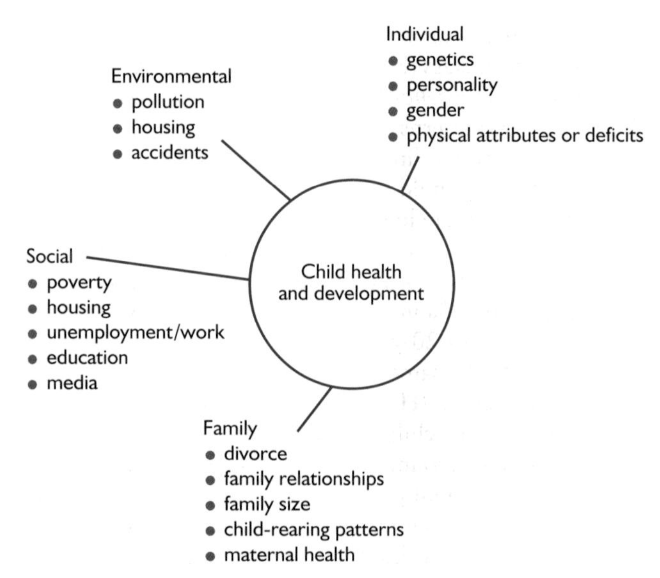

Figure 10.5 Overview of factors affecting health.

exist, for example, in old buildings. Other sources of lead include motor vehicle exhaust fumes. While the levels of lead in the air are decreasing due to the introduction of lead-free petrol, exhaust fumes still remain a major source of lead. In particular, high levels of lead are found near motorways and in large urban areas (especially during the rush hour). The findings of a report by the World Health Organization (WHO, 2004) suggest that lead is the single most important damaging chemical for children. In 2001, the estimated percentage of European children in urban areas with elevated blood levels (above 10 μg/dL) ranged from 0.1 to 30.2%. Globally, the WHO says, 15–18 million children in developing countries suffer permanent brain damage from lead poisoning. Other threats to children's health include methylmercury, dioxins, furans, polychlorinated biphenyls (PCBs), pesticides, nitrites and nitrates, and benzene.

'Vastly increasing numbers of people, on a vastly increasing scale, now dig the earth to take and make what they want: they cut down forests, breed animals, grow crops and fish the seas: and from everything that is made or eaten pollution is generated.'

(Government White Paper on pollution control, 1970)

Other sources of air pollution are industry and agriculture. The link between air pollution and lung disease has been acknowledged since the 1930s. The latter poses a serious health threat. The long-term effects of a high exposure to motor fumes are thought to include asthma, chronic obstructive airways disease, coughing, wheezing and chest pain.

The 1980s saw the emergence of concerns related to excessive exposure to sun in childhood and the links to skin cancer in later life. Children and adolescents who have frequent and long periods of exposure to intense rays causing painful blistering sunburn are at risk from developing malignant melanoma later in life. Malignant melanoma is largely preventable and curable if recognised early. Children and carers should therefore be educated about safety in the sun, including the use of hats and sunscreens.

poverty
Peter Townsend (1979, p. 31) offers a definition of poverty:

'Individuals, families, and groups in the population can be said to be in poverty when they lack the resources to obtain the types of diet, participate in the activities and have the living conditions and amenities which are customary or are at least widely encouraged and approved, in the societies in which they belong.'

Social issues

There is an ongoing debate about the definition of poverty and how to measure it. Poverty can be measured either *directly*, through income or material circumstances, or *indirectly* using proxies such as benefit/tax credit receipt or social class (Flaherty *et al.*, 2004). The most commonly used measure is the *Households Below Average Income* (HBAI) measure, which analyses patterns of low income. Families are said to be living below the 'poverty line' when the household income is 50% below the average household income (Flaherty *et al.*, 2004). The proportion of children living in low-income households more than doubled between the late 1970s and mid-1990s (HM Treasury, 2004). In 2003, 3.5 million children (28% of all children) were living in poverty; this was an increase from 13% in 1979 (Flaherty *et al.*, 2004). In 1999 the government announced a 20-year mission to eradicate child poverty for ever (Blair, 1999). In the same year a comprehensive survey of poverty in the UK was conducted (Health Statistics Quarterly, 1999). Parents defined 30 necessities for children, through which child poverty could be measured. The report found that children are least likely to go without the items that the largest proportion of parents thought were necessary: food, environmental and developmental items. Nearly all parents thought that 'new, properly fitted shoes', 'a warm waterproof coat' and 'fresh fruit and vegetables at least once a day' were necessities and yet 1 child in 50 goes without these due to lack of money. One child in 25 goes without 'celebrations on special days such as birthdays', 'educational games', 'meat, fish or vegetarian equivalent at least twice a day' and a 'garden to play in'. Over one-fifth of children go without a 'holiday away from home at least once a year' (Health Statistics Quarterly, 1999). Under this definition 18% of all children are deprived.

Low-income households are frequently workless, lone parents, members of an ethnic minority or disabled parents who are out of work. Of all children in poverty, 57% are in households that are workless, with one or more disabled adult, where the head of the household is from an ethnic minority group (Flaherty *et al.*, 2004). Children living in local authority housing are most likely to be deprived (Health Statistics Quarterly, 1999).

A report by the charity group Shelter found that more than 900 000 children living in run-down housing were suffering from serious and prolonged illnesses exacerbated by the appalling conditions in which they lived (Shelter, 2003). The report found that many were suffering in damp, mouldy and overcrowded homes, which are linked to health problems ranging from gastro-enteritis and skin disorders to chronic asthma. Shelter also found that, at the end of 2003, there were approximately 47 000 families with children living in temporary accommodation provided by local authorities (Shelter, 2003). The insecurity and disruption of living in temporary accommodation, often in cramped conditions, clearly has a damaging effect on children's health and well-being. A Barnardo's survey in 1997 found that although children of homeless families living in temporary accommodation face acute problems, a much more serious problem is presented by the plight of children who are housed but whose homes are damp, infested, overcrowded or in some other way unfit. The report stated that the home conditions of some children constitute serious impediments to learning, help to lower health standards and therefore increase absences from school, contribute continually to low self-esteem and lack of confidence (Barnardo's, 1997).

gene

'. . . a large complex molecule of a protein compound (deoxyribonucleic acid – DNA) which is capable of self-duplication. Genes contain information necessary for controlling the development and activity of cells.'

(Watson, 1979)

Examples of chromosome disorders

- Down's syndrome (trisomy 21)
- fragile-X syndrome
- Klinefelter's syndrome
- Turner's syndrome

Examples of single-gene disorders

- Autosomal dominant:
  - Marfan's syndrome
  - achondroplasia
  - Huntington's chorea
- Autosomal recessive:
  - cystic fibrosis
  - phenylketonuria
  - galactosaemia
- X-linked recessive:
  - Duchenne muscular dystrophy
  - haemophilia
- X-linked dominant:
  - hypophosphataemic vitamin D-resistant rickets

Genetic Factors

Each of us has our own individual genetic make-up, the only exception being identical twins. Recent advances in biochemistry, molecular genetics and cytogenetics have raised awareness of the importance of hereditary influences on health. Many disorders and diseases in children have a genetic link. In some there is a definite genetic cause, which is known (cystic fibrosis and Down's syndrome are just two examples) and the disorder is apparent at birth. In others the effects of the disorder do not become apparent until some months or even years after birth (for example sickle cell anaemia, phenylketonuria). There are three broad categories of genetic disease: chromosome (cytogenic) abnormalities, single-gene (monogenic) disorders and multifactorial disorders.

Chromosome abnormalities occur when there is a deviation in the number or structure of one or more chromosomes (*see also* Heredity p. 54).

In single-gene disorders there is a definite single-gene mutation. The consequences of such a mutation can be mild, with no effect on the child, or can lead to serious disability or be incompatible with life. Genes are classed as either dominant or recessive in their effect. For a dominant gene to be passed on, only one parent need carry the gene. For a recessive gene to be passed on, both parents must carry the gene. This latter scenario is less likely than the first unless the parents are blood relatives, when the likelihood increases.

Multifactorial disorders show an increased incidence in some families but do not show a definite inheritance pattern. Individuals appear to have a genetic susceptibility for a certain disorder – for example, some congenital abnormalities (such as spina bifida), diabetes and hypertension.

As research into genetics increases it is becoming more possible to identify those fetuses that have abnormalities. This, in turn, poses ethical and moral questions, because one has to deal with the consequences of finding out that a child carries a genetic disorder. Some would argue that knowing about problems enables early detection and subsequent treatment (of phenylketonuria, for example) or termination of pregnancies should that be an alternative. Others show concern about genetic screening in that, in some instances, it is difficult to know the extent to which a child will be disabled and that terminating abnormal fetuses is a contradiction of human rights. Nevertheless genetic screening is offered to families who have reason to believe they may be carriers of certain genes. This must only be done against the backdrop of an effective counselling service, the purpose of which must be to help the family or individual to:

- understand the facts – the diagnosis, course of the disorder and available management
- appreciate how heredity contributes to a disorder and how it may affect specified relatives
- choose an appropriate course of action in view of the risks and family situation
- adjust as well as possible to the disorder in an affected family member and/or the risk of re-occurrence

Study activity

The ethical and moral issues related to genetic screening are huge, so we suggest that you explore this area more fully. Try discussing issues with your colleagues, either on the ward or in college. Remember to make notes of any references. They could be useful to you in the future.

Summary

The health of the nation's children has improved in many ways, but there remain children whose health status is compromised by a poor environment, inadequate diet and inequalities. Health in a child's early years is of paramount importance and these issues must be addressed if all children are to be given the best possible chance of a healthy future. As the patterns of illness and disease change, so children's health needs will change. An increasing prevalence of chronic disease will require a reallocation of resources into the community. Debates will continue over the moral and ethical issues related to the treatment of low birthweight infants and of those children requiring multiple organ transplants. Many factors influence the health of our children today, both before and after birth. By being aware of these factors it may be possible to address some of them and contribute to the future health of all children.

Key Points

1. The infant mortality rate has fallen dramatically since the 1940s and continues to fall.
2. The survival rates for some cancers are improving.
3. One in every four children in England is overweight.
4. The number of accidents in children is declining steadily, although accidents are still the major cause of death in boys under 15 years of age.
5. There is a rising trend in the numbers of children with disabilities and long-standing illness.
6. Marked inequalities exist in nearly all areas of child health.
7. A variety of factors influence the health of children today, including environmental issues, social issues and individual factors.

Chapter 11
Health

Introduction

To consider the theoretical aspects of health promotion and education, we should first consider the meaning of health.

Study activity

Consider what the term 'being healthy' means to you. List all the factors that contribute to your health.

Many people have attempted to define health over the years and the only concrete notion to emerge is that there is no simple, obvious definition. Health is a complete, multidimensional idea, the interpretation of which differs from person to person. The word is derived from the Old English term *hoelth* meaning 'a state of soundness' and has been used to refer to soundness of the body. One commonly quoted definition is that from the WHO (1946:2), which states that health is 'characterised not only by the absence of disease but also by a state of complete physical, mental and social well being'. This definition describes an ideal state.

More recently various definitions have been proposed. A few will be offered here for the reader to consider. The definitions fall into three categories:

- Definitions that emphasise actualisation. These stress the realisation of human potential through purposeful action. Health is seen not merely as a state free from illness but as a much more dynamic, emergent process. Among the nurse theorists who hold this view is Orem (2001). In her self-care theory she describes health as consisting of two characteristics. The first is soundness of human structures and bodily functions. The second is movement towards fulfilment of one's self-ideal and personalisation.

- Definitions that emphasise adaptation. These view health as being concerned with the ability of the individual to adapt to the environment. Neuman (1982) describes health as being a condition in which the physiological, psychological and sociocultural systems are in balance. The central concept of Roy's model of nursing (Roy, 1984) is one of adaptation, and she defines health as a state and process of successful adaptation.
- Definitions that embrace both actualisation and adaptation. The definition that demonstrates this view is that of King (1981:5). King sees health as a dynamic process that involves 'continuous adaptation to the internal and external environment through the optimum use of one's resources to achieve maximum potential'.

Further reading

Naidoo, J. and Wills, J. (2000) *Health Promotion: Foundations for Practice*, 2nd edn. London: Baillière Tindall.

Hanna (1989) explored student nurses' views of health, describing it as an awareness of physical abilities, appearance and energy level as well as a mental state of happiness, contentment and clarity of thinking.

One idea that has been proposed by several authors is that the same person can view health in many different ways. Individuals can change their perception of health depending on the situation in which they find themselves at any given time. Health could therefore be defined as being what the individual says it is. This can present difficulties for health professionals when trying to implement health-promotion activities.

Study activity

Analyse each of the definitions given above. Identify the strengths and weaknesses of each. Talk to friends and patients about what health means to them. Then try to write your own definition of health.

Health Promotion and Education

Until the 1980s, health education was the main way in which individuals were encouraged to adopt healthy behaviours. Health education arose out of the traditional concern with the treatment of illness rather than with its prevention. Much of the activity in this area took on an individualistic approach. It used as its basis the assumption that individuals have control over their own health. This approach has been criticised for failing to acknowledge the social influences on health and for assuming that individuals have free choice. It has engendered a tendency towards victim blaming. In reality there is much to suggest that there are often factors mitigating against personal change. The health of people in Britain has generally been improving since the 1980s but inequalities in health still exist. According to Acheson (1991) there is a limit to the extent to which individuals can change their behaviour in the absence of wider strategies to reduce deprivation and improve the environment.

Health promotion

One of the major contributing factors in the development of the concept of health promotion has been the Health for All movement initiated by the WHO in 1977. This enabled a culture shift towards prevention rather than cure and strengthened the idea that the promotion of health was much more than an individual responsibility. It led to the development of the New Public Health movement. This emerged as an approach that embraces environmental change *and* individual responsibility, thereby seeking to avoid victim blaming. Underlying many of today's health problems are issues of local and national public policy that the New Public Health seeks to address. The motivation for the government to change the focus of health towards prevention came from a number of reports that spelt out the need for a society more 'fully engaged' in health (Wanless, 2004). Wanless informed the government that the UK would no longer be able to afford a National Health Service unless the public was encouraged to improve its own health.

It is in this culture of empowerment and personal responsibility for health that the first ever White Paper on public health was produced in 2004. The development of *Choosing Health: Making Healthier Choices Easier* (DH, 2004a) consisted of a public consultation, which asked the public what it considered to be important in terms of health improvement. The result was that people wanted to make their own choices about health issues but wanted the government to support them in making those choices. They wanted clear and credible information and expected support to help them make changes.

While the infectious diseases that used to kill people have now been eradicated or controlled, the biggest killers are now diseases that are preventable (DH, 2004a):

- smoking remains the biggest preventable cause of ill health and death in the UK
- one in 10 sexually active young women may be infected with chlamydia
- since 1974 there has been an increase in the number of mental health problems experienced by young people
- suicide is the most common cause of death in men under 35
- around 1 in every 10 attendances in A&E departments is alcohol related

Various definitions of health promotion have been proposed over recent years. All have as their core the view that health promotion is a global term that incorporates the promotion of health through a wide range of initiatives, policies and campaigns. Emphasis is placed on putting energy into dealing with the underlying problems, which lead to negative health behaviours. This is achieved by building healthy public policy and empowering individuals and groups within society. Some of the views of health promotion are considered in more detail.

The WHO (1986) defines health promotion as '. . . the process of enabling individuals and communities to increase control over the determinants of health and thereby improve their health'. Five principles underpin this definition:

- health promotion focuses on the population as a whole rather than on individuals who are at risk
- health promotion should be aimed at the factors that influence health
- health promotion must combine a wide variety of complementary approaches including education, legislation and organisational change
- health promotion requires full community participation
- health professionals have a key role to play in nurturing and promoting health through education and advocacy

New public health – to find out more about this you should look at:

Orme, J., Powell, J., Taylor, P. and Grey, M. (2007) *Public Health for the 21st Century*, second edition. Maidenhead: Open University Press.

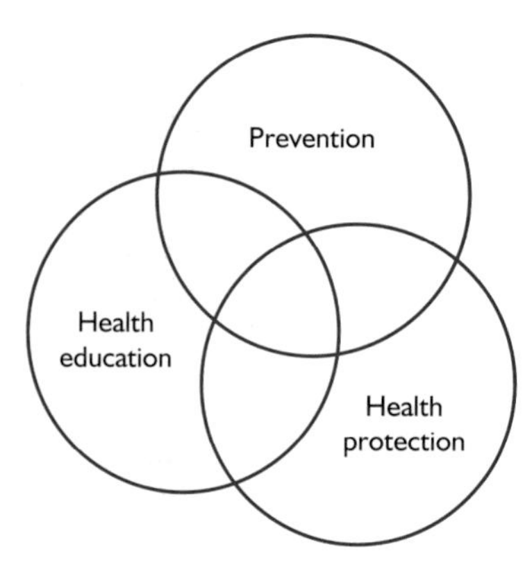

Figure 11.1 A model for health promotion (from Downie *et al.*, 1990; reproduced by permission of Oxford University Press).

Tannahill's model of health promotion

One widely acknowledged model is that of Tannahill (1985). Tannahill's model sees health promotion as consisting of three overlapping activities (Figure 11.1):

- preventive care
- protection
- education

Preventive care is aimed at reducing the likelihood of the onset of a disease process, illness or disability (or some other unwanted state). Individuals are provided with information and advice to enable them to avoid health-damaging behaviours. It is an area with which the nurse should be familiar and is of particular importance to the community team. It is generally taken to consist of intervention at three levels:

- Primary prevention. This includes immunisations and specific actions to prevent accidents, curb smoking and encourage a balanced healthy diet.
- Secondary prevention. This is concerned with the early detection of disease or illness *before* it manifests itself. This then allows early treatment to be initiated. Screening plays an important role in the prevention of disease and illness in children. One example is the routine test for phenylketonuria. This is test is carried out on all babies at 10 days of age. It has been instrumental in detecting the condition early so that effective treatment can be started as soon as possible. Developmental surveillance is another example of secondary prevention. Every child is seen at regular intervals. Checks are made on developmental progress and deviations from the norm are identified.
- Tertiary prevention is concerned with curing disease, preventing complications and the prevention of spread of disease. Action at this level includes medical and surgical interventions and rehabilitation. Specialist nurses work at this level to teach individuals how to cope with a disease or illness so as to limit the development of complications.

phenylketonuria
A relatively rare autosomal recessive metabolic disorder. The conversion of phenylalanine to tyrosine is blocked. Increased levels of phenylalanine lead to severe mental deficiency and seizures.

According to Downie *et al.* (1990:51), health *protection* comprises 'legal or fiscal controls, other regulations and policies, and voluntary codes of practice aimed at the enhancement of positive health and the prevention of ill-health'. The aim is to make it less likely that individuals will meet hazards in the environment and behave in an unhealthy way. It is about making the healthy choices the easy ones:

- Legal control – this is concerned with legislation, for example the use of child and infant restraints in cars.
- Fiscal control – this is concerned with the imposition of healthy monetary policies by the government, for example the imposition of more tax on leaded petrol to make unleaded petrol cheaper and therefore more attractive.
- Other policies – these are implemented by agencies other than the government. One example is the implementation of no-smoking policies in the workplace.
- Voluntary codes of practice – these are agreed codes, as in the advertising of tobacco products. However with no legal back-up these can be broken with no redress.

Health education is the third activity in Tannahill's model. It is a long-established activity that has been defined by many authors over recent years. Within the new concept of health promotion, education is seen as being aimed at influencing behaviour, promoting positive health and preventing ill health. It is important that education takes into account people's backgrounds, including their social and cultural situations. Thus it moves away from the victim-blaming approach and acknowledges the underlying influencing factors.

The model suggests that each of the three activities can occur in isolation. Examples of these have been given previously. However, in reality they overlap, giving rise to a further four health promotion activities (Figure 11.2):

- *Preventive health education.* Education related to available preventive measures. Immunisations are a valuable preventive measure but without education parents may not realise the benefits of taking up the programme. Thus education is aimed at parents and carers. One

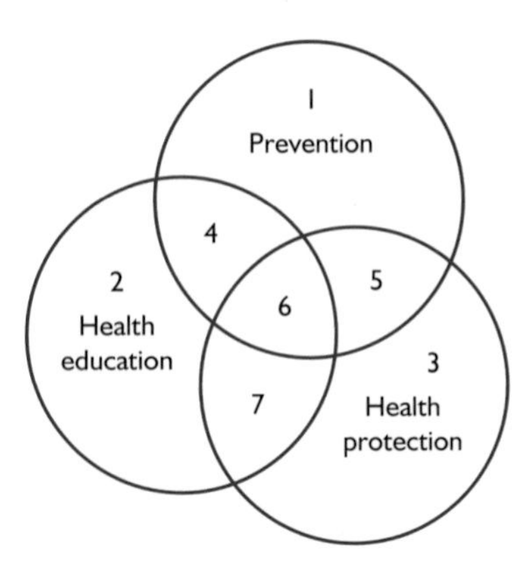

Figure 11.2 Health education activities (from Downie *et al.*, 1990; reproduced by permission of Oxford University Press).

recent example of this has been the Web site set up to promote uptake of the MMR vaccine. Education is also carried out with the use of posters and leaflets.

- *Preventive health protection.* This includes legal, fiscal or other policies that are preventive in nature. One example of this is the fluoridation of water supplies to promote healthy teeth.
- *Health education for preventive health protection.* Although many preventive policies exist, individuals need to be educated about them so as to gain the maximum benefit. Using the above example, parents and carers need to be given the facts about fluoridation and its benefits. In this way more will be enabled to make informed choices about their child's care.
- *Health education aimed at health protection.* This entails raising the public's and policymakers' awareness of the need for protection measures. One recent example of this has been the lobby for the introduction of traffic-calming measures outside schools. As a result of public pressure in many areas, speed restrictions have been imposed outside schools.

MMR the facts

You can find information and resources for parents about the MMR vaccine on:

www.mmrthefacts.nhs.uk (accessed 30 April 2006).

health education

'Health education is communication aimed at enhancing positive health and preventing or diminishing ill health in individuals and groups, through influencing beliefs, attitudes and behaviours of those with power and the community at large.'

(Smith, 1979)

Beattie's model of health promotion

Beattie (1991) suggests that there are four paradigms of health promotion. He identifies two factors, which he sees as fundamental to health promotion, namely the *mode* and the *focus* of intervention (Figure 11.3).

The *mode of intervention* is where ownership of the appropriate knowledge in health promotion, and therefore the control, lies. At point A, control lies with the expert. It is the expert who decides what it is that the client needs to know. At point B, clients determine control. Clients identify what it is that they wish to learn, taking into account their needs, circumstances and beliefs. The importance of this mode is stressed as it contributes to a feeling of empowerment.

The *focus of intervention* is concerned with the targets of the education. At point C, the education is aimed at the individual – the *individualistic approach.* At point D the focus is the roots of ill health, the community, an institution or even society – the *collective approach.*

Beattie shows these factors as two intersecting lines giving rise to four paradigms of promotion (Figure 11.4):

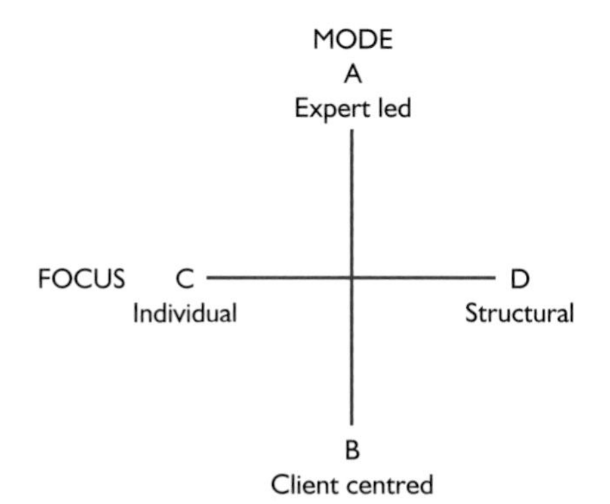

Figure 11.3 Factors fundamental to health promotion (adapted from Beattie, 1991).

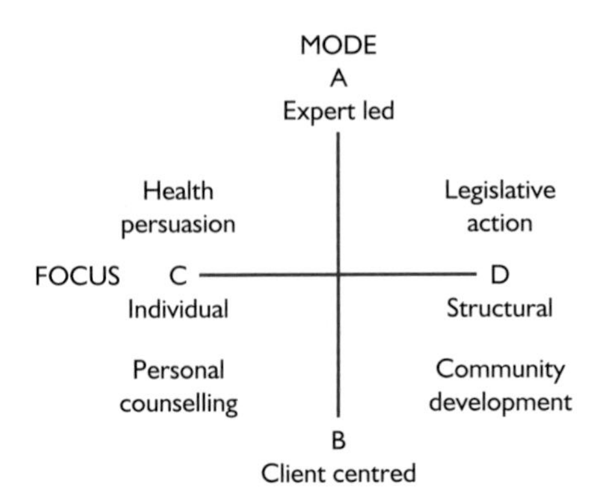

Figure 11.4 Four categories of health promotion (adapted from Beattie, 1991).

- *Health persuasion* – this is expert led and is directed at the individual. An example is a health visitor encouraging a mother to allow her child to have the MMR vaccination.
- *Personal counselling* – a young mother realises she does not know enough about weaning and feeding her son. She asks the health visitor for advice. The health promoter is a facilitator rather than an expert. This is client led and client centred and encourages a feeling of being in control.
- *Legislative action* – a group of experts agrees on the need for a plan for education related to HIV and AIDS. They attempt to educate the policy formers and decision makers. This is expert led and collective in its focus.
- *Community development* – parents lobby their MP regarding the need for traffic-calming methods outside a local school. This is client led and collective in its focus and encourages empowerment.

Study activity

Take each paradigm shown in Figure 11.4 and identify an example from your own field of work.

The health-oriented approach (Downie *et al.*, 1990)

This model is based on two main principles, namely the prevention of ill health and the enhancement of positive health (Figure 11.5).

It acknowledges the underlying factors that influence health. Action is aimed at the risks and is applicable at both the structural and the individual level. It is not merely led by professionals but involves public (and group) participation, especially in identifying the risks, thus highlighting the importance of empowerment.

The three views on health promotion described here have certain similarities, which can act as principles:

- They all acknowledge that individual approaches have a role to play, provided that the individual's circumstances are taken into consideration. It is important to start where the client is and to consider his or her social circumstances, beliefs, values and culture.

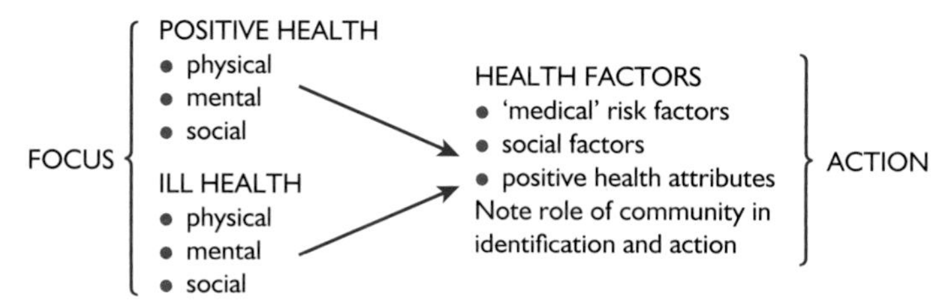

Figure 11.5 Health-oriented approach (from Downie *et al.*, 1990; reproduced by permission of Oxford University Press).

- They each see a role for public agenda-setting and for involving individuals and communities in securing action.
- Finally, they each have the concept of empowerment as a central theme.

Tannahill and Beattie offer traditional methods of health promotion, however. *Choosing Health* states that many traditional methods of improving health are no longer effective and a new approach is needed. The latest approach to health improvement recognises and utilises approaches used to good effect in the business world.

Social marketing (French and Blair Stevens, 2005)

Social marketing is a flexible and adaptable approach to health promotion that draws on marketing techniques and approaches used in the commercial world. Some of these approaches are being used in the commercial sense to promote unhealthy lifestyles, for instance fast food companies have been very successful in promoting food that is unhealthy for children. However, where marketing is used in the commercial world for financial gain, in social marketing, market approaches are used for social gain. The definition of health-related social marketing is:

> . . . the systematic application of marketing concepts and techniques to achieve specific behaviour goals relevant to improving health and reducing health inequalities.
>
> (French and Blair Stevens, 2005:31)

Social marketing has three key elements:

- *a systematic approach:* phased to address short-, medium- and long-term goals
- *a marketing mix:* using a range of marketing techniques and approaches
- *based on social good:* rather than commercial benefit

It is based on three core principles:

- *Behaviour and behaviour goals.* The driving purpose is to achieve tangible and measurable impact on actual behaviour. It moves beyond communicating information of health messages and focuses on understanding existing behaviour and the key influences behind that behaviour. It works to establish specific behavioural goals, not to simply change behaviour.

- *Voluntary actions.* Social marketing is focused on how to encourage and achieve voluntary action, starting from where people are now and where they might want to be.
- *Audience segmentation.* Avoiding the approach of sending blanket health messages, social marketing looks at ways to segment and differentiate audiences.

It has three core concepts:

- *Insight.* Developing genuine insight into the reality of everyday life, avoiding professional assumptions about what people need, want and think.
- *Exchange.* Fully understanding what the person has to give in order to get the proposed benefit; for example, time, money, social consequences, loss of pleasure and so forth. Understanding how to maximise the benefits and minimise the barriers to new behaviours.
- *Competition.* Recognising that whatever is being offered will always face both external and internal competition – for example, the power of pleasure, habit or addiction, peer or media pressure. Moving beyond seeing competition as 'goodies' or 'baddies'.

In social marketing the 'four Ps' of the traditional market approach are used, but in a different sense:

- *Product.* What do the customers get? What is being offered to them?
- *Price.* How much will it cost them? (Not just money but also time, effort, emotional cost.)
- *Place.* Where does the relevant behaviour happen? Where are there opportunities to reach the customers?
- *Promotion.* What package of incentives can be put in place, which will be valued by the customer?

Social marketing
For more information and resources visit http://www.nsms.org.uk (accessed 30 April 2006).

With smoking as an example, social marketing would start with a whole population analysis, looking at people's relationship to smoking. Who is most at risk from smoking? People could fall into different categories:

- 'never smoked and never will'
- 'susceptible to pressure to smoke'
- 'recent quitter – potential to restart'
- 'would like to quit but find it hard'
- 'strong entrenched resisters'

The focus would fall on those with the most potential for change and would recognise the limitations to change. Particular attention would be paid to how certain audiences think or feel about smoking in relation to where they sit within these categories. Marketing would then be targeted to have specific influences on the different audiences. A traditional approach to smoking cessation may have as its goal the cessation of a number of people smoking in a specific time frame. However, in that time frame 1000 younger smokers may have taken up smoking. A behaviour goals approach would recognise that changing established behaviours is generally harder than helping prevent them in the first place. A major part of this approach to smoking would be to explore the key influences to starting smoking and influences that reinforce smoking behaviour.

Study activity

Explore some of the market techniques used by commercial firms and the media to sell products and ideas to children. Think about how the same techniques could be used to sell healthy messages.

Empowerment

Empowerment is a popular term in use today in many different arenas. This makes it difficult to simply define the term, as it can take on different meanings for different people in different contexts. The word is derived from the Latin *potere* meaning 'to be able'. Today the term is particularly relevant to the current health promotion movement and can be defined as the social process by which people are enabled to take control of their own health. It involves helping people to take a critical look at a situation and facilitating a realistic plan of action. In doing this, health educators need to be aware of the complex array of political, social, economic and demographic factors that influence health and illness. However, it is necessary to attempt to change the conditions that create powerlessness at the same time, and to be proactive. An example of this is installing a suggestion box on the ward, and encouraging children and parents to participate in the improvement of the environment. Thus the process of empowerment must include not only individual change but also change in the social setting itself (Wallerstein, 1992).

Within the arena of childcare, obstacles to the empowerment of children exist. The first is to do with the developmental stage of children and the second with the social context in which children live.

The amount of responsibility that children can assume for their own health must be considered. Too much too soon can create demands that children are not developmentally ready to meet. However, it is important to acknowledge that children have their own views and ideas about health, and to accept these as valid. The children's nurse, therefore, needs an understanding of the changing perceptions that children have of health as they develop. This then enables the nurse to promote empowerment where appropriate (*see also* The role of the nurse pp. 165 and 222 and Children's perceptions of health p. 141).

Within the social context children are assumed to be cognitively and socially immature. While the health needs of children are recognised in policy and planning documents, their role is one of passive recipient (Kalnins *et al.*, 1994). Children are not generally given the opportunity to participate in health-making decisions. Factors that act against empowerment include:

- Parental attitudes – while many parents are willing to involve their children in the decision-making process, they can feel threatened by the competence of their children (Lewis and Lewis, 1990).
- Non-participation in clinical interviews – interactions between doctors and carers can often ignore the child. Attitudes of health professionals can influence the child's perceptions of his/her role and can lead to silent cooperation rather than questioning.

empowerment

'. . . a social process of recognising, promoting and enhancing people's abilities to meet their own needs, solve their own problems and mobilise the necessary resources in order to feel in control of their own lives'.

(Gibson, 1991)

- Professional jargon – this can exclude children and carers from participation in decision making. Language must be interactive and encourage open participation both by carers and children.

It is important that children have a voice in their future health. They often have very firm views on health issues and will participate in community projects with great enthusiasm. It is necessary to encourage a shift in thinking as children are encouraged to participate in health promotion. Empowerment is for all, not just for the adults in society (*see also* Empowerment p. 170).

Study activity

How feasible is the boxed definition of empowerment? What are your reasons for your conclusions?

Study activity

Set yourself the task of analysing each of the views covered above. Explore any other theories and/or models that you find in your reading.

Summary

It is essential that you have an understanding of the theoretical basis of health promotion if you are to fulfil your role as a health promoter. This section has given you an overview of theories and you should now read further to expand your knowledge and understanding. Material in this section will help you to look critically at some of the health promotion interventions related to child health.

Key Points

1. Defining health is complex. The concept is viewed in different ways by the same person. Everyone will have their own views about what it means to be healthy.
2. The health promotion movement incorporates promotion of health through a wide range of initiatives and activities. Building a healthy public policy is one of the central concepts.
3. Traditional methods of improving health may no longer be effective and a new approach is needed.
4. Empowerment of people and of communities is central to all health promotion. People need to feel in control of their own lives and need to be enabled to make healthy choices. This concept is applicable to adults and children alike.

Chapter 12

Children's Perceptions of Health

Introduction

As we have seen, it is difficult to define health. Each of us has our own definition based on experience, knowledge and developed concepts, and influenced by culture, society, family and personal beliefs. The concepts that we have as adults are formed from our experiences during the maturation process and then refined and adapted as we grow and mature. Children's ideas about the world in which they live change and develop as these concepts are formed. Hence their ideas about health change. To meet the healthcare needs of children, nurses must understand how these ideas change with age. It is essential that health promotion activities are pertinent to a child and are related to the way in which he or she interprets health. Only then can the promotion of healthy behaviours begin to be successful. Knowledge of how children view health can also be useful when caring for them during periods of ill health. Their ideas may affect how they interpret information about disease and can lead to alarming misconceptions. Take, for instance, a child who is told that his tonsils will have to be removed from his throat. He becomes quite frightened as he thinks that his throat will be cut to remove the tonsils. Compliance with treatment may also be affected by a lack of understanding. For example, a young child who does not understand the function of the gastro-intestinal tract may be reluctant to take an oral pain killer for a headache (*see also* Children's concepts of illness p. 205 and Children's perceptions of pain p. 354).

The fact that children's perceptions change as they grow and develop presents us with a challenge – to understand each child and to value his or her beliefs and ideas, acknowledging that what they believe is important.

Developing Ideas about the Human Body

Studies that explore children's beliefs about the human body are limited. Table 12.1 draws on some of the studies and shows how a child's ideas might develop.

Table 12.1 Children's developing ideas about the human body

Age	Knowledge of inside of body	Knowledge of function of organs
3–5 years	Draws pictures that show food, bones and sometimes blood. These are all things that the child can 'see' or 'feel'.	Limited understanding of body functions. Unclear about body boundaries.
5–10 years	Drawings often include the heart and brain. Not until 10 years are children likely to regularly include the stomach and the lungs.	Believe that organs can only have one function, e.g. the heart is for loving, the brain is for thinking. Do not identify the role of the brain in the senses or motor behaviour. Not able to relate the various parts of the body together.
Adolescence	Now aware of liver, kidneys and the internal reproductive organs.	Understand that organs can have more than one function. Relate parts of the body together so would understand the workings of the digestive system.

McEwing (1996) and Gaudion (1997) concur that young children have more knowledge about the heart, bones and brain than other parts of the anatomy and that as cognitive ability develops children are more able to understand more abstract concepts. Some studies have suggested that children with chronic conditions may not follow the normal developmental progression in developing schema of the internal body (Neff, 1990; Neff and Beardslee, 1990). To explore this idea more fully Vessey and O'Sullivan (2000) carried out a study to compare the knowledge of children with and without congenital heart disease. They found no differences between the two groups and point out that knowledge about the body's interior cannot be presumed.

Developing Ideas about Health

It is interesting to note that there is less research available about health beliefs than there is about illness beliefs. Perhaps this is because of the traditional ideas that put more emphasis on cure and treatment than on prevention and health. As the importance of promoting health in childhood is recognised, and as the views of children are acknowledged, we may be more interested in finding out what they have to say about health.

Two major approaches to the study of children's health beliefs are evident from the available literature.

Cognitive developmental approach

This approach is based on the belief that the development of concepts follows the same pattern in all children, albeit at different rates. It assumes that, as children mature, they gradually develop expanding and more differentiated concepts. It would seem that the formation of many concepts, for example time, space and number, follow the patterns outlined by cognitive psychologists. The approach questions 'how' behaviour comes about, analysing the thinking, cognitive processes of children. It relies on the interviewer probing children's minds to find out reasons for saying what they say about health. The difficulty here is that

Cultural perspectives

Despite general agreement that cross-cultural research is needed, most existing investigations of children's development of health and illness-related concepts have involved samples from developed countries. A study by Boruchovitch and Mednick (1997) examined the development of the concepts of health and illness in a Brazilian sample of 96 elementary and junior high-school students. The study showed a predictable relationship between subject's age and school grade level and increasingly more highly differentiated and multidimensional concepts of health and illness. This investigation suggests that, for the most part, cross-cultural similarities in children's concepts of health and illness may be more striking than the differences.

Table 12.2 Changes in children's concepts about health (adapted from work by Bibace and Walsh, 1980; Natapoff, 1982)

Age	Cognitive development	Concept of health
Up to 7 years	Pre-operational – egocentric, present-oriented, intuitive, magical thinking, unable to reverse processes.	Find health difficult to define – tend to list activities and behaviours centred on self. Health in others judged by external cues (rosy cheeks, clear eyes). Health and illness unrelated. Rely on others to tell them when they are sick. Health vulnerable to external forces, e.g. magic.
7–11 years	Concrete operational – begin to consider causal relationships. Develop reversibility and conservation. Can think through a chain of events. Classify objects and concrete ideas. Able to shift from part to whole and back again. Remain present-oriented until about 9 years.	Health viewed as a broad whole body concept – feeling good, being fit and strong. Possible to be part healthy, part not healthy. Still see health vulnerable to external forces but see that ill health can be caused by physical contact, e.g. with dirt. Understand that illness can be prevented to some degree.
11–16 years	Formal operations – future-oriented, can formulate hypotheses, consider abstractions. Develop deductive reasoning.	Aware of problems associated with defining health. Use internal cues as well as external ones to judge people's health – consider the abstract points. See health and sickness as related. Consider mental health important.

the results of such an interview are affected by the effectiveness of the interviewer. If he or she does not probe well enough, insufficient information may be gained on which to make a judgement. The interviewer may also misinterpret what the child says. The technique really calls for an ability to interpret what children say. This can be difficult as no adult can really know exactly what is going on inside a child's head. However, it is an approach that is used frequently, perhaps because of the popularity of cognitive psychologists in child development. The framework that has been used most frequently by researchers in this area is based on Jean Piaget's work. Studies show that the quality of children's thoughts about health do change developmentally, reflecting the stages of cognitive development as described by the Swiss psychologist Piaget, and that their ideas become more complex and abstract as they mature (Table 12.2).

Pre-operational stage (up to age 7)

Children at this stage of cognitive development find it difficult to define health. Eiser *et al.* (1983) asked 6-year-olds 'what does it mean to be healthy?' Sixty-five per cent of them were unable to answer the question. Natapoff (1982) found that children in the pre-operational stage gave general, undifferentiated answers to questions about health and had to use visual cues to judge whether somebody was healthy or not. However, when it came to judging their own health they often relied on other people to tell them if they were ill. They based their own health on what they were able to do: play outside, go to school. Health at this age is seen as a series of unrelated activities of which eating the right food is seen as important. So children at this age tend to list things that make them healthy. According to Piaget, children in this stage are unable to reverse processes. This is evident in their inability to see health and ill health as part of a continuum or existing together. They see health as an absolute and believe that if you are healthy you cannot get sick. The maintenance of health relies on external forces. Explanations for the cause of illness are often magical in nature (Bibace and Walsh, 1980) and so it is not surprising that children have little perception or understanding of illness prevention (Eiser *et al.*, 1983). The future is too abstract for children of this age to think about, so any discussion about the consequences of non-healthy behaviours would be meaningless.

Concrete operational stage (7–11)

As children develop their cognitive abilities they begin to be able to classify pieces of information into a whole. Therefore they define health as a total body state. Being healthy is feeling good, being in good condition, fit and strong (Natapoff, 1982). Health is seen as a broad concept developed from an integration of learned material and information. As children of this age have learned to conserve, they see the possibility of being part healthy and part not healthy. They can shift from the whole to part of the whole. Therefore somebody with a broken leg can still be healthy. Operational children still see health as being vulnerable to external forces but are beginning to understand that illness can be contracted through physical contact with a source, for example dirt (Bibace and Walsh, 1980). They therefore understand that illness can be avoided and can identify rules for maintaining health. Myant and Williams (2005) found that the children in their study defined health as being free of illness and linked to eating healthy food and being happy.

Formal operations stage (11–16 onwards)

Young people at this stage of development are aware that it is very difficult to define health. They can now see that it is possible to be part healthy and part sick at the same time. The children in Natapoff's study (1982) described health as 'lasting a lifetime' and involving both the body and the mind. This was the first time that children had mentioned the importance of mental health. They saw sickness as something temporary and therefore something that it was possible to avoid and/or prevent by taking proper care of oneself and by avoiding certain behaviours that were unhealthy (Bibace and Walsh, 1980). Children in the formal stage are becoming capable of abstract thinking and now do not rely on visual cues to judge health in other people. They acknowledge the importance of questioning individuals to find out how they feel about their health. There has been a shift from the use of external cues to the use of internal ones.

The developing complexity of cognitive processes identified above enables adolescents to engage in self-care and to take more responsibility for their own health, taking actions and making decisions about health behaviours. This has implications for health promoters as it is vital to find the right time in a child's development to use initiatives that focus on healthy behaviours and the prevention of ill health.

Health belief model approach

The health belief model (Rosenstock, 1974) was developed to attempt to explain why individuals differ in their health-related behaviours. The model starts from the premise that any actions will be influenced at the outset by age, sex, social and cultural factors. These factors, in turn, influence individuals' perceptions of their vulnerability to ill health. Together with their reception of the benefits of health-related actions, this will then influence the degree to which they intend to take actions.

The use of this model in the study of children's concepts of health addresses the action component of that concept. It concentrates on the child's beliefs about one or more aspects of health and does not try to look at the underlying causal relationships between action and thought. Instead it studies actions that children take. The advantage of this approach is that it is easy to implement. Children of different ages are asked a series of questions to determine their beliefs about particular health issues in relation to:

- perceived vulnerability
- perceived benefits of healthy behaviours and/or illness-avoiding behaviours
- intentions to take actions

The frequency with which certain beliefs are held is then analysed.

In the 1970s, Gochman (1970, 1971a, b) carried out a number of studies using this approach. He developed a series of tools that measured:

- salience – the degree to which children were aware of health issues
- vulnerability – how vulnerable the children thought they were to 16 health problems, including fever, rash, sore throat and dental problems
- motivation
- potential behaviour – measured children's awareness behaviours that were beneficial to health

The results of these studies suggested that children are not generally motivated by health and that their perceived vulnerability is low. Beliefs about vulnerability become stable at around 10–11 years of age. Only a small number of children perceive themselves as vulnerable to various health problems. Perhaps this relates to the fact that young children can only deal with the present and the future is too abstract a concept to deal with. If this is so, then promoting illness-avoiding behaviours may be ineffective in children unless their perceived vulnerability can be increased. Gochman's studies also showed that children's perceived vulnerability and their potential for health behaviours are influenced by age, sex, class and locus of control. Boys in the study had a lower level of expectancy of health problems than the girls, as did the younger children compared with the older children. Children living in inner city areas had a higher level of expectancy of health problems than did children living in rural areas. Dielman *et al.* (1980) found that young children's beliefs about health and illness differed more among them than in older children. This finding relates well to findings from the cognitive developmental studies and serves to suggest that health teaching should begin early before a differentiated belief system is established at the age of about 12.

Further reading

France, A., Bendelow, G. and Williams, S. (1999) A risky business: researching health beliefs of young people. In McWhirter, J. (ed.), *Researching From Children's Perspectives.* Milton Keynes: Open University Press.

Further research

Malcarne, V. L., Drahota, A. and Hamilton, N. A. (2005) Children's health-related locus of control beliefs: ethnicity, gender, and family income. *Children's Health Care,* **34** (1), 47–59.

Young people's views

A Web site for young people based on research at Oxford University and launched on 22 March 2006, Youth Health Talk (http://www.youthhealthtalk.org, accessed 30 April 2006) is a site where young people talk about their experiences of health and illness. It covers teenage cancers and sexual health and will include diabetes, epilepsy, chronic fatigue, obesity and issues such as bereavement, as well as issues such as bullying, self-esteem, smoking, taking drugs and being a young carer. Short video diaries made by the young people themselves will also be used on the site.

Study activity

Take an opportunity to talk to well and sick children of different ages about health. Ask them questions such as:

- What does being healthy mean to you?
- What food is healthy?
- What things do you do that are not healthy?
- How do you know when you are ill?

Ask them to draw pictures about health. Analyse what they say and what they draw. How does it compare to the findings from the above studies?

Whichever approach is used to assess children's concepts of health, it is important to remember that all children are individuals and are influenced by their families, peers and significant others. Williams *et al.* (2003) carried out a study to examine how attitudes, beliefs and behaviours of young people regarding health, risk and lifestyles vary according to factors such as age and socio-demographic characteristics. They concluded that young people's concepts of health are multi-dimensional, a complex mixture of personal and expert knowledge and beliefs. In addition, health is not necessarily a key priority in these basically 'healthy' young people's lives. The study also found that the young people's beliefs and behaviours are influenced by a variety of media. Lewis and Lewis (1974) showed that television advertisements had a considerable impact. Children aged 10–13 years of age thought that 70% of advertisements relating to health were true. Nearly half of the children believed all the messages conveyed in advertisements.

Further reading: effects of the media

H J Foundation (2005) *The Effects of Electronic Media on Children Ages Zero to Six: A History of Research. The Henry J Kaiser Family Foundation.* http://www.kff.org (accessed 30 April 2006).

This is a review of the history of research and summarises the findings of major studies from the 1960s through to the 2000s.

Further reading

Shucksmith, J. and Spratt, J. (2002) *Young People's Self-identified Health Needs.* Aberdeen: University of Aberdeen, The Rowan Group.

http://www.hebs.scot.nhs.uk/researchcentre/pdf/RE06220012002Final.pdf (accessed 30 April 2006).

This review looks at recent (mainly post-1997) qualitative research undertaken with young people in the age range 11–25 years, and concentrates on those pieces of work that give voice to young people's own concerns about their health and well-being.

Social and cultural factors must also impact on children's beliefs about health. For example, the Romany rituals of body cleanliness and the system of wash bowls are introduced to children from an early age and are strictly adhered to from puberty (Taylor, 1991). Williams *et al.* (2003) found that Asian young people in their study were far less likely than those from other ethnic groups to engage in smoking, drinking and drug taking. Children vary in their cognitive abilities and it would be dangerous to assume that all children of a particular age hold the same views and beliefs. It may be useful to try to put the two approaches reviewed here together. It would seem that 'what' children believe about a certain health issue must be influenced by 'how' they think. This in turn depends on the complexity of their cognitive processes. Generally, researchers have found that there is a distinct change in the way children perceive health (and illness, their bodies and treatment) at around the age of 8–9 years, with an improved ability to think in a reality-oriented causal manner.

It is important that children's nurses, who are in an ideal situation to influence the health beliefs and behaviours of children, understand the development of the concept of health through the ages. In order to empower children and to encourage them to take responsibility for their own health, their views and ideas about health must be acknowledged by other people as being valid. Spend time talking to children to find out what they believe and understand about health. Then you can begin to incorporate your findings into the care that you implement.

Key Points

1. Children's ideas about the world in which they live change and develop as concepts are formed.
2. This presents children's nurses with a challenge – to understand *each* child and value his or her beliefs about health, acknowledging them as valid.
3. Cognitive development theorists suggest that beliefs about health develop in an orderly, staged manner. The approach questions how behaviour comes about.
4. Studies based on the health belief model are more interested in the action component of the concept of health and concentrates on what children believe about various aspects of health issues.
5. The importance of a variety of influences (social, cultural, environmental) on children's beliefs about health is acknowledged.

Chapter 13

Developing Strategies for Health

Introduction

Putting effective health promotion into practice presents a challenge for all professionals. Strategies need to be appropriate for the audience, stimulating, educative and empowering. This section examines some important child health issues and looks at the way in which health promotion has been implemented and evaluated.

Study activity

Take a few minutes to list the child health issues that you believe to be particularly important today. Your list may include some of the following issues:

- smoking
- obesity
- teenage pregnancy
- childhood poverty
- accidents
- skin care in the sun
- respiratory diseases such as asthma
- drug and alcohol abuse

The following chapter will explore how the health service can contribute to some of the outcomes set out in *Every Child Matters* (DfES, 2004). It will concentrate on three of the five outcomes:

- being healthy
- staying safe
- achieving economic well-being

These three outcomes were chosen because the health service is most likely to play a major role in achieving them for children and young people. The outcomes for children and young people are central to the programme of change for services and have been given a legal force as a part of the Children Act 2004. The outcomes are interdependent and demonstrate the links between educational achievement and well-being. In the document *Every Child Matters: Change for Children* (DfES, 2004) the outcomes have each been given specific aims. Some of these aims link to standards 1 to 5 of the *National Service Framework (NSF) for Children, Young People and Maternity Services* (DH, 2004a) and to targets set in the White Paper *Choosing Health: Making Healthier Choices Easier* (DH, 2004a). We will concentrate on issues highlighted in all three documents pertinent to children and young people today.

Under 'being healthy' the discussion will examine and analyse interventions related to *childhood obesity*, focusing on diet and exercise as two linked major interventions; *smoking*, focusing on interventions to protect children from other people's smoke and to prevent the uptake of smoking in young people; and *teenage sexual health*, exploring and analysing interventions.

As accidents remain the biggest cause of death in children and young people in the UK, 'staying safe' will discuss *accident prevention.* The chapter will begin by exploring the outcome *achieving economic well-being* as it examines childhood poverty and the contribution the health service can make towards increasing the life chances of children and young people in the UK.

Every Child Matters: Change for Children. Aims and Outcomes (DfES, 2004)

Being healthy means:

- being physically healthy
- being mentally and emotionally healthy
- being sexually healthy
- leading healthy lifestyles
- choosing not to take illegal drugs

Staying safe means:

- being safe from maltreatment, neglect, violence and sexual exploitation
- being safe from accidental injury and death
- being safe from bullying and discrimination
- being safe from crime and anti-social behaviour
- having security, stability and being cared for

Achieving economic well-being means:

- engaging in further education, employment or training on leaving school
- being ready for employment
- living in decent homes and sustainable communities
- having access to transport and material goods
- living in households free from low income

National Service Framework (NSF) for Children, Young People and Maternity Services (DH, 2004b)

Standards 1–5:

- Standard 1: Promoting health and well-being: identifying needs and intervening early
- Standard 2: Supporting parenting
- Standard 3: Child, young-person and family-centred services
- Standard 4: Growing up into adulthood
- Standard 5: Safeguarding and promoting the safety of children and young people

Achieving Economic Well-being

Mitigating the effects of poverty

The facts (Child Poverty Action Group; Flaherty *et al.*, 2004)

- The UK has one of the worst rates of child poverty in the industrialised world.
- Over 3.5 million children live in poverty in the UK.
- The proportion of children living in poverty has increased from 1 in 10 in 1979 to 1 in 3 in 1998. Today 28% of children in the UK live in poverty.
- The majority of poor children (52%) live in a household where at least one adult works.
- Forty-five per cent of poor children live in a single-parent household; the majority (55%) live in a household headed by a couple.
- One-fifth of the workforce, 6 million people, in the UK has a low-paid job; this has doubled since 1977.
- Since the government pledged to end child poverty in 1999, 700 000 children have been lifted out of poverty.

The effects (Gordon *et al.*, 2000)

- One in three poor children does not have three meals a day.
- One in three poor children misses out on toys, school trips and out-of-school activities.
- One in three poor children lacks adequate clothing, particularly shoes and winter coats.

Poverty and life chances (ECPC, 2005)

- Poverty shortens lives: a boy in Manchester can expect to live 7 years less than a boy from Barnet. A girl in Manchester can expect to live 6 years less than a girl in Kensington, Chelsea and Westminster.
- Poor children are born smaller. Birth weight is on average 130 g lower in children from social classes IV and V. Low birth weight is closely associated with infant death and chronic disease.
- Poverty shapes children's development. Before reaching their second birthday, children from poorer homes are more likely to demonstrate a lower attainment than children from more affluent homes.
- A child from a poor family is more likely to leave school at 16 with fewer qualifications.

Interventions

Sure Start

Sure Start is a government programme designed to offer the best start in life for every child by bringing together early education, childcare, health and family support. There are 524 local programmes working across England. Sure Start local programmes form the cornerstone of the government's drive to tackle child poverty and social exclusion. Programmes are concentrated in neighbourhoods where high proportions of children are living in poverty. Sure Start local programmes (SSLPs) are area-based interventions, with all children under 4 years of age and their families living in a prescribed area serving as 'targets' of intervention. SSLPs offer a flexible programme developed to meet the needs of the local area. Services are evidence based and a wide and varied range of services are delivered. An evaluation of SSPLs showed that they are having a limited effect on family functioning and tend to benefit families who are moderately disadvantaged rather than those who are severely disadvantaged (Sure Start, 2005). The report also showed that programmes led by health agencies had some advantages over those led by education.

Study activity

Find out about the local Sure Start programme in your area. Log on to the Web site http://www.surestart.gov.uk (accessed 30 April 2006) and find out what your local programme consists of. Do you think that Sure Start can be effective in dealing with child poverty and its effects on children and young people? Critically examine the evaluative study.

Being Healthy

Obesity

The facts

- In 2000, 27% of girls aged 2–19 years were overweight, compared with 20% of boys.

- In the same year, 7% of girls were obese compared with 5% of boys (ONS, 2004a).
- Since 1994 there has been an increase in the proportion of all children spending less than 1 hour per week on physical education, from 5% in 1994 to 18% in 1999 (MORI, 2001).
- In 1999, 11.4 hours per week were spent watching television or videos compared with 7.5 hours of physical activity (MORI, 2001).
- The number of children walking to school has declined from 63% in 1992 to 54% in 2001 (ONS, 2004a).
- Increased media attention on 'stranger danger' and bullying, increasing traffic and the availability of cheap, accessible electronic equipment has made the home an attractive environment.

The effects

- Obesity can negatively affect children's physical and mental health.
- Fatter children are much more likely to become fatter, less healthy adults.
- Children between 11 and 18 years have a poor vitamin intake (ONS, 2004a).

Obesity and life chances

- There is clear evidence that inequalities exist in the consumption of fruit and vegetables, with lower consumption in children from lower socio-economic households (ONS, 2004a).
- The combination of an unhealthy diet and sedentary lifestyle could have a significant effect on children's health and well-being, which increases the risk of disease into adulthood. This could severely affect opportunities for further education, future training and employment.

Interventions

Childhood obesity is a complex public health issue. It threatens the health of British children but also poses a threat to NHS resources. It is estimated that obesity already costs the NHS directly around £1 billion a year and costs the UK economy a further £2.3 billion indirectly (National Audit Office, 2006). Interventions aimed at prevention have included environmental changes (changes to school meals), behaviour techniques and education related to exercising and healthy eating. However, there is no evidence that this has been successful (Sahota *et al.*, 2001). The *National Service Framework for Children, Young People and Maternity Services* (DH, 2004b) states that health promotion involves every level in society and stresses the responsibility of health services and schools, as well as individuals. The European Childhood Obesity Group (ECOG) identifies six levels that could be involved in the prevention of childhood obesity: family, schools, health professionals, government, industry and the media (Flodmark *et al.*, 2004). Schools are in a good position to promote healthy eating and increased activity in children and young people, particularly with the implementation of the Healthy Schools Initiative in 2005 (DH, 2004b). School nurses will play a pivotal role in the programme and are well placed to identify and help individual children at risk of obesity. We will now look at a small, multi-agency promotion project to treat obesity in young people.

Jump Start – Daventry and Northants PCT

This is a multi-agency project developed to address the issue of excess body weight, develop a positive self-image, promote behaviour change and encourage a more healthy and active lifestyle to identified young people aged 13–16 years. Referrals are made from a number of agencies, including the young people themselves. The intervention consists of 10 weekly, 2-hour sessions for 8–10 young people, involving health education and physical activity. Each week the group walked to the local supermarket to choose a piece of fruit to eat during the session. The physical activities included taster sessions of t'ai chi and kickboxing. A 3-day residential element involved a stay at a nearby country park, where young people cooked for themselves and meals were taken together, sitting around a table, which was a new experience for many. The 3-day session included activities and workshops looking at issues important to the young people such as bullying and coping strategies. The stay also included a 'pamper session' with face packs, foot spas and relaxation, which provided opportunities to talk about body image and self-esteem. The final day concluded with a 'ready steady cook' session where the group prepared a healthy meal for themselves and their families from a few ingredients. The project was evaluated in a qualitative way. Young people were not weighed or measured at the beginning of the programme as this was felt to be negative and could further reduce self-esteem. Instead, the participants were asked to describe themselves before and after the programme. Before the programme the descriptions included 'bigger than my friends', 'not confident', 'fat', 'very sad' and 'ugly, down and conscious of my weight'. In evaluation after the programme the descriptions included 'more confident', 'happy', 'in a better place than before', and 'very happy with self, mainly inside'. The young people paid £2.00 per session and £45.00 towards the residential stay. All of the participants made new friends and now meet regularly for social occasions (Evans, 2005).

Study activity

There has been some debate about the best way to measure childhood obesity. It is now recommended that primary care trusts (PCTs) will be responsible for collecting the height and weight of all children in reception class and year 6 (National Audit Office, 2006). The data will be used to calculate the children's body mass index (BMI). Consider this action in light of the decision taken not to weigh and measure young people for the 'Jump Start' programme. Could weighing and measuring children in school lower self-esteem? Would the data collected tell us as much as the rich, qualitative data collected as part of the 'Jump Start' evaluation?

You may consider that children and young people will not feel happy about being weighed and measured in school and question whether they will have a choice about whether they are weighed or not. Just weighing obese children could lower self-esteem, particularly in the school setting, where they may be subject to ridicule and bullying. Health professionals would need to be sensitive to this situation. Taking height and weight measurements would provide a good baseline to evaluate interventions aimed at combating obesity in children and would provide a good national picture. However, it will not tell us why children are obese or how they feel about their body. It will not tell us if we are raising self-esteem or empowering children to make healthier choices. It is difficult to gather good qualitative data, such as those collected for the 'Jump Start' programme, for large groups of children. One important aspect of health promotion is that it should be accessible to all. The fact that 'Jump Start' charges for its programme could detract from its effectiveness.

Smoking

The facts

- Three out of four children are aware of cigarettes before they reach the age of 5 years, whether their parents smoke or not (ASH, 2005).
- Around 450 young people start smoking every day.
- In England the number of children who regularly smoke (defined as usually smoking at least one cigarette per week) reached 10% in 2000 (ONS, 2004a).
- In 2000, 29% of 16- to 19-year-olds in the UK were defined as current smokers (ONS, 2004a).
- Children are three times more likely to smoke if one or both of their parents smoke (ASH, 2005).
- In 2002, 18% of children aged 11–15 tried to buy cigarettes from shops. Only 23% of these found it difficult to do so (DH, 2004a).

The effects (ASH, 2005)

- Children who smoke are 2–6 times more susceptible to coughs and increased phlegm, wheeziness and shortness of breath than those who do not smoke.
- Bronchitis, pneumonia, asthma and other chronic respiratory illnesses are significantly more common in infants and children who have one or two smoking parents.
- Children of parents who smoke during the child's early life run a higher risk of cancer in adulthood.
- A clear association has been found between maternal and other passive smoking and sudden infant death syndrome (Golding, 1993).

Smoking and life chances (ASH, 2005)

- There is a clear class gradient in smokers in the UK.
- People on low incomes are more likely to start smoking at a younger age, be nicotine dependent and be exposed to other people's tobacco smoke.
- In 2003, the poorest 10% of households spent 2.43% of their income on cigarettes per week whereas the richest 10% of households spent 0.52%.
- Among the most deprived groups – including lone parents in receipt of state benefits – three out of four families smoke and spend a seventh of their disposable income on cigarettes.
- In 2000, 20% of mothers smoked throughout pregnancy and 36% of mothers classed as 'never worked' smoked throughout pregnancy

compared with only 8% of mothers in managerial and professional occupations (Hamlyn *et al.*, 2002).

- Children who smoke are three times more likely to have time off school.
- Eighty per cent of adult smokers start smoking during adolescence and continue into young adulthood.
- Fifty per cent of young adult smokers will still be smoking at 60 years of age.

Development of smoking in children and young people

Study activity

List the factors that you think may influence children to smoke. Reflect on your own experiences of childhood and the extent to which you were persuaded to smoke, or not as the case may be.

You may have listed some or all of the following factors that have been shown to influence smoking in children:

- personality – risk-taking, rebelliousness, poor self-image
- perceptions of smoking as 'fun' combined with a disregard for the long-term effects of smoking
- young people are more likely to smoke if other people at home smoke
- siblings seem to be more influential than parents
- best friends who smoke
- social activities, for example dancing, discos, parties
- teachers smoking at school
- smoking in public places where smoking is seen as the norm
- availability of tobacco – illegal sales to children under 16 persist
- advertising in magazines, films, soap operas, sports sponsorship publicity, billboards

Interventions

Considering the numerous and varied factors that influence smoking in young people, it is necessary to use a number of different approaches to:

- improve knowledge
- develop personal skills to resist social pressures
- create supportive environments within the family and within the wider community
- strengthen community action
- raise public awareness and promote non-smoking among adults
- build healthy public policy

Many projects have been or are being implemented that attempt to address some of the issues and topics mentioned above. One such initiative is 'The Teenage Health Freak' Web site – www.teenagehealthfreak.org (accessed 30 April 2006). This Web site provides a wide range of information and advice about health issues for young people, such as stress, alcohol, drugs, smoking, sex and relationships. This is an interactive Web site that includes a section answering commonly asked questions and a range of quizzes to check young people's knowledge on health issues. There is a virtual surgery, where specific questions can be put to Dr Ann. Over 1000 questions are sent to the site every month and a new question goes on the site every day. Questions that are not answered receive an automated response based on a key word search, informing young people where to look on the site and linking them to information already available on the site. Over 1 million hits were received in July 2004 with teenagers staying online for an average of 10 minutes (DH, 2004a).

Another project is Smoke Free Hampshire and Isle of Wight. This project includes a number of measures developed to take a whole area approach to smoking in and around children and young people. The aims of the project include promoting smoke-free workplaces and public areas, preventing young people from starting and helping them to stop, and promoting specialist help for smokers who want to quit. It includes:

1. Infant and primary smoke-free zones for kids:
   (a) children aged between 4 and 8 years are offered education about smoking
   (b) children negotiate a smoke-free area in their homes
   (c) children receive a smoke-free door 'wobbler'
   (d) parents can join a 'stop smoking' group
2. Secondary and colleges QUIT breakfree programme:
   (a) presentations are lively and energetic
   (b) the approach is non-patronising
   (c) the programme encourages young people to develop skills to make their own choices
   (d) the presentation is adapted to the needs of the year group
   (e) there is a QUIT Web site
3. 'Too young to die, too young to buy' – underage sales initiative
   (a) this is led by Trading Standards and supported by primary care trusts and health promotion services
   (b) it has a responsible tobacco retailers award scheme

Study activity

Look at the two interventions described above with reference to Beattie's model of health promotion on page 135. Which paradigm does each intervention fall into? What is the mode and focus of intervention for each project?

You may have discovered that the 'Teenage Health Freak' Web site falls into the 'personal counselling' paradigm. In this intervention the health promoter acts as a facilitator, providing information and support when requested by the user of the Web site. However, the questions to be answered are selected by the health professional, which could be considered health persuasion rather than health empowerment, as the professional is in control. The group of interventions in Hampshire fall into two paradigms: health persuasion and legislative action. Both are expert led. On a personal level young people and parents of children are encouraged to stop smoking or provide smoke-free areas. Collectively, legislative action is taken to control cigarette sales.

Study activity

Explore in more detail the programmes identified above. Have they been evaluated? What are the findings? In your reading you may come across other interventions – make a note of them. Try to analyse the interventions to identify what area of the curriculum they address and how they aim to contribute to a decline in teenage smoking. Look for other interventions aimed at reducing smoking in children and young people and critically evaluate their effectiveness.

Sexual health

The facts

- Young people are having sex earlier. The average age of first sexual activity for both men and women is 16, with over a quarter of young people becoming sexually active under the age of 16.
- Condom use has increased in recent years. However, young people under the age of 16 are most likely to have unprotected sex (Thistle, 2003).
- Conception in teenagers under 16 is more likely to be unintended and to end in termination than in older age groups (ONS, 2001a).

The effects

- The UK has the highest rate of teenage pregnancy in Europe and the second highest in the world (UNICEF, 2001).
- While birth rates across most of Europe fell during the 1970s, they have remained relatively stable in the UK since 1969 (Swann *et al.*, 2003).
- Around half of new HIV infections occur in young people aged 15–24 years (Thistle, 2003) (*see also* Caring for children with HIV disease p. 507).
- In 2001, 36% of all females with genital chlamydia in the UK were under the age of 20.
- In the UK between 1994 and 1999 the rate of gonorrhoea among females under 16 years doubled (ONS, 2004a).

Sexual health and life chances (ONS, 2004a)

- Teenage mothers are more likely to be from a lower socio-economic background.
- They are likely to have a lower level of education.
- They are also likely to have parents who were teenagers at the time of their conception.

The interventions

Adolescence is a transition between childhood and adulthood and as such brings with it curiosity, not least in the area of sexual activity. Young people need opportunities to gain knowledge and skills within a supportive environment so that they can make informed choices about their sexual relationships and promote their sexual health. Sexual health is about being empowered to make choices – to say no if that is what you want. It is about being free of disease but also being autonomous and respecting one's rights and those of others (Massey, 1990). One way of promoting sexual health is through sex education.

Sex education

Sex education in school remains a very controversial issue and views are polarised. The largest body of evidence comes from the US, which has suggested that sex education in schools does not delay the initiation of sexual activity or improve the use of contraception (Wight, 1996). However, the situation is unclear because there is some evidence that sex education is related to early initiation of sexual activity, some that sex education makes no difference to the initiation of sexual activity or contraception use, and some that it does delay initiation (Wight, 1996).

In Sweden, sex education has been compulsory in schools since the 1950s. Health and education have worked in partnership with shared aims and joint funding. Sexual health services have been developed in tandem with sex education in schools. The result was a country with one of the lowest teenage pregnancy and sexually transmitted infection (STI) rates and the virtual elimination of chlamydia (Jackson and Plant, 1997). However, following a cutback in the budget for sex education in schools, Sweden's teenage pregnancy rate is now rising (Jackson, 2004).

The Sex Education Forum is an independent body representing organisations involved in providing support and information to those who provide sex education to young people. The Sex Education Forum (1992) recommends that sex education should:

Sex Education Forum

http://www.ncb.org.uk/sef
Tel: 020 7843 6051

- be an integral part of the learning process for all children, young people and adults, including those with physical, learning or emotional problems
- encourage exploration of values and morals, consideration of sexuality and relationships, and the development of decision-making skills
- foster self-esteem, self-awareness, a sense of moral responsibility and the skills to resist unwanted sexual experiences

Legislation has an important bearing on the way in which sex education is carried out in schools today.

- The 1996 Education Act requires that the sex and relationships elements in the National Curriculum science orders are compulsory across all primary and secondary schools and that all schools should have sex and relationships education (SRE).
- A controversial part of this act is the right of parents to withdraw their children from sex education that is taught outside the science curriculum. This even applies to people over the age of 16 years.

Realcare baby programme

The Realcare baby programme is a part of a programme of sexual health promotion run by school nurses and health promotion advisors in Dumfries and Galloway (Currie and Lyttle, 2004). The wider health promotion project consists of a youth clinic operated within a purpose-built youth facility. The management of the facility has been given over to the young people themselves, who have decorated and furnished it to their own taste. As a part of the programme, volunteer year six pupils, trained and supported by a GP and school nurse, deliver sex education sessions to third and fourth year pupils. The programme also has a Web site that has become very popular and helps disseminate information. In the Realcare baby programme, a group of girls aged between 13 and 15 years become a 'parent' of an interactive doll for the weekend (McKie, 2005). The programme is designed to help students understand the full-time commitment and responsibility of parenting. The programme begins with a session of theory in which students learn about pregnancy, STIs, contraception and the effects of drugs and alcohol on the fetus. The babies are designed to cry and demand attention at random times during the day and night. Like real babies, they deprive the students of sleep, disrupt their social life and attract disapproving looks from members of the public. The girls are given an emergency telephone number in case they really cannot cope, but the vast majority of students do manage the weekend. On evaluation, the girls enjoyed the role-play, but found it much harder than they expected. For a full report visit http://www.think4urself.com (accessed 30 April 2006).

Contacts

Brook Advisory Centre
421 Highgate Studios
London NW5 1TL
Tel: 020 7284 6040
http://www.brook.org.uk
(accessed 22 May 2006)

Contraceptive Education Service
Helpline: 020 7837 4044

Study activity

Arrange visits to your local schools. Talk to the headmaster and school nurse about their sex education policy. Perhaps you could arrange to observe a sex education session.

Staying Safe

Accidents

The facts (CAPT, 2006)

- The number of deaths due to accidents has been steadily declining. In 1997, 2.5 million children under 15 years were taken to hospital following an accident. In 2002 the number was 2.01 million.
- Over 40% of all childhood accidents occur at home or in the garden. In 2002 nearly 480 000 children injured accidentally at home were under 5 years old.
- In 2002, almost 900 000 children under 15 visited hospitals with accidental injuries that had happened in the home.
- The largest number of non-fatal injuries happen when children fall. In 2002, 390 000 children aged under 15 were taken to hospitals following a fall. Under-fives are most at risk from falls.
- In 2002, 37 000 children were taken to hospital after a burn or scald. Scalds are more common and hot drinks are the major cause.
- Road accidents are the major cause of death and injury outside of the home. Sports, cycling and road-traffic accidents are most to blame.
- House fires cause the most accidental deaths of children in the home. Thirty-two children died in house fires in 2002.
- The second most common causes of hospital attendance in children are choking incidents or the need to remove a foreign body that has been swallowed, inhaled or stuck.

The effects (CAPT, 2006)

- In the UK in 2004, 275 children under the age of 15 died as a result of an accident. This is many more than died from cancer or meningitis.
- Accidental injury is one of the biggest causes of death in children over the age of one in the UK.
- Accidents were the most common form of death in boys of the same age, accounting for 27% of deaths (ONS, 2002a).
- The type of accidents that occur in any age are generally related to the child's developmental stage (see Table 13.1).

Accidents and life chances

- The decline in child death rates from injury in road accidents over time has been less for children in the manual social classes than for children in the non-manual social classes.
- Children in the lowest socio-economic group are over four times more likely to be killed as pedestrians than children in the highest socio-economic group.
- Significant differences in child pedestrian injury rates based on ethnicity have been identified, particularly for younger non-white children.
- On journeys to and from school, deprived children are exposed to greater risk than more affluent children as they are less likely to travel to school by car or to be accompanied by an adult.
- Restricted access to play space and proximity of housing to busy roads, compounded by a lack of supervision in younger children, appear to exacerbate road accident rates in disadvantaged areas.

Study activity

Analyse the possible reasons for social class variations in the accident rates for children. To help you do this, carry out a literature search for any research or papers that might relate to the subject.

Some of the points you may have analysed might have included:

- Children in the lower social classes are perhaps more likely to live in poor-quality housing in which they are more at risk from fire and burns, unsafe and faulty electrical wiring, injury from non-safety glass in windows, and hazardous forms of heating such as paraffin stoves.
- It is perhaps likely that children in working-class families live in a more dangerous physical environment than middle-class children, leading to the risk of injury from deserted canals, railway lines, derelict houses, factories, rubbish tips and busy streets.
- There tends to be a lack of safe areas to play.
- Poverty could lead to an inability to afford to buy expensive safety equipment, such as car restraints. It may also be that second-hand safety devices are used which may be broken and unsuitable.
- Differences in child-rearing patterns. Mothers who work and who cannot afford appropriate childcare may leave their older children

Table 13.1 Developmental factors and associated accidents

Age group	Significant development factors	Related accidents
Infants 0–1 year	Increasing locomotor skills: rolling, sitting, crawling, cruising Unsteady in locomotion Improving manipulative skills	Falls, e.g. off beds, down stairs
	Curiosity about the environment	Burns, e.g. from unguarded fires; drowning in baths, toilets; suffocation, e.g. from plastic bags
	Mouthing of objects	Aspiration and choking, e.g. from small toys
Toddlers and preschoolers	Unrestricted freedom through locomotion Unaware of dangers Undeveloped visual field – limited peripheral vision	Motor vehicle accidents, e.g. caused by running into the road, misjudging speeds
	Can open some doors and gates Explores, curious Climb up and down stairs, limited depth perception	Falls, e.g. down stairs, from windows, off climbing frames
	Helpless in water, unaware of depth	Drowning
	Able to reach heights by climbing, standing on tip-toe and/or on objects Unaware of potential sources of heat	Burns, e.g. by pulling at pan handles, flexes
	Explore objects by putting them in their mouths (becomes less likely through this age group)	Choking, poisoning
	Generally clumsy	General bodily injury
School age	Achieving social acceptance, peer pressure	Ingestion of poisonous material, e.g. glue sniffing, tablets
	May attempt hazardous feats without planning or realising consequences	Falls, e.g. from trees, walls; drowning, e.g. when playing near rivers, canals
	Becoming more independent in daily activities, e.g. walking/cycling to school Limited understanding and application of road safety measures, misinterpretation of traffic signs, speed of traffic Lack of concentration when playing, limited range of vision	Motor vehicle accidents, e.g. crossing busy roads; cycle accidents
Adolescents	Clear physical, sensory and psychomotor function Feelings of strength and confidence Increased energy that must be released through action often at the expense of common sense	Motor vehicle accidents as a passenger or driver; moped and/or motorbike accidents; sporting injuries
	Propensity for risk taking, especially among boys Access to more complex tools, objects, locations	Drowning
	Stress from peer pressure, exams, social acceptance	Suicide

Module 3

unattended after school. Possible different parental perceptions about what is safe and how much supervision children need (*see also* Child-rearing practices p. 34).

How many of these factors did you examine? Are there many studies that corroborate them or disprove them?

	Education	Engineering	Enforcement	Equity
Primary prevention				
Secondary prevention				
Tertiary prevention				

Figure 13.1 Accident prevention matrix (from Mackie, 1993; reproduced by permission of PMH Publications).

Accident prevention

To prevent accidents in childhood, interventions need to concentrate on changing children's behaviour and the environment in which they live using a multi-agency approach. Mackie (1993) suggests the creation of an accident prevention matrix (Figure 13.1) in which he identifies four types of intervention, namely:

- education – increasing knowledge of problems and their solutions
- engineering – changing the design and construction of products
- enforcement – using regulations, standards and legislation
- equity – ensuring equal access to accident prevention activities

These can occur at three levels:

- primary – actions to prevent accidents occurring, for example the fitting of stair gates
- secondary – actions to decrease the severity of an accident, for example the wearing of cycle helmets
- tertiary – actions to limit the severity of the final outcome of an accident, for example teaching first aid

These types of interventions clearly relate to some of the ideas and concepts that we have already examined in looking at theories and models. This will become evident as we move on to examine some of the initiatives that have been implemented within these four areas at various levels.

Education

The Children's Traffic Club (http://www.trafficclub.co.uk, accessed 30 April 2006), aimed at preschool children and their carers, is an example of education at the primary level. The idea originated in Scandinavia and aims to teach children and their carers about road safety, using activities designed to involve children in learning by 'doing'. The material consists of booklets, each designed by teachers and psychologists to meet the developmental needs of a specific group. Each page of the booklet concentrates on a particular aspect, giving things to do at home and things to do outside. Brightly coloured pictures encourage discussions about the road and the traffic on it. A checklist enables carers to evaluate their children's progress. Activity cards in each book give games to play, cut-out vehicles to make and pictures to colour. There are many clubs across England and in 1995 the scheme was rolled out across the whole of Scotland. In 2003, an evaluation reported a 20% increase in children holding hands when out, an 18% increase in children 'stopping' when told and a 47% reduction in children playing out in the street. Over 98% of parents felt that the club helped them teach their children road safety skills.

Study activity

How does this programme relate to the various ideas and models of health promotion discussed earlier in this module?

You may have picked up the following points:

- Education is one of the activities that contribute to health promotion (Tannahill, 1985). This particular programme is at the primary level in that it attempts to reduce the number of road accidents by influencing children's behaviour. It therefore falls into the category of preventive education. By giving information to carers it could promote empowerment and help them to feel more in control over their child's safety on the roads.
- According to Beattie's model of health promotion this programme fits into the category of health persuasion. The club was designed by professionals (teachers and psychologists) and is aimed at the individual.
- As the programme is aimed at the individual it is possible that it could be seen as 'victim blaming' in that it sees carers as being responsible for their children's safety on the roads. It is not easy to judge how the individuals' social and cultural situation can be taken into account in such a broadly aimed programme.

Study activity

Another example of the educative approach to the reduction of accidents is the Play It Safe television campaign that ran in the early 1980s and again in 1991. Find out about this campaign and its effectiveness. Analyse it in relation to theories and models.

Engineering

Educating individuals about safety, be it inside the home or outside, is insufficient by itself. Children are at the mercy of their environment and so the products and the environment must be designed with safety in mind. This involves alliances between designers, politicians, architects, health professionals, businessmen and the children and carers themselves. Improvements in product design have been numerous in recent years. It has been shown that changes in design can have positive effects on injury reduction (Towner *et al.*, 1993).

Study activity

Search for examples of this type of intervention. Some are given in the box to the right to get you started. Is there any evidence to show how effective these interventions have been in preventing accidents?

Enforcement

It is often not enough to advocate changes in design and to try to educate people about safety. Laws are needed to try to enforce measures to protect children from the dangers in our everyday lives. Legislation relevant to child safety exists in many areas, for example:

- Toy safety – the Toy (Safety) Regulations (1995) govern the design of toys made specifically for use by children.
- Safety at school – several Acts cover the safety of children at school, for example the School Standards and Framework Act 1998.
- Children in cars – in 1989 legislation was passed which made it compulsory for children under 14 to be restrained in the rear seats. New regulations for 2007 require that children under 135 cm (4 ft 5 in) use booster seats or booster cushions.

Study activity

In what other areas does legislation exist that is designed to protect children from accidental injury? How easy is it for this legislation to be upheld? Next time you are out for a drive, see how many children are properly restrained in vehicles. Have a discussion with a colleague as to why children may not be restrained adequately.

Equity

Equity is about ensuring that health promotion reaches everybody. Many of the activities related to accident prevention call for resources; for example, the fitting of smoke alarms and the purchase of safety items, many of which are expensive. This can mean that not all families can have access to these resources – particularly those that live in poverty. Several schemes have been set up that make it easier for carers to borrow or buy safety equipment at cost price. Crew and Fletcher (1995) have described one such scheme in Stockport. The Brinnington Action for Safety Equipment (BASE) scheme was set up in a socially deprived area of Stockport in January 1994. It sold safety equipment at cost price to families who would otherwise not be able to afford it. Crew and Fletcher identify the advantages of the scheme as:

- making equipment available at affordable prices
- raising awareness of safety issues
- making equipment accessible
- empowering people to have more control over the safety in their homes
- improving community networks by healthy alliances
- spreading payment over a number of weeks

Safety

Domestic engineering to improve home safety:

- prohibition of open-tread stairs
- installation of regulation safety glass
- compulsory handrails on stairs

Improved product design:

- redesign of front-loading washing machines
- warnings on plastic bags
- redesign of pen tops to prevent asphyxiation when swallowed
- coiled kettle flexes
- safety devices for use around the home
- childproof packaging

Toy safety

The DTI's guide to the regulations can be downloaded from:

http://www.dti.gov.uk/strd/toy99.pdf (accessed 30 April 2006).

You should make yourself familiar with the 'Amendment to the Seat Belt Wearing Regulations' which you can find at

http://www.dft.gov.uk/stellent/groups/dft_rdsafety/documents/page/dft_rdsafety_611256.hcsp (accessed 22 May 2006).

Module 3

Study activity

Using the accident prevention matrix in Figure 13.1, identify alternative health promotion activities for accident prevention in each of the boxes. They can be ones that you know of or ideas for activities that you have developed.

Summary

This part of the module has attempted to give you some insight into the types of health promotion activities that have been introduced for children and young people. You should now read and explore how health promotion can influence children's lives with regard to some of the other health issues that you identified earlier on.

Key Points

1. Health promotion aimed at children and young people must be appropriate to their developmental stage and to their particular needs.
2. A number of different approaches to health promotion must be used to enhance health for young people.
3. It is vital that the public become aware of the risks to the health of the young people of today so that they can be influential in bringing about change.
4. Health promotion requires a multi-agency approach – child health is everybody's business.
5. Children and young people must be allowed and encouraged to participate in health promotion programmes.
6. Health promotion activities for children and young people must promote empowerment, thus enabling them to make healthy choices about their future lifestyles.

Chapter 14

Role of Children's Nurses in Child Health Promotion

Introduction

The promotion of child health is everybody's business if children are to reach their full health potential. All professionals who have contact with children have a responsibility to identify opportunities for the implementation of health promotion activities, not only with individuals but also in the context of the community and society (*see also* The role of children's nurses as health educators p. 675 and The teacher p. 626).

Study activity

Take a few minutes to identify the professionals who come into contact with children and whom you believe have a role to play in promoting child health.

You may have listed the following:

- children's nurses – in hospital and in the community
- public health nurses (health visitors)
- school nurses
- general practitioners
- practice nurses
- social workers
- teachers
- dentists
- nursery nurses, playgroup leaders

The discussion here will concentrate on the role that nurses can play, with particular reference to children's nurses in hospital and in the community. The role of other community nurses will also be explored.

Background

The idea that nurses were potential leaders in the new health promotion movement was first proposed by Hafdan Mahler (WHO, 1986), then the WHO Director General. He recognised that nurses were in an ideal position to influence health, not only with individual patients but also on a more global level. The role of the nurse in child health has come under scrutiny recently as part of the outcomes set out in *Every Child Matters* (DfES, 2004). In order to achieve the outcomes, *Every Child Matters* focuses on four main areas:

- supporting parents and carers
- early interventions and effective protection
- accountability and integrations
- workforce reform

The proposals for workforce reform included a chief nursing officer (CNO) review of the contribution that health visitors and other nurses and midwives can make to the health and well-being of children and to protect children at risk. The CNO's review stated that nurses, midwives and health visitors play a key role in children's and young people's services and therefore have a responsibility to become the lead professional for children and families with health and development needs (DH, 2004c). The review spelt out a major change in the role of health professionals who come into contact with children and their carers and families, and a need for greater integration.

Changing Role of Nurses

Traditionally the nurse's role has been illness-orientated, with goals aimed at treating and caring for sick individuals. Little emphasis was placed on teaching about health and, when it was, the outcome was often prescriptive and expert led. Professional dominance was evident, leaving no room for patients to participate in decision making. This approach often failed to recognise the social and environmental background of the individual, and health education was often unsuccessful. The style of ward management, task-orientated and hierarchical, did not allow for trusting, supportive relationships between staff and patients to be built up. Moving from this state to one where health promotion is seen as an integral part of a nurse's role, in whatever setting, requires a shift in thinking.

Some studies have looked at how this changing role has been incorporated into the nurse's function. Bjorklund and Fridlund (1999) state that nurses' cognisance, knowledge and competence in health promotion vary widely. They suggest that nurses' demeanour and understanding of health promotion are important in enabling individuals to cope with their illness and the hospital environment, in order to develop a sense of well-being. However, Callaghan (1999) states that nurses often adopt fewer health practices than lay people. His study demonstrates an empirical link between nurses' own health beliefs and their effectiveness as health promoters. He suggests that influencing nurses about their own health behaviours can have a positive effect on their ability to empower others. Bjorklund and Fridlund (1999) state that by using health promotion programmes, such as the empowerment model, nurses can encourage individuals to adopt healthier lifestyles.

Factors Facilitating or Inhibiting Health Promotion in Hospitals

Before looking at how nurses can effectively incorporate health promotion into their work, it is useful to examine some of the factors that inhibit and facilitate health promotion (*see also* Team nursing p. 741 and Primary nursing p. 742).

Study activity

Read the activity, then close the book before you do it. Think for a few minutes about your own health promotion activities with children or adults. Then jot down all the factors that you think influence this part of your work. Which inhibit and which facilitate your health promotion? Compare your thoughts with those presented in Table 14.1.

Now let us examine in more detail why these factors might inhibit or facilitate health promotion. Lack of time is often a factor used to explain non-events. How many times have you used this excuse for not doing something? Linked to heavy workloads and staff shortages it serves as a plausible excuse. The 'care' of patients is of the utmost importance and therefore only what has to be done is done. However, promoting health should be an integral part of caring for sick children. All too often it is seen as an extra role and therefore it is argued that there is no time to 'do it'. Next time you are looking after a child see if you can incorporate some health promotion into your work. Even discussing health issues with a child or carer while you perform a dressing or monitor an infusion is health promotion.

The method of management can influence the extent to which health promotion is carried out on a ward. The traditional hierarchical structure often leaves staff feeling disempowered and unable to take decisions for themselves. If the staff are disempowered, they are not in a position to empower the child or carer. Once the structure changes

Table 14.1 Factors that inhibit and facilitate health promotion

Inhibiting factors	Facilitating factors
Lack of time	Team nursing or primary nursing
Heavy workload	Supportive ward environment
Staff shortage	Appropriate skill mix
Traditional hierarchical ward management	Provision of sufficient health promotion resources
Disempowered staff	Empowered, autonomous staff
Lack of knowledge	Enhanced knowledge
Short length of patient stay	Facilitative sisters/charge nurses

to a more democratic one, with team nursing or primary nursing, staff become more autonomous, decision making is devolved, giving a better basis for the formation of trusting, supportive relationships between the nurse and the child or carers. This, in turn, can facilitate health promotion. Even children and their carers can then be involved in promoting health by giving suggestions on how to improve the ward environment. Supportive, facilitative ward managers can encourage staff to be proactive and to identify health-promoting opportunities.

Study activity

Analyse the style of management in your own area of work. Do you feel empowered and autonomous? Identify where changes could be made to improve opportunities for health promotion by adapting the style of management.

Lack of knowledge of health promotion can lead to reluctance on the part of the nurse to engage in activities. Enhanced knowledge therefore can facilitate the nurse's role in promoting health, as can the provision of sufficient resources.

The Role in Perspective

We have identified the need for health promotion to be an integral part of the nurse's work. Achieving this will need a shift in thinking, a change in attitudes and enhanced knowledge about health-related issues. How can you begin to incorporate health promotion into your roles? Using health-promotion models can help to see where you might start.

Tannahill's (1985) model of health promotion identifies three overlapping health-promoting activities, as we have already seen:

- preventive care
- protection
- education

Beattie's (1991) model identified four categories of health promotion:

- health persuasion
- personal counselling
- community development
- legislative action

By integrating these two models it is possible to see the huge potential for health promotion within the nurse's work (*see also* Beattie's model p. 135 and Tannahill's model p. 133).

Preventive care/education–health persuasion

This is led by the expert and aimed at the individual. Here nurses are the experts and use their knowledge to provide information, give advice, teach and take action aimed at the individual in relation to the three levels of prevention (Table 14.2).

Table 14.2 Levels of preventive care/education–health persuasion

Primary	Explain the importance of protective precautions to a child and carer confined to a cubicle because of an infectious disease Give out a leaflet on immunisation to a young mother
Secondary	Carry out a routine test for phenylketonuria on a 10-day-old baby in your care Relay your concerns over a baby's developmental progress to the health visitor
Tertiary	Teach a newly diagnosed diabetic youngster about the complications of diabetes and how to avoid them

Study activity

Using Table 14.2, identify health promotion opportunities within your own field of work related to each level of prevention.

Preventive care–personal counselling

This type of health promotion is still individualistic but the children/carers are the experts. In other words, the activities are centred around what they think they need, not what the nurse *believes* they need. This can be a difficult thing for the nurse to do, as the tradition has been for the nurse to be the expert and to prescribe care. However, with the advent of family-centred care and partnerships in care, the children's nurse should be ready to take this aspect of health promotion on board. Assessment of need, negotiation, an understanding of the child's/carers' perceptions of health and empowerment are the key to making this aspect of health promotion successful.

Study activity

Using Table 14.2, explain how each situation would be different were it to be child/carer centred rather than expert led.

Preventive care/protection/education–community development

This is expert led, but this time the activities are not aimed at the individual but at communities and/or society in general. You may think that you have a minimal role to play here, but in fact children's nurses could and should work together to influence the policy makers and decision makers. To do so you need to recognise the consequences on health of political forces and policies. The issues relating to health and its promotion must be explored and understood if you are to use your skills to convince others that health is important and that it can be improved by community and social programmes. You and your colleagues, either individually or as a group, can influence health at varying levels, from within your own cohort of students to a national level. Working as a

Table 14.3 Ways of influencing health at various levels

Within your cohort	A small group of students in your cohort smoke; the rest of you decide to use your knowledge and experience to put together a package aimed at changing your colleagues' habits
Within your hospital	You notice that the food presented to the children at meal times is inappropriate and unhealthy; using your knowledge of children and healthy eating you draw up a letter to the catering manager; you get the support of the Ward Manager and other staff

group will probably hold more sway at all levels. Table 14.3 gives you some ideas of how you might achieve action.

One way of becoming politically active and of influencing health at a local level is to send your concerns, as a knowledgeable professional, to your local councillor or MP. The following activity makes you think about this.

Study activity

You decide to write to your local councillor regarding the lack of safe and appropriate play areas in your town. What main points would your letter contain and how would you back up your arguments? Who is your local councillor? You could check your answer by arranging an appointment with him/her to discuss ways of influencing action.

Preventive care/protection/education–legislative action

This type of activity is led by the client and aimed at groups or society. The people themselves identify health issues that need to be addressed and they lobby the appropriate individual/group. As a children's nurse you may well find yourself joining other members of your community in lobbying for change. While you are using your professional knowledge you are also acting as a consumer/client. Examples include joining action groups for safer packaging of dangerous products, for a reduction in the sugar content of yoghurts or for a change in the law regarding the wearing of cycle helmets by children.

The potential role of the children's nurse in health promotion has been examined and shown to be quite wide. You may find yourself working with the individual child/carer or becoming involved in a much wider arena. Whichever it is, you should be actively concerned with the empowerment of children and their carers.

Empowerment

Empowerment is a valuable tool in the fight for children's health. If, as nurses, we want to increase children's responsibility for their own health then we must make them feel more in control. How can you help to empower the children and carers you work with? (*See also* Empowerment p. 140)

- You must take into account the developmental age and stage of the child and his/her perceptions of health.
- The clinical environment needs to encourage children's participation.
- Acknowledge the important role of the child's carers and ensure that partnership in care actually happens and is not just an ideal theoretical concept.
- Acknowledge children's concerns about their health as valid.
- See children as partners in health promotion – accept that children are capable of representing themselves, making decisions about health and participating in their health care.
- Exchange medical and nursing jargon for a more mutually interactive style of communication that children can actually understand.
- Make children aware of their role and responsibilities within the healthcare system.
- Be proactive in encouraging empowerment. You should not wait for reaction from the children but should take actions to stimulate response. For example, you could allow the children to be involved in teaching each other about healthy lifestyles. Ask children what they want, rather than telling them. Involve them in the decision-making process.

Study activity

Look around the clinical area in which you are working for aspects that (a) encourage participation from children/carers and (b) dissuade participation.

Some research exists showing that children are capable of taking an active role in health and that they actually respond very well. The 'healthy schools' campaign led to empowered children making changes in schools, including recycling programmes and efforts to reduce alcohol, drug abuse and smoking (Kalnins and Love, 1982). The campaign strove to give children the opportunity to make decisions and demonstrated that children often address health issues that have been ignored by adults. Early evaluation of the Food in Schools programme (DH, 2005) shows that children can be empowered to adopt a healthy lifestyle. Perhaps you are required to undertake a research project in your studies. This may be one of the areas that you could consider.

Ideas for research

- Children's views about health in the context of everyday life
- Children's level of participation in health care
- Children's perceptions of health promotion activities
- Children's understanding of health issues

The Role of the Health Visitor (Public Health Nurse)

Health visitors have a long history of working with children and families. The concept of the health visitor originated from recognition of poor health in disadvantaged children and families. There are four core principles of health visiting:

- the search for health needs
- the stimulation of an awareness of health needs
- the facilitation of health-enhancing activities
- the influence on policies affecting health

These principles have underpinned the public health role of the health visitor. However, since the mid-1970s health visiting has become tied into child-structured child health programmes, such as screening and immunisations, which have rendered health visiting inflexible and unable to take up its public health function.

More recently, there has been a recognition of the public health role of the health visitor, with government policy driving changes in practice, but also an increasing recognition by health visitors themselves that in order to deal with inequalities they will need to return to their public health roots. The health visitor is in an ideal position to contribute to the new public health, particularly in relation to children and families.

Important aspects of the health visitor's role include:

- leading and overseeing the delivery of the child health programme
- encouraging the use of personal health guides (PHGs) as part of family health plans
- bringing a specialist public health nursing role to integrated children's services such as Sure Start, children centres and general practice
- preventative work with families and communities, to safeguard and promote the health of children and young people
- delivering measurable health outcomes, focusing on the vulnerable and disadvantaged

Personal health guides (PHGs)

As part of the new child health promotion programme set out in the *National Service Framework for Children, Young People and Maternity Services* (NSF), children's health guides will be introduced. Building on and developing the existing Child Health Record, the children's health guides will form the foundation for personal health guides for life. For more information, look on the DH Web site: http://www.dh.gov.uk (accessed 30 April 2006).

The Role of the School Nurse

School nurses play a key role in supervising the health care of children at school, liaising with teachers, parents and healthcare professionals. They play a central role, within the school health team, in promoting children's health and taking forward the government's health agenda. The school nurse can be highly influential in broadening a school's approach to health, developing trusting and confidential relationships with children. The early interventions of school nurses can be vital in the detection of disabling health problems, for example asthma and anorexia, and they play a vital role in identifying child abuse.

The importance of the school nurse was recognised by the United Kingdom Central Council (UKCC) in its 1994 strategy for post-registration education and training, meaning that school nurses take their place alongside other specialist community healthcare nurses. The review by the chief nursing officer (CNO) emphasised the key role that school nurses could play in working with children and young people, parents, carers, teaching staff and others to support the use of children's PHGs, and to provide information and support towards promoting a healthy lifestyle and the development of healthy choices and risk management (DH, 2004a). The review suggested the need to work towards having a minimum of one full-time, whole year, qualified school nurse for each cluster or group of primary schools and its secondary school, taking account of health needs and school populations (DH, 2004c). The school nurse is in an ideal position to empower children within the healthy schools campaign. In many instances school nurses have been involved with setting up support groups for teachers who want to give up smoking, promoting healthy eating policies and encouraging exercise among children.

The role of the school nurse involves:

- health promotion, normally integrated naturally into the curriculum – for example, sex education, HIV and AIDS, family planning, smoking and health, alcohol and drugs, exercise
- participating in immunisations – the use of the school nursing system to immunise children against a threatened measles epidemic in 1994 helped to flag up the importance of having a service that reaches all schoolchildren quickly, although practice nurses could be taking over the role in future
- participating in investigating communicable diseases in the school
- participating in surveillance programmes
- acting as an advocate for the children and enhancing empowerment
- fulfilling an occupational health role with education staff

Like health visitors, school nurses can play a vital role in influencing health policies that affect children in today's society, particularly at a local level but also at national level.

Study activity

Analyse changes in the school nurse structure and the effects on the service that have occurred in recent months and years.

Key Points

1. The nurse is in an ideal position to influence health on an individual and global level.
2. Health promotion needs to be an integral part of a nurse's role.
3. The factors that facilitate health promotion within the nurse's role should be identified and enhanced.
4. Empowerment is a valuable tool in the fight for children's health.
5. Health professionals working with children must be proactive in empowering children and families.

Chapter 15

Aspects of Health in Childhood

'Children are people. They grow into tomorrow only as they live today'.

John Dewey

Introduction

In order for the children's nurse to promote health and healthy behaviours in children it is important to understand some of the key issues related to such behaviours. The purpose of this part of the module is to examine some of these issues in relation to:

- nutrition
- dental hygiene
- immunisation

Nutrition

A healthy, balanced diet is a good foundation for improving the health and well-being of children. Dietary patterns in childhood and adolescence have an influence on dietary preferences and eating habits in later life. It is well known that eating habits and food preferences are firmly established during childhood and can have a major influence on health in later life. So infancy and childhood are a critical time for promoting growth and development by encouraging healthy eating (*see also* Nutrition pp. 56 and 120).

Infant Nutrition

Breast milk is the best source of nourishment in the early months of life (DH, 1994) but it must be recognised that there are mothers who, for many reasons, are unable to breastfeed. Every effort should be made to encourage mothers to breastfeed for at least 4 months, but those who choose not to should be supported in carrying out successful bottlefeeding and should not be made to feel inadequate or guilty.

Breastfeeding

In encouraging mothers to breastfeed, consideration should be given to the following points:

- Babies should be put to the breast immediately after birth.
- Breastfed babies should be left with their mothers and not removed to the nursery at night. However, it is important to be available to give support during the night. Personal experience of being left with a new baby in the middle of the night without any support served to stress the importance of this for the author.
- Breastfed babies should not normally be given complementary bottle feeds. This will only serve to lessen the supply of breast milk. Remember the more a baby sucks, the more milk will be produced. So, if the milk supply is inadequate, increase the frequency of feeding and ensure the mother's intake of fluid and nutrients is adequate.
- Additional water is rarely needed by breastfed babies, even in hot weather.
- The mother must be shown how to position the baby for feeding ensuring that the whole of the nipple and areola is taken into the baby's mouth. The baby must be facing the mothers breast (chest to chest) not looking upwards (Figure 15.1). Painful nipples can be avoided if this position is adopted.
- Allow the baby to feed on demand. This increases the supply of milk.
- It is a fallacy that breastfed babies do not get wind. Some may, and will need winding in the normal way.

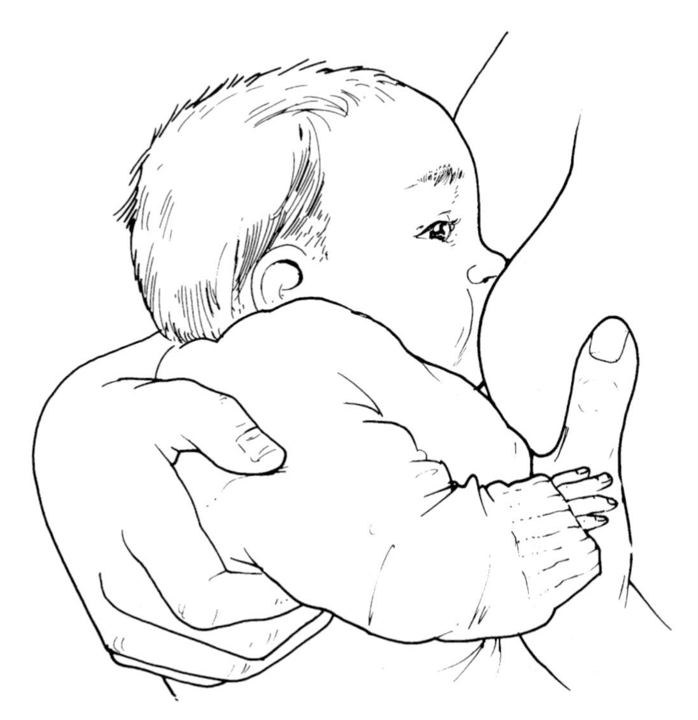

Figure 15.1 Correct position for breastfeeding.

Ten facts about breast milk

1. The fat content of breast milk increases as the breast empties.
2. The composition of breast milk is influenced by the stage of lactation.
3. The mean energy value of human milk is 60–70 kcal/100 ml.
4. The fat in human milk is well absorbed.
5. Breast milk has a lower concentration of protein than other milks with low casein.
6. A high proportion of the whey fraction contains immunologically active proteins, which enable the absorption of iron and inhibit the growth of micro-organisms.
7. Passive transfer of immunoglobulins G and M occurs during feeding and breastmilk cells produce immunoglobulin A.
8. Breast milk alone does not provide sufficient iron, copper and zinc from 6 months of age.
9. Breast milk is easily digested and contains enzymes that reduce the risk of gastrointestinal and respiratory infections (Renfrew *et al.*, 2005).
10. Breast milk possibly reduces the risk of gastro-intestinal disorders (for example Crohn's and coeliac disease).

Further reading

Royal College of Midwives (2001) *Successful Breastfeeding*, 3rd edn. Edinburgh: Churchill Livingstone.

This small book contains a wealth of well-researched information and many excellent references for further reading. It would be useful to have it on your ward.

Useful addresses

La LECHE League (GB)
Helpline 0845 120 2918
http://www.laleche.org.uk (accessed 30 April 2006).

National Childbirth Trust
Alexandra House, Oldham Terrace, Acton, London W3 6NH
Tel: 0870 7703236. Enquiry Line: 0870 444 8707
http://www.nctpregnancyandbabycare.com (accessed 30 April 2006).

Association of Breastfeeding Mothers
Helpline 0870 401 7711
http://www.abm.me.uk (accessed 30 April 2006).

Scientific Advisory Committee on Nutrition
http://www.sacn.gov.uk (accessed 22 May 2006).

Department of Health
http://www.dh.gov.uk/infantfeeding (accessed 30 April 2006).

NHS
http://www.breastfeeding.nhs.uk (accessed 30 April 2006).

UNICEF
http://www.unicef.org/programme/breastfeeding/baby/htm (accessed 30 April 2006).

WHO
http://www.who.int/topics/breastfeeding/en/ (accessed 30 April 2006).

- Support for breastfeeding mothers is always available from the National Childbirth Trust, the La Leche League (GB) and the Association of Breastfeeding Mothers.

Bottlefeeding

Infants who are not breastfed should be given infant formula or follow-on milk, although follow-on milk is not recommended for the first 6 months (DH, 1994). The range of available infant formulas is wide, with the choice of dry powder or ready-made bottles/cartons.

In teaching mothers about bottlefeeding and supporting them, consideration should be given to the following points:

- The preparation of infant formulas must be explained, with special emphasis on the importance of hygiene. Bottles and teats must be washed carefully to remove all traces of milk before being immersed in a sterilising solution. If salt is used to wash the teats, care must be taken to ensure that all traces of salt are removed in order to avoid hypernatraemia.
- Enough bottlefeeds for 24 hours can be made up in one batch if they are cooled immediately and placed in the refrigerator.
- Once heated, milk must not be reheated but should be discarded.
- In making up the feeds care must be taken to ensure the correct amount of boiled water is added to the appropriate amount of powder. The general rule is one scoop of formula to 1 fl oz of water. If the concentration of formula is too high, hypernatraemia can result. A weak solution will lead to failure to thrive.

Ten facts about infant formulas

1. Guidelines for the composition of infant formulas were agreed in 1991 in a European Commission Directive.
2. Alpha-linoleic acid, an essential fatty acid, is added to infant formulas in the UK.
3. Absorption of some minerals from infant formula is less efficient than from human milk, therefore levels of iron, zinc and vitamin D are increased to overcome poor bioavailability.
4. The carbohydrate most commonly used is lactose.
5. Whey-dominant formulas have a whey : casein ratio similar to that of human milk. Examples include Cow & Gate Premium, Farley's First Milk, Milupa Aptamil and SMA Gold.
6. In casein-dominant formulas the whey : casein ratio is approximately the same as in cow's milk. Examples include Cow & Gate Plus, Milupa Milumil and SMA White.
7. Infant formulas provide a satisfactory sole source of nutrients in the first 4–6 months of life.
8. Follow-on milks generally have higher concentrations of protein than infant formulas and are therefore not suitable for the younger infant.
9. Soya infant formula can be used in cases of cow's milk protein allergy, lactose intolerance, and for vegan/vegetarian diets. Examples include Cow & Gate Infasoy, Mead Johnson Prosbee, SMA Wysoy.
10. Lactose-free formulas are available and may be used in a variety of conditions, for example gastro-enteritis. Examples include Mead Johnson Nutramigen.

- Freshly boiled water should be used. Using water that has been repeatedly boiled can result in an over-concentration of minerals.
- Babies must never be left alone with a bottle because of the danger of choking. Encourage mothers to hold babies for bottlefeeding just as they would if they were breastfeeding.
- Bottles of milk should not be warmed in a microwave oven. The distribution of heat is uneven and the baby can be severely burnt by the milk.
- When feeding with a bottle ensure that the teat remains full of milk to avoid the ingestion of too much air.
- Babies will probably need winding during feeds, although this will depend very much on the individual baby. Simply sitting the baby up and gently massaging the back is generally all that is needed. Avoid banging the baby's back; this is not necessary.

The Department of Health recommendations on feeding infants

- Breast milk is the best form of nutrition for infants.
- Exclusive breastfeeding is recommended for the first 26 weeks of an infant's life.
- Six months is the recommended age for the introduction of solid food for infants.
- Breastfeeding (and/or) breast milk supplements should continue beyond the first 6 months, along with appropriate types and amounts of solid foods.

(Infant Feeding Recommendations, DH, 2003)

Weaning

Weaning is defined by the DH (1994) as the 'process of expanding the diet to include food and drinks other than breast milk or infant formula'. It enables infants to meet their changing nutritional requirements at a time of rapid growth. *Guidelines for Infant Feeding* (DH, 2002) recommend that weaning should begin at 6 months but no earlier than 4 months. However, introduction to solid foods should not be delayed any longer than 6 months as, by this time, the infant's nutritional requirements can no longer be met by milk alone, which gives

Weaning

Start weaning no earlier than 4 months because before this age:

- babies have poor head control and effective positioning for feeding is difficult
- babies cannot easily form a bolus to move solid food from the front of the mouth to the back
- limited renal function means that water is not conserved efficiently and large solute concentrations cannot be dealt with
- the secretion of intestinal and pancreatic enzymes is not fully developed in the young infant

Weaning

Start weaning no later than 6 months because after this time:

- it may be difficult to teach the baby to chew lumpy foods
- the baby is more likely to refuse foods
- the baby will become underweight and fail to thrive as nutritional needs will not be met

insufficient energy, protein and vitamins A and D. The infant's iron stores also become depleted at this age and additional sources are needed. By the age of 6 months infants have developed sufficient neuromuscular coordination to allow them to eat solid food and the renal and digestive systems have matured enough to cope with a varied diet.

The 1994 Coma Report (DH, 1994) made several recommendations regarding the content of the weaning diet:

- The provision of adequate dietary energy is essential to ensure normal growth and development – Table 15.1.
- An adequate intake of protein with a proper balance of amino acids is essential – Table 15.2.
- As fat provides the major energy source for infants, any reduction is likely to give rise to a diet of lower energy density. It is therefore advised that fat reduction should not be considered for children under 2 years. Semi-skimmed milk can be given after 2 years and skimmed milk after the age of 5 years. The report recommends a flexible approach to the reduction of fat between the ages of 2 and 5 years.
- The intake of non-milk extrinsic sugars (added sugars, sugars in fruit juices and honey) should contribute no more than about 10% of total dietary energy. Sugars provide energy but make no other contribution to nutritional needs.
- If energy intake is adequate the amount of starch in the diet should increase as fat decreases.
- Adequate intakes of iron and calcium are essential. The report acknowledges that iron deficiency is the most commonly reported

Table 15.1 Energy requirements for children aged 0–24 months (adapted from DH, 1994)

Age (months)	Energy intake per kg body weight (kJ (kcal)/kg/day)
1	480 (115)
3	420 (100)
6	400 (95)
9	400 (95)
12	400 (95)
18	400 (95)
24	400 (95)

Table 15.2 Recommended protein intake for children aged 0–24 months (adapted from DH, 1994)

Age (months)	Protein intake (g/day)
0–3	12.5
4–6	12.7
7–9	13.7
10–12	14.9
13–24	14.5

nutritional disorder during early childhood in the UK and other countries. Iron deficiency anaemia is associated with psychomotor delay, apathy and reduced exercise capacity.

- Adequate vitamin intake should be encouraged through a varied diet and moderate exposure to summer sunlight. Vitamin A and D supplements should be given:
  - from 6 months of age where breast milk is the main drink
  - to bottlefed babies if intake is less than 500 ml per day
  - to bottlefed babies on cow's milk
  - to all infants aged 1–5 years unless it is certain that vitamin status is adequate
  - milk or water should constitute the majority of drinks given

Table 15.3 gives a guide to the foods to use during weaning. It must be remembered that each child is an individual and the diet will need to be flexible in order to meet nutritional requirements as well as any cultural, religious beliefs.

Practical hints for successful weaning

- Be flexible, patient and calm. Allow infants to progress at their own rate in a relaxed and happy environment. Do not force an infant to eat solids but be encouraging and supportive. Do not be afraid to backtrack. Pick meal times when other members of the family are not demanding attention. Introduce one new food at a time. Avoid undue praise or punishment during the weaning process. Above all try to make meal times enjoyable.
- Show tolerance. Accept that infants are individuals and do not impose your tastes on them. Do not force infants (or children) to 'eat up'. Accept food refusal without fuss or try to ignore it. Do not expect a high standard of table manners. Instead prepare the eating area appropriately – for example, put a plastic cloth under the high chair. Try to tolerate the mess and spills but gently encourage good eating habits as time progresses.
- Use appropriate utensils. Ensure that the infant is sitting comfortably in a chair (restrained) or on your knee. Use plastic teaspoons. Offer finger foods. Use cups with lids. Do not add solid foods to bottles. Never leave an infant alone at mealtimes.
- Offer variety from the four main food groups (in a texture appropriate for the infant's age): meat, fish, eggs, beans, pulses; bread, cereals, rice, pasta; fruit and vegetables; milk and milk products. Giving a range of foods, either home prepared or commercially produced, broadens the infant's experience of tastes and will encourage acceptance of a varied diet.

Study activity

Making use of the above points, plan a day's menu for:

- a 5-month-old infant
- an 11-month-old infant whose parents wish to bring him up as a vegetarian
- a 2-year-old toddler

Religious, cultural beliefs and diet

Judaism

- avoidance of pork, shellfish
- foods prepared by special 'kosher' methods
- meat products kept separate from dairy products at all stages of preparation, eating and cleaning up

Islam

- avoidance of pork
- foods either 'haram' (unlawful) or 'halal' (lawful).
- food prepared by 'halal' methods
- Ramadan – month-long abstinence from food during daylight hours – not practised by children

Hinduism

- may be strict lactovegetarians
- pork (unclean) and meat from cows (sacred) avoided
- milk and ghee (clarified butter) sacred foods
- dairy products usually important part of diet

Rastafarianism

- variable dietary restrictions
- may follow vegan diets
- preserved foods are chemical and avoided

Sikhism

- sometimes vegetarians
- pork and beef usually avoided
- meat if eaten must NOT have been bled but killed by stunning 'jhatka'

Table 15.3 A guide to foods during weaning (adapted from DH, 1994)

Food	4–6 months	6–9 months	9–12 months	After 1 year
Milk	Breast or infant formula	Breastmilk, infant formula or follow-on milk	Breast milk, infant milks	Whole milk as a drink
Dairy products and substitutes	Cow's milk in weaning, e.g. yoghurt, custard	Hard cheese cubed or grated as finger food		Soft cheese; low fat milk in cooking
Starchy foods	Low fibre smooth cereals Mash or pureed starchy vegetables	Two to three servings daily Introduce wholemeal bread and cereals Foods with a 'lumpier' texture Toast as finger food	Three to four servings daily Encourage wholemeal foods Discourage biscuits and cakes Starchy foods can be normal adult texture	Minimum of four servings daily At least one serving at each mealtime Discourage high fat starchy foods, e.g. crisps and pastry
Vegetables and fruit	Smoothly pureed soft cooked vegetables and fruit	Two servings daily Introduce raw soft fruit, e.g. bananas, melon, tomato Cooked vegetables can be coarser	Three to four servings daily Encourage lightly cooked or raw fruit and vegetables Unsweetened orange juice with meals	Minimum of four servings daily Foods can be adult texture though some fibrous foods may be difficult, e.g. celery
Meat and meat alternatives	Soft cooked meat/pulses Add no salt or sugar to food during cooking or after	One serving daily Soft cooked minced or pureed meat/fish/pulses	Minimum of one serving daily from animal source OR two from vegetable source In vegetarian diet use mixture of vegetables and starchy foods, e.g. macaroni cheese	Minimum of one serving daily or two from vegetable source Encourage low fat meat and oily fish (sardine, herring) Liver pâté after 1 year
Occasional foods	Low sugar desserts, e.g. yoghurts Avoid high salt foods	Encourage savoury rather than sweet foods Fruit juice not necessary; try to restrict to mealtimes – offer water or milk	Moderate amounts of butter, margarine Small amounts of jam on bread Limit salty foods	Limit crisps and savoury snacks Give bread, fruit between meals Do not add sugar to drinks Limit soft drinks to mealtimes Encourage pattern of three meals a day Discourage frequent snacking on fatty or sugary foods

Healthy eating during childhood

Children's diets are influenced by many factors including their attitude to food, knowledge and understanding of food and nutrition, parental attitudes to eating and media advertising. If they are to develop healthy eating habits in adulthood, they must be given the opportunity to learn and explore the requirements of a healthy diet. The general advice to young people regarding their diet should be:

- enjoy your food
- eat a variety of different foods, including starchy foods; meat/alternatives, fish and eggs; fruit and vegetables; dairy products
- eat the right amount to be healthy
- do not eat too much fat
- do not eat sugary foods too often
- eat plenty of foods rich in fibre and starch
- meals should be based on fibre-rich starchy foods: bread, pasta, potatoes, rice
- ensure that there are sufficient minerals and vitamins in your food
- girls particularly need good sources of iron and calcium (HEA, 1995)

Dental Hygiene

Recent reports show a continued improvement, with dramatic falls in the prevalence of dental caries (ONS, 2004a). The improvement was particularly strong among 15-year-olds, with the proportion having decay into dentine falling from 42% in 1983 to 13% in 2003. It also showed a fall in the proportion of 5- and 8-year-olds with filled primary teeth. However, dental caries is preventable and children's nurses are in an ideal position to give advice and education regarding dental health, in hospital or in the community. Dental caries can be prevented by:

- A diet low in sugar. It has been shown that the frequency of consumption of non-milk extrinsic sugars is the most important factor in the development of dental disease (HEA, 1982). Every time that sugar is consumed, acid is generated in dental plaque within seconds. Within 1–2 minutes the pH has fallen, allowing enamel dissolution to occur. The return to a neutral pH can take from 20 minutes to 2 hours. Therefore if consumption of sugars occurs frequently, there is no time for the plaque pH to recover. It is therefore advisable to limit sugary foods and drinks to mealtimes and to avoid sugary snacks in between meals. Children should be encouraged to quench their thirst with water (*see also* Dental health p. 119).
- Effective teeth cleaning. Teeth are at risk of dental decay as soon as they appear. Plaque can form readily, covering the teeth with a sticky bacterial coating. The first tooth generally appears between 6 and 9 months and it is vital that effective tooth cleaning begins straight away. The role of toothbrushing is to remove the plaque. In the young infant this can be done with special toothbrushes and a pea-sized amount of fluoride toothpaste. This can easily be carried out by holding the infant on the lap with his back resting on the carer's chest. Hold the chin gently with one hand and brush with the other.

Approximate ages at which teeth emerge

Deciduous teeth

- incisors 6–9 months
- canines 16–18 months
- 1st molars 12–14 months
- 2nd molars 20–30 months

Permanent teeth

- lower incisors 6–8 years
- upper incisors 7–9 years
- lower canines 9–10 years
- upper canines 11–12 years
- premolars 9–12 years
- 1st molar 6–7 years
- 2nd molar 11–13 years
- 3rd molars 17–21 years

Dental health resources

British Dental Health Association
Eastlands Court, St Peter's Road, Rugby, Warwickshire CV21 3QP
Tel: 01788 546365
http://www.bda-dentistry.org.uk (accessed 30 April 2006).

Brochures:
Caring For Your Teeth and Gums
Don't Be Afraid
Your Guide To a Better Smile

Leaflets:
Dental Care for Mother and Baby
Preventive Care and Oral Hygiene
Visiting the Dentist

General Dental Council
37 Wimpole Street, London W1M 8DQ
Tel: 020 7887 3800
http://www.gdc-uk.org (accessed 30 April 2006).

Leaflets:
Diet and your Child's Teeth
Healthy Mouth, Happy Smile
Danger Mouse, Tooth Sleuth

Packs:
Dental Discovery Kit Teaching Pack for 12–15 Year Olds

Wallcharts and posters

Every surface of every tooth must be brushed with special attention to the area between the tooth and gums. Children generally need assistance with brushing until about 8 years of age. Brushing should be done twice a day but particularly at night.

- The use of fluoride. Fluoride is a mineral that inhibits the demineralisation of enamel and can strengthen teeth against caries, making them more resistance to acid attack. Fluoride is present in drinking water in some areas. Fluoride can also be used topically with fluoride toothpaste or can be given as a supplement in the form of drops or tablets. However, these supplements must be taken daily from the age of about 6 months through to adolescence and compliance with this may be difficult. The amount of supplement given will depend on the amount of fluoride in the water supply and advice should always be sought from the dentist. If the local water supply is already well fluoridated, overdosage of fluoride can occur, giving rise to staining of the teeth.
- Encouraging regular dental attendance. Babies can be registered with a dentist from birth. Mothers should be encouraged to take babies and children with them when they attend for check-ups to help build up confidence and trust in the dentist. Regular attendance also makes the detection of problems easier.

Study activity

Find out the level of fluoride in your local water supply by contacting the relevant water authority. Do children in your area need fluoride supplements?

Immunisation

In 1994, immunisation uptake rates were at an all-time high and accompanied by an overall reduction in the incidence of infectious diseases. However, as infectious diseases become less prevalent carers may become more concerned with the possible associated risks of immunisation. These may appear to be greater than the risk of contracting a relatively rare disease. If this occurs, immunisation uptake rates may well fall with a subsequent increase in the incidence of diseases again. It is essential, therefore, that children's nurses are able to contribute to the maintenance of the uptake rates by giving accurate and knowledgeable information to parents. Immunisations are available against nine infectious diseases:

- diphtheria
- measles
- polio
- tetanus
- pertussis
- rubella
- mumps
- *Haemophilus influenzae* type B infections (Hib)
- pneumococcal meningitis

Immunisation against tuberculosis depends on local policy (*see also* Immunisation p. 122 and Immunisation schedule p. 512).

Answering questions commonly asked by parents

- *What is the possibility of my child having a severe reaction to immunisation?* Severe reactions are rare. Between 1997 and 2003 there were 130 reports of severe reaction following immunisation. No deaths from reactions were reported. In that time 117 million doses of all vaccines were supplied to hospitals and GPs. This rate of around one in a million doses is similar to that reported in other countries (DH, 2006a).
- *My child is adopted and we do not know his family history – should we have him vaccinated?* Yes, he should receive all vaccinations appropriate to his age unless there is reason to believe that he may be HIV positive. In this case contact the adoption agency.
- *I had a bad reaction to my vaccinations – should my daughter still be vaccinated?* There is no real evidence to suggest that reactions run in families, therefore you should go ahead with vaccination.
- *My child has had an infectious disease – should he still be vaccinated against it?* There is no harm in him being vaccinated against a disease that he has already had.
- *My baby was born prematurely – should the timing of his vaccinations be altered to compensate?* No. The timing of vaccinations starts from birth, not the expected date of delivery.

Contraindications

There are very few contraindications to vaccination and it is important to dispel any myths that surround this subject. The true contraindications are:

- Acute illness with fever or systemic upset. Vaccination should be postponed until the child is well. Minor illness without a fever is *not* a reason for withholding vaccination.
- Children who have previously had an anaphylactic shock should only be given vaccinations under hospital supervision, if at all. Minor allergic reactions to eggs or antibiotics are *not* relevant.
- If children are immunocompromised or are HIV positive, they should be referred to their consultant for advice.
- Household contacts of children who are immunosuppressed should be given inactivated polio vaccine instead of the oral vaccine because the former is not transmissible.
- Pertussis vaccine should not be given to children who have had a severe systemic or local reaction to a previous dose.
- Children with cerebral damage, idiopathic epilepsy or convulsions have an increased risk of a febrile convulsion after vaccination against pertussis, measles, mumps and rubella. However, they are not at any greater risk for severe reactions and should be vaccinated.

Vaccinations should not be withheld due to asthma, eczema, hay fever, snuffles, failure to thrive, cerebral palsy, Down's syndrome or history of neonatal jaundice (DH, 2006b).

Key Points

1. Children's nurses have a major role to play in promoting healthy behaviours in children and as such need to keep abreast of issues relating to health.
2. Dietary habits formed in childhood may be a factor contributing to the onset of diet-related disease in adulthood.
3. The message to carers and children about healthy eating should be 'eat a variety of foodstuffs from the four main groups, cut down on sugar and fat and ensure adequate intakes of fibre, starch and vitamins'.
4. Although the dental health of children is improving, many children have experienced dental decay by the time they are 15.
5. Dental caries can be prevented by:
   - low-sugar diet
   - effective teeth cleaning
   - fluoridation
   - regular dental checks.
6. Children's nurses play a major role in maintaining high uptake rates of vaccinations by giving accurate and informed advice to parents and carers.

References

Acheson, D. (1991) The health divide. *Guardian*, 13 September 1991.

ASH (2005) *Young People and Smoking.* Factsheet No. 3. http://www.ash.org.uk/html/factsheets/html/fact03.html (accessed 22 May 2006).

Barnardo's (1997) Children in care left with no qualifications. http://www.literacytrust.org.uk/Database/housing.html#The%20Real (accessed 22 May 2006).

Beattie, A. (1991) Knowledge and control in health promotion: a test case for social policy and social theory. In Gabe, J., Calnan, M. and Bury, M. (eds), *The Sociology of the Health Service.* London: Routledge.

Bibace, R. and **Walsh, M. E.** (1980) Children's concepts of illness. *Pediatrics*, **66**, 912–917.

Bjorklund, M. and **Fridlund, B.** (1999) Cancer patients' experience of nurse behaviour and health promotion activities: a critical incident analysis. *The European Journal of Cancer Care*, **8**, 204–212.

Blair, T. (1999) *End Child Poverty.* http://www.ecpc.org.uk.

Bornam, R. and **Prior, G.** (1999) *Health Survey for England: The Health of Young People '95–97.* London: TSO. http://www.archive.official-documents.co.uk/document/doh/survey97/hs00.htm (accessed 22 May 2006).

Boruchovitch, E. and **Mednick, B. R.** (1997) Cross-cultural differences in children's concepts of illness. *Revista de Saude Publica*, **31** (5), 448–456.

Britton, M. (1989) Mortality and geography. *Population Trends*, **56**, 16–23.

Callaghan, P. (1999) Health beliefs and their influence on United Kingdom nurses' health-related behaviour. *Journal of Advanced Nursing*, **29** (1), 28–35.

CAPT (Child Accident Prevention Trust) (2006) *Child Accident Factsheets.* http://www.capt.org.uk/FAQ/default.htm (accessed 22 May 2004).

Crew, K. and **Fletcher, J.** (1995) Empowering parents to prevent childhood accidents. *Health Visitor*, **68** (7), 291.

Currie, J. and **Lyttle, P.** (2004) Teenage sexual health promotion: the Dumfries and Galloway perspective. *Community Practitioner*, **77** (12), 450–452.

Cystic Fibrosis Trust (2006) *What is Cystic Fibrosis?* http://www.cftrust.org.uk/scope/page/view.go?layout=cftrust&pageid=28 (accessed 30 April 2006).

Davey Smith, G., *et al.* (2000) Height and risk of death among men and women: aetiological implications of associations with cardiorespiratory disease and cancer mortality. *Journal of Epidemiology and Community Health*, **54**, 97–103.

DfES (2003) *Every Child Matters: Green Paper.* Nottingham: DfES Publications. http://www.everychildmatters.gov.uk/_files/EBE7EEAC90382663E0D5BBF24C99A7AC.pdf (accessed 22 May 2006).

DfES (2004) *Every Child Matters: Change for Children.* Nottingham: DfES Publications. http://www.everychildmatters.gov.uk/_files/F9E3F941DC8D4580539EE4C743E9371D.pdf (accessed 22 May 2006).

DH (1994) *Weaning and the Weaning Diet: Report of the Working Group on the Weaning Diet of the Committee on Medical Aspects of Food Policy.* London: HMSO.

DH (2002) *Infant Feeding 2000.* London: The Stationery Office. http://www.dh.gov.uk/PublicationsAndStatistics/Publications/PublicationsStatistics/PublicationsStatisticsArticle/fs/en?CONTENT_ID=4079223&chk=UpJ4Sr (accessed 22 May 2006).

DH (2004a) *Choosing Health: Making Healthier Choices Easier.* London: The Stationery Office. http://www.dh.gov.uk/PublicationsAndStatistics/Publications/PublicationsPolicyAndGuidance/PublicationsPolicyAndGuidanceArticle/fs/en?CONTENT_ID=4094550&chk=aN5Cor (accessed 22 May 2006).

DH (2004b) *National Service Framework for Children, Young People and Maternity Services.* London: The Stationery Office. http://www.dh.gov.uk/PolicyAndGuidance/HealthAndSocialCareTopics/ChildrenServices/ChildrenServicesInformation/fs/en (accessed 22 May 2006).

DH (2004c) *Review of the Nursing, Midwifery and Health Visiting Contribution to Vulnerable Children and Young People.* London: HMSO. http://www.dh.gov.uk/PublicationsAndStatistics/Publications/PublicationsPolicyAndGuidance/PublicationsPolicyAndGuidanceArticle/fs/en?CONTENT_ID=4086949&chk=4jYqAb (accessed 22 May 2006).

DH (2005) *Food In Schools Programme.* www.dh.gov.uk/PolicyAndGuidance/HealthAndSocialCareTopics/FoodInSchools/fs/en (accessed 30 April 2006).

DH (2006a) *Planned Changes to the Routine Childhood Immunisation Programme.* Press release, 8 February 2006. http://www.dh.gov.uk/PublicationsAndStatistics/LettersAndCirculars/DearColleagueLetters/DearColleagueLettersArticle/fs/en?CONTENT_ID=4128120&chk=pbquLY (accessed 22 May 2006).

DH (2006b) *Immunisation against Infectious Diseases (The Green Book).* London: HMSO.

Dielman, T. E., Leech, S. L., Becker, M. H., Rosenstock, I. M. and **Horvath, W. J.** (1980) Dimensions of children's health beliefs. *Health Education Quarterly,* **7**, 219–238.

Downie, R. S., Fyfe, C. and **Tannahill, A.** (1990) *Health Promotion Models and Values.* Oxford: Oxford University Press.

ECPC (End Child Poverty Campaign) (2005) *Children and Poverty.* London: ECPC.

Eiser, C., Patterson, P. and **Eiser, J. R.** (1983) Children's knowledge of health and illness: implications for health education. *Child Care, Health and Development,* **9** (5), 285–292.

Evans, S. (2005) *Jump Start: Evaluation Report.* Daventry: Daventry and South Northants PCT.

Fitzpatrick, J. and **Cooper, N.** (2001) *Patterns and Trends in Stillbirths and Infant Mortality, Geographic Variations in Health.* Decennial supplement DS16. http://www.statistics.gov.uk/downloads/theme_health/DS16/DS16_cap06.pdf (accessed 22 May 2006).

Flaherty, J., Veit-Wilson, J. and **Dornan, P.** (2004) *Poverty: The Facts,* 5th edn. London: Child Poverty Action Group.

Flodmark, C. E., Lissau, I., Moreno, L. A. and **Widhalm, K.** (2004) New insights into the field of children and adolescents' obesity: the European perspective. *International Journal of Obesity,* **28** (10), 1189–1196.

French, J. and **Blair-Stevens, C.** (2005) *Social Marketing, Pocket Guide.* National Social Marketing Centre for Excellence. London: Department of Health and National Consumer Council. http://www.nsms.org.uk/images/CoreFiles/NSMCNationalSocialMarketingPOCKETGUIDEDec2005.pdf (accessed 22 May 2006).

Gaudion, C. (1997) Children's knowledge of their internal anatomy. *Paediatric Nursing,* **9** (5), 14–17.

Gibson, C. (1991) A concept analysis of empowerment. *Journal of Advanced Nursing,* **16**, 354–361.

Gochman, D. S. (1970) Children's perceptions of vulnerability to illness and accidents. *Public Health Reports,* **85**, 69–73.

Gochman, D. S. (1971a) Some correlates of children's health beliefs and potential health behaviour. *Journal of Health and Social Behaviour,* **12**, 148–154.

Gochman, D. S. (1971b) Children's perceptions of vulnerability to illness and accidents: a replication, extension and refinement. *HSMHA Health Report,* **86**, 247–252.

Golding, J. (1993) Parental smoking and sudden infant death syndrome. In Chief Medical Officers Expert Group (eds), *The Sleeping Position of Infants and Cot Death.* London: HMSO.

Gordon, D., *et al.* (2000) *Poverty and Social Exclusion in Britain.* Ref. 930. London: Joseph Rowntree. Available at http://www.jrf.org.uk/bookshop/details.asp?pubID=302 (accessed 20 April 2007).

Hamlyn, B., Brooker, S., Oleinkiova, K. and **Wands, S.** (2002) *Infant Feeding Survey 2000.* London: The Stationery Office.

Hanna, K. M. (1989) The meaning of health for graduate nursing students. *Journal of Nursing Education,* **28** (8), 372–376.

Harper, S. (2003) *Changing Families as Societies Age.* Oxford: Oxford Institute of Aging.

HEA (1982) *The Scientific Basis of Dental Health Education,* 3rd edn. London: Health Education Authority.

HEA (1995) *Diet and Health in School Age Children.* London: Health Education Authority.

Health Statistics Quarterly (1999) Office for National Statistics. Autumn 1999. http://www.statistics.gov.uk/downloads/theme_health/HSQ3Book.pdf (accessed 22 May 2006).

Health Statistics Quarterly (2003) Office for National Statistics Winter 2003. http://www.statistics.gov.uk/downloads/theme_health/HSQ20.pdf (accessed 22 May 2006).

HM Treasury (2004) *Child Poverty Review.* http://www.hm-treasury.gov.uk/spending_review/spend_sr04/associated_documents/spending_sr04_childpoverty.cfm (accessed 22 May 2006).

Jackson, P. (2004) Sexual health and young people. *Community Practitioner,* **77** (8), 287–288.

Jackson, P. and **Plant, Z.** (1997) Mock sexual health clinics for school pupils. *Health Education,* **1**, 6–18.

Jarvis, S.,Towner, E. and **Walsh, S.** (1995) Accidents. In Botting, B. (ed.), *The Health of our Children.* OPCS decennial supplement. London: HMSO.

Kalnins, I. and **Love, R.** (1982) Children's concepts of health and illness – and implications for health education: an overview. *Health Education Quarterly*, **9**, 104–115.

Kalnins, I., McQueen, D. D., Backett, K. C., Curtice, L. and **Currie, C. E.** (1994) Children, empowerment and health promotion: some new directions in research and practice. In Gott and Maloney (eds), *Child Health – A Reader*. Oxford: Radcliffe Medical Press.

King, I. M. (1981) *A Theory for Nursing: Systems, Concepts, Processes*. New York: Wiley.

Lewis, C. E. and **Lewis, M. A.** (1974) The impact of television commercials on health-related beliefs and behaviours of children. *Pediatrics*, **53**, 431–435.

Lewis, M. and **Lewis, C.** (1990) Consequences of empowering children to care for themselves. *Pediatrician*, **17**, 63–76.

Macdonald, H., Henderson, R. and **Oates, K.** (2004) Low uptake of immunisation: contributing factors. *Community Practitioner*, **77** (3), 93–100.

Mackie, P. (1993) Health of the nation targets: 1. Reducing accidents locally. *Professional Care of Mother and Child*, April, 105–109.

Massey, D. (1990) School sex education: knitting without a pattern? *Health Education Journal*, **49**, 134–142.

Matheson, J. and **Babb, P.** (2002) Social Trends. No. 32. http://www.statistics.gov.uk/downloads/theme_social/Social_Trends32/Social_Trends32.pdf.

McEwing, G. (1996) Children's understanding of their internal body parts. *British Journal of Nursing*, **5** (7), 423–429.

McKie, K. (2005) Realcare Baby: Evaluation of the Programme, 2005. http://www.think4urself.com/pro_realcareeval05.php (accessed 22 May 2006).

MORI (2001) *Young People and Sport in England*. National Survey commissioned by Sport England. London: MORI. http://www.sportengland.org/downloads/Young-People-and-Sport-2002-report.pdf (accessed 22 May 2006).

Myant, K. and **Williams, J. M.** (2005) Children's concepts of health and illness: understanding of contagious illnesses, non-contagious illnesses and injuries. *Journal of Health Pyschology*, **10** (6), 805–819.

Natapoff, J. N. (1982) A developmental analysis of children's ideas of health. *Health Education Quarterly*, **9** (2 and 3), 34–45.

National Audit Office (2006) *Tackling Obesity: First Steps*. London: The Stationery Office. http://www.nao.org.uk/publications/nao_reports/05-06/0506801.pdf (accessed 22 May 2006).

Neff, E. J. and **Beardslee, C. I.** (1990) Body knowledge and concerns of children with cancer as compared with the knowledge and concerns of other children. *Journal of Pediatric Nursing*, **5** (3), 179–189.

Neff, J. A. (1990) Body knowledge and concerns. *Nursing Times*, **86** (20), 67–71.

Neuman, B. (1982) *Neuman's Systems Model: Application to Nursing Education and Practice*. Norwalk, CT: Appleton Century Croft.

ONS (2001a) *Abortion Statistics*. Series AB No. 27 TSO London: ONS. http://www.statistics.gov.uk/downloads/theme_health/AB27/AB_No27_V1.pdf (accessed 22 May 2006).

ONS (2001b) *Living in Britain 2001*. http://www.statistics.gov.uk/lib2001/index.html (accessed 22 May 2006).

ONS (2002a) *Children in the UK*. London: Stationery Office. http://www.statistics.gov.uk/downloads/theme_social/social_focus_in_brief/children/Social_Focus_in_Brief_Children_2002.pdf (accessed 22 May 2006).

ONS (2002b) *Mortality Statistics: Childhood, Infant and Perinatal*. Series http://www.statistics.gov.uk/StatBase/xsdataset.asp?vlnk=7976&Pos=1&ColRank=2&Rank=272 (accessed 22 May 2006).

ONS (2004a) *The Health of People and Young Children*. London: The Stationery Office. http://www.statistics.gov.uk/children/ (accessed 22 May 2006).

ONS (2004b) *Survey of the Mental Health of Children and Young People in Great Britain, 2004*. London: The Stationary Office. http://www.statistics.gov.uk/cci/nugget.asp?id=1229 (accessed 22 May 2006).

Orem, D. E. (2001) *Nursing: Concepts of Practice*, 6th edn. New York: McGraw-Hill.

Reading, R. (1997) Poverty and the health of children and adolescents. *Archives of Diseases in Children*, **76**, 463–467.

Renfrew, M. J., Dyson, L., Wallace, L. M., D'Souza, L., McCormack, F. and **Spilby, H.** (2005) Breastfeeding for longer: what works? *Journal of the Royal Society for the Promotion of Health*, **125** (2), 61–62.

Rosenstock, I. M. (1974) Historical origins of the health belief model. *Health Education Monograph*, **2**, 328–335.

Roy, C. (1984) *Introduction to Nursing: an Adaptation Model*, 2nd edn. New York: Prentice Hall.

Sahota, P., Rudolf, M. C. J., Dixey, R., Hill, A. J. and **Cade, J.** (2001) Randomised controlled trial of primary school based intervention to reduce risk factors for obesity. *British Medical Journal*, **323**, 1029–1032.

Sex Education Forum (1992) *A Framework for School Sex Education*. London: Sex Education Forum.

Shelter (2003) *Children and Families*. http://england.shelter.org.uk/policy/policy-967.cfm (accessed 22 May 2006).

Smith, E. A. (1979) In Sutherland, I. (ed.), *Health Education, Perspectives and Choices*. London: George Allen & Unwin.

Sure Start (2005) *National Evaluation Report*. http://www.ness.bbk.ac.uk/documents/Methodology.pdf (accessed 22 May 2006).

Swann, C., Bowe, K., McCormick, G. and **Kosmin, M.** (2003) *Teenage Pregnancies and Parenthood: a Review of the Reviews*. London: Health Development Agency.

Tannahill, A. (1985) What is health promotion? *Health Education Journal*, **44**, 167–168.

Tannahill, A. (1990) Health education and promotion; planning for the 1990s. *Health Education Journal*, **49** (4), 194–198.

Taylor, J. (1991) Health behaviour and beliefs. *Health Visitor*, **64** (7), 223–224.

Thistle, S. (2003) *Secondary Schools and Sexual Health: Forging the Links*. London: National Children's Bureau.

Thompson, N. P., Montgomary, S. M., Pounder, R. E. and **Wakefield, A. J.** (1995) Is measles vaccination a risk factor for inflammatory bowel disease? *Lancet,* **345**, 1071–1074.
Tones, K. and **Telford, S.** (1994) *Health Education: Effectiveness and Efficiency and Equity.* London: Chapman & Hall.
Towner, E., Dowswell, T. and **Jarvis, S.** (1993) *Reducing Childhood Accidents. The Effectiveness of Health Promotion Interventions: A Literature Review.* London: Health Education Authority.
Townsend, P. (1979) *Poverty in the United Kingdom: A Survey of Household Resources and Standards of Living.* Harmondsworth: Penguin.
Townsend, P. (1980) *Inequalities in Health: the Black Report.* Harmondsworth: Penguin.
UNICEF (2001) A league table of teenage births in rich nations. *Innocenti Report Card,* (July), 3.
Vessey, J. A. and **O'Sullivan, P.** (2000) A study of children's concepts of their internal bodies: a comparison of children with and without congenital heart disease. *Journal of Pediatric Nursing,* **15** (5), 292–298.
Wallerstein, N. (1992) Powerlessness, empowerment and health: implication for health promotion programs. *American Journal of Health Education,* **6** (3), 193–205.
Wanless, D. (2004) *Securing Good Health for the Whole Population.* London: The Stationery Office. http://www.hm-treasury.gov.uk/consultations_and_legislation/wanless/consult_wanless04_final.cfm (accessed 22 May 2006).
Watson, J. E. (1979) *Medical–Surgical Nursing and Related Physiology.* London: W. B. Saunders.
WHO (World Health Organization) (1946) *Constitution.* New York: WHO.
WHO (World Health Organization) (1986) *Ottawa Charter for Health Promotion.* Geneva: WHO.
WHO (World Health Organization) (2002) *WHO Information Fact Sheet Number 104: Tuberculosis.* http://www.who.int/mediacentre/factsheets/fs104/en/ (accessed 22 May 2006).
WHO (World Health Organization) (2004) *The Future of our Children.* http://www.euro.who.int/mediacentre/PR/2003/20030404_1 (accessed 22 May 2006).
Wight, D. (1996) Does sex education make a difference? *Medical Research Council News,* (Spring), 29–32.
Williams, S. J., Bendelow, G. A. and **France, A.** (2003) *Beliefs of Young People in Relation to Health, Risk and Lifestyles.* http://www.dh.gov.uk/PolicyAndGuidance/ResearchAndDevelopment/ResearchAndDevelopmentAZ/MotherAndChildHealth/MotherAndChildHealthArticle/fs/en?CONTENT_ID=4015169&chk=CfroCg (accessed 22 May 2006).
Woodroffe, C., Glickman, M., Barker, M. and **Power, C.** (1993) *Children, Teenagers and Health.* Buckingham: Open University Press.

Part 2

Health and Deviations in Childhood

Module 4
Understanding Families in Stress

Joan Ramsay

Learning Outcomes

The material in this module and the references should enable you to:

- appreciate the effect that stress within the family has upon the child
- discuss children's perceptions of death
- explore how chronic illness and disability affect the child and family
- consider how the stress of hospitalisation affects the child
- examine the effects of violence upon the child and understand the role of the nurse in recognising and reporting child abuse
- appreciate the role of the nurse in helping children and families to cope with stressors

Introduction

Children's health depends not only upon their physical health but also upon their individual psychological, social and spiritual lifestyle. This module explores how stress within these aspects of family living impacts upon children. It discusses how stress and illness within the family has an effect upon the physical and mental health of the child. It also explores how families cope with disability, violence and death, and the effect that these stressors have upon children.

Chapter 16

The Influence of Family Stress upon the Child

Introduction

Children are born with very few innate behaviours and they rely on their parents to provide the necessary factors for their continued growth and development. Although the structure of the family has changed in recent years and no longer consists of only a man, his wife and his children, who live in a common household, it is generally responsible for the child's physical and psychological health.

In 1946 the World Health Organization redefined health as the state of complete physical and social well-being, and not merely the absence of disease or infirmity. More recent definitions see health and illness in relative rather than absolute terms. This means that children's state of health will not only depend on their biological fitness but also on personal, psychosocial and spiritual factors.

How much does the family influence these factors? The Chinese calculate the age of their children not by the child's date of birth but by the date of its conception. This seems appropriate when studying the family's influence on the health of the child, as some behavioural problems have their origin before birth and even before conception (*see also* Family structures p. 5, Health p. 130, Role of the family in child development p. 29 and Factors affecting child health p. 125).

Maternal Health

Studies have shown that pregnant women under excessive stress have more complications during pregnancy, labour and delivery, and are less likely to have healthy babies than those mothers not under stress. Arehart-Treichel (1980) reported that negative emotions such as grief, fear and anxiety during the last 3 months of pregnancy appear to give rise to irritable, hyperactive children who feed badly. The same author found that a high percentage of mothers of autistic children had been subject to disharmony during pregnancy. Many children who were born to mothers in Central London during the early years of World War II showed a high incidence of delinquency (Stott, 1962). Gunther (1963) found a significant association between psychosomatic symptoms and crises during pregnancy and premature delivery, which is one of the most crucial factors contributing to infant mortality. The Avon Longitudinal Study (2005) showed that children born to mothers who experienced extreme stress during pregnancy experience long-lasting mental health problems, particularly depression and anxiety. These children demonstrated high levels of the stress hormone cortisol up to 10 years after their birth, suggesting that stress in pregnancy increases the mother's cortisol levels and that these high levels are then passed on to the unborn baby (O'Connor *et al.*, 2005). It has also been shown that fetuses grow more slowly in mothers who are subject to stress (Paarlberg *et al.*, 1995). Maternal depression and other severe mood disorders also slow intrauterine growth and can cause premature labour (Weinstock, 1999). It is yet to be determined how much these effects are due to increased cortisol levels or to the indirect effect of the mothers' emotional state.

Maternal health also influences the unborn child. It is well known that smoking retards fetal growth and increases the stillborn and neonatal death rate (Fourn *et al.*, 1999). Tomblin *et al.* (1997) also suggest that children of mothers who smoked heavily during pregnancy have higher rates of learning and behavioural disorders. Smoking in pregnancy also affects subsequent psychological development. Women who smoke and cough heavily during pregnancy have been found to have more nervous and insecure infants than non-smokers (Butler and Goldstein, 1973). In 1979, Brown and Cooper found that maternal malnutrition could cause cerebellar dystrophy and predispose to clumsiness, hyperactivity and learning disorders. They also discovered that disorders of pregnancy, such as toxaemia, hypertension and hyperemesis or prolonged labour, showed a correlation with a variety of childhood behaviour problems such as hyperactivity, defective concentration, tics and emotional instability. These studies do not clarify whether the effect on the child is due to the physiological effects of stress on uterine function or the attitude of the mother towards the child who has caused the difficult pregnancy or labour.

Study activity

Find a child with a behaviour problem such as those described above and discover whether the mother's obstetric history reveals any problems. Talk to the mother about her feelings about the baby during the time of the problems.

Parent–Child Relationship

Parental attitude towards a child is an important pre-conceptual factor, as wanted children are more likely to be happy and healthy. A 1975 Czech study cited by Arehart-Treichel (1980) found that unwanted children, especially boys, are liable to experience more acute illness, hospitalisation and antisocial behaviour than wanted children.

Conversely, Illingworth (1983) describes a very-much-wanted child, born after 17 years of marriage, developing hypochondria as a result of his parents' overanxiety and overprotection (*see also* Roles and relationships p. 17).

Overprotection or smother-love can also occur for other reasons. It may occur as the result of the birth of a healthy child after a series of miscarriages, or following the birth of a child of a particular sex after a series of children of the opposite sex. It may occur if the baby is premature or handicapped, especially if initially it was not expected to live. It may also be due to the mother's personality. A mother who had an unhappy childhood or is unhappily married may smother her child to meet her own needs for affection. A child who is overprotected is insecure, does not react well to others, lacks confidence, is accident prone and has a tendency towards sleeping and eating problems (Illingworth, 1983).

The parents' desire for a child also affects their ability to relate to their newborn baby. Much has been written about the importance of the reciprocal relationship between parent and child and the adverse effects of separation of the two because of pre-term delivery or illness. Lynch and Roberts (1977) found that children who had been taken away from their mothers to be nursed in intensive care units showed a higher incidence of child abuse than those cared for immediately by their mothers. Bonding may not occur because of rejection of the child, which might occur because the child is not the preferred sex or has congenital anomalies; it might be the result of an accidental pregnancy, or it might have caused a difficult pregnancy or labour. Parental attitudes may range from excessive criticism to neglect and cruelty. The rejected child tends to be excessively shy and fearful, more aggressive and quarrelsome, and demonstrates severe behavioural problems such as enuresis, head banging, truancy and stealing (Illingworth, 1983). Rejection can also cause physical problems. McCarthy (1974) made a special study of children with stunted growth and concluded that children who eventually show physical signs of this syndrome have suffered from rejection from an early age, probably from birth or even before birth.

Separation

Physical and psychological problems might occur if the bonding relationship is broken by separation of the child from one or both parents later in childhood. Initial studies by Bowlby (1973) indicated that severe long-lasting emotional problems could result from hospitalisation. Separation anxiety is now a well-known complication in preschool children who have been separated from their mothers for long periods of hospitalisation. Regression and emotional instability may continue for some time after the child has returned home. The crucial factors appear to be the length of the separation and the continuity of care, as there is no indication that daily separation of children from their mothers is harmful, provided the children are cared for in a consistent way by a known carer (Wallston, 1973) (*see also* Attachment pp. 86 and 87 and Family break-up and its effects on children p. 13).

Permanent separation from a parent may be the result of separation, divorce or bereavement. The child's consequent behaviour depends upon the reason for the separation and the quality of the relationship with the remaining parent. Rutter (1971) concluded that although children's behaviour tended to deteriorate immediately after a divorce or separation, severe problems such as delinquency were more likely to occur within a discordant family life than a stable one-parent home. Discord also seems to affect the child more than the actual loss of a parent. Waterhouse (1993) found that marital breakdown causes children much unhappiness and may lead to long-term emotional harm. Analysis of the studies into the characteristics of adolescents who take overdoses show a significant number of these children are from families who have split up (Kingsbury, 1993). Children living in step-parent families tend to have higher rates of delinquency, behaviour problems, and perform less well at school than those from intact families (Pagani *et al.*, 1997).

Many studies have been performed on the effect of being part of a non-traditional family on the child. Schaffer (1988) describes studies that compare children from single-mother families, social contract families, families living in communes and traditional two-parent nuclear families. Any problems were found to be independent of the type of family group.

The child–parent relationship can also be disturbed by the birth of a sibling. The first child is likely to become more tearful, have difficulty in sleeping and show a regression in toilet habits (Dunn, 1981).

Aetiology of deliberate self-harm in children

- Single-parent family
- Under the care of social services
- Psychiatric disorder and previous overdose among family members
- Not living with either parent
- Significantly high rate of arguments with parents
- Difficulty in communicating with fathers
- Parents seen as controlling

(Russell-Johnson, 1997)

Family Disability and Illness

Chronic physical illness or prolonged severe illness in one parent, which affects family life and relationships, may also cause behaviour problems in the children but, generally, mental illness in the parents has been found to have a more disturbing effect. Parental depression appears to have the more damaging effect. Preschool children and schoolchildren of mothers who are depressed show a high incidence of psychiatric problems. Children who have siblings with a chronic illness or handicap generally show more disturbed behaviour than the affected child. The child may feel guilty or fearful and demonstrate behavioural problems in order to regain parental attention (Gath, 1980).

However, there are also positive effects from living with a family member who is disabled. Faux (1991) showed that siblings of a disabled child can demonstrate a greater degree of empathy and kindness than children with healthy siblings (*see also* Living with a disability p. 224).

Study activity

Talk to a sibling of a child with a chronic illness or disability and find out the effect this has had upon the sibling's lifestyle. Consider what effect this has had upon the sibling's character.

Parental Behaviour

In Western societies the cultural values of independence and relating well to others usually underpin the way in which parents raise their children. Swanwick (1996) suggests that undue pressure on children to develop autonomy and social skills may result in separation fears and nightmares (*see also* Parenting styles p. 36).

In any kind of behavioural problem the attitude of the parent will determine the extent and spread of the behaviours. Patterson (1982) has investigated the acquisition of problem behaviours in children. As a result of his work he developed the coercion theory. Coercion theory suggests that unskilled parents permit young children to use aversive techniques such as crying, demanding and having tantrums to achieve their needs. Without effective and consistent intervention the child continues the aversive behaviour to manipulate the environment. Such children tend to be more aggressive and resort to lying and stealing.

Parental behaviour will also affect their child's behaviour – children are natural imitators. Social learning theory considers that aggression is learnt through observation, and the more such behaviour is reinforced the more likely it is to occur. Bandura (1973) showed that nursery school children readily imitated aggression following either filmed or live models of aggression. Children who watch violence on television are more aggressive and are more likely to think that aggression is a good way to overcome problems (*see also* The media p. 59).

Study activity

Watch a children's TV cartoon and consider what children may learn about verbal and physical violence from seeing this type of programme. Also watch an early evening adult film or comedy and assess what influence this may have upon children.

Study activity

Considering your findings from the previous activity; what rules or limits (if any) would you place on children watching TV?

Type A
Behaviour includes such characteristics as impatience, ambitiousness, competitiveness, hostility and achievement-orientated behaviour. These individuals are easily stressed.

Type B
People with a Type B personality are more relaxed and laid back.

If there is violence in the home, the children (especially boys) will be more aggressive. Girls from such homes tend to grow up to be violent and neglectful mothers. Illingworth (1983) describes an Australian study of parental alcoholism where the irrational and violent behaviour of fathers tended to lead to depression, hostility and aggression in the children.

Some studies have also investigated whether parental behaviour can cause children to develop type-A behaviour and thus a predisposition to coronary heart disease. Rosenman *et al.* (1975) found that hard-working boys had fathers with the same traits. Further studies seem to show that type-A behaviour is more likely to develop in children whose mother and father were achievement- and competition-oriented.

Parental Attitude and Physical Illness

Other physical illnesses may be exacerbated by parental attitudes. Arehart-Treichel (1980) reports that the underlying cause of ulcerative colitis, asthma and anorexia nervosa may be related to family influences. Her studies have shown that children with ulcerative colitis have domineering mothers and passive, remote fathers, neither of whom are able to express their emotions freely. Like ulcerative colitis, anorexia nervosa often has origins in a dominating mother and in a family where emotions are usually repressed. However, mothers of anorexics tend to be preoccupied with food and may use food as a way of showing affection. Obesity also seems to stem from overprotection and dominating parents. Obese children are often the only or youngest children, with a pathological dependence on their parents. A similar situation is seen in the origins of asthma, which commences during childhood. Retrospective studies suggest that many children with asthma have dominating mothers and ineffective fathers. Childhood asthma is twice as common among boys as girls, and the affected boys, who are usually only children or the youngest child, tend to have been overprotected and overindulged by their mothers and rejected by their fathers. However, these studies have been largely unsupported as it is always difficult to know whether parental behaviour is the cause or effect of the child's chronic condition (*see also* Parenting styles p. 36).

Juvenile rheumatoid arthritis also shows origins in family influence but in a different way to those discussed above. Arehart-Treichel (1980) suggests that children with rheumatoid disease tend to be first-born children who have one parent who is rejecting, aggressive and punitive. An American study in 1979 showed that nearly a third of children with rheumatoid arthritis had lost a parent through death, divorce or separation, compared with 11% in the control group. Parental loss or separation also appears to be a predisposing factor in mental illness. A 1965 study showed that 38% of suicides had experienced the death of one or both parents during childhood and a further 34.5% had parents who had separated or divorced. A 1975 German study found that over 25% of schizophrenics had lost a parent by death or divorce while young. Reactive depression appears to correlate with strict unemotional fathers and mothers who are intrusive and perfectionists (cited by Arehart-Treichel, 1980).

Studies have also been carried out to discover if events in childhood can predispose individuals to cancer. The New York Longitudinal Study, an American study that has been ongoing since the 1940s, found that 30% of cancer patients report a lack of warm, loving parental relationships (Chess and Thomas, 1984). Most significantly, none of these patients were only children. Further studies have suggested that early frustrations in childhood due to the birth of a sibling correlate with the later development of cancer (*see also* Mental health pp. 59 and 120).

Study activity

Study the family background of a child with one of the above disorders and see what evidence you find for the link between physical illness and parental attitude.

Relationships Between Stress and Disease

Why do childhood experiences cause a person to develop a disease? Although little research has been done in this area, there seem to be three factors involved. Increased levels of adrenal steroid hormones have been found in adults whose mothers had died when they were young. Elevation of adrenal steroid hormones have been found to depress the immune system. Depression and grief also result in a rise of steroid hormones, whereas repressed emotions reduce antibody levels (Arehart-Treichel, 1980). Studies of 100 children by Meyre and Haggerty in 1962 seem to give strength to this theory. Throat swabs of each child were taken every 2 weeks and cultured for streptococci. The family kept a diary of events, particularly noting upsetting events and illnesses. The researchers found that 25% of the children showed positive throat swabs 2 weeks after stressful events. This does not totally explain why children develop physical or psychological problems related to stressful lifestyle events. Not all only children develop juvenile rheumatoid arthritis and not all unwanted children have behavioural problems. This difference may be due to personality or the individual differences between the children. Psychologists do not agree about the way in which personality develops but, one way, social learning theory, indicates that individual differences result from variations in learning experiences. Some personality characteristics such as moods are inherited biological factors, so it is possible that the family still plays a part in influencing the child.

Factors protecting children from the effects of stress

- A good relationship with at least one parent
- Effective supervision and security
- Clarity and consistency of rules
- Respect as an individual
- Recognition of effort and achievement
- Gradual increase of responsibility and independence
- Good relationships with siblings
- Own adaptable and sociable temperament

Lask and Fossen (1989)
(***See also*** Development of personality p. 83 and Social issues p. 126)

Social Class and Environment

It is also known that there are many other predisposing factors that influence the development of mental and physical illness. One great influence is social class. In the Newcastle study of 1000 children (Miller *et al.*, 1974) it was shown that effective parental skills increased with social class, due to better education and health services. Accidents are more common and more severe in poorer families, especially if there is maternal neglect or an overcrowded home (Miller *et al.*, 1974). Overcrowding tends to give rise to infection more readily, and poor children catch these diseases earlier in life when they have less mature body defences (*see also* Development of personality p. 83 and Social issues p. 126).

Environmental factors may also influence behaviour. Rutter *et al.* (1975) compared children from a stable and cohesive community with a comparable group of children from an inner London borough. He showed how the unsettling influences of city life gave rise to a greater incidence of delinquency.

The availability of social support is also of importance. In a study of battered children and their parents (Smith *et al.*, 1974), social isolation and loneliness were as important as environmental problems such as cramped conditions and lack of amenities.

Thus it appears that although the family does have an important influence on health, there are also other factors to consider. This is perhaps best summarised by the National Child Development Study (Wedge and Prosser, 1973). Ten thousand children were studied from birth until the age of 11. The results showed clearly the interrelationship between physical development, ill-health, accidents, maladaptive behaviour, with social and environmental disadvantages and parental interest.

Study activity

Do a literature search to discover more recent research to support or dispute the findings cited in this module. Make a note of your findings.

It seems to follow that there is an increased need for health practitioners to look at the whole family and not just the child. Any action relating to the prevention, maintenance or improvement of children's health should take into account the children's relationship with their carers as well as their home setting and family structure. McMahon (1995) states that it makes sense to use family therapy and work with the family rather than the individual child because the causes of so many childhood problems are found within the families' relationships with each other. Preconceptual advice and education about the factors affecting child health may also help to reduce the psychological and physiological disorders of childhood as well as promote mental and physical health through positive family influences.

Key Points

1. Certain characteristics of parental behaviour towards children, such as emotions, controlling methods and communication patterns, significantly influence psychological development.
2. Families who provide warmth and affection have children who develop better and more secure social relationships than those who are cold and rejecting.
3. The structure of the family affects family functioning. Changes in family structure are associated with significant stress and adversely affect child-rearing patterns.
4. The overall level of poverty or affluence of the family influences family interactions and relationships by affecting health, discipline and levels of stress and support.
5. Authoritative parents who provide warmth, control, communication and security while responding to their children as individuals produce children who are more confident, competent, independent and affectionate.
6. Family therapy can be used as a way of gaining insight into the cause and nature of children's psychological problems.

Chapter 17

Hospitalisation and Illness

Introduction

Hospitals are strange and frightening environments for everyone. They are associated with real and imagined fears, and actual and potential threats. Since Bowlby and Robertson's studies in the 1950s, hospitalisation is known to cause particular anxiety for children and can lead to short- and long-term emotional and behavioural problems. For children, the unfamiliar environment, numerous strangers, peculiar equipment and the sight and sound of other distressed children is confusing and frightening.

Study activity

Take some time to look at your own place of work from a child's viewpoint. Crouch down and consider how it looks for a small child. What changes might make it more welcoming from this view?

It is not only the strange environment of hospital that children find stressful. Bossert (1994) discovered that hospitalised children could identify a range of stressful events. She categorised these stressors into six main areas: intrusive events, physical symptoms, therapeutic intervention, restricted activity, separation and environment. She also found that children with short-term acute illnesses were more likely to name physical symptoms as most stressful. Children with chronic illness had a greater number of stressors and found intrusive events the most stressful.

Children's reactions to hospitalisation are influenced by several factors and are known to be reduced by preparation and explanations. However, familiarity with hospital, for those children with chronic illness, does not reduce fears (Hart and Bossert, 1994). For these children fears may be worse because they know the reality of being in hospital. Although most children experience some stress when in hospital, it can also be a positive experience. It can give children the opportunity for further social interaction and it may help them to cope better with future illness or stressors.

Illness and hospitalisation in childhood affects the whole family and, as family stress has its impact on the ill child, the children's nurse should be aware of these effects. Other sections discuss the ways of minimising the traumatic effects of hospitalisation for the child, so this section will concentrate mainly on the reactions of the child and family to this trauma (*see also* Creating an appropriate hospital environment for children p. 257 and Preparation for hospital and procedures p. 267).

Separation Anxiety

Infants appear to be fearless for the first 6–8 months of life and the startle reflex of the young baby, which occurs in response to a sudden noise or movement, is probably the nearest reaction to fear (Marks, 1987). After about 6 months the infant or child becomes wary of strangers and may show anxiety, depending on age and previous experience. At the same time as the development of this stranger anxiety, children show evidence of separation anxiety when their usual caregiver is absent. Kagan (1979) explains that this reaction is due to the child losing the usual source of physical and emotional comfort and not understanding the reason or the temporary nature of the loss. The understanding that people and things still exist even though they cannot still be seen does not develop until 10 months of age. However, separation anxiety occurs after this age and is exacerbated by other unfamiliar events, such as hospitalisation. The amount of distress is determined by parenting styles. Main *et al.* (1985) found that parents who were easily accessible and responsive to their children increased the children's confidence and enabled them to accept brief separations. Children with affectionate parents who are used to being comforted by them tend to be more confident and able to tolerate brief separations (Ainsworth, 1982). The amount of distress is also affected by the parents' response to the separation; if parents are calm and happy with the situation, it is likely that the child will be less anxious. This is an important issue for nurses who need to be able to reassure parents at least as much as the child.

Regardless of influencing factors, some separation anxiety will always occur and should be accepted as a normal display of grief at the loss of someone who is important to the child. Children should be comforted and reassured so they still feel secure and loved. If the manifestations of separation anxiety are ignored or punished, children may develop long-term consequences. Ainsworth (1973) suggests that the feelings of insecurity and loss of confidence and trust that the child experiences during separation can result in difficulty in developing and maintaining relationships in adulthood.

Bowlby (1953) observed children in foster care and discovered that, when young children were separated from parents for any length of time, they demonstrated three distinct phases of separation anxiety: protest, despair and detachment. His observations centred around children between the ages of 8 months and 3 years, but older children can also display some signs of anxiety on being separated from their home

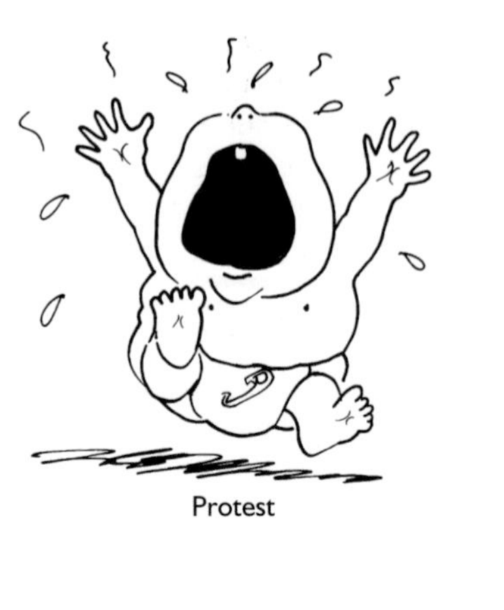
Protest

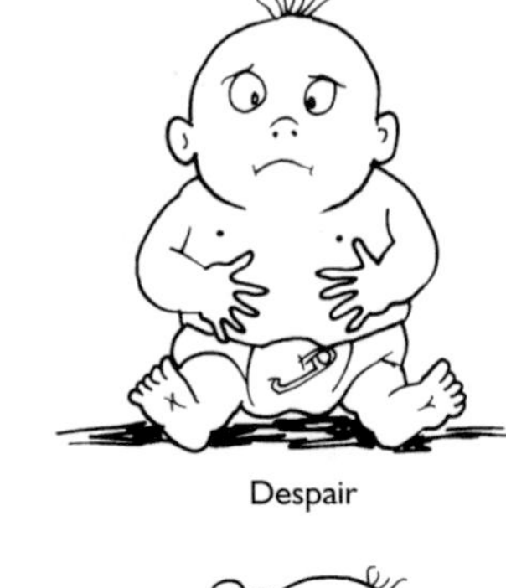
Despair

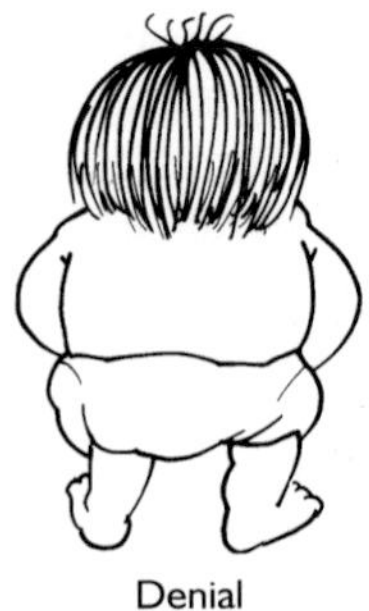
Denial

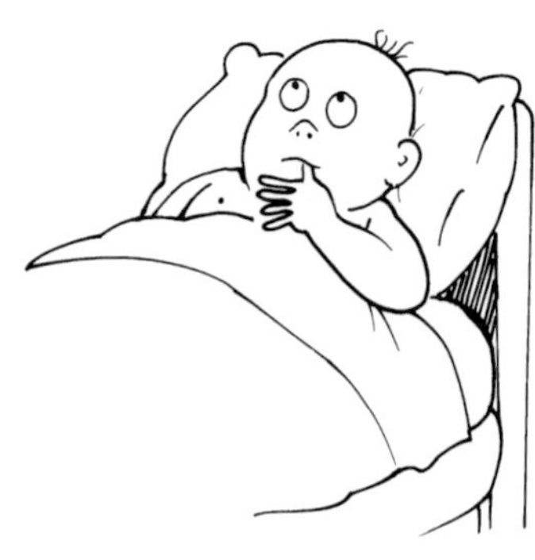
Regression

Figure 17.1 Separation anxiety.

Module 4

Separation anxiety – influencing factors

- Sex of the nurse and usual caregiver
- Parental response to the separation and the nurse
- Familiarity of the environment
- Friendly attitude of the nurse
- Distance of nurse from the child
- Amount of physical contact by the nurse
- Child used to other carers
- Child's personality – anxious versus confident
- Parenting styles

Children's reactions to hospitalisation
Depend upon:

1. Developmental age
   - infancy
   - preschool
   - school age
   - adolescence
2. Previous experience
   - illness
   - family separation
   - hospital
3. Available support
   - resident parents
   - family and friends
   - named nurse
4. Seriousness of the illness

and parents. Detachment is uncommon because most children stay in hospital for only short periods and any parental separation is only brief. However, the protest and despair phases can occur after only a brief separation and it is important that nurses recognise and react to these so that long-term effects of separation are avoided (Figure 17.1) (*see also* Vertical relationships p. 87).

Protest

The child first demonstrates separation anxiety by protesting. Protest may be shown in many ways, according to the age of the child. Infants and young children will cry loudly for their parents and will be inconsolable, refusing comfort from anyone else. This phase can last for several days and small children may only sleep when they are exhausted by crying.

Older children may express their protest by anger and may be aggressive to other children and anyone who tries to console them. Adolescents may show anger and frustration and be generally uncooperative. They do not cry or express their concerns because they do not want to appear weak, childish or dependent, but Hart and Bossert (1994) discovered that the fear of being separated from the family was schoolchildren's greatest cause for concern about hospitalisation.

Despair

At this stage of separation, the young child appears to accept that parents are not returning and shows features of depression. This behaviour can go unnoticed and the child can be labelled as quiet and good. The child is withdrawn, sad and apathetic, showing no interest in toys, food or other children. Usually when parents visit, the child cries bitterly and nurses have used this as evidence that parental visiting is upsetting to children in hospital. However, Robertson (1970) showed that these children were crying to relieve their tension and not because the presence of their parents upset them.

Older children's despair may be demonstrated by stoicism, withdrawal or passive acceptance. They also lose interest in activities and food.

Detachment

At this stage the child appears to have adjusted to the new situation and becomes more active and interested in the surroundings. Detached children will play, eat and sleep as usual and will accept care from anyone. In reality, they have coped with their separation by unattaching themselves from their parents. As a result they lose interest and no longer relate to their parents. Robertson (1970) suggests that at this stage the child represses the fear, sorrow and loneliness and tries to make the best of the alternative situation. Although this stage is rarely seen now, because children stay in hospital for shorter periods than previously, it is perhaps not recognised because it is less common.

Regression

Children in hospital who feel insecure often display attention-seeking behaviour, which may continue on discharge home. This behaviour usually relates to the characteristics of a younger child. If this regression is not recognised and managed appropriately by nurses or parents the child will suffer further stress and insecurity.

There are three important ways of preventing regression: getting to know the child as an individual, being able to anticipate needs, and minimising stress. If the nurse knows and maintains normal home routines and does not expect behaviour beyond the child's developmental abilities, the child's security is upheld. The nurse who knows the child's preferences and abilities can anticipate needs, which provides added security. Further stress can be minimised by consistency of care given by familiar staff. These named nurses can provide cuddles and comfort in the family's absence as well as explanations and preparation for procedures which are adapted to meet the individual child's needs. They can also establish a relationship and work in partnership with the parents to care for the child. The child will also feel more secure if parents appear calm and relaxed.

If a child does show regressive behaviour, the nurse should not insist upon usual behaviour. The situation should be accepted calmly and the reasons for insecurity explored. Parents should be warned that children sometimes show regression once they return home, even if they appeared to adjust well to hospital. They also need to know that if regression is recognised and managed appropriately immediately following their return home, normal behaviour will gradually return.

Regressive behaviour

- Clinging to parents
- Persistent comfort-seeking behaviour
- Temper tantrums
- Unusual aggressiveness
- Refusal to associate with other children or siblings
- Refusal to eat
- Refusal to go to bed
- Waking and crying in the night
- Soiling or wetting although toilet trained

Parental Concerns

It is never easy for parents whose child is in hospital. Even if there are no siblings, parents have other concerns. They tend to feel fearful, anxious and guilty. Fear and anxiety is often related to their lack of knowledge about the illness and its treatment, which may be exacerbated if they had frightening experiences themselves as children in hospital. Remember that resident parents and dedicated children's wards are a relatively new concept, which may not have been available when some parents were small. Guilt is a common reaction of most parents to any child's illness; they always wonder if any action or omission could have caused or prevented the illness.

As with any crisis, parents often report feelings of depression after hospitalisation. They may have been so busy supporting the ill child in hospital as well as managing the home that it is not until they return home that exhaustion occurs. It is then difficult to manage any emotional and behavioural changes that the child or siblings may exhibit. In addition, they now have concerns about the child being at home and whether they have the necessary skills to provide continuing care. Bailey and Caldwell (1997) found that parents always want more discharge information than they receive and suggest that nurses need to look at the effectiveness of their communication and discharge planning.

Parental reactions to hospitalisation

Depend upon:

1 Parental temperament
- adaptable
- confident

2 Previous experience
- illness
- hospitals

3 Available support
- communication within family
- personal coping mechanisms
- cultural and religious beliefs
- other stresses within the family

4 Seriousness of the illness
- degree of threat to the child
- medical procedures involved

Module 4

Siblings of Hospitalised Children

The effects of childhood chronic illness upon siblings has been widely studied (Morrison, 1997). However, until recently the effect upon siblings of short-term hospitalisation for acute illness has not been considered. Yet, the feelings of loneliness, fear and anxiety still occur. Simon (1993) found that the stress of siblings was equal to the stress experienced by the ill child, with those siblings who visited daily experiencing the most stress. These findings were replicated by Morrison (1997), who found that this stress was demonstrated by feelings of sadness, nervousness and difficulty in sleeping and concentrating at school. The reasons for this stress have not been proven, but are thought to relate to parental separation, as one parent is likely to remain with the hospitalised child (*see also* Sibling relationships p. 22).

Study activity

Consider how you could minimise stress for the child whose sibling is in hospital for 48 hours.

Morrison (1997) suggests that family-centred care should not centre around the parents but should involve siblings. The same methods that have been developed to reduce the stress of the hospitalised child can be used for siblings. Initiatives have taken place to provide siblings of children with cancer the opportunity to learn more about the care of cancer (Woodhouse, 1996) and this idea could be extended. The siblings of those children coming into hospital for a planned admission could also be invited to the pre-admission club, and siblings of long-term hospitalised children could be invited to a special open day. Nurses can also explain sibling stress to parents so that they can appreciate the need to keep siblings informed. Evidence shows that parents do not realise that healthy siblings also have concerns about hopitalisation (Craft, 1986) and it seems likely that siblings either do not talk to parents about their concerns or do not have the opportunity to discuss problems with them.

Children's Concepts of Illness

Carson *et al.* (1992) believe that children's adaptation to hospitalisation can be determined by their concept of illness. Studies into children's understanding of illness rely heavily on Piaget's theory of cognitive development but recent studies suggest that young children are able to understand more than Piaget's cognitive levels imply (Meadows, 1993). Bird and Podmore (1993) suggest that small children's limited knowledge of illness is more likely to be due to poor or inadequate explanations than to their inability to understand the concept. Although nurses are taught to explore children's existing level of knowledge and intellect before any explanation or teaching, it would appear that in practice they accept cognitive development theory and prevent children's understanding of illness through their inadequate information (Alderson, 1993). Rushford (1996) found that most nurses aimed their information-giving at mid school-age level regardless of the child's actual age, intellect or previous knowledge and experience (*see also* Children's perceptions of health p. 143).

Concepts of illness begin at preschool age. These young children tend to accept what they have been told about illness and their lack of experience with language causes them to interpret what is said literally. Because of this, common nursing expressions such as 'taking a temperature' may be viewed with alarm. Equally, their lack of knowledge about body functioning means that explanations need to be carefully phrased and thorough to prevent fear and confusion. They are often told at this age that colds are caught and they may use this rationale for all illnesses unless told otherwise.

School-age children are more concerned about the consequences of the illness than its causation. They usually know that some outside factor causes illness but are not very clear about the exact explanation, although school, television, books and life experience have now given them more information about the body and its illnesses. Because of this, they are aware of, and worry about, disability and death, and their greatest fear is being told that they have a chronic illness (Hart and Bossert, 1994). They become frustrated when illness prevents their developing independence and physical activity. At this age they have a thirst for knowledge and take an active interest in finding out about their illness. They cope better with the illness and hospitalisation by finding out as much as possible about it. Given appropriate information, most children of this age can give a good account of their illness, which would appear to support the idea that children's cognitive abilities are not limited to their age.

The stressful effects of hospitalisation

1 *Bobby*, aged 2. Bobby has been admitted to hospital after a car accident in which his father was seriously injured. His mother is trying to divide her time between Bobby, his siblings at home and her husband. She cannot be resident with Bobby and her visits can only be brief. She is distressed by the situation and worried about its effect on Bobby
2 *Jane*, aged 4. Jane is at home following a brief stay in hospital following a febrile convulsion. Her mother asks you for advice about her behaviour since their return home. Jane, who always went to bed with no fuss, is now refusing to settle and wakes constantly during the night. She is very clingy during the day and making a terrible fuss about leaving her mother to go to nursery
3 *Rosie*, aged 8. Rosie was admitted earlier today with appendicitis. She is shortly going to theatre. Her mother needs to stay at home with Rosie's twin brothers, aged 6 months, and her father is out of the country. Rosie is in pain and is frightened and very upset at her mother's absence
4 *Mark*, aged 14. Mark has been in hospital for 3 weeks. He fractured his femur in a road accident on his way to school and is now in traction. He is becoming more and more rude and uncooperative to the nurses. His mother, a single parent, can only visit in the evenings after work. During her visits he is often rude and uncommunicative and she is very upset by his behaviour

Study activity

Ask a school-age child to tell you about his or her chronic illness and consider whether the explanation is related to the child's cognitive age or ability.

Independence, individuality and freedom are important for adolescents. Illness and hospitalisation may take all of these away. Adolescents may further isolate themselves from peers and family as they strive to maintain some independence. They are then left with no support mechanisms. Thus illness is seen as a loss of control and power. To help them regain control they also want to know as much as possible about their illness. They now know about the physical and psychological causes of disease and expect to be given information as adults. They will not tolerate or value being treated as a child or having information hidden from them. They are aware of potential problems of illness and treatment, and will expect to be told about these. Appearance is important to this age group and they worry about alterations such as scarring and deformity.

Minimising Separation Anxiety

Study activity

Read the case studies entitled 'The stressful effects of hospitalisation' and suggest ways in which these problems could be overcome.

Ideally, admission to hospital for children between 6 months and 4 years of age should be avoided. If hospitalisation is essential, then day care is less traumatic than an in-patient stay. Allowing a close family member (preferably a parent) to be resident with the child is the best way to overcome separation anxiety, but it may not always be possible. Parents with other children have the unenviable task of deciding which child benefits from the parental presence and there may not be other family members around to help. Harris (1993) suggests that, when this is not possible, a soft article of clothing belonging to the parent provides the young child with a constant and comforting reminder of the parent. Any other comforters (teddy, blanket, dummy) should also be left with the child. To try to prevent the child from feeling unloved and insecure, a consistent figure other than the parent should be available and should follow the child's home routine wherever possible. If parents or family cannot stay with the older child, links with home may be provided by photographs and a clock to denote times of visits.

Older children's fears of loss of control may be minimised by explanations and involvement with treatment or care, and being allowed a choice as much as possible. Burr (1993) believes that despite the fact that adolescence is known as a period where independence and self-control develop, little consideration is given to enable these older children to be independent in hospital. Although conflicts with parents tend to occur at this age, parents are still very important, especially at times of stress. Greenberg *et al.* (1983) found that the quality of adolescents' relationships with their parents was central to their sense of well-being and happiness. Therefore, it is important not to presume that hospitalised children in this age group do not need their parents.

The effects of hospitalisation on the older child can be minimised by preparation for the strange environment of hospital and any associated procedures, and this helps to overcome some fears of the unknown.

Key Points

1. Hospitalisation is traumatic for children of any age, but it particularly affects children between the ages of 6 months and 4 years.
2. When a child is in hospital it affects the whole family and family-centred care should take this into account.
3. Nurses should take care not to mistake the features of separation anxiety for the characteristics of a good child who is settling well into hospital.
4. If separation anxiety is not recognised or managed well, the child can have problems maintaining relationships in later life.
5. The behaviour of children who have been discharged from hospital can regress. This can be very distressing for parents if they are not warned of this and given advice on its management.
6. Admission to hospital for very young children should be avoided whenever possible. If hospitalisation is essential, procedures should be in place to minimise the traumatic effects for the whole family.

Chapter 18

Death and the Family

Introduction

Death is a necessary and natural part of human life. Hiding death in a shroud of mysticism will not change the inexorable fact that death is the end of the line for every living thing. There is therefore a need to discuss death to rid society and ourselves of the myths and superstitions that surround it. This section aims to help you to begin to examine your own ideas, feelings and beliefs about death, so that any fears, anxieties or conflicts that you may have can be diminished. As a result, it should begin to enable you to talk openly about death and accept it as part of life. It is only when you can do this that you can hope to help others cope with death. Parents of children who are dying need help to come to terms with this and also need help to explain what is happening to the child and the siblings. The role of the nurse in this situation will range from giving information and practical advice to providing emotional support for the whole family. Effective psychological care requires the nurse to be aware of personal feelings about death (McKerrow, 1991).

A century ago, people were exposed to death earlier and more often throughout their lifespan. The extended family meant that children were more likely to observe death and that they participated in the emotional and ceremonial aspects. Today, children are often shielded from the trauma of death. Improved living conditions, health care and highly skilled medical and surgical interventions have contributed to longer lifespans, which mean that death becomes a distant event that seems too far away to consider. The breakdown of the extended family and the tendency for more people to die in hospital or residential homes means that children are less likely to encounter death. Their grief for a lost pet is often tempered by a replacement. If children are not involved in the reality of death, the development of a realistic concept of death is inhibited and thus, in adulthood, death is surrounded by fear and myths.

Death attitudes

1. How would your personal lifestyle change drastically if you discovered you had a terminal illness?
2. Are you afraid of death? What do you think has influenced your answer?
3. What are your personal beliefs about death?
4. Do your family and friends discuss death openly? Why do you think this is so?
5. What are your plans for your own death?
6. What things would you like to do before you die?
7. What sentiments would you want to express to your family and friends before you die?
8. What experience of death have you had to date? How much has this influenced your answers to the previous questions?

Study activity

Consider your ideas and beliefs about death by answering the 'Death attitudes' questions.

Children's Feelings about Death

Children's perceptions of death depend upon their age and, in general, their understanding parallels their cognitive and psychological development. They encounter death in various ways and at different ages. This encounter is most likely to be on television, or in games and fantasies, which may not give them a realistic idea of death. Some children may have experienced the death of a pet or a grandparent, but their understanding of this event may be influenced by their parents' explanations. As Lovell (1987) notes, many adults are too confused about death to be able to give their child a rational explanation (*see also* Caring for the dying child and family p. 400).

Study activity

Billy, aged 4, tells you about the death of his cat. He asks: 'If Kitty is in heaven and heaven is in the sky, why did Daddy bury her in the garden?' How should you reply?

Lovell (1987) suggests that for younger children, such as Billy, death can be explained by relating it through nature and the life cycle of flowers and trees. The concept of heaven is confusing for children who are not able to think in the abstract. It is also difficult for preschool children to appreciate the permanency of death. Michael and Landsdown (1986) found that children wanted to talk about death, and those who were not allowed to do so were those who had more difficulty in adjusting to their loss. Extreme fear and phobic behaviour can result from the exclusion of children from family discussions about death (Bentovim, 1986).

Study activity

Samantha is 8 years old and her grandmother, of whom she was very fond, has just died. Samantha's parents want your advice about whether she should attend the funeral. What advice should you give?

Children in this age group are often excluded from mourning. Randall (1993) believes that young children grieve differently from adults. In reality, the difference lies not in the grief process but the way in which children express their grief. For young children, whose bereavement occurs at the stage of development when they cannot properly understand the meaning of death or the meaning of their loss, loneliness and fear may be immediate reactions. Their inability to communicate can lead to misunderstandings about the level of grief they feel. This situation, and the exclusion from any involvement in the death, can cause them more distress. This distress may manifest itself in regressive or aggressive behaviour. Pettle and Landsdown (1986) found that children who were able to participate in the events surrounding the death of a sibling were less disturbed than those who did not. The death of a parent has been found to have long-reaching psychological effects among children (Randall, 1993) and Lovell (1987) suggests that these reactions could be minimised by allowing the child to spend time with the dying parent and to help with his or her care, and by giving the child the opportunity to discuss what is happening.

Talking about Death

Talking with parents and children is an emotional, difficult thing to do. Often a nurse is reluctant to approach a dying child and the family because she does not know what to say. Nurses worry about answering questions wrongly. There can be no set procedure for this situation and the most appropriate way of learning to cope with this problem is to use role play and discussion.

Study activity

You are looking after Bobby, aged 6, who has been admitted for investigations because of a severe headache, dizziness and vomiting. Investigations indicate an inoperable cerebral tumour but parents have not yet been told. Suddenly, Bobby's mother asks: 'Is Bobby going to die?' Consider your response.

Listening is the most important skill for the nurse. It may be difficult for an experienced nurse to answer direct questions about whether a child is dying, but parents will only choose a nurse whom they can trust to ask such crucial questions. The nurse can accept that trust by enabling them to talk more generally about the issue. Faulkner (1995) suggests such responses as: 'What do you already know about the condition?' or 'Is that what is worrying you?' In this way the nurse can listen to the parents' real concerns and fetch appropriate help if unable to answer all questions personally.

Families' emotions affect the care and support they can give to the dying child. They are in great need of understanding and support from the nurses they meet. Parents need time as individuals and together to work through their reactions to knowing their child is going to die. They will not always feel the same emotions at the same time. Anger, guilt, resentment, and blame of the other parent are all common reactions. Hill (1994) recognises that mothers find it easier to express these emotions and that healthcare professionals expect fathers to cope. Consequently, fathers' needs are often not adequately met.

Children may be well aware of their own death, but choose not to discuss it with their parents because they have learnt that this is not a topic with which the family feels at ease. Children as young as 4 or 5 can usually sense when they are seriously ill and they need simple, honest answers to their questions.

Study activity

Peter is a 14-year-old who is dying from an inoperable cerebral tumour. His parents have remained adamant throughout his illness that he should not be told of diagnosis and prognosis. During his bath he suddenly asks you: 'Am I dying?' How should you reply?

There is no easy answer to whether parents can override the rights of dying children to be told the truth. Peck (1992) discusses the factors involved in this difficult situation. The need to be honest with the child must be considered alongside the needs of the parents and the legal issues. Ideally, this dilemma should be discussed with parents who wish to withhold information from the child.

Nurses worry about how to answer direct questions about death but Hill (1994) advises that a response such as 'Is that something that worries you?' enables the child to discuss his feelings, gives the nurse an idea of the child's concerns and provides time to alert others of the child's readiness to explore death.

Parents often ask for guidance about what to tell children and siblings. As with any person, it is useful to listen to what is being said and only to answer the question that is being asked. Long and complicated answers may confuse the child even further. Simple answers may be all the child needs. They may give the impetus for further questions but they allow the child to dictate the pace. It is useful to remember the anecdote about the small boy who asked his mother where he came from. Mother gave a detailed account of the facts of life only for the small boy to explain that his friend came from Scotland and she still had not answered his question!

Children's questions about death

- How do you die?
- Will you and I die one day?
- Will I be able to see Granny again when I am dead?
- Can nurses make dead people come alive again?
- How do dead people on TV come alive again?
- Why do people die?

Study activity

Read 'Children's questions about death' and consider how you would answer these.

Children's questions are always asked for a good reason and they should be treated with sincerity (Lindsay, 1994). Discussions about death with young children, when death has affected their family, are possible and may be very helpful to them (Meadows, 1993).

Grieving

Grieving means feeling and expressing all the emotions related to the death and the deceased person. It is not about forgetting what has happened but about slowly accepting it and adjusting to it. It is about

Table 18.1 A generalised pattern of bereavement

Time	State	Behaviour	Helpful responses
1–14 days	Shock	Crying/inability to cry	'Permission' to cry
	Disbelief	Refusal to accept	Accept feelings
	Relief	Emotionless	Listen
After 14 days	Fear	Fearful of leaving house	Acknowledge fears
	Anger	Resentment, allocating blame	Reassure 'normal' reaction
	Guilt	Self-reproach	Listen
	Denial	Enshrining	Be non-judgemental
2–3 months	Yearning	Repetition of death	Allow to talk
	Searching	Fear of forgetting, visiting old haunts	Listen
			Be patient
3–12 months	Depression	Withdrawal	Allow to share despair
	Loneliness	Clinging to grief	Be tolerant
1–5 years	Acceptance	Recall deceased happily	'Allow' grief to stop
	Adjustment	Find 'new' life	Encourage
	Healing	Renewed self-image	Acknowledge

finding a way to remember the person with love rather than pain. Rather like pain, the intensity of grief is difficult to describe and cannot be compared with the grief of another person. Everyone is different, and one person's grief may be as painful as another's, whatever the circumstances. Feelings of grief may last for a long time and may change from day to day.

There is no right way to grieve and, although there is a generalised pattern of behaviour that all bereaved people exhibit, the time scale is widely variable and there may not be a steady progression to acceptance. Many bereaved people will move backwards as well as forwards between these generalised patterns (see Table 18.1).

Study activity

Read the accounts illustrating the stages of grief below. For each one consider why the characters are behaving in this way and how you could help.

Grieving does not always begin at death. For many families this process starts at the moment when they know that the person is going to die. In this situation, there are intense feelings of grief at diagnosis, which may reach a plateau or even decline if there is any length of time between the bad news and the death. In some cancers these feelings may fluctuate with remissions and relapses. Grief rises again at the actual death but the worst point for many people is during the first 6 months following the death. Grief tends to be at a high level throughout the first year of bereavement. During this time every day is an anniversary of a significant event. The first Christmas, wedding anniversary or birthday can be particularly difficult to cope with.

After the first year, grief usually begins to lessen in intensity but it never goes away; it just becomes more manageable with the passing years. Even then, it may resurface at specific times of the year which are emotive for the family.

Providing Support

The exact needs of those who have been bereaved depend upon their individual feelings and personalities, but there are many general needs that nurses can meet. Bereaved parents and children are very sensitive at the time of death and during the early months after the death. Although it is difficult to know what to say, it is important that words are carefully chosen. Brewis (1995) gives examples of statements that were probably meant well but left bereaved parents with negative memories of the carers:

- I know how you feel
- Never mind, it's for the best
- You can always have another child

The bereaved do not want to be told how they feel – only they can know this. But they do sometimes need the opportunity to talk about their needs and feelings. It is important to listen to what they have to say and be sensitive to the thoughts they cannot express. Remember that it is sometimes as difficult for them to express themselves as it for you to know what to say. It may help if you can share your own feelings about the death, always taking care not to overwhelm them with your grief.

Study activity

Write a letter of condolence to a friend whose child has just died after a road traffic accident. Afterwards consider the following:

- Did you use platitudes?
- Did you communicate your honest feelings and beliefs?
- Were you tempted to put off writing the letter?

The bereaved often relate how other people avoid talking to them, or talk about everything except the death, when what they want is to feel comfortable with someone who will talk about their loved one and listen to their feelings of grief. For this reason many parents are comforted by others who have had a similar experience to their own. There are many statutory and voluntary agencies offering emotional support and counselling for bereaved children and parents. Families need to be able to choose how they wish to be supported, but information should be readily available for them.

Stages of grief

1. *Mrs James.* Mr and Mrs James' 5-year-old daughter Sally died suddenly following a road traffic accident one month ago. They have come to the local bereavement group. Mrs James has not been out of the house until now and her husband says that she will not allow Sally's room to be touched. She is ignoring day-to-day life and their other two children.
2. *Jason.* Jason is a 14-year-old in the terminal stage of cystic fibrosis. While caring for him you have found conversation difficult – his answers are monosyllabic. Eventually you ask him what he would like to do during the afternoon. He retorts, 'What can I do? There is little point in me getting interested in anything – all I can do is lie here and wait to die.'
3. *Mr Graham.* You are looking after Emily, a 5-year-old with acute myeloid leukaemia. Emily was diagnosed a year ago and initially responded well to treatment. She was re-admitted to hospital a week ago, following a fairly sudden relapse. Her poor prognosis has been discussed with her parents and they have agreed that she should have no further active treatment. When you introduce yourself to Emily and her parents, Mr Graham shouts, 'I don't want you to look after Emily. She needs a more experienced nurse who knows what to do in these situations.'

Supporting the bereaved

Do

- Let your concern and caring show
- Be available to listen, run errands, help with the children
- Say you are sorry about the death and about their distress
- Allow them to share their grief
- Encourage them to be patient with themselves
- Allow them to talk about the dead person
- Talk about the special qualities of the dead person
- Reassure them that they did all they could
- Give extra attention to children who are often forgotten by grieving adults

Don't

- Avoid them because you feel uncomfortable
- Say you know how they feel
- Tell them what they should feel or do
- Avoid mentioning the dead person's name
- Try to find something positive about the death
- Suggest that other members of the family can replace the dead person
- Indicate that the care given before death was inadequate
- Let your own feelings of helplessness stop you from offering support

Practical Arrangements

When someone dies the bereaved often do not know what practical arrangements have to be made. Often they are too upset to take control of such matters. It is often the nurse that people turn to for advice about such arrangements. Some parents may want advice about planning the funeral service before the death and may find these decisions easier when the child is still alive (Walter, 1990). It is also useful for the nurse to discuss any religious traditions before death to ensure that no beliefs are ignored and to avoid any confusion.

Study activity

Find out the answers to the questions listed in the section titled 'Death – the practical details'.

Faulkner (1995) recommends that, if the death occurs in hospital, a small quiet room be available for the bereaved to receive information about registering the death and finding a funeral director. She stresses the importance of this formality being carried out by a nurse who knows the family well to add the personal element and to provide emotional support. It is useful also to be able to give this information in written form as it is likely that the shock and grief felt at this time will prevent retention of facts.

Parents report that being able to see and hold their dead child has helped them to grieve. The nurse should prepare them for this experience and be present to offer support if needed (Thompson, 1992). After their child has died parents sometimes need to feel that they have some lasting memory and may be helped by photographs, hand or footprints or a lock of hair.

Death – the practical details

Do you know:

- When a cremation can take place?
- What practical decisions have to be taken when planning a funeral and who can advise on these?
- How much a funeral costs?
- What sort of financial help is available for low income families?
- How to find out about local support groups for the bereaved?
- The circumstances under which an inquest may be held?
- The names of three national organisations which provide support for the bereaved?
- The circumstances under which the doctor must report a death to the coroner?
- The time period within which a child's death should be registered?
- Which services should be notified of a death?
- Who provides what kind of certificate following an expected death?

Key Points

1. Nurses need to come to terms with their own beliefs and emotions about death if they are able to talk openly about it with parents and children.
2. Children's perceptions of death are more likely to have been gained from the media than any direct experience. As a result, they may have developed unrealistic and confusing ideas.
3. Children need to be involved in the care of the dying sibling or parent and need to be allowed to discuss their thoughts and fears. Exclusion only distresses them further and may cause long-term psychological problems.
4. There is no right or wrong way to answer children's and parents' questions about death. Listening and providing simple and honest answers are the most helpful ways of dealing with awkward questions.
5. The grief of bereavement is a long and complicated process that is different for each individual and never passes. However, there is a gradual adjustment to a new life which can be helped by a patient and understanding listener.
6. Nurses can help parents after the death by being able to give advice about the practical issues which distressed parents do not have the energy or desire to manage.

Chapter 19

Chronic Illness – Family Stress and Coping

Introduction

When a child has a chronic and debilitating disorder, the ongoing feelings of grief, guilt and sorrow experienced by the parents have been defined as chronic sorrow (Myer, 1988). The intensity of these feelings depends on the family's developmental stage, the age of the child at diagnosis, communication between spouses and the degree of support available from family and physician (Burr, 1985). Mothers often feel guilty at producing a child with a chronic problem and this may cause them to become overprotective while resenting the time involved in the child's care and feeling uncertain and anxious about the child's future. In comparison, fathers often feel excluded by the relationship between mother and child. Both parents may feel socially isolated due to their child's condition or time-consuming treatment. Thus parents of a child with a chronic condition often have to cope with their own emotions about the implications of the disorder as well as a complex treatment regime. The affected child and siblings also have to cope with conflicting emotions, often without the support of their parents who are too distressed themselves to provide the usual comfort.

Parental knowledge of a chronic childhood illness is considered important for its effective treatment. Education usually begins as soon as the condition is diagnosed, but this is a stressful time and many parents are too anxious to be able to fully comprehend the significance of information given at this time. Studies suggest that parental knowledge and understanding of their child's illness contributes to the development of independence for the child, treatment compliance, control of the illness and maintenance of appropriate family relationships and lifestyle. However, it has also been suggested that parents of children with life-threatening illnesses resist information about the condition because such knowledge will destroy their denial mechanisms with which they cope with the threat of the potentially fatal outcome. The chronic uncertainty of an unknown outcome is responsible for much of the stress experienced by parents which, in turn, affects their coping strategies (Cohen and Martison, 1988).

Psychosocial stresses of chronic illness affecting the children

Schooling

- disruption due to hospitalisation, out-patient appointments
- learning difficulties, due to excessive disruption or treatment

Relationships

- jealousy with siblings
- disruption of social life

Uncertain future

- employment prospects
- marriage and fertility
- genetic implications of illness

Body image changes

- directly related to the condition
- subsequent to surgery
- retarded growth/puberty
- side effects of treatment (alopecia, weight loss or gain)

Frequent hospitalisation

- pain and discomfort from procedures
- disruption of normal routine
- feelings of dependency

Lazarus and Cohen (1977) define coping in terms of the strategies used in the face of different kinds of threat. Leventhal (1986) identifies three important processes involved in coping. The individual needs to:

- understand the threat
- compare self with others exposed to the same or similar threat
- acquire a sense of hope

There appear to be two main methods of coping with the threat. *Approach coping* is concerned with doing something directly about reducing the threat and *avoidance coping* relates to taking palliative action to avoid confronting the threat.

Approach Coping Methods

Gibson (1988) found that parents of children with a chronic illness used three main approach coping strategies: social support, problem-solving skills and a belief in the efficacy of medical care. Social support is usually gained from healthcare professionals or other parents in similar circumstances and enables parents to feel a sense of control. Problem-solving skills and having a system of beliefs are intra-psychic methods of coping that also give parents a personal sense of control, which in itself is rewarding.

Support groups can provide social support that reduces the problems of isolation as well as providing emotional and practical support. However, Llewelyn and Haslett (1986) warn that support groups can have a negative influence by imposing the views of dominant members of the group. Isolation tends to be self-imposed because of society's attitude to disability. These negative attitudes have an impact on the family's coping skills (Geen, 1990). This sense of isolation is heightened by 20th-century social factors. Families are now smaller and nuclear and more geographically separated, making family support less available than previously. Affluent families have more resources to overcome these social factors and Macaskill and Monach (1990) note that these families are more likely to adjust to the stress of living with a chronic illness.

The need for social support varies within cultures. In cultures where the family is important their own support networks enable them to cope well and they may resist help from healthcare professionals or other parents. Conversely, Spinetta (1984) found that Mexican and Vietnamese families cope with difficulty because their culture does not value close communication and sharing of emotions. Similarly, the British culture still tends to consider that males should keep a stiff upper lip, and Faulkner *et al.* (1995) describe how fathers found it particularly difficult to share their emotions and felt they should remain unemotional to support the rest of the family.

Problem-solving skills and a belief in the efficacy of health care depends largely on adequate information being available to all the family. Yet, Whitehead (1995) concludes from studies of parents and children's knowledge of diabetes that there is little relationship between parent and child knowledge of the condition; the length of time since diagnosis does not increase the amount of knowledge and knowledge

Psychosocial stresses of chronic illness for the parents

Finances

- frequent hospital trips
- loss of employment and income

Relationships

- meeting the needs of the affected child and the siblings
- social isolation due to child's treatment needs, finding responsible carer
- decreased time for usual family activities
- role changes

Communication

- ability to share feelings with spouse
- coping with the affected child's questions and fears
- ability to explain to siblings

Maintaining discipline

- treating all the family equally
- avoiding overprotective behaviour

Psychosocial stresses of chronic illness for the siblings

Relationships

- resentment towards ill sibling
- loss of contact with parents
- isolation

Role change

- extra responsibilities
- support for parents

Changes in beliefs

- concerns about infection/inheritance
- feelings of guilt about the cause of the condition
- fear of own death

does not relate to management skills. My own studies of parents of children with cystic fibrosis had similar findings. My own conclusions were that, although families needed more information and advice, they also required a structured teaching programme to help them analyse and evaluate their knowledge to aid their problem-solving skills and management of the condition. Similar programmes have been carried out for families of children with asthma, with significant positive effects (Pinkerton and Kieckhefer, 2002). This teaching needs to take into account the physical and psychological problems of the condition. Local initiatives such as asthma camps have been shown to improve children's physical and psychological status as well as educating them and helping them to cope with their condition (Hodges, 2004).

In 2005 the NHS developed the Expert Patients Programme, 'a self management course to provide patients the confidence, skills and knowledge to manage their chronic condition better and be more in control of their lives'. This concept is criticised by Bury and Pink (2005) who do not believe there is sufficient evidence to show this approach remains effective over time. Interestingly, this debate about self-management does not include children and yet it is particularly relevant to them as they have to learn to manage their chronic condition independently as they grow older.

Study activity

Talk to a teenager with a chronic illness and discuss what has been most helpful in learning to manage the condition

Studies indicate that healthcare professionals tend to ignore the psychological concerns and need to be taught to identify and manage them (Faulkner *et al.*, 1995). Black (2005) describes how she did not feel confident or comfortable enough to discuss self-esteem and body image with a disabled teenager. The inability of healthcare professionals to give bad news in a sensitive way and to address the psychological concerns of the whole family does not help the family to have trust and confidence in them. Farrant and Watson (2004) found that teenagers with chronic diseases and their families valued most health professionals who could demonstrate honesty, confidentiality and good medical knowledge, and who were good listeners. This same study revealed that 25% of young people did not trust their health professional because of concerns about confidentiality and 10% of them withheld information because of this lack of trust.

Avoidance Coping Methods

Denial is a common emotion during the time of diagnosis of a chronic illness and is often seen as a maladaptive reaction to stress. However, parents have to come to terms with the loss of their 'perfect child' and Whyte (1992) argues that the defence mechanism of denial is a necessary response to reduce the impact of the diagnosis and all its consequences, and allow life to continue. Prolonged use of denial can prevent long-term adaptation to the situation and may cause parents to overprotect and overindulge their child and neglect treatment (Tropauer *et al.*, 1970).

Jennings (1992) found that many parents of chronically ill children felt intense anger during the period of adjustment to the condition and demonstrated this by crying, screaming and slamming doors. While these reactions can be helpful in the short term, they do not help long-term adaptation and may cause further stress for other members of the family. Anger often results from the frustration of trying to cope with all the consequences of the illness and maintaining a normal lifestyle, especially when no one seems to recognise these stresses. Beth, the mother of Tom, who died from a chronic neurological condition, remained angry with the healthcare professionals 2 years after Tom's death: 'I am still cross that so much of my energy had to be used to get the help and support I needed, when I could have used it to be with Tom.'

Other reactions include shame, guilt, uncertainty and depression. Generally, mothers appear to take on the burden of caring for the affected child as well as for the rest of the family, and this responsibility often becomes too overwhelming. I remember one mother who refused to talk to me about her child's illness 'because I cry whenever I talk about it'. This reaction is not unique; Shapiro (1983) found that mothers often experience depression which inhibits their talking to others about their child. This is a very difficult problem as it is likely that these mothers are the very people who need help to talk. Difficulty in open communication often impairs parents' management of the child's condition (Faulkner *et al.*, 1995) and may cause marital difficulties. Evidence of marital breakdown is conflicting. Some authors believe that existing difficulties will be exacerbated (Jennings, 1992), but others have shown that couples feel closer because of the experience (Macaskill and Monach, 1990).

The sheer physical demands of the child's treatment may cause emotional and physical exhaustion. Families will react to this stress in different ways, by an alteration in thoughts, emotions and behaviour. Some of these changes represent attempts to cope but may in themselves become secondary causes of stress and result in physical or mental ill-health (Figure 19.1).

Adaptation

McCollum and Gibson (1970) studied families of children with a chronic condition and identified four phases of adaptation:

- pre-diagnostic
- confrontational
- long-term adaptive
- terminal

In the pre-diagnostic stage parents, especially mothers, felt guilt, despair and even hostility towards the child, whom they were unable to rear successfully. There may be conflicts with others over the reality of the child's symptoms. At the confrontational stage, when the diagnosis was

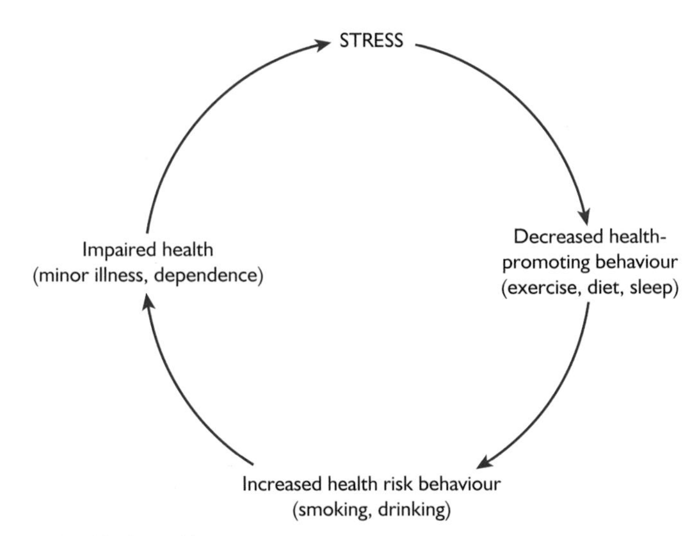

Figure 19.1 Coping with stress.

> **Positive adaptive responses to chronic illness**
>
> - Acceptance of the child's condition
> - Realistic expectations for the child
> - Day-to-day management of the condition
> - Meet the child's normal developmental needs
> - Meet the developmental needs of the other family members
> - Assist family members to express their feelings
> - Educate others about the child's condition
> - Establish a support system
>
> (Canam, 1993)

confirmed, parents felt initial disbelief followed by intense grief, anxiety and depression. Faulkner *et al.* (1995) found that the way in which health professionals handled this stage clearly affected parents' ability to adapt to the situation. Inept handling can cause such intense fear and anxiety that adaptation to reality is delayed. Diagnosis is often associated with the family's search for a reason why the illness has occurred to them. Faulkner *et al.* (1995) argue that families need to have a belief in a pattern of life events to help them adapt. As parents come to terms with the diagnosis they fluctuate between denial and optimism, grief and chronic anxiety. During this long-term adaptation phase they also reported problems in managing the treatment regime and admitted repressing and forgetting information. The success of the final stage of adaptation seems to depend upon the family's ability to cope positively with the condition. Parents in my own study revealed the problems of the early years after diagnosis and stressed the importance of their own resources and those of other parents in finding solutions (Ramsay, 1990). At this stage, when contact with healthcare professionals has decreased, help is less available and families feel that they have full responsibility; as one parent described it: 'You either sink or swim.'

Compliance

Survival into adulthood and beyond for children with chronic illnesses is associated with the avoidance of not only the medical complications of the condition but also the psychological effects of living with a chronic condition. Poor psychological adjustment to the condition often results in depression and poor compliance (Goodchild and Dodge, 1985). There is increasing evidence that compliance with regimens for chronic illnesses is less than optimal. Compliance with treatment regimens for children obviously involves parents until the child is old

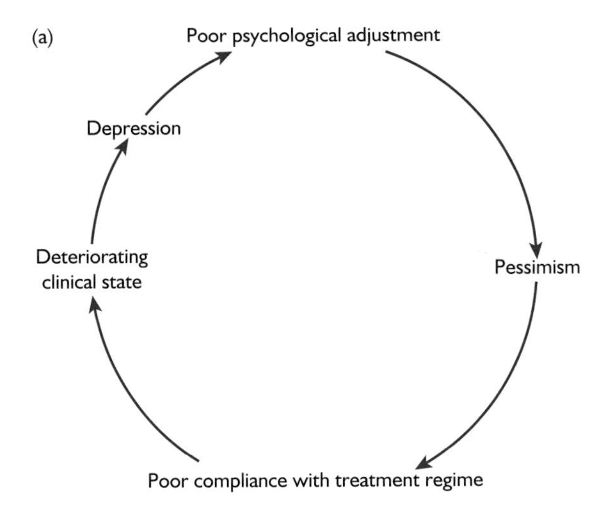

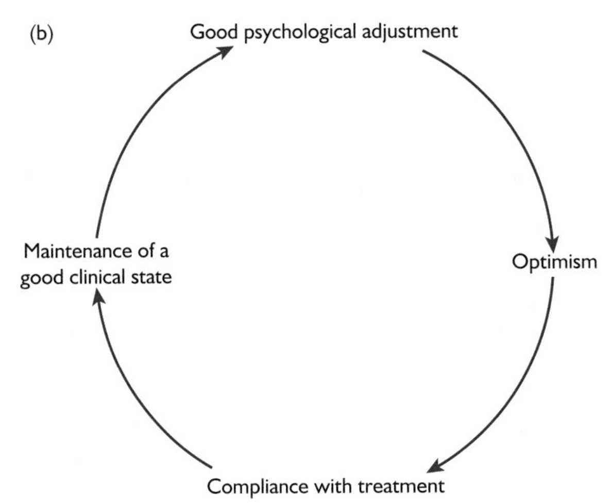

Figure 19.2 Psychological factors and compliance. (a) Poor compliance. (b) Good compliance.

enough to provide self-care independently. Even then, parental attitude and management of the condition during young childhood are likely to shape the way the older child behaves in relation to the illness (Figure 19.2a, b).

Compliance can be defined as a disposition to act in accordance with rules, wishes; to be obedient. Studies on the identification of factors that influence compliance have revealed that compliance behaviour is affected by several issues. Psychological characteristics such as attitudes and perceptions of health and illness affects the individual's concepts of the severity of the disorder and thus the importance and necessity of complying with treatment. Environmental factors such as social support, socio-economic status and education affect the individual's ability and desire to comprehend the treatment regimen. Physician–patient interaction also influences the acceptance and understanding of the illness and its treatment. Ley and Llewelyn (1995) discuss the importance of

Improving compliance by communication

Improving oral communication:

- using shorter words and sentences
- avoiding jargon
- stressing the importance
- breaking down information into categories
- using specific statements
- repeating information
- arranging follow-up visits to test recall

Providing written information

- using symbols, graphics, colour to ensure it is noticed
- ensuring legibility
- using simple terms in short sentences
- explaining technical terms
- stressing relevance
- highlighting areas of specific importance
- addressing counter-arguments

oral and written communication for understanding and compliance. They stress the need for health professionals to ensure that their communication is effective, memorable and given in a sensitive way. Finally, the therapeutic regime itself will affect compliance. It appears that the more complex and lengthy the treatment, and the more changes to usual behaviour it involves, the less likely compliance will occur (Ley and Llewelyn, 1995). Again, improved methods of communication can help families to remember and manage complex regimens.

Compliance may be a specific problem in adolescence when chronic illness may be most detrimental to normal growth and development. Illness interferes with the adolescent's need for autonomy and a positive self-image. The adolescent tendency for rebellion and risk-taking may manifest itself in non-compliance with treatment regimens. However, Auslander *et al.* (1991) found that poor compliance in diabetic adolescents was related to stress in the family so it may be that positive adaptation of the family to the condition determines the older child's ability to manage it.

The Role of the Nurse

Robinson (1993) has noted that nurses can play a negative role in helping families to adapt to chronic illness. Others believe that the caring, competent and committed attitude of most nurses is enough to support parents to cope positively with the situation (Ray and Ritchie, 1993). Given the importance of social support and the need to believe in the effectiveness of the healthcare professionals, it seems important that the nurse has the skills to help the family to:

- understand the condition and treatment
- live as normal a life as possible
- discuss their feelings with each other
- include the child and siblings in decision making
- meet their practical needs
- establish realistic goals for the future

How does the nurse learn these skills? Faulkner *et al.* (1995) believe that a thorough understanding can only be gained by working with and listening to families who live with a child with a chronic illness. Certainly, this will add a depth of understanding that teaching alone cannot impart, but they propose that nurse education becomes more interactive and experiential so that nurses can role play stressful situations and learn to identify psychological problems. Faulkner *et al.* (1995) also suggest that a named practice nurse, who has been taught these skills of working with families with chronic illness, be assigned to the family at diagnosis. This nurse can identify concerns and help the family to deal with them. This method would provide the family with immediate and long-term credible support.

Key Points

1. Having a child with a chronic condition changes the lives of the whole family and threatens their plans for the future.
2. Families use a variety of adaptive and maladaptive behaviours during their adjustment to the situation.
3. The family's acceptance of the condition and their adjustment to it is associated with appropriate adaptive behaviours in response to the psychological and physiological management of the condition.
4. Positive adaptation is associated with social support, belief in the efficacy of healthcare and the ability to solve problems.
5. Postitive adaptation is aided by open and honest communication between all the members of the family and between the family and the healthcare professionals.
6. Nurses can help families to cope by providing information and recognising psychological and practical problems.

Chapter 20
Living with a Disability

Introduction

Having a child with a disability can be a positive or negative experience for the rest of the family. Some families gain strengths from the experience, but for others it causes disharmony and distress. Negative attitudes and labelling children with disabilities seem to pervade society and affect service quality (Holmes, 1999) and the general view is that parents with a disabled child can never recover from this tragic burden (Chappelle *et al.*, 2001). Nurses can do much to help families cope with the disability and meet the challenge of living with a disabled child.

It is also not easy for the affected child to live with a permanent disability and overcome prejudice, ridicule and discrimination as well as physical problems that influence roles, relationships and life experience. The nurse can help these children to maximise their abilities and to overcome their disability. With the appropriate treatment, education and support disabled children may reach the same goals in adulthood as their 'normal' peers. However, even this does not prevent the disabled child from a constant feeling of being different (Harrison, 1997).

Thus, the role of the nurse is complex. Families need help with the practical issues relating to caring for a child with a disability but they also need counselling and sympathetic and uncritical support. The child also requires emotional and physical help to be able to live as normal a life as possible.

impairment
A stable and persisting defect in the individual . . . which stems from known or unknown molecular, cellular, physiological or structural disorder.

disability
A stable and persisting physical or psychological dysfunction at the personal level, by necessity again confined to the individual; this dysfunction stems from the limitations imposed by the impairment and by the individual's psychological reaction to it.

handicap
Persisting social dysfunction, a social role assumed by the impaired or disabled individual that is assigned by the expectations of society. Handicap stems not from the individual but from social expectations; it follows from the manner and degree in which expectations alter the performance of social roles by impaired or disabled persons.

(WHO, 1980)

Adjustment to Disability

Moos and Tsu (1977) found that six factors were associated with adjustment to disability. Positive adjustment was aided by the ability to:

- change beliefs and goals for the future
- accept responsibility for the disability
- seek information about overcoming the disability
- contain negative feelings

Poor adjustment was associated with anger and blame directed at others as the cause of the disability, and time-consuming fantasies about recovery. Small children growing up with a disability usually take their cues from their parents about their disability. Parents who are able to help their child to live as normal a life as possible will enable their child to adjust and overcome their disability better than the child who is protected from reality (Russell, 1989). Denial of the disability and unrealistic expectations about the future are natural at times but are dangerous if allowed to develop. These fantasies can be accidentally promoted by hospitalisation for surgery or treatment, which the child may think will restore normality. If the nurse does not give an honest explanation, the child can feel devastated when the anticipated improvement does not occur. Children with Down's syndrome are now having plastic surgery to correct the characteristic facial features associated with this condition. Some may argue that this provides children with the best chance of normal socialisation but others suggest that such surgery is an unnecessary discomfort for the children, for the purpose of appeasing society's expectations of what is normal.

Adjustment is also related to health locus of control. Disabled adults have been found to cope better with their disability if they have an internal locus of control, they have more knowledge of their condition, and practise more self-care. Wilkinson (1995) suggests that developing an internal locus of control in disabled children could enhance their satisfaction with life and psychological well-being. It could also help their level of self-care and independence.

Often the care of a disabled child is mainly the mother's responsibility. Complicated, time-consuming and onerous care may use up all her physical and mental resources, leaving little energy for the rest of the family. This can result in social isolation for all the family, loss of maternal care for any siblings and feelings of resentment. This negative scenario does nothing for the disabled child's self-esteem. Maternal reaction to the disability, which appears to be related to adequate support, has been found to significantly influence siblings' acceptance of disability in the family. Inadequate support is associated with neglect of the needs of siblings, and especially with girls being given more responsibility for care of the disabled child (Atkinson and Crawford, 1995). The Carers National Association estimates that 40 000 to 50 000 children in the UK provide care for a disabled friend or relative. This can be a positive experience but they are at risk from unrecognised stress and isolation (Syverson, 1997).

Attitudes to Disability

Wright (1983) suggests that the general population assumes that physically disabled people also have a mental disability and tend to treat the disabled with a patronising and pitying manner. Wilkinson (1995) considers that these attitudes arise from idealised images of normality with body image being associated with status, achievement and success. The experience of living with a disability allows some families to reconsider these attitudes to illness and disability. Peace (1996a) cites a mother who said that her definition of disability before she had a child

Factors that influence adjustment to disability

- Age of acquisition
- Insidious versus traumatic onset
- Stability of condition
- Severity of disability
- Degree of dependency
- Intellectual functioning
- Associated pain or illness

Supporting siblings

Communication

- inform them about the disability and update them as appropriate
- listen to their ideas and concerns
- discuss the future with them

Involvement

- include them in the care of the disabled child
- let them teach their life skills to the disabled sibling
- do not overburden them with responsibility for care

Appreciation

- treat all children the same in relation to discipline, attention and resources
- provide all children with their own special time alone with parents
- value all children equally
- allow all children to have privacy and solitude
- permit sibling squabbles and disputes

with cerebral palsy was unhappiness. Since her personal experience she now realised that everyone was an individual and no one was perfect.

Although personal attitudes may change, the family still has to cope with others' misconceptions. Atkinson and Crawford (1995) found that 70% of siblings had been bullied, teased or avoided because of their brother's or sister's disability. Over half of these children admitted that they were embarrassed, upset or angry by the effect of their sibling's disability on their relationships.

The attitudes of health professionals to disability have also been criticised. Mikulic (1971) found that nurses tended to reinforce dependency rather than independent behaviour. They do not tend to promote normal lifestyles, often seeing such tactics as evidence of the denial of the disability (Robinson, 1993). In this way they may actually prevent families from developing ways of coping (Ray and Ritchie, 1993). Purssell (1994) suggests that such attitudes are due to a lack of education and that nurses need more input about disability and the importance of maximising normalisation.

Adaptations to the home

Communications

- intercom system
- telephone modifications (amplifier, headset)

Mobility

- wheelchair/adapted pushchair
- hoist
- stair lift
- ramps
- standing frame

Rest and sleep

- bean bag
- support chair
- adjustable height bed
- pressure area aids

Hygiene needs

- bath/shower seat
- bath handles
- lever taps
- thermostatic control shower
- wall-hung basin
- toilet seat

General safety

- fire guards
- non-slip floors
- hand rails
- wide doorways
- toys stored at waist level
- waist-height switches/cords

Utensils

- lengthened handles
- pick-up gadgets
- lever handles
- adhesive place mats
- plate guards

Disabled Living Foundation

380–384 Harrow Road, London W9 2HU
Tel: 020 7289 6111
www.dlf.org.uk

Caring Needs

Wilkinson (1995) argues that hospitals are for sick people and are not best suited to learning to cope with a disability. Rehabilitation and disability management learnt in hospital is not easily transferred into the home. Transitional areas, sometimes found in maternity units, which are more like the home environment, could enable the disabled child and family to develop independence in the skills needed for successful discharge. It would be easier for families to rediscover normality in this kind of environment, giving them a better chance of overcoming the feelings of being different and taking control of their lives. To enable this control the family need to have a suitably adapted environment to encourage the child's independence. Many aids and adaptations are available for the disabled and the Disabled Living Foundation can provide useful information about these. Practical advice about clothing for the older child can help the child's independence and still enable them to be fashionable.

Before discharge, parents also need advice about minimising the effect of the disability on family life. Robinson (1993) advocates that the child and family should live a normal family life and that the child should be exposed to the reactions of others so that they can learn to accept these. The family should be encouraged to treat the disabled child as a child and not as a disability. The development of any child is individual and, like any child, the disabled child needs stimulation to aid this development, minimise the disability and maximise abilities. Although parents find it difficult to be strict with their disabled child, it is important to maintain discipline or the child may develop into an immature and spoilt adolescent. Ignoring bad behaviour may also lead to behaviour problems in siblings who will be jealous of what appears to be favouritism. As with any child, the disabled child will need to be able to interact with others as an adult and socialisation should be encouraged. A variety of leisure activities is available for disabled children and participation in these helps socialisation as well as being part of normal childhood.

Study activity

Find out what leisure activities are available for disabled children in your locality.

Professional intervention in the care of the disabled child cannot cure the physical problems but it can add to the child's quality of life. Parents of children with disabilities often come into contact with a great variety of healthcare professionals and are frustrated by the lack of continuity and coordination of care (Peace, 1996b). Peace suggests that a key worker could help to overcome these problems which result in criticisms of inappropriate or duplicate care or none at all. A children's community nurse could be the ideal key worker in these situations and could do much to coordinate care while enabling the family to take overall control. In addition, a children's nurse would have the skills that families value: an appreciation of the reality of living with a child with a disability and easy accessibility for advice and support (Peace, 1996b). Thorne (1993) also found that families had most confidence and trust in those professionals who could demonstrate competence and effective communication skills.

Farrell (1996) believes that disabled children and their families can benefit from hospice respite care. The huge physical and emotional demands for these families mean that they can become completely physically and emotionally exhausted. This can affect their own physical and mental health as well as the care they provide for their child. Respite care aims to give a supportive environment where the hospice team will share the care usually given solely by the family. It provides an opportunity for the family to rest and to participate in family activities, which may previously have been impossible because of the care demands of the disabled child. Moreover, respite care may be able to provide the child with new experiences; new treatments or trips out may be possible because the hospice may have access to more resources and skilled help than the home environment. But is this what families really want? There are few examples of families being asked specifically about their needs and expectations of support (Read, 2000). Brett (2004) found that parents experienced difficulty in acknowledging that they needed support. In her study she found that parents viewed support and respite care as a measure of their failure and vulnerability.

Educational Needs

Learning disability/difficulty are now the terms to describe children with an intellectual impairment who were once said to have a mental handicap. Earys *et al.* (1993) found that this term was prejudicial and did not recognise the specific problems of the child. While some children may only be intellectually disabled, many of them also have associated physical and sensory disabilities. Children with only a physical or sensory disability may have special educational needs in terms of the school environment or the specialist equipment they require.

Practical advice – clothing

- Avoid back fastenings which are awkward to fasten and may cause sores for children in wheelchairs
- Separates can be bought in different sizes and are easier to put on and take off. Velcro strips can be used to hold tops and bottoms together
- Sturdy material which stretches is likely to prolong the life of the clothing
- Bra slips or brassieres which fasten at the front are easier than traditional brassieres
- Capes are more convenient than coats for children in wheelchairs
- Boots and shoes are easier to manipulate if they are elasticated or have laces which open the shoe to the toes
- Most large shoe manufacturers operate an odd-shoe scheme for children with different-sized feet. They have to be ordered at an additional charge
- Over-the-knee socks or hold-up stockings are easier to manage than tights, but care should be taken to ensure that these do not compress the top of the leg

The Warnock Committee on Special Education Needs did much for the educational rights of disabled children. It made 250 recommendations about the care of children with disabilities, including the abolition of the term 'handicap' and the recognition that parents should be partners in their child's care and education. The 1981 Education Act, which arose from the Warnock report (DES, 1978) and has since been supported by the Children Act (DH, 1989), stressed the importance of multi-agency cooperation to identify and meet the needs of disabled children. It promoted the concept of assessment of needs rather than determining requirements by diagnosis, IQ or physical abilities. The Act also enabled children to receive special education in a variety of settings, including ordinary schools. The importance of integration into ordinary schools is emphasised and defined in many different ways; it can mean a place in an ordinary class, a special unit in an ordinary school or sharing of some facilities between an ordinary and a special school (*see also* Educational provision for children with special needs p. 104).

Study activity

Consider the advantages and disadvantages for a disabled child in an ordinary school.

When I consider this issue I am reminded of the quotation 'Better to reign in hell than serve in heaven' from John Milton's *Paradise Lost*. Is integration really the answer for disabled children? The theory behind integration is that disabled children can gain in self-confidence and independence by associating with able-bodied children in the usual environment of childhood. Evidence of these positive effects have been shown by the National Foundation for Educational Research (Russell, 1989). However, this is not true for all children and there are wide variations between the attitudes of local educational authorities towards resourcing disabled children in ordinary schools.

Roger was diagnosed with a degenerative sensory disorder at the age of 8 years. Initially, he was educated at his usual primary school but he became sullen and withdrawn and his previously good schoolwork deteriorated. On investigation, it was found that even with special aids to compensate for his disability, he could not keep pace with his peers. To use his aids he had to sit separately from the rest of the class and he was not allowed to join sports activities, in which he previously excelled, because it was thought to be unsafe. He was eventually transferred to a residential school for the sensory impaired where he has thrived. He integrates with children with a variety of degrees of disability which has helped him appreciate their needs as well as realising that he is not unique. He is able to participate on equal terms with his school friends in a variety of educational and sports activities and, because he is also learning specific life skills for his disability, is able to make realistic future plans.

The Education Act 1981 made provision for the assessment of children's learning needs based on the child's abilities rather than their disabilities. The Act also placed a duty on health authorities to inform the parents and the LEA of any child who has, or is likely to develop, special educational needs. Formal assessment can take place from the age of 2 years, but assessment can take place earlier than this at parents' request. If the LEA considers that a child over 2 requires special educational facilities outside those that are usually available through the school services, formal assessment procedures may be initiated. The end product of this assessment is the statement, which includes educational, medical and psychological opinion about the child's educational needs and ways of meeting these. Parents have a right to contribute to this written assessment and to use other representatives to provide evidence if they wish. Parents have argued that although they have an opportunity to query the draft statement and appeal about the outcome, it is only those who are vocal and able to express themselves well who can make a real impact on the statementing process.

Growing Up

Adolescence is a difficult time for most children as they struggle to achieve social acceptance as well as independence, self-esteem and autonomy. It is an even more difficult struggle for the disabled adolescent who already has a feeling of being different. Adolescence is often a challenging time for parents who may be reluctant to release responsibility for their child. Parents of disabled children feel this more acutely and are more concerned about the child's ability to be independent.

Leisure facilities for the disabled

- *Opportunity playgroups* – for children with any type of disability are available in some parts of the country
- *Toy libraries* – loan toys and play equipment for disabled children
- *Handicapped adventure playgrounds* – throughout greater London and elsewhere
- *Pets* – trained to assist the blind, deaf or disabled
- *Swimming* – advice from the Swimming Teachers Association Guidelines for teaching the disabled to swim. Many pools have special sessions for the disabled
- *Holidays* – suitable accommodation listed by the Royal Association for Disability and Rehabilitation. Voluntary organisations often have schemes to provide holidays for disabled children. Social Services may help with costs
- *Duke of Edinburgh Award Scheme* – open to disabled and able-bodied children
- *Music* – Disabled Living Foundation has information about courses, teachers and orchestras for the disabled
- *Riding* – The Riding for the Disabled Association has 330 branches throughout the country
- *Sports* – Information from the British Sports Association for the Disabled
- *Scouts and Guides* – County advisor can offer opportunities for disabled children
- *Youth club activities* – organised by the National Physically Handicapped and Ablebodied (PHAB) Association for disabled and able-bodied children over 13

The Warnock Committee of Enquiry (1978)

Recommended that the:

- Single categories labelling a child as handicapped be abolished and replaced by detailed descriptions of the child's special educational needs
- Rigid demarcation between the handicapped and non-handicapped be abolished
- Term sub-normal be replaced by the new descriptive phrase child with special learning difficulties
- Handicapped child should be integrated into normal schools to benefit both the handicapped and the normal child by providing a better opportunity for the development of a constructive attitude to disability

Based on the principles that:

- Handicapped children should be regarded as children first, some having special needs
- A suitable educational programme best suited to the individual child's particular needs should be established
- Children may have several needs which must all be met. One single handicap should not obscure other needs
- Handicap is not static and the child's needs may change over time

Local authorities have a statutory obligation to provide special accommodation for the disabled and if the adolescent wishes to live away from home parents need to make sure their name is on the waiting list for this accommodation. A number of surveys now exist to provide information about the available facilities for disabled students within universities. These can be obtained from the National Union of Students. Education authorities are required to award full-time disabled students an additional grant to meet the cost of special equipment related to the disability, but the student is expected to apply and explain the need for this extra money.

The Disablement Resettlement Officer (DRO) is employed by the Employment Service specifically to encourage employers to find suitable work for the disabled. Some big companies employ their own DRO. The DRO assesses each disabled person's abilities and compares these with the local job vacancies and the vocational and professional training opportunities. There are also local day facilities for the disabled that may offer some kind of paid employment. These centres tend to be for those who are too disabled to work and can be seen to further segregate the severely disabled.

Study activity

Find out what opportunities there are for further education, training or employment for the disabled teenager in your own locality.

Society often considers that sexual relationships for the disabled are inappropriate. Children with a disability may have little understanding of sex and sexuality. By the time they reach school-leaving age they may have had little opportunity for privacy with other adolescents or to observe the development of usual boy–girl relationships that occur during adolescence. Their ability to get professional advice may be hampered by the constant presence of a carer. Support groups for teenagers with disabilities can help them to overcome this and other problems. Nurses may be able to provide clear explanations in an uninhibited way, and provide information about contraception and other practical issues. However, this is not a subject with which all nurses feel at ease and they tend not to assess or plan care around the issue of sexuality (Van Ooijen and Charnock, 1994). Van Ooijen (1996) suggests that this is because nurses are not at ease with their own sexuality and are uncomfortable listening to others discussing sexual matters.

Study activity

Discuss with a colleague your feelings about talking to a disabled teenager about potential sexual problems. Discuss also the reasons for your feelings and the amount of knowledge you have about such problems.

Statementing

General advice for parents providing evidence:

- Describe the relevant aspects of the child's functioning at home and at school which contribute to or lessen needs
- Include the child's physical and psychological strengths and weaknesses
- Enclose any relevant aspects of the child's past history (e.g. environments which enabled or prevented the child's development)
- Explain the necessary aims to enable the child to achieve educational development and increased independence
- Describe how the recommended facilities and resources will promote the aims explained above

Key Points

1. Living with a disabled child can be a positive or negative experience for the family.
2. Children's nurses have an important role in providing families with the necessary skills to accept the disability and adjust to it in an appropriate way.
3. Society holds negative views towards disability and tends to equate a less-than-perfect body image with failure and loss of status.
4. Children's nurses can act as a resource to provide the practical advice that will help the disabled child to maximise abilities and reach independence.
5. Living with a disabled child can be a huge physical and emotional strain for parents. Respite care can provide them with a rest from their responsibilities while helping the child to experience new pursuits.
6. Integration of education can have advantages and disadvantages that depend upon the individual child, the degree of disability and the available facilities. Disabled adolescents need advice and support about all the usual issues related to growing up and the children's nurse may be the most appropriate person to provide this.

Chapter 21

Violence in the Family

Introduction

Violence can be defined as behaviour that is intended to hurt another person or to destroy property. Psychologists disagree about the causes of the development of violence. Freud believed that it was a basic instinct and could not be eliminated – only modified by other activities such as sports. Other early psychologists suggested that violence had a biological basis and that frustration induced an aggressive drive that motivated violent behaviour. Social learning theory proposes that violence is no different from any other learned response. It can be learnt by observation or imitation. Bandura (1973) showed that nursery school children learnt violence by imitation and were more likely to repeat the aggressive behaviour if such actions were reinforced. This raises the question of the effect of violence watched on television or in films. Most studies agree that viewing violence increases aggression, particularly in young children by:

- teaching aggressive types of behaviour
- increasing arousal
- desensitising people to violence
- reducing restraints on aggressive behaviour
- distorting views on the resolution of conflict (Bee, 1989)

Violence or abuse in the family falls into five main categories: physical, emotional, neglect, sexual and financial. It can be inflicted against children, young adults and the elderly, and occurs in both the community and in institutional settings. Gelles and Cornell (1985) note that persons who observe violence or who are victims of violence in childhood often become abusers themselves. Additionally, McKibben *et al.* (1989) found that an abused spouse was often an abusing parent.

This section will briefly discuss violence in the family, because of its impact upon any children who are present, but will mainly explore child abuse. It is vital that any professional working with children is able to recognise actual and potential child abuse, and that they know how to react to their findings.

Definitions

Abuse is difficult to define precisely but may be described as physical and/or psychological harm to another person, either temporarily or over a period of time, and may be inflicted intentionally or unintentionally, or be the result of neglect.

Physical abuse usually means that the attacker causes physical hurt, injury or even kills the subject. It can involve hitting, shaking, squeezing, burning or biting. It also involves the administration of poisonous substances, inappropriate drugs and alcohol, and attempted suffocation or drowning. It includes use of excessive force when carrying out tasks like feeding or washing a dependent person. Physical abuse includes the fabrication or induction of illness by a carer (previously termed Munchausen's syndrome by proxy or factitious illness by proxy), where the abuser induces an illness in another person, usually a child. In children, it is usually the mother who contrives to produce features of illness in the child to gain medical attention (Jones *et al.*, 1987). The fabricated illness can take many forms from suffocation to produce apnoeic attacks to chronic poisoning. Meadow (1989) suggests that this form of abuse continues to affect the children as adults, when they often adopt Munchausen's syndrome.

Sexual abuse involves adults seeking sexual gratification by using others against their will. This may be by having sexual intercourse or anal intercourse (buggery), engaging with the person in fondling, masturbation or oral sex, and includes encouraging them to watch sexually explicit behaviour or pornographic material, including videos. Kempe and Kempe (1984) provide the most commonly encountered specific definition of sexual abuse in children: '. . . the involvement of dependent, developmentally immature children and adolescents in sexual activities they do not truly comprehend, to which they are unable to give informed consent, or that violate the taboos of family roles'. This definition includes the following:

Munchausen's syndrome

Munchausen's syndrome and Munchausen's syndrome by proxy are named after Baron von Munchausen, a legendary 16th-century story-teller who told amazing and incredible tales.

- *Munchausen's syndrome.* Habitual seeking of hospital treatment for an apparent acute illness, the patient giving a false but plausible dramatic history and presentation of the features of the illness. Some patients may add blood to their urine or ingest poisons to create a more realistic picture. Such patients often undergo many invasive investigations and surgery before a true diagnosis is made.
- *Munchausen's syndrome by proxy.* An illness that one person fabricates for another. This is commonly a mother who concocts clinical features of an illness in her child or proxy, to gain the attention of healthcare professionals or to gain recognition as a dedicated carer who has saved the child's life. Affected children have been known to have been poisoned, to produce chronic diarrhoea and vomiting, or suffocated causing apnoeic attacks, to necessitate medical intervention.

Definitions of child abuse

Though child abuse defies precise definition, *Working Together*, the guide to inter-agency cooperation in child protection, offers the following definitions:

- *Neglect.* The persistent or severe neglect of a child, or the failure to protect a child from exposure to any kind of danger including cold or starvation, or extreme failure to carry out important aspects of care resulting in the significant impairment of the child's health or development including non-organic failure to thrive
- *Physical injury.* Actual or likely physical injury to a child, or failure to prevent physical injury or suffering to a child including deliberate poisoning, suffocation and Munchausen's syndrome by proxy
- *Emotional abuse.* Actual or likely severe adverse effect on the emotional and behavioural development of a child, caused by persistent or severe emotional ill-treatment or rejection. All abuse involves some emotional abuse
- *Sexual abuse.* Actual or likely sexual exploitation of a child or adolescent. The child may be dependent and/or developmentally immature

(DHSS, 1988)

Features of neglect
Behavioural observations

- constant hunger
- constant tiredness
- frequent lateness or non-attendance at school
- destructive tendencies
- low self-esteem
- neurotic behaviour
- no social relationships
- running away
- compulsive stealing or scavenging

Physical observations

- poor personal hygiene
- poor state of clothing
- emaciation
- untreated medical problems

Features of physical abuse
Physical observations

- black eyes without gross bruising of forehead
- bruises on trunk
- bruises on upper arm consistent with gripping
- fingertip bruising – finger marks
- cigarette burns
- human bite marks
- burns caused by lengthy exposure to heat
- scalds with upward splash marks or tide marks
- fractures, particularly spiral fractures
- swelling and lack of normal use of limbs
- any serious injury with no explanation or conflicting explanations, inconsistent accounts

Behavioural observations

- unusually fearful
- unnaturally compliant
- frozen watchfulness
- refusal to discuss injuries – fear of medical help
- withdrawal from physical contact
- aggression towards others
- wearing clothing which covers arms and legs in all weathers

- incest
- sexual intercourse with children in other relationships not covered by current incest legislation, including adopted and step-children
- other forms of sexual activity

Neglect is a more difficult area to define but is usually described as a failure to meet the basic essential needs of dependants, like adequate food, clothes, warmth and medical care. Leaving young children or dependent adults alone and unsupervised is another example of neglect. Refusing or failing to give adequate love and affection is a case of emotional neglect.

Emotional abuse occurs when a constant lack of love and affection, or threats, verbal attacks, taunting or shouting causes psychological problems. This type of abuse can also take the form of constant ridicule, intimidation or swearing at the victim.

Financial abuse, which occurs mostly in the elderly, is the withdrawal of finances so that the person becomes totally dependent on the abuser. The victim cannot buy basic necessities, such as food and clothing, and continually worries about money.

Epidemiology

It is difficult to give statistics about violence as much abuse is subtle and many of the abused are too frightened or embarrassed to reveal what is happening. Abuse of adults is usually termed domestic violence and in 95% of cases the abuse takes the form of physical abuse committed by men against women (Smith, 1987). Most abused older people are also women, with the majority of their abusers being men. However, abused men may be less inclined to report violence inflicted upon them by women. In child abuse the abuser is more often female (Stier *et al.*, 1993). Consequently, there is no 'typical' abuser or abused person and everyone has the potential for either of these roles (Pritchard, 1996). Nurses also have to accept that some colleagues abuse patients, as incidents such as those which occurred at Glasgow's Victoria Infirmary (Clark, 1996), Bassettlaw Hospital (Kenny, 1996) and Grantham and Kesteven District General Hospital (Clothier, 1994) sadly reveal.

No single aetiological factor seems to be responsible for abuse, as it is more likely to occur when several variables are involved. The most significant of variables appear to be low wages, poor housing, lack of facilities outside the home, social isolation and overcrowding (Smith, 1987). Recent studies show that domestic violence often begins or increases when the wife is pregnant and that this abuse during pregnancy often continues into child abuse once the baby is born (Bewley and Gibbs, 1994). Waterhouse (1993) found that children who regularly see their parent being beaten suffer as much as they would if they are being frequently and severely hit. However, although social factors are linked with abuse, violence is not confined to the lower socio-economic classes. Personality also predisposes people to violence. Those who are aggressive, easily stressed and frustrated have a need to control and are accustomed to violence being used freely are more likely to abuse (Dale *et al.*, 1986). Negative parenting, often described as low on warmth and high on criticism, places children at a higher risk of abuse (DH, 1999).

Domestic Violence

In 1999, 4.2% of females had experienced domestic violence (DH, 2000a). Half this number had children living with them and just under a third of these recognised that the children were aware of the violence. As acknowledged above, these figures are likely to be a understatement of the true picture because domestic violence is often hidden and not usually explored by professionals when taking histories. Domestic violence can be an important factor in determining the aetiology of psychiatric problems in childhood (DH, 2000a). Evans (2005) studied 33 children referred to the Child and Adolescent Mental Health Services (CAMHS) and found that 27% of these lived in families where there had been domestic violence. The two main presenting features were anxiety and behavioural problems. The Department of Health now recommends routine screening of women by health professionals to help uncover instances of domestic violence. Little (2000) suggests a routine screening policy for all female patients over 14 years enables the identification of victims, assessment of immediate danger and effective safety planning. This view is not held by all health professionals or supported by all women. A 1999 study of midwives' attitudes towards domestic violence found that 55% did not think questions should be part of antenatal assessment and Bacchus *et al.* (2002) found that not all women benefited from such screening. The authors concluded that routine screening was only useful with the right training for the health professionals and effective support mechanisms for those women who revealed abuse.

Child Abuse

The exact incidence of child abuse is not known but each week at least one child is killed by a parent or carer. During the year ending March 2004, the names of almost 30 000 children in the UK were placed on child protection registers, having suffered abuse or considered to be at significant risk of abuse (NSPCC, 2004). It is essential that children's nurses are alert to the signs of child abuse (see Figures 21.1 and 21.2) and that any concerns are shared with the appropriate people. Wherever you work as a children's nurse you should have access to your local Trust's child protection policies and procedures and also your Local Safeguarding Children Board (LSCB) procedures. LSCBs were created in 2005 (having previously been known as Area Child Protection Committees – ACPCs) to monitor agencies' responsibilities for safeguarding and promoting the welfare of children, as required by the Children Act 2004.

Study activity

Locate, read and identify your own responsibilities in relation to:

- your own Trust proceduress for recording and referring suspected child abuse
- your LSCB manual of policies and procedures

Predisposing factors for child abuse

- Parental indifference, intolerance, overanxiousness towards the child
- History of family violence/socio-economic problems
- Infant premature, low birth weight
- Parent abused or neglected as a child
- Step-parent or cohabitee present
- Single or separated parent
- Mother less than 21 years old at the time of the birth
- History of parental mental illness, drug/alcohol addiction
- Infant separated for more than 24 hours post-delivery
- Infant mentally or physically handicapped
- Less than 18 months between birth of children

(Browne and Saqi, 1988)

Myths about child abuse (NSPCC, 2004)

- Children are usually abused by strangers
- Females do not sexually abuse children
- Some cultures believe that child abuse is acceptable
- Children often lie about abuse
- Disabled children are less likely to be abused
- Child abusers are usually of low intelligence and from deprived backgrounds
- Children are always safe in groups
- Children abused by their parents are always taken into care

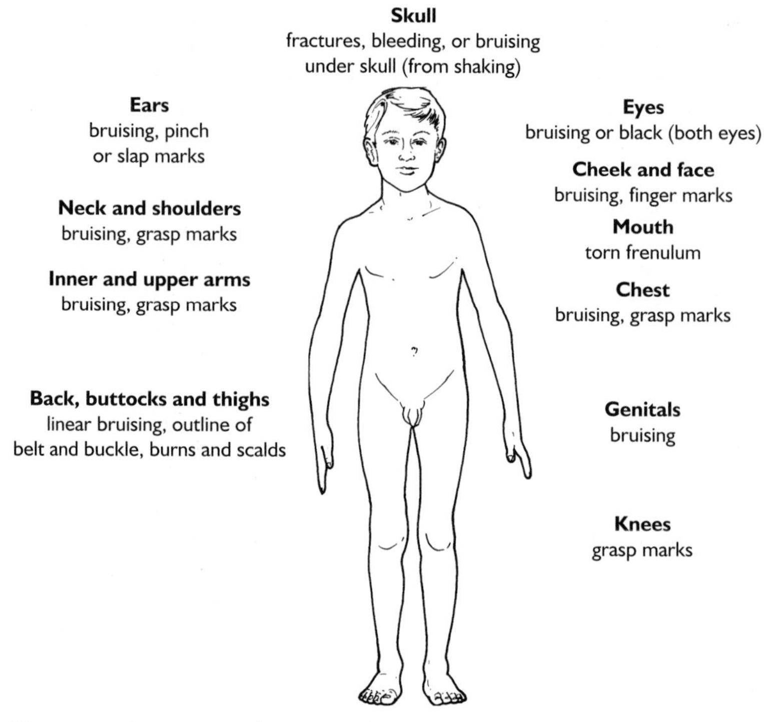

Figure 21.1 Common sites for non-accidental injuries.

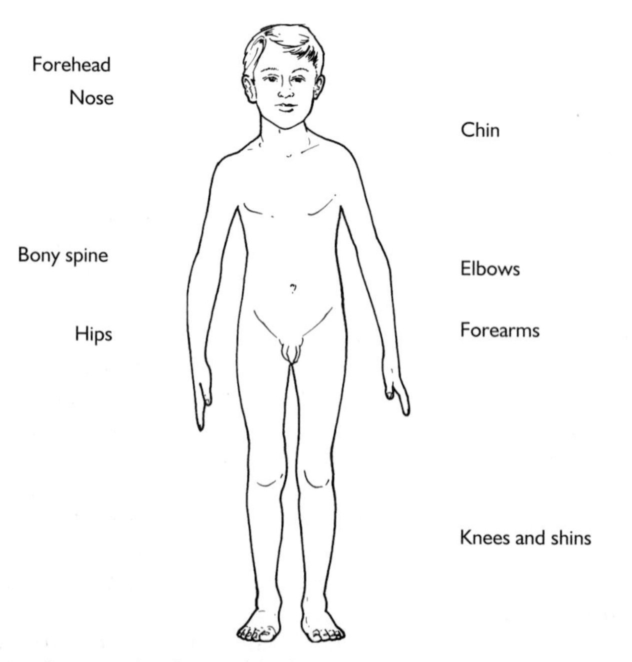

Figure 21.2 Common sites for accidental injuries.

Most children have falls or knocks that cause minor bruising and grazing, and children of school age, who tend to be the most active, are rarely without some mark that has been gained by accident during play. These accidental injuries are usually easily explained, whereas non-accidental injuries are often unexplained and characteristic. There are also characteristic predisposing factors of child abuse. Bannister (1992) warns against the uncritical acceptance of these predisposing factors. First, there is a danger of only recognising these conditions in families where abuse has occurred and not responding to other factors, perceived as insignificant but in reality more crucial. Secondly, some children in high-risk families are well cared for and not abused. However, Bannister still recommends that all professionals who work with children are aware of the warning signs that can lead to abuse, as well as being able to identify the characteristic features of abuse.

Small children have fundamental needs that may not be perceived by some parents. Parents are often unaware of normal child development and expect too much from their children. Some children are vulnerable to abuse merely because their mother cannot bond with them after an unwanted or difficult pregnancy and labour, or she simply cannot cope with another child (Reder *et al.*, 1993). Other children may be at risk because they have additional needs due to a demanding temperament, chronic illness or disability. Although child abuse is never restricted to an isolated episode of violence, there is usually a precipitating incident that initiates the abuse.

Study activity

Think about the day-to-day activities of babies and children. Consider which of these could stress parents, particularly those parents who are already under some other strain.

Many parents can recall how a particular episode of prolonged crying or naughtiness brought them to the brink of violence. The difference between these parents and those who physically abuse their children is the knowledge of methods other than violence to discipline their child and their ability to recognise and manage their own stress appropriately. Young mothers are a predisposing factor in child abuse because they often lack an understanding of the realities of being a parent. An initiative that commenced in the USA to reduce teenage pregnancies involves providing simulator babies for young teenagers to take home from school at weekends in an effort to show that caring for a baby has no resemblance to playing with a doll! Children's nurses should appreciate the stresses and strains of parenthood and not make judgements about abusers. Most parents in this situation need to be able to trust the nurse to support them and help them to avoid a recurrence. Their feelings of guilt, inadequacy and isolation may be exacerbated by the nurse who tries to exclude them from their child's care. Instead, the nurse should provide a role model for parents and work with them to support the child.

Abused children rarely accuse their abuser. They are too often frightened of the consequences if they reveal what has happened. They may

The child's fundamental needs

- Basic physical care
- Affection
- Security
- Stimulation of innate potential
- Guidance and control
- Responsibility
- Independence

Vulnerability of the child

- A difficult pregnancy and/or birth may make it hard for mother to relate to the child
- A premature birth or low birth weight may lead to frustrations and anxieties which are displaced on to the child
- One child too many may create maternal overload
- Chronic disappointment about the sex of the child
- A stressful time of day – meal times with children who are slow or fussy eaters, bedtimes, middle of the night, a child who refuses to sleep

Characteristics of parents who abuse

- Hostile background
- Excessive dependency needs
- Role reversal
- Blind to developmental needs
- Rigid, obsessive
- Power, powerlessness
- The saviour
- Stereotyped helplessness
- Violence
- Morbid jealousy
- Drug or alcohol dependency

(Altmeier *et al.*, 1982)

have been threatened with further violence if they name their abuser. They may also fear that they will be taken away from their parents. Many children blame themselves for the abuse. Even when children have been sexually abused, home may still represent affection and security because they do not know that there are other ways of expressing love and affection.

Study activity

Consider how you might encourage an abused child to talk freely to you.

Abused children should be treated like any other children in hospital. They should not be pressurised into talking about the abuse and any revelations about the abuse should be accepted with equanimity and without criticism of the child or the abuser. The key is to listen to them and take what they say seriously. They may need time and more than one opportunity to develop sufficient trust to share any concerns. Reassure them that the abuse is not their fault and that they are right to tell someone about it. Do not promise not to share the information, as the courts may require it. Do not ask leading questions or attempt to investigate any allegations of abuse, as you may jeopardise any police investigation.

Child Protection

Child protection is the specific action taken to protect children from abuse (Home Office, Department of Health and Welsh Office, 1991) (Figure 21.3). The concept of strategies to protect children was initiated in the UK in 1985, when social services became responsible for investigating allegations of child abuse. Nurses working with children have a responsibility to report to social services all concerns about children whom they suspect are at risk of significant harm (DfES, 2005). The Children Act 2004 defines significant harm as that which prevents the child's health or development from meeting the usual standards for a child of similar age and circumstance. If, after an initial investigation, social services decide to pursue concerns, the nurse may be expected to:

- provide a written report about the concerns
- provide copies of relevant nursing records for any court proceedings
- attend a child protection conference
- join the inter-agency group to produce a child protection plan
- attend reviews as necessary

The Department of Health (2000b) stressed the need for inter-agency liaison in child protection work, and any child protection issue usually involves representatives from social services (the key agency), education, health, police and in some areas the National Society for the Prevention of Cruelty to Children. In an emergency, concerns can be reported to the police, who have powers to ensure the child's safety. The Children Act 1989 enabled the police to take children at risk into their protection as well as identifying three new child protection orders:

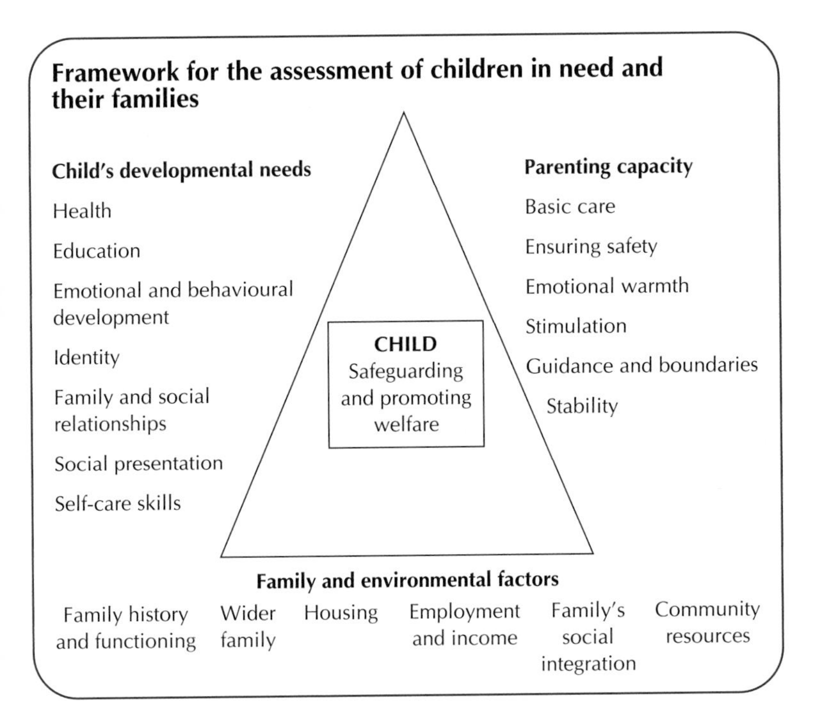

- child assessment order (CAO)
- emergency protection order
- recovery order

The child assessment order can be obtained by social services when a child is not at immediate risk but significant harm is suspected. It is a time-limited order that allows for an assessment of a child's health, development and treatment, which might not otherwise be possible due to parental refusal (Stower, 2000). The emergency protection order enables a child to be made safe when there is reasonable cause to suspect that the child would be at risk if not removed from the present environment. The recovery order can be made by the courts to discover the whereabouts of a child who has been removed from care.

The Children Act, which took effect in 1991 and was updated in 2004, was seen at that time to be an important influence in promoting the rights of the child. However, it has been criticised because it does not balance children's wishes with their needs. Dorrell (1997) indicated that although it is important to listen to children's views, it is equally important not to expect them necessarily to make mature judgements about their interests. He believes these judgements are best made by adults.

Study activity

Read the other sections relating to the Children Act (p. 692) and the role of the nurse as an advocate for the child (p. 625) and discuss Dorrell's point of view with some colleagues.

Characteristics of accidental injuries

BRUISES are likely to be:

- few and scattered
- no pattern
- frequent
- same colour and age

BURNS and SCALDS are likely to be:

- treated
- easily explained

INJURIES are likely to be:

- minor and superficial
- quickly treated
- easily explained

FRACTURES are likely to be:

- arms and legs
- seldom to the ribs except for road traffic accidents – rare in very young children
- rarely due to brittle bone syndrome

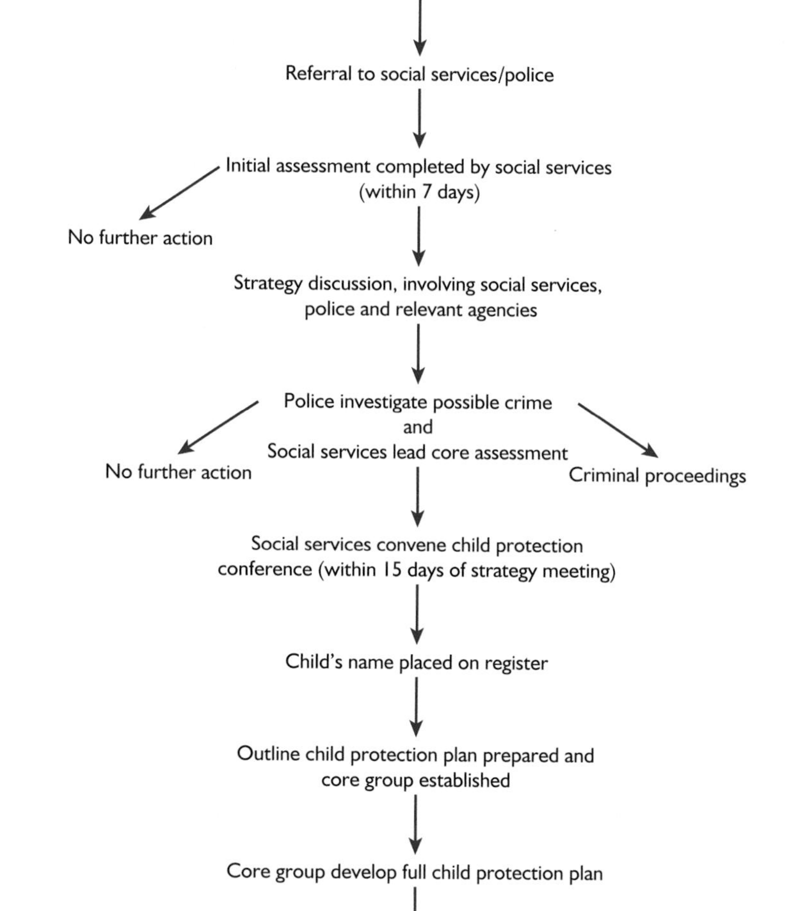

Figure 21.3 Child protection process.

Characteristics of non-accidental injuries

BRUISING is likely to be:

- frequent
- patterned, e.g. finger and thumb marks
- old and new in same place (note colour)
- in unusual positions (see Figure 21.3)

BURNS and SCALDS are likely to have:

- a clear outline
- splash marks around burn
- unusual position, e.g. back of hand
- indicative shapes, e.g. cigarette burns, bar of electric fire

SUSPICIOUS INJURIES are likely to be:

- bite marks
- fingernail marks
- large and deep scratches
- incisions, e.g. from razor blades

FRACTURES are likely to be:

- numerous and healed at different times
- always suspicious in babies under 2 years of age

SEXUAL ABUSE may result in:

- unexplained soreness
- bleeding or injury to genital or anal areas
- sexually transmitted diseases

Prevention of Child Abuse

Study activity

Consider what part you can play in the prevention of child abuse.

Children's nurses can play an important part in the prevention of child abuse. In the neonatal unit separation of the mother and baby can be kept to a minimum and bonding encouraged. Children's community nurses (CCNs) can help new parents to appreciate the developmental needs of young children and help them to overcome problems. Studies have shown that this kind of help is more likely to have an impact on reducing child abuse if aimed at the parents of children under 2 years old (Olds *et al.*, 1994). Children's community nurses can also refer parents who have no family close by to community services such as mother and toddler groups, which can help to provide social support to isolated families. They can also be alert to parents who need help. Jones *et al.* (1987) found that frequent visits to the clinic, GP or hospital with apparently minor problems might indicate parental anxiety and insecurity and represent a cry for help. Some areas have initiated schemes to help parents under stress who can call a 24-hour helpline for advice if they feel unable to cope.

All nurses can be alert to altered relationships between children and parents and listen carefully to children's concerns. They can also teach parenting skills to meet children's fundamental and developmental needs and give advice about protecting and educating children about sexual abuse. They can be alert to stressors in the home environment, which may cause the child to be neglected. For instance, when a parent is caring for another dependant or suffering from mental health problems. In a study of 100 reviews of child death where abuse and neglect had been a factor in the death, around 33% showed clear evidence of parental mental illness (DH, 2000a). When parents are mentally or physically ill, the eldest child may have to be the main carer for the family, restricting his social and recreational development. The role of the nurse in the prevention of child abuse is strengthened by findings about the long-term consequences of child abuse.

Adult Survivors of Child Abuse

Cloke and Nash (1997) stress the need for services to support the adult survivors of child abuse so that the experience does not adversely affect the relationship they have with their own children. The National Commission of Inquiry into the Prevention of Child Abuse (1996) found that only around 30% of child abuse is reported and, while all survivors need support in adulthood, serious long-term consequences are more likely in those where the abuse had not been recognised or treated. The Commission found that these adults were often dependent on alcohol or drugs and that pregnancy and childbirth could cause acute distress. In their conclusion, the Commission recommended that existing child surveillance programmes should include the assessment of the general welfare of the child and family, thus identifying children at risk and parents in need of advice and support. This could be difficult to implement in view of the lack of recognition given to preventative health in the NHS (Cloke and Nash, 1997). Although the *Children's National Service Framework* (DH, 2004) stresses the importance of safeguarding children, it seems to have missed this preventative opportunity.

Record Keeping

Clear, concise, accessible and comprehensible records are an essential part of good child protection processes. In 2000 the Department of Health introduced the *Framework for the Assessment of Children in Need and their Families* (DH, 2000b) to provide a multidisciplinary tool, which guided the collection and analysis of information and

Laming recommendations (Mulholland, 2003)

The Laming recommendations arose from an inquiry into the death of Victoria Climbié. Victoria died after a catalogue of neglect and abuse that took place between 1998 and 2000. Lord Laming who led the inquiry concluded his report by stating that: 'Sadly, the report is a vivid demonstration of poor practice within and between social services, the police and the health agencies.' He made a total of 108 recommendations to improve this poor practice, 27 of which related to health professionals. Ten of these related directly to nursing:

- any suspicion of deliberate harm should be fully recorded in the child's notes on admission
- health professionals should work from a single set of records for each child
- a record must be made of all face-to-face discussions – including medical and nursing handovers – and telephone conversations relating to the care of the child
- a record must be kept of all decisions made; a note should also be made of who is responsible for carrying out any action noted
- frontline health professionals coming into regular contact with families with children must ensure that basic information about the child is recorded:
  - name and address
  - age
  - name of the child's GP, primary carer and school
- nurses admitting children with suspected deliberate harm must enquire about any previous admissions
- health professionals involved in child protection must be trained in hospital and community service liaison
- staff involved in caring for children should be kept up to date with child protection training

Module 4

helped all agencies to make decisions about how to help those children and families. The framework is a useful tool for guiding the assessment of all children and families (DH, 2000b). Other hospital records should include records of all face-to-face and telephone conversations between the child, family and other agencies, as recommended by the Victoria Climbié Inquiry (2003). This report also recommended that the nursing care plan must take full account of the diagnosis of possible abuse whenever a child is admitted to hospital with suspected deliberate harm. This poses a challenge to nursing staff to document all their concerns while ensuring that they distinguish between their personal values and beliefs and their professional responsibilities. It may also pose a challenge in determining whether the nursing records are kept at the bedside, although the Department of Health (DH, 1999) recommends that professionals are open, honest and explicit with children and families.

Study activity

Ellie is a 2-year-old who has been brought to the accident-and-emergency department by her mother. Ellie has bruises on the side of her face which her mother says were caused by her walking into a door.

- What immediate nursing interventions/observations should the nurse make?
- What could facial bruising indicate in this child?
- What other signs could indicate long-term abuse in a 2-year-old child?

Mandy is a 17-year-old mother of Kylie, aged 3 weeks. Kylie was born at 32 weeks' gestation and is being cared for on the neonatal unit. Mandy is a single mother and estranged from her parents. She lives in a bedsit and rarely visits Kylie. As the named nurse for Kylie, you want to make sure her future discharge is well planned.

- What risk factors for child abuse exist in this situation?
- What other factors should you take into account to help you determine the degree of risk?
- What actions can you take to help minimise the risk?

Bobby, aged 2 years, is admitted via his GP with numerous bruises to his back and abdomen. Other marks are suspected to be cigarette burns. He was taken to the GP as his grandmother was concerned about him. The GP has informed social services of his suspicion that Bobby is a victim of abuse.

- Write a care plan for this child.

Key Points

1. There is no accepted single cause for violent behaviour.
2. Violence in the family falls into five main categories of abuse: physical, emotional, neglect, sexual and financial.
3. Violence may be inflicted against and by anyone of any age.
4. It is difficult to give precise statistics about abuse as much of it goes unreported by those who are too embarrassed or frightened to reveal it.
5. Nurses have a responsibility to recognise and report any concerns that a child may be at risk of abuse.
6. There is now a need to have strategic programmes for the prevention of child abuse, including the support of adult survivors of abuse.

References

Ainsworth, M. (1973) The development of infant–mother attachment. In Caldwell, B. and Ricciuti, H. (eds), *Review of Child Development and Research, Vol. 3: Child Development and Social Policy*. Chicago: University of Chicago Press.

Ainsworth, M. (1982) Attachment: retrospect and prospect. In Parkes, C., Atkinson, N. and Crawford, M. (1995) *All in the Family: Siblings and Disability*. London: Action for Children.

Alderson, P. (1993) *Children's Consent to Surgery*. Milton Keynes: Open University Press.

Altmeier, W., *et al.* (1982) Antecedents of child abuse. *Journal of Pediatrics,* **100**, 823–827.

Arehart-Treichel, J. (1980) *Biotypes*. London: W. H. Allen.

Atkinson, N. and **Crawford, M.** (1995) *All in the Family: Siblings and Disability*. London: Action for Children.

Auslander, W., *et al.* (1991) Predictors of diabetes knowledge in newly diagnosed children and parents. *Journal of Paediatric Psychology,* **16** (2), 213–228.

Bacchus, L., Mezey, G. and **Bewley, S.** (2002) Abuse screening may backfire. *British Journal of Obstetrics and Gynaecology,* **11**, 451–457.

Bailey, R. and **Caldwell, C.** (1997) Preparing parents for going home. *Paediatric Nursing,* **9** (4), 15–17.

Bandura, A. (1973) *Aggression: A Social Learning Theory*. Englewood Cliffs, NJ: Prentice-Hall.

Bannister, A. (1992) *Child Abuse and Neglect: Facing the Challenge,* 2nd edn. Milton Keynes: Open University Press.

Bee, H. (1989) *The Developing Child,* 5th edn. New York: Harper & Row.

Bentovim, A. (1986) Bereaved children. *British Medical Journal,* **292**, 1482.

Bewley, C. and **Gibbs, A.** (1994) Coping with domestic violence in pregnancy. *Nursing Standard,* **8**, 25–28.

Bird, J. and **Podmore, V.** (1993) Children's understanding of health and illness. *Psychology and Health,* **4**, 175–185.

Black, K. (2005) Disability and sexuality. *Paediatric Nursing,* **17** (5), 34–37.

Bossert, E. (1994) Stress appraisals of hospitalised school-aged children. *Children's Health Care,* **23** (1), 33–49.

Bowlby, J. (1953) *Child Care and the Growth of Love*. Harmondsworth: Penguin.

Bowlby, J. (1973) *Attachment and Loss: 2. Separation, Anxiety and Anger*. London: Hogarth Press.

Brett, J. (2004) The journey to accepting support: how parents of profoundly disabled children experience support in their lives. *Paediatric Nursing,* **16** (8), 14–18.

Brewis, E. (1995) Issues in bereavement: there are no rules. *Paediatric Nursing,* **7** (9), 19–22.

Brown, K. and **Cooper, S. J. (eds)** (1979) *Chemical Influences on Behaviour*. London: Academic Press.

Browne, K. and **Saqi, S.** (1988) Approaches to screening for child abuse and neglect. In Browne, K., Davies, C. and Stratton, P. (eds), *Early Prediction and Prevention of Child Abuse*. Chichester: Wiley.

Burr, C. (1985) Impact on the family of a chronically ill child. In Hobbs, N. and Perrin, J. (eds), *Issues in the Care of Children with Chronic Illness*. San Francisco: Jossey-Bass.

Burr, S. (1993) Adolescents and the ward environment. *Paediatric Nursing,* **5** (1), 10–13.

Bury, M. and **Pink, D.** (2005) Self-management of chronic disease doesn't work. HJS debate. *Health Service Journal,* **115**, 18–19.

Butler, N. R. and **Goldstein, N. R.** (1973) Smoking in pregnancy and subsequent child development. *British Medical Journal,* **4**, 573–577.

Canam, C. (1993) Common adaptive tasks facing parents of children with chronic conditions. *Journal of Advanced Nursing,* **18**, 46–53.

Carson, D., Gravely, J. and **Council, J.** (1992) Children's pre-hospitalisation conceptions of illness, cognitive development and personal adjustment. *Child Health Care,* **21** (2), 103–110.

Chappelle, C., *et al.* (2001) Making connections: the relevance of the social model of disability for people with learning disabilities. *British Journal of Learning Disabilities,* **29,** 45–50.

Chess, S. and **Thomas, A.** (1984) *Origins and Evolution of Behaviour Disorders*. New York: Raven Press.

Clark, G. (1996) Internal conflicts. *Nursing Times,* **92** (40), 16–17.

Cloke, C. and **Nash, J.** (1997) Save the children. *Nursing Times,* **93** (14), 34–37.

Clothier, C. (1994) *The Allitt Report*. London: HMSO.

Cohen, M. and **Martison, I.** (1988) Chronic uncertainty: its effect on parental appraisal of a child's health. *Journal of Pediatric Nursing,* **3** (2), 89–96.

Craft, M. (1986) Validation of responses reported by school-age siblings of hospitalised children. *Children's Health Care,* **15**, 13–16.

Dale, P., *et al.* (1986) *Dangerous Families*. London: Tavistock.

DES (1978) *Special Educational Needs – Report of the Committee of Inquiry into the Education of Handicapped Children and Young People (Warnock Report)*. London: HMSO.

DfES (2005) *What to Do if You are Worried a Child is Being Abused*. London: Department of Health Publications.

DH (1989) *An Introduction to the Children Act*. London: HMSO.

DH (1999) *Working Together to Safeguard Children*. London: HMSO.

DH (2000a) *Domestic Violence: A Resource Manual for Health Care Professionals*. London: HMSO.

DH (2000b) *Framework for the Assessment of Children in Need and their Families*. London: HMSO.

DH (2004) *Children's National Service Framework*. London: Department of Health.

DHSS (1988) *Working Together: A Guide to Inter-agency Co-operation for the Protection of Children from Abuse*. London: HMSO.
Dorrell, S. (1997) *Social Services: Achievement and Challenge*. London: HMSO.
Dunn, J. (1981) *Sisters and Brothers*. London: Fontana.
Earys, C., Ellis, N. and **Jones, R.** (1993) Which label? An investigation into the effects of terminology on the public perception of and attitudes toward people with learning difficulties. *Disability Handicap Society*, **8** (2), 114.
Evans, N. (2005) Domestic violence: recognising the signs. *Paediatric Nursing*, **17** (1), 14–15.
Expert Patients Programme (2005) *Moving from Patient to Person*. www.expertpatients.nhs.uk.
Farrant, B. and **Watson, P. D.** (2004) Healthcare Delivery: perspectives of young people with chronic illness and their parents. *Journal of Paediatrics and Child Health*, **40** (4), 175–179.
Farrell, M. (1996) The role of a children's hospice. *Paediatric Nursing*, **8** (4), 6–8.
Faulkner, A., Peace, G. and **O'Keefe, C.** (1995) *When a Child has Cancer*. London: Chapman & Hall.
Faulkner, E. (1995) The importance of communications with the patient, family and professional carers. In Robbins, J. and Moscroft, J. (eds), *Caring for the Dying Patient and the Family*, 3rd edn. London: Chapman & Hall.
Faux, S. (1991) Sibling relationships in families with congenitally impaired children. *Journal of Pediatric Nursing*, **6** (3), 175–184.
Fourn, L., Ducic, S. and **Seguin, L.** (1999) Smoking and intauterine growth. *Journal of Epidemiology and Community Health*, **53**, 432–433.
Gath, A. (1980) How illness in one member of the family affects the children in that family. *Journal of Maternal and Child Health*, **12**, 6–8.
Geen, L. (1990) The family of a child with cancer. In Thompson, J. (ed.), *The Child with Cancer – Nursing Care*. London: Scutari Press.
Gelles, R. and **Cornell, C.** (1985) *Intimate Violence in Families*. Beverly Hills: Sage.
Gibson, C. (1988) Perspectives of parental coping with a chronically ill child. *Issues in Comprehensive Pediatric Nursing*, **11**, 33–41.
Goodchild, M. and **Dodge, J.** (1985) *Cystic Fibrosis*, 2nd edn. Sussex: Balliere Tindall.
Greenberg, M., Siegel, J. and **Leitch, C.** (1983) The nature and importance of attachment relationships to parents and peers during adolescence. *Journal of Youth and Adolescence*, **12**, 373–386.
Gunther, L. M. (1963) Psychopathy and stress in the life experience of mothers of premature infants. In Illingworth, L. S. (ed.), *The Normal Child*, 8th edn. Edinburgh: Churchill Livingstone.
Harris, A. (1993) *Child Development*, 2nd edn. Minneapolis: West.
Harrison, C. (1997) Wax, sunlight and X-rays. *Nursing Times*, **93** (22), 52–53.
Hart, D. and **Bossert, E.** (1994) Self-reported fears of hospitalised school-aged children. *Journal of Pediatric Nursing*, **9** (2), 83–90.
Hill, L. (1994) *Caring for Dying Children and their Families*. London: Chapman & Hall.
Hodges, B. (2004) Asthma camp. *Paediatric Nursing*, **17** (6), 20–22.
Holmes, L. (1999) Nurses' attitude to disability. *Paediatric Nursing*, **11** (10), 18–20.
Home Office, DH and Welsh Office (1991) *Working Together under The Children Act 1989: A Guide to Arrangements for Inter-agency Co-operation for the Protection of Children from Abuse*. London: HMSO.
Illingworth, L. S. (1983) *The Normal Child*, 8th edn. Edinburgh: Churchill Livingstone.
Jennings, P. (1992) Coping strategies for mothers. *Paediatric Nursing*, **4** (9), 24–26.
Jones, T., *et al.* (1987) *Understanding Child Abuse*, 2nd edn. London: Macmillan.
Kagan, J. (1979) Overview: perspectives on human infancy. In Osofsky, J. (ed.), *Handbook on Infant Development*. New York: Wiley.
Kempe, R. and **Kempe, C.** (1984) *The Common Secret: Sexual Abuse of Children and Adolescents*. New York: Freeman.
Kenny, C. (1996) Jailed nurse lied to bosses about psychiatric past. *Nursing Times*, **92** (45), 5.
Kingsbury, S. (1993) Parasuicide in adolescence: a message in a bottle. *ACCP Review and Newsletter*, **15** (6), 253–259.
Lask, B. and **Fossen, A.** (1989) *Childhood Illness – The Psychosomatic Approach*. Chichester: Wiley.
Lazarus, R. and **Cohen, J.** (1977) Environmental stress. In Altman, J. and Wohlwill, J. (eds), *Human Behaviour and Environment*, vol. 2. New York: Plenum.
Leventhal, H. (1986) Health psychology: a social psychological perspective. In Berkowitz, L. (ed.), *A Survey of Social Psychology*, 3rd edn. Japan: CBS.
Ley, P. and **Llewelyn, S.** (1995) Improving patients' understanding, recall, satisfaction and compliance. In Broome, A. and Llewelyn, S. (eds), *Health Psychology*. London: Chapman & Hall.
Lindsay, B. (1994) Like skeletons or ghosts. Developing a concept of death and dying. *Child Health*, **2** (4), 142–146.
Little, K. (2000) Screening for domestic violence. *Postgraduate Medicine*, **108** (2), 135–141.
Llewelyn, S. and **Haslett, A.** (1986) Factors perceived as helpful by members of self-help groups: an exploratory study. *British Journal of Guidance and Counselling*, **14**, 252–262.
Lovell, B. (1987) Sharing the death of a parent. *Nursing Times*, **83** (42), 36–39.
Lynch, M. A. and **Roberts, J.** (1977) Predicting child abuse; signs of bonding failure in the maternity hospital. *British Medical Journal*, **1**, 624–627.
Macaskill, A. and **Monach, J.** (1990) Coping with childhood cancer. The case for long-term counselling help for patients and families. *British Journal of Guidance and Counselling*, **18** (1), 13–26.

Main, M., **Kaplan, N.** and **Cassidy, J.** (1985) Security in infancy, childhood and adulthood. *Monographs of the Society for Research in Child Development,* **50** (1/2), 66–104.
Marks, I. M. (1987) The development of normal fear. *Journal of Child Psychology, Psychiatry and Allied Disciplines,* **28** (2), 667–697.
McCarthy, D. (1974) Physical effects and symptoms of the cycle of rejection. *Proceedings of the Royal Society of Medicine,* **67**, 1057–1060.
McCollum, A. and **Gibson, L.** (1970) Family adaptation to the child with cystic fibrosis. *Journal of Pediatrics,* **77** (4), 571–578.
McKerrow, L. (1991) Dealing with the stress of caring for the dying in the intensive care unit. *Intensive Care Nursing,* **7** (4), 219–222.
McKibben, L., **Devos, E.** and **Newberger, E.** (1989) Victimisation of mothers of abused children: a controlled study. *Pediatrics,* **83** (2), 531–535.
McMahon, B. (1995) A family affair – understanding family therapy. *Child Health,* **3** (3), 100–103.
Meadow, R. (1989) Munchausen syndrome by proxy. *British Medical Journal,* **299**, 248–250.
Meadows, S. (1993) *The Child as a Thinker: The Development and Acquisition of Cognition in Childhood.* London: Routledge.
Meyre, S. and **Haggerty, A.** (1962) Stress and physical illness. *Journal of Pediatrics,* **29**, 539–561.
Michael, S. and **Landsdown, R.** (1986) Adjustment to the death of a sibling. *Archives of Disease in Childhood,* **61**, 278–283.
Mikulic, M. (1971) Reinforcement of independent and dependent patient behaviours by nursing personnel: an exploratory study. *Nursing Research,* **20**, 148–155.
Miller, F. J. W., *et al.* (1974) *The School Years in Newcastle-Upon-Tyne.* London: Oxford University Press.
Moos, R. and **Tsu, V.** (1977) The crisis of physical illness; an overview. In Moss, R. (ed.), *Coping with Physical Illness.* New York: Plenum.
Morrison, L. (1997) Stress and siblings. *Paediatric Nursing,* **9** (4), 26–27.
Mulholland, H. (2003) Child protection: the nurse's role. *Nursing Times,* **99** (18), 22–24.
Myer, P. (1988) Parental adaptation to cystic fibrosis. *Journal of Pediatric Health Care,* **2**, 20–28.
National Commission of Inquiry into the Prevention of Child Abuse (1996) *Childhood Matters.* London: HMSO.
NSPCC (2004) *Child Protection Awareness Programme.* London: NSPCC.
O'Connor, T. G., *et al.* (2005) Prenatal anxiety predicts individual differences in cortisol in pre-adolescent children. *Journal of Biological Psychiatry,* **58**, 211–217.
Olds, S. D., **Henderson, C.** and **Kitzman, H.** (1994) Does pre-natal and infancy nurse home visitation have enduring effects on qualities of parental caregiving and child health at 25–50 months of age? *Pediatrics,* **93** (1), 89–98.
Paarlbergk, P., *et al.* (1995) Psychosocial factors and pregnancy outcome. *Journal of Psychosomatic Research,* **39**, 563–595.
Pagani, L., *et al.* (1997) Behavioural development in children of divorce and remarriage. *Journal of Child Psychology and Psychiatry,* **38**, 769–781.
Patterson, G. (1982) Coercion theory. In Lachenmeyer, J. and Gibbs, M. (eds), *Psychology in Childhood.* New York: Gardner Press.
Peace, G. (1996a) Living under the shadow of illness. *Nursing Times,* **92** (28), 46–48.
Peace, G. (1996b) Chronic complements. *Nursing Times,* **92** (41), 46–47.
Peck, H. (1992) Please don't tell him the truth. *Paediatric Nursing,* **43** (2), 12–14.
Pettle, M. and **Landsdown, R.** (1986) Adjustment to the death of a sibling. *Archives of Disease in Childhood,* **61**, 278–283.
Pinkerton, C. and **Kieckhefer, G.** (2002) Educating children with asthma. The nurse practitioner. *American Journal of Primary Healthcare,* **27** (3), 12–14.
Pritchard, J. (1996) Darkness visible. *Nursing Times,* **92** (42), 26–27.
Purssell, E. (1994) The process of normalisation in children with chronic illness. *Paediatric Nursing,* **6** (10), 26–28.
Ramsay, J. (1990) *Parental understanding and management of cystic fibrosis.* Unpublished MSc dissertation, City University.
Randall, P. (1993) Young children grieve differently from adults. *Professional Care of Mother and Child,* February, 36–37.
Ray, L. and **Ritchie, J.** (1993) Caring for chronically ill children at home: factors which influence parents' coping. *Journal of Pediatric Nursing,* **8** (4), 217–225.
Read, J. (2000) *Disability: The Family and Society: Listening to Mothers.* London: Sage.
Reder, P., **Duncan, S.** and **Gray, M.** (1993) *Beyond Blame: Child Abuse Tragedies Revisited.* London: Routledge.
Robertson, J. (1970) *Young Children in Hospital,* 2nd edn. London: Tavistock Press.
Robinson, C. (1993) Managing life with a chronic disability: the story of normalisation. *Qualitative Health Research,* **3** (1), 6–28.
Rosenman, R., *et al.* (1975) Coronary heart disease in the Western Group study. *Journal of the American Medical Association,* **233**, 872–877.
Rushford, H. (1996) Nurses' knowledge of how children view health and illness. *Paediatric Nursing,* **8** (9), 23–27.
Russell, P. (1989) *The Wheelchair Child,* 3rd edn. London: Souvenir Press.
Russell-Johnson, H. (1997) Deliberate self-harm in adolescents. *Paediatric Nursing,* **9** (1), 29–36.
Rutter, M. (1971) Parent–child separation: psychological effects on the children. *Journal of Child Psychology and Psychiatry,* **12**, 233.
Rutter, M., *et al.* (1975) Attainment and adjustment in two geographic areas: III: Some factors accounting for area differences. *British Journal of Psychiatry,* **126**, 520–533.

Schaffer, H. R. (1988) Family structure or interpersonal relationships. *The Context for Child Development,* **2**, 91–94.
Shapiro, J. (1983) Family reactions and coping strategies in response to the physically ill or the handicapped child: a review. *Social Science and Medicine,* **17** (14), 913–931.
Simon, K. (1993) Perceived stress of non-hospitalised children during the hospitalisation of a sibling. *Journal of Pediatric Nursing,* **8** (5), 298–304.
Smith, L. (1987) *Domestic Violence: An Overview.* London: HMSO.
Smith, S. M., Hanson, R. and **Noble, S.** (1974) Social aspects of the battered baby syndrome. *British Journal of Psychiatry,* **125**, 568–570.
Spinetta, J. (1984) Measurement of family function, communication and cultural effects. *Cancer,* **53**, 2230–2237.
Stier, D., *et al.* (1993) Are children born to young mothers at increased risk of maltreatment? *Pediatrics,* **91** (3), 642–648.
Stott, D. H. (1962) Evidence for a congenital factor in maladjustment and delinquency. *American Journal of Psychiatry,* **118**, 781–785.
Stower, S. (2000) The principles and practice of child protection. *Nursing Standard,* **14** (17), 48–55.
Swanwick, M. (1996) Child rearing across cultures. *Paediatric Nursing,* **8** (7), 13–17.
Syverson, C. (1997) The young ones. *Nursing Times,* **93** (24), 28–29.
Thompson, D. (1992) Support for the grieving family. *Neonatal Network,* **11** (6), 73–75.
Thorne, S. (1993) *Negotiating Health Care – The Social Context of Chronic Illness.* London: Sage.
Tomblin, J., Smith, E. and **Zhang, H.** (1997) Epidemiology of specific language impairment: prenatal and perinatal risk factors. *Journal of Communication Disorders,* **30**, 325–344.
Tropauer, A., Neal-Franz, M. and **Dilgard, V.** (1970) Psychological aspects of the care of children with cystic fibrosis. *American Journal of Diseases of Childhood,* **119**, 424–431.
Van Ooijen, E. (1996) Learning to approach patients' sexuality as part of holistic care. *Nursing Times,* **92** (36), 44–45.
Van Ooijen, E. and **Charnock, A.** (1994) *Sexuality and Patient Care.* London: Chapman & Hall.
Victoria Climbié Inquiry (2003) *The Victoria Climbié Inquiry: Report of an Inquiry by Lord Laming.* London: HMSO.
Wallston, B. (1973) The effect of maternal employment on children. *Journal of Child Psychology and Psychiatry,* **14**, 81–85.
Walter, T. (1990) *Funerals and How to Improve Them.* London: Hodder & Stoughton.
Waterhouse, L. (1993) *Child Abuse and Child Abusers.* London: Jessica Kingsley.
Wedge, P. and **Prosser, H.** (1973) *Born to Fail.* London: Arrow Books.
Weinstock, L. (1999) Gender differences in the presentation and management of social anxiety disorder. *Journal of Clinical Psychiatry,* **60**, 9–13.
Whitehead, N. (1995) Behavioural paediatrics and childhood cancer. In Broome, A. and Llewelyn, S. (eds), *Health Psychology.* London: Chapman & Hall.
Whyte, D. (1992) A family nursing approach to the care of a child with a chronic illness. *Journal of Advanced Nursing,* **17**, 317–327.
Wilkinson, S. (1995) Psychological aspects of disability. In Broome, A. and Llewelyn, S. (eds), *Health Psychology.* London: Chapman & Hall.
Woodhouse, S. (1996) Do siblings need a special day? *Paediatric Nursing,* **8** (3), 8–9.
World Health Organization (1980) *International Classification of Impairments, Disabilities and Handicaps (ICIDH).* Geneva: WHO.
Wright, B. (1983) *Psychosocial Aspects of Disability.* London: Harper & Row.

Module 5

Principles of Caring for Sick Children

Joan Ramsay

Learning Outcomes

The material in this module and the further reading/references should enable you to:

- evaluate the suitability of hospital environments for children
- discuss the value of different types of preparation of children for hospital and procedures
- appreciate the importance of the assessment process
- explore the process of day surgery for children and families
- consider the care of children in the accident-and-emergency department
- appreciate the differences between the administration of medicines to children and their administration to adults
- consider how to provide adequate nutrition and maintain fluid balance for children in hospital
- discuss the problems associated with caring for children in pain
- examine the surrogate role of the nurse
- explore the provision of paediatric community nursing in the UK
- discuss the specific pre- and post-operative care of children
- explore the provision of paediatric intensive care in the UK
- consider how to meet the psychological and physical needs of the dying child

Introduction

Sick children need the care and skills of a specially trained nurse who has a clear understanding of the particular needs of children and their families and can therefore assess, plan, implement and evaluate appropriate family-centred care. This module examines the principles of caring for sick children to provide you with the necessary understanding that children are not just small adults but are unique individuals with specific needs of their own. The module begins by exploring the requirements of an appropriate hospital environment for children. It also considers the care of children in particular areas of the hospital – the day care ward, the intensive care unit and the accident-and-emergency department. It discusses the particular need of children for clear and age-appropriate preparation for hospital and hospital procedures to help to allay their fears and to promote their cooperation. Children's fears and lack of understanding of hospitals make the care of their pain, meeting their pre- and post-operative needs and the administration of medicines a particularly challenging part of nursing children, and this module looks at these issues. It also considers how the differences between the structure and function of children's bodies and those of adults are particularly relevant when assessing sick children and providing nutrition and maintaining fluid balance. Much of the nurse's role for sick children in hospital and at home involves working with parents to adapt family routines and to include specific nursing care, and the module examines this surrogate role in hospital and in the community. As more children are being cared for at home, the module explores the provision of children's community nursing and the development of this role. Finally the module looks at the physical and psychological needs of the dying child.

Chapter 22

Hearing Children's Voices in NHS Service Delivery and Evaluation

Participation

Since the beginning of the 1990s there has been a drive towards involving children and young people more in the development and delivery of services. This drive is supported by a range of policy documents that emphasise the importance of involving children in decisions affecting their lives. Possibly the most significant contribution to this movement was the ratification by the United Nations of the UN Convention on the Rights of the Child in 1989 and its subsequent ratification by the UK government in 1991. A number of Articles in the Convention reflect the rights of children and young people to participate but Article 12 summarises participation in this way:

> States' parties shall ensure to the child who is capable of forming his or her own views the right to express those views freely in all matters affecting the child, the views of the child being given due weight in accordance with the age and maturity of the child.

Rights and the law

For comprehensive information about various laws pertaining to children's rights see the material at http://www.crae.org.uk/cms/index.php?option=com_content&task=view&id=76&Itemid=103 (accessed 19 May 2006), on the Web site of the Children's Rights Alliance for England.

Module 5

Policy background

Recognition of the importance of acknowledging the participation rights of children and young people is evident in government policy:

- The Department of Health consultation draft on child health in the community (DH, 1995) stressed the importance of taking into account the provisions of the UN Convention on the Rights of the Child when considering the principles on which to base services.
- The Department of Health specifies the role children and young people can play and commits itself to 'ensuring that the voice of the child is heard and correctly acted upon' in its introduction to the *Children's Taskforce*. See http://www.dfes.gov.uk/qualityprotects/pdfs/taskforce.pdf (accessed 19 May 2006).
- The Every Child Matters: Change for Children programme aims to ensure that policies and services are designed around the needs of children and young people, and that they are involved in decision

Policy documents and where to find them

- The DH consultation draft on child health in the community (DH, 1995).
- Children's Taskforce – DH (2001) and http://www.dfes.gov.uk/qualityprotects/pdfs/taskforce.pdf (accessed 20 May 2006).
- Every Child Matters: Change for Children (DH 2004). Find this and all the other publications related to Every Child Matters at http://www.everychildmatters.gov.uk/publications/ (accessed 20 May 2006).
- The Children Act (2004) http://www.opsi.gov.uk/acts/acts2004/20040031.htm (accessed 20 May 2006).
- *The National Service Framework for Children, Young People and Maternity Services* (DH, 2004).

making with regard to service planning and delivery at a local and national level. See the documents at http://www.everychildmatters.gov.uk/publications/ (accessed 19 May 2005).

- The Children Act 2004 provides the legal framework for the programme of reform outlined in Every Child Matters. The Act relates to *all* children regardless of need, with participation of children at its core.
- *The National Service Framework* (NSF) *for Children, Young People and Maternity Services* (DH, 2004) is part of the government's wider Change for Children programme and stresses the importance of involving children in the improvement of their services.

Study activity

You should familiarise yourself with all of the above policy documents. Search them to find out more about what they say with regard to children's participation in decision making.

Why should children participate?

Willow (1997) suggests that failing to involve children or consult with them means that one does not take into account their specific views and experiences and that one fails to recognise them as future citizens. It can be argued that if they have no voice, children and young people may feel that they have no duty to contribute to society's norms or abide by its rules. Promoting the participation of children and young people increases their visibility, brings their needs to the attention of adults and can lead to better decision making. The adults in a survey conducted by Lightfoot and Sloper (2001) drew attention to the potential benefits for children of being consulted about health services. These benefits included the development of confidence, improvements in compliance with treatment and an increased feeling of being cared for. Sinclair and Franklin (2000) identified the reasons for participation as being to:

- uphold children's rights
- fulfil legal responsibilities
- improve services
- improve decision making
- enhance democratic processes
- promote children's protection
- enhance children's skills
- empower and enhance self-esteem

Children and young people themselves give a variety of reasons why they believe they should participate in decision making. It

- offers them new skills, builds their self-esteem and leads to better outcomes (Lansdown, 2001; Kirby *et al.*, 2003)
- gives them a chance to make a difference
- enhances personal development
- makes them feel valued and respected
- is useful in a CV

- is an opportunity to have fun and meet people (Lightfoot and Sloper, 2003)

Study activity

Talk to children and young people in hospital about why they think they should participate in decision making. How do their reasons compare with those above? What decisions would they like to participate in?

Defining participation

Study activity

Before reading on stop for a minute to think about the term 'participation'. What does it mean to you?

Various authors have attempted to define participation:

- Cutler and Taylor (2003:14) define it simply as 'taking part in decision making'. They use the terms 'participation' and 'involvement' interchangeably. They recognise a spectrum of degrees of power in taking part, ranging from giving opinions on a predetermined issue upon which adults decide, to young people choosing their own agenda and taking their own decisions.
- The Children and Young People's Unit (2001:4) use participation to cover 'the whole range of activities' (from consultation to active participation in decision making or service delivery) recognising that no one focus or method will be appropriate in all cases.
- Lansdown (2001) gives no clear definition of participation but distinguishes between 'consultative processes', where children have no control, activities are initiated, led and managed by adults, and 'participatory processes' involving collaboration with adults, necessitating sharing of power.
- Hart (1992) states that participation refers to the process of sharing in decisions that affect one's life and the life of the community in which one lives.

We need to ensure that participation is meaningful for children and young people. When participation is done badly it can act against the interests of the child and can suggest a low value being placed on the child's views (Phillips, 2000). Expectations can be raised and then dashed, leading to disillusionment and further isolation. Participation is about finding ways of incorporating children's views into decision-making processes within the context of what is possible both institutionally and culturally.

Models of participation

There are a number of models of children's participation for you to explore:

- Hart's (1992) 'ladder of participation'
- Shier's (2001) 'pathway to participation'
- Chawla's (2001) 'forms of participation'
- Treseder's (1997) 'degrees of participation'

Study activity

Find out about each of the models identified here. Compare and contrast them. How might each of them be useful in your practice?

In analysing the models, you might deduce that participation can mean different things in different contexts and that no one model or form can be applied across all settings and in all situations. Each model has its strengths and limitations and each might be appropriate for use in different contexts and situations. What is important, and is acknowledged by many authors, is that children's participation should be fostered across a wide range of settings. Formal structures that facilitate children and young people's participation should be created by adults and a balance sought between guidance and independence in step with growing levels of competence. Roche (1999:487) neatly sums it up by saying that 'it is about respecting and valuing the contribution children can make and have to make to the world children and adults share'.

Children's Voices – Some Practical Examples

Prior to the mid-1990s, although children's views were sought informally, few formal consultations were evident in the literature. Where consultations were carried out, the respondents tended to be parents and/or carers rather than children. Children and young people with an acute illness, a chronic illness or physical disability are likely to be both long-term and heavy users of a wide range of NHS services. However, an inquiry by the House of Commons Health Committee (1997, para. 120) found that 'health services for children and young people do not always focus on and are not always designed to meet the needs of children and young people'. The mid-1990s saw an increase in the extent to which children and young people were asked their views about hospital experiences and some examples are given for you to consider here:

- In 1995 Doorbar involved more than 700 children and young people (mean age 13 years) in a qualitative study to find out what children and young people thought about the healthcare services they received in a particular health authority. Nurses who were friendly, who took time to listen and to give explanations that were honest and clear, who treated children and young people with respect and made them feel more comfortable were more likely to produce positive responses. Nurses who were 'grumpy' led to negative responses. The importance of carrying out treatments with skill was also identified from the data and those who reported a painful experience tended to complain about the quality of their treatment. A follow-up to the initial project (Doorbar, 1996) found that a number of changes in the presentation and practice of services had taken place as a direct result of the feedback given by children and young people.

- A report by Lightfoot and Sloper (2001) noted an apparent increased interest among NHS organisations in involving children and young people in service development. This national survey of health authorities and NHS Trusts in England revealed a limited but growing range of initiatives involving children and young people with chronic health problems in decisions about service development. The survey identified 27 initiatives that concentrated on the involvement of children and young people. These initiatives focused mainly on practical aspects of service provision and in 17 cases children's views were sought on hospital in-service. They found that, although all the initiatives included consultation with children and young people, the majority of initiatives were characterised by limited involvement of the children, and in only 11 cases were the children actually involved in the process of decision making.
- During 2002, as part of the development of the Children's National Service Framework, several consultations with children and young people aged 5–16 years were carried out across the UK. An analysis of five of the consultations, involving a total of 91 children and young people, identified a number of themes (in no order of priority) as being important to children when using healthcare services.
- Curtis *et al.* (2004) used a qualitative approach to identify what children and young people identified as positive and not so positive about their local health services. The study included a total of 149 children and young people aged between 4 and 19 years from across a range of community and clinical settings. Positive aspects included the presence of friendly staff who took efforts to make hospital experiences as good as they could be, continuity of care and good resourcing of waiting areas for young children. Issues that the young people raised as being problematic were more numerous. They included a need for greater privacy and cleanliness in the wards, better food, better information and the need to be treated with courtesy and respect.
- Moules (2005) carried out participatory research with 138 children and young people aged between 9 and 16 years, exploring how they could be involved in monitoring quality in hospital. The study found that young people tend to value qualities related to characteristics of the provider as more important than those relating to the physical environment. They want staff to be technically skilled, friendly, caring, respectful and able to assist them in making healthcare choices, where possible, by giving them information. Furthermore, it was possible to present these five quality criteria in some order of priority. Omission of any of the first three – technical expertise, friendly staff and respect – during clinical interventions or during general care is likely to lead to care being rated as poor. Though the latter two – choice and explanations – are important, their omission would not necessarily lead to the children rating care as poor.
- In October 2005 the new Evelina Children's Hospital (http://www.guysandstthomas.nhs.uk, accessed 19 May 2006) opened in London. Children who were treated at Guy's were consulted about the layout, design, colour schemes and themes for the interior of the hospital. As

Important themes for children and young people in hospital – an analysis from five NSF consultations

- The need to feel at ease and comfortable – related to the need for friendly, welcoming staff.
- The need to be treated with care and understanding.
- Confidentiality is a key issue.
- The need to feel listened to and talked to, with facts being explained clearly in language they can understand.
- The need to build up relationships with mutual respect, trust and understanding.
- Continuity of care.
- Taking part in making plans – playing a role in improving services.
- Not too much waiting.

a result children chose everything, from the menus and furnishings to the design of the building itself.

Study activity

Carry out a search to find more examples of where children's voices have been heard in relation to NHS service delivery and evaluation. Critically analyse each example. Were children's voices heard and actively listened to? What evidence is there to support your conclusions? Here are two references to get you started:

Horstman, M. and Bradding, A. (2002) Helping children speak up in the health service. *European Journal of Oncology Nursing*, **6** (2), 75–84.

Carney, T. *et al.* (2003) Children's views of hospitalisation: an exploratory study of data collection. *Journal of Child Health Care*, **7** (1), 27–40.

Hearing Children's Voices – Building a Culture of Participation

Meaningful participation is a process and is not simply about implementing isolated events or activities. It needs to be about developing child/youth–adult relationships that are rooted in mutual trust and respect. The appropriate degree or level of participation depends on a number of factors, including the type and content of decisions, the context and on the children/young people themselves. So for participation to be meaningful, the organisation you work in needs to reflect the government's *Core Principles for the Involvement of Children and Young People* (Children and Young People's Unit, 2001).

Core principles for the involvement of children and young people (Children and Young People's Unit, 2001)

- A visible commitment is made to involving children and young people, underpinned by appropriate resources to build a capacity to implement policies of participation.
- Children and young people's involvement is valued.
- Children and young people have equal opportunities to get involved.
- Policies and standards for the participation of children and young people are provided, evaluated and continuously improved.

Kirby *et al.* (2003) identify three cultures of participation, which can be present in organisations that involve children and young people in decision making:

- Consultation-focused – where children are consulted to inform the development of services and policies.
- Participation-focused – where children are consulted and involved in making decisions within higher-level participation activities which are usually time bound. Usually a sample of children is involved.
- Child/youth-focused – where participation is central to all practice. There is a culture in which it is assumed that *all* children and young people will be listened to about all decisions – personal and public – that affect their lives.

Kirby *et al.* stress that the boundaries between these are blurred and non-hierarchical. Organisations can move from one to another and different departments within an organisation can adopt different types of culture. However, they suggest that organisations that deliver services to children and young people should always be child/youth focused.

Study activity

Reflect on the ward/hospital/Trust in which you work. Should hospital services always be child/youth focused? When would it be appropriate for one of the other cultures to be adopted?

In building a culture of participation it is necessary to take the following steps. These can apply to a whole organisation, to a ward or department or even to you as an individual:

- *Assess what is already happening.* One tool for self-assessing is Shier's (2001) 'pathways to participation'. At each level of participation, individuals and organisations may have different degrees of commitment to the process of participation. Shier (2001:110) identifies these 'three stages of commitment to the process of empowerment' as openings (where there is an intent to commit), opportunities (where the resources are available to enable to commitment) and obligations (where there are agreed policies). Each level poses questions for you, or the organisation, to assess the level and stage reached. Responses provide a guide as to what can be achieved and what may need to change to enable child participation. As a consequence the model is an extremely useful tool for practitioners and, like other models, can force adults to check their own motivations for implementing participatory activities with children and young people.
- *Develop clear aims and values.* There is a need to be clear about why children should be involved, what values underpin participation work and what will be achieved.
- *Identify what needs to change for participation to be meaningful.* All levels of staff need to be willing and able to listen to children and to act on what they say. This may require a shift in attitudes and most certainly requires a supportive child-focused infrastructure.
- *Develop a common vision and communicate this across the ward/hospital/Trust.* Staff need to be supported in understanding what participation means in practice; staff need the knowledge and skills to make participation meaningful.
- *Choose ways of involving children in decision making.* This will depend on whether the decision is related to personal care or public issues, level of influence they can have, the context of the decision making and the children themselves.
- *Reflect on and evaluate participatory practice.* This should be ongoing and should identify what works well or not so well. Are children's voices being heard? Is what they say being acted upon? Remember to ask children how they think participation is working.

What do young people say about participation and how it can be done effectively?

- Make sure there is flexibility about meeting times so that they can happen at times that suit young people.
- Staff with the right skills need to be specifically dedicated to support young people's participation.
- Make sure a range of methods is used for communicating with young people in ways they will find easy, such as text messaging.
- Make sure you give good feedback to young people about how they have contributed.
- Make sure you provide clear, ongoing communication about how the participation process will develop and what concrete action has been taken.
- Always provide clear, relevant information.
- Be prepared to take feedback about yourselves from young people.
- Make sure you get the atmosphere right and use methods and approaches that don't exclude particular groups of young people.
- Make sure you are always culturally inclusive.
- Make sure participation is enjoyable for all concerned.

http://www.everychildmatters.gov.uk/participation/faq/ (accessed 19 May 2006).

Study activity

Take some time to talk to children and young people in hospital to assess to what degree they feel their voices are heard within the decision-making process.

Study activity

Reflect on your own practice. To what extent do you ensure the voice of the child is heard and acted upon? Observe other staff at work. Identify examples of good and poor practice. Discuss ways of improving practice with your colleagues.

Further reading/information/guidance on involving children and young people in decision making

Participation Works – http://www.participationworks.org.uk/ (accessed 20 May 2006).

This is an online gateway to the world of children and young people's participation. With one click you can access policy, practice, networks and information from across the UK. You can share resources, learn about children's rights, search the knowledge hub or find out about innovative practice and new ideas.

Hear by Right (2005) – http://www.nya.org.uk/hearbyright.

This is a tried and tested standards framework to assess and improve practice and policy on the active involvement of children and young people. It relies on self-assessment, divided into three levels of 'emerging', 'established' and 'advanced', with each level building on the last. This ensures that young people's involvement is built in and not just bolted on.

Lina Fajerman – *Children are Service Users Too.* A guide for consulting children and young people. Available from Save the Children Publications, c/o Plym-bridge Distributors Ltd, Estover Road, Plymouth, PL6 7PY.
Tel: 01752 202301; fax: 01752 202333; email: orders@plymbridge.com

This practical guide is aimed at all organisations that are looking for ways to consult children and young people. The guide can be used to draw up a strategy for consulting children and young people. There are checklists and question and answer sections to help you get started and there is a selection of tried and tested consultation methods that can be used with children and young people of all ages.

Phil Treseder – *Empowering Children and Young People Training Manual Promoting Involvement in Decision Making.* Available from Save the Children Publications, c/o Plymbridge Distributors Ltd, Estover Road, Plymouth, PL6 7PY.
Tel: 01752 202301; fax: 01752 202333.

A manual to help professionals empower children so that they can contribute to the decisions that affect them as individuals and as a group, at unit, local and national levels. It examines the importance of empowerment to children and young people, the benefits of empowerment to children and professionals alike, the barriers to empowerment, and the need for workers and organisations to understand their own intentions. All the material is photocopiable and, in particular, the checklists and exercises have been designed to be photocopied as handouts.

Alison Clark and Peter Moss – *Listening to Young Children – The Mosaic Approach.* Published for the Joseph Rowntree Foundation by NCB. Available from: NCB Book Sales, 8 Wakley Street, London EC1V 7QE.
Tel: 020 7843 6029; fax: 020 7843 6087.

This report looks at how young children's views and experiences can become the focus for reviewing services. The Mosaic approach is a multi-method approach in which children's own photographs, tours and maps can be joined to talking and observing to gain a deeper understanding of children's perspectives.

Key Points

1. A drive towards involving children and young people more in the development and delivery of services is supported by a range of policy documents that emphasise the importance of involving children in decisions affecting their lives.
2. Promoting children's and young people's participation increases their visibility, brings their needs to the attention of adults and can lead to better decision making.
3. Participation is about finding ways of incorporating children's views into decision-making processes within the context of what is possible both institutionally and culturally.
4. Participation can mean different things in different contexts and no one model or form can be applied across all settings and in all situations.
5. Meaningful participation is a process and is not simply about implementing isolated events or activities.

Chapter 23

Creating an Appropriate Hospital Environment for Children

Introduction

In 1859 Florence Nightingale believed that hospitals should do the sick no harm. Although she was primarily concerned with nursing adults, she was stressing the importance of meeting the physiological and psychological needs of patients to avoid them physical or mental stress. This belief is still the concern of nurses over a century later and is a particular issue for nurses caring for hospitalised children (*see also* Hospitalisation and illness p. 200).

Children in hospital have different needs from adult patients because their physical and emotional development is still ongoing and they are still dependent on their parents. Jolly (1981) describes the uniqueness of children's nursing as caring not only for children's physical problems but also responding to their thoughts, feelings and the need for their families. It has been accepted for some time that the physical well-being of children must be assured if they are to reach their maximum potential as adults (Illingworth, 1975). However, it is only comparatively recently that the importance of attending to children's psychological needs in hospital has been recognised as being of equal value. Robertson and Robertson (1952) clearly identified the severe psychological disturbances that occur during the hospitalisation of young children. Such bad experiences can slow children's recovery and impair their psychosocial development to such an extent as to affect adulthood behaviour (Audit Commission, 1993). Do hospitals in the 21st century take children's needs into account and do them no harm?

In 1993 the Audit Commission undertook a study of over 200 hospitals and found significant concerns related to the care of children. They recommended that the care of children in hospital should be based on the following six principles. These six principles have been recognised since the Platt Report (Platt, 1959), which was based on the work of Bowlby (1953) and Robertson (1958) and recognised the psychological trauma caused by hospitalisation (Nichols, 1993):

The NSF for Children, Young People and Maternity Services (DH, 2004)

Part 1

Consists of five standards to help the NHS, local authorities and partner agencies to achieve high-quality service provision for all children, young people, and their parents or carers:

- *Standard 1*: Promoting health and well-being, identifying needs and intervening early.
- *Standard 2*: Supporting parents.
- *Standard 3*: Child-, young person- and family-centred services.
- *Standard 4*: Growing up into adulthood.
- *Standard 5*: Safeguarding and promoting the welfare of children and young people.

Part 2

Contains six standards addressing specific needs of children and young people and their parents or carers:

- *Standard 6*: Children and young people who are ill.
- *Standard 7*: Children in hospital.
- *Standard 8*: Disabled children and young people and those with complex needs.
- *Standard 9*: The mental health and psychological well-being of children and young people.
- *Standard 10*: Medicines for children and young people.
- *Standard 11*: Maternity services.

- child- and family-centred care
- specially skilled staff
- separate facilities
- effective treatments
- appropriate hospitalisation
- strategic commissioning

Unfortunately, these were only recommendations and they were not implemented nationally. In 2004, in recognition of the gaps in the care of children and, in particular, to respond to the Bristol Royal Infirmary Inquiry (2001), which concluded that the needs of sick children in the 1980s and 1990s were not given a high priority, the Labour government produced the National Service Framework (NSF) for children. This set of standards aimed to ensure that health and social services were designed around children and families, rather than around organisations and professionals. Standard 7 of the NSF relates to hospital services for children in order to 'deliver hospital services that meet the needs of children, young people and their parents, and provide effective and safe care, through appropriately trained and skilled staff working in suitable, child-friendly, and safe environment'. The standard has three parts, which reflect the six principles of the 1993 Audit Commission recommendations:

- child-centred hospital services
- quality and safety of care provided
- quality of setting and environment

Child-centred Hospital Services

Children, young people and parents as partners in care

For over 50 years it has been suggested that parents should be involved in the care of children in hospital (Spence, 1947). The UK has led the way in allowing parents to stay with their children in hospital and most children's wards nowadays do recommend parental presence throughout the child's stay in hospital, but the degree of acceptance by staff is still variable. The National Association for the Welfare of Children in Hospital found that whereas staff welcomed 67% of parents, 24% were only accepted and 9% were tolerated. Many wards also practise family-centred care, but 32% of parents consider that their involvement in care is a substitution for the lack of staff. Care must be negotiated with parents for them to appreciate that their involvement is important, otherwise they may well feel abused and frightened. These feelings may then be transmitted to the child. The importance of parental presence and involvement in care is often not recognised in other hospital units/departments (Audit Commission, 1993). Family-centred care can pose difficulties for some staff who may fear loss of control (Bishop, 1988). Children's nurses may need to be more active in communicating the advantages of family-centred care to staff throughout the hospital if the concept is to be accepted more widely and psychological harm to the children is to be minimised. The Children's NSF appreciates that a parent's presence is beneficial in aiding the child's recovery and can be essential to provide practical care. It emphasises that parents and the family as a whole should be treated with respect and their expertise in the care of their own child recognised.

Study activity

Analyse the degree to which child- and family-centred care is practised in your own hospital. Investigate the views of staff, children and parents in all areas of the hospital where children are nursed.

Sharing information with children and parents

The Children's NSF believes that real choice about aspects of treatment and a true partnership in care with children, young people and parents can only really occur if they are provided with accurate information that is 'valid, up-to-date, timely, understandable and developmentally, ethically and culturally appropriate'. Information should be available in a range of formats, media and languages.

Study activity

Within the area where you work, take a selection of information available for children, young people and parents and critically evaluate how it meets the above criteria.

The NSF supports previous Department of Health guidance on providing information and choice to children and parents. In 2002 the Department of Health issued guidance on consent, which required Trusts to specifically take into account the needs of children and young people. It suggests that best practice for children under 16 years, who cannot by law give their own consent for treatment, is to provide them with the opportunity to countersign the consent form. It stresses the above need for clear information that facilitates properly informed consent.

From 2004, all NHS Trusts were required to copy clinicians' letters to patients and were given guidelines to enable clinicians to produce letters that the lay person could understand (DH, 2003a). Unfortunately this proposal did not take into account the cost of reproducing all the correspondence or the difficult dilemma of corresponding directly with a younger person who may not wish parents to be involved.

One of the findings from the Bristol Royal Infirmary Inquiry (2001) was the unsatisfactory way in which bad news was sometimes conveyed. The NSF seeks to address these shortcomings by providing guidance about the most sensitive way to deliver bad or difficult news, so it is received, understood and dealt with as easily as possible.

Considering the 'whole' child

The NSF stresses the need to make hospitalisation as normal an experience as possible for children and to recognise that health

Family-centred care – parents' views

Families of children with chronic health problems often feel:

- their role on the ward is unclear
- uninvolved in decisions about their child's care
- their experience in caring for their child was often ignored
- their role is to substitute for lack of staff
- unsure of the staff's attitude towards their participation in care
- their role is to provide support and reassurance for their child
- they provide continuity of care for their child in a frightening situation

The Bristol Inquiry (The Kennedy Report)

An inquiry into the excessive number of deaths of children receiving open heart surgery at the Bristol Royal Infirmary from 1991 to 1995. During this time 30–35 more children died than might have been expected in a typical paediatric cardiac surgery unit. The government set up a review group to make recommendations for the safe organisation of the paediatric cardiac service. This review concluded that 'the failure to accord children's services a sufficient priority in Bristol and elsewhere in the NHS resulted in the death and damage of a number of very young children'. The report of the group made nearly 200 recommendations for change, involving the:

- development of child-centred health care
- promotion of safe care
- maintenance of the competence of healthcare professionals
- comparable terms of employment for all healthcare professionals
- development of agreed standards of clinical care
- openness of clinical performance
- monitoring of clinical performance

(Bristol Royal Infirmary Inquiry, 2001)

protection and promotion and disease prevention are integral to hospital care. Marriott (1990) states that it is essential for children's nurses to be part of clinical directorates to put forward the special needs of children. Without this representation at directorate level it appears that hospital managers also do not recognise the importance of play and education for children in hospital. Thirty per cent of wards surveyed by the Audit Commission (1993) had less than 50% full-time equivalent trained play staff. If play in hospital enables children to restore normality, relieve anxieties and aid understanding (Kitchener, 1993), hospitals may be harming children by not facilitating such diversion.

The 1944 Education Act stated that all children had the right to receive education, which was appropriate to their age, ability and aptitude. It also enabled children to receive education in areas other than school. Schooling in hospital provides children with diversion and also provides continuity of the child's usual home routine. It is therefore an important aspect of hospital life for children but it requires appropriate facilities and the appointment of a flexible teacher who can meet the needs of different age groups and abilities. Hospital teachers often only cater for younger children and are not usually available outside children's wards.

The NSF recommends that hospitals play an active role in the prevention of ill health and inequalities. It suggests that staff working with children require a change of attitude to think beyond the presenting problems and consider whether the illness or injury could have been avoided and/or a recurrence prevented. This includes making opportunity for health education for parents and children. These are sensitive areas, which some healthcare professionals steer clear of to avoid distressing or antagonising parents who are already distressed by their child's illness or injury.

Quality and Safety of Care Provided

Clinical governance systems with a focus on children

The NSF recognises that hospital procedures and systems can put the safety and well-being of children at risk. It states that all Trusts should give the care of children a specific focus within their clinical governance arrangements. This includes appointing a children's lead at Trust board level and producing an annual report to the Trust board on children's services within the Trust.

Effective and efficient hospital services for children rely on clear hospital policies and standards based on children's needs. Few commissioning authorities identify children's services separately from those of adults or show any evidence of the specific health needs of children within their district (Audit Commission, 1993). Consequently, strategic plans rarely identify precise developments to meet the needs of children in hospital or provide examples of child-specific quality monitoring. This is another area where children's nurses could be more active in research to identify children's needs clearly and to pinpoint areas that need development and evaluation.

Study activity

- Obtain a copy of your hospital's business plans for the next year. Assess how much these plans take children's needs into account.
- Find out who the children's lead is for your Trust. Is this post well known within the Trust?
- Read the latest annual report for children's services within your Trust. Does it reflect a recognition that children are a separate and vulnerable client group?

Appropriately trained and skilled staff

Specially skilled staff who can provide specific care for children and their families are necessary in every part of the hospital that provides health care for children. According to the 2005 Dr Foster hospital guide (http://www.drfoster.co.uk/public.asp, accessed 19 May 2006) there is considerable variation throughout the UK. On average, 61% of district general hospitals have 24-hour cover from a specialist paediatrician but this varies from 43% in Northern Ireland to 84% in England. Nationally only 59% of surgeons undertaking paediatric surgery have spent at least 6 months training in a specialist unit, as recommended by the Kennedy Report (Bristol Royal Infirmary Inquiry, 2001). Fifty-six per cent of anaesthetists in the UK undertake at least one paediatric list per week. Although there is no research to substantiate this, it may be that these anaesthetists are those who cause unnecessary psychological trauma to children by continuing to prescribe intramuscular pre-medication and do not encourage parental presence in the anaesthetic room.

Medical staff who have insufficient experience in caring for children often do not have the special skill necessary to treat children with the less common childhood illnesses. Stiller (1988) has shown that survival rates of children with cancer are significantly higher when they are treated in a paediatric oncology centre. This may also be true for children treated in paediatric intensive care units as opposed to a general intensive care unit. The psychological stress of these children and their families must be less in a specialised unit with known successful outcomes. Parents also gain much psychological support from meeting other parents in similar stressful situations (Ramsay, 1990). Unfortunately, the Audit Commission (1993) found that referral to specialist centres is decreasing as hospitals try to lower costs and expand services.

The Audit Commission (1993) found that even paediatric units lacked sufficient numbers of registered sick children's nurses (RSCNs) (*see also* Caring for children in pain p. 351). Hutt (1983) noted that one reason for this was that general managers did not perceive a need for RSCNs. Since the Platt Report (Platt, 1959) it has been accepted that RSCNs/RNs (child) have specialist knowledge, skills and attitudes. In 1991 the DH set a target standard for 1995 of 'two registered sick children's nurses – or nurses who have completed the child branch of Project 2000 – on duty 24 hours a day in all hospital children's departments and wards . . . and a RSCN on duty 24 hours a day to advise on the nursing of children in other departments' (see Figure 31.1, p. 353).

The Allitt inquiry (Clothier, 1994) recommends that these standards should be more closely monitored. It is interesting to note that there were significant shortcomings in the RSCN staffing levels at the time

Surgeons' and anaesthetists' practice with children

The Audit Commission (1993) found that many surgeons and anaesthetists had little experience with children. Each year:

- over 50% of surgeons perform fewer than 10 operations on babies under 6 months
- only 30% of surgeons performed over 50 operations per year on children aged 3–10 years
- over 90% of surgeons perform fewer than 50 operations per year on children between 6 months and 2 years
- only 10% of anaesthetists deal with more than 50 babies under 6 months each year
- less than 75% of anaesthetists annually deal with more than 50 children aged between 6 months and 2 years
- 45% of anaesthetists deal with fewer than 50 children aged 3–10 years each year

Recommendations from the Allitt inquiry

- Entrants to child nursing should have at least a record of sickness from their most recent place of employment
- Candidates with a history of major personality disorder should not be employed in children's nursing
- Consideration should be given to how GPs might certify that a candidate for employment in the NHS has no excluding medical history
- Consideration should be given to making a candidate's sickness records available to occupational health departments
- All nurses should undergo formal health screening before their first appointment after registration
- Procedures for management referrals to occupational health departments should clarify the criteria which trigger such referrals
- Coroners should send copies of post-mortem reports to every consultant involved in the patient's care
- The provision of paediatric pathology services should be available whenever a child's death is unexpected or unaccountable
- The DH should take steps to ensure that the recommendations of *Welfare of Children and Young People in Hospital* are more closely observed
- When alarms on monitoring equipment fail, an untoward incident report should be completed and the equipment serviced before it is used again
- Reports of serious untoward incidents should be made, in writing, to District and Regional Health Authorities through a single channel
- That the Allitt disaster heightens awareness of the possibility of malevolent interventions as a cause of unexplained clinical events

(Clothier, 1994)

of the Allitt murders. Although this was obviously an exceptional situation, it is certainly an instance of where a hospital did harm the patient. Another issue of concern raised by the Allitt inquiry is the supervision of non-RSCNs. Tucker (1989) questions the ethics of exposing general students to the need to care for children. This question becomes even more pertinent when it becomes apparent that such students do not always have the supervision of registered children's nurses. An appropriately qualified children's nurse at management level may help to ensure that sufficient attention is given to recruiting and retaining appropriate numbers of such nurses (Audit Commission, 1993). At this level an RSCN/RN (child) can also ensure good practices in the care of children throughout the hospital.

The 2004 Children's NSF does not address these issues in depth. Although it makes reference to the need for staff working with children to have had appropriate training in the physical and psychological needs of children, it describes this training as perhaps leading to a National Vocational Qualification or similar rather than a professional registration. Perhaps because of the difficulties in meeting previous recommendations, it makes no clear definition of the numbers of specialist children's nurses required per shift or the amount of experience required by medical staff working with children. This is an interesting omission given that the Bristol Royal Infirmary Inquiry (2001) revealed that this specialist children's hospital had no full-time paediatric cardiac surgeon and too few registered children's nurses.

Study activity

Look at the staffing in your own hospital in all the areas where children are nursed. How far does it meet the DH guidelines? Is there a named children's nurse to provide advice about the care of children outside the children's ward?

Separate facilities

Children in hospital also need separate facilities that are attractive, bright and age related (Muller *et al.*, 1994). Such surroundings reassure children and parents and minimise the trauma of hospitalisation (Rodin, 1983). A separate area for play also helps to minimise the stress of hospitalisation and provides a secure place for children to act out their fears. In 1991 the Department of Health recommended that all children staying in hospital should have daily access to a play specialist to support them at each stage of their journey through the period of hospitalisation. A separate treatment room where clinical procedures can be carried out enables the child to keep the bed and play area as secure places. Most children's wards have these facilities and are bright and cheerful, but they do tend to only attract the younger children. Areas outside children's wards where children are treated (for example, X-ray, and accident-and-emergency departments) often lack specific facilities for any age group. Teenagers are probably most disadvantaged in hospital as appropriate facilities are largely lacking (National Association for the Welfare of Children in Hospital; NAWCH, 1986). Some hospitals have no policy for adolescents in hospital, who are consequently sometimes admitted to adult wards where they can feel anxious and isolated (Miller, 1991). Even when they are admitted to children's wards they can still feel out of place and concerned about the lack of privacy in a mixed-sex ward.

In 2004 NHS Estates published *Design for Health*, which documents the experience of involving children, families and staff in the building of a new purpose-built children's hospital in Bristol. The study shows how the child's experience in hospital can be enhanced by the right environment. It also demonstrates how the right working environment can increase job satisfaction for staff (*see also* Play and education p. 95).

Study activity

Take a critical look at how your hospital defines children. What is the hospital policy with regard to admitting adolescents to adult or children's wards?

In an English National Board (ENB) study in 1992, over 25% of hospitals did not use separate facilities for any children admitted for ophthalmic, ear, nose or throat surgery because of consultants' preferences. In 2003 this had not changed significantly, with 38% of hospitals in the UK that had paediatric inpatients still admitting them to adult wards (Royal College of Paediatrics and Child Health, 2003). Many hospitals also have no separate outpatient or accident-and-emergency facilities for children (ENB, 1992). These areas may be children's first contact with hospital and these initial impressions are important influences on any subsequent reaction to hospital. Apart from the unsuitability of adult wards and departments for children, these areas also lack facilities for parents. Parents require time, provision and support for their needs if they are to be fully involved in the care of their child. If parents are anxious, tired or uneasy, children will sense this and also become alarmed (Muller *et al.*, 1994). In contrast, 60% of paediatric units usually provide parents with facilities for sleeping, washing, eating and drinking, and relaxing that are close to their child (Audit Commission, 1993) (Figure 23.1). An added anxiety for parents in recent years has been the introduction in many hospitals of prohibitive parking costs. An Australian study (Shields and Tanner, 2004) found that financial barriers such as the cost of parking and meals hinder parents from staying with their children. Shields and Tanner (2004) recommend that all parents staying with their children have three free meals per day, which the family can eat together, and that there should be free parking. Rising healthcare costs in the UK, which are leading Trusts to introduce many ways to generate income, may make this difficult to achieve.

Study activity

- Analyse the separate facilities for children and their families in your own hospital. Consider how far these facilities meet the needs of different age groups as well as the needs of parents.
- Find out the costs for parents staying with their children in hospital or attending outpatient departments. Does your hospital have any separate policy for parents in relation to payment for parking or meals?

Functions of play in hospital

- Provides diversion from pain and fear
- Enables relaxation
- Helps to reduce the stress of hospitalisation
- Provides a link with normal home routines
- Enables expression of feelings
- Encourages interaction with others
- Allows the child some control over the environment
- Encourages creativity
- Helps to prepare and teach about hospital and related procedures

Functions of education in hospital

- Links with home and usual school
- Stimulation and motivation to learn
- Continuity of education
- Therapeutic learning activities which also promote overall development
- Opportunities for acting out fears and anxieties
- Career advice, especially for disabled children

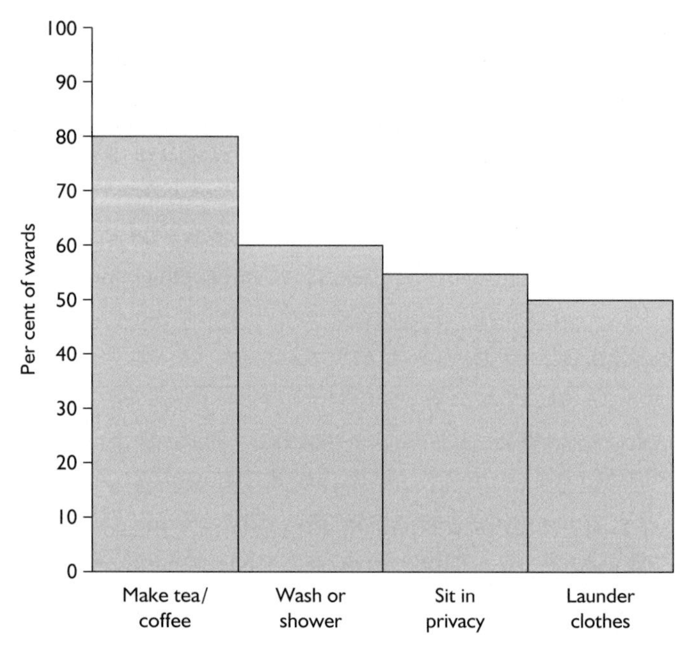

Figure 23.1 Parents' facilities in children's wards (Audit Commission, 1993). $N = 41$ wards in 5 hospitals.

Facilities for children in hospital also have to take into account children's special needs for safety. In 1992 the Child Accident Prevention Trust and the Royal College of Nursing discovered that accidents to children in hospital were largely preventable (Child Accident Prevention Trust, 1992). The children's area itself should be safe, with high door handles or childproof catches to prevent toddlers wandering away. Windows, lifts and stairs should be secure and all electrical points should be covered. Furniture in a children's ward should be sturdy and of an appropriate size to minimise the danger of falls. Beds should be lowered and cot sides kept raised at all times when children are unattended. Falls from cots mostly occur when cot sides have not been raised (Banco and Powers, 1988). Safety straps for seats should be used for small children (*see also* Developmental factors and associated accidents p. 160).

Stock lotions, cleaning fluids and medicines should be kept in a securely locked cupboard or trolley and medicines should never be left at the bedside. Treatment rooms, sluices and kitchens should be kept securely fastened when not in use. Electrical equipment should be serviced regularly and there should be a clear policy for the identification of out-of-order apparatus (Clothier, 1994). Special care should be taken with equipment used at the bedside; infusion pumps should have a child-locking device, plugs and fans should be placed out of reach and any tubing should be carefully secured so that it cannot pose any danger to the child.

Toys should be unbreakable, non-allergic and washable, and appropriate for the child's age and condition. Small toys can be swallowed by small children and can cause pressure sores when left in the beds of paralysed or immobile children.

Children also have special needs for safety in relation to infection control. Infants under 6 months have little natural immunity from infection and need to be nursed in protective isolation. Older children may need to be protected from children admitted with an infectious illness. Bathrooms should provide appropriately sized facilities to promote good hygiene after toileting.

Study activity

Take a critical look at a children's ward and identify any areas where the children's safety may be compromised.

Effective treatments

In the present climate of cost-effective care, hospitals may find it difficult to rationalise expenditure on separate facilities. However, this money may be gained by savings on inappropriate or ineffective treatments. Lous *et al.* (2005) found no evidence that myringotomies performed for the insertion of grommets, one of the most common procedures performed in children, helped speech and language development and recommended a watchful waiting strategy for children with glue ear. Couto (2004) suggests that the effects of the very expensive intensive care of newborn babies may not always be appropriate and should be monitored. Although such care has significantly reduced the mortality rate in low birthweight babies, the infants who survive are often disabled. This can cause great psychological trauma to the growing child and the family. Monitoring the treatment of such infants would enable staff and parents to make informed decisions about the suitability of such intensive care. Glasper (1993) stresses the need for children's nurses to become involved in practice-based research to enhance child and family care. Perhaps this is one area that would benefit from this type of investigation. (*See also* Ear surgery p. 475.)

Appropriate hospitalisation

In addition to the evaluation of treatments, it may also be useful to study whether hospitalisation is always necessary. The National Association for the Welfare of Children in Hospital (NAWCH) (1986) found a considerable expansion in day care surgery for children, but the Audit Commission (1993) noted that some children were still experiencing an excessive stay in hospital due to administrative or organisational inefficiency. Earlier discharge from hospital may help to reduce the harmful effects of separation and hospitalisation for children and their families.

Study activity

Find out the average length of stay for children in your hospital. Consider the appropriateness of the reasons why some children stay longer than average. Has the hospital made sufficient arrangements for day or short-stay care to meet local need?

In the future it should be possible to see a more active interest in the development of services for children. In 1995 the government produced a draft children's charter for discussion. This document listed some of the rights expected by children in hospital (*see also* Children's Charter p. 268).

Summary

Since the 1950s there have been many innovations and changes to provide appropriate care for children in hospital. However, it would appear that hospitals still have the potential to harm children. Children's nurses should be more assertive and active in trying to establish and maintain recommended standards of care for children. They need to promote their specialist knowledge and skills so that they can be accepted as the specialists in childcare. Swanwick and Barlow (1993) have begun to investigate the uniqueness of this branch of nursing. More research is needed in this area to strengthen the rationale for the need for more RSCNs/RNs (child). This research should to be related to the benefits of meeting needs. Possibly the evidence that the lack of psychological care causes harm has lost its impact over time. It may be that now there is a need to show that such care reduces parental complaints and enables earlier discharge, as parents who have been fully involved in their child's care are happy to take the child home knowing that they have access to specialised help and support. Such research would also help to provide research-based standards relating to the specialist care of children. These could then form the basis of audits and quality assurance programmes, which could be applied specifically to paediatrics. In these ways an argument can be put forward for the cost effectiveness of providing psychological care, enabling future league tables of hospital performance to include some measurement of this, and thus improving the present situation so that the hospital really does do the patient no harm.

Key Points

1. Hospitals still do not always meet the psychological needs of children in hospital.
2. Children's nurses are necessary to promote these needs in all areas of the hospital.
3. More research is needed to strengthen the importance of the role of the children's nurse.
4. The importance of psychological care should be part of any evaluation of hospital performance.
5. Patients' charters should include the rights of the child in relation to health care.

Chapter 24

Preparation for Hospital and Procedures

Introduction

One of the unique roles of the children's nurse is the preparation of the child for hospitalisation or procedures. Children find illness and hospitalisation extremely stressful and frightening and if these feelings are not allayed, the child is at risk from developing behavioural changes and a long-term fear of hospital and medical intervention.

Any preparation has to be adjusted to suit the individual child, whose personality and past experiences may all influence the reaction to hospital and understanding of procedures. Carson *et al.* (1992) believe that the child's conception of illness and hospital is the most important factor in determining how well the child will adjust. Other studies have discovered further factors influencing adjustment to illness and hospitalisation. Gillis (1990) found that children from rural areas responded less well to hospital than those in urban areas, perhaps because children in urban areas have more day-to-day contact with the local hospital. However, it appears that intimate knowledge of hospital and procedures is not helpful. Hart and Bossert (1994) discovered that prior experience and familiarity with hospital did not reduce children's fears. They suggest that fear of the unknown is replaced by fear of reality.

One of the most important strategies children use for coping with stress is play. In 1991 the Department of Health issued guidelines on the welfare of children in hospital and stated that play: '. . . can help them to resolve stressful situations like admission to hospital where they have to undergo painful procedures . . .' Using play to prepare children for the unknown reduces their fears and enables them to develop a feeling of control over the event, thus helping them to cope better. Many types of play materials can be used to prepare children, and studies have not shown any method to be more effective than another. Becker (1972) even suggests that some of these methods may actually increase stress and anxiety. However, the age of the child does appear to influence which method is most effective. Bates and Broome (1986) found that small children reacted better to involvement in active play, whereas

Children's reactions to hospital – influencing factors

- Personality – ability to cope with stress
- Conception of illness and hospital
- Age (especially preschool age)
- Intelligence
- Parental reactions
- Type and length of illness

older children preferred age-appropriate videos. Broome and Lillis (1989) discovered that the main benefit of preparation was increased cooperation from the child, but they also found a significant reduction in the amount of pain the children reported and in their heart and respiratory rates.

Parents need preparation too. Parents do not always know what to do or how best to support their child during hospitalisation or procedures. Children readily sense parental anxiety and this can increase their fears and resistance to the event. Some parents may be undecided about staying with their child during hospitalisation or a specific procedure, and will need help and support from the nurse to make this decision.

Principles of preparing children for procedures

- Assess the child's present level of understanding
- Find out parental wishes about presence and involvement
- Prepare the teaching and visual aids
- Use concrete terms and familiar words
- Explain any unfamiliar terminology
- Emphasise body parts and functions not involved
- Be honest
- Explain how the child will feel
- Demonstrate and practise any coping mechanisms
- Include negative information carefully
- Emphasise the positive aspects
- Evaluate learning and allow time for questions

Preparing Children for Hospital

The preparation for children having a planned admission to hospital is often well organised. Several hospitals run pre-admission clubs for children on the waiting list. These clubs usually provide children with an opportunity to visit the ward, meet some of the staff and play with equipment. These clubs tend to be arranged to primarily meet the needs of younger children. There is some justification in this, as this is the age group known to be most traumatised by hospitalisation. However, this does not mean that older children do not also require information. The Children's Charter (DH, 1995) recognised this and recommended that adolescents should have the chance to visit adult and children's wards, and be able to make a choice about where they are nursed. Parents also require information. Accompanying their children to a pre-admission club will provide them with increased knowledge but it will not tell them about the normal and expected behavioural responses of children to hospital. Vulcan and Nikulich-Barrett (1988) found that parents who were told about such behaviour were less anxious and managed it better. Parents also need advice about the hospital routine and their role. Although many children's units claim to believe in the partnership with parents' philosophy, few of them explain to parents what this means (Audit Commission, 1993; Darbyshire, 1994) (*see also* Pre- and post-operative care p. 384).

Principles of preparing parents for their child's hospitalisation

- Show around ward
- Indicate parents' facilities
- Explain ward philosophy
- Outline ward routine and staffing
- Explain children's physical and psychological reactions to hospital and illness
- Warn of siblings' reactions
- Clarify nurses' role in providing care, support and teaching
- Provide opportunity to discuss issues, ask questions
- Consolidate verbal information with a written account

Study activity

Ask some parents and children in hospital about their preparation and consider how useful it was in meeting their needs.

Siblings are often missed out in the preparation of a child for hospital. Siblings can feel neglected by the absence of parents or fear that they too may have to be admitted to hospital. At times they may feel guilt that they are somehow responsible for the hospitalisation. As a result, they often demonstrate feelings of anger and resentment towards the ill child or their parents. Even when these feelings are not exhibited, the repressed emotion may result in other types of problem behaviour. Morgan (1990) found that even siblings of children admitted to hospital for short periods demonstrated behavioural changes when the hospitalised child returned home. It is obviously difficult to meet all the needs of children of various ages, their siblings and parents in terms of preparing them for hospitalisation. The efficacy of pre-admission clubs depends upon their ability to respond to these varying needs.

Study activity

Think about how you could plan a pre-admission facility to meet the needs of siblings.

It is important not to overload the family with information at the pre-admission visit. However, it is unlikely that everything will be remembered. For this reason it is useful to have the information in a written format, which can then consolidate the advice given on the day. This written information could also address the needs of the different members of the family. Parents can also be given a resource list of books and play items useful for preparing children for hospital. Adams *et al.* (1991) found that a preparation booklet reduced children's anxieties on admission, reduced the number of behavioural problems occurring after discharge, and increased parental satisfaction when compared with verbal preparation alone. Hall (1996) describes how storytelling prior to hospitalisation helps children gain confidence about going to hospital and Clough (2005) describes the success of an individualised story to prepare an 8-year-old for surgery.

Study activity

- Visit your local children's library and see what books are available to prepare children of different ages for admission to hospital. Take a critical look at these books and consider how useful they are.
- Write an individualised short story for a child you are nursing to explain an aspect of their care.

Children on the waiting list for planned admission are usually well catered for in terms of preparation, but can the same be said for children entering hospital as an emergency? Every year, 25% of children in the UK between the ages of 0 and 16 years will visit an accident-and-emergency (A&E) unit and the majority of these will be preschool children (Campbell and Glasper, 1995). This visit is likely to be their first contact with hospital and it can affect their future response to any further contact. Accident-and-emergency departments can be frightening and children taken there are often already stressed because of pain and fear. Much can be done to alleviate the stress of the A&E department but it would be much better if children could become familiar with the environment before they needed to use the facility. Hospital tours alone are known to be ineffective in relieving anxiety (Peterson *et al.*, 1990) but in the 1990s a group of hospitals in Northern Ireland set up a Well Teddy Clinic to reduce children's anxiety about A&E. Children bring their teddies to hospital for a check-up and, through play, become familiar with the equipment used in hospital. Evaluations of this facility have been very positive (Burton, 1994). Other innovations to prepare children for emergency admission to hospital are visits by ambulance staff to nurseries and infant classes, giving the children a chance to see inside an ambulance and handle some of the equipment (*see also* A&E p. 298).

Study activity

Investigate what strategies are used in your area to prepare children for emergency admission to hospital.

Role of the nurse in caring for children before, during and after procedures

- *Be confident.* Even babies can sense anxiety in adults and will react by resisting
- *Provide realistic choices.* Allow children some control over events by offering choices, but only offer realistic choices. Children may not have any control over the timing of the procedure but they may be able to choose a toy to cuddle
- *Allow participation.* Providing children with something to do during the procedure will also help them to feel in control. They may like to hold the sticking plaster and help to apply it after the procedure
- *Help with coping strategies.* Remind the child of methods practised before the procedure. Join in breathing or singing
- *Accept child's response.* Small children usually react to stress by crying, shouting or hitting out. Older children may cry or swear. They should not be punished for reacting in this way to procedures
- *Give praise.* Help children's self-image by praising their coping skills whatever the outcome. They need to know that their reactions were acceptable in the circumstances and not to feel that they have failed. Rewards for bravery provide evidence of their ability to cope with the situation and may help to boost confidence
- *Provide comfort.* Give hugs and cuddles during and after the procedure

Preparing Children for Procedures

Children of any age need preparation for any procedure. They need to know what is going to happen and what they will need to do. Parents also need information about the procedure and their role. Care must be taken to give the information at an optimum time to reduce rather than heighten anxiety. Generally, small children can best deal with this sort of information as close as possible to the event. Older children manage better if given time between the preparation and the implementation of the procedure to allow them to absorb the information and ask questions. The preparation needs to take into account the child's age, stage of development, temperament, previous experiences and coping strategies, and the individual's need to know. Like adults, children vary in the amount of information they want to know (Peterson and Toler, 1986) and the nurse can be guided by the parents and the child's reaction to the preparation. The actual procedure is best carried out away from the bed area. Even babies can associate objects or places with painful experiences and protest when meeting them again. For all children, it is useful to have prepared the necessary equipment prior to the procedure so there is no added distress for the child by having to wait and watch this happen.

A child who has a distressing experience during a procedure will develop a long-lasting fear of the procedure and is likely to become more and more resistant to it. To prevent this negative cycle of events, it is important to try and ensure that the child receives the optimum psychological and physical preparation.

Psychological Preparation

The nurse preparing the child for the procedure ideally needs to be someone who has had time to build up a rapport with the child and family. The child needs to be able to trust the nurse to have confidence in what is said. Babies are usually wary of strangers and have a strong attachment to their parents. They are too young for an explanation of the procedure but can be helped by parental presence during the procedure. If parents are unable to be present, a familiar object may help. Infancy is the period of sensori-motor learning and, although most babies are likely to actively withdraw from pain and need to be effectively restrained during procedures, the nurse or parent can still provide comfort by gentle massage, talking or singing quietly or providing a dummy.

Toddlers are egocentric with limited communication skills. They attribute lifelike behaviour to inanimate objects and often believe that thoughts can cause events. They enjoy imitating adult behaviour but can also be very negative as they try to develop some autonomy. They need to be told in very simple terms what they will experience during the procedure and have time to play with equipment so they are not frightened of it. They should be given some opportunity for autonomy, perhaps by having a choice of toy to accompany them, so that they do not feel totally out of control. Toddlers also need very careful restraint but may be reassured by distraction, storytelling or singing. The preschool child is still egocentric but has developed more communication skills. At this age children are very conscious of their bodies and worry about the effect of any injury. Having now developed an independent personality, these children now try to take further control of situations by using their initiative. They can now understand that pain is not a punishment and the nurse can use simple terms to explain the reason and the effects of the procedure. They should be allowed to take part in the procedure, perhaps by holding equipment.

The school-age child is beginning to develop concrete thinking skills and is described by Erikson as having a sense of industry. In other words these children have an interest in learning and are keen to use their increased language and thinking skills to gain a greater understanding of the world. They need to have the reasons for procedures clearly explained and to understand the purpose and effect of the equipment involved. At this age children can relate to their peers and may be able to help each other prepare for a procedure. Their developmental need for industry should be satisfied by allowing some participation in the procedure and an active coping strategy.

Adolescents are concerned with developing their autonomy and are capable of abstract thought. They need to know the reason and consequences of the procedure and any effects it may have on their appearance. Their need for autonomy can be helped by enabling them some choice in the timing and place for the procedure. Peer groups are important to this age group and they may gain more benefit from preparation by another adolescent. The nurse may need to accept that the adolescent may refuse to consider a specific coping strategy and may resort to more childish ways of coping.

Use of Play

Dolls can be used to explain exactly what the procedure entails. Some children may like to act out procedures on the doll, which also provides them with an opportunity to handle the equipment. Dressing up as nurses or doctors enables children to act out feelings towards these people and may help them to come to terms with medical interventions. Drawing or colouring in pictures of the event may also help children to

Table 24.1 Books available for preparing children for hospital

Age	Books
Ages 3–4 years	Norman Bridwell (2000) *Clifford Visits the Hospital* Bridwell Cartwheel Books Ann Civardi and Stephen Cartwright (2002) *Going to the Hospital* Usborne Books Liesbet Slegers (2005) *Kevin Goes to the Hospital* Frances Lincoln Publishers Dick Bruna (2003) *Miffy in Hospital* Egmont Books Ltd Barbara Cork (2002) *Katie goes to Hospital* Waterbird Books
Ages 5–8 years	Russell Hoban and Ian Andrew (2001) *Jim's Lion* Candlewick Press Fred Rogers and Jim Judkis (1987) *Going to the Hospital* GP Putnam's Sons H.A. Rey and Margaret Rey (1995) *Curious George goes to the Hospital* Houghton Mifflin Juvenile Books
Ages 9–12 years	Diana Kimpton and Peter Kavanagh (1994) *The Hospital Highway Code* Macmillan Children's Books

talk about any fears. Photographs or videos of other hospital departments and equipment will help to remove the fear of the unknown and play equipment can then be used to give children some appreciation of procedures such as X-rays or scans (a rigid play tunnel can make a realistic scanner).

Older children may prefer to read about the procedure. There are children's books which provide information about medical procedures (Table 24.1) and, in addition, some hospitals provide information leaflets for children about specific investigations (*see also* Functions of play in hospital p. 263).

Study activity

Visit some departments in your hospital where children undergo investigations and explore what specific preparatory information is available for them. Consider what additional information may be useful.

Coping Strategies

Teaching coping strategies before a procedure helps to give children some control of the event. When procedures are to be repeated, successful strategies such as relaxation instructions or favourite music can be put on tape as a reminder of the technique. The most effective strategies are based on behavioural therapies and produce feelings of calmness and relaxation in situations that would otherwise provoke stress and maladaptive behaviour. This new behaviour weakens the connection between anxiety and its stimulus. The most appropriate strategy for the individual depends upon choice and the discomfort of the procedure. Children experiencing severe discomfort may not be able to concentrate wholly on a complicated coping strategy. Most children will benefit best by being able to choose the method most appealing to them.

During the past 20 years, hypnosis has been developed to deal with children's psychological problems. Hypnotherapy is often successful in children because their high imaginative skills make them easily susceptible candidates. Self-hypnosis can be taught to individuals so that the technique can be used independently. Cohen *et al.* (1984) suggest that children as young as 3 years can use this technique and it is particularly useful for adolescents and for children who require repeated painful procedures. Its success appears to relate to the child's control and mastery of the situation.

Relaxation and guided imagery (see box to the right and over the page) are techniques similar to hypnosis and are also well accepted by children with good imagination skills. Even small children can be helped to relax by rocking and quiet, soothing words. Older children can be helped to relax by controlled breathing and progressive relaxation of different parts of the body. This can be combined with a discussion of an enjoyable event, which can be enhanced by music or pictures of the event. Some children may cope better by being more active and controlled breathing may be used as a way of pretending to blow the pain away. Singing or even shouting can help children distract themselves from the reality of the procedure. Distraction can also be provided by storytelling or a favourite video. The child usually needs help to use these methods and parents who have also been taught the strategy can often provide this support.

Children who are very uncooperative may benefit from some kind of positive reinforcement. Stars or tokens or a bravery certificate can be offered for cooperation. In addition, praise for coping well will provide the child with intrinsic reinforcement.

Relaxation exercise for children

Ensure that the child is lying or sitting down in a comfortable position and in a quiet, even voice say the following:

- put your hands on your tummy so that the tips of your fingers are just touching
- feel your fingertips moving apart as you breathe
- see how your tummy goes up and down as you breathe

Allow the child to experience this for 10–20 breaths. Then say:

- put one hand on your chest
- feel your hand going up and down as you breathe

Allow the child time to recognise this feeling and then say to the child:

- put one hand on your tummy and one hand on your chest and feel your tummy and chest going up and down. When I say 'down' let your tummy and chest go down and when I say 'up', let your chest and tummy lift up

Keep your voice quiet and even, giving your instructions at a suitable pace to ensure a deep, relaxing breathing rate with a slightly longer exhalation period. Remember that the child's respiratory rate is likely to be faster than your own.

Physical Preparation

Consideration should be given to the most appropriate means of physical preparation prior to distressing procedures. Sedation, analgesia or local anaesthetic may help to make the procedure more bearable but may need to be given 1 to 2 hours before the procedure. Whenever possible, injections should be avoided as most children regard these as painful procedures and their fear may actually be increased. Sometimes it is useful to give heavy sedation for the first of several procedures to enable to child to realise that the procedure is not to be feared. Once the child is more relaxed it may be possible to gradually reduce the medication.

Summary

One of the unique roles of the children's nurse is the preparation of children for hospital and procedures. Children cannot be expected to accept strange interventions passively and children who are unprepared will be unable to cooperate and are likely to become progressively more upset and scared with subsequent contacts with health care. Children's nurses working with healthy children should consider how their patient group can be introduced to the hospital environment before they have a need to use these facilities. Children's nurses working with sick children should be able to use a range of techniques to prepare children

Guided imagery for children

Guided imagery attempts to help children to concentrate on an image other than the one that is disturbing to them. It can also be used as an aid to relaxation by helping the children to imagine they are elsewhere. Children tend to have good imaginations and usually respond well to this technique. Individuals all have their own idea of pleasure and the imagery needs to be negotiated with them first. The following is only an example which will only be successful if the child is able to associate this scenario with relaxation.

As with any strategy for relaxation the child should be in a comfortable and relaxed position. Spend a short time ensuring that the child is relaxed and breathing evenly – you could commence by using the breathing exercise described above. Then commence your description in a quiet and even tone:

Imagine you are lying on the beach. The sun is hot and the sand is warm. You can feel the sun on your skin making you warm and sleepy. The sand is so soft and warm that it is as if you were lying in bed. As you gently move your feet and hands you can feel the warm grains of sand between your toes and fingers. You can smell mummy's perfume and you can hear her turning the pages of her book as she sits beside you reading. In the distance you can hear the sound of the sea as it gently moves up to the beach and away again. You feel too tired to move and your arms and legs feel very, very heavy. It is difficult to keep awake so you make yourself more comfortable on the sand and listen to the sounds of the sea. You count the gentle waves as they come into the shore . . . 1 . . . 2 . . . 3 . . . 4 . . . 5. Think about the warmth of the sun . . . the feel of the sand . . . the smell of mummy's perfume . . . how heavy your legs and arms feel . . . and the sound of the sea . . .

Continue with the description with pauses to enable the child to really imagine the scenario.

When the procedure is finished, gradually talk the child into a more wakeful situation.

of different ages and experiences for a variety of interventions. They should make themselves aware of the different interventions performed on children and the different departments in which these are performed so they can give truthful and informed preparation. Nursing assessment should include an assessment of the child and family's previous experiences and their individual need for information and preparation.

Key Points

1. Children who are exposed to unresolved stress and fear in hospital are likely to undergo long-term behavioural problems as a result of this experience.
2. Preparation for hospital or procedures should suit the individual child's age, stage of development, temperament and previous experience.
3. Parents and siblings should also be given information about the ill child's treatment and their supportive role.
4. Children need preparation for emergency admission as well as planned hospitalisation.
5. Behavioural therapies are useful strategies for helping children to cope with the discomfort of procedures.

Chapter 25

Assessment of the Sick Child

Introduction

Assessment of the child involves a knowledge and appreciation of usual child growth, development and behaviour as well as the skills of communication and observation. Assessment should be an ongoing process but is particularly important during the admission of the child to hospital. At this time assessment performs a number of functions. It primarily enables the nurse to make a systematic collection of information about the child to identify the child and family's individual needs for nursing care. However, it also provides an opportunity for the nurse to form a therapeutic relationship with the child and family and to develop a partnership with them in providing the care.

During the nursing assessment, the nurse will interview the child and family to discover their:

- usual home routines to help promote a more familiar environment in hospital
- previous experience of illness or hospital and understanding of this admission
- needs and concerns

During the interview, observation skills will enable the nurse to identify physical and psychological problems. Measurement of vital signs and information from other health professionals will provide more detail.

The use of an appropriate nursing model for the care of children will provide structure for the assessment and ensure that all areas are explored in a holistic way (*see also* Models of children's nursing p. 635).

Preparation for Assessment

First impressions are often very important on admission to hospital when children and families may be very anxious. Their first need is often to feel more at ease, and preparing for the admission assessment may help to provide that reassurance. Arriving on a busy ward and being left alone will not help to relieve the anxieties of the child or family.

Study activity

Consider how you might prepare for an admission assessment to provide a welcoming and reassuring atmosphere.

Even when nurses are busy, it is possible to provide a friendly and reassuring atmosphere. If possible, the child should welcomed by name and the nurse should introduce himself or herself and find out the names of the family present. If the nurse is too busy to interview the parents at that moment, the child and family should either be taken to the bed area, which has been prepared with a few suitable toys, or shown to the playroom. The child and family can be introduced to other families or the play therapist and the nurse can promise to return.

Ideally, the admission assessment should be undertaken in a quiet, private area, which is free from distractions. If an interview room is not available, an empty side room may be used for this purpose. Otherwise, curtains round the bed area may provide some psychological privacy. The area should be prepared with suitable toys to occupy the child, with the nursing charts and equipment kept to a minimum to avoid making the assessment seem too clinical.

In most settings the nurse undertaking the assessment will be the child and family's named nurse for that admission. The nurse should explain the relevance of this concept as well as the purpose of the assessment. The child and family should understand that the assessment is as much for them to obtain information as it for the nurse to collect data. Parents and older children may also be reassured by a promise of confidentiality.

The child and family need time to adjust to their surroundings. An interview that commences with probing questions is unlikely to be successful. Similarly, an assessment that commences with a physical examination of the child is likely to end in tears. The nurse needs to build up a rapport with the child and family before trying to make in-depth investigations. This rapport is probably best developed by casual conversation, giving the child and family time to assess and be confident with the nurse.

Family Routines

Study activity

What will you need to ask the child and family to find out as much as possible about their usual home routines?

Family routines can be ascertained by asking the child or family to complete a 24-hour diary of usual home events (Figure 25.1). This

Please complete this diary with as much information as you can about your child's normal daily activities. This will help us to try and keep to this same routine while your child is in hospital			
Time	**Meals**	**Activity**	**Parental care**
01:00			
02:00			
03:00			
04:00			
05:00			
06:00			
07:00			
08:00			
09:00			
10:00			
11:00			
12:00			
13:00			
14:00			
15:00			
16:00			
17:00			
18:00			
19:00			
20:00			
21:00			
22:00			
23:00			
24:00			

Figure 25.1 Assessment of the child – 24-hour diary.

information can then be built upon by asking specific questions relevant to the child's age and condition.

Health problems

The nurse needs to be aware of any health problem for which the child is currently receiving treatment. This may be a long-term problem, such as asthma, which may be unrelated to this admission, or a new problem which initiated the admission. The usual routine for medication and any other treatment should be ascertained.

Eating and drinking

It is important to know about the child's usual nutrition, meal and snack times, and appetite so that appropriate food and drink can be offered in hospital. Information about any special cups, bowls or cutlery and help required can also be used to help the child maintain usual nutrition.

Elimination

Information about the child's usual bowel and bladder habits will help the nurse to identify any changes and any problems the family may have. To avoid confusion it is also useful to know small children's stage of potty training and the family words used for toilet habits. The stress of hospitalisation can disturb menstruation so it is important to ask older girls about their periods and what sanitary protection they use.

Rest and activity

Individual children have very different patterns of rest and activity and the nurse needs to be aware of these to be able to identify what is normal for a particular child. The nurse needs to discover the child's usual bedtime and time of waking. If the child wakes in the night how does the family react? Special routines before bed such as a bedtime story, favourite toy or comforter, or nightlight are particularly important to know if the parents cannot be resident. Smaller children's nap times need to be known if this routine is to be continued in hospital.

An outline of the child's usual level of activity can be gained from the diary, the nurse can then ask about favourite pastimes or TV programmes, which may help to relieve boredom in hospital.

Washing and dressing

The nurse needs to know how much help children require with washing and dressing, as well as their usual routines. What is the family schedule for washing and is the child used to a bath or shower? If there is any aspect, such as hair washing, which the child finds distressing, the nurse needs to discover how the family deals with this. If the child has a skin problem there may be special bathing creams or lotions and the nurse needs to know about them.

Communication

To communicate with the child it is useful for the nurse to know who is important to the child at home. This information may include the names of pets, teachers, aunts, uncles and friends. It is also useful for the nurse to have an appreciation of the child's usual temperament so any changes can be quickly identified. For instance, is the child usually quiet and shy or very active and talkative? What tends to upset the child and what does the child do when tired or upset? What comforting methods work best?

Religion

The nurse needs to appreciate the importance of religion to the child and family, as there may be religious practices that they would like to be continued in hospital. Parents may also wish to discuss baptism if this has not been performed before admission.

Identification of Needs and Problems

Once the nurse has gained an idea of the usual home routine, the needs and problems of this admission should be identified. Actual needs and problems can be discovered by asking how the reason for this admission has affected or changed the child's usual behaviour. The knowledge and experience of the nurse will help the identification of potential needs and problems. The extent to which the child and parents understand the health problem can be discovered at this time, and the nurse should also

Table 25.1 Assessment of a child's needs and problems

Jamie is an 8-year-old who was diagnosed with asthma when he was 2 years old. He has been admitted with an acute attack. On admission he is very wheezy and cyanosed. He is also very scared as he has been in hospital many times before and hates it. He misses his two brothers, especially at night as he shares a room with them, and dislikes the 'pins' in his arm and the oxygen mask. During his assessment the needs and problems shown below were identified.

Activity	Needs	Problems
Breathing	Provide oxygen Avoid over-excitement	Unable to breathe with wheeze and cough
Eating and drinking	Maintenance of fluids and encouragement to return to normal after the asthmatic attack	Unable to eat or drink
Play	Provide reassurance (Teddy Edward is his special toy) Provision of more active play when able	Unable to get out of bed to play
Rest and sleep	Reassurance and company	Exhausted but too frightened to sleep
Hygiene	Help with washing while breathless	Unable to meet own hygiene needs
Elimination	Record all output	Has not passed urine for 7 hours – may be dehydrated
Concerns	Reassurance re. needles and oxygen masks – use EMLA cream and nasal cannulae	Fear of IV and oxygen mask
Communication	Anticipate needs with help from parents	Too breathless to talk

be able to identify any learning needs the child or family have in relation to the hospitalisation.

For example, a child who has been newly diagnosed with asthma may report that exercise is a problem due to breathlessness. The parents may express sorrow that the child will probably need to give up sports. The nurse will recognise that one of the child's problems is being unable to play sport without becoming breathless and that the parents need teaching about asthma and exercise. If the nurse does not recognise these concerns, acceptance of the condition and compliance with treatment could become a potential problem; see the case history in Table 25.1.

It is important to identify needs and problems in negotiation with the child and family, otherwise a solution might never be found! Sometimes the parent may identify a problem that the nurse cannot appreciate. The nurse should probe gently to find the reason for the problem so that appropriate care can be given to overcome it. On occasions the nurse will identify a problem that the parent denies. In these situations the nurse may need to seek help from another colleague or approach the problem at a later time. Reasons for potential problems should be explained so that the child and family fully understand their care and treatment and feel part of the assessment process.

Interview Technique

It is apparent that the nurse needs to ascertain a great deal of information and without careful attention to a good interview technique the assessment process may become more like an interrogation.

Study activity

What communication techniques can the nurse use to ensure that the assessment interview does not intimidate the child and family and encourages them to talk?

Communication can be transmitted by non-verbal means and the nurse should make sure that her posture or facial expression does not reveal disinterest, superiority, authority or insensitivity. A relaxed but alert sitting position facing the parents will facilitate communication. Writing down everything the child or parents say can prevent a dialogue and hinders listening as the writer cannot pay close attention to the speaker's words or behaviour. In Western cultures eye contact is a sign of interest and paying attention, but in other cultures this direct approach may be considered rude and hinder communication.

The nurse should address family members by their names to convey interest and respect for them as individuals. Parents should be addressed as Mr, Mrs, Miss or Ms, as they prefer, until such time as they request to be called by their first names. The nurse should also be careful not to use jargon or medical terminology that the child or family do not understand, and the use of open-ended questions provides a non-threatening way of gaining more information than the use of direct questions. Ley and Llewellyn (1995) report that healthcare professionals often use vocabulary with which they presume patients are familiar. The nurse should include the child whenever possible and be alert when older children may want to share information without their parents' presence.

Active listening can also encourage others to talk. The nurse, although providing information, does not want to monopolise the conversation. Parents who are hesitant to talk may be helped by the accepting behaviour of the nurse, indicated by nodding or a murmur of assent. Sometimes the child or parent may be silent while they consider the best way to express what is possibly a difficult area for them. The nurse should allow this period of silence, as a rush to continue the discussion may destroy the moment at which a crucial problem was to be revealed.

Communicating with the Child

Whatever the child's age, the assessment interview should be directed at the child and the parents. However, at the end of the interview the nurse needs to examine the child and by this time it is helpful for the child to feel comfortable with the nurse. Children generally need time to evaluate strangers and do not respond well to rapid advances of friendship. They are also very sensitive to non-verbal communication and soon become anxious if they sense fear, hesitancy and concern in others. Many parents will exhibit just these emotions when bringing their child into hospital and the nurse needs to be able to dispel these attitudes and gain their confidence if the child is to be approached easily. A knowledge of the development of children's communication and thought processes can aid this approach (*see also* Language development p. 77).

Study activity

Consider how communication can be facilitated between the nurse and an infant, toddler, schoolchild and adolescent.

Pre-verbal children rely on non-verbal communication to make their needs known and to understand others' behaviour. They readily respond to their parents' anxiety, often transmitted by a change in voice or the way in which they are held. They can be reassured if their parents show signs of relaxing and by a quiet, calm voice and gentle, but firm, handling. Older infants who have begun to recognise the individual characteristics of their parents are best held in a position where they can still see them.

Preschool children only see events from their own perspective and can only understand things explained in concrete terms. Children at this age tend to give lifelike qualities to inanimate objects. This animism can cause them to be very fearful of medical equipment that they can believe is capable of causing them pain because of their naughtiness. However, Flavell (1985) has shown that animism usually occurs when the child has no information about the characteristics of the object. If the nurse can allow the child to play with the equipment and explains in simple terms how the equipment is used, the child's fears may be overcome. Any explanation also needs to include how the individual child will be affected. Preschool children have limited understanding and cannot differentiate between fact and fantasy, so they are very fearful of the unknown. Parents are still important to preschool children and in times of stress they still need the physical presence and comfort of their parents. Harris (1993) suggests that the best way of managing these children's fears is to provide the child with parental support. Thus, communication with these children can often be facilitated by first gaining the acceptance and trust of the parents and talking to the child in their presence.

The schoolchild has begun to explore the environment and is interested in finding out the reasons for everything around them. Giving them opportunity to question events before they happen helps them to communicate. They can interpret the meaning of words and are quicker to acknowledge when they do not understand. They are able to express their concerns and feelings about hospitalisation but need encouragement to do so. As schoolchildren grow older parents become less important to them but they still need parental support, comfort and advice in a strange environment. If the nurse includes school-aged children in the interview, they will feel accepted as an active participant and be more able to express their own thoughts.

Erikson describes adolescence as a phase of 'identity versus role confusion'. Adolescents find themselves changing physically and psychologically from children to adults, and this can be a difficult phase for them. They want to have autonomy but at the same time want help and support at times of stress. They tend to reject others' beliefs and values because of their need to make their own decisions. They can avoid conversation if they feel insecure or sense disapproval. The nurse probably

Communicating with children

Infants

- handle firmly but gently
- avoid sudden movements and loud noises
- allow the parents to remain in sight
- discover the infant's preferred position

Toddlers

- position yourself at the child's level
- focus on the child
- use simple language and short sentences
- use only concrete terms

School-age children

- allow time for questions, give honest answers
- facilitate expression of fears
- explain everything
- use previous experiences

Adolescents

- expect mood changes
- treat as autonomous individuals
- accept hostility, anger, non-cooperation
- provide privacy, reassure about confidentiality
- be non-judgemental
- do not pry
- avoid giving advice unless asked

needs to interview adolescents and parents separately, making it clear that any information will be treated confidentially. Talking to adolescents first may help them to feel that they are important. Keeping to casual conversation initially may help to give adolescents a sense of security. The nurse needs to show respect, interest and acceptance by avoiding any indication of surprise, judgement or disapproval and by not offering advice unless asked (*see also* Erikson p. 85).

Using Interpreters

Study activity

Consider the disadvantages of using interpreters for the assessment interview.

On occasions it may be necessary to use an interpreter to carry out an assessment of a child and family. This can pose communication, cultural, ethical and legal difficulties. It is difficult for the nurse to show respect, concern and empathy when communicating via an interpreter, and it is not always easy to know if certain Western expressions can be translated directly into another language. The child and family may have difficulty talking to an interpreter, who may be a stranger of another class or gender, particularly if the questions are of a personal and confidential nature. This may be overcome partly by allowing the family time to meet the interpreter before the assessment interview (Slater, 1993). Legal and ethical issues arise when the nurse cannot be certain that all the necessary information has been given or understood to enable the child and family to make informed choices about care and treatment. The nurse can watch the non-verbal behaviour of the family in response to questions to try to assess understanding, but if such direct observation is seen as threatening, this is not an easy or foolproof way of determining concern.

Physical Assessment

It is preferable to be able to talk to the child and family and gain their trust and acceptance before trying to make any assessment of the child's physical state. If the nurse makes an immediate move to examine the child before doing anything else, it is likely that the child will cry or refuse to cooperate, making this assessment impossible. However, during the interview phase the nurse can learn much about the child's physical condition by just observing the child.

Study activity

Take time out to observe a child and consider how much you can learn about his condition by just looking and listening.

Table 25.2 Observing the sick child: looking at skin colour

Observation	Significance
Pallor	Shock, anaemia or cold
Flushed	Possible pyrexia
Cyanosis	Cardiac or respiratory problem
Jaundice	Physiological or hepatic infection or obstruction
Bruising	Accidental or non-accidental injury or clotting disorder
Diaphoresis	Cardio-respiratory distress
Rash	Infectious disease or allergy

Although first impressions of a child and family must be used with caution, it is likely that at the first meeting the nurse will gain an immediate idea about the child's development and hygiene. An experienced nurse will be able to see if the child's weight, height and head circumference is within the normal range for that age. Obvious neglect of hygiene will also be immediately apparent. The child's colour will give information about fever, shock, jaundice or cardiac problems (Table 25.2). Difficulty in breathing can be seen from flared or blocked nostrils or sweating. Rashes, cuts, bruises or swellings will also be obvious, as will any infected areas of the skin. The child's mobility, posture and behaviour will give some clue about the severity of the child's condition and the degree of anxiety. Dehydration may be apparent by the dryness of the mouth and, in babies, sunken fontanelle. Swollen fontanelle may indicate raised intracranial pressure. The characteristics of any vomit or sputum will also provide clues about the child's condition (Table 25.3) (*see also* Growth p. 67).

Listening will give the nurse even more information. Respiratory problems can be heard by grunting, stridor, wheeze or cough (Table 25.4). The child's cry may reveal fear, hunger, exhaustion, pain or cerebral irritation (Table 25.5).

Once the initial information has been gained by interview and observation, the nurse should be able to examine the child. The less invasive techniques should be used first to avoid alarming the child and to enable the nurse to continue to gain the child's trust and confidence. The child should be involved in the examination process by being able to choose to sit on a parent's lap or on the bed and by handling the equipment (*see also* Urine testing pp. 490–4).

The measurement of growth in children is one of the most important areas in the assessment of their health. Weight (Figure 25.2), height or length (Figure 25.3) and head circumference (Figure 25.4) should be measured and recorded on an appropriate percentile chart for all admissions. The percentile charts used in the UK use the third and 97th percentiles to indicate those children who are outside the normal growth parameters. However, such evaluations should be made with caution as small or large size may be genetic and the charts do not take into account the growth of children from different ethnic backgrounds.

Table 25.3 Observing the sick child: looking at excreta

Excreta	Observation	Significance
Vomit	Undigested food/milk	Overindulgence, feeding too fast, gastric irritant
	Bile stained	Stomach is empty
	Blood stained	Following swallowed blood (dental extraction, epistaxis, tonsillectomy), oesophageal varices or stress gastric ulcer
	Projectile	Pyloric stenosis
Sputum	Mucous	Respiratory tract inflammation
	Yellow/green	Respiratory tract infection
	Blood stained	Trauma of coughing
Urine	Polyuria	Drinking heavily or diabetes mellitus/insipidus
	Oliguria	Dehydration, renal problem
	Dark coloured	Dehydration or biliary obstruction
	Pale coloured	Drinking heavily
	Blood stained	Urinary tract infection/trauma or renal problem
	Cloudy	Urinary tract infection
Faeces	Soft and yellow	Normal infant stool
	Watery	Gastro-enteritis
	Soft and green/brown	Gastro-enteritis
	Hard and green/brown	Hunger or constipation
	Mucus or blood	Inflammation of the bowel
	Black	Meconium of newborn or digested blood
	Undigested food	Intestinal hurry
	Pale and bulky	Undigested fat

Table 25.4 Observing the sick child: looking and listening to respirations

	Observation	Significance
Rate	Tachypnoea	
	Dyspnoea	Cardiac or respiratory problem
Movements	Nasal flaring	Respiratory distress
	Sternal retraction	Respiratory distress
	Intercostal recession	Respiratory distress
	Tracheal tug	Respiratory distress
Noise	Sighing, yawning	Shock, blood loss
	Stertorous	Altered conscious level
	Wheeze	Inflamed and narrow lower airway
	Cough/whoop	Irritation of upper respiratory tract
	Bark	Inflamed and narrow upper airway
	Stridor	Obstruction of upper airway
	Grunting	Respiratory distress (infants)

Table 25.5 Observing the sick child: listening and looking at the child's behaviour

	Observation	Significance
Cry	Shrill/high pitched Whimpering Lusty	Cerebral irritation Pain and/or fear Anger or hunger
Position	Limp/flaccid Head/neck retraction Knees drawn up	Toxicity Cerebral irritation Abdominal pain
Behaviour	Unresponsive Lethargy or irritability	Neurological deficit Toxicity
Relationship with others	Watchful	Pain/fear

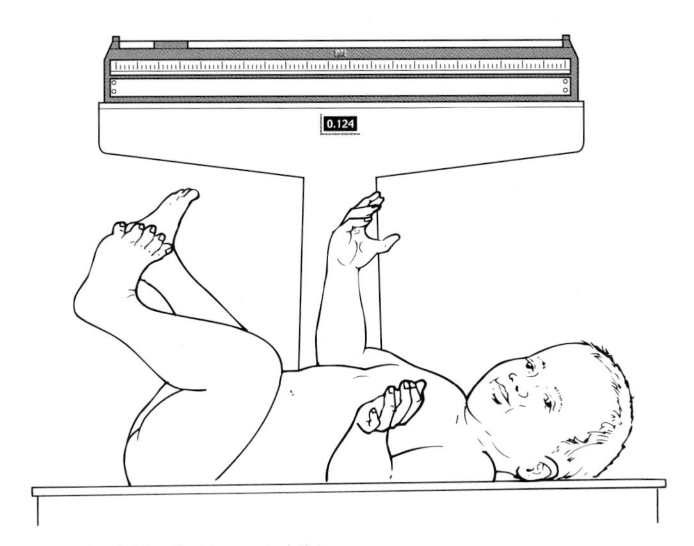

Figure 25.2 Weighing babies and children.

Children under 36 months of age should have their length and head circumference recorded. A paper or metal tape measure should be used as false small recordings may be made with a stretchy cloth tape.

Young children have difficulty maintaining body temperature and this is a useful measurement to assess the child's condition. However, there has been much controversy about the optimum route and most accurate method of obtaining this recording. In the UK the digital thermometer or the Tempadot are mostly used for an initial temperature recording, as both methods have the advantage of measuring temperature quickly without invading either the mouth or rectum. Morley *et al.* (1992) found that these axillary measurements tend to underestimate core temperature and are easily affected by the environmental temperature, but they are probably useful for an initial determination of body temperature. This measurement also brings into question the normal temperature. Once thought to be 37°C, the mean body temperature is now recognised to be 36.8°C, with a variable fluctuation between individuals

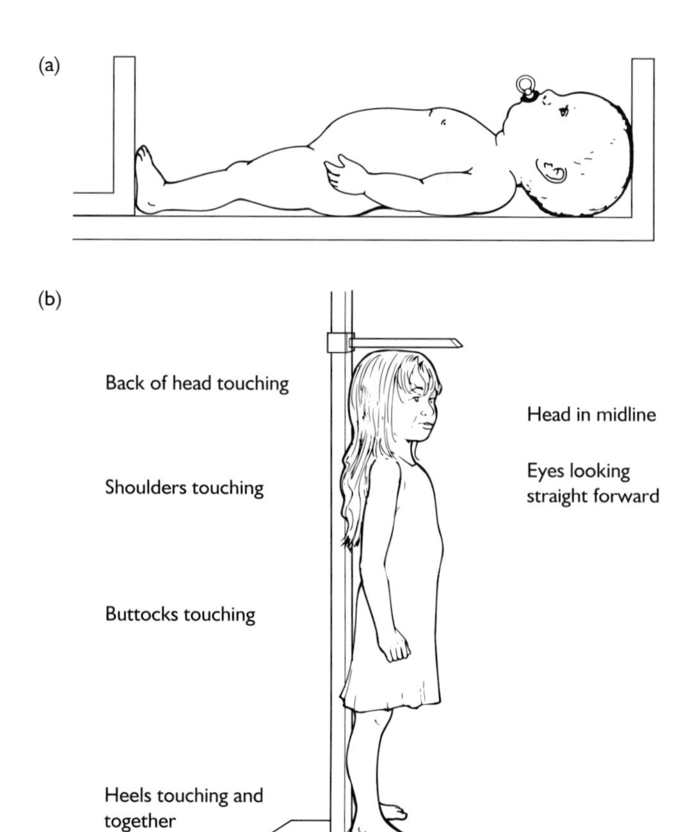

Figure 25.3 (a) Measuring length. (b) Measuring height.

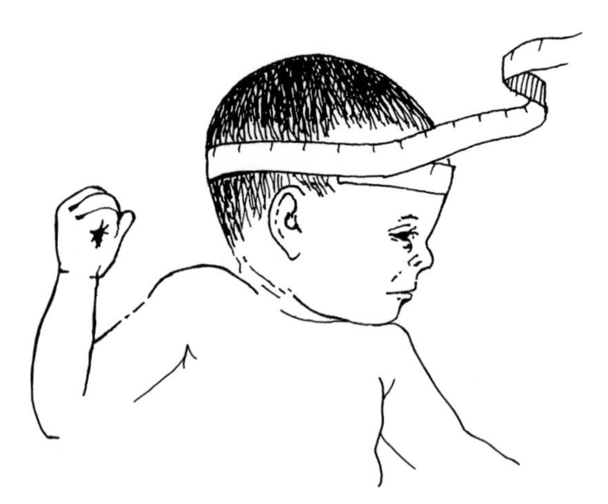

Figure 25.4 Measuring head circumference.

of 0.5°C (Mackowiak *et al.*, 1992). In addition, Pontious *et al.* (1994) suggest that the difference between axillary and oral temperature is considerably less than the traditionally assumed 1.0°C.

An accurate pulse should be measured for a full minute and should be measured using a stethoscope placed over the apex of the heart in children under 2 years. Respiratory rates in young children should also

Table 25.6 Recording children's blood pressure

Method	Rationale
Wrap the cuff snugly round the limb	A loose cuff will give false high recordings; a cuff which is too tight will also record inaccurately
Ensure that the lower edge of the cuff is 2–3 cm above the artery to be palpated; place the tubes superiorly	To prevent interference with auscultation
Place the sphygmomanometer at eye level on a flat surface	To facilitate accurate pressures
Palpate the chosen artery and inflate the cuff until pulsation disappears	To estimate systolic pressure; auscultatory gaps in phase 1 sounds can cause underestimation of systolic pressure unless already determined in this way
Place the stethoscope gently over the artery at the point of maximum pulsation	If the stethoscope is pressed too firmly or touches the cuff, the diastolic pressure may be underestimated
Inflate the bladder to 30 mmHg above the estimated systolic pressure. Reduce the pressure by about 2 mmHg/second	Releasing the pressure too quickly will underestimate systolic pressure
Note the point at which repetitive clear tapping sounds first appear for at least two beats	This is the systolic pressure
Continue to gradually reduce the pressure and note the point at which the repetitive sounds become muffled	Releasing the pressure too quickly will overestimate the diastolic pressure; the point of muffled sounds is taken to be the diastolic blood pressure in children

be measured over a full minute and can be gained by watching abdominal movements as their respirations are diaphragmatic.

Blood pressure (BP) should be measured routinely in children to identify essential hypertension (Portman and Yetman, 1994). It can be measured manually or with an electronic device, but either method can be inaccurate if not used correctly (Tables 25.6 and 25.7). The most important factor in accurate BP recording is the correct size cuff. Cuffs that are too narrow or too wide produce inaccurate measurements.

De Swiet *et al.* (1989) recommend a cuff width equal to two-thirds limb length. Accuracy is further aided by positioning the limb at the level of the heart and holding it in position. Careful preparation and reassurance will help to minimise the child's anxiety, which will produce an elevated BP.

Table 25.7 Blood pressure norms in children

Age	Systolic blood pressure (mmHg)	Diastolic blood pressure (mmHg)
0–1 month	65–85	53–55
1–3 months	85–90	50–53
6–12 months	90–92	53–56
1–5 years	90–95	54–56
6–10 years	96–102	56–62
11–16 years	101–115	62–67

Note: Blood pressure for children over 1 year may be approximated as follows: Systolic pressure (50th percentile) = 90 mmHg + (age in years × 2)

Summary

The assessment process is one in which the nurse aims to develop a rapport with the child and family that will facilitate data collection by communication and observation. The nurse needs to have communication skills that encourage the parents to share information and enable children of different ages to express themselves and lose their anxieties about the strange hospital environment. This will enable the nurse to establish an appreciation of the family's usual home life, identify the child's and family's needs and problems, and formulate a care plan. Nurses' observation skills enable them to form an overall impression of the child's physical condition, state of nutrition, behaviour and stage of development. Accurate measurements of growth and vital signs provide more objective assessments of the child's condition and provide a baseline for future observations.

Key Points

1. Assessment of a sick child enables the nurse to develop a relationship with the child and family while identifying the child's nursing problems.
2. A successful assessment requires careful preparation, a welcoming environment, time and privacy.
3. An assessment of usual home routines enables the nurse to adhere to these as far as possible, thus minimising the disturbance of hospitalisation for child and family.
4. Good communication skills are vital for an accurate assessment. These should be adapted according to the individual child and family's needs.
5. The need and problems of the child should be identified in negotiation with the child and family.
6. Much of the assessment of a sick child can be gained by looking and listening to the child.

Chapter 26

Day Care

Introduction

The Platt Report (Platt, 1959) first recognised the value of minimising the stress of hospitalisation for children by shortening the amount of time they spent as inpatients. Gradually the concept of day care arose to provide essential medical interventions for the child while eliminating the need for an overnight stay in hospital. Apart from reducing the stress of a stay in hospital, day care also has the advantages of decreasing the chance of a hospital-acquired infection, being a less expensive way of providing medical care and enabling a reduction in waiting list time (Campbell and Glasper, 1995). However, it can also have disadvantages and it is important to recognise that it might not be suitable for all children or beneficial for all families.

Advantages and Disadvantages

Study activity

Jamie, aged 3, is to be admitted for circumcision as a day case. His father, a single parent, is self-employed. Jamie usually goes to a nursery during the day. Consider the disadvantages of day care for Jamie and his father.

When children are admitted for day care, a member of their family needs to be able to take them into hospital and be available for the discharge later in the day. In many instances, the parent then has to take on the role of carer at home. Some parents may feel unable or unwilling to do this. Providing care for the child during this period may necessitate taking time off work. Depending on the employer, this may have to be unpaid leave, which may lead to financial difficulties or even the loss of the job.

Cases suitable for day surgery

- Hernia repair: epigastric, femoral inguinal, umbilical
- Hydrocele/varicocele: repairs or ligation
- Orchidopexy: unilateral >5 years
- Circumcision: meatotomy, separation of preputial adhesions
- Minor hypospadias
- Cystoscopy
- Division of tongue tie
- Proctoscopy, sigmoidoscopy, sphincter stretch
- Examination under anaesthetic (EUA)
- Excision of skin lesions
- Lymph node biopsy
- Brachial sinus
- Thyroglossal cyst
- Correction of prominent ears
- Excision of superficial accessory auricles
- Minor orthopaedic surgery: manipulations, plaster change, release of trigger thumb, excision of ganglion, arthroscopy
- Dental surgery: extractions, excision or biopsy of oral lesions and cysts
- ENT surgery: EUA of ears, post nasal space, removal of foreign bodies, myringotomies, grommets, reduction of nasal fracture
- Sub-mucosal diathermy, electrocautery of epistaxis, antrum wash-outs
- Ophthalmic surgery: correction of strabismus, EUA

(Royal College of Surgeons of England, 1992)

Day care also has the disadvantage that the nurse does not have the time to develop a relationship with the child and provide individualised care. Many day care units also use core care – plans that can impede individualised care. Children being admitted for surgery are often admitted early in the morning, for an operation 1 or 2 hours later, giving the nurse little time to get to know them.

Pre-admission Information

This short assessment time may be partially overcome by inviting the child to a pre-admission club (Figure 26.1). At this time the child and parents have an opportunity to visit the ward, meet the staff and have an outline of the day case routine explained to them. This means of preparation relies on a member of the family being available to accompany the child. Pre-admission clubs are usually held during the week prior to the child's admission but this may be too long for the younger child who may forget or misinterpret the information before admission.

These disadvantages can be overcome by sending the parents and child clear information with the date of admission. This can be in the form of a puzzle or colouring book for the child. Parents can also be advised of other useful resources to help prepare them and their child, which are often available from children's libraries.

Before admission it is important that the parents are aware of any possibility that the child may have to stay in overnight, so they can make

INVITATION TO THE PRE-ADMISSION CLUB

Woodlands Children's Unit
St. Someone's Hospital
Anywhere, County.

Dear

Please come to our special club meeting on ....

at ....

You will be able to find out all about the hospital and what will happen when you have your operation next week. You will be able to see:

- the ward where your bed will be
- a video about your operation day
- the theatre where your operation will take place
- our playroom and toys
- the nurses who will be helping mummy or daddy to look after you

Please bring mummy or daddy with you. Brothers, sisters and toys can come too if you would like them to. Please ring and tell us if you can come.

From all the nurses

Figure 26.1 Invite to club.

provisional arrangements for this before the day of admission. They also need advice about taking the child home so they do not have unrealistic plans to go home by public transport.

All this information can be given at the pre-admission visit, but it needs to be consolidated into written form. This helps those who are unable to attend a pre-admission session.

Study activity

Consider ways of encouraging parents and children to attend a pre-admission club.

Day care often has the disadvantage of expecting parents to make arrangements to visit the hospital on three occasions: the initial outpatient appointment, followed by a pre-admission session and then the actual day of admission. An eye-catching, multilingual poster or display in the outpatient department would provide the means of explaining the purpose and function of the pre-admission club and could be supported by leaflets for parents to take home (Figure 26.2). Parents need to be

Is your child booked for surgery?

Not sure what to expect or how to answer questions?

Help to reassure your child and yourself and come to the:

CHILDREN'S PRE-ADMISSION CLUB

- Held every Saturday morning 10–11 am
- Run by children's nurses and play staff
- Includes a tour, video and question time
- You and your child will have the opportunity to find out what the operation day entails

Figure 26.2 Poster for club (picture reproduced from Beaver *et al.*, 1994).

Advice about transport

- Private transport or taxi
- An adult, other than the driver, should be available to sit with the child
- Have a pillow and blanket in case the child wishes to lie down
- Take a bowl in case of vomiting
- Do not make precise arrangements about timing – these may change

Preparation for hospital – resources available

Toys

- anatomically correct dolls
- anatomy aprons
- nurse's or doctor's outfits
- play people hospital
- 'Lego' hospital
- 'Sindy' hospital set
- jigsaws about hospital

Books

- see Table 24.1 – page 272
- colouring books

aware of the dates and contents for these visits, and to realise the benefits to them and their children (James, 1995).

Programme for the pre-admission club

Registration (5 min)

- children and families are welcomed
- children are given colour-coded name badges according to the type of planned surgery
- drinks and biscuits available

Introduction (5 min)

- all children and families are told the outline of the day

Video (15 min)

- shows the process of day care from admission to discharge

Visits (15 min)

- tour of the ward and theatres

Question time (15 min)

- the play leader takes the children to play and ask questions
- the nurse gives parents an opportunity to ask questions, clarify issues

Departure (5 min)

- children are given a booklet about coming into hospital
- parents are given an advice sheet about the ward, fasting and further age-related preparation for their child

On admission: actual and potential health problems

- Pyrexia
- Cough, cold, sore throat
- Heart problems
- Respiratory problems
- Contact with infectious disease
- Length of fasting time
- General health

Day Care Admission Assessment

One of the other disadvantages of day care is that the nurse has little time to develop a relationship with the child and parents. As a result of this the admission assessment is particularly important in day care.

Study activity

Amy, aged 5, has been admitted as a day case for an adenoidectomy. What would you need to know from Amy and her mother on admission?

First, the nurse needs to be aware of what the child and parents already know about the proposed surgery and the ward. If the child and parents have attended the pre-admission club, this is an opportunity to check their understanding and consolidate information. If not, the nurse may need to begin preparation by showing them around the ward. Assessing previous knowledge is useful to correct misbeliefs. Jolly (1981) recalls a 5-year-old who, despite careful preparation for his tonsillectomy, believed his throat would be cut during the operation.

The aim of any pre-operative care is to ensure the child is not only prepared psychologically, but also physically. Some children have been fasted at home prior to admission; the nurse needs to check the parents have understood this instruction and that the child has obeyed it. It is not always easy for parents to comply exactly with the hospital's requirements. For instance, they may have been told that the child may have nothing to eat or drink for at least 4 hours prior to the operation. If the child goes to bed after an evening meal at 19:30, is woken at 07:00 and arrives at the hospital at 07:30 for an operation at 09:00, then the actual period of fasting has been for a period of over 12 hours and on admission the nurse may find the child is dehydrated. Alternatively, the nurse may discover that the child has been given a drink of water because the parents thought clear fluids were acceptable.

On admission the nurse needs to check that the child has no actual or potential health problems that could be exacerbated by surgery. Recording the child's vital signs not only gives the nurse an indication of the child's current health status, it also gives the child an opportunity to become familiar with these procedures.

The admission assessment is also an opportunity for the nurse to discover the family's usual home routine. Being aware of the child's likes and dislikes in relation to fluids and diet may help to encourage the child to return to normal eating and drinking habits after an anaesthetic. A knowledge of the child's behaviour and comforters will enable the nurse to recognise and respond appropriately to any signs of distress at an early stage. James (1995) suggests that much of the information required at the admission assessment can be gained by asking the parents to complete a pre-admission questionnaire (Figure 26.3).

Your child may go to theatre soon after admission which may not give us much time to get to know you. You can help us by completing the following questionnaire so that we can learn about your child and help you to look after your child in the same way as you do at home.

Previous experience of hospital/illness
Has your child been in hospital before? . . . . When? . . . .
What was the reason for this? . . . .
How did s/he react to this? . . . .
How have you explained the reason for this admission? . . . .
. . . .
Please tell us about any special worries your child has . . . .
. . . .
How does your child react to pain? . . . .
What method do you find best relieves their pain? . . . .
. . . .
If your child is taking any medicines please state what these are and the reasons for their use . . . .
. . . .
. . . .

Eating and drinking
What does your child use for drinking? bottle/cup/trainer beaker
What does s/he prefer to drink? . . . .
We usually offer toast or biscuits as the first solids after the anaesthetic.
Does your child have any preferences for these? . . . .

Toileting
What help does your child need to go to the toilet? . . . .
Does your child ever wet or soil her/himself? . . . .
Toddlers: When does your child wear nappies? . . . .
What words does s/he use to indicate the need for the toilet? . . . .
. . . .
Teenage girls: Has your daughter started menstruating? . . . .
When is her next period due? . . . .
Does she use pads or tampons? . . . .

Play and comfort
Please tell us about any special toy/comforter your child has with them . . . .
. . . .
If your child is bored before or after surgery, what quiet forms of play would interest them? . . . .
. . . .

***Please use the back of this form to tell us anything else you think is important**

Figure 26.3 Pre-admission questionnaire.

Pre-procedural Care

Study activity

Once the admission assessments have been completed, consider how the child's preparation for the day care procedure should continue.

Module 5

When the initial assessment is complete the nurse should ensure that the final preparations for the child's procedure are made. Simultaneous preparation of a favourite toy may be appreciated by some children. James (1995) advocates that children should be able to choose what they wear, arguing that theatre gowns are not always necessary. The removal of underwear is often the most distressing and bewildering aspect for children, and should not be necessary except for procedures involving the genital area. In these cases cotton underwear may be an acceptable alternative.

If cannulation is required, local anaesthetic cream can be applied to the selected site 1 or 2 hours before the procedure. Children who have been adequately prepared should not need pre-medication (James, 1995) but the nurse should assess each child's need for such medication, recognising that the aim of pre-medication is to allay anxiety, facilitate induction of anaesthetic and provide an analgesic effect. If a pre-medication is required, it should be given in an oral form as most children's anxiety will only be heightened by an intramuscular injection.

Pre-medication

Aims

- to alleviate anxiety
- provide pre-emptive analgesia
- facilitate the induction of anaesthesia

A typical pre-medication usually comprises a sedative, analgesic and anticholinergic, and should not in itself cause anxiety or distress.

Elective procedures

Age	Recommended pre-medication
<6 months	Nil
>6 months	Trimeprazine 1.5 mg/kg* + orally Atropine 30 mg/kg

*Alternative sedatives:

- temazepam 0.5–1 mg/kg
- diazepam 200–300 mg/kg
- chloral hydrate 30–50 mg/kg

(*Guys, Lewisham and St Thomas Paediatric Formulary*, 1994)

Transport to theatre

If the child has not had pre-medication:

- walking
- trike or pedal car

If the child has had pre-medication:

- carried by parents
- decorated theatre trolley

Anaesthesia

The child should also be able to choose the mode of transport if the procedure is to be carried out away from the day care ward. Small children often prefer being carried by a parent or to use a pedal car or bike. In recent years, there has been much discussion about the presence of parents in the anaesthetic room. The nurse should be aware of the benefits and drawbacks of parental presence at this time so that parents can be given appropriate advice.

Study activity

What are the benefits and drawbacks of having parents present in the anaesthetic room?

Gauderer *et al.* (1989) found that most parents, although anxious, were grateful to have been able to provide support for their child during induction. Most children also expressed a need for parental presence at this time. However, Vessey *et al.* (1990) discovered that a few parents became obviously distressed at the induction procedure and were unable to support their child or the healthcare professionals. Understandably, it is these latter reactions that concern the anaesthetic team, whose aim is to ensure a smooth and effective induction. Therefore, although most authors (Coulston, 1988; Glasper, 1990) found that the advantages of the presence of a parent in the anaesthetic room outweigh the disadvantages, it is important that this issue should be discussed fully with parents. If they feel that they would not be able to remain calm, they should not be made to feel guilty. Instead, they may accompany their child to the door of the anaesthetic room and the child's named nurse should provide the necessary psychological support during induction.

Recovery from Anaesthesia

Parents should also be given the opportunity to be with their child in the recovery area following the procedure. Again, they should be well prepared for this and know their child's likely condition as well as their role in this situation. Staff in recovery areas have found that children who woke to a parent's presence were far less disturbed than those who woke alone in a strange environment. Distressed children tend to cry and this can often result in increased pain or post-operative bleeding.

If there are no specific contra-indications, as soon as the child is awake and able to swallow he/she should be able to drink and eat. Diet and fluids should usually be encouraged 1 to 2 hours following the procedure to reduce the risk of dehydration and hypoglycaemia.

Appropriate analgesia should be prescribed to enable the child to remobilise without fear of pain. Ibuprofen syrup or paracetamol suspension are appropriate oral analgesics, and are usually well accepted by children who have undergone minor procedures. Alternatives may be paracetamol suppositories or a local anaesthetic gel.

Discharge Home

Study activity

What criteria would you use to determine a child's suitability for discharge after day surgery?

All day case children should meet given criteria before being discharged home. They should be able to eat and drink without vomiting, walk unaided and should have passed urine without difficulty. Their pain should be controlled with an appropriate analgesic and they should be apyrexial. Any unexpected or excessive bleeding is reason enough for an overnight stay. Parents need general and specific advice about their child after day care procedures. They need to have these details explained to them and to have time in which to consider any questions. Written instructions will help them to remember what they have been told. These written instructions should be expressed in simple language and be available in a bilingual form. Ley and Llewellyn (1995) cite many studies showing that written instructions for patients were too difficult for them to understand and comply with. Written discharge information should have been distributed at the pre-admission visit, to give parents time to assimilate and question the information. Before the child goes home this information should be reiterated. Parents worry most about being able to manage effectively their child's pain (Kankkunen *et al.*, 2003), so it is important that discharge advice includes guidelines for the administration of analgesia, alternative ways of managing pain, and positioning and handling the child.

Any other specific advice, such as wound care, should also be explained carefully. This advice appears to be best given by nurses in a specific day care facility (Jonas, 2003).

Discharge criteria

Before discharge all day case children should:

- be apyrexial
- not have experienced any unexpected complications or excessive bleeding
- be able to eat and drink without vomiting
- have passed urine
- be able to walk unaided
- have their pain controlled

Discharge advice

Questions most commonly asked by parents:

- when can the dressing be removed?
- are there stitches to come out?
- when can the child have a bath?
- when can the child return to nursery/school?
- should activity be restricted in any way?
- what can be given to eat and drink?
- what should be given for pain?
- is there a review appointment?

(Norris, 1992)

Paediatric Community Support

Even with discharge advice, parents can feel overwhelmed and anxious about providng post-operative care at home (Bastable and Rushford, 2005). In some areas the children's community nurse (CCN) will continue the child's care after discharge. In these instances it is ideal if the CCN can meet the child and family before discharge. Where a CCN is not available, it is useful if the day care nurse can telephone at a pre-arranged time to check on the child's progress. This support has been shown to be welcomed by parents who often just want reassurance that they are caring for their child correctly (Higson and Bolland, 2000). It has also been shown to increase compliance with discharge advice (Spicher and Yund, 1989) (*see also* Community nursing p. 375).

Summary

In 1991, it was suggested that the health care of children could be improved by following a comprehensive set of standards for pre-admission and discharge care (Thornes, 1991). This report, titled *Just for the Day*, has formed the basis of the operational policy of the many day care units.

In 1992, the Royal College of Surgeons published guidelines to facilitate more day care surgery. These guidelines do not take into account that surgery on children is not always undertaken by surgeons and anaesthetists who are experienced in paediatric surgery (Audit Commission, 1993). Markovitch (1991) found that children having day care surgery were often seen as a lower priority by inexperienced medical staff. Nevertheless, the number of day care units continues to increase, and their success is determined by the degree of preparation and planning that occurs before admission. These pre-admission arrangements should take into account the multicultural needs of the population, to ensure that all children are treated equally. With careful preparation and planning the potential risks and disadvantages can usually be overcome.

Cases unsuitable for day surgery

- Operations >1 hour
- Uncontrolled asthma, epilepsy, blood disorders
- Under 46 weeks' gestational age (gestation + age)
- Ex-premature infants <6 months
- Infants <5 kg
- Respiratory tract infection in past 2 weeks
- Cardiac, hepatic, renal or endocrine insufficiency

(Bradshaw and Davenport, 1989)

Key Points

1. The individual child's and family's suitability for day care should be assessed as it is not always beneficial.
2. Children having day care need to have fears allayed by careful pre-admission preparation.
3. Fasting times, pre-medication and anaesthesia should be adjusted to meet the individual child's needs.
4. Parents need careful preparation for the discharge of their children to enable them to continue care with confidence and recognise and react to complications.
5. Children should meet given criteria before discharge to minimise the possibility of complications.
6. Parents benefit from support in the community after their child has been discharged.

Chapter 27

Emergency Care

Introduction

In the UK approximately 25% of all patients seen in the accident-and-emergency (A&E) department each year will be children (DH, 1991a). This effectively means that about one in four children under the age of 16 years will attend an A&E department at some time in their childhood. A high proportion of these children will be under the age of 5 years and about 65% of them will have sustained some kind of trauma (Figure 27.1).

Most of these children will be seen in a busy adult A&E department as there are only about 40 dedicated paediatric A&E departments in the UK (Royal College of Paediatrics and Child Health, 2003). Collins

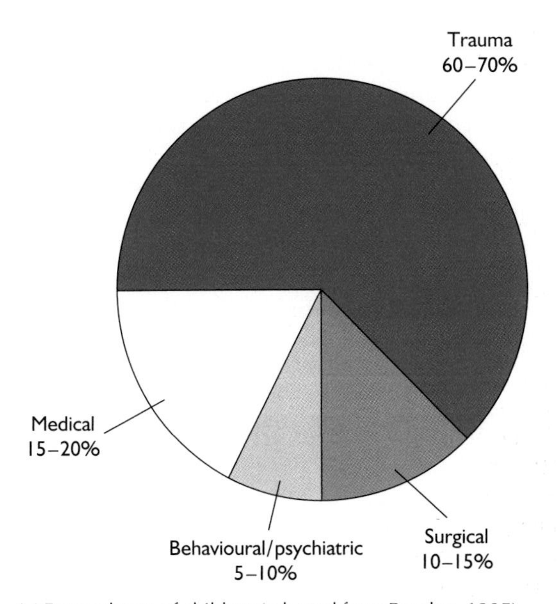

Figure 27.1 A&E attendance of children (adapted from Bentley, 1995).

Minimum requirements for children in A&E

- A consultant paediatrician with specific responsibility for liaison with the A&E consultant regarding the care of children
- Nursing establishment to include at least one registered children's nurse
- A liaison health visitor to provide a link between hospital and community services
- Separate waiting area from adult area with facilities for play
- Separate child-friendly treatment area with appropriate equipment
- Private room available for distressed family

(Morton and Phillips, 1992)

(1995) suggests that the two disciplines of children's nursing and A&E nursing have opposing philosophies, and that these differing beliefs add to the unsuitability of general A&E departments for the care of children.

The need for children to be treated in a different way began to be recognised in the 1980s, and in 1988 the British Paediatric Association (BPA), British Association of Paediatric Surgeons (BAPS) and Casualty Surgeons Association (CSA) produced a joint statement that identified the optimum requirements for the care of children in A&E (Morton and Phillips, 1992). Although these indicators of good practice have not been universally adopted (McConichie, 2005), there are many exciting developments and innovations in the field of paediatric emergency care in relation to preparing children for admission to A&E, staffing the unit appropriately and the triage of children in a specific area of the department.

The A&E Environment

Study activity

Imagine the busy A&E department of your local general hospital. Consider what a small child's reaction to this environment might be.

The A&E department is most children's first contact with hospital so it is important that this first experience is made as reassuring as possible. The A&E environment has traditionally been designed to provide fast and effective immediate care and the need to make the department welcoming and attractive has not always been a priority. A separate waiting area with play facilities is recommended, but many A&E departments do not have the space or financial resources to develop such an area. However, even with these limitations, it is important to ensure that the admission area has some decoration at the child's height and that children do not have to observe the physical and mental stress of other acutely ill patients. Often the treatment area has more medical equipment than pictures and toys. An area that has a few familiar pictures and toys can help to relax the child and reduce anxiety. Child-sized trolleys and seating also help to make the environment safer as well as more friendly. Even the nurses' uniforms and doctors' white coats may be threatening to a child who has no previous experience of hospital (McMenamin, 1995). A nursery print tabard for the nurse looking after the children may help to make her appear less frightening.

The family also have special needs in the A&E department. They will feel anxious and possibly guilty about their child's condition and may have had to bring other children with them to the department. They need space and facilities to feed a baby, and change nappies. A pushchair to soothe a fractious toddler or to lay a baby down is a useful addition.

The A&E Staff

Meeting the needs of the family and the child is the basis of children's nurse education and this is the reason why it is recommended that every

A&E department has at least one RSCN or RN(child) on its staff (DH, 1991a). Children have physiological and psychological needs that are different from those of the adult patient, and an appropriately qualified and experienced nurse is required to assess and meet these needs in a stressful situation. Recruiting an experienced children's nurse who also has A&E experience is not easy. To overcome this shortage of appropriate staff, some units have made the most of flexible rostering to ensure that their RSCN/RN(child) is on duty during their recognised peak periods for children attending the department. At other times a named nurse is identified from the paediatric unit to provide specialist advice. In 2005, 23% of A&E departments seeing 18 000 children per year did not have appropriately qualified nurses (McConichie, 2005).

A play leader or nursery nurse is also a useful addition to an A&E department. The use of therapeutic play to prepare children for procedures will decrease anxiety as well as making the wait for treatment less stressful.

Thornes (1993) suggests that the A&E department is no longer merely the provider of emergency health care but has to respond to the changing provision of health care by also providing primary and secondary health care. The children's nurse in the department can be actively involved in health promotion and provide display material and advice for parents, but there needs to be a formal means of communication between the hospital and the community staff if continuing care is to be effective. It is suggested that a liaison health visitor can provide this continuity.

Accident-and-emergency medical staff need to have experience of the emergency care of children and be able to handle them and their families when they are frightened and distressed. The first consultant in paediatric A&E medicine was appointed in 1971, although it was not until 1988 that this was recognised as a unique speciality. Morton and Phillips (1992) recommended that every A&E department had a paediatric A&E consultant. To gain such a post applicants must have had experience in general and A&E paediatrics, as well as paediatric anaesthesia, orthopaedics, surgery and intensive care, and are best able to manage paediatric medicine, surgery and trauma. This recommendation has not had much effect in A&E departments, and in 2003 17% of hospitals seeing children in A&E still had no resident paediatric cover (Royal College of Paediatrics and Child Health, 2003).

Study activity

Consider whether children should only be seen in purpose-built paediatric A&E departments.

The advantage of children being seen only in specific paediatric A&E units would be that the environment would be child oriented and that all the staff would be experienced in assessing and treating children. However, the disadvantage could be that specialist services are not readily available 24 hours a day. In addition, staff would not necessarily gain the wide experience in trauma available in a large general A&E

department, and injured families would have to be separated. The optimum arrangements for children may therefore be integrated or adjacent children's departments within the general A&E complex.

Triage

Triage means assessing and prioritising patients according to their medical needs. The use of triage in A&E departments has enabled staff to meet Standard 5 of the Patient's Charter (DH, 1991b), which states that patients in A&E departments should be seen and assessed within 5 minutes of admission. This immediate assessment is even more important for children, who should be seen as a priority because of their age. Children need continuous supervision as their clinical condition can deteriorate much quicker than that of an adult. Action for Sick Children supports DH guidelines (1991a) which state that A&E departments should have effective procedures to prioritise waiting children and ensure that they are seen promptly. In spite of these recommendations, McConichie (2005) found that only 25% of A&E departments in England had formal triage arrangements for children. Ten per cent of departments gave no priority to children and the remaining 70% mostly left triage decisions to the discretion of the individual nurse.

The nurse involved in the triage of children needs to understand the developmental differences in the anatomy and physiology of the 0–16 age group (*see also* Maturation p. 65).

Study activity

How would you make an immediate assessment of any child entering the A&E department? What specific differences need to be taken into account when making an immediate assessment of children?

The ABC criteria for the assessment of a patient are useful in any circumstance (Lloyd-Thomas, 1990).

A = airway

Children's airways are much more easily compromised than that of the adult. They have comparatively large tongues and their airways are much narrower, shorter and straighter than those of adults. As a result, upper respiratory tract infections soon affect the lower airways, where a small amount of mucus or swelling can easily cause obstruction.

B = breathing

Unless the child has a congenital cardiac problem, breathing problems are likely before circulatory problems. The small child has a soft cartilaginous thorax and the intercostal muscles are underdeveloped, causing the chest to retract inwards when lung compliance is decreased by a respiratory obstruction. Nasal flaring, intercostal or substernal retractions are signs of respiratory distress. In addition, noisy respirations will

Table 27.1 Respiratory rates in childhood

Age	Range	Average
Neonate	30–50	35
1–11 months	25–40	30
1–3 years	20–30	25
4–5 years	20–30	23
6–7 years	18–25	21
8–9 years	18–25	20
10–13 years	16–24	19
14–16 years	12–20	18

be heard: wheezing and grunting are signs of lower respiratory obstruction, stridor indicates upper respiratory tract obstruction. Children have a high metabolic rate and therefore a comparatively high oxygen need; if this is compromised, they easily become hypoxic resulting in agitation and bradycardia.

Cyanosis is a late sign in children, who are more likely to become pale.

C = circulation

Children naturally have a comparatively high pulse rate and a pulse of 60 or less in an infant is sufficient reason to commence cardiac arrest procedures, as this pulse rate is insufficient to provide an adequate circulation. Circulation is affected by the volume of circulating fluid. Children's fluid balance, in comparison to that of an adult, has been likened to a kettle with a large spout and a small lid! In other words, their ability to lose fluid is much higher than their ability to gain it, because of their large surface area to volume ratio. They can rapidly become hypovolaemic due to diarrhoea, vomiting or inability to drink. A small blood loss can also be catastrophic for an infant who may only have 240–300 ml of circulating blood volume (Figure 27.2). Colour, capillary refill and skin turgor are quick ways of making a cardiovascular assessment.

C can also stand for conscious level. Small children's neurological status is never easy to assess and an adapted form of the Glasgow Coma Scale is needed for pre-verbal children (Figure 27.3). The following

Table 27.2 Pulse rates in childhood

Age	Range	Average
Neonates	100–180	140
1–11 months	100–160	120
1–3 years	80–130	100
4–5 years	80–120	95
6–7 years	75–115	90
8–9 years	70–110	85
10–13 years	70–110	80
14–16 years	60–100	72

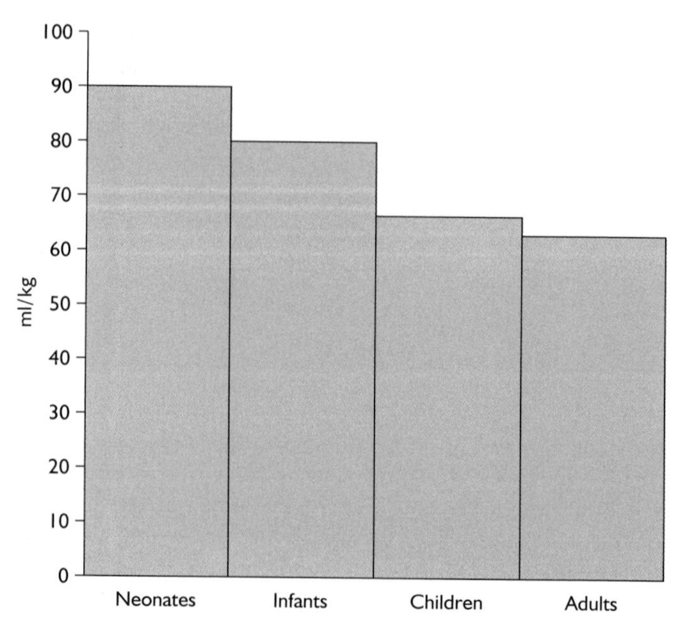

Figure 27.2 Circulating blood volumes.

Rapid cardiopulmonary assessment

A = Airway patency
- Able to maintain independently
- Requires assistance to maintain

B = Breathing
- Rate
- Mechanics
  - retractions
  - grunting
  - accessory muscles
  - nasal flaring
- Air entry
  - chest expansion
  - breath sounds
  - stridor
  - wheezing
  - paradoxical chest movements
- Colour

C = Circulation
- Heart rate
- Blood pressure
  - volume/strength
- Peripheral pulses
  - present/absent
  - volume/strength
- Skin perfusion
  - capillary refill time
  - temperature
  - colour
  - mottling
- CNS perfusion
  - responsiveness
  - recognises parents
  - muscle tone
  - pupil size
  - posturing

(American Academy of Pediatrics, 1994)

is usually used to make a rapid initial assessment of the level of consciousness:

A – awake
V – non-verbal, quiet, calm, opens eyes to voice
P – only responds to pain
U – unresponsive

For children, the Glasgow Coma Scale scores (Figure 27.3) are usually interpreted as:

13–15 – mild neurological deficit
9–12 – moderate neurological damage
<8 – severe neurological damage

(*See also* Neurological assessment p. 517.)

Study activity

Once these immediate assessments have been carried out, what other observations may be useful to determine the severity of the child's illness?

The mnemonic DEF can be a useful way of determining the other useful observations to make of a child during triage.

D = diet and fluids

A clear history of the child's recent intake may help to determine the possibility of dehydration, the likelihood of an infective type of gastroenteritis or the possibility of an allergic reaction.

Module 5

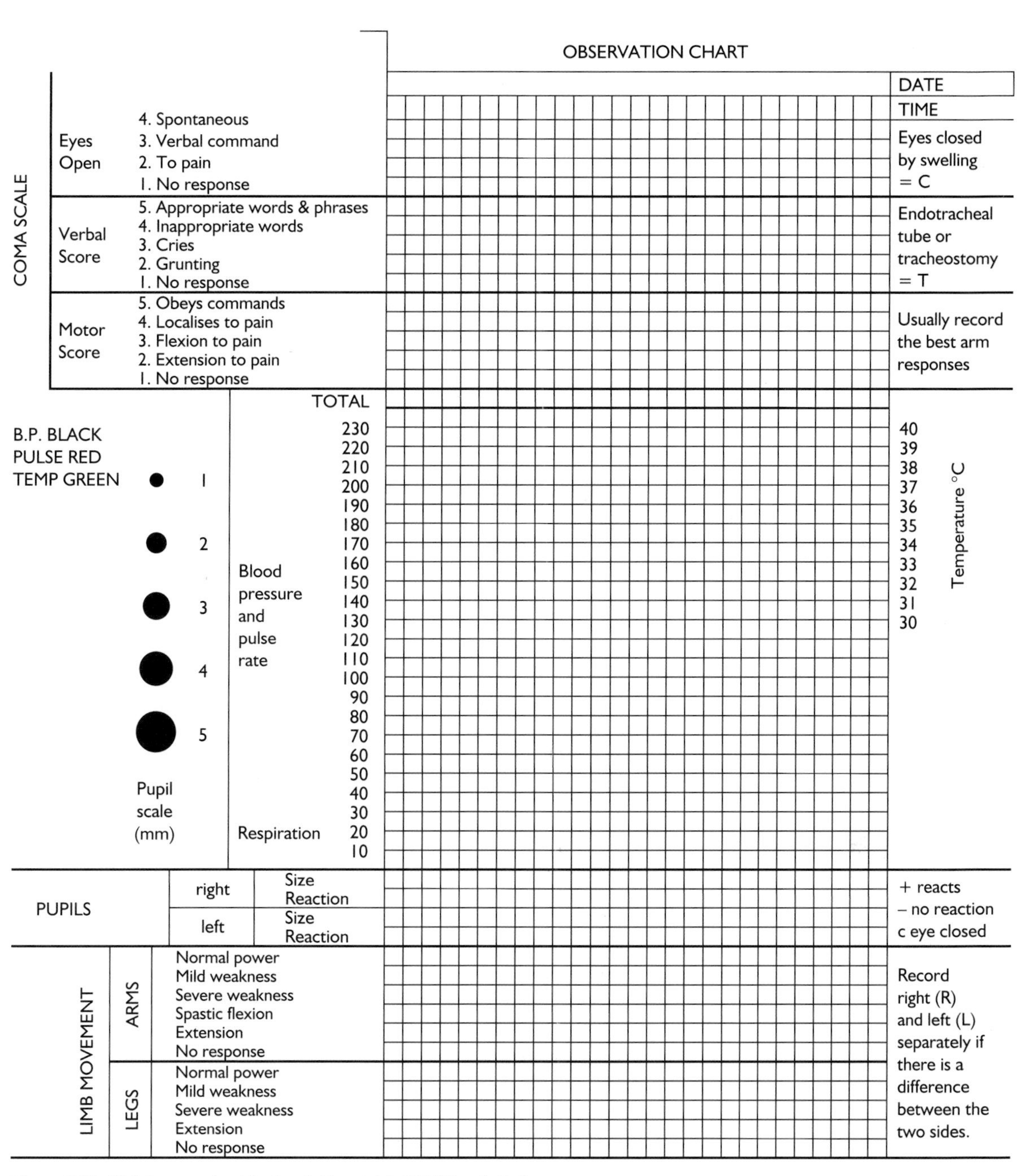

Figure 27.3 Child neuro chart (Luton & Dunstable NHS Trust), 2–5 years.

E = evidence of infection

Children can quickly become severely ill due to infection, and temperature control is poor in children under 5 years. Any small child presenting with a pyrexia over 38°C should be given an antipyretic as soon as possible to prevent a febrile convulsion. The history from the parents may give a clue to the site of infection by revealing that the child has been reluctant to drink or has been rubbing the ears, but there may be no obvious clues. Always look for skin rashes, a child with an infectious disease will need to be kept away from other patients.

F = fontanelle

Looking at an infant's fontanelle may provide some indication of the diagnosis. In dehydration, the fontanelle becomes depressed, while a bulging fontanelle is an indication of raised intercranial pressure. The anterior fontanelle usually closes at the age of 18–24 months while the posterior fontanelle does not close until 2–3 months. These closures are not solid until the age of 10–12 years and it may still be possible to identify changes in an older child.

Resuscitation of Children

In infants and children, prevention is the recognised management of respiratory and cardiac arrest. Early recognition of the child at risk may prevent an arrest from occurring (Smith and Wood, 1998). Survival is low for children who suffer a cardiopulmonary arrest and the risk of neurological impairment for survivors is high (Zideman, 1999).

Although the principles of basic life support for adults and children are the same, there are some important differences because of certain variations in the anatomy and physiology of children (Simpson, 1994). There is evidence to indicate that these differences are not always appreciated and that nurses have poor knowledge and understanding about paediatric arrests (Tume and Bullock, 2004).

Cardiac arrest in the child is rarely a primary event. The child is likely to have a cardiac arrest secondary to hypoxia and respiratory acidosis. If there is no response from a child and cardiac arrest is suspected, a quick assessment of airway, breathing and circulation (ABC) should be carried out. An infant's responsiveness is best checked by flicking or gentle shaking.

Respiratory movement in children aged 0–6 years is mainly abdominal, so respirations should be assessed by observing the rise and fall of the abdominal region. As respirations are likely to be shallow the child will need to be undressed to do this accurately.

Infants' necks are short and chubby so the brachial pulse is used to check circulation. A pulse rate of 5 beats or fewer in 5 seconds is an indication to commence cardiac massage as an infant's normal pulse rate is 150–160 per minute. Sixty beats or fewer indicates that circulation is severely compromised.

The 2005 resuscitation guidelines provide two definitions for the purpose of resuscitation:

- an infant is a baby under 1 year
- a child is between 1 year and puberty

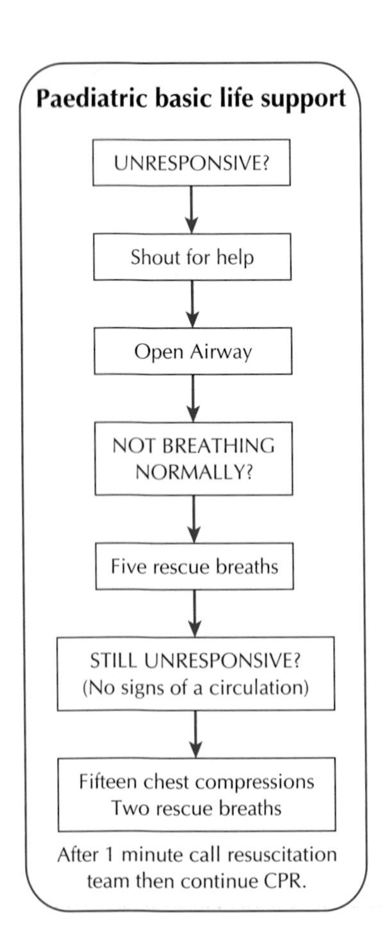

Airway management

Obstruction by the relaxed tongue is common in children as their tongues are relatively large. In addition, because infants' upper airways

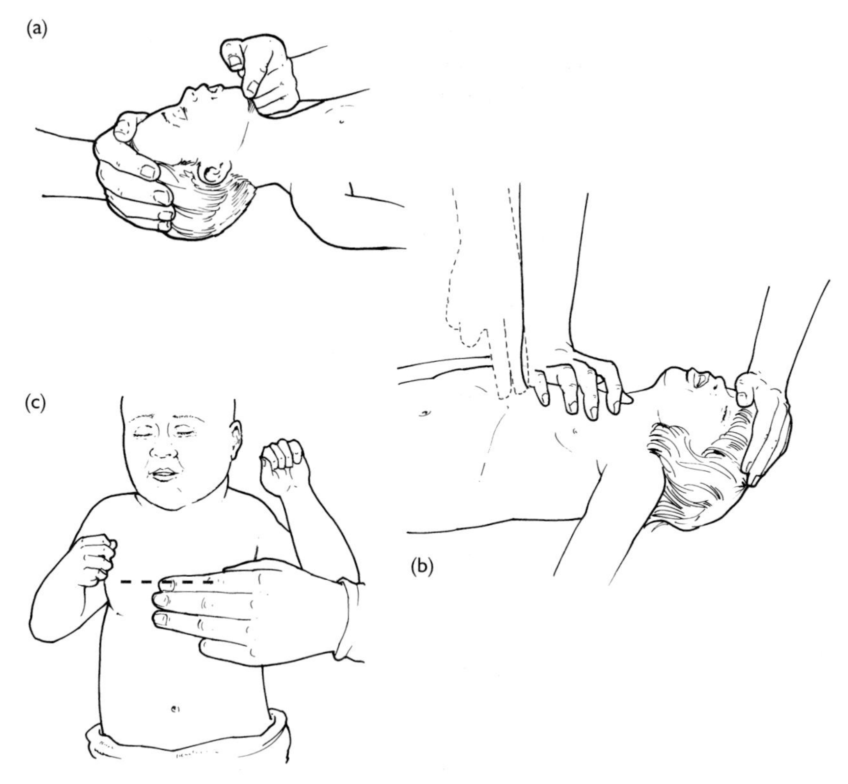

Figure 27.4 Infant and child resuscitation: (a) the sniffing position; (b) child compressions; (c) infant compressions.

are relatively narrow and short, extending the neck will obstruct the airway. To open the airway the infant's head and chin should be tilted to the 'sniffing position' (Figure 27.4a). The hand should not push on the soft tissues under the chin as this may block the airway. The airway should only be cleared manually if the obstruction can be observed. Use the little finger to hook it out. Finger sweeping can cause damage to the delicate childhood soft palate. In infants it can also push the obstruction further down as their pharynx is funnel-shaped.

Breathing

Infant artificial respiration is given by small breaths or puffs from the cheeks, given steadily over 1–1.5 seconds to inflate the lungs every 3 s. Such low-pressure breaths minimise the risk of gastric distension. If resistance is felt during artificial respiration, it is most likely that the airway position is incorrect. If a change of position is unsuccessful, the airway may be blocked by a foreign body, which is one of the main causes of arrest in children (Woodward, 1994).

If an infant's airway is occluded:

- support the baby in the prone position over the forearm
- give five back blows (Figure 27.5b) between the shoulder blades with the heel of the hand
- if this fails, turn the baby over and administer five chest thrusts (place two fingers on the sternum, one finger breadth below the nipple line, and push upwards)

Never administer abdominal thrusts to a baby as the stomach and liver lie below the rib region.

If a child's airway is occluded:

- perform back blows with the child over the lap (Figure 27.5a), in the upright position

or

- perform the Heimlich manoeuvre (Figure 27.5c)

Circulation

In an infant, the lone rescuer should locate the xiphisternum by finding the angle where the lowest ribs join in the middle, and place two fingers on the sternum, one finger's breadth below this line. If there are two or more rescuers, the baby can be encircled in the hands with both thumbs placed side by side on the lower third of the sternum. Compress

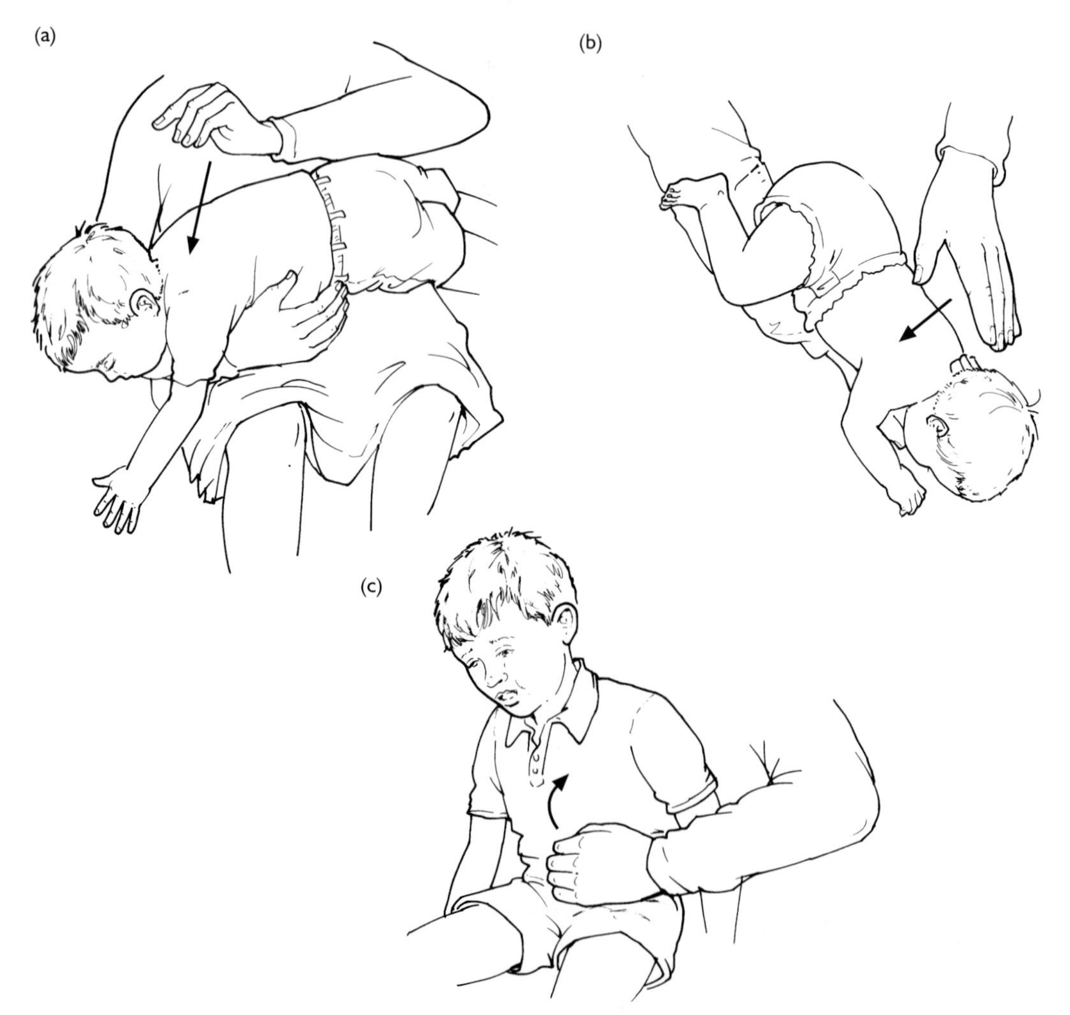

Figure 27.5 Management of choking: (a) child back blows; (b) infant back blows; (c) Heimlich manoeuvre.

the sternum approximately one-third of the depth of the infant's chest (1.3–2.5 cm) at a rate of at least 100 compressions per minute (Figure 27.4c).

In a child, locate the site of compressions and use the heel of one hand to compress the sternum by 2.5–3.8 cm at a rate of 80 per minute (Figure 27.4b). In larger children or with small rescuers, it may be easier to use both hands with the fingers interlocked.

In any paediatric resuscitation the ratio of respirations to cardiac massage should be 2 : 15 whether or not the rescuer is accompanied, although lone rescuers can use a ratio of 2 : 30 if they are having difficulty with the transition between giving respirations and compressions (Resuscitation Council, 2005).

Advanced life support

Cardiac arrest in children does not follow a prescribed pattern and is dictated by the individual child. Once basic resuscitation techniques have commenced, electrocardiogram (ECG) leads should be positioned to aid further diagnosis and treatment. The Resuscitation Council UK (2005) has set out algorithms to guide advanced resuscitation.

Asystole is the most common arrest situation in children and is treated initially by ventilation and intubation followed by adrenaline, 10 mcg/kg (Figure 27.6). Electro-mechanical dissociation, which is the absence of a palpable pulse while the ECG monitor shows acceptable complexes, is commonly caused by severe shock. It is also treated initially with

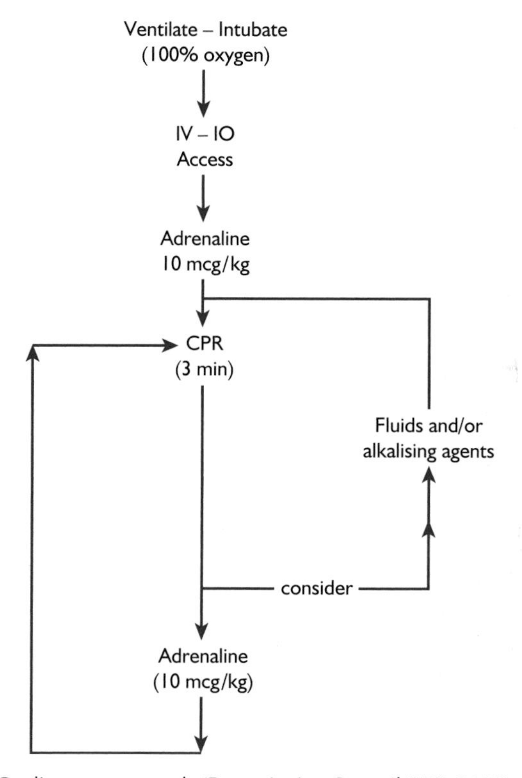

Figure 27.6 Cardiac arrest: asystole (Resuscitation Council (UK), 2005).

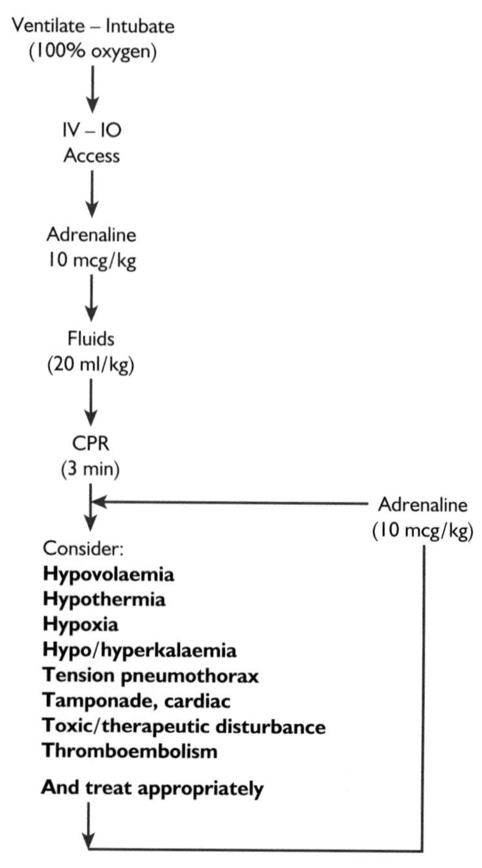

Figure 27.7 Cardiac arrest: electro-mechanical dissociation (Resuscitation Council (UK), 2005).

ventilation, intubation and adrenaline (10 mcg/kg). This is followed by a rapid infusion of 20 ml/kg crystalloid or 10 ml/kg plasma (Figure 27.7).

Ventricular fibrillation (VF) is seen in fewer than 10% of paediatric arrests (Somes, 1991). If VF is seen developing, a precordial thump can be given (using two fingers for infants). Otherwise it is treated by defibrillation (using infant paddles for babies under 10 kg) at 4 J/kg (Figure 27.8). A standard automated external debribrillator (AED) can be used in children over 8 years but purpose-made pads, or programmes that attenuate the energy output, are recommended for children aged between 1 and 8 years. If no such machine is available, an adult AED can be used for children over 1 year. There is no evidence for or against the use of AEDs for infants and therefore the UK Resuscitation Council (2005) recommends manual defibrillation for this age group.

Access for drugs during advanced resuscitation can be:

- intravenous (IV)
- intraosseous (IO)

Drugs can be given via an endotracheal tube, but this is not the most favourable route as evidence shows that there may be a paradoxical effect.

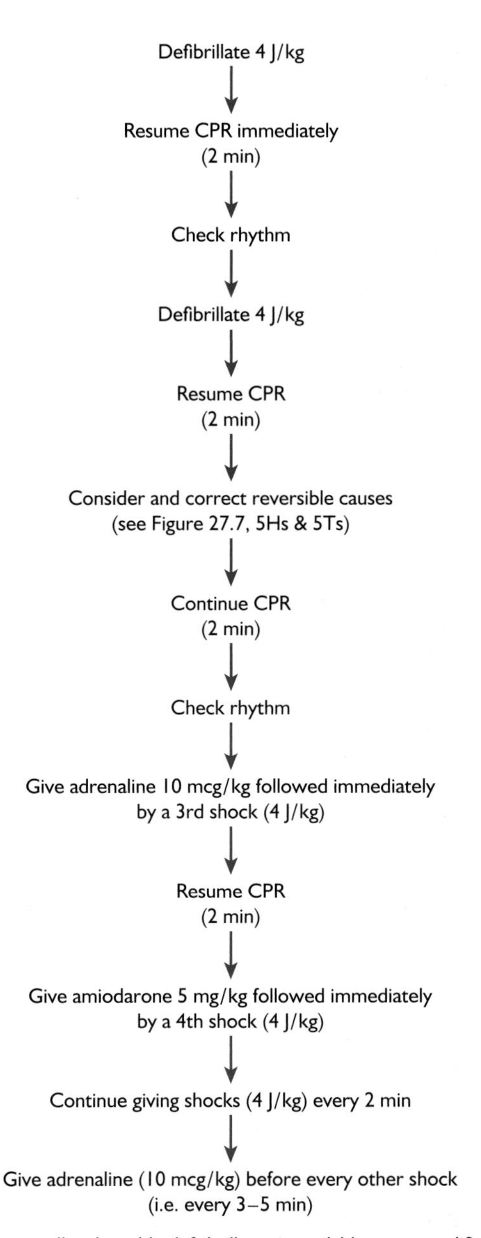

Figure 27.8 Cardiac arrest: ventricular fibrillation (Resuscitation Council (UK), 2005).

As children quickly become peripherally constricted, IV access may be impossible. In such cases an intraosseous (IO) line can be inserted into the tibial or femoral medullary cavity (Lawrence, 1993).

Unless the child is hypothermic or has had an overdose of a cerebral depressant drug, Ziderman (2003) recommends that resuscitation attempts should stop after 25 minutes with no evidence of cerebral activity or cardiac output. Once cardiac arrest occurs the survival rate is only 3–17%. Some of these resuscitated children then die later of multi-organ failure, or survive with significant neurological impairment (Zideman, 2003). The team leader should decide when resuscitation efforts should be abandoned. This should be done in a sensitive manner and a debriefing session should be held soon after the event to enable the team to reflect on the situation and their practice in a supportive environment (Resuscitation Council UK, 2005).

Parental Presence

The Resuscitation Council UK (2005) report that many parents would prefer to be present during resuscitation so they can be reassured that everything possible is being done for their child. Studies show that parents who have had this opportunity show less anxiety and depression after the death. An experienced member of staff must be allocated to support the parents by explaining what is happening if parents are to find the experience beneficial.

Problems in Paediatric Resuscitation

There is little research evidence to indicate the success or failure of particular ways of managing paediatric cardiac arrest situations (Resuscitation Council UK, 2005). However, there is evidence to indicate that there are three main factors that hinder paediatric arrests:

- Drugs and fluids have to be given to children according to their body weight and surface area. These precise measurements are often not known in an emergency.
- The equipment used for paediatric arrests varies in size. Staff must be able to identify the correct-sized equipment and know how to use it.
- Accident-and-emergency staff are largely inexperienced in the management of paediatric emergencies (Hughes, 1990) and Collins (1994) showed that many RSCNs were unable to demonstrate competence in resuscitation.

Cole (1995) suggests that some of these problems may be overcome by the use of the Broselow paediatric resuscitation system. The Broselow tape measure, designed in the US, aims to provide information about the correct-sized equipment and appropriate drug dosage for individual children. It is laid alongside the child and the colour segment that corresponds with the child's length gives the necessary information. The correctly sized equipment for that child is stored in a colour-coded pack. Research into the accuracy of the Broselow system shows that it greatly facilitates decision making but care must be taken when using it for obese or emaciated children (Cole, 1995).

Methods of determining equipment of appropriate size and drug dosages in the UK are the BMA reference chart (Oakley, 1988) and the modified paediatric resuscitation chart (Burke and Bowden, 1993) (Figures 27.9 and 27.10). Burke and Bowden modified the BMA reference chart after they found it to be of dubious benefit because of the time and complexity of its use. However, these charts rely on age-specific weights and no research has been done to determine their accuracy.

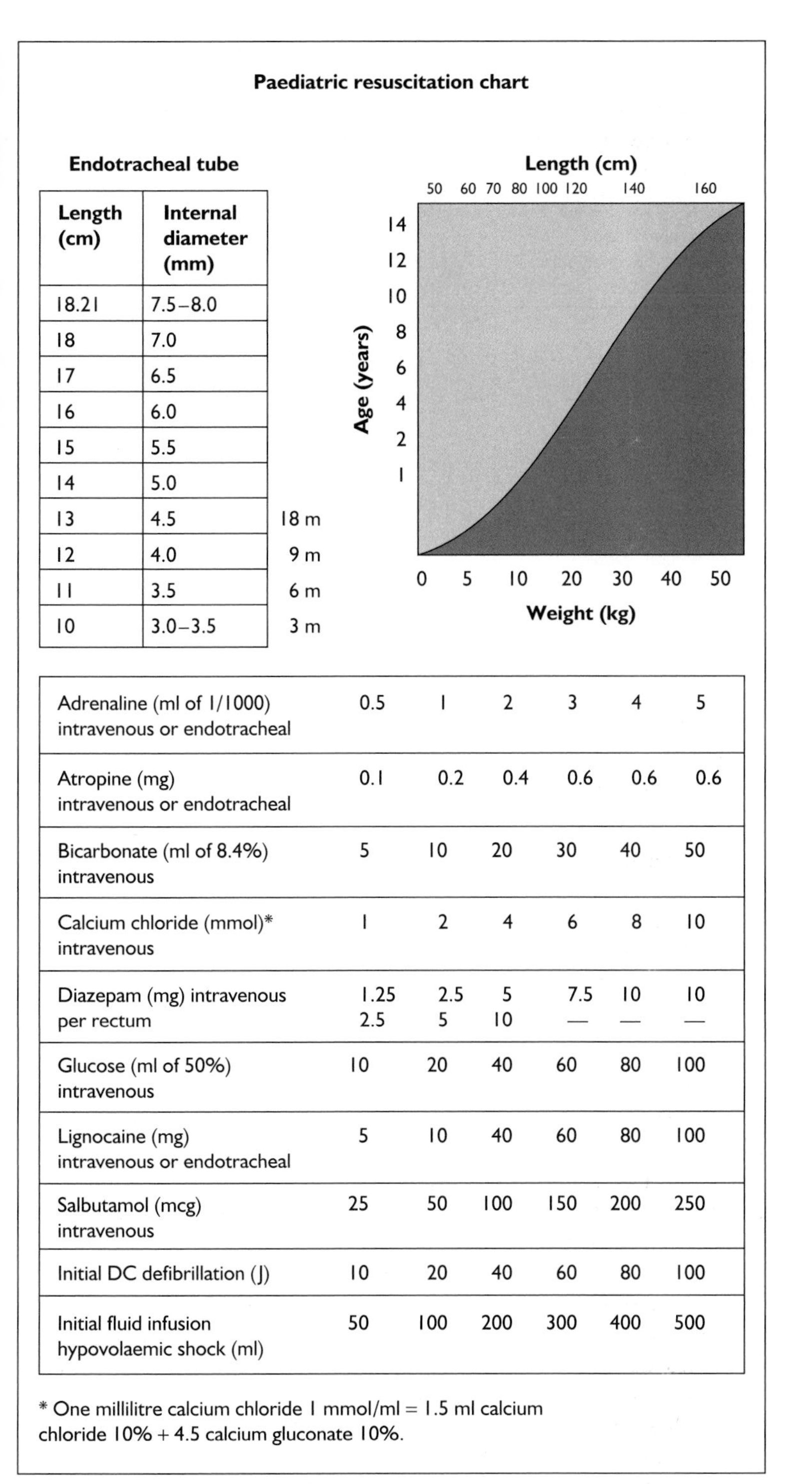

Paediatric resuscitation chart

Endotracheal tube

Length (cm)	Internal diameter (mm)	
18.21	7.5–8.0	
18	7.0	
17	6.5	
16	6.0	
15	5.5	
14	5.0	
13	4.5	18 m
12	4.0	9 m
11	3.5	6 m
10	3.0–3.5	3 m

Adrenaline (ml of 1/1000) intravenous or endotracheal	0.5	1	2	3	4	5
Atropine (mg) intravenous or endotracheal	0.1	0.2	0.4	0.6	0.6	0.6
Bicarbonate (ml of 8.4%) intravenous	5	10	20	30	40	50
Calcium chloride (mmol)* intravenous	1	2	4	6	8	10
Diazepam (mg) intravenous	1.25	2.5	5	7.5	10	10
per rectum	2.5	5	10	—	—	—
Glucose (ml of 50%) intravenous	10	20	40	60	80	100
Lignocaine (mg) intravenous or endotracheal	5	10	40	60	80	100
Salbutamol (mcg) intravenous	25	50	100	150	200	250
Initial DC defibrillation (J)	10	20	40	60	80	100
Initial fluid infusion hypovolaemic shock (ml)	50	100	200	300	400	500

* One millilitre calcium chloride 1 mmol/ml = 1.5 ml calcium chloride 10% + 4.5 calcium gluconate 10%.

Figure 27.9 The BMA paediatric resuscitation reference chart (Oakley, 1988).

Paediatric resuscitation chart

All doses are expressed as volumes (ml) and to be given intravenously unless stated otherwise.

Endotracheal tube • internal diameter (mm) • length (cm)	3 10	3.5 12	4 13	5 14	5.5 15	6.5 17	7.5 18	8 21
Maximum age	2	6	1	3.5	6	10	13	14
	Months		Years					
Maximum length (cm)	55	70	75	90	115	135	155	160
Maximum weight (kg)	5	7.5	10	15	20	30	40	50
Adrenaline (1/10 000)*	0.5	0.75	1	1.5	2	3	4	5
Atropine (600 μg/ml)*	0.2	0.25	0.3	0.5	0.7	1	1	1
Bicarbonate (8.4%)	5	7.5	10	15	20	30	40	50
Calcium chloride (1 mmol/ml)	1	1.5	2	3	4	6	8	10
Diazepam (5 mg/ml) • intravenously • per rectum	0.25 0.5	0.4 0.75	0.5 1	0.75 1.5	1 2	1.5 —	2 —	2 —
Glucose (50%)	5	7.5	10	15	20	30	40	50
Lignocaine (1% = 10 mg/ml)*	0.5	0.75	1	1.5	2	3	4	5
Salbutamol (50 μg/ml)	0.5	0.75	1	1.5	2	3	4	5
Initial fluid bolus (ml) • colloid • crystalloid	50 100	75 150	100 200	150 300	200 400	300 600	400 800	500 1000
Initial DC defibrillation (J)	10	15	20	30	40	60	80	100

All intravenous drugs may be given intraosseously at the same dose.
* May be given by the endotracheal route at the same dose.

Figure 27.10 Modified resuscitation chart (Burke and Bowden, 1993).

Sudden Death in A&E

The sudden death of a child is an overwhelming event for the family. They need time to come to terms with the event, express their grief and ask questions. Even children who are already dead on arrival to A&E should be brought into the department and the family shown to a private room. To avoid false hope, they need to have the death confirmed as soon as possible in an honest but sensitive way. Some professionals try to avoid the term 'death' but sometimes by using euphemisms the family will not appreciate exactly what has occurred.

Parents' reactions will vary according to their personality, culture, previous experience and the circumstances surrounding the death. The nurse will need to accept parents' reactions and demonstrate empathy

Further reading
Randle, H. (1998) What happens now? Information for parents whose child has died in A&E. *Paediatric Nursing*, **10** (4), 22–23.

and support. Parents will need to ask questions about the death and the nurse should be prepared for these. Once the child has been made presentable, parents should be given the chance to see and hold their child, but they also need to know that they can inform the hospital mortuary at any time should they want to return to do this. They may also wish to be involved in washing their child. Some A&E departments will take a Polaroid photograph of the child or take hand- or footprints. These may be appreciated by the parents, especially if the child is very young.

Parents also need advice about what will happen next. They need to be advised of the coroner's role in sudden or unexplained death without being made to feel that they are suspected of some crime. A post-mortem is often requested in these cases and they need to understand this procedure and the reasons for it. The nurse will need to appreciate that some religions do not permit post-mortems.

Practical advice about funeral arrangements, the death certificate and registration of the death should be discussed before the family leaves the department. Written information booklets, such as those available from the Department of Health, provide a useful resource to shocked parents, who will not remember all that they have been told. Liaison with the family GP or health visitor will enable continued advice and support on their return home. A code of practice is now available from the Department of Health to guide clinical staff in the communication with parents about the need for a post-mortem (DH, 2003b).

The Future

While advances have been made in the care of children in A&E departments, there is still scope for further developments. In Nottingham, an emergency children's nurse practitioner post has been in operation since 1991 and is able to take total responsibility for the assessment and treatment of about 5% of children seen in the department (Kobran and Pearce, 1993). As nurses continue to develop their roles, as prescribers for instance, this type of emergency practitioner may become more common, with a greater scope of practice.

Another recent development in A&E nursing practice is telephone triage. Many parents call A&E departments for advice about their children's symptoms (Campbell and Glasper, 1995) and Burton's 1989 study revealed that some parents attend A&E for reassurance rather than treatment. Areas that have developed a formal telephone triage system have found this to be cost-effective and that it helps to reduce the number of inappropriate visits to the A&E department. This formal system needs an experienced and suitably qualified children's nurse available 24 hours a day. Calls need to be well documented in case of further problems as well as providing a means of referral and auditing the effectiveness of the service.

The introduction of NHS Direct has provided parents with another source of telephone advice. However, there is evidence that it may not be accessed equitably by those with the greatest need for healthcare services. Ring and Jones (2004) found that its use is widespread among carers of preschool children unless they are from ethnic minorities, lower socio-economic groups and those with chronic ill-health problems.

Key Points

1. A significant number of children are seen in A&E departments in the UK yet few departments have dedicated facilities for them.
2. Many A&E departments do not have nurses or medical staff who have specific qualifications in the care of children.
3. Specific differences in paediatric anatomy and physiology need to be taken into account when undertaking an initial ABC assessment.
4. In infants and children, the recognised management of cardiac arrest is prevention of the two main causes: hypoxia and respiratory acidosis.
5. Specific differences in paediatric anatomy and physiology give rise to important variations in basic life support between adults and children.
6. The management of paediatric arrests is hindered by the need for varied dosages of fluid and medication and different-sized equipment according to the size and weight of the child.

Chapter 28

Administration of Medicines

Introduction

The administration of medicines has always been an integral part of nursing care, but when caring for children it involves several problem areas. The responsibility of the children's nurse in ensuring that the correct medication is safely and appropriately administered to the correct child is a huge undertaking that requires many different skills.

Children are at particular risk from medication for a number of reasons. Their immature body systems make them less able to absorb, metabolise and excrete drugs (Figure 28.1). Their age, weight and surface area varies widely, making standardised dosages impossible. In addition, many children dislike taking medication, so the nurse has to be able to find an acceptable method of administration for each individual child to promote compliance. This may be further aided by

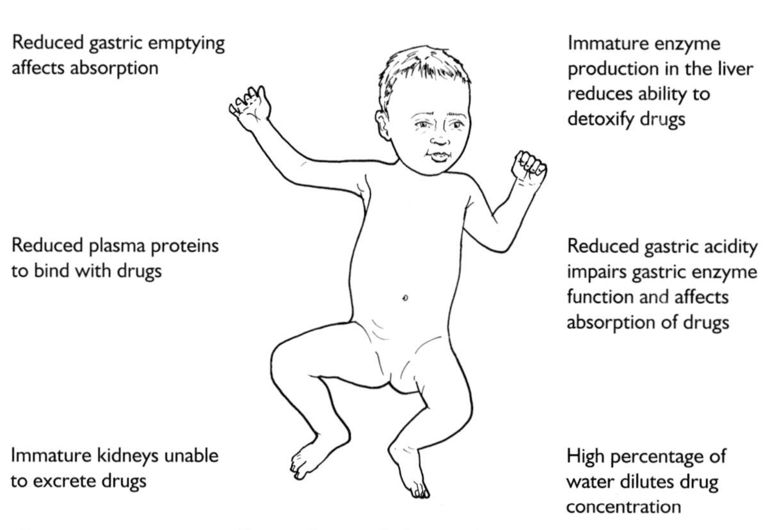

Figure 28.1 Immaturity affecting the metabolism and excretion of medication.

the nurse's knowledge of alternative preparations available for each medication.

Although it is mostly the doctor's responsibility to prescribe appropriate medication, the nurse who will be administering the prescription should have an understanding of the appropriate dosage, route of administration, desired action, possible side-effects and contra-indications of each medication to be given (UKCC, 1989). The nurse will also need to be able to explain most of these aspects to the child and family to ensure continued acceptance of the regimen.

The nurse has a professional responsibility to question any drug prescription that appears inappropriate and may be justified in refusing to administer a medication when there are clear contra-indications to any part of the prescription.

Absorption, Metabolism and Excretion of Drugs

Babies and children need a different dose of drugs than adults because of their comparatively low body weight and because of the differences in the distribution of body fluids and in the developmental stage of their body organs. These latter differences are complex and mean that a child cannot just be given a smaller proportion of the adult dose (*see also* Body water p. 67).

Water is the largest constituent of the body but the actual percentage varies according to age and the amount of body fat (Figure 28.2). About 85% of a premature baby's weight consists of water, compared with an adult whose water content averages 55% of body weight. In an infant water is about 70% of the body weight.

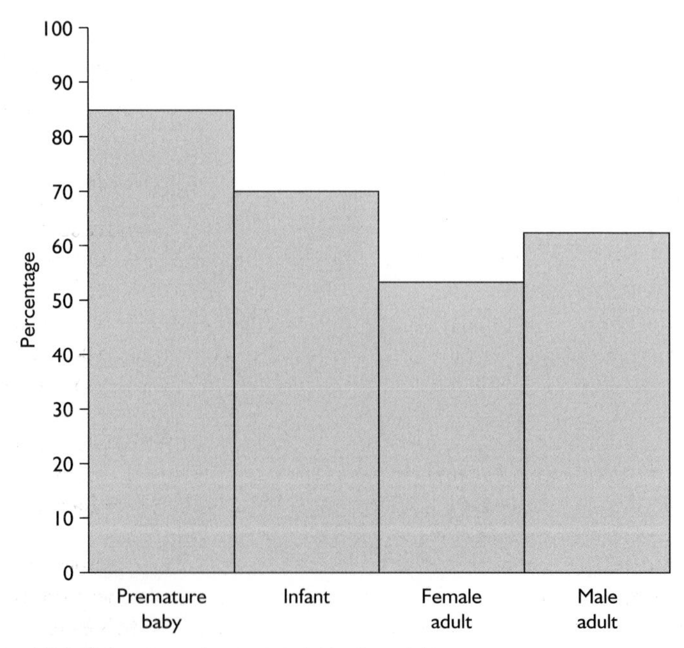

Figure 28.2 Percentage of water to total body weight.

This means that certain drugs, which are water soluble, are less concentrated in a small baby than they would be if taken by an adult. Consequently, higher doses relative to the baby's weight may need to be given initially.

Children under 3 years of age have a round stomach, which is slow to empty. The secretion of gastric acid is also reduced, which is believed to impair the function of the gastric enzymes and alter the absorption rate of oral medications.

The mature liver can detoxify or excrete into bile certain drugs such as antibiotics. It can also chemically alter or excrete steroids. However, these functions are not fully developed in infancy and, as a result, some drugs could reach a dangerous concentration unless prescribed in a very reduced dosage. In older children, the opposite applies as the liver becomes relatively large in comparison with body size.

Complete maturity of the renal system does not occur until the child is about 3 years old. Before this age the glomerular filtration rate is much reduced, resulting in an inability to excrete drugs as efficiently as the older child and adult. This may lead to the accumulation of high concentrations of drugs in the bloodstream and the dosage of certain drugs therefore needs to be comparatively low (*see also* Maturation of renal system p. 65).

Nurses also need to be aware of these differences when breastfeeding mothers have been prescribed medication. Small molecules of drugs can pass from the bloodstream into the milk-producing cells of the breast, causing the breastfed baby to also receive a small dose of the drug. Drugs that are fat soluble pass across in greater concentrations than other drugs, and are more likely to produce unwanted effects in the baby.

Safety of the Drug

Apart from the differences in drug dosages because of the different and immature body systems of the small child, some drugs are contra-indicated for children because there is some evidence that they are harmful when used during childhood.

Aspirin- or salicylate-containing medication is contra-indicated in children under 12 years of age because it was thought to have some role in the development of Reye's syndrome. Although this link is now being questioned (Casteels-Van Daele, 1993) aspirin is still not advised for children. Reye's syndrome is a degenerative condition characterised by cerebral oedema and liver dysfunction and has also been linked with the administration of anti-emetics to children during viral illnesses (Whaley and Wong, 2002).

Alimemazine (trimeprazine), an antihistamine that may also be used as a pre-medication for children because of its sedative action, is not advised for infants under 6 months as it has been shown to have a possible link with cot death (Ellis, 1995).

The Children's National Service Framework (NSF) recommends that the use of medicines in children should be guided by the best available evidence of clinical effectiveness. In practice, most medicines for children have not been formally researched with children (DH, 2003c).

Some drugs are only licensed for adults and must be used 'off-label' as they have not proven to have a therapeutic use for children. Other 'unlicensed' drugs do not have a licence at all. This is obviously not ideal and best practice is currently to use medicines that have been proved to work well in adults and where there is a good theoretical basis for believing they will work equally well for children. When the prescribed drug is unfamiliar, the nurse should always check the drug data sheet or a paediatric formulary, or ask their pharmacologist for advice.

Clearly, research into the use of medicines for the different ages of childhood is a huge ethical and practical dilemma. The Children's NSF (DH, 2004) recommends that hospitals routinely use a paediatric formulary to aid prescribing, and have policies and procedures in place relating to safe medicines practice for infants and children, which include:

- preparation of IV injections and infusions centrally under controlled conditions in the pharmacy
- inclusion of sufficient trained pharmacy staff to cater for the needs of children as part of the multidisciplinary team
- reporting, investigating and monitoring of all medication errors
- controls assurance standards to include weighing children and checking dosages before administration
- monitoring that formulations of medicines are appropriate to the age and ability of the child

Study activity

Investigate your own hospital's policies and procedures. Is there a policy to encompass the above recommendations? Are these practices in place in all areas where children are seen?

The Effects of Medication

Medication is obviously prescribed to achieve a positive result, but most drugs also have other effects in addition to the beneficial effects. Before administering any medication, the nurse should be aware of the desired effects as well as the possible side-effects and adverse effects.

Side-effects are the frequently experienced, expected reactions to a drug. It is almost inevitable that a drug taken for its beneficial effect on one part of the body will have other effects on other organs. For instance, salbutamol, given to reduce bronchospasm, has the common side-effect of tachycardia. Antibiotics often affect the normal flora in the rest of the body and may lead to oral thrush or diarrhoea. Side-effects can be trivial or so serious that they require the cessation of treatment, but their severity is usually determined by the individual child's condition.

Adverse effects are unusual and unexpected reactions to a drug. They can be predictable or unpredictable. Predictable adverse effects are often due to a child's known medical history. For example, propranolol, a beta-blocker that can be prescribed for migraine to dilate cerebral blood vessels, also dilates bronchioles and can trigger an asthmatic attack in known asthmatics. It also suppresses the body's response to hypoglycaemia, which is a potential danger to a diabetic child. Unpredictable adverse effects are abnormal allergic reactions, which can occur at any time during the administration of the drug and can range from skin rashes, urticaria, wheezing or tachycardia to anaphylactic shock.

The effects of any medication may be altered if it is taken in combination with certain other drugs, food or drink. Some of these interactions may be desirable, but others may be unwanted and harmful. Two or more drugs that depress the central nervous system, such as codeine and an antihistamine, should not be given in combination as they will cause dangerous oversedation. Theophylline and salbutamol can cause cardiac arrhythmias when given in combination. Tetracycline and iron combine in the intestine to make a non-chelated mixture that is not readily absorbed, reducing the effect of both drugs. In a similar way, milk also reduces the effect of some drugs and this should be considered with any medication prescribed for infants.

Sometimes an interaction can be beneficial. Naloxone, when given with morphine, blocks the receptors used by narcotics to reduce respirations and is thus used as an antagonist for morphine overdosage. Antibiotics are given in combination so that a smaller dose of each may be prescribed, not only reducing side-effects but lessening the risk of bacterial resistance.

Monitoring the Effect of Drugs

Drug administration includes the observation of the child for any effect of the prescribed medication. Evaluation of the response to drug therapy is not always easy, especially in very young children, and a knowledge of the child's usual behaviour is vital. Parents should be encouraged to share any changes they have noticed.

To accurately monitor the effect of any drug the nurse needs to appreciate its reaction and duration time. Whereas salbutamol can take effect within 5–15 minutes and be effective for up to 6 hours, metronidazole starts to work within an hour of administration but beneficial effects may not be apparent for 24–48 hours. Parents need to be advised of reaction times as this may affect their compliance.

Observations of vital signs may also help to indicate the effects of the medication. Monitoring the temperature of a child being treated with an antipyretic and checking the peak flow readings before and after administration of a bronchodilator will help to determine the efficacy of these drugs. Checking the pulse rate of a child taking frequent doses of salbutamol or regular doses of digoxin will help to ensure that they are not receiving too much of the drug. Certain drugs, such as gentamicin and sodium valproate, are very toxic when they reach a certain concentration in the bloodstream. Gentamicin is nephrotoxic and sodium valproate can cause liver damage, so blood levels are checked periodically to ensure that safe concentrations are maintained.

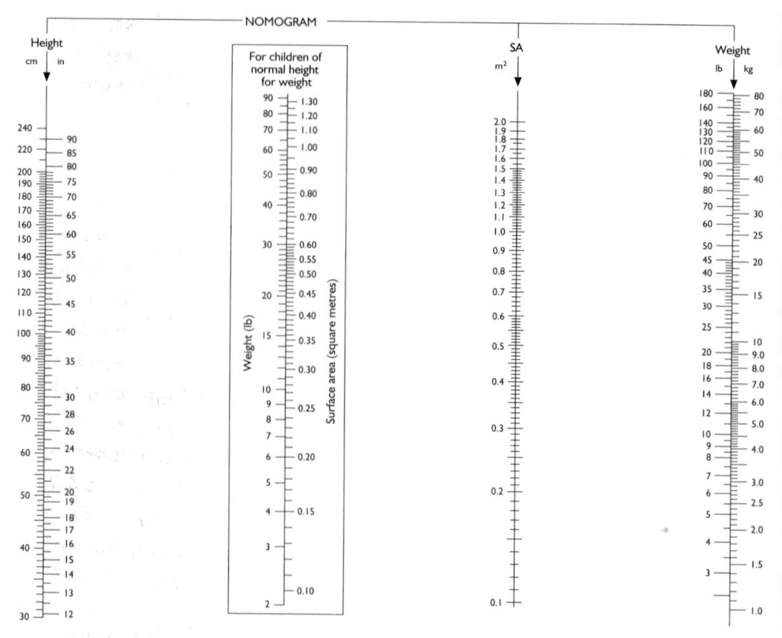

Figure 28.3 Nomogram (Whaley and Wong, 2000). Surface area (SA) is calculated by drawing a straight line to connect the child's height and weight. Surface area is given at the point where this line crosses the SA column. If a child is thought to be an average size, weight alone may be used to calculate SA (second column).

Calculating Drug Dosages

The dosage of any medication must be carefully calculated to ensure that the required site of action receives the drug at the appropriate concentration to achieve a therapeutic effect. The appropriate dose for an individual child can be calculated by age, weight or body surface.

The use of age to determine drug dosage is not to be recommended except in an emergency, as there is a huge range in children's body weight at any age. The most commonly used method in the UK is by weight, with most drugs for children giving a recommended dose per kilogram body weight. In the USA, the most commonly used method involves the calculation of the child's body surface area (BSA), which is estimated by the child's weight and height using the West nomogram (Figure 28.3). The drug dosage is then determined by:

child's BSA (m^2) × dose/m^2 = child's dose

At present, this method is only used in the UK when the margin between the therapeutic and the toxic dose is very small, for example with cytotoxic agents.

Before administering any medication the nurse should be aware of the correct range of dosage for the specific child. Each child is likely to require a different dose corresponding to their individual weight. Because most drugs are prepared and packaged in adult-dosage strengths, the ability to calculate fractional drug dosages from larger amounts is essential to the children's nurse. Such calculations may also involve the conversion of grams (g) to milligrams (mg) or micrograms (mcg).

Study activity

Consider the following prescriptions and determine the correct amount to be given.

(a) Stock drug contains 30 mg/5 ml. The child has been prescribed 21 mg.
(b) Stock drug contains 1 g/2 ml. The prescription asks for 375 mg to be administered.
(c) A child has been prescribed 4 mcg of a drug that is available as 0.006 mg/ml.

Answers at end of this chapter.

Although some nurses may be able to use mental arithmetic or calculators to determine the answers, to justify the answer it is necessary to be able to demonstrate the calculation used. Brains and calculators are not infallible! A rough idea of the correct answer is an additional check of accuracy. For instance in problem (a) in the study activity it can easily be seen that 21 mg is over half of 30 mg and that the required dose will be more than 2.5 ml. The calculation that should be used is:

dose required ÷ dose available × dilution = amount to be given

Calculations of dosages are further complicated if reconstituting drugs for injection. Many of these are prepared in powder form and have to be reconstituted with sterile water, which often causes a displacement value that must be taken into account if only part of the reconstituted solution is to be used. The calculation in these situations is:

dose required ÷ dose available × dilution + displacement value = amount

The drug data sheet or your pharmacy department will be able to give advice about specific displacement values.

Metric conversions

Metric units of mass

- 1 kilogram (kg) = 1000 g
- 1 gram (g) = 1000 mg
- 1 milligram (mg) = 1000 mcg

Conversions

- kilograms to grams = multiply by 1000
- grams to milligrams = multiply by 1000
- milligrams to grams = divide by 1000
- grams to kilograms = divide by 1000

Calculations

1 Bobby is prescribed 0.6 mg atropine. The ampoule of atropine states that it contains 600 mcg/ml. How much does Bobby need?

0.6 mg × 1000 = 600 mcg (decimal point moved three places to right)

Bobby needs 1 ml of atropine.

2 Jane is prescribed 250 mcg Lanoxin. The stock elixir is 0.25 mg/ml. How much does Jane need?

250 mcg ÷ 1000 = 0.25 mg (decimal point moved three places to left)

Jane needs 1 ml of Lanoxin.

Now try the following:

- Convert 300 g to kg
- Convert 5 kg to g
- Convert 0.3 mg to mcg
- Convert 20 mcg to mg

(Answers overleaf)

Routes of Administration

Oral administration

The preferred route of administering drugs to children is by mouth. Most paediatric medications are dispensed in palatable and colourful preparations to make them attractive and acceptable for children. However, this may not be the most appropriate route and it does have some disadvantages. The absorption of oral drugs is variable, there may be a risk of gastric irritation, small children can aspirate oral medication given too quickly and discoloration or destruction of tooth enamel can be caused by very sugary solutions.

The most accurate method for administering oral drugs to children is the plastic disposable syringe. Measured plastic cups and spoons are less accurate as some of the liquid tends to adhere to these devices. The child should always be prepared for medicine. Forcing a crying child to take medicine may result in aspiration and the child is likely to resist further doses (Figure 28.4). Orenstein *et al.* (1988) suggest that swallowing can be induced in infants by blowing a small puff of air into their face.

Drug calculations

How to calculate the amount needed

- What you want ÷ what you have × the dilution = the amount needed
  (a) Tom is prescribed 42 mg Vallergan. The stock bottle contains Vallergan 30 mg per 5 ml. How much should you give Tom?

  what you want = 42 mg
  what you have = 30 mg
  dilution = 5 ml
  $\frac{42}{30} \times 5 = \frac{42}{6} = 7$ ml

  (b) Emma is prescribed 64 mg of gentamicin. The stock ampoule contains 80 mg in 2 ml. How much should you give?

  $\frac{64}{80} \times 2 = \frac{64}{40} = \frac{16}{10} = 1.6$ ml

Answers to calculations in activity on p. 321

(a) $\frac{21}{30} \times 5 = \frac{7}{10} \times 5 = \frac{35}{10} = 3.5$ ml

(b) 1 g = 1000 mg

$\frac{375}{1000} \times 2 = \frac{750}{1000} = \frac{3}{4} = 0.75$ ml

(c) 0.006 mg = 6 mcg

$\frac{4}{6} \times 1 = \frac{2}{3} = 0.66$ ml

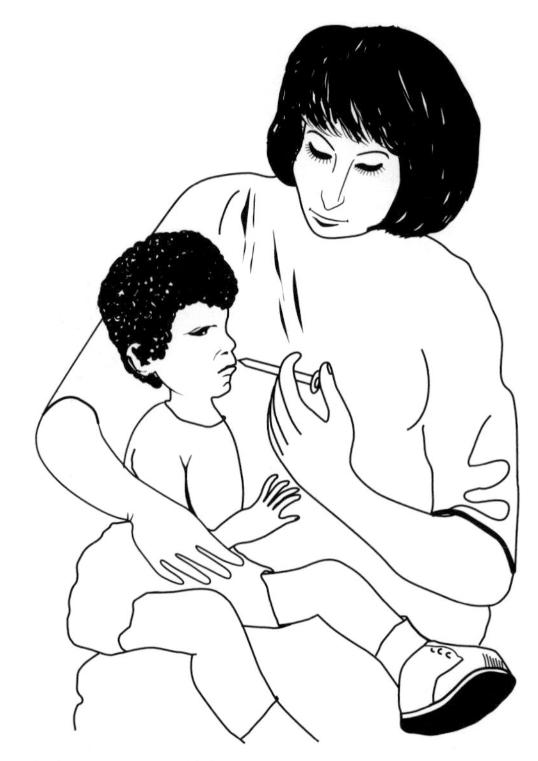

Figure 28.4 Infant restraint – oral drug.

Oral medicines should not be added to drinks as there is no guarantee that the child will finish the drink and any change in the taste may then cause the child to refuse drinks. However, it is acceptable to offer the child a favourite drink or foodstuff once the medication has been taken. It is often useful for the nurse to sample a small amount of the medication and therefore appreciate when its taste needs to be camouflaged.

Most young children have difficulty swallowing tablets, and preparations that are not available in liquid form may need to be crushed. Some tablets have a protective coating to facilitate slow release so it is always advisable to check that breaking or crushing the tablet does not affect the action of the drug.

Rectal

The rectal administration of medication, usually in the form of suppositories, can be a very effective route for children, especially if they are nauseated or cannot have anything orally. Sedatives, analgesics and anti-emetics can be given in this way, but the absorption and action of the drug can be slowed or impaired by a rectum loaded with faeces. To ensure acceptance of the drug the suppository needs to be placed beyond both rectal sphincters and held in place until the danger of reflex expulsion has passed. Abd-el-Maeboud *et al.* (1991) suggest that insertion of the suppository blunt end first reduces the risk of expulsion but no study is available to determine if the discomfort of insertion is affected by this method.

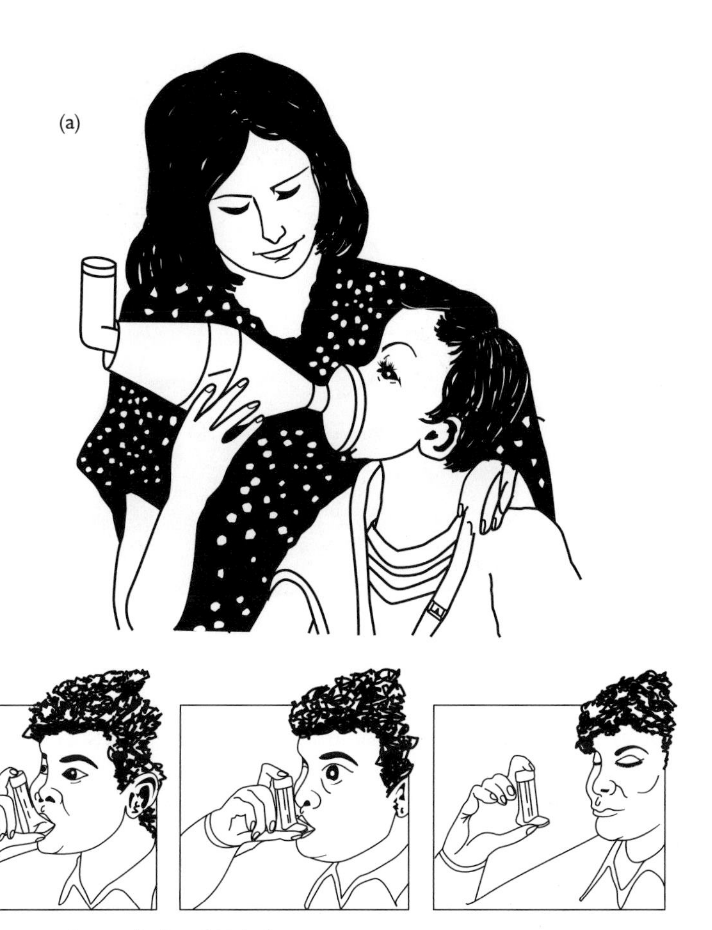

Figure 28.5 (a) Spacer device. (b) Inhaler.

Inhalation

Bronchodilators, steroids and antibiotics, suspended in particulate form, can be inhaled directly into the airway using a nebuliser or a metered dose inhaler. Nebulisers can be used with air or oxygen and metered dose inhalers are available in a range of different formats. Children and parents need to be prepared for the use of inhalants to ensure the maximum effect is gained from the drug. The noise of the nebuliser can be frightening for the unprepared child, who may be further scared by the mask. Metered dose inhalers can be used successfully by children over 5 years of age but they need to be able to coordinate their breathing with the administration of the drug and to hold their breath for about 10 seconds after inhalation. A spacer device makes inhalation techniques easier for younger children but again careful preparation will facilitate acceptance of the mask and device that can otherwise appear alarming (see Figure 28.5).

Topical

Topical medications are used for their local effect and can be applied to the skin, eyes, ears or nose. Although this route minimises systemic

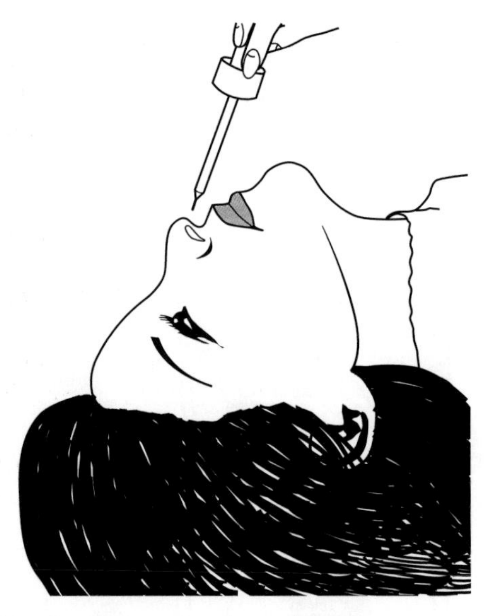

Figure 28.6 Position for adminstration of nose drops.

side-effects of the drug, it should be remembered that such effects can occur if the drug is given over a long period of time.

To ensure cooperation, children need preparation for topical administration but all discomfort can be eliminated by careful technique. A small child will need to be restrained to avoid sudden movements. To prevent the child from being able to taste eye drops, apply gentle pressure to the lacrimal punctum for 1 minute after administration to prevent the medication from draining into the nasopharynx. Ear drops should be allowed to warm to room temperature before being instilled, to prevent the discomfort and shock of cold fluid in the ear. The unpleasant sensation of nose drops trickling into the throat can be avoided by placing the child in a head downwards position (Figure 28.6).

Subcutaneous and intradermal injections

Insulin and hormone replacements are the drugs commonly given subcutaneously. These injections can be given wherever there is subcutaneous tissue, and the injection given with a short needle at an angle of 90° to avoid giving an intradermal injection. Pain is reduced by not injecting more than 0.5 ml fluid.

Intradermal injections are commonly used for local anaesthetics, or tuberculin or allergy testing. The preferred site is the forearm but the medial aspect should be avoided as this is the most sensitive. The needle should be $\frac{3}{8}$ to $\frac{1}{2}$ inch long and inserted at an angle of 10° to 15°.

Intramuscular injections

Most children are frightened of injections, which can often be painful. The use of intramuscular (IM) injections should be avoided in children and only given when there is no alternative route. A topical local anaesthetic can be given prior to the procedure (*see* Caring for children in pain p. 351) but these usually require some time to take effect. The use of ice or a freezing spray may be more appropriate, to reduce anticipatory fear.

The discomfort of IM injections can be minimised by selecting the most appropriate equipment and injection site. The needle length can be estimated by pinching a fold of lateralis or deltoid muscle between the thumb and index finger. The appropriate needle length is half the length between the finger and thumb in this position. Hicks *et al.* (1989) have shown that a 1-inch needle is necessary to penetrate the muscle in 4-month-old infants and Whaley and Wong (2002) suggest that 0.5–1-inch needles are necessary for most IM injections, with 1.5-inch needles used for injections into the gluteus maximus muscle in older children. Needle gauge should be the smallest that will deliver the drug safely, with the usual range being 22–25 gauge.

Injections must be given into muscles large enough to accept the amount of medication to be given (Figure 28.7). There is no research

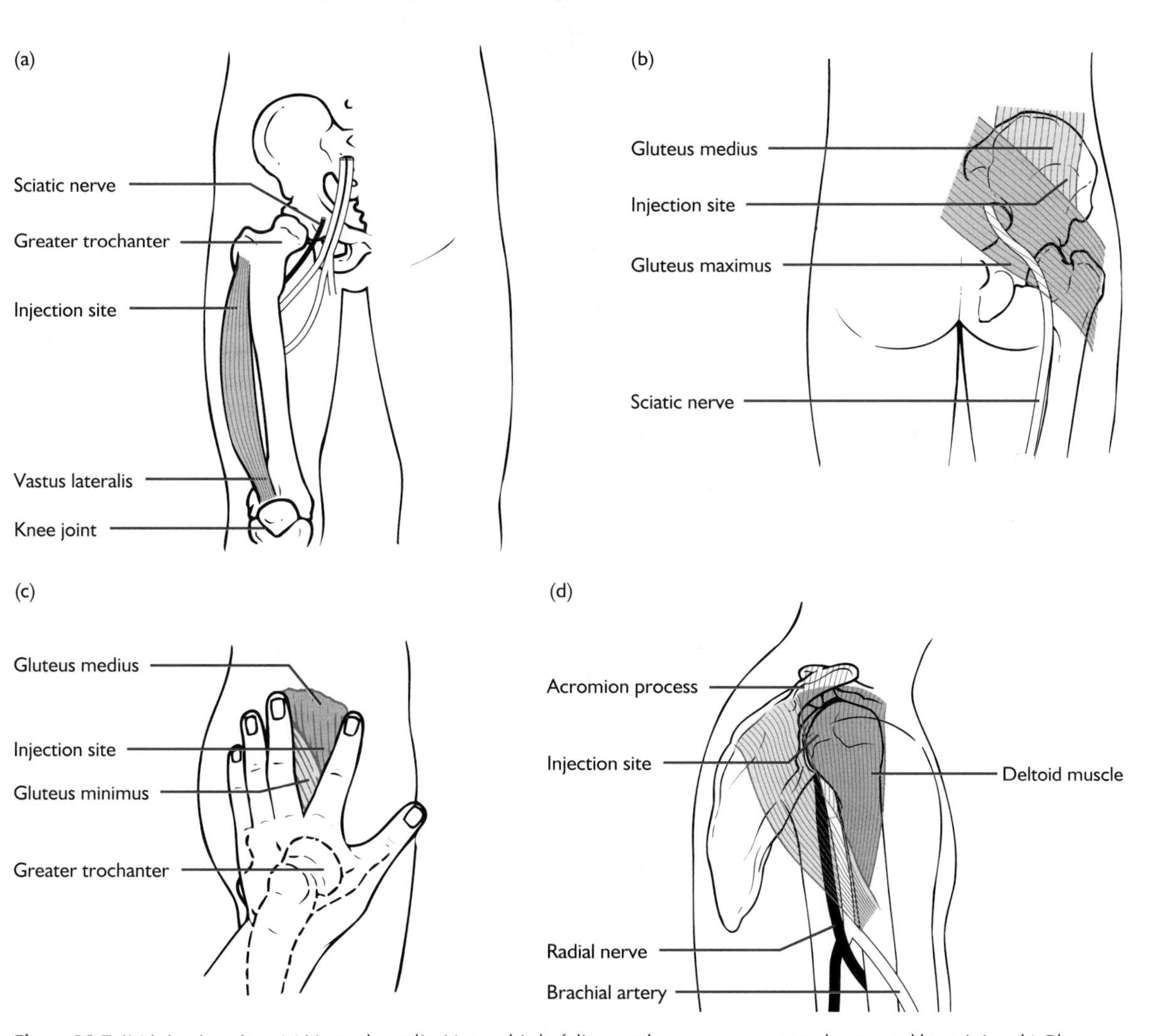

Figure 28.7 IM injection sites. (a) Vastus lateralis. Upper third of distance between greater trochanter and knee joint. (b) Gluteus maximus. Upper outer quadrant of buttock. (c) Gluteus medius. Centre of 'V' formed by index and middle finger when palm placed over greater trochanter. (d) Deltoid. Upper third of muscle which begins two finger breadths below acromion process.

to identify the optimum IM injection site for children but it is recommended that the gluteus maximus muscle should not be used until the child has been walking for at least a year, since this muscle only develops with locomotion. The preferred site for infants is usually the vastus lateralis but Beecroft and Reddick (1990) recommend the use of the gluteus medius muscle for all ages of child as it is a safe, easily accessible site and injections here are less painful than those given into the vastus lateralis muscle. This muscle can be located by placing the palm over the greater trochanter, the index finger over the anterior–superior iliac spine and the middle finger over the posterior iliac crest. The gluteus medius muscle is then between the V formed by the fingers. The deltoid muscle is also easily accessible and a relatively painless injection site and has the added advantage that medications injected here have a faster absorption rate. However, as it is a small muscle, only small volumes of fluid (0.5–1.0 ml) can be given.

Intramuscular injections can cause complications. Injections close to the sciatic nerve can cause permanent disability and repeated use of a site may result in fibrosis and contracture of the affected muscle. Unless the child is held securely, sudden movement once the injection is in progress can cause the needle shaft to break. Preparation for IM injections should be given briefly and immediately before the event. One nurse should hold the child gently but securely so that no movement of the chosen area is possible, and reduce discomfort by giving the child some distraction.

Intravenous injections

If a rapid action is required, the intravenous (IV) route will be chosen. The drug enters the bloodstream directly and a higher serum concentration is possible, allowing for a constant therapeutic effect if the drug is given regularly. However, there is a higher risk of complications for drugs administered by this route. There is a higher risk of toxicity, allergic reactions and, because the normal body protective systems are bypassed, infection. Mixing more than one drug in a syringe or infusion can lead to instability and precipitation, especially if those drugs or fluids contain calcium or magnesium or have very different pH values (for example, gentamicin and penicillin). Saline flushes should be given between two IV drugs and should also be used prior to IV administration to ensure venous access, and following the procedure to flush the cannula.

Drugs can be given IV by bolus, intermittent or continuous infusion. Bolus injections should generally be given over 2–3 minutes but some drugs (e.g. Tazocin) require a specific rate. If the drug is to be given by intermittent infusion, it is diluted in a specific volume of a specific fluid and infused over a given time using a syringe or infusion pump. A continuous infusion may be necessary if the drug has a short life in the body or when the clinical effect needs careful control by adjusting the infusion rate.

Intravenous drugs are mostly given for a short period via an intravenous cannula, but for a few children, who need venous access for a period of time, other devices may be more appropriate. If IV drugs are required for a week or more, a long line inserted into a major vein, usually the subclavian, is more appropriate than a short cannula inserted into a peripheral vein, which tends to become dislodged after 48–72

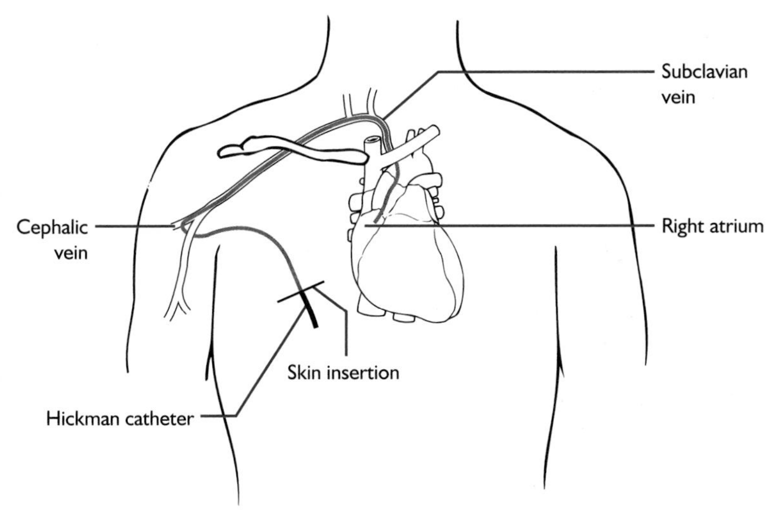

Figure 28.8 Hickman line.

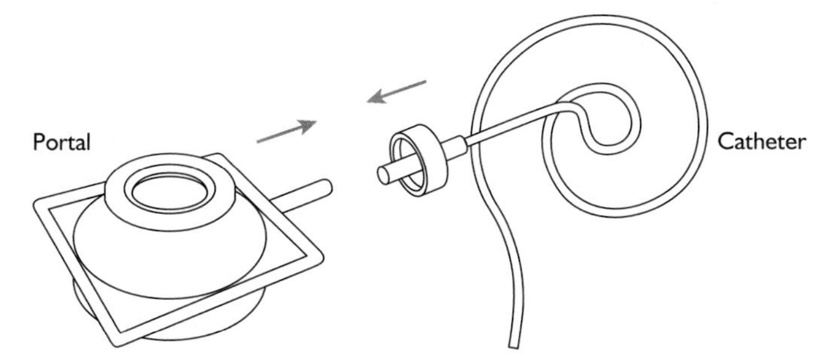

Figure 28.9 Port-a-cath. Portal is placed under the skin and sutured to the chest wall. The catheter is tunnelled as the Hickman line with the tip resting within a major vein or right atrium.

hours of use. Long lines are kept patent with the use of heparin after each episode of drug administration. Children with chronic health problems (cystic fibrosis, leukaemia) who need long-term IV drug therapy usually have either an indwelling central venous catheter (Broviac or Hickman, see Figure 28.8) or an implanted infusion port (Mediport, Port-a-cath, see Figure 28.9). Special care must be taken when administering drugs by these routes to avoid infection and clotting (*see also* Uses, risks, principles of care and advantages and disadvantages of central venous devices pp. 347–50).

Study activity

What would be the most appropriate route of drug administration for the following children?

- Tom, aged 4, who is vomiting post-operatively after repair of an inguinal hernia and is complaining of pain.
- Lucy, aged 6, who has cystic fibrosis, needs to achieve long-term control of her repeated chest infections.

Checking Drugs

Before checking the drug to be administered, the nurse should ensure that the appropriate drug has been prescribed correctly.

Study activity

What should the nurse check to ensure that the prescription is correct?

The prescription should be legible and written in a way that complies with local policy. The nurse should check that the drug is suitable for the individual child's age and condition, and that the dosage and the route is appropriate.

Study activity

Having decided that the prescription is correct, what precautions should the nurse now take to ensure the administration is carried out safely?

The nurse is responsible for ensuring that the correct child receives the correct dose of the correct medication at the correct time and by the correct route. Most hospital drug policies state that two nurses must check and administer all drugs to children, but in certain circumstances it may be permissible for named nurses to give specified drugs on their own. Before dispensing the drug, the details of the prescription should be double-checked against the details of the bottle or vial. The expiry date of the drug should be checked as well as any special instructions (for example, to be given with food). Finally the child's identity should be checked by comparing the hospital identification band with the prescription chart. The child may prefer a parent to give the medication, but the nurse is responsible for ensuring that the drug is taken.

Parental Education

Study activity

Consider what parents may need to know about their child's medication before going home.

Parents will need to know the reasons for the medication being prescribed as well as the likely effects of the drug. They need to know the amount, frequency and length of time of the drug's administration. They may need to know how to measure up the drug and how best to give it to their child. They may need help to organise a schedule which best fits into their home routine. This advice and teaching is ideally performed before discharge to give parents time to assimilate the information and practise new skills.

Needle Phobia

Needle phobia is the term used to describe an anticipatory fear of needles that results in such high levels of fear and distress that a procedure might have to be postponed or abandoned. Some anxiety is experienced by at least 80% of preschool children and over 50% of primary school children (Humphrey *et al.*, 1992). Negative experiences may affect the child's future behaviour when faced with the procedure again but the parents' fears and anxieties may also be conveyed to the child (Smalley, 1999). Modern medicine is increasingly reliant on blood tests and cannulation prior to IV drugs or fluids so it is important to overcome any fears around venepuncture (Gaskell *et al.*, 2005). Thurgate and Heppell (2005) describe the successful implementation of a three-step approach to preparing needle-phobic children for needle procedures: relaxation, control and graded exposure.

Summary

Drug administration is not a role to be taken lightly. The children's nurse needs to have a good understanding of drugs to be able to administer them safely and accurately. Doctors outside the paediatric team often have little experience of prescribing drugs for children and the nurse should be alert to recognise any prescriptions that appear inaccurate. For this reason, drugs should be given by qualified children's nurses with appropriate knowledge and experience, whenever possible. The administration of IV drugs is usually considered to be outside the usual scope of nursing practice, and nurses should ensure that they gain the additional knowledge and skills required for this role before accepting accountability and responsibility for it.

Key Points

1. Children's immature body systems and wide variations in age, weight and body surface cause them to be at risk from medication.
2. Children's nurses need to be skilled at promoting compliance for each individual child.
3. Children's nurses have a professional responsibility to be aware of the appropriate medication and dosage for each child for whom they are caring.
4. Some drugs, used commonly in the treatment of adults, are contra-indicated for use in children.
5. Children's nurses should be aware of the different routes for medication and be able to identify the most appropriate route for the children in their care.
6. Children's nurses need to be able to explain the purpose and the administration of medication to the child and the family if compliance is to be maintained.

Chapter 29

Providing Nutrition

Introduction

Effects of protein and energy malnutrition for children

- Growth deviations
- Development delay
- Mental retardation (infants)
- Muscle atrophy
- Gastrointestinal disturbances
- Reduced resistance to infection
- Behavioural changes (irritability, apathy, lethargy)
- Delayed puberty

Childhood diseases can often be complicated by poor nutrition. Babies with respiratory problems may find it difficult to suck; ill toddlers and small children often suffer from accompanying anorexia. Older children may be fussy eaters and this fussiness may be exacerbated by illness. The disease process may prevent adequate nutrition. As a result of any of these situations the child may be unable to consume, absorb or use sufficient energy and nutrients to grow.

Providing adequate nutrition for sick children is a challenge for children's nurses. Recent surveys appear to suggest that this challenge is not always recognised or responded to. These studies reveal that children can actually suffer from malnutrition while in hospital (Moy *et al.*, 1990; Cross *et al.*, 1995). Protein and energy malnutrition have serious effects for children who are still growing and developing.

Study activity

Consider the reasons why children may not be able to consume, absorb or utilise energy and nutrients.

Mechanical problems which prevent normal sucking, chewing and swallowing prevent children from being able to consume sufficient energy and nutrients. An adequate intake is also impaired by respiratory and cardiac problems as the child is unable to breathe and eat simultaneously. Anorexia, which may be the result of chronic illness or a psychological problem, will also prevent an adequate intake.

Metabolic disorders prevent the absorption and utilisation of nutrients, as do problems of the digestive tract resulting in protracted vomiting or chronic diarrhoea. Some children have increased metabolic rate and require increased energy and nutrients. In such cases nutritional support may be implemented to meet these additional needs. When children are unable to maintain an adequate oral intake of energy and nutrients, support must be provided enterally or parenterally.

Booth (1991) recommends careful evaluation of the need for enteral or parenteral nutrition as an alternative to oral feeding, because resistance to normal feeding results from any long-term feeding method that bypasses the mouth. This evaluation should consider whether the child is:

- unable to consume high energy supplements to maintain an adequate energy intake
- demonstrating severe and worsening effects of protein and energy malnutrition
- exhibiting a downward growth deviation

Enteral feeding can be defined as any method of providing nutrition using the gastro-intestinal tract. It includes the oral route as well as the alternative methods of naso-gastric, gastrostomy and jejunostomy feeding.

Parenteral nutrition is also known as intravenous (IV) alimentation or hyperalimentation, involving IV infusion of highly concentrated solutions of protein, glucose and other nutrients. It is used to maintain the nutritional needs of those children in whom it is impossible to use the gastro-intestinal route.

Reasons why children cannot maintain an adequate oral intake of energy and nutrients

REDUCED INTAKE

Mechanical problems

- gastro-oesophageal reflux
- mental retardation/unconsciousness
- oro-facial injuries/malformation
- tracheo-oesophageal fistula

Breathlessness on feeding

- respiratory problems
- cardiac failure

REDUCED ABSORPTION

- chronic diarrhoea
- glycogen storage disorder
- short bowel syndrome

FAILURE OF UTILISATION

Increased requirements

- cystic fibrosis
- metabolic disorders
- chronic infection

Food intolerance

- reduced appetite
- chronic illness
- malignancy
- anorexia nervosa

Oral Feeding

Once a child has been identified as having poor nutrition it is useful to obtain a full dietary history. Remember that poor nutrition can result in obesity as well as decreased weight gain.

Study activity

Consider the information you would need to obtain a detailed picture of the child's dietary and feeding routines.

Careful questioning of the family is required to establish a child's dietary and feeding routines. It does not just involve information about the child's exact intake. It is also important to discover times and places of meals and snacks and the family's involvement in these feeding routines. Failure to meet nutritional needs may not be related to an organic cause. Psychosocial factors may be the only reason for poor nutritional intake and should be excluded before investigations for organic problems.

Study activity

Think about the psychological factors that could lead to a child having inadequate nutrition.

Poor nutritional intake – psychosocial factors

Poverty

- insufficient food
- cheap foodstuffs, low in nutrients

Health beliefs

- fad diets
- excessive concern with health

Nutritional ignorance

- cultural confusion
- lack of parental dietary knowledge
- immature, inexperienced parents

Psychological stress

- emotional deprivation
- family dysfunction
- maternal depression
- school, peer pressures
- need for attention

Lack of feeding pattern

- inconsistent meals, snack routines
- inconsistent carers

When the dietary history is completed it is possible to analyse the child's nutritional intake with dietary reference values and estimated average requirements for age and sex. The history will also provide information about the family's beliefs and routines in relation to food.

Janes (1996) believes that in the majority of situations the problem may be overcome by adapting the child's usual diet to include high-energy and nutritious versions. Snacks between meals will provide extra calories. It is important that families understand the rationale for such interventions, which contradict usual healthy eating advice.

If such interventions do not lead to a sufficient increase in energy requirements, additional dietary supplements may be used. As far as possible the child should always be enabled to maintain the usual feeding routine so that this normality is not lost. To ensure that the normal routines can be maintained, supplements should be given at a time when the appetite for a meal is not suppressed, for example at bedtime.

In some situations, parents may also require advice about the management of their children's eating habits. When a child's eating habits become the focus of attention the child can use this to manipulate the situation. The child then becomes in control and will only eat certain foods at chosen times.

Study activity

Think about your own meal times. What factors may help or hinder a child's eating habits?

Enteral Feeding

Naso-gastric feeding

Infants and children can be fed by naso-gastric tube for years (Holden *et al.*, 1996). A polyvinyl, silicone or polyurethane tube is passed into the stomach via the nose. It can be left in place after feeding or removed and reinserted before each feed. The main disadvantages of this route of feeding are psychological. The insertion of the tube is usually very distressing for the child and family as well as the nurse. When the tube is left *in situ* the child and family can become upset by the attention it attracts in others.

Naso-gastric tubes are chosen according to the child and the frequency and length of time required for an alternative method of feeding. Polyvinyl tubes quickly lose their flexibility when in contact with gastric secretions and need to be changed at least weekly. Polyurethane and silicone tubes do not harden, but their softness and flexibility make them more difficult to insert and easier for the child to dislodge. Their small lumen makes them unsuitable for use with thick feeds (Table 29.1).

The length of tube is usually estimated by measuring from the nose to the bottom of the earlobe and then to the end of the xiphoid process. Ellet *et al.* (1992) suggest that using the child's height is a more reliable way to judge the distance from nose to stomach.

Table 29.1 Principles of tube feeding

Principle	Rationale
Check placement of tube and flush with sterile water	To ensure tube is in stomach
Warm feed to room temperature	To prevent discomfort and maintain body temperature
Allow feed to flow into stomach by gravity at a rate of 5 ml/5 minutes for infants and 10 ml/1 minute for children	To prevent nausea, ingestion and regurgitation
Replace aspirate in infants	To prevent electrolyte imbalance
Flush the tube with sterile water	To clear the tube and encourage patency

Study activity

Consider how you could check the correct placement of a naso-gastric tube and check your local procedure for the recommended method in your area of work.

Care must be taken when inserting a naso-gastric tube to ensure it passes into the oesophagus and stomach and not into the bronchial tree. Naso-gastric tubes can also become displaced after insertion. For this reason it is essential to check the placement of the tube before and after each feed. In 2005 the National Patient Safety Agency alerted all NHS organisations that conventional methods for checking naso-gastric tube placements could be inaccurate. They cited 11 deaths and one case of serious harm over the previous 2 years.

Aspiration of gastric contents has always been accepted as a safe method of checking tube placement, but Metheny (1998) suggests that stomach contents can be mistaken for respiratory secretions. However, Metheny *et al.* (1989) found that respiratory, gastric and intestinal secretions all had different pH values and that pH testing of aspirate (rather than simply testing for acidity or alkalinity) correctly identified the whereabouts of the tube in about 80% of cases. If the tube is correctly placed, the aspirate will have a pH of 5.5 or below. Some medications will affect pH and the nurse should be alert to these, especially if the aspirate consistently has a pH of over 6.0.

When there is no aspirate it is difficult to ascertain whether the tube is displaced or the stomach is empty. A small amount of air injected into the tube results in gurgling on auscultation. However, it is possible to hear this when the tube is sitting at the cardiac sphincter of the stomach. In addition, copious respiratory secretions can transmit sound to the epigastric area. Therefore this method of testing placement is now banned.

If doubt exists about the correct placement of the tube, X-rays should be taken. This is obviously not practical before each feed or when naso-gastric feeding occurs at home. There are several ways to manage the situation when there is no aspirate:

Additional dietary supplements

Glucose polymer
- Amount of nutrient: 15 g carbohydrate per 100 ml
- EXAMPLES: MAXIJUL POLYCAL and CALOREEN
- USE: Add to soups, drinks and desserts
- Available on prescription: YES

Glucose drinks
- Amount of nutrient: 30 g glucose per 100 ml
- EXAMPLES: HYCAL and LIQUID MAXIJUL
- USE: Dilute with water or squash
- Available on prescription: YES

Milk shake drinks
1. Amount of nutrient: l kcal/ml
   EXAMPLES: 200 ml CARTONS: FRESUBIN
   USE: Ready made drinks in various flavours
   Available on prescription: YES
2. Amount of nutrient: 1.5 kcal/ml
   EXAMPLES: 200 ml CARTONS: FORTISIP and ENSURE PLUS
   USE: Ready made drinks in various flavours
   Available on prescription: YES

Fortified juice drinks
- Amount of nutrient: 1.25 kcal/ml
- EXAMPLES: 200 ml CARTONS: PROVIDE and FORTIJUCE
- USE: Ready made drinks in various flavours
- Available on prescription: YES

Fortified puddings
- Amount of nutrient: 250 kcal/142 g
- EXAMPLES: FORMANCE and FORTIPUDDING
- USE: Ready made mousse style pudding
- Available on prescription: YES

Milk shake products
- Amount of nutrient: 4.5–5.0 kcal/mg
- EXAMPLES: BUILD UP and COMPLAN
- USE: Added to milk
- Available on prescription: NO

Behavioural management of nutritional problems

- Establish regular meal times
- Offer snacks only as a complement to meals
- Make meal times a social, family event
- Praise eating successes, ignore poor eating
- Ensure meal times are free of distractions
- Maintain calm and peaceful environment for meals
- Avoid force-feeding

Disadvantages of indwelling naso-gastric tubes

- Aspiration
- Gastric perforation
- Nasal airway obstruction
- Ulceration/irritation of mucous membranes
- Epistaxis
- Displacement into bronchial tree
- Embarrassment about appearance

- turn the child onto the side
- inject 1–5 ml air into the tube using a 20 ml or 50 ml syringe
- wait for 15 minutes to 30 minutes
- advance the tube by 1–2 cm

Feeding should not commence if there is any uncertainty about the placement of the tube. The NPSA produced a parent and carer briefing sheet in 2005, which should be given to all carers involved in naso-gastric feeding.

Nurses need to be aware of the shortcomings of existing methods of checking tube position, and that this is a significant disadvantage of this method of feeding.

Naso-jejunal feeding

For some children naso-jejunal feeding is more appropriate than the naso-gastric route. The tube is passed via the nose into the stomach and time is allowed for gastric emptying to enable it to pass through the pylorus. This can be aided by positioning the child on the right side or by medication that increases gastric emptying.

The position of the tube is then checked by radiography by performing abdominal postero-anterior and lateral X-rays. Naso-jejunal tubes can return spontaneously to the stomach and before feeding the position must be confirmed by checking the pH of the alkaline aspirate.

The naso-jejunal route minimises the aspiration risk of naso-gastric feeding but many of the other disadvantages of naso-gastric tube feeding still apply. In addition, abdominal pain and diarrhoea can occur with bolus feeding because the stomach's natural reservoir and anti-infective properties are bypassed.

Gastrostomy feeding

Feeding via a gastrostomy tube is used for children who require a long-term means of complementary feeding to increase energy and nutrient intake (for example, children with cystic fibrosis) or whose anatomy does not allow the passage of a tube through the mouth, pharynx or oesophagus (for example, children with oesophageal atresia). A contra-indication to gastrostomy feeding is gastro-oesophageal reflux, which may be exacerbated by feeding directly into the stomach (Table 29.2).

A gastrostomy tube is inserted surgically or percutaneously into an opening through the abdominal wall giving direct access into the stomach. Both these procedures are carried out under general anaesthetic for children. There are many different types of tube for gastrostomy feeding but the main types are balloon catheters and button devices. Balloon catheters have a balloon at the distal end, which is inflated with a prescribed amount of water and pulled up against the wall of the stomach thus maintaining its position as well as preventing the leakage of gastric contents into the peritoneum. The sterile water in the balloon should be changed weekly, checking that no leakage has occurred and that the balloon is still patent. Some of these catheters have a securing device that lies flush against the skin to prevent excessive traction on the tube causing soreness and widening of the opening. If such a device is absent, the tube should be taped securely on to the surface of the abdomen.

Table 29.2 Gastrostomy tube replacement (balloon catheters)

Method	Rationale
Loosen securing device	To free catheter
Stabilise site and gently pull catheter out	To minimise trauma to the stoma
Clean and dry site	To avoid entry of bacteria
Lubricate tip of replacement tube	To facilitate entry
Guide tube through stoma to a depth of 1–1.5 inches	To ensure tube reaches stomach
Inflate balloon with sterile water (amount prescribed by manufacturer) and pull up until resistance is felt	To ensure balloon fits snugly against stomach opening to prevent leakage of gastric contents
Slide locking disc down tube until snug against abdominal wall	To prevent undue friction of tube

Button devices can be inserted via percutaneous endoscopic gastrostomy (PEG), usually after an established tract has been created. Button devices are better in appearance than balloon catheters as the button is positioned at skin level and no tubing is visible, but they are more expensive than balloon catheters. These devices incorporate a one-way valve at the proximal end, which prevents the leakage of gastric juices when the button is open. However, if displacement occurs they require a general anaesthetic for replacement, whereas balloon catheters can be replaced immediately.

Because of the danger of displacement of the tube, its position should be checked before feeding. Gastric fluid should be easily aspirated and its acidity can be checked with litmus paper. Displacement into the peritoneum or duodenum will make the tube difficult to aspirate and will cause abdominal pain, vomiting and diarrhoea. Gastrostomy tubes can be accidentally removed and should be replaced within 4–6 hours or spontaneous closure of the stoma will occur. Blockage of the tube can be avoided or overcome by flushing the tube with lemonade or inserting a pancreatic enzyme solution. Any artificial material inserted into the body can cause irritation and inflammation. Localised infection can occur around the gastrostomy site unless it is kept clean and dry. Granulation of tissue around the stoma can also lead to infection.

Jejunostomy feeding

Jejunal feeds are administered via a jejunostomy (surgical incision through the abdominal wall into the jejunum). Such feeding is necessary for children with severe reflux, in whom other methods of enteral feeding would carry a significant risk of reflux and aspiration. However, because this method of feeding bypasses the reservoir and anti-infective functions of the stomach, there is always a risk of gastro-intestinal infection and an aseptic technique and sterile feeds should always be used. The lack of a reservoir function of the jejunum means that feeds should be given continuously, as bolus feeds by this route can cause abdominal distension and diarrhoea. The tube should be flushed every 4 hours to prevent blockage, stasis and infection. As with other methods of enteral feeding, the tube can become dislodged and its position should be checked prior to feeding by using blue litmus paper to verify the alkalinity of the aspirate.

Parenteral Feeding

Total parenteral nutrition (TPN)

Total parenteral nutrition is usually administered via an established central venous or long line into a central vein with a high blood flow. It is used to maintain nutrition for children who are unable to use their gastro-intestinal tract to ingest and/or absorb their nutritional needs. It can be used as a long-term treatment for children with structural gastro-intestinal anomalies, such as short bowel syndrome, or as a temporary measure to allow an inflamed or diseased gastro-intestinal tract to rest and heal (necrotising enterocolitis, Crohn's disease).

Parenteral nutrition solutions mainly consist of glucose and amino acids. Electrolytes, vitamins, minerals and trace elements can be added according to individual need. Lipids may also be given as a separate solution. The exact amount of nutrients will be calculated according to the individual child's growth pattern, health problem and age (Table 29.3). High concentrations of glucose (over 12.5%) are very irritating to vessels and therefore need to be infused into wide-diameter veins, which have sufficient blood volume and pressure to enable rapid dilution and absorption. However, it is possible to use lipids as the main source of calories and these, together with dilute glucose and amino acid solutions, can be infused into peripheral veins. In principle, the care of children undergoing TPN is the same as the care of any intravenous therapy, but the result of any complication is potentially more severe because major vessels are being used. Major problems can result from displacement of the central catheter or long line. Central catheters can migrate into the right ventricle, causing cardiac dysrhythmias, and haemothorax or pneumothorax can be caused by migration of a subclavian catheter.

There are also potential problems caused by the content of the infusate. The high concentration of glucose in TPN solutions makes it an excellent medium for bacterial growth. In addition, this high level of glucose can cause hyperglycaemia, and the rate of the infusion must be gradually increased to allow the child's natural production of insulin to accommodate this change in glucose load. Sudden changes in the rate of infusion can cause hyperglycaemia or hypoglycaemia and the child

Complications of TPN

- Infection
- Hepatic dysfunction
- Hyperglycaemia
- Hypoglycaemia
- Hypomagnesaemia
- Hyperlipidaemia
- Acidosis
- Trace element deficiencies
- Cardiac dysrhythmias
- Air or fat emboli
- Phlebitis
- Tissue necrosis
- Liver failure
- Migration of central catheter/long line

Table 29.3 Guidelines for providing daily TPN for children

Amino acids	1.5–3.0 g/kg
Glucose	20–30 g/kg
Lipids	20–30 g/kg
Potassium	2–4 mEq/kg
Sodium	3–8 mEq/kg

should be observed for features of these conditions. Acidosis can occur in vulnerable children if immature or diseased kidneys cannot excrete all the ammonia created by the breakdown of amino acids. Trace element deficiencies are common in neonates or children receiving long-term TPN. The infusion of lipids creates the risk of fat emboli when prolonged contact with the amino-acid solution causes emulsification. To minimise this risk, lipid solutions are usually joined to the amino-acid infusion at the nearest point to the infusion entry site.

Some children develop reactions to lipid infusions and complain of breathlessness, nausea, headache, dizziness, chest or back pain. Lipids bind with albumin to displace bilirubin and cannot be given to children with known liver disease. Cholestatic jaundice is a common complication of long-term TPN and raises ethical issues about using TPN to maintain nutrition in children with no functional gastro-intestinal tract, although at present the alternative of gastro-intestinal tract transplant is not widely available or successful. Increased serum conjugated bilirubin results in bile-duct proliferation and bile stasis, eventually causing liver failure.

Study activity

From the information given above, draw up a plan of care for a child receiving TPN.

Principles of Providing Enteral or Parenteral Nutrition

There are certain common principles of care when providing enteral or parenteral nutrition. Whatever the feeding route, the aims of care are to:

- facilitate adequate nutrition
- enable desired growth and development
- maintain the child's safety during the period of alternative feeding
- maximise normal lifestyle
- enable the child and family to manage the feeding

The dietician should be involved in planning feeds that provide the correct amount of energy and nutrients to ensure that the child can reach and maintain average growth parameters (Table 29.4). Regular developmental assessments should be performed to monitor development; Booth (1991) found that gross motor and language skills are most likely to be delayed in children undergoing alternative methods of feeding. If oral feeding is not possible, babies should be given a dummy to enable them to associate sucking with feeding and encourage oro-motor skills. Holden *et al.* (1996) advocate the use of oral feeds whenever possible to enable the development of chewing and swallowing. The speech therapist and physiotherapist will advise on facial movements to develop the muscles involved with chewing and speech.

The nurse and family should be aware of the likely problems and complications of the chosen method of feeding and how to deal with and recognise these. Bacterial contamination of enteral feeds prepared

Care of children requiring TPN

Prevention of infection

- aseptic technique for: preparation of solutions, changing bags and giving sets, and changing occlusive dressing site
- infuse solutions via micropore filter
- change bags and giving sets every 24 hours
- perform routine blood cultures
- observe infusion site for erythema or exudate
- record 4-hourly temperature, pulse and respirations

Prevention of vascular injury

- monitor site hourly for extravasation, phlebitis
- infuse using electronic pump to enable constant rate of infusion
- monitor rate hourly
- do not increase rate if infusion behind time
- avoid air embolus or haemorrhage by ensuring connections are secure
- maintain line patency with heparin if intermittent TPN

Prevention of electrolyte and glucose imbalance

- check solutions with daily prescription before administration
- measure blood glucose 2–4-hourly
- test urinary glucose, ketones, protein and pH 4-hourly
- do not stop infusion suddenly
- monitor for hypoglycaemia if TPN stopped
- weekly checks of serum magnesium, phosphate and calcium
- weigh daily
- record strict intake and output chart

Table 29.4 Nutrient requirements of normal children (adapted from DH, 1991b)

Age	Energy (kcal/kg/day)	Protein (g/kg/day)
0–6 months	115	2.2
6–12 months	95	2.0
1–3 years	95	1.8
4–6 years	90	1.5
7–10 years	75	1.2
11–14 years	55–65	1.0
15–18 years	40–60	0.8

at home is common (Anderton *et al.*, 1993) and parents need to be taught how to avoid this. Bags of feed should not be allowed to hang for more than 6 hours and pre-prepared feeds should be kept refrigerated for no more than 24 hours. If children are having enteral feeds overnight, they should be positioned in bed with the head end raised to encourage gastric emptying and minimise the risk of aspiration. To minimise their different lifestyle, children having bolus feeds should have feeds at family meal times and be allowed to sit at the table with the family. They should be involved with normal family activities as much as possible. School-age children can often attend school as usual, with the school nurse or family member administering a bolus feed at lunchtime. If oral feeding is continued, the child should be involved in the choice of complementary foods and/or drinks. Children unable to have an oral intake should be encouraged to brush their teeth and rinse their mouths regularly to avoid infection of the oral mucous membranes caused by lack of saliva. Total parenteral feeding further dries mucous membranes because of the hyperosmolarity of the infusate (*see also* Dental hygiene p. 181).

Family Teaching and Home Care

When alternative feeding is required for a long period of time the family may wish to learn the necessary techniques to enable them to continue care at home. The decision to continue treatment at home should be a joint decision between parents and nursing, medical and dietetic staff.

Study activity

Consider what criteria you would use to determine the appropriateness of any family for managing enteral or parenteral feeding at home.

Casey (1988a) describes the role of the children's nurse as one who provides family care as well as nursing care, and also acts as a teacher, supporter and resource person. In the preparation for home feeding the nurse will use all these roles. The nurse can show the family how to adapt usual family care and routines to incorporate the chosen method of feeding, as well as demonstrating the specific nursing care required.

The family will need teaching about the specific feeding method and its complications, and will require support to come to terms with providing such care at home (Figure 29.1). Planned support should be available from community or hospital staff with written advice available for schools. The family will also be grateful for advice about other resources available to them. A social worker may be able to help with financial allowances and a list of parenteral support groups such as Half PINNT, a sub-group of Patients receiving Intravenous and Naso-gastric Nutrition Therapy (PINNT).

Patient name .... Hosp No .... Ward ....

Named name .... Dietitian ....

Goal	Demo/ Discuss (date)	Comments Sign
When discharged from hospital the patient or carer will know:		
• The principles of normal gastro-intestinal tract function and how this has changed for the individual patient		
• The principles of enteral nutrition		
• How to set up a feed using an enteral infusion pump*		
• How to manage a pump and its alarms*		
• Negotiate appropriate equipment for home with dietitian and Nutrition Nurse Specialist		
• Ayliffe's handwashing technique		
• Aseptic preparation of feed		
• Correct hang time for feed		
• Correct use of enteral feed sets, adaptors and syringes		
• Prevention, recognition and action to take in the event of: – infection of the gastro-intestinal tract – infection of the stoma site – chest infection (aspiration of feed) – occlusion of tube – misplacement of tube – malfunction of tube		
• How to irrigate a blocked tube		
• How to change or repair the tube as appropriate		
• How to store enteral feeds and equipment and how they will be delivered		
• The names and telephone numbers of healthcare professionals available to provide advice 24 hours a day		

Figure 29.1 Home enteral feeding learning goals.

Goal	Demo/ Discuss	Comments	
• Of the existence (including name, telephone number) of a patient support gruop e.g. PINNT or the paediatric subgroup of PINNT (Half PINNT)			
• The follow-up arrangements – NNS dietitian consultant			
• The social security benefits to which he/she may be entitled (refer to Medical Social Worker if appropriate)			
The patient/carer (e.g. parent or guardian in the case of a child) will be able to:		*Practice under supervision*	*Practice unprompted*
• Check the tube position			
• Secure the tube adequately			
• Prepare the feed ready for administration			
• Connect the feed to the feeding tube			
• Programme the feeding pump for continuous feeding*			
• Administer a bolus feed down the tube*			
• Administer medications down the tube			
• Disconnect the feed and flush water down the tube			
• Contact the appropriate health professional when necessary			
** delete as necessary*			
The patient or carer will state or indicate that he/she feels:	*Discuss*	*Comments*	
• Confident in his/her ability to self-care or in the ability of a carer			
• That expression of physical, emotional or social discomfort, when shared with the hospital staff, will be treated with respect and an appropriate intervention			
• Trust in his/her General Practitioner's knowledge of home enteral tube feeding (HETF)			
• That he/she is one of many patients receiving HETF in the United Kingdom			

Figure 29.1 *(continued)*

Study activity

Compare one child's nutritional intake for 24 hours while in hospital and at home. Compare your findings with Table 29.4 to assess whether these intakes meet recommended energy and protein requirements.

Key Points

1. Sick children do not always receive adequate nutrition in hospital.
2. Inadequate intake of nutrition and energy causes mental and physical problems for growing children.
3. Careful evaluation should be made before commencing alternative methods of feeding.
4. The advantages and disadvantages of the different methods of enteral feeding should be explained to the child and/or family before any choice is made.
5. The chosen alternative method of feeding should enable the child to carry out as normal a lifestyle as possible.
6. The use of TPN as a long-term method of feeding involves ethical decision making.
7. Home enteral or parenteral feeding needs careful preparation and teaching.

Chapter 30

Maintaining Fluid Balance

Introduction

Fluid balance is the term used to mean that the various body compartments contain the required amount of water for the body's needs. Because electrolytes are dissolved in body fluids it is impossible to separate fluid balance from electrolyte balance.

Water is the largest single constituent of the body, the actual percentage of total body weight varying with the age and fat content of the body. An infant has the highest proportion of water compared with body weight. This fact, together with the inability of the physiologically immature small child to react to changes in fluid intake and output, make the maintenance of fluid balance crucial in the care of children.

The main sources of fluid intake are ingested fluids and food and that produced by energy released from chemical reactions within the body. The main routes of fluid output are the skin and the renal, gastrointestinal and respiratory systems. Dehydration resulting in sensations of thirst controls fluid intake, while fluid output is mostly under hormonal control (*see also* Body water p. 67).

Daily fluid requirements

Adults

2500 ml/day

Children

1–10 kg	100 ml/kg
11–20 kg	1000 ml + 50 ml/kg per kg over 10 kg
>20 kg	1500 ml + 20 ml/kg per kg over 20 kg

Study activity

Infants and small children have a greater need for water and are more vulnerable than adults to fluid and electrolyte imbalances. Consider why this is so.

Insensible fluid losses are controlled by heat, humidity, body temperature and respiratory rate. An immature hypothalamus makes children unable to regulate body temperature until about 5 years of age. Until this age body temperature responds readily to changes in environmental temperature and increases with any activity. Infections cause a more rapid and higher increase in temperature than in adults. For each degree of temperature above the norm, the basal metabolic rate increases by 10% with a corresponding increase in the need for extra fluid.

Whaley and Wong (2002) estimate that the surface area in relation to weight of the premature neonate is five times greater than that of an adult and that the newborn has a surface area two to three times greater. This allows a greater proportion of fluid to be lost by insensible means. In addition, infants lose a greater proportion of fluid via the gastro-intestinal tract, which is proportionally longer than in the adult. The larger surface area of the growing child results in a high metabolic rate which creates a greater amount of waste for excretion by the kidneys. Unfortunately, these organs are not fully efficient in childhood and cannot concentrate or dilute urine according to the body's need for water.

Dehydration is a common problem in babies and small children and occurs whenever the total output of fluid exceeds the total intake. This can occur as a result of a decreased intake or an increased output. Such disturbances occur more often and more rapidly than in adults and small children are not able to adapt to these changes as readily as adults. Therefore one of the most important aspects of caring for sick children is maintaining an accurate record of fluid balance.

Measuring Fluid Balance

Study activity

List the situations when it would be important to record fluid balance for a sick child.

If an accurate fluid balance record is to be kept it is important to measure all intake and output. This may not be easy with children who have not learnt to control any elimination. Urine collection bags can be used but frequent application and removal may cause excoriation of the skin. Nappies can be weighed before and after use and the amount of urine passed estimated by the difference in weight. (The volume of fluid in millilitres is equal to the weight in milligrams.) However, this method has disadvantages. If stool is mixed with urine it is impossible to be accurate about the type of loss, and additional losses may occur because of evaporation and/or leakage. Any other form of output (vomit, wound drainage, naso-gastric aspirate) must also be measured and recorded. If a child's only intake is fluid this can be easily measured but it is not easy to estimate the amount of fluid in a mixed diet. Because of the difficulties in ensuring the accuracies of all intake and output measurements a daily weight is often the preferred method of determining fluid balance. This also has potential problems. To ensure accuracy, the scales should be regularly serviced and the child weighed at the same time of day in the same clothing (*see also* Weighing children and babies p. 285).

Older children may like to help in the recording of fluid balance and may enjoy recording details or drawing pictures of their intake. They and their parents should be reminded of the importance of saving all excreta for measurement. Parents may be happy to keep records of intake and output.

Restricted Intake

Children with renal problems or following surgery to the gastro-intestinal tract may need a restricted intake. Children having surgery or certain investigations may need a period of time with no intake. Such restrictions pose a challenge for the children's nurse as many children may be too young to appreciate the reasons for the restrictions or may simply forget that they have been told not to have anything to eat or drink. Periods of starvation before surgery or investigations should be kept to a minimum. Children can easily become dehydrated or hypoglycaemic if left for too long without fluid or food, but many studies show that children are sometimes starved for unnecessary lengths of time (While and Crawford, 1992a). Most research indicates that the maximum starvation period for food or milk is 6 hours but that juice or glucose drinks can be given up to 2 hours before a general anaesthetic (Meakin *et al.*, 1987; Splinter and Schaeffer, 1990).

Study activity

Look at your hospital policy for the pre-operative fasting of children and critically evaluate it in relation to the above research findings.

To inform others about restrictions a notice needs to be attached to the child and many children enjoy wearing a special badge. Drinks and sweets should be removed from the bedside to help the child avoid temptation. Small children need close attention as their thirst may cause them to drink straight from the tap or to take another child's drink. Children who are starved for a longer period post-operatively will have intravenous fluids to overcome dehydration and hypoglycaemia but this will not prevent the discomfort of being unable to eat or drink. In these situations the mouth should be kept clean and moist and lip salve applied to prevent the lips from cracking. A dry mouth may also pose a problem for children on restricted intake. These children have the additional difficulty of trying to eke out their allotted amount of fluid throughout the day and often need help to do this and not drink the whole amount in the morning leaving nothing for later.

Study activity

Think out a strategy to help a 5-year-old child maintain a restriction of 500 ml fluid/day without becoming too distressed or uncomfortable.

Intravenous Fluid Therapy

Children with problems maintaining fluid and electrolyte balance are often given intravenous (IV) fluids. Livesley (1993) suggests that specific guidelines are needed for the management of IV fluids in the treatment of children because of the unique problems. To maintain the child's safety during IV therapy the nurse should be aware of all the associated risks and their prevention.

Site and equipment

In most children the IV cannula of choice is a 22–24 gauge over-the-needle catheter. The insertion site should be chosen with the child's age and development in mind (Figure 30.1). Using a non-dominant arm allows older children to be able to continue most of their normal activities with the minimum of help. Avoiding the use of a vein at a joint prevents accidental dislodgement as the child tries to use the limb as normal. A scalp vein can be used in babies under 9 months as, at this age, these veins are prominent and easily accessible. They also do not interfere with the baby's movement. However, they do require part of the head to be shaved, which may distress the parents.

Small children cannot understand the need for IV fluids or the need to keep the site relatively still. The cannula should be secured in such a way that the insertion site is easily visible and the cannula is stable. The cannula site is an open wound and should be managed aseptically and therefore sterile dressing or tape should be used to protect the site. Cannula-related sepsis is associated with the proliferation of skin flora at the insertion site so any sterile transparent dressings used should allow the escape of moisture from the skin to prevent this occurrence. To ensure that the insertion site remains visible, splints and bandages are not usually used for adults but these items are usually necessary for children to prevent interference and to provide extra stability for the insertion site. Splints should be washable and padded to avoid the risk of pressure sores over bony prominences. Stickers can be applied to make them more acceptable to children. A plastic gallipot can be cut to shape to provide protection for a scalp vein site.

An infusion pump is nearly always used in the care of children to reduce the risk of circulatory overload and speed shock. The nurse

Calculation of IV fluid rates

Replacement of fluid is essential if 10% of the child's total body weight is lost.

Bobby is 4 years old and has been vomiting for 24 hours. His normal weight is 17 kg. He is unable to take anything orally at present and it is estimated that he is 10% dehydrated:

- calculate his daily fluid requirement
- add 10% to overcome his dehydration
- calculate the hourly rate of his infusion

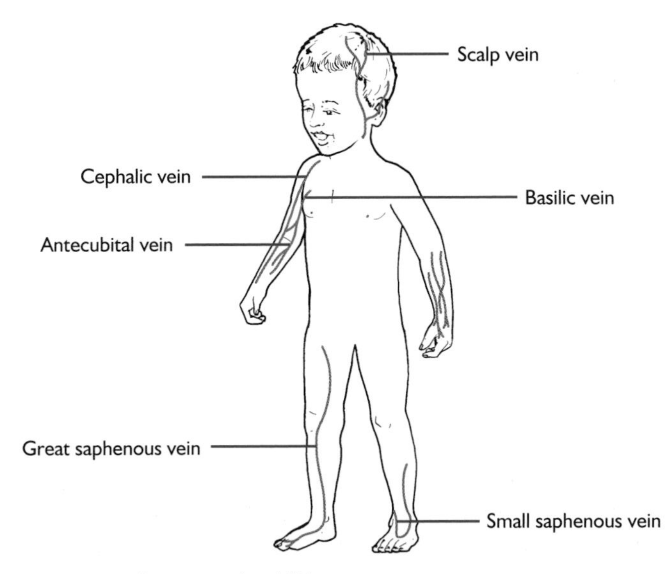

Figure 30.1 Cannulation sites for children.

should not presume the accuracy of the pump. Any electronic device depends upon the competency of the operator. The nurse should check that the prescribed rate is appropriate for the child before setting the pump. The pump should then be checked every 1–2 hours to ensure the fluid is running as programmed. Most infusion pumps will alarm when the infusion stops for whatever reason but it is possible for pressure to build up if the rate exceeds the capacity of a small vein. Hecker (1988) suggests that a build-up of pressure can cause hyperplasia of the vein lining, which can lead to phlebitis. Many pumps also have a tamper-proof facility to prevent mischievous children from interfering with the device.

Prevention of infection

Phlebitis or inflammation of the vein can result from sepsis, chemicals or mechanical trauma (Table 30.1). It can often be misdiagnosed (Griffiths-Jones, 1990), but it should be noted and reported quickly as, if untreated, it can lead to septicaemia. It may be recognised by erythema, pain, swelling or inflammation around the insertion site.

Table 30.1 The prevention of complications of IV therapy

Complication	Prevention
Phlebitis	Aseptic technique for all associated procedures Inspection of infusates for contamination Secure cannula to prevent movement Inspect insertion site 1–2 hourly for inflammation, erythema and pain Dilute additives as per manufacturers' instructions Change infusates and lines every 24 hours Maintain a closed infusion system
Extravasation	Secure cannula Inspect insertion site for local oedema, leakage of infusate
Circulatory overload/ under-infusion	Check prescribed rate Monitor rate of infusion 1–2 hourly Monitor intake and output hourly Report any dyspnoea, cough
Allergic reaction	Check allergy history Report any rashes, itching, dyspnoea
Air embolism	Clear all air from infusion set when commencing infusion Do not allow infusion to run dry – ensure rate does not exceed amount of fluid Check all connections are air-tight Maintain a closed infusion system
Occlusion of IV line	Maintain limb in optimum position Ensure line not kinked or compressed Ensure line is free of air Maintain flow of infusate to prevent fibrin formation Treat fibrin formation with saline flush
Venous spasm	Keep affected limb warm Do not administer refrigerated medication until at room temperature

Septic phlebitis is associated with contaminated cannulae or infusates. The insertion of cannulae should be a speedy, aseptic procedure preceded by effective skin cleansing. The infusate should be checked for signs of contamination before administration and any breakage of the infusion line to change infusates or administer drugs should include disinfection at the point of insertion. In long-term infusions, IV tubing and solutions should be changed daily to prevent bacterial growth. In adult nursing the rotation of cannula sites every 48–72 hours is recommended but this is a debatable practice in children's nursing where it is known that children and their families experience a great fear of cannulation. In addition, there is now evidence to suggest that after 72 hours there is actually less risk of complications in children with peripheral IVs (Garland *et al.*, 1987). The risk of septic phlebitis is also reduced if a closed infusion system can be maintained. Weinbaum (1987) identified that three-way taps provided a reservoir for micro-organisms. Removal of the IV cannula should be performed with an aseptic procedure. The cannula should be removed gently and firm pressure applied to the site immediately to prevent haematoma formation and potential infection. Once the bleeding has ceased a sterile dressing can be applied.

Chemical phlebitis is related to IV fluids that have a high osmolarity and low pH and some IV medications. Intravenous medication such as potassium chloride and antibiotics should always be diluted according to manufacturers' instructions and compatibility with the IV fluids checked.

Mechanical phlebitis is caused by the presence of a foreign body in the vein. This problem is exacerbated if there is movement of the cannula within the vein. It can be prevented by careful fixation of the cannula and the infusion giving set. Effective methods of securing the line also help to prevent the cannula from becoming dislodged from the vein and slipping into the surrounding tissues (extravasation). Extravasation of some infusates can cause necrosis of surrounding tissues and can result in severe injuries and long-lasting consequences (Wehbe and Moore, 1985). The increased subcutaneous fat found in children tends to make infiltration difficult to identify. The site and nearby dependent areas (palms, soles, behind the ears) should be examined for coolness, hardness and swelling and the infusion stopped if these features are found.

Prevention of mechanical problems

Mechanical problems can also cause serious complications. Air in any part of the infusion set may result in an air embolism. The child will become cyanosed, tachycardic and shocked. If this occurs the infusion should be stopped, a doctor informed and the child should be laid in a head down position on the left side to prevent the air from entering the pulmonary artery. Most infusion pumps are programmed to detect air but air can enter below the detection chamber when connections are broken. All connections should be checked when the nurse checks the infusion site.

Care of the child

The reason for the IV therapy and the need to protect the site can be explained to most older children whose mobility need not be impaired. If these children feel well they should be allowed to walk around and join in play as far as possible. Small children can only be allowed to mobilise with supervision as they will not understand or remember the need to care for their IV infusion. When children are confined to bed their personal belongings should be placed within easy reach on the side without the infusion so they do not dislodge the cannula by stretching. They will also require help with most of their activities of daily living. The type of play should be chosen with care to maintain the integrity of the infusion. To prevent accidental damage water play and the use of scissors are probably contra-indicated. Care should be taken with placing the infusion tubing. While the child needs to be able to move freely there have been incidents of small children getting tubing caught around their necks.

Study activity

Consider what help will be required by an adolescent with an IV infusion sited in the non-dominant hand. Try putting your own non-dominant hand in your pocket and seeing what can be done single-handed.

Study activity

Plan suitable play for a 5-year-old with an IV infusion sited in his left (non-dominant) arm.

Central venous devices

Peripheral cannulae have a relatively short lifespan and children are easily distressed by repeated cannulation. When long-term venous access is required to maintain fluid and electrolyte balance, an indwelling central venous catheter or implanted infusion port may be sited within the superior or inferior vena cava or right atrium via a large vein (Figure 30.2). There are a range of devices for central venous use, which all have their advantages and disadvantages (Table 30.2). The choice depends on the age of the child, the reason for the device and the amount of available access. McInally (2005) suggests that the selection of the most appropriate device will minimise trauma and discomfort and enhance acceptance of the device, and should be based on the child's

- diagnosis and treatment regimen
- age and maturity
- physical condition, weight and stamina
- lifestyle and perception of body image

There are many complications associated with the insertion of a central venous catheter and for this reason the insertion is usually performed in a clean environment under heavy sedation or a general anaesthetic. Implantable ports carry fewer risks but do require surgery and a general anaesthetic for their insertion. Correct placement requires radiological confirmation. Hickman, Broviac or Groshung catheters are made of clear, radiopaque, flexible silicone and designed to remain in place indefinitely. They are tunnelled subcutaneously for a short way before entering a large vein, thus reducing the risk of infection of having

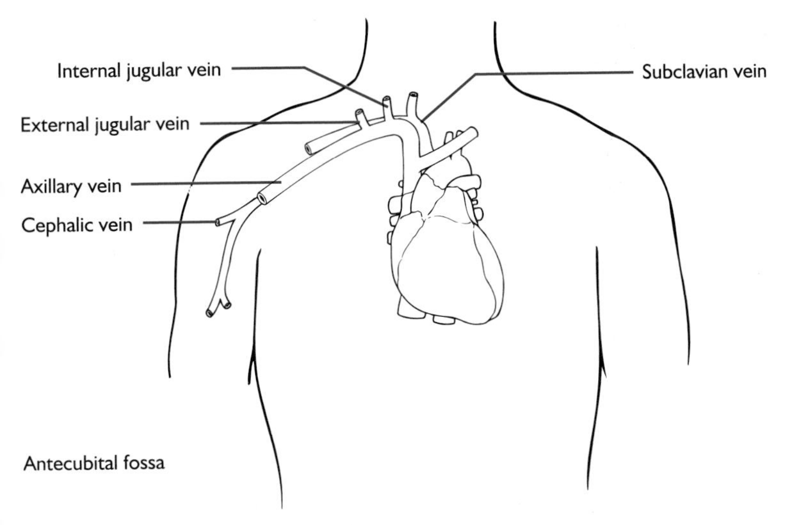

Figure 30.2 Sites for central venous devices.

long-term access directly into a main vein. Implanted ports are metal or plastic devices that lie under the skin and are sutured to the chest wall. The port is attached to a silicone catheter, which is tunnelled subcutaneously into a large vein. All catheters which are tunnelled into place have a Dacron cuff sited part way along their length which promotes tissue ingrowth and prevents bacterial migration. Although these tunnelled catheters have a reduced risk of infection, that risk is still present and exit site infections can result in septicaemia and removal of the device. At present no study has been able to clearly identify a strategy for managing the exit site to reduce the incidence of such infection. Lucas and Attard-Montalto (1996) found that dressing the site actually increased the incidence of infection, although they recognise the limitations of their small study. Ports still require needle access, although some surgeons deliberately sever some of the subcutaneous nerves to make the area over the port permanently numb (Liossi, 2002). McInally (2005) found that children found the pushing, prodding and holding of the port septum by less confident staff more uncomfortable than the actual needle insertion (*see also* Hickman line p. 327 and Port-a-cath p. 327).

These long-term devices were introduced primarily to allow patients having long-term treatment to return home between treatments. To ensure the child's safety, the family should have the opportunity to learn, practise and feel confident in the care of the device before discharge.

An alternative to the above devices is the safer and cheaper peripherally inserted central (PIC) catheter or long line which is a central venous catheter usually sited within the axillary or subclavian vein via the antecubital vein (Rountree, 1991). These lines have their entry point directly into a vein and therefore are not usually suitable for care at home. They are usually used for medium-term access (7–10 days).

One disadvantage of intermittent access to central venous catheters is occlusion of the line as a result of clot formation. Groshung catheters have a two-way valve to minimise this problem but still require weekly saline flushes to ensure patency between uses. Other catheters should be

Uses of central venous catheterisation

1. To monitor central venous pressure in acutely ill children
2. To replace large amounts of IV fluids or blood in cases of severe shock and/or haemorrhage
3. To provide long-term venous access for:
   - fluid and electrolyte maintenance
   - long-term IV cytotoxic therapy
   - long-term IV antibiotic treatment
   - regular blood tests
4. To administer total parenteral nutrition

Risks of central venous catheterisation

- Sepsis
- Haemorrhage
- Thrombosis
- Cardiac dysrhythmias
- Haemothorax
- Hydrothorax
- Pneumothorax
- Cardiac tamponade
- Air embolism
- Catheter embolism
- Misplacement
- Brachial plexus injury
- Thoracic duct injury

Principles of care for central venous catheter devices

Prevention of infection

- strict aseptic technique for all procedures
- observe exit site for erythema, discharge or swelling
- apply dressing after insertion until sutures removed

Prevention of haemorrhage or air embolism

- maintain a closed system
- use luer locks for all equipment
- clamp lines securely

Prevention of clot formation and occlusion

- flush catheter when not in use
- flush catheter between medications to prevent precipitate formation
- ensure line does not become kinked or compressed by clothing
- retain fluid in the catheter by using a positive pressure injection technique

Prevention of damage to the catheter

- avoid the use of sharp-edged forceps/clamps
- use no smaller than 10 ml syringes to access the line
- only allow the child to use scissors under close supervision

Table 30.2 Advantages and disadvantages of long-term central venous access devices

Device	Advantages	Disadvantages
Hickman/Broviac	Dacron cuff reduces risk of bacterial migration Self-administration easy	Exit site must remain dry Must be clamped Protrudes outside body Heavy activity restricted Daily heparin flushes May affect body image Difficult to repair
Groshung	Low maintenance two-way valve: • no clamping • backflow unlikely • air entry unlikely Easy to repair Self-administration easy Dacron cuff reduces risk of bacterial migration	Weekly saline flush Exit site must remain dry Heavy activity restricted Protrudes outside body May affect body image
Implanted ports (Port-a-cath, Infus-a-port)	Low infection risk Lies under skin Activity less restricted No dressing required Monthly heparin flush Body image less affected	Port accessed by injection Difficult to self-administer Special equipment needed to access port

flushed with 2.5–5 ml heparinised saline between uses and weekly when the device is not in use. If occlusion does occur, gentle flushing and aspiration with saline should dislodge the clot. Silicone catheters expand on pressure and will allow the saline to pass around the clot and dislodge it. If a larger thrombus has formed, it may be necessary to administer prescribed urokinase or streptokinase. Excessive pressure to dislodge an occlusion is not recommended as silicone is prone to cracking and splitting (Marcoux *et al.*, 1991).

Key Points

1. Differences in children's physiology make the maintenance of fluid balance one of the most important aspects in the care of the sick child.
2. Children and their families can be involved in the measurement and recording of intake and output.
3. Periods of fasting should be kept to a minimum and the child carefully monitored to ensure dehydration does not occur.
4. Children receiving IV therapy have unique problems and require specific care.
5. The use of central venous access devices enables the child to go home between long-term treatments but the family needs careful teaching about the care of the device to avoid complications.

Chapter 31

Caring for Children in Pain

Introduction

All children have a fundamental right to have their expressions of pain recognised, believed and managed appropriately. Unfortunately, the difficulties inherent in responding to children in pain in this way represents a major challenge to children's nursing practice. The Children's National Service Framework (DH, 2004) recognised that dealing with children's pain is one area that still needs improvement, requiring better assessment, planning and treatment.

Pain is not an easy topic for any healthcare professional to understand. As McCaffery (1983) rightly stated, 'Pain is what the patient says it is and exists when he says it does'. Pain is unique to the individual and it is impossible for the nurse to be able to recognise the experience for anyone else. Consequently, nurses need to be able to appreciate the various factors that affect the individual's perception and reaction to pain. They also have to be able to identify the varied manifestations of pain, especially when children are too ill, too young or too frightened to verbalise their pain. It is important that the nurse does not dismiss such communications. Finally, it is crucial that the nurse is able to offer pain management strategies that take into account the impact that pain is having on the child's physical and psychological state (*see also* Neonatal pain p. 572).

Standards for managing children's pain in hospital (DH, 2004)

- Children have the right to appropriate prevention, assessment and control of their pain.
- Clinical staff should receive training in the prevention, assessment and control of children's pain.
- Children can expect the management of pain to be a routine part of any treatment or procedure, in any part of the hospital. They can also expect to be involved as active partners in pain management.
- Pain should be assessed and reviewed in all children and monitored after all procedures.
- Protocols and procedures should support the safe use of pain-controlling medicines.
- Children's pain management should be demonstrated by regular audit.
- Trusts should support and coordinate activities and resources to ensure that children's pain is recognised and addressed.

Factors Affecting Pain

Sociological factors

The word pain is derived from the Latin *poena* meaning penalty. Historically the experience of pain was thought to be beneficial to the individual as it helped to strengthen the character. This belief is still held by some cultures, particularly in relation to the male sex.

Children learn by others' behaviours and will soon recognise the accepted response to pain. Depending upon their childhood experiences

Definitions of pain

- Suffering or distress of body (from injury or disease) or mind (*Concise Oxford Dictionary*)
- Range of unpleasant bodily sensations (*Oxford English Dictionary*)
- An unpleasant sensation, occurring in various degrees of severity, especially as a consequence of injury, disease or emotional disorder
- Suffering or distress (*Reader's Digest Universal Dictionary*)
- Hurt, distress, discomfort, anguish, misery, agony, suffering, ordeal, torment, torture (*Roget's Thesaurus*)

they learn to bear pain with stoicism or to display overt expressions of distress. Bond (1979) reports frequent complaints from children whose home environment is stressful. Budd (1984) dealt with more frequent complaints of pain among children from large families whose parents argued and used physical abuse, or whose siblings exhibited pain as part of a neurotic behaviour pattern. Children from Italian and Jewish families may learn to respond openly and emotionally to pain, whereas British children may believe it should be borne quietly (Bond, 1979).

Pfefferbaum *et al.* (1990) support the idea that cultural factors affect responses to pain but warn that this influence is probably minimal.

Study activity

Think about your own childhood and what you learnt about the expression of pain. Consider what effect this may have had on your nursing care.

Most adult values and beliefs about pain have originated from childhood experiences. Nurses who, as children, were expected not to make a fuss about their pain probably still manage their own pain quietly and without reliance on others. Such nurses probably find it more difficult to respond to a child who screams loudly at any discomfort than the nurse who was brought up to vocalise pain.

Political factors

The United Nations (UN) Convention on the Rights of the Child (1989) provides minimum standards for the care and treatment of children. It recognises that children are still discriminated against because of their immaturity, and recognises that children have a right to the highest attainable standards of health care (Newell, 1991). Although the UN cannot enforce the convention, governments that ratified the convention are required to submit a progress report (*see also* UN Convention on the Rights of the Child (1989) p. 684).

Despite repeated government and pressure group reports recommending improvements in childcare, the UK is still struggling to ensure that these rights are met. Platt (1959) realised that children in hospital have special needs that are best met by nurses and other healthcare professionals who have had specific training and education. This is particularly true in the care of children in pain. Other reports (Court, 1976; National Association for the Welfare of Children in Hospital (NAWCH), 1986; DH, 1991a; Audit Commission, 1993) reiterate this point. Studies into the care of children in hospital consistently reveal that there is still a concerning lack of specialist nurses in children's wards (Figure 31.1).

Such reports, as mentioned above, also recognise the important contribution that parents make to a sick child's care. Parents are able to recognise when their child's behaviour is different. They often know their child's way of expressing pain and they also understand the best comforting measures for their child. In partnership with the nurse they can help to provide the optimum pain management. However, many hospitals still do not cater well for parents, who are sometimes still left

(a)

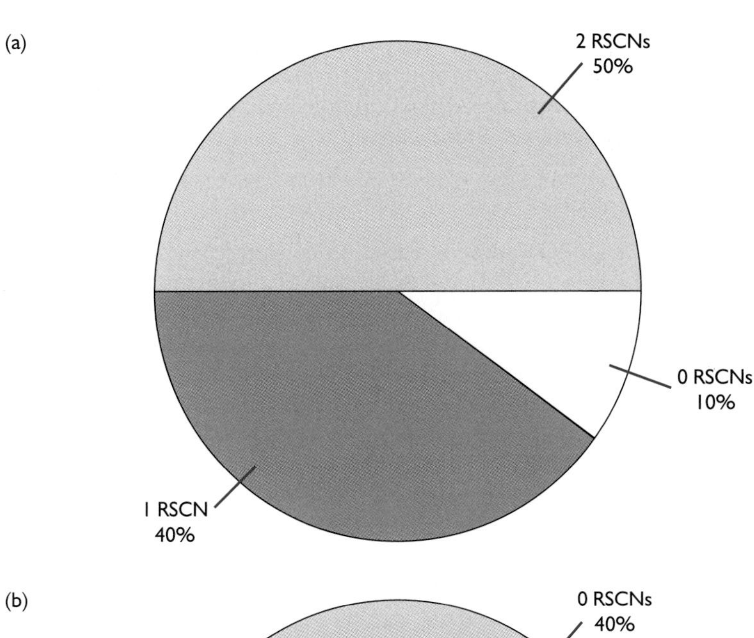

(b)

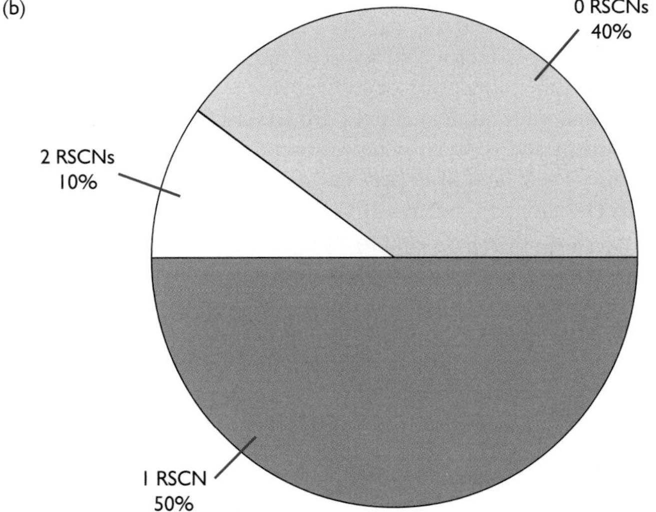

Figure 31.1 Number of registered children's nurses on duty: (a) day duty; (b) night duty. $N = 31$ wards in seven hospitals (adapted from Audit Commission, 1993).

to feel 'in the way' or 'interfering' and are at best 'tolerated' (Audit Commission, 1993). Instead of being able to help care for their child's pain, many parents become helpless witnesses and feel as anxious and fearful as their child (Carter, 1995).

Government initiatives to improve standards of care, such as the skill mix review and the named nurse concept, may have been designed to help these problems. Using one nurse skilled in pain management to supervise others giving care to children could prove useful. In addition, if each child and family had a named nurse accountable for their care, that nurse could appreciate their individual reactions to pain. However, in reality, these initiatives have been slow to develop. Nurses want to be able to give individualised, holistic care but the separation of nursing into specialist skills can appear a retrograde step and a return to

Parents' view of partnership and pain control

- Parents are usually familiar with their own child's responses to stress but nurses rarely use this expertise (O'Brien and Konsler, 1988)
- Parents are able to recognise their own child's non-verbal cues of pain (Elander *et al.*, 1991)
- Parents prefer to remain with their child during painful procedures (Dearmun, 1992)
- When given appropriate information, parents can help their child cope with pain (Schepp, 1991)
- Parents can feel powerless if their child is in pain and they do not know how to cope (Wyckoff and Erickson, 1987)
- Parents find that the central part of their child's anxiety in the first 3 post-operative days is the management of their pain (While and Crawford, 1992b)
- Parents believe that nurses tend not to prepare children for post-operative pain (Gillies *et al.*, 1995)

task allocation. At the same time, the lack of appropriately qualified children's nurses makes it difficult to provide children and families with an individual named nurse. Often the named nurse is the senior nurse on duty who provides little clinical care.

Economic factors

Health provision nowadays is based on consumerism and the market economy (Langdon, 1995) and as a result quality assurance is emphasised. Written polices and measurable standards of care to ensure a high quality of care for children in hospital were recommended by the Audit Commission (1993) but have been slow to develop. Llewelyn (1991) suggests that pain is one area where a written standard would be invaluable to ensuring that children's needs are met in a knowledgeable and consistent way; perhaps because of the subjective and individual nature of pain, such standards are rare.

The marketplace approach to health care may also provide nurses with a moral dilemma in relation to pain control. It may be difficult for them to offer a wide range of pain control methods if constrained by cost. The way in which nursing care is organised in the UK relates to political and economic factors. In spite of the introduction of Project 2000 (UKCC, 1986) student nurses still provide much of the direct care to children in hospital. Student nurses are less aware of the influences of pain assessment and so may be more susceptible to the myths about children's pain. Their lack of experience also means that they are less likely to detect certain pain behaviours (Read, 1994).

Direct care is also often provided by nurses who are not qualified children's nurses and lack the special skills needed to assess children in pain.

Many authors advocate that the initial nursing assessment of any child coming into hospital should include an assessment of the child's perceptions and experience of pain (Hester, 1979). Such specific areas are not usually investigated, which may also be due to the fact that this initial assessment is allocated to the less qualified members of the ward team.

Children's Perceptions of Pain

In addition to family and cultural influences, children's individual perceptions of pain are also affected by their age, cognitive and linguistic ability, neurological development, experience, personality and family and cultural beliefs. Assessing pain in pre-verbal children is difficult, especially in the neonatal period, and evaluation is thus based on behavioural and physiological changes such as crying, diffuse body movements, facial expressions and increased heart rate. However, these are not exact indicators, as an infant who is lying still with his/her eyes closed may still be experiencing pain (Shapiro, 1989) (*see also* Children's perceptions of health p. 141 and Children's concepts of illness p. 205).

Communicating with toddlers (1- to 3-year-olds) is also difficult; their language is largely imitative and they are egocentric, often believing that doctors and nurses deliberately set out to hurt them (Perry, 1994).

School-age children can consider viewpoints other than their own but still think mostly in concrete terms and can believe that pain is a punishment for their misdeeds. They cannot understand words such as 'pain' and 'anxiety', and may deny pain for the fear of the consequences, such as having an injection or staying in hospital. Adolescents are capable of fairly mature reasoning but their lack of experience of pain may make it difficult for them to cope with it. McCaffery and Beebe (1989) report a 17-year-old in pain saying: 'Tell the nurses we're younger than adults and more scared, so we need more attention'.

Study activity

Question some children of different age groups who have never been in hospital about the meaning of pain and anxiety. Consider carefully some the reasons for their answers.

Experience of pain alters infants' and children's perception of it. A study of behavioural responses in infants during subsequent visits to an immunisation clinic showed that a significant number cried in anticipation (Levy, 1960). Older children who have had previous experiences of illness and pain may become stoic in painful situations, whereas others with no experience may become terrified when they first feel a significant amount of pain (Eland, 1985). Fear and anxiety heighten pain (Alder, 1991), and Bond (1979) suggests that children with emotional personalities report greater levels of pain than more placid individuals. First-born and only children seem to be more anxious about pain, possibly because they have not been able to observe siblings (Eland, 1985). The context of pain also affects perception (McGrath, 1990): children who have been distracted from their pain often report less discomfort, while those who have seen a cannula during insertion, or blood spillage, generally complain of more pain (Johnson *et al.*, 1993).

Study activity

Now question some children who have had painful procedures about the meaning of pain and anxiety. Are their answers significantly different from those children of similar ages whom you questioned earlier?

Nurses' Perception of Pain

Nurses are as vulnerable as their patients to the psychological and sociocultural factors that influence the perception of pain. Bradshaw and Zeanah (1986) suggest that health professionals have additional biases from working with patients in pain. Their study indicated that many nurses still rely on intuitions, assumptions, personal beliefs and knowledge about pain related to specific diagnoses to assess children's pain. Nethercott (1994) found that nurses still rely on physiological

Myths and misconceptions about children's pain

- Infants do not feel pain
- Infants do not expect pain
- Children tolerate pain better than adults
- Children cannot accurately locate their pain
- Children become used to repeated pain
- Children are always truthful about their pain
- Children's behaviour accurately determines the degree of their pain
- Children are more susceptible than adults to the side-effects of narcotics

The use of narcotics for children

- The administration of narcotics for pain is no more dangerous for children than it is for adults (Burrows and Berde, 1993)
- Respiratory depression as a side-effect of opiates is rare in children (Paice, 1992)
- Addiction to opiates used to treat children's pain is extremely rare in children (Morrison, 1997)
- By 3–6 months of age children can metabolise narcotics in the same way as adults (Koren *et al.*, 1985)
- Increased doses of opiates for increased pain do not increase the side-effects (Paice, 1992)
- Continuous infusions of opiates provide more constant analgesia for post-operative children

(Dilworth and MacKellar, 1987)

measurements and verbal expressions as indicators of pain, although it has been shown consistently that these are not reliable indicators. I once saw a teenage boy who had received no analgesia during his first 12 hours following a splenectomy because he did not appear in pain or ask for pain relief. In reality, he was frightened of any intervention and was lying rigid to avoid further pain. In another situation, a neonate with intracerebral haemorrhage following a traumatic delivery whimpered whenever handled, yet received no analgesia for 24 hours, 'because he was not pyrexial'.

Read (1994) found that more experienced nurses had a higher perception of children's pain. Gadish *et al.* (1988) suggested that nurses who were mothers themselves often provided better pain measurement. They also found that graduate nurses had a better understanding of the assessment and management of pain than those nurses with a basic nurse education.

Nurses are also affected by the misconception about the effects of analgesia on children. Controversy still exists over the safety of pharmacological interventions and children's ability to feel pain. In addition, it has been noted that nurses give less priority to relieving pain than to more measurable nursing duties (Baillie, 1993). To enable nurses to identify their own beliefs and values about pain, which may interfere with their ability to make a subjective assessment, Whaley and Wong (2002) advise nurses to reflect on their answers to a series of questions about children's pain.

Study activity

Answer the questions in the box 'Reflection about views regarding children's pain' and consider the reasons why you have made your responses.

Pain Assessment

Pain assessment aims to identify all the factors that affect a child's perception of pain (Pritchard and Davis, 1990). Pain is both a sensory and emotional experience, so a multidimensional approach to assessment is preferable. One such approach is QUESTT (Baker and Wong, 1987):

- question the child
- use pain rating scales
- evaluate behaviour and physiological changes
- secure the parents' involvement
- take the cause of pain into consideration
- take action and evaluate results

Where it is possible to communicate with children, verbal statements and descriptions of pain are vital sources of information.

Question the child

On admission or pre-operatively when the child is able to communicate, questions such as those in the box at the foot of page 357 may help to

Table 31.1 Pain rating scales

Rating scale	Principles	Age of use
FACES pain rating scale (Whaley and Wong, 2002)	Facial expressions to represent degrees of pain	3 years +
Oucher (Beyer, 1989)	Photographs of children's faces showing degrees of pain	3–13 years
Numeric scale	Straight line marked 0 (no pain) to 10 (worst pain)	5 years +
Poker chip tool	Four counters given to child to represent 'pieces of hurt'	4 years +
Word graphic scale	Horizontal line marked at intervals with descriptions of pain intensity	8 years +
Colour tool (Eland, 1993)	Child constructs own colour tool choosing different colours to represent degrees of pain	4 years +
Liverpool Infant Distress Score (LIDS) (Horgan *et al.*, 1996)	Eight behavioural categories each with a 0–5 score enable carer to calculate pain score	Neonates
Pain Assessment Tool for Children (PATCh) (Quershi and Buckingham, 1994)	Combines face scale, body outline and numeric scale with descriptions of pain and behavioural changes	All ages

ascertain the child's understanding of pain. Children under the age of 6 may not understand the word 'pain' (Eland and Anderson, 1977) and may be more familiar with terms such as 'hurt' or 'sore'.

Use of pain rating scales

Pain rating scales (Table 31.1) should ideally be selected with this prior knowledge about the individual child, who should be shown how to use the scale before any pain occurs. However, few reliable tools are available for assessing children's pain. Jackson (1995) and Ellis (1988) believe that pain measurement should be based on behaviour, physiological measurements and the child's own report. However, self-assessment of pain in children relies on children's participation and upon their communication, numerical or drawing skills.

Evaluating behaviour and physiological changes

Buckingham (1993) has designed a pain scale for pre-verbal toddlers that combines assessment of physiological changes with changes in behaviour and body language. This could be adapted for use in neonates. The faces scale (Wong and Baker, 1988) can be used for children as young as three; studies show it is one of the most accurate pain assessment tools for children and is well received by them (Wong and Baker, 1988). Older children can usually use a numerical scale, which may range from 1 (no pain) to 10 (worst pain); some children can relate to the intensity of their pain better if these numbers appear on a vertical line (Beyer and Ardine, 1988). The Eland colour scale seems to

Reflection about views regarding children's pain

Do you believe that:

- infants and children feel pain in the same way as adults?
- infants and children forget the pain caused by procedures?
- children who are easily distracted from their pain have only minor pain?
- parents find it difficult to assess their child's pain accurately?
- nurses should be the child's advocate if pain control seems inadequate?
- nurses have the right to withhold analgesia if they think the child is not experiencing pain?
- sleep may be the result of exhaustion from pain?
- children should be woken if analgesia is prescribed on a regular basis?
- analgesia should reduce pain to a manageable level?
- nurses' assessment of vital signs and behaviour is a more reliable way of determining pain than the child's own account?
- post-operative analgesia which is prescribed whenever necessary should be given only on request?
- nurses can estimate the amount of pain caused by a specific procedure, illness or operation?

Assessing a child's knowledge of pain

- What is pain?
- What pain have you had before?
- What do you do when you have pain?
- What helps to make the pain go away?
- What makes the pain worse?

be the most accurate assessment tool for the location of pain. The child locates the pain on a body outline and represents its severity with different colours (Eland, 1985). The Hester poker chip scale can be used with children as young as 4 years. The child is given four or five counters (chips) and asked to display none or all of them to represent the amount of pain felt (Hester, 1979). McCaffery and Beebe (1989) gave a selection of assessment questions and tools that can be duplicated for use in practice. There is, however, a lack of research about the reliability of these scales and many authors have criticised their use (Wilson, 1993), so it is advisable to combine the use of pain scales with an objective form of measurement.

Study activity

Use a variety of these assessment tools with children of different ages. Consider their ease of use and effectiveness.

Secure parental involvement

Parental involvement is crucial when children are unable to communicate. They can be questioned on admission to ascertain the child's knowledge of pain and reaction to it. It is also useful to question parents wherever possible about the child's usual patterns of behaviour *before* any pain occurs; parents often find it difficult to make a subjective assessment of their child when he or she is distressed, as their own distress, anxiety and sometimes guilt interfere with their ability to judge behaviour (McCaffery and Beebe, 1989). It is also important to discuss the parents' role in pain assessment with them if they are to be partners in their child's care. Parents are, too often, unaware of their role when the child is in hospital (Audit Commission, 1993). If they are helped to work in partnership with the nurse, they will be alert to manifestations of pain and can help in controlling the pain. In a similar way, they can help an older child to express pain and make a choice about its management.

Study activity

Talk to some parents about their child's pain. How does their information add to your knowledge and care of the child?

Taking the cause of the pain into account

The cause of potential pain should not be forgotten. Children may deny pain because of a lack of understanding or fear of intervention. Eland (1985) describes a teenager with chronic pain who denied any discomfort because he had forgotten what it was like to be pain free. A knowledge of disease pathology offers a clue to the type of pain being experienced. Whaley and Wong (2002) suggest that nurses should accept that whatever is painful to an adult is painful to an infant or child unless proved otherwise. This is particularly pertinent to A&E work, where it is not always possible to undertake a detailed assessment of the child's and family's previous experience of pain. Children in A&E departments often present in pain and this can be heightened by the fear and anxiety caused by the strange and stressful situation, while painful and frightening procedures are undertaken to aid diagnosis and treatment. Gay (1992) and Read (1994) found that nurses tended to underestimate actual and potential pain in these situations. Gay (1992) also found that preparatory information about procedures and equipment alleviated children's stress and pain. Nurses may need to give more consideration to finding out about procedures in order to prepare children in a more realistic way.

Taking Action and Evaluating Results

The aim of caring for a child in pain should be to provide total pain relief. This may be done using a variety of methods suitable for each individual child's pain. Both pharmaceutical and non-pharmaceutical interventions can be used. If the nurse is familiar with a range of such interventions, the child and/or parents can select the one that seems most suitable.

The most suitable method for relieving pain often depends on the child's personality and participation. It also relies upon a therapeutic relationship between the child, parents and the nurse. The child and parents need to be able to trust the nurse to believe their concerns about the pain and to react accordingly. Whatever the method used, the nurse should teach the child and family about the pain while trying to avoid words that may describe the type of pain. In the same way, the nurse should prepare the child and family for painful procedures. If the nurse is not evaluative about the type of pain experienced, the child does not anticipate pain and may be able to give a clearer description of it as an individual experience. Parents who are well prepared can often lessen a child's anxiety and therefore pain by their presence. They can also be taught non-pharmacological techniques and can help the child in their use.

Non-pharmacological methods of pain relief are best taught to the child and family *before* the child actually experiences pain. Some techniques can be put on audiotape or video tape and used again at a later date. Cleeland (1986) suggests that this type of pain control is best used for children with mid-range pain. Children with severe pain often cannot relax sufficiently to make best use of these methods and children with little pain may not be motivated to learn the technique. Massage can be used to enhance relaxation and abdominal massage has been reported to be effective in reducing the discomfort of colic in small babies (Lorenz *et al.*, 2005).

When nurses are first taught about the administration of medicines, they learn that it is the responsibility of the nurse to ensure that the patient receives the *right drug* in the *right dose* at the *right time* and by the *right route*.

Although the nurse is not responsible for the prescription of medicines, a knowledge of these principles in relation to the pharmacological management of pain enables the optimum pain relief to be used.

non-pharmacological
Relating to the use of strategies to minimise the perception of pain which do not involve the administration of drugs; these strategies should not be seen as an alternative to drugs but as a means of enhancing the effectiveness of pharmacological interventions

pharmacological
Relating to the use of medicinal drugs

Non-pharmacological interventions

General strategies

- reassurance
- parental presence
- explain reason for pain
- emphasise positive information

Distraction

- play
- singing or shouting
- stories

Relaxation

- rocking
- deep breathing
- muscle relaxation

Guided imagery

Use of heat or cold or massage

Table 31.2 Non-steroidal anti-inflammatory drugs

Drug	Recommended dose	Precautions
Ibuprofen	5–10 mg/kg 6–8 hourly	Can cause gastric irritation if given on an empty stomach
Aspirin	300–2600 mg 4 hourly	Not recommended for under-12s
Naproxen	5 mg/kg 12 hourly	Children older than 2
Diclofenac sodium	0.5–1 mg/kg 8–12 hourly (orally or rectally)	Maximum dose 3 mg/kg/day (enteric coated – do not crush)

Table 31.3 Use of opioids for children

Drug	Route	Recommended dose
Morphine	Oral	0.2–0.4 mg/kg 3–4 hourly
	Sustained release	200–800 mcg/kg 12 hourly
	Intramuscular	0.1–0.2 mg/kg 3–4 hourly
	Continuous IV infusion	Loading dose 50–100 mcg/kg Hourly dose 10–30 mcg/kg
	Patient-controlled IVI	Loading dose 50–100 mcg/kg Background infusion 2–8 mcg/kg Bolus dose 10–20 mcg/kg/5–15 minutes
Pethidine	IV or IM injection	500 micrograms–2 mg/kg/dose
	IV infusion	Loading dose 1 mg/kg Background 100–400 mcg/kg/hour
Codeine phosphate	Oral (1–12 years) IM injection	3 mg/kg/day, doses every 4 hours 1 mg/kg/dose every 4–6 hours

In discussion with medical colleagues the nurse can advise the most suitable intervention for each individual child.

Ensuring that a child receives the right drug depends on an accurate assessment of the pain. Non-opioids and non-steroidal anti-inflammatory drugs (NSAIDS) are suitable for mild to moderate pain (Table 31.2). Opiates are needed for moderate to severe pain (Table 31.3). The 'analgesic' ladder is a useful way to determine the right medication, as the child and parents may lose confidence in the nurse if the wrong medicine is prescribed. If the chosen drug is too mild, the child may refuse further doses because it is not having any effect. If the chosen drug is too strong, the child may suffer severe side-effects and again refuse further doses.

Distressing side-effects of inadequate pain control may also occur if the dosage of the drug is wrong or if it is given at an inappropriate time. Dosages should be carefully calculated according to the age, height and weight of the child. In chronic pain, analgesia should be given regularly to ensure continuous pain relief. Mild analgesics given regularly can often be more effective than infrequent doses of strong opioids.

Table 31.4 Routes of administration for analgesia

Route	Advantages	Disadvantages
Local	Ease of administration Usually well accepted	Slow onset of action Cannot be used under 6 months of age
Oral	Ease of administration Usually well accepted	Inappropriate in the post-operative period Absorption and action may be slow Gastric irritation Danger of aspiration for infants Discoloration of tooth enamel
Rectal	Useful if child is vomiting or unable to swallow	Social acceptability? Ineffective in loaded rectum
IM	Rapid onset of action	Disliked by children: 'The worst hurt ever'
IV	Rapid onset of action Continuous action if infusion	Discomfort of IV cannula Potential hazards of IV therapy
Inhalation (Entonox)	Child can self-administer	Needs careful preparation Child needs to understand use

Once the right dosage and frequency of the medicine has been decided, the most appropriate route must be chosen (Table 31.4). Although the oral route is often the first choice, it is not always the most appropriate for frightened toddlers and children who are nauseated. Intramuscular injections are not well tolerated by most children and many children will deny pain if they think an injection will follow.

Infusions are a more effective way of providing continuous pain relief and if the child and parents are prepared well, they can be given some control over the dosage and frequency. Llewelyn (1991) found that children as young as 3 years could use patient-controlled analgesia (PCA) well. Morphine at 1 mg/ml is the choice of drug for PCA as it is considered to provide significantly more pain relief and fewer side-effects than other opioids (Vetter, 1992).

Morphine, in conjunction with a long-acting anaesthetic, is also the choice of drug for the epidural route. It can be given continuously or intermittently via an infusion and acts directly upon opiate receptors in the spinal cord. This lessens the risk of sedation and respiratory depression, which can occur from the effect of opioids on the brain. A small dose of morphine can be used nasally, when it acts almost immediately, to reduce pain from relatively short procedures such as applying traction.

Prior to potentially painful procedures involving punctures of the skin, a topical local anaesthetic cream can be used. Eutectic mixture of local anaesthetic (EMLA) is approved for children over 1 year in age. It takes 60 to 90 minutes to numb an area of intact skin for up to 4 hours after application (see overleaf). Topical amethocaine (Ametop) gel can be used for children over 6 months. It takes 30 to 45 minutes to act and its effect can last for 4 to 6 hours. Although EMLA cream can cause

Patient-controlled analgesia

Definition

Patient-controlled analgesia (PCA) is a technique which was developed in the 1970s to enable adult patients to have some control over the dose and frequency of their analgesia. Its use began to be extended to children in the 1980s.

Variations

The PCA pump can be programmed to deliver an opioid analgesia in three different ways:

- *bolus dose* – the child can press a button to deliver a bolus pre-programmed dose of analgesia as required. A lock-out device prevents this dose from being repeated so often that the child receives an overdosage. However, the pump records every request for analgesia so that the nurse can assess how often the child is requiring analgesia and adjust the dose if necessary. The nurse or parent can use this method on the child's behalf.
- *continuous background infusion* – delivers a continuous pre-programmed dose of analgesia.
- *continuous background infusion and bolus doses* – a combination of the above, allowing the child to receive an extra dose of analgesia as required.

All children receiving a form of PCA should be regularly observed for the side-effects of opioids and have their respiratory rate, depth and pattern monitored to detect any complications.

Side-effects of opioids

- *Depresses central nervous system* – sedation, drowsiness, mental clouding
- *Action on the respiratory centre in the brain stem* – respiratory depression
- *Stimulation of the chemoreceptor trigger zone which activates the vomiting centre* – nausea and vomiting
- *Release of histamine* – pruritus, flushing and sweating
- *Increase of smooth muscle tone* – urinary urgency or retention
- *Decrease of peristalsis and intestinal secretions* – constipation

Administration of Ametop cream

Used to numb pain from the following procedures:

- lumbar puncture
- finger or heel pricks
- arterial or venous access
- implanted port access
- superficial skin biopsies
- removal of chest tubes
- bone marrow biopsy
- SC or IM injections

Procedure

- not recommended for children under 1 year
- use on intact skin
- apply thickly to area 1 hour before procedure (90 minutes for dark skin when absorption is slower, 2 hours for deep procedures)
- apply occlusive dressing
- pallor or erythema indicates local anaesthetic effect
- wipe off remaining cream 5 minutes before procedure to allow vasoconstrictive effect to reverse

constriction of blood vessels, Ametop dilates them. However, Ametop can cause blistering or skin discoloration if left in position for longer than 45 minutes (Hewitt, 1988). Patient-controlled inhalation devices such as Entonox, due to the advantage of its almost immediate effect, can be useful prior to more invasive painful procedures when used by a health professional trained in its use. Smith and Kanagasundaram (2002) suggest that its use is more effective with older children, and pre-procedural education is vital if the child is to use the mask correctly. All medicines have undesired as well as desired side-effects and the nurse needs to be aware of these so that a careful evaluation of the medication can be made. This evaluation of the medication needs to also include the child's and the parents' views of the efficiency of the method used. Evaluation of care is not understood or undertaken well by nurses, and more consideration needs to be given into incorporating this aspect of care into care plans.

Study activity

Compile your own list of analgesia for children, finding out the dose range, method of action, use, side-effects and variety of routes for each medication listed.

Summary

Primary nursing may be a way of providing more individualised and effective pain control. One nurse acting as a key figure for a child throughout the hospital stay will be able to establish a close therapeutic relationship with the child and family (Binnie *et al.*, 1988). Providing care in this way calls for good interpersonal skills, and one of the crucial elements of such a nurse–patient relationship is self-awareness – being honest about personal thoughts and emotions. It also requires the nurse to evaluate the relationship and care given. As yet this type of nursing is not widely practised in the UK, but now the focus of nurse education has changed, it may be possible to provide individualised pain management within such a therapeutic relationship.

The introduction of a systematic method of pain assessment such as that suggested by Baker and Wong (1987) could also improve pain management, especially if introduced before the pain occurs. The use of such methodology would give the nurse more experience on which to base the assessment of children admitted in acute pain. However, further research is required on the validity and reliability of pain scales to ensure that children are able to define their pain in meaningful ways.

Children continue to suffer unnecessary and treatable pain (DH, 2004). Nurses need increased education about pain, while improved methods of assessing pain are crucial to identifying and managing pain effectively. Nurses should consider how best to incorporate specific pain assessment tools into their care and how children's care can best be organised to enable consistency of care and an individualised approach. Further research into the accuracy of children's pain assessment will also help to improve this area of practice.

Key Points

1. Nurses need more education about pain assessment in children.
2. Children's perceptions of pain are influenced by many factors.
3. It is important to be aware of one's own beliefs and values about pain to prevent them from interfering with one's professional judgement.
4. Wherever possible, it is advisable to question children and their families about pain before it occurs.
5. The organisation of care may need to change to enable the effective assessment of children's pain.
6. The use of both pharmacological and non-pharmacological interventions will enhance pain control.

Chapter 32

The Role of the Nurse as a Surrogate

Introduction

Peplau's (1952) model of nursing, created initially to define mental health nursing, describes six roles of the nurse. One of these roles is described as the surrogate role. Peplau defines this role as helping the patient to become aware of the nurse as an individual and thus promoting an interpersonal relationship between them to enable the nurse to take over roles that the patient is unable at present to fulfil. If the term 'patient' is seen as the child and family, this role becomes the development of the partnership relationship with the child and family.

The children's nurse does not want to take over the role of the parent when caring for children but there is sometimes a need for the nurse to take on aspects of care that the parents would usually provide. Casey (1988b) describes this as family care, in contrast to nursing care, which relates to the technical care the nurse provides because of the child's health problem. The nurse adopts the role of surrogate carer when the parents are unable to perform their usual role (*see also* Peplau's interpersonal relationships model p. 638 and Casey's partnership model p. 640).

Parents may be unable to perform their usual role because they are unable to be resident in hospital with their child. Although most children's wards encourage parents to stay with their child in hospital it is not always possible for all parents to do so. Parents who have other children, are self-employed or are single parents and have no close family nearby may be unable to be resident. Other parents may stay with their child but, for a number of reasons, may find it difficult to carry out their child's usual care. As one parent of a 6-year-old admitted for revision of a hypospadias repair said: 'I want to be with Richard to support him, but do not ask me to help with his care because I am too squeamish'. Parents who are unable to carry out family care should not be made to feel guilty but should be supported in their decision and enabled to take their chosen responsibility. Ahmann (1994) suggests that parents should be reassured that they have an essential role in the care of their child in hospital, but such reassurance can cause stress to parents who cannot provide that care.

Parents who are resident and take on most of their child's care are often abandoned by the nursing staff. These parents are often anxious about this responsibility and feel obligated to stay with their child for fear that no care will be given in their absence. They become exhausted with lack of adequate nutrition, rest and sleep. The nurse should not let this situation develop and should be available to take on the family care to give parents a respite.

Ideally, a named nurse is assigned to each child and family. This nurse can provide family and nursing care as necessary to meet the needs of the child and family. This surrogate role requires a detailed knowledge of the child as an individual as well as the family's usual daily routine.

Family Care

Family care for the child in hospital should be as similar as possible to the care that the family would give their child at home. Times of waking, eating and resting should be adhered to as closely as possible. Hospitalisation is not an appropriate time to try and change family routines that do not meet with the nurses' approval, unless these are putting the child in danger. However, helping with family care can give the nurse an opportunity to advise the family about health education.

Washing and dressing

Bath time is often also playtime for younger children. The nurse should recognise this and spend time playing with the child as well as ensuring cleanliness. To avoid frightening the child the big bath should only be used if this is what the child normally uses. All children should be supervised in the bath but some children may need help with aspects of washing.

Any specific lotions or creams should be used as at home. The stress of the hospital environment can be minimised by encouraging the child to wear clothes from home. Help should be given according to the child's level of independence. Children under 8 years usually require help with teeth cleaning. Hair should be cared for as at home, which may include shampooing.

Eating and drinking

Children often react to illness or hospitalisation by loss of appetite and the named nurse needs to appreciate the child's usual likes and dislikes to encourage eating and drinking. Bottles, teacher beakers and toddler cutlery should be available as at home. If possible, a normal family mealtime can be simulated by having the child eat at the table with others. The times and content of meals should correspond to the home routine as far as possible, with cooked meals provided at midday or evening according to the family's usual practice (*see also* Nutition p. 330).

Play

Play is an important part of a child's usual home routine and should not be forgotten when the child is in hospital. The nurse providing surrogate

Encouraging the ill child to eat and drink

- Use attractive eating utensils – bowls and plates with familiar characters on the surface, coloured mugs, curly straws
- Arrange the food attractively on the plate (make a picture of a face or garden with the food, cut sandwiches into shapes (boat, teddy, star, etc.))
- Serve small portions – an overloaded plate can be off-putting
- Provide the child's favourites – bring from home if necessary
- Serve the food imaginatively, e.g. in a paper bag for a picnic, use straws as skewers to eat sausages, etc., by hand
- Make meal times into social events by gathering children together
- Involve the child, e.g. filling in food/fluid chart, choosing from a menu, etc.

care should provide for play as the parents would do at home. Favourite toys or stories brought from home can be included. Storytime may be an important part of the child's day at home; time for a cuddle on mother's lap or a quiet time before sleep. Letting the child play in the playroom with other children cannot replace this and the named nurse should organise to spend one-to-one time with the child so that this special time is not lost (*see also* Play p. 95).

Elimination

Children in hospital can find it difficult to maintain their usual elimination patterns because of their anxieties, the strange environment and lack of privacy. The nurse can help by ensuring that the child is given the opportunity to go to the toilet in the same way as parents will usually ask small children to go to the toilet, for instance, on waking, after breakfast and before going to school. This routine may help to avoid constipation or urinary tract infections caused by ignoring the desire to eliminate. The nurse should provide the same amount of help as the parents usually provide. A knowledge of the child's usual bowel habits will help to alert the nurse to any problems.

Usually toddlers begin toilet training at around 2 years. Some parents will sit the younger child on the potty at set times to familiarise the child with the pot. Although children often regress in hospital, the surrogate nurse should keep to home potty routines so that training is not interrupted and can continue on discharge.

Mobility

Children who are ill rarely want to be as active as usual. However, as they recover they will regain this and it is useful to know the child's usual level of activity to be able to cater for this. The surrogate nurse needs to be aware if the 1-year-old can walk unaided or if the child with special needs requires assistance to mobilise. This knowledge will also help to maintain children's safety as they become more active.

Rest and sleep

Often children sleep more when they are feeling unwell, but they need to feel safe in order to relax and rest. If parents are unavailable, the nurse should ensure that home routines are maintained. This will require careful organisation of work to ensure that the nurse is able to settle the child for a nap or for bed at the usual time. Any special routines like drawn curtains, nightlight, cuddly toy or blanket or night-time drink should be followed (*see also* Sleep pp. 40–41).

Communication

Infants' communication is largely non-verbal, by touch and tone of voice. Even with such limited communication an infant is usually aware of strangers. The surrogate carer cannot explain this temporary role and can only provide security for this age group by following home routines. As children's vocabulary and understanding increase it is important that the named nurse has an idea of the common words and expressions used. To prevent accidents it is particularly important to understand the words used by the child to communicate elimination needs. A knowledge of the family and those close to the child, including pets, enables the nurse to talk with the child about home (*see also* Language development p. 77).

Communication may also include the need for prayer. Family routines in relation to this should be noted and respected so that the child may be given time and, if necessary, privacy to pray.

If the nurse is to identify stress in hospital, it is also important to know the child's usual personality. Is the child normally talkative and friendly or shy and uncommunicative? The surrogate carer needs to know how the child usually reacts to stress and the most comforting way to respond as the parents would. For example, Alex, a 3-year-old, is best comforted by having his feet stroked. Fergus, aged 6, prefers to hide behind the door and to be left alone to talk to his teddy.

Providing family care is not always easy in a hospital environment and the nurse may have to be flexible and imaginative and use skills of advocacy to enable children to follow home routines.

Study activity

Compare the usual routine of a children's ward with the usual home routine of a child known to you. Consider how the hospital day might be adjusted to meet your child's usual routines. Identify any areas of difficulty and consider how you might be able to change these.

Care of the Child Confined to Bed

On occasions family care has to be adapted because of the child's condition. The named nurse has a carer/surrogate role in this situation in helping the family to adjust their routines to meet these changed circumstances. The nurse can also offer advice to parents caring for children at home who are temporarily confined to bed.

Study activity

Consider the aspects of family care which will need adaptation for the child who is confined to bed.

Washing and dressing

The child confined to bed should be bathed at the usual times for washing at home. If the bed linen and any wound dressings are protected with plastic, bed baths can still provide an opportunity for play, boats or ducks can swim in the washing bowl and the child can splash the water around. It is important to ensure that teeth, nails and hair still receive attention. Hair may become very matted and difficult to brush if the child is unable to move, and this problem will only worsen if brushing is neglected. Shampooing should be considered if the child is confined to bed for longer than a week.

Eating and drinking

The child confined to bed may find it difficult to eat and drink because the recumbent position hinders normal digestion. This position also impairs elimination and can result in constipation due to sluggish peristalsis and urinary tract infections because of inadequate bladder emptying. It is therefore particularly important to encourage fluids. Favourite fluids should be offered at regular intervals and the use of bendy straws or dolls' teacups may promote cooperation. Food should be easily digestible and provided in small and attractive servings, making full use of the child's likes. Food from home may be more acceptable than that provided by the hospital.

Study activity

Consider ways in which you could encourage the child confined to bed to eat and drink.

Play

Play is still important for the child in bed but will have to be adapted to meet the child's altered abilities, medical equipment and their position. Generally, children who feel unwell will have reduced levels of concentration. As a result, a range of different types of play must be organised to respond to this. For example, allowing a child with a plaster of Paris to play with water may be hazardous! Equally, unsupervised cutting out with scissors may be risky for any age of child with an intravenous infusion or traction, who may, by accident or design, cut through their equipment. Children who have to lie flat will need particular attention. Travel games, which can be played on a magnetic board, are useful, as is a slanting easel for drawing, painting or just supporting reading books.

Elimination

It is difficult to maintain a home routine for toileting when the child is confined to bed, and potty training may have to be delayed until this period of immobility has ceased. However, because of the complications of constipation and urinary tract infection associated with immobility, it is important to retain some semblance of routine. If a child defecates at a specific time of day bedpans should be offered at this time. If a child is used to going to the toilet at set times in the day (on waking, before school, midday), this routine should continue. In the hospital setting privacy for toileting must be ensured as some children may be very self-conscious about such activity. Small children may wet the bed during illness because they are less aware of the need to urinate, are scared of using bedpans or because of an urinary tract infection. It is important not to punish them but to analyse why it happened and try and prevent a reoccurrence.

Mobility

Children who are immobile are at risk from pressure sores, stiff joints, wasted muscles and joint deformities. Changes of position and physiotherapy are required to minimise the risk of these complications.

Table 32.1 Preventing the complications of immobility

Complication	Nursing care
Pressure sores	Encourage movement of mobile limbs Encourage change of position Observe pressure areas for redness Avoid pressure, shear or friction
Circulation problems (deep vein thrombosis, pulmonary embolus)	Encourage movement as able Encourage deep breathing exercises to aid venous return Note complaints of calf or chest pain
Chest infection	Encourage deep breathing Record temperature and respirations Note chestiness, cough, pyrexia
Elimination problems (constipation, urinary tract infection)	Encourage good fluid intake Enable usual routine and privacy for toileting Monitor urine output and bowel action
Anorexia	Encourage appetite
Boredom and depression	Provide daily programme of activity Encourage family and friends to visit
Joint stiffness/deformity/ muscle weakness	Encourage active exercises for mobile limbs Provide passive exercises for immobile limbs
Difficulty in resting and sleeping	Provide daily programme of activity Keep to home bed-time routines

Although the incidence of pressure sores in children is less than in adults because children tend to have healthier skin and a vigorous circulation, immobile children are at risk and preventive care should be taken. Pressure sores can develop when the pressure on the skin and underlying tissues is greater than the pressure within the underlying capillaries. If this degree of pressure is maintained, the capillaries collapse, the underlying tissues become ischaemic and eventually necrose. The primary causes of pressure sores are direct pressure, friction and shearing forces. The immobile child should be positioned carefully to ensure that bony prominences are not under pressure from other limbs or medical equipment. Change of position is the most effective way of preventing pressure sores but care should be taken to ensure that the child is moved without causing friction or shearing. Pressure-relieving devices should be used for children who are at risk from pressure sores. Although there are several well-researched tools for assessing adults' risk of pressure sores, this is a poorly explored area of children's nursing. Risk-assessment tools need to take into account all the secondary factors that predispose to pressure sores. These factors are those that make the skin less healthy and more liable to the effects of pressure.

Study activity

Consider which secondary factors would cause a child to be more at risk from pressure sores.

Extrinsic causes of pressures sores

- *Pressure.* The blood pressure at the arterial end of capillaries is approximately 32 mmHg. At the venous end this pressure is about 12 mmHg. The mean capillary blood pressure is around 20 mmHg and any external pressure higher than this will cause capillary obstruction. Tissues usually served by these capillaries will be deprived of their blood supply and will eventually die from ischaemia
- *Shearing forces.* When the child slips down the bed or is dragged into a new position, the skeleton moves over the underlying tissues and the circulation of these damaged tissues is destroyed
- *Friction.* Friction and stripping of the upper layer of the epidermis also occurs when children slip down the bed or are dragged. This results in a superficial break in the skin rendering it more prone to further damage

Prevention of pressure sores

- *Assessment.* All children should have a risk assessment calculated on admission and this should be updated regularly as their condition changes significantly
- *Plan of care.* Care plans should incorporate specific measures to combat pressure sores according to child's degree of risk
- *Careful positioning.* Children should be positioned to avoid pressure. Care should be taken that all traction equipment and infusion, feeding, oxygen, or urinary or wound drainage tubing is not causing pressure. The use of bean bags rather than angled bed rests reduces friction and shearing forces
- *Good bed making.* Beds should be made with taut bottom sheets to prevent pressure from creases. Crumbs and small toys are also risks for small children who are immobile
- *Hygiene.* Pressure areas should be kept clean and dry. The affected area should not be rubbed as this action macerates the subcutaneous skin which degenerates
- *Nutrition.* The child should receive a nutritious diet and adequate fluids to prevent excessive weight loss or gain and dehydration while promoting a healthy skin. Vitamins A and C and zinc are especially useful for maintaining healthy skin
- *Patient lifting and handling.* The most effective treatment and prevention of pressure sores is the relief of pressure. If a child is unable to move and change position the nurse must help. Nurses should have short fingernails and no rings which may damage the child's skin during repositioning. Incorrect lifting will result in the child being dragged up the bed, causing damage to underlying tissues
- *Pressure-relieving devices.* A wide variety of pressure-relieving devices are available but their efficacy is not always research based. Nurses should be aware of their use, function, disadvantages and advantages and base their choice according to the specific child's needs
- *Patient/family education.* The older child and family should be told about the risk of pressure sores and how to prevent their occurrence so that they can cooperate with the care prescribed

Intrinsic causes of pressure sores

- *Weight.* Reduced subcutaneous fat causes an increased localised pressure over bony prominences. Extra subcutaneous fat does not combat the increased pressure caused by the extra weight of the obesity (Waterlow, 1988)
- *Temperature.* An increase in temperature causes a rise in basal metabolic rate and a greater need for oxygen to maintain healthy tissues. It also causes sweating
- *Moisture.* Moisture increases the risk of pressure sores by 5%. Perspiration, wound drainage and incontinence result in waterlogged skin which is softer and weaker than healthy skin. Faecal incontinence further damages this fragile skin by exposing it to bacteria and toxins (Wyngaarden and Smith, 1988)
- *Nutrition.* Oedematous and adipose areas are poorly vascularised, causing the skin to become thin and fragile. Dehydration leads to dry, wrinkled and withered skin which breaks down relatively easily (Waterlow, 1988)
- *Mobility.* Lack of mobility impairs the ability to change position, thus relieving pressure and improving the circulation to the tissues (National Pressure Ulcer Advisory Panel, 1989)
- *Circulation.* Low diastolic blood pressure (BP) (below 60 mmHg) indicates poor peripheral circulation and therefore poor tissue perfusion
- *Neurological factors.* Sensory loss due to paralysis, coma, sedation or analgesia decreases or prevents the awareness of pressure and the ability to react to it (Waterlow, 1988)
- *Age.* Increasing age causes a decrease in tissue elasticity, texture and cell replacement. The healthy skin of a baby or young child helps to counteract many of the intrinsic causes of pressure sores but care should be taken to protect it from damage as pressure sores can still occur (National Pressure Ulcer Advisory Panel, 1989)
- *Emotional stress.* Raised glucocorticoids produced by stress result in decreased collagen formation. Stressed individuals may also have a low self-concept and neglect to take care of their skin

Joint stiffness, muscle wastage and joint deformities may be prevented by exercise and position. Depending on the child's condition, these may be passive or active exercises. All limbs should be put through a range of movements at least twice a day. Active exercises can be incorporated into play. Immobile children should have their limbs placed in a natural position that maintains body alignment (Table 32.1, Figure 32.1 and 32.2).

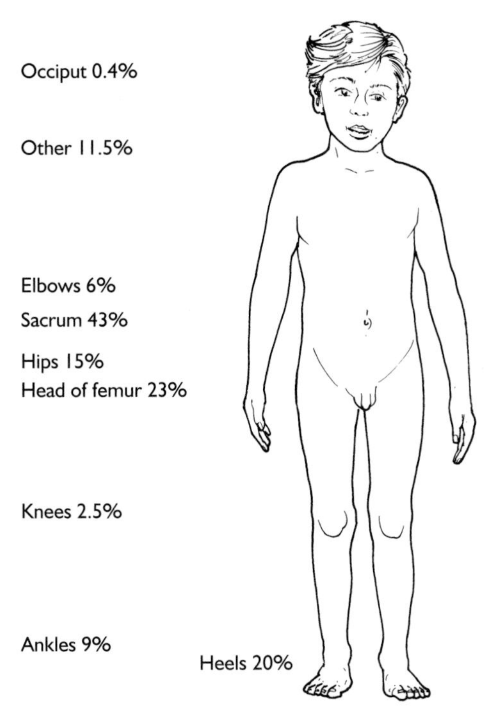

Figure 32.1 Pressure areas at risk. Torrance (1983) revealed those areas of the body most at risk from the effects of pressure. A sample of 1000 people found the percentage risk to be as shown. This study also showed that when in the sitting position the pressure on the ischial tuberosities was 300 mmHg, and when supine the pressure on the buttocks was 70 mmHg.

Study activity

Make up a list of games that would enable a child on traction to exercise the unrestricted limbs.

Rest and sleep

Rest and sleep are often difficult for children confined to bed as their usual mobility is severely curtailed. This is a particular problem for children on traction who do not feel ill but are forced to be immobile for long periods of time. Such children need to have their days planned carefully to ensure that they are as mentally and physically active as possible during the day, with a planned routine of events just as they would have at home. These activities should be as close as possible to the normal home routine. For instance, if a boy plays football after school, a game of blow football may take its place. In this way the nurse can endeavour to ensure that the child is tired by bedtime and will sleep as well as usual.

Study activity

Rashid, aged 8, is being nursed on traction for a fractured femur. Plan a day's activity for him for a Friday and a Saturday.

Date			
Weight			
Average according to age	0	0	0
Below birth weight	2	2	2
Below weight according to age	3	3	3
Overweight	3	3	3
Continence			
Continent	0	0	0
Catheterised	1	1	1
Incontinent for children >4 years	2	2	2
Nappies	2	2	2
Nappy rash	3	3	3
Enuretic	3	3	3

Date			
Skin types			
Dark	0	0	0
Fair	1	1	1
Sensitive	2	2	2
Broken/spot	3	3	3
Mobility			
Fully	0	0	0
Restless/fidgety	1	1	1
Sedated/non-walker restricted	2	2	2
Paralysed	4	4	4
Appetite			
Average/good	0	0	0
Poor	1	1	1
NG tube			
Fluids only	2	2	2
Malabsorption	3	3	3
Failure to thrive	3	3	3
Nil by mouth dehydrated	3	3	3

Date			
Age			
Neonates	3	3	3
Infant	1	1	1
Toddler	1	1	1
Pre-school (2–5)	1	1	1
6 years plus	1	1	1
General assessment			
Severe cyanosis and clubbing	5	5	5
Moderate cyanosis	3	3	3
Mild cyanosis	1	1	1
Asymptomatic	0	0	0

Date			
Special risks			
Tissue malnutrition e.g. terminal cachexia	8	8	8
Circulatory/vascular disease	5	5	5
Diabetes	4	4	4
Hypoxaemia	5	5	5
Inotropic support	3	3	3
Known infection, e.g. MRSA, *Pseudomonas*	2	2	2
Neurological deficit			
Unconsciousness	5	5	5
Developmentally delayed	2	2	2
Normal milestone achieved	0	0	0
Major surgery/trauma			
On table > 2 hours	5	5	5
On table > 5 hours	7	7	7
Medication			
Antibiotic-induced diarrhoea /thrush/rashes	3	3	3

Total score at end of each assessment

Significant event	Date	Score	Name of nurse
Admission			

Score classification	10+ At risk	15+ High risk	20+ Very high risk

Figure 32.2 Pressure sore risk assessment chart for children (Bedi, 1993).

Communication

Children are normally active so a period of forced immobility is particularly frustrating. If clear explanations are not given to rationalise the need for immobility small children can believe that it is a punishment for bad behaviour. Immobilisation alters the number of environmental stimuli that active children receive and affects their growing need for autonomy and independence, leading to feelings of boredom, frustration, depression and isolation. Children of varying ages and personality will respond differently, but young children tend to become more attention seeking and may regress to earlier behaviour such as thumb sucking or bed wetting. Older children may become aggressive, irritable, argumentative or uncooperative in an attempt to assert some control over the situation. Boredom tends to decrease communication, concentration and problem-solving skills. These types of behaviour are not usually acceptable but in difficult situations such as immobility children need to be able to express their anger without fear of further punishment. They need to be helped to act out this anger appropriately in play and given a full and varied programme of activity to avoid boredom and its consequential maladaptive behaviour changes.

Study activity

Check your answer to the previous activity and assess whether you have enabled Rashid to overcome his frustration and boredom.

Breathing and circulation

Immobility can lead to a sluggish circulation and clotting problems, as well as stasis of respiratory secretions and chest infections. Chest physiotherapy should be included in the day's planned activities to improve venous return and breathing and avoid these complications. Chest physiotherapy that consists of deep breathing exercises can be incorporated into play.

Study activity

Consider what play to use for an immobile child, which would also provide chest physiotherapy.

Maintaining body temperature

Ill children may have a pyrexia that interferes with their usual ability to be alert and active. Pyrexia can be relieved simply by pharmacological intervention or cooling measures such as minimal clothing and reducing the circulating air temperature. Cooling measures should not induce shivering as this is the body's compensatory mechanism and will increase metabolic requirements even further. Antipyretic drugs include paracetamol and non-steroidal anti-inflammatory drugs, such as ibuprofen, but there is considerable debate whether such drugs are

The debate about the use of antipyretics

In favour of antipyretics	Against antipyretic use
Beliefs that fever is harmful	Fever by itself is self-limiting and rarely harmful
Untreated fever may rise to a dangerous level, causing CNS damage	Fever, unlike hyperthermia, is regulated by an effective thermoregulatory centre
Relieves parental anxiety	Educating parents may reduce use
Risk of febrile convulsion	No scientific evidence that antipyretics prevent febrile convulsions
Fever has a protective role against infection	Antipyretics may interfere with characteristic fever patterns, which have a diagnostic value
	Antipyretics can have adverse effects

(Sahib el-Radhi, 2004)

harmful or beneficial. Pyrexias are thought to be incidental in enhancing immunity and recovery from infection, so treatment should be aimed at reducing the child's discomfort rather than the fever itself. If antipyretics are used, the child's temperature should be checked approximately half an hour after administration. Traditional methods of reducing fever such as tepid baths are now known to be infective and generally add to the child's discomfort (Sahib el-Radhi, 2004).

Key Points

1. The children's nurse has to take on the role of the surrogate carer when parents are unable to give their child the usual family care due to other commitments, the nature of the child's illness or the need for a break from the demanding hospital routine.
2. Providing family care as a surrogate carer requires the nurse to have an intimate knowledge of usual family routines.
3. The child's usual activities of normal living may need adaptation to be continued in hospital and to fit the child's altered abilities.
4. Children confined to bed are at risk from complications of immobility and their care needs to take the prevention of these into consideration.

Chapter 33

Community Nursing

Introduction

Nursing children at home is not a new concept. Before the Industrial Revolution sick children were cared for at home by their mothers or siblings and rich families employed a physician or nurse to care for the child in the home. It is only since the development of scientific medicine, and the emergence of the National Health Service (NHS) in 1948, that hospital care has become the accepted place for the sick. This shift to institutional care occurred despite evidence from psychologists and government recommendations that children may become traumatised by hospitalisation and are best nursed at home. It is only within the past 25 years that schemes have emerged to provide care and support in the community for ill children to avoid hospital admission or to shorten their hospital stay. However, the type and degree of specialist services to assist children to be nursed at home vary considerably throughout the country.

Study activity

Find out what facilities there are in your area for nursing children at home.

Background

It appears that in some areas of the UK, children's community care does not have a high priority despite the recognition by the government that children should be nursed at home whenever possible (RCN, 1994). This recognition largely developed from the work of psychologists who were able to demonstrate the adverse effects of hospitalisation for children. However, it must not be forgotten that long before this some doctors and nurses were aware that hospitalisation was inappropriate for some children. In 1909, Nichol reported on a day surgery scheme in

Glasgow and suggested 'that with a mother of average intelligence and assisted by advice from the hospital sister, the child will fare better at home than in the hospital'. The following year, Boge recognised that the value of children's nurses in the community had not been fully realised and that some nurses could help 'people to keep crippled children at home'. However, wider recognition of the need to minimise hospitalisation for children did not occur until the 1950s. In 1953, Bowlby identified that after admission to hospital young children suffered 'maternal deprivation' and as a result became depressed, withdrawn and failed to thrive. His findings were supported by Robertson and Robertson (1952). These findings initiated the Platt Committee's report (Platt, 1959), which recommended the creation of a specialist community nursing service for the home care of ill children to prevent or minimise the need for admission to hospital. Very few health authorities responded to this recommendation, but specialist services were introduced in Rotherham (Gillet, 1954), Paddington (Lightwood *et al.*, 1956) and Birmingham (Smellie, 1956). The children's community nurses (CCNs) involved mostly cared for children with infectious diseases (Whiting, 1994). This poor response needs to be considered alongside children's services generally in the 1950s. Most general hospitals did not have any registered sick children's nurses (RSCNs) and the concept of involving the family in care was largely unknown. Many of the hospitalised children at this time were admitted with complications following infectious diseases such as measles, chickenpox, whooping cough or tuberculosis (Conisbee, 1982), and parents were only allowed to visit twice weekly for 1 hour because of the fear of the spread of infection (Currie, 1982). Therefore, it is not surprising that many health authorities did not respond to the Platt Report.

From the 1960s the government began to emphasise the importance of community care generally (MoH, 1962). In 1971 they again specifically investigated children's community services and found them lacking. Further emphasis was placed on the importance of caring for children in their own homes (MoH, 1971). In 1976, the Court Report recommended the development of nursing advice and support for sick children in the community by child health nurses (DHSS, 1976a). Children were identified as a priority group and it was suggested that an increase in the provision of community and preventive care for children would reduce spending on acute and institutional care areas (DHSS, 1976b). However, major reorganisation of the Health Service was occurring at this time and was repeated in 1982. These changes in Health Service management resulted in health authorities no longer being obliged to have a senior nurse and medical officer responsible for child health (Graham, 1987). Some areas showed a decline in childcare services because of the loss of such posts and the consequent lack of commitment to the care of children from the health authority. Children continued to be nursed mainly in hospital by general nurses.

In the 1990s government reports and policies continued to stress that children should only be admitted to hospital if their needs cannot be met at home or on a day-care basis (DH, 1991a; Audit Commission, 1993). Pressure groups also campaigned for the expansion of children's community nursing services so that children could be nursed in their own homes (British Paediatric Association, 1991b; Caring for Children in the Health Service, 1993; Action for Sick Children, 1993).

These had little impact on the provision for community care for children in many areas. Whiting (1989) reported that there were 24 children's community nursing teams across the UK at this time. Some NHS Trusts employed a liaison health visitor who took responsibility for informing the community nurses and/or health visitors of all children discharged from hospital, all new births and all children seen in the A&E unit. In these areas, any nursing care required at home was performed by community nurses who were not RSCNs/RNs(child). Their job descriptions stated that they would provide care for patients of all ages. As Kitchener (1993) indicated, the competence of these staff was not in question, but the inability to provide care by registered children's nurses did not give those children receiving care at home the same rights and specialist care that they could receive in hospital. It also did not meet the Court Report (Court, 1976) recommendations that paediatric skills and knowledge be applied in the care of all children whatever their age or disability and wherever they live. Fradd (1990) recognised that most general trained district nurses are not experienced in the care of sick children, were inappropriately equipped and often frightened by this involvement. The Audit Commission (1993) discovered that many children have a prolonged period of hospitalisation if there is no specialised community care available. Certainly, children with asthma, diabetes and fractures, conditions that the Commission suggest could be mainly cared for at home with appropriate support, tended to stay in hospital for at least 7 days in areas where there were no specialist community children's nurses (Kitchener, 1993).

In other areas there was only one CCN who liaised directly with the wards and neonatal unit as well as receiving referrals from other clinical areas. These post holders found it impossible to take on the responsibility of actual nursing care for a large number of acutely ill children and could only provide a Monday-to-Friday office hours service. Instead they taught the family and/or district nurses the necessary care and provided them with specialist support. They also provided liaison with school nurses and teachers. Patel (1990) agreed that one of the advantages of community care to the child is the ability to continue school. When Fradd (1990) set up a CCN service in Nottingham she quickly realised that one nurse could not cope with the workload, but even this minimum service meets the needs of mothers as identified by McDonald (1988). Although a small study, this research discovered that over 50% of parents whose children had been discharged from hospital would have appreciated more support and information for care continuing at home. The Audit Commission (1993:54) reports similar responses; for instance, one parent in their survey stated: 'I was terrified of doing something wrong and could never have come out of hospital without the paediatric nurse'. A single CCN can enable children with asthma and fractures to go home earlier than similar children in areas where there is no CCN service.

Children's Community Nursing in the 21st Century

How has children's community nursing progressed? In recent years there has been recognition of the need for more community care for children and significant investment has been made. In 1998 the Department of Health provided funding for the establishment of 52 projects to enable the care of children with life-threatening illnesses (NHS Executive, 1998). In 1999 further funding was made available to create eight Diana, Princess of Wales, CCN teams (DH, 1998). In 2002 the New Opportunites Fund donated £48 million to enable the creation of 71 teams to provide palliative care for children with life-threatening and life-limiting illnesses. In 2005 the RCN directory of services showed that there were almost 240 CCN teams across the UK. The majority of areas without a CCN team cite finance as the main reason for this lack (Catchpole, 1986; Whiting, 1989).

However, the teams that are in place have developed to meet local need rather than having been strategically planned or commissioned (RCN, 2000). As a result, the teams work in different ways and provide care in a variety of ways for children with acute and chronic needs and for children with complex needs. There are at least six different models of providing the service and many different philosophies and referral criteria (Eaton, 2001). There are also significant gaps in provision of care. Many of the children who are technology dependent require intensive support and expensive equipment to enable them to be cared for at home and CCN teams support them with limited resources (Kirk and Glendinning, 1999) so that social support and respite care is often lacking (Heaton *et al.*, 2003). In 2000 the Department of Health recognised that there was no equity of care across the UK for children in the community and recommended that CCN services should have an investment plan for reform. This recommendation is supported by the Bristol Royal Infirmary Inquiry (2001), the Laming report (Victoria Climbié Inquiry, 2003) and the Department for Education and Skills. The Audit Commission (2003) found that services for disabled children in the community were fragmented and that the needs of families were rarely taken into consideration in any provision of health or social care. In part, this picture may have developed as a result of different funding arrangements. In recent years Primary Care Trusts have taken on the commissioning role for health care and are the sources of funding. With so many demands on their restricted funds it is hardly surprising that the healthcare needs of a child with complex needs, whose care package may cost between £10 000 and £25 000 a year, may not always be totally met.

Standards 6 and 8 of the National Service Framework (NSF) for children recognises the opportunities to develop CCN services to improve the current situation. Standard 6 aims to develop integrated services to provide coordinated care for those children who need care outside the hospital setting. Standard 8 relates specifically to disabled children and those with complex needs. This standard emphasises the need to provide coordinated, high-quality child- and family-centred services to enable these children and their families to live ordinary lives as far as possible. The Children Act 2004 provides the legislative framework to enable these reforms to take place. It strengthens the need for effective integration of all the agencies involved in the care of children and requires local authorities to bring together local partners through the development of Children's Trusts. The development of Trusts aimed to delegate functions and pool resources to provide integrated delivery, processes, strategy and governance to enable better inter-agency partnership working in the delivery of services for children. To aid this integration, Trusts are required to develop a national common assessment framework and enable information sharing between agencies.

Thirty-five Children's Trusts were created in 2004 as pilot sites with the aim that all areas of England would have Trusts by 2008. The government did not prescribe the model for the pilot Trusts that link health, education and social services to enable guidance for the most successful way of working to steer the development of future Trusts. However, the expectation that Trusts will be created rapidly has not allowed time to evaluate the pilot sites. Consequently there are local variations and the emphasis has moved from Trusts being providers of all services to a commissioning model. They integrate local education, social care and some health services. This may not solve the funding issues for health. Spending for education and children's social care is significantly greater than health and it is difficult to see how priorities will be determined (Moore, 2004). There are also problems of territory. The boundaries of county councils are not always the same as the boundaries of healthcare providers and commissioners. The involvement of healthcare professionals varies across the country. In some areas health visitors have moved from health centres and GP attachments and are working from the newly created children's centres. Will CCN teams be following this pattern? There is concern about professional leadership in these situations with directors of children's services mostly coming from a local authority background (Moore, 2004).

The role of the children's community nurse

Neonatal care

- care of babies with home oxygen
- management of babies with physiological jaundice

Care of children with acute problems

- respiratory tract infections
- gastro-enteritis
- constipation

Post-operative care

- ear, nose and throat surgery
- wound dressings
- circumcisions
- hernia repairs

Follow-up and support following trauma

- fractures stabilised in plaster of Paris
- children discharged on traction

Support and teaching for families of children with long-term health problems

- chronic respiratory problems (asthma, cystic fibrosis)
- skin disorders (eczema, psoriasis)
- haemoglobinopathies (including administration of blood)
- alternative methods of feeding
- taking blood/administering IV medication from established lines
- peritoneal/haemodialysis

Care and support for families of terminally ill children

- cytotoxic therapy
- palliative care

Study activity

Find out about the Children's Trust in your own area. How does it work and to what extent are healthcare professionals part of the Trust?

The Advantages and Disadvantages of Nursing Children at Home

Study activity

Is nursing children at home always beneficial? Consider if there are any disadvantages to this service and whether these drawbacks outweigh the benefits.

It should be appreciated that home care may cause problems for some children and their families (Table 33.1). Although children who have day care avoid the traumatic effects of hospitalisation (Visintainer and Wolfer, 1975), they can become fearful at home if their parents are anxious about home care and are not confident in their own caring abilities (Glasper *et al.*, 1989). There is evidence that parents can cope better with children's impending death if they can care for them at home, but not all parents feel able to take on this responsibility (Sidey, 1990). Siblings of children cared for at home sometimes suffer as a result of reduced attention to their needs (Bluebond-Langer, 1989). These

Table 33.1 Advantages and disadvantages of home care

Advantages	Disadvantages
Child feels safe in familiar environment	May associate parts of home with painful procedures
Reduced risk of cross infection in own home	Home may not be suitable for aseptic procedures
Parents may feel more in control	Nurse must respect family values
Nurse has fewer distractions than in a busy ward	Parents may feel unsupported when nurse not there
Nurse able to know child and family better as individuals	Nurse may find the closer relationship stressful
Increased bed availability in hospital	Increased patient dependency in hospital wards
Nurse has more autonomy in care	Nurse may feel unsupported by colleagues

problems cannot be ignored but they can be overcome by the careful assessment of families before discharge by an experienced children's nurse. A CCN, who will be used to working in partnership with parents, can also be alert for signs that home care is becoming too stressful for the family.

Although there is little research to show the benefits of a CCN service, Stein and Jessop (1984) found that home care for children with chronic illness was effective in improving the satisfaction of the family with care and the child's psychological adjustment. It also reduced maternal stress. However, this was an American study, which may not compare with health care in this country. The researchers also used lay interviewers who may have unknowingly confounded the results. In 1985, Atwell and Gow found that the CCN service in Southampton reduced patient stay by 3.2 days, increased patient turnover, reduced waiting lists and saved £215 000 a year. The Kennedy Report (Bristol Royal Infirmary Inquiry, 2001) greatly supported the need for nurses with specific training in the care of children. Although Kennedy was describing the care of children in hospital the working parties preparing the Children's NSF found that his recommendations applied equally to services in the community (DH, 2003c). The RCN cited the lack of children's diabetic nurses as a major contributing factor for 80% of diabetic children not reaching recommended blood glucose levels (RCN, 2004).

The Role of the CCN

The aims of many community children's services include parental support and the avoidance of hospitalisation for children by preventing admission or enabling early discharge. The early services were set up to provide community care for children with acute illnesses who would otherwise be admitted to hospital. However, the number of children now being discharged from hospital with long-term needs is increasing, and their care and support is beginning to form a considerable portion of the CCN's caseload. As a result, the care of acutely ill children at home is decreasing. In 1954, the first recorded RSCNs were appointed to care for children in the community and the Paddington Home Care Unit was established. At this time GP referrals formed 60% of the caseload. In 1994, this proportion had decreased to six referrals per year. In response to this trend, Hospital at Home schemes have developed. These schemes provide an integrated service between hospital and home. Nurses rotate from ward to community, enabling them to transfer their skills in acute care to the child's home while helping them to appreciate discharge planning when working in the ward area. The child and family are visited by the nurse while the child is still in hospital, and they remain in the care of this nurse and the hospital consultant until discharged from the scheme.

Different roles for CCN teams have emerged over the years. As the integration of children with disabilities into mainstream schools increases, many teams are involved in teaching education staff about these children's healthcare needs. As part of this role they often become involved in health education and promotion. Leask (2005) describes a scheme where a CCN team helps to improve the health of those children who are persistently absent from school. In 2006, the government began to discuss increasing GP services and the reintroduction of GP-led 'cottage' hospitals, where GPs would care for patients with short-term problems and perform minor surgery. This could result in further changes in the admission of children to hospital and the role of the CCN.

Since the growth of the children's community nursing service, the question of specific preparation for CCNs has arisen. All CCNs are registered children's nurses but many of them do not have a specific children's community nursing qualification. Some services make the community nursing course an essential prerequisite for applicants. The validity of this course as a means of preparation for a CCN has been debated, as the theory and practice relate mostly to adult nursing with the emphasis on the care of the elderly (Godman, 1994). However, at present, there are still very few courses designed specifically for the CCN. As the present RN(child) course prepares the nurse to work in hospital and community settings it may be argued that such preparation is not necessary.

Independent nurse prescribing may also help to advance the CCN service by preventing fragmentation, duplication and unnecessary delays in care (Peter and Flynn, 2002). Currently the approved course is adult focused and effective support by a paediatrician and paediatric pharmacist in the candidate's own Trust is required if practitioners are able to function safely.

The Future?

Campbell (1987) suggests that the reason why community services for children vary across the country is that local services develop to meet local need. This is not always the case. Some areas where there is a large child population and a known increase in childhood diabetes, asthma and accidents (Kitchener, 1993) still lack an effective CCN service to meet all needs. This may be because the needs of children in such regions have not been specifically identified. There may be no senior nurse to provide a focus for children's services as recommended by the Audit Commission (1993) and, apart from childhood accidents, public health reports often do not relate to children specifically. This is in spite of the opening statement of the Court Report: 'We want to see a child and family-centred service'. This omission may be because the local health plans are based on the government's *Health For All* targets, which also do not relate specifically to children. It may be that children's nurses have not been proactive enough to promote the advantages of their unique skills and to actively support these recommendations (*see also* The future of children's nursing p. 669).

Study activity

Take time to discuss with others the possible reasons government policies such as this have not always supported recommendations for improving children's services. Consider if this is beginning to change.

The children's NSF makes it clear that healthy children have more chance of becoming healthy adults. It aims to ensure that children have services in place to have a fulfilling and enjoyable childhood, laying the right foundations for a healthy adult life. The present government appears to be committed to improving the health of children and young people but the NSF is a 10-year programme that lacks measurable goals.

Summary

It seems likely that nursing children in the community will continue to be a developing service. It not only meets parents' and children's wishes but relieves the pressure on hospital beds. However, as more children are nursed at home there is a great need for more specialised and integrated support for the parents. They need specialised nursing support as well as a respite service to enable them to spend uninterrupted time with the rest of the family. To meet this need, more community nursing programmes are required for children's nurses and all community nurses need to emphasise the importance of having the specific community nursing preparation for caring for their own client group and working in partnership with other agencies. In this way these nurses can recognise and act as advocates for their client group in urging for other forms of support in the community.

Key Points

1. The provision of community children's care in many areas is still poor. There has been little recognition of government reports that recommend such services and there is no senior children's nurse to promote the development of the services.
2. The type of service available to provide care for children at home is very variable across the UK.
3. The role of the CCN is varied and has changed over time to meet the changing health needs of the population.
4. There needs to be more research into the benefits and drawbacks of home care for children.
5. Children's nurses need to be more assertive and active in trying to establish and maintain recommended standards of care for children. They need to promote their specialist knowledge and skills so that they are accepted as the specialists in child care.

Chapter 34

Pre- and Post-operative Care

Tina Moules

Introduction

Expertise is required when caring for children undergoing surgery to ensure that the experience is as positive as it can be. Hospitalisation can be traumatic for any child but the added stress of surgery may cause considerable anxiety for the child and his carers. Personal experience has shown that even minor surgery can be distressing to a parent who, for a period of time, has no control at all over what happens to their child. It is vital, therefore, that the surgical experience is managed effectively and with a degree of empathy in order to achieve a successful outcome.

Study activity

Critically reflect on experiences that you may have had – perhaps you had surgery as a child, or perhaps you have a child who has required surgery at some time. Were the experiences positive? What were the negative aspects (if any)?

The nurse's role before and after surgery is to ensure that:

- the child and family are helped to cope with the experience in a positive manner
- the child is adequately prepared physically
- the child's safety is not compromised
- the likelihood of post-operative complications is minimised and the child's recovery is uneventful
- the child and family are adequately prepared for discharge home

Surgical interventions can be divided into two groups:

- *Planned or elective procedures*. In this case surgery can take place when the child is in the best possible condition physically. Much of the preparation can take place before admission and the child and his carers can be given opportunity to come to terms with the forthcoming surgery. Children can be admitted in good time to allow physical preparation to be carried out. Admission to hospital can sometimes be arranged on a day-care basis so that the effects of hospital are minimised. However, even planned short-stay surgery can cause distress and anxiety and so care must be implemented accordingly.

- *Emergency or unplanned procedures*. Emergency surgery is carried out when the severity of the child's condition may be life threatening or disabling. In these cases preparation time is much reduced for the child and his carers, who have to cope not only with sudden illness or trauma but also the uncertainty of emergency surgery. It is important therefore to ensure that all essential preparation is done and that the child and carers are given sufficient information on which to base any decisions. This can be a difficult time and decisions may have to be taken quickly. You should ensure that carers are given support and someone to talk to, especially while the child is in theatre (*see also* Day care p. 289).

Examples of procedures which may be done on an elective basis

- Adenotonsillectomy
- Insertion of grommets
- Correction of squint
- Circumcision
- Correction of orthopaedic deformities
- Some heart surgery
- Orchidopexy
- Dental extractions

Examples of procedures which may be done on an emergency basis

- Appendicectomy
- Some neurosurgery
- Hernias
- Pyloric stenosis
- Stabilisation of fractures
- Surgery for abdominal trauma

Study activity

Try to put yourself in the following situation (if possible try role-playing it with some colleagues – use any experiences that you have had to help you). Make a list of all the feelings you might have and consider what support you would like. You are the young parent of a 4-year-old daughter, Sarah, who has been admitted following a road traffic accident in which she was knocked over by a speeding car. The driver of the car is suspected of being under the influence of alcohol. Sarah is your only child and she requires emergency life-saving surgery within the next 2 hours. Your partner is working away from home and will not be with you until the next day.

Whether surgery is planned or not, you must endeavour to ensure that the child and family are helped to cope with the experience of surgery in the best way possible. Activities to achieve this may include the following:

- Arrange to talk to groups of young children in a variety of settings (for example, play groups and schools) about hospital and surgery. Preparing children in this way can promote understanding of hospitals and help to dispel misconceptions. Rodin (1983) found that children who had this sort of preparation and who were subsequently admitted to hospital were less anxious and more cooperative than other children.
- Ensure that preparation is geared towards the child's cognitive and emotional level. Using inappropriate words can cause more distress than they are meant to alleviate. Young children think literally and those under 7 years may take analogies literally (*see also* Language development p. 77, Preparing children for procedures p. 270 and Day care p. 289).

Study activity

Consider how a young child might interpret the following – in each case think of a more appropriate way to explain: (a) 'I am just going to suck out your mouth to take away all the spit', (b) 'I am going to take your blood pressure', (c) 'your lungs are like balloons' and (d) 'your heart is like a pump'.

Further reading

Oster, G. D. and Gould, P. (1987) *Using Drawings in Assessment and Therapy*. New York: Brunner/Mazel.

Factors influencing body image

These factors include:

- social class
- skin colour
- culture
- physical attractiveness
- weight and height
- speech
- puberty
- congenital abnormalities
- learning disability
- life-limiting illness
- chronic illness
- physical disability

(White, 1995)

- Organise 'Saturday Clubs' or pre-admission sessions – many wards and units have set these up as a way of preparing groups of children for planned surgery.
- Encourage children to draw in the pre-operative period. O'Malley and McNamara (1993; see also Oster and Gould, 1987) describe the use of drawing as a means of assessing children's understanding of forthcoming surgery and of highlighting their fears and anxieties. Drawing allows children to express feelings and ideas. Artwork can reveal concerns such as loss of control, body changes and mutilation. Personal use of this technique demonstrated how effective this can be. A young boy had been admitted to my ward for tonsillectomy. His mother was unable to stay and after she left he became withdrawn and displayed signs of extreme anxiety. He would talk to no one and concerns about his psychological state prompted the Sister to ask for help from the psychologist. She asked the boy to draw a picture of himself after surgery – his picture showed himself with only one leg. On further investigation it was discovered that the boy's uncle had recently been in hospital for amputation of his leg. The boy was under the misconception that his surgery would be the same – his fears were allayed.

Study activity

Try this technique out on some children waiting for surgery. What do their pictures tell you?

- Consider the possible effect surgery may have on the child's body image (for example plastic surgery, stoma formation, limb surgery). Art therapy may highlight any fears that the child may have. Many factors influence a child's perception of their body image. A concern with appearance is part of physical development (particularly during adolescence) and therefore the implications of surgery need to be discussed. Often a child's fears can be allayed through detailed explanation. Where physical deformity is a likely outcome of surgery time must be made to ensure counselling from specialist nurses (such as the stoma nurse).
- Encourage the presence of parents in the anaesthetic and recovery rooms where appropriate (*see also* Anaesthesia p. 294).

Preparing Children Physically for Surgery

The aim of pre-operative preparation is to ensure that the child is well enough for surgery and to obtain relevant information in order to plan and implement care appropriately. A general assessment should be done and the following specific interventions carried out:

- Accurate weight – the dosages of anaesthetic drugs are generally calculated according to the child's weight. The importance of this cannot be stressed enough. The child should be weighed wearing the minimum of clothing and in some units the weight must be checked

by two people (check your hospital policy on weighing children). The weight should be displayed prominently on the relevant documentation (*see also* Weighing babies and children p. 285).
- Urine test – a routine urinalysis should be carried out on all children having surgery. Testing the urine will identify children who may have undiagnosed renal disease or diabetes.
- A discussion about pain control – prior to surgery it is useful to discuss pain with the child and his carers.
- Ensure that consent for surgery has been given and that the consent form is attached to the child's notes. This is the responsibility of the surgeon but the nurse should check that the parents and child have been fully informed and that all relevant information regarding surgery has been explained. The consent form should meet 2002 Department of Health guidelines and best practice would enable the child to give a consenting signature too. The information given to parents should provide them with details of the benefits and risks of the procedure as well as the alternative treatments. Where possible it is advisable for a nurse to be present when consent is gained to ensure misconceptions are avoided.
- Implement pre-operative fasting – children who are 'nil by mouth' must be clearly identified.
- Administration of pre-medication – prior to giving the pre-med it is useful to encourage the child to visit the toilet to pass urine. This enables the last passage of urine prior to surgery to be noted and reduces the need for the sedated child to be disturbed.
- Children from certain ethnic groups (of Asian, North African, Mediterranean and Afro-Caribbean origins) will require assessment of sickle-cell or thalassaemia status. Surgery on a child with an undiagnosed abnormality may provoke a crisis.

(*See also* Urine testing pp. 490–92, Caring for children in pain p. 351, Informed consent p. 683, Restricted intake p. 294, Pre-medication p. 344 and Management of sickle-cell crisis p. 425.)

Study activity

- Find out the Department of Health guidelines for consent and see how your unit's consent process follows these.
- Investigate the pre-medication protocol in your children's surgical unit. Discuss with the anaesthetist.

Safety of the Child

To ensure that the child's safety is not compromised you should take the following actions:

- Check all notes and other relevant documentation are in order.
- Ensure that the child is wearing a correct identification band.
- Ensure that the child removes all jewellery – diathermy is used to cauterise blood vessels during surgery and any contact with metal objects can cause diathermy burns.

- Ensure that the child is not wearing any make-up or nail varnish – this is so that the child's skin and nailbeds can be monitored for signs of hypoxia during surgery.
- Check for loose teeth and make appropriate note on child's records. Loose teeth can become dislodged during intubation.
- Ensure that the child is transferred safely to and from theatre.
- Ensure that the child's condition is stable before leaving the recovery area. It is the anaesthetist's responsibility to ensure that full recovery is assured (Simpson, 1977). This responsibility can be delegated to the nurse in recovery provided that proper training has been given. It is therefore important that the nurse collecting the child from theatre checks all aspects of the child's surgery and recovery before taking the responsibility of escorting the child back to the ward. If you are in doubt you should ask for the child to be checked by the anaesthetist.
- Prepare for the child's return to the ward – prepare the bed area – oxygen and suction equipment should be close by, along with any other specific equipment.
- Implement post-operative care.

Post-operative Care

The purpose of care during this period is to monitor the child's recovery and detect signs of any complications. The frequency of observations will depend on the child's general condition and will be decreased or increased accordingly. The observations made post-operatively can help to detect complications.

Potential hypoventilation and asphyxia

Hypoventilation is common in the immediate post-operative period and can lead to serious respiratory complications (hypoxaemia, hypercarbia, collapsed segment of the lung, pneumonia). Hypoventilation can occur as a result of (Watson, 1979):

- central nervous depression by anaesthetic agents
- respiratory muscle depression by muscle relaxant
- partial airway obstruction by tongue or lower jaw
- laryngeal oedema following endotracheal intubation

Observe the child for signs of hypoventilation, which include: abnormally slow or shallow respirations, excessive secretions, wheezing, restlessness, cyanosis and rapid pulse rate.

Asphyxia can occur if the relaxed tongue and lower jaw 'fall back' blocking the pharynx, or following aspiration of mucus and vomit, which can occur due to loss of the swallowing reflex. Measures should be taken to promote adequate ventilation as follows:

- The child should be nursed in the lateral or semi-prone position until a gag reflex is well established. If necessary the position can be maintained by the use of pillows.
- Remove excessive secretions as necessary using pharyngeal suction.
- Administer oxygen by nasal cannulae or mask as directed.
- Once the child has recovered, encourage deep breathing and coughing to remove secretions and expand lungs. Assist to the sitting position.

Small children will assume the most comfortable position for themselves, which often means lying flat. In this instance therapy from the physiotherapist may be required.

Shock

Shock is defined as circulatory failure that leads to inadequate perfusion of body tissues and organs. It can develop immediately after surgery, or slowly, becoming evident several hours after surgery. It is important that signs of shock are identified early so that treatment can be implemented. One of the most important observations to make is that of the general appearance of the child. Often a child will 'look bad' before there are any measurable changes in vital signs. A child who is in shock will have pale mucous membranes, mottled cold extremities, irritability, then lethargy. Other signs include weak, thready, rapid pulse (bradycardia is a dangerous sign and should be reported immediately), tachypnoea and temperature instability. Hypotension is a late sign of shock in children. Report any signs of shock promptly. Support a child who is shocked by keeping the surroundings calm, treating pain (which reduces the demand for oxygen), keeping the child warm and administering oxygen as needed.

Types of shock

- *Hypovolaemic* – 'a compromise in systemic perfusion resulting from inadequate intravascular volume relative to the vascular space'.
- *Cardiogenic* – caused by impaired myocardial function which compromises cardiac output.
- *Septic* – that which occurs 'when an infectious organism triggers a host response which compromises cardiovascular function, systemic perfusion and oxygen delivery and use'.

(Hazinski, 1992)

Haemorrhage

Haemorrhage following surgery (reactionary) may occur as a result of a slipped ligature or an increase in blood pressure, which dislodges a clot that plugged a severed vessel. Haemorrhage may be visible at the wound site or may be internal, in which case it can only be recognised by a change in vital signs. These include rapid, thready pulse, fall in blood pressure (a late sign in children), rapid respirations, pallor, apprehension, restlessness and weakness. Report any suspicion of haemorrhage promptly. Secondary haemorrhage can occur several days or weeks after surgery and parents should always be warned of this and given information as to what action to take.

Nausea and vomiting

Post-operative nausea and vomiting (PONV) are important complications of surgery in children. Many of the common surgical procedures in childhood are associated with a high incidence of PONV (Patel *et al.*, 1995). The highest incidence occurs in the 5–12 age group. Factors affecting the degree of PONV include the type of surgery, history of motion sickness, excessive pre-operative fasting, anaesthetic technique used, too rapid mobilisation after surgery (stimulates the vestibular system which may have been desensitised by opioids – White *et al.*, 1988) and early oral intake after surgery. Nursing actions should therefore be implemented to take account of these factors. Any nausea or vomiting should be reported immediately so that treatment with an anti-emetic can be implemented.

Urine retention

Urine output may be reduced due to the effects of anaesthetic gases. This can be complicated by the stress response to surgery, which increases ADH from the anterior pituitary, which in turn acts on renal tubules

Stages of wound healing

- *Inflammatory stage* – initial bleeding when incision made stops after diathermy and during the clotting phase. Vasodilation and oedema result
- *Destructive stage* – polymorphs and macrophages clear dead tissue and debris. The formation of fibroblasts stimulates angiogenesis. This stage can be delayed by vitamin C, iron or oxygen deficiency
- *Proliferative stage* – fibroblasts produce collagen to promote tensile strength of the wound
- *Maturation stage* – wound contracts, collagen fibres reorganised, tensile strength gradually returns

(Galvani, 1997)

Wound cleansing agents

- Tap water (Angeras *et al.*, 1992)
- Saline
- Antiseptics

Dressings

According to Turner (1985) dressings should have the following characteristics to promote optimum healing – they should:

- maintain a high humidity between the wound and the dressing
- remove excess exudate and toxic compounds
- allow gaseous exchange
- provide thermal insulation to wound surface
- be impermeable to bacteria
- be free from particles and toxic wound contaminants
- allow removal without causing trauma

Module 5

increasing permeability and reducing/preventing the excretion of water. The child's urine output must be monitored and the first passage of urine following surgery noted. Normal excretion is considered to be 0.5–1.0 ml/kg/hour. Anything less than this should be reported. Anxiety, fear of pain and/or recumbent position can all contribute to urine retention. Therefore actions can be taken to reduce all of these to encourage the child to pass urine. One favourite trick is to take the child to the bathroom and run the tap – try it yourself!

Wound complications – infection, dehiscence

Surgical wounds in children rarely become infected (Foale, 1989) and are commonly closed using dissolvable sutures. However, it is important to be vigilant for signs of wound infection, which include redness, swelling, pain at site and oozing. Any suspicion of infection should be reported and a wound swab taken. Dressings, where they are used, need to be changed using aseptic technique to avoid introducing infection. When changing dressings the nurse may have to use distractive techniques to avoid the child interfering with the procedure. The use of play and music is helpful as is the assistance of another person. Where possible encourage children not to explore underneath the dressing. This can be made harder to do if the dressing is taped all round with appropriate tape. A variety of dressings and cleansing agents are available and their use will depend on the type of wound and local policy.

Study activity

Critically explore your local policy on wound care and the use of particular types of dressing.

It is common for many surgical wounds to be left uncovered after the first 48 hours. The use of leeches is becoming more common, particularly in the management of reconstructive surgical wounds and in plastic surgery. Godfrey (1997) suggests that children take to the use of leeches quite readily while parents need a little more persuasion.

Wound breakdown (dehiscence) can occur as a result of infection, excessive coughing and general debilitation. Immediate action should be taken and the wound covered with a sterile pad. Resuturing is usually carried out.

Pain

The child should be monitored using an appropriate pain assessment tool and nursing actions implemented accordingly (*see also* Caring for children in pain p. 351 and Relieving pain pp. 356–62).

Other

Other care that may need to be considered includes:

- management of fluid balance
- positioning and handling the child
- mobilisation/physiotherapy

Study activity

Critically reflect on a child you have nursed following surgery. Which of any of the above complications occurred? What actions were taken? Do the same activity with children of differing age groups. Make notes of any research-based care that was implemented.

Planning for discharge

The aim of care is for the child to be discharged home as soon as possible following surgery. This has implications for the family and any decisions must be made with their full cooperation (*see also* Discharge home p. 295 and Management of fluid balance p. 342).

Key Points

1. The role of the nurse before and after surgery is vital to ensure optimum recovery.
2. Care of the child and family must be adapted to suit the needs of children undergoing planned or emergency procedures.
3. The safety of the child must not be compromised.
4. The nurse must understand the potential complications of surgery and their management, to promote uneventful recovery.

Leeches

Leeches are parasites that feed on the blood of mammals. The leech breaks the skin by sawing through it with minute teeth and then attaches itself with a sucker. The leech secretes a local anaesthetic (to avoid detection by the host) and an anti-coagulant (to keep blood running freely so that it can feed efficiently). The blood-sucking power of the leech is used to relieve venous congestion which can cause delicate tissues to die.

(Godfrey, 1997)

Chapter 35

Aspects of Paediatric Intensive Care

Introduction

The relatively small number of paediatric intensive care beds in the UK means that many critically ill children undergo treatment in general intensive care units, which cater predominately for adults. In these units children may be nursed in an open area alongside adults undergoing intensive care. Alternatively, critically ill children may be nursed in part of a general children's ward. Neither arrangement is satisfactory and both have serious disadvantages. First, staff involved in the care of these children may not have sufficient experience or training in paediatric intensive care, and the required skills cannot merely be extrapolated from the knowledge of the care of critically ill adults or the care of less acutely ill children. Secondly, equipment for monitoring and treating children may be inadequate and, because children's wards are often located some distance from the main hospital facilities, specialist assistance in an emergency may not be immediately available. Thirdly, critically ill children need unrestricted access and visiting from their family, and this may not be possible or appropriate in an adult intensive care unit.

In 1991 the British Paediatric Association (BPA, 1991a) set up a working party to conduct a national survey into hospital inpatient and intensive care services for children in the UK. The BPA drew attention to the lack of available information on the numbers of critically ill children, referral patterns, illness severity measures and outcomes, but concluded that

- the great majority of adult intensive care units were clearly neither staffed nor equipped to care adequately for critically ill children
- availability and staffing of facilities for children's intensive care were severely deficient
- provision of paediatric intensive care varied widely between regions
- area of major deficiency was the provision of facilities to transport sick children
- provision of intensive care on children's wards was a most unsatisfactory standard of care

Framework for the future: proposed organisation structure (for a hypothetical geographical area)

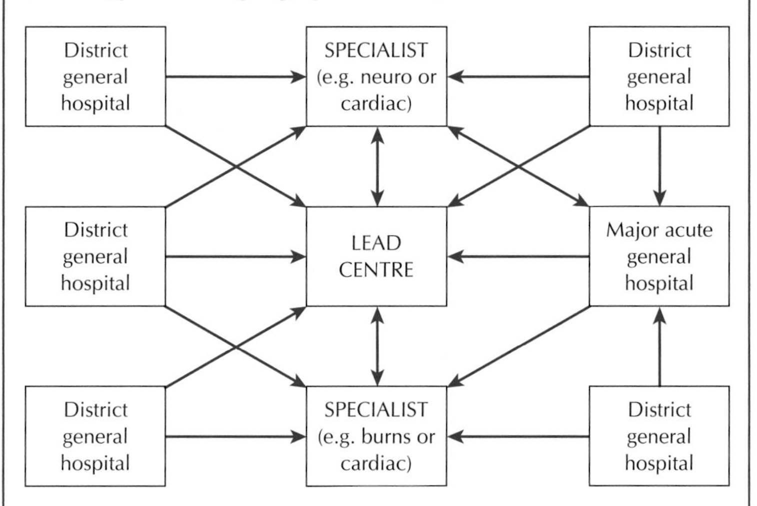

- *Lead centre*: provides all general and emergency level 3 care and most level 2 care and the retrieval service.
- *Major acute general hospital*: with a large general intensive care unit and with paediatric provision. This will already provide a considerable amount of level 2 care and will be able to initiate level 3 care.
- *Specialist centre*: providing paediatric intensive care only in association with the speciality.

(DH, 2001)

Rationale for centralising paediatric intensive care unit services (DH, 2001)

- Children in the highest risk groups are unlikely to die if treated in a PICU within a tertiary centre.
- Mortality is lower in large tertiary centres with a full complement of trained specialist staff.
- The number of critically ill children requiring level 2–3 care is small (approximately 13 000 per year in England as a whole).
- Expertise in treating these children should be concentrated to maintain skills and develop best practice.
- To maintain expertise the large centres should cover a population of at least 500 000 children aged between 0 and 16 years.

As a result of the survey the BPA recommended that:

- virtually all critically ill children should be cared for in a designated paediatric intensive care unit (PICU)
- there should be regional networks of PICUs with adequate facilities for the safe transfer of critically ill children
- a national initiative should develop PICU services
- a national mechanism be established to collect information about the need for and the provision of PICU beds

The Demand for Paediatric Intensive Care

The BPA (1993) estimated the need for PICU beds as 1 : 48 000 children, but it also recognised that seasonal variations may increase this demand in the winter months to 1 : 26 000 children. In 1993 it estimated that the national shortfall was at least 72 beds.

Study activity

Find out the child population in your own county and use this figure to calculate the county's need for PICU beds.

Definitions of levels of high dependency and intensive care

- *High dependency care (Level 1).* Those children needing close monitoring and observation, but not requiring assistance from life-support machines. For example, the recently extubated child; the child undergoing close post-operative supervision with ECG, oxygen saturation or respiratory monitoring and who may be receiving supplementary oxygen and intravenous fluids or parenteral nutrition. *This level of care requires a nurse to child ratio of at least 0.5 : 1*
- *Intensive care (Level 2).* The child requiring continuous nursing supervision who is intubated and is undergoing intermittent positive pressure ventilation or continuous positive airways pressure. Some non-intubated children may also fall into this category if their airway is unstable. For example, the child with acute upper airway obstruction requiring nebulised adrenaline. *Requires a nurse to child ratio of at least 1 : 1*
- *Intensive care (Level 3).* The child who needs intensive supervision at all times requiring additional complex and regular nursing and therapeutic procedures. This would include ventilated children undergoing peritoneal dialysis or receiving intravenous infusions of vasoactive drugs or inotropes, and children with multiple organ failure. *Requires a nurse to child ratio of at least 1.5 : 1*

(BPA, 1993)

Study activity

Take a critical look at your local provision for the care of acutely ill children and consider if it is sufficient and whether it meets the BPA (1993) recommendations.

In the winter of 1996/7 the media highlighted a number of disturbing cases of severely ill children being transported long distances in the search for a PICU bed. As a result of this growing problem, government ministers agreed to provide additional funds totalling £5 million to help maintain momentum on improvements to PIC in 1997/8. These funds were designated according to the main priorities:

- recruitment and training of nurses with specialist PIC skills
- recruitment and training of medical staff with specialist PIC skills
- enhancing retrieval services
- opening new beds in lead centres to allow care to be moved out of inappropriate areas (such as general children's wards)

However, 1997 research appears to indicate that other factors are involved in the lack of PICU beds. Fraser *et al.* (1997) questioned all PICUs in England and Scotland and discovered that children requiring long-term ventilation were occupying 12% of the available beds. During the 3-month period of the study 267 critically ill children were refused admission to these units because no beds were free and the authors estimate that an additional 273 beds could have been available if these children could have been cared for more appropriately. They suggest that prioritisation be given to:

- enabling children requiring long-term ventilation to be cared for at home or at their local hospital
- providing community rehabilitation centres or hospital long-term ventilation units for children
- clarification about which authority has the financial responsibility for such children, thus enabling funds for alternative care arrangements to be readily available

(*See also* Resources and rationing p. 709.)

Interhospital Transfers

One of the BPA's 1993 recommendations was that the care of critically ill children should be centred around designated PICUs. The NHS criticised the BPA for basing their recommendations on opinion rather than evidence, but two independent reviews commissioned by them agreed on the need for severely ill children to be cared for in dedicated PICUs (De Courcey-Golder, 1996). In 1998, in response to the 1996/7 media reports, the Department of Health produced a report suggesting a framework for the future of paediatric intensive care (DH, 1998). The report supported the centralisation of services and estimated that the number of children needing this level of care in England was around 1000 per year. The centralisation of PICUs increases the need for acutely ill children to be transported long distances to access these services.

Barry and Ralston (1994) indicated the dangers of non-specialised transfers of critically ill children between hospitals. Their study, undertaken at Birmingham Children's Hospital, indicated that almost 75% of children who were transferred suffered serious complications, with nearly 25% of these adverse events defined as life threatening. On arrival at the referral unit 11% of children needed immediate intubation and 9% were hypotensive. In most of these children monitoring of vital signs was not possible during transfer. Kanter and Tompkins (1993) estimated that at least 10% of episodes of physiological deterioration and adverse events were related to the lack of monitoring equipment during transportation.

In 1991, about 33% of PICUs provided specialised retrieval services (BPA, 1993). A study by Britto *et al.* (1995) of 51 critically ill children transferred from hospitals in and around the London area to a PICU at a tertiary centre concluded that a specialist retrieval team could deliver intensive care rapidly to children awaiting transfer. They can also transfer these children to PICU with minimal morbidity and mortality. This opinion is supported by Edge *et al.* (1994) and Logan (1995), although Logan (1995) recommends careful costing and evaluation of newly established retrieval teams to ensure a more evidence-based approach for future developments. The children's NSF (DH, 2004) recommended that each tertiary service had reliable arrangements for paediatric intensive care retrieval. The Department of Health estimated the need was for around 170 journeys per million children per year.

The provision of an effective retrieval team relies upon the availability of appropriate transport to transfer the PICU team to the referring hospital as well as returning the team and the child. It also requires a specifically trained transport team, which usually consists of a senior registrar and senior intensive care nurse. Kelly *et al.* (1996) emphasise the importance of communication between the referral hospital, PICU and the retrieval team, and recommend the use of a portable telephone to enable the retrieval team to remain in contact with the referring hospital and PICU throughout the transfer. A dedicated retrieval team requires preparation and training. After the initial training, an in-house education programme can continue to train and update staff and provide opportunities for other staff to accompany the team to gain supervised experience.

Study activity

Find out the retrieval arrangements in your own area.

High-dependency Care

In 1998 the Department of Health recognised that there was poor differentiation between high dependency and intensive care. In 2001 it commissioned a report to address this. The report found that of all children admitted to district general hospitals:

Disorders most likely to require high-dependency care (DH, 2001)

- Prolonged (over 1 hour) or recurrent convulsions
- Bacterial meningitis
- Glasgow coma score 8–12
- Circulatory instability due to hypovolaemia (other than that caused by meningococcal disease)
- Diabetic ketoacidosis with drowsiness
- Patient with uncontrollable pain
- Meningococcal septicaemia – stable state
- Intravenous fluid resuscitation >10 ml/kg and <30 ml/kg
- Acute renal failure (urine output <1 ml/hour)
- $FiO_2 > 0.5$ via headbox or facemask or nasal continuous positive airways pressure (CPAP) for bronchiolitis
- Recurrent apnoeas
- Upper airway obstruction requiring close observation
- Asthma on IV drugs or hourly nebulisers
- Poisoning/substance misuse with potential for significant problems
- After/during sedation for procedures
- Pre- or post-operative patients with complex fluid management, analgesia, bleeding, complex surgery (elective or emergency)
- Cardiac arrythmia that has responded to first-line therapy (other than cardioversion)
- Stable long-term ventilation

Module 5

- 5–15% will require high-dependency care
- 0.5–1% will require transfer to a paediatric intensive care unit

It recommended that all hospitals providing acute care for children had arrangements for high-dependency care.

Study activity

Find out the arrangements for children requiring high-dependency care in your own area.

The PICU environment

Children over 4 weeks requiring intensive care in a general hospital are often admitted to adult intensive care units (Audit Commission, 1993). Although there is no evidence from UK studies about the efficacy of such care, studies from the USA suggest that survival rates may be four times higher in a tertiary unit (Pollack *et al.*, 1991). This, with other evidence discussed above, seems likely to perpetuate the concept of centralisation of PICUs. Although centralisation has disadvantages of cost and travel it is probably the most realistic option given the limited specialist resources available. Centralisation also meets the needs of the two key principles in the care of children endorsed by government guidelines (DH, 1991b, 1995):

- infants, children and young adults have a right to safe and competent care, especially when they are critically ill and requiring intensive care
- sick children have a right to be cared for by appropriately qualified nurses

Who can provide safe and competent nursing care for children requiring intensive care? Atkinson *et al.* (1996) argue that critically ill children are not just biophysical beings requiring a high degree of technical care. They believe that registered children's nurses are essential for the care of these children who, more than ever, need their carers to recognise their unique developmental needs as children. The Audit Commission (1993) highlighted the importance of the play therapist, who can help the child to overcome the stresses of hospitalisation. The play therapist is therefore of particular importance in the PICU. Children who are in adult intensive care units often do not have children's nurses or play staff available to them.

Paediatric intensive care units are busy, clinical environments, which are stressful for the children and their families. Parents often find their altered parental role, as well as their children's behavioural and emotional responses, the most stressful aspects (Miles and Manthes, 1991). Children's stressors in the PICU environment vary according to their developmental age, but a high level of parental anxiety will lead to a high level of anxiety in the child, whatever his age. Hughes *et al.* (1994) advocate asking parents what they find most stressful and then helping them to cope with these specific stressors rather than presuming all parents have the same perceptions.

When a stay in PICU is anticipated, such as after major surgery, the parents and child can be prepared for the experience.

Study activity

Arrange to visit your local intensive care unit and consider the impression such a unit might make upon parents who have never visited such an area. How could you prepare them for the unfamiliar sights and sounds? Consider if the area is child friendly and the possible changes you could make to enhance this aspect.

The PICU provides a physical environment of constant noise, light and activity (Redman, 1994). Weibley (1989) compares noise in an intensive care unit from rubbish bins, monitor alarms, telephones and staff voices with that of road traffic and industrial machinery. Christenson (2004) found that the main source of noise in a PICU was staff conversation. My personal recollection of my first 2 days working in a PICU is hearing monitor alarms constantly, even when off duty! Extensive and continuous monitoring makes it difficult to differentiate between day and night. As a result, the child's usual waking and sleeping routine is destroyed by constant noise, light and/or stimulation. Movement and positioning are likely to cause pain and discomfort to children attached to ventilator circuits and multiple lines. Such intensive care is known to cause pain in adults (Calne, 1994) and, as suggested by Whaley and Wong (2002), 'what causes pain to adults will cause pain to children unless proven otherwise'. While frequent handling of critically ill children can increase stress and cause abrupt changes in arterial blood pressure, therapeutic touch can aid relaxation. Weibley (1989) advocates the use of stroking, cuddling and gentle touch, which also provides the most fundamental form of communication.

Lack of meaningful stimuli causes sensory deprivation and enhances the stress of an intensive care environment. Psychological stress can lead to physiological complications and impair growth and development (Mann *et al.*, 1986). In addition, constant light for infants in an intensive care environment may disturb the development of circadian rhythms and result in poor nocturnal sleep patterns in childhood.

Study activity

Consider how these PICU stimuli can be reduced and the child's usual routine enhanced while maintaining the child's safety and care.

In recognising the adverse effects of PICU, Weibley (1989) identified factors that would provide a 'growth enhancing critical care unit'. White (1997) introduced the use of *Snoezelen* as a relaxation technique within the PICU environment. *Snoezelen* incorporates the use of sight, hearing, touch and smell to provide gentle stimulation that leads to relaxation. White (1997) suggests that this technique can involve the whole family and enable them to relax, reduce feelings of helplessness and humanise intensive care.

In addition to physiological and psychological stress to patients, staff would also benefit from a quieter environment. Morrison *et al.* (2003) suggest that noise-induced stress is a good predictor of 'burn-out' for

Disorders most likely to require intensive care (DH, 2001)

- Arrythmia that fails to respond to first-line therapy
- Post-cardiac surgery
- Possibility of progressive deterioration to the point of needing ventilation (e.g. recurrent apnoeas, airway obstruction)
- The need for IV infusion of vasoactive drugs to support cardiac output or control blood pressure
- Nebulised adrenaline for upper airway obstruction after two doses or more
- Patients recently extubated after prolonged ventilation
- Post-operative patients with multiple chest drains requiring hourly fluid replacement
- Any airway intervention (e.g. tracheal intubation)
- Ventilated or assisted respiration (e.g. bag and mask) other than during recovery from anaesthesia
- Cardiopulmonary resuscitation
- Central nervous system depression sufficient to compromise the airway protective reflexes/respiratory drive or potential to progress
- Uncontrolled shock needing repeated volume or inotropics or greater than 30 ml/kg resuscitation volume
- Diabetic ketoacidosis with deteriorating level of consciousness after start of therapy
- Tracheostomy for acute illness

PICU staff as it causes negative effects on performance, attention and cognitive tasks.

Family Support

Parents can feel confused, anxious and bewildered about what is happening to their child in PICU. It is vital that staff recognise this and help them to interact and care for their child. If parents do not have this opportunity, problems such as inadequate parenting and family breakdown can occur (Shellabarger and Thompson, 1993). Continuity of carers is useful for parents, who are then able to gain confidence and trust in a consistent approach. Weibley (1989) suggests that primary nursing is crucial in optimising individualised family care in a critical care environment.

Parents should be encouraged to stay with their child in the PICU to provide the child with the comfort and security of their presence. Despite this beneficial effect, the nurse should not forget the stresses of the critical care environment and the constant anxiety that parents feel when their child is critically ill. Sometimes parents become exhausted by their constant vigil and the sensitive nurse needs to recognise this and suggest periodic respites. Darbyshire (1994:99) describes this vigil as a way of parents 'dwelling attentively and receptively with their child' which gives some indication of the fatigue caused by such watchfulness.

Siblings should not be forgotten. Siblings provide each other with companionship and emotional support, and the loss of these can make hospitalisation for a critical illness particularly stressful for the well sibling. Simon (1993) advocates early visiting by siblings to prevent the well sibling from imagining and magnifying fears. However, Morrison (1997) found that siblings who visited most frequently demonstrated the most stress. It would appear that this issue is best discussed and explained carefully to siblings and parents to enable them to make an informed decision. Then the timing and length of sibling visits can be well prepared and planned in advance. Haines and Childs (2005) found that, while most parents were satisfied with most aspects of PICU, they thought that more could be done to provide privacy, comfort and care to siblings.

The family and child can experience further stress when the time comes for transfer back to the general ward. They have gained confidence and trust in the close monitoring strategy within the PICU environment and the 1 : 1 nursing they have received. The sudden loss of this intensive care can make them feel very insecure. Dissatisfaction lies mostly around concerns with the level of staffing, supervision and safety in ward environments (Haines and Childs, 2005). Transfers should be carefully planned to enable gradual deintensification and ensure that families continue to feel that their child is being appropriately managed for the next stage in his care.

Supporting the family

- Provide encouragement to continue their important role in the child's life
- Assist them to participate in their child's care
- Encourage them to teach the staff about their child's individual needs and behaviour
- Share all information
- Ensure explanations are consistent and recognise the need to repeat these
- Stress the importance to their child of a familiar touch and voice
- Help them to understand the important issues necessary to make informed decisions
- Recognise signs of stress and exhaustion
- Help them to feel able to take a break and remind them of their need for food, drink and rest

Study activity

Prepare a plan to transfer a school-aged child and family from a central PICU back to the general paediatric ward of his or her local hospital.

The growth-enhancing critical care unit

The PICU which avoids stress and enhances the growth of the children is that in which staff:

- provide care, concern and gentleness
- give psychological care the same priority as physical care
- make the unique needs of children and families the focus of attention
- organise care and procedures with consideration of the child's needs
- address the child and family by name
- are constantly alert for features of distress and provide relief
- comfort and reassure the children with touch and positive contact to counterbalance the unpleasant treatments
- teach and help the child to use positive coping strategies
- acknowledge the child as an individual and include the child in age-appropriate conversation
- make full use of toys and play and encourage parents to bring in the child's favourite objects from home
- make parents welcome and rarely ask them to leave their child's bedside
- never leave a dying child alone

(Weibley, 1989)

Providing play in PICUs

- Low volume, low pitch music is relaxing
- Make use of familiar toys and comforters from home
- Audio cassettes of familiar voices or songs can be comforting and provide security
- Make use of all the senses to stimulate play – rotating mirrors, familiar perfumes, different fabrics
- Allot a specific time for play
- Use the expertise of hospital play therapists to create a plan of play
- As the child improves encourage him to initiate play

Supporting the Staff

Staff in an intensive care environment are subject to many stresses, which can be overcome by a supportive relationship with other staff members. Foxall *et al.* (1990) found that intensive care nurses were more likely to be stressed as a result of death and dying than nurses working in general wards were to be stressed as a result of work overload. Benner and Wrubel (1989) recognise the temporary benefit of laughter and detachment for ICU staff in overcoming their stress, but suggest that acknowledgement of the stress and support from one's colleagues are a much more effective long-term strategy. Support groups can help this sharing of feelings and encourage communication between the multidisciplinary team.

Stresses for PICU nurses

Ethical dilemmas

- withdrawal of life support
- use of technology for severely injured children
- conflicts between family and staff values
- scarcity of resources

Death and dying

- supporting the family
- organ donation
- personal feelings

Interpersonal relationships

- conflict with medical opinion
- lack of positive feedback from senior staff
- difficulty in relationships with parents

Key Points

1. Critically ill children should be nursed by registered children's nurses in a designated PICU.
2. More evidence is required about the national need for and provision of PIC.
3. Transfers of children from general hospitals to designated PICUs are more safely undertaken by specialist retrieval teams.
4. The role of the PICU nurse is to allay parental anxiety and provide a growth-enhancing environment for the critically ill child.
5. The whole family can benefit from careful preparation for the admission, stay and discharge from the PICU.

Chapter 36

Caring for the Dying Child and the Family

Introduction

The child is not a small adult and this concept is especially true when caring for the dying child. More than ever, in this situation the nurse should be able to recognise children's different levels of understanding according to their age and experience. This appreciation will enable the nurse to be able to talk to the child about death and dying in a meaningful way and be able to identify physical and psychological needs. A knowledge of how children respond to their illness will aid the planning and implementation of specific care to meet these needs (*see also* Death and the family p. 208).

Family-centred care provides the children's nurse with the additional roles of educator and support person for the parents as the nurse helps to care for their child. The nurse has to be able to appreciate and respond to the various emotions displayed by the parents whose child is dying. The situation will also have a psychological impact on the child's healthy siblings and they will need help and support to cope with this trauma. Often families in such severe turmoil have difficulty in recognising and dealing with each other's grief and the nurse may be the person who can help them communicate and share their thoughts and worries. Last but not least, the nurse needs to be able to recognise that providing such support for the whole family is not easy, to be aware of personal values and beliefs concerning death and to have a strategy for releasing their stress.

Differences in care for dying adults and dying children (Papadatou, 1997; DH, 2001)

- Ethical and legal issues of self-determination, which are very different for the dying child.
- The parents, multidisciplinary team and young patients perceive and interpret the child's condition and palliative status in a very different way than occurs in the care of the dying adult.
- The need for professionals caring for children to have specific training to develop the skills to relate and communicate effectively with children.
- Parents are more likely to be directly and actively involved in the care of their dying child than the next of kin for adults.
- Grief over the death of a child is known to be more intense, long-lasting and complicated than the grief process for the death of an adult.
- The dying process and the death of a child tends to have an unique impact on the professional care providers.

Meeting Psychological Needs

Children's perceptions of death

Most children have some ideas about death. Their games often involve death, usually in a violent way, probably as a result of television and cartoons. Some children have also had some experience of the reality of death because of the death of a grandparent or family pet. These ideas about death will be different for every child because of their individual experiences but also according to their stage of cognitive development.

Study activity

Consider your own experiences of death as a child. Have these had any effect on your adult views?

The work of Piaget demonstrates that children's understanding varies between different age groups and that this variation is largely predictable. Several researchers have found that these development changes can also be seen in children's understanding of illness. Children's understanding of death has not been studied extensively, possibly because it is a more difficult topic to explore ethically with young children. The few studies that are available indicate that this understanding is also linked to age. These studies relate to children over the age of 2 years. It is difficult to know whether children under this age have any awareness or understanding of death. Preschool children (2–5 years) are described by Piaget as being at a pre-operational (or pre-logical) stage. During this stage children do not think logically and tend to view ideas from their own perspective. At this age they are unable to accept the irreversibility of death and can only relate it to their understanding of sleep which is only a temporary process. This may be partly due to the influence of cartoon characters who always return to normal after violent occurrences (*see also* Children's perceptions of health p. 141 and Children's concepts of illness p. 205).

Study activity

Watch a cartoon with a preschool child and discuss the violent episodes. Find out how this child perceives them.

These young children usually consider a dead person as being somewhere else (for example, in heaven or under the ground). Often death is associated with darkness, which may be connected with the child's experience of sleep, which mostly occurs at night, in the dark. Vidovich (1980) reports that a 5-year-old who was dying was heard to ask: 'When will it be dark? Will mummy be there when it gets dark?'

The egocentricity of young children may cause them to feel responsible in some way for the death of a loved one. They consider it as a punishment for being naughty. They may have wished that a sibling would go away because of jealousy or anger and when this becomes a reality they may see themselves as having caused it to happen. These feelings may be perpetuated if they find themselves neglected because the rest of the family are overcome by grief. They also find it difficult to perceive death as a normal event which happens to everyone, including themselves.

Children between the ages of 5 and 8 years are beginning to understand that death is a natural event. Lansdown and Benjamin (1985) found that 60% of children in this age group had realistic ideas about the finality of death, although they were still largely unaware that it could happen to them during childhood. This reasoning is more sophisticated than that of the younger child, but the cause of death is still generally seen as external and they may still be concerned about death being infectious, occurring at a certain age or after a specific event. Lucy, aged 7, was terrified of going to hospital after a leg injury and it was eventually ascertained that granny had died in hospital following a fractured femur and Lucy thought that everyone with an injured leg died in hospital. It is also difficult for a child at this age to perceive the future and therefore they do not have the ability to recognise gradual deterioration in themselves or others, or to consider what may follow this deterioration.

During middle childhood, children acquire an even more realistic picture of death and recognise it as an inevitable and universal process. They are also able to gather information together and make reasoned judgements about that information. Thus, children who are terminally ill can come to realise that death is imminent. Piaget terms adolescence the formal operational stage of cognitive development. This is the age at which children can think beyond the present and conceptualise the future. They can imagine processes such as death, even if they have not directly experienced such events. They also appreciate that emotions can affect body functions. The adolescent is able to visualise the future and has goals and aspirations for adulthood, so anger and resentment often occur because death has interfered with these.

Communicating with the Dying Child

The use of Piaget's stages of cognitive development is a useful guide when caring for dying children but the nurse also needs to consider the individual child. Reilly *et al.* (1983) discovered that children who had had personal experience of death generally had an accelerated understanding of death. It is therefore important that the nurse knows as much about the child as an individual as possible so that she can communicate at an appropriate level. This understanding of the child as an individual will also help her to become aware of the child's willingness or otherwise to talk about dying. (*See also* Jean Piaget p. 74.)

Bluebond-Langer (1989) suggests that children often appreciate the seriousness of death even when they have not been told of their condition. They often choose not to discuss their fears of dying because they have learnt from the behaviour of others that death is not something that is spoken about openly. Lansdown (1980) summarises the stages children pass through when recognising the inevitability of their own death:

- 'I am very sick.'
- 'I have an illness that can kill people.'
- 'I have an illness that can kill children.'
- 'I may not get better.'
- 'I am dying.'

Thus the pretence that the child is not fatally ill and the unwillingness to pursue difficult questions about the nature of dying is an affront to children's intelligence. A tendency to avoid the issue may lead to the child losing trust and confidence in the nurse. Communication with the dying child is discussed further elsewhere.

Paediatric Palliative Care

Palliative care for children is a relatively new speciality (Davies, 2003) and in most industrialised countries the care of the dying child is rarely encountered (Papadatou, 1997). Palliative care focuses on providing holistic care to maximise the quality of life for the child and support for the family. It includes management of distressing symptoms, provision of respite and care throughout the dying process and ongoing bereavement support for the family (Matthews *et al.*, 2006).

In developing countries it is estimated that one child aged up to 19 years from every 1000 will require palliative care each year. One child per 10 000 aged up to 17 years will die from a life-limiting illness each year. Hynson (2003) estimate that each year in a district with a child population of 50 000 there are likely to be:

- five children dying from a life-limiting illness
- two children dying from cancer
- one child dying from heart disease
- two children dying from other causes

Fifty children will require palliative care for a life-limiting illness.

As it is relatively rare to find instances of care for children who are dying, it is a challenge to find evidence for best practice in this area of nursing. Integrated care pathways that are developed with current best practice guidelines and evidence enable a competent, integrated and multidisciplinary approach to care (Selwood, 2000). The Liverpool Care Pathway (LCP) for the dying patient was developed to guide appropriate palliative care for the adult patient. It has achieved this so well that it is now highlighted by the National Institute for Health and Clinical Excellence (NICE) as the recommended way of providing best care at the end of life for adults (Ellershaw and Wilkinson, 2003). Work is now under way to adapt this template of best care to enable the delivery of optimum care for all dying children and their families (Matthews *et al.*, 2006).

Involving Parents in Care

When they have a child who is dying, parents may feel they are losing control and they may see the nurse as taking over that control. A supportive relationship with the parents should enable the nurse to help them maintain their role as decision makers and carers. All care should be negotiated and the nurse's and parents' roles clearly defined. At the same time, the nurse should be alert to parental needs, abilities and stresses. Parental involvement can range from a presence at the bedside to total care of the child under supervision from the nurse (Evans, 1991). Parents may need support from the nurse to take time away from the dying child and not to feel guilty at the need for sleep, relaxation or time for home or work.

To provide the parents with both physical and psychological support the nurse needs to be available to answer questions, explain care and to respond to spoken and unspoken fears, anxieties, stresses and strains.

Support for the Family

Children's nursing is concerned with supporting the family as much as it is about caring for the child. This is particularly pertinent when caring for the dying child. Studies, as well as personal accounts, have shown that this support is often lacking for parents whose children have died (Bennett, 1984). Davies (1979) voices parents' reactions very succinctly when she describes her feelings when her daughter, Sarah, was dying: 'You feel totally inadequate, lost, helpless and stupid.'

Other emotions experienced by parents caring for a dying child are shock, confusion, fear, anger and guilt. Parents are often so shocked at being told their child is dying, even if this is confirmation of their own suspicions, that they do not hear any further explanations. The nurse needs to give parents time to come to terms with this news and then provide opportunities to answer questions. Following the initial shock parents then feel confused about their parental role; they no longer feel able to care for their child and they do not know how to divide their time between the dying child and the other members of the family. Their lives have been completely altered by this event and they do not know how to cope. Mothers, particularly, experience a loss of control or mastery, perhaps because they tend to bear the burden of the caring role (Jennings, 1992). The nurse can help both parents rediscover their role, involve them in the care of their child and support them in making decisions about sharing their time and presence amongst other family members. Kitchener (1993) suggests that this is best achieved by a primary nurse who can get to know the family's values, beliefs and relationships.

Confusion can also be due to fear. Many parents are frightened by their perceptions of the actual death and often visualise that this will be violent and painful for the child. They are also frightened that they will not be able to cope with the physical care or be able to control their emotions. Like nurses, they often have difficulty in communicating with their child about dying and they sometimes dread the questions that the child might ask because they fear they will be unable to respond in an appropriate way. The nurse needs to be able to give the parents the time and opportunity to express these fears and provide them with simple guidelines on how to deal with the child's questions.

Anger may arise from their fear and confusion, often as a result of their need to understand the situation and control it. This anger can be directed at the nurse. It is not easy for the nurse to accept such emotions but as Wright (1991) acknowledges, the verbal expression of anger can often aid catharsis. If the nurse can accept the anger and remain supportive, she can strengthen her relationship with the family. Often an angry outburst will cause the parents to feel guilty at causing distress to others. Guilt is a common reaction amongst parents of dying children, they may feel guilty because the illness is hereditary or because their behaviour (for example, smoking) somehow triggered the illness. Even if there is no obvious cause, parents can always imagine that some action or omission on their part is the reason for their child's illness. The nurse should be alert to parental expressions of guilt or self-blame and assist parents to examine the validity of their apportionment of blame. If necessary, this may also involve helping them to forgive themselves or others.

These emotional reactions to the dying child are not confined to the parents. Bluebond-Langer (1989) recognises that the destructive effects of terminal illnesses involve the whole family. In particular, siblings of the dying child may feel rejected and neglected as the sick child become the centre of attention (Collinge and Stewart, 1983). Healthy siblings may feel anxiety about their own health (Cairns *et al.*, 1979). In addition, jealousy and resentment may result from parental preoccupation with the dying child. This, in turn, may lead to feelings of guilt as the siblings try to direct attention upon themselves (Burton, 1975). If these effects are not recognised and/or managed, behavioural problems such as enuresis, school phobia, depression and abdominal pain may ensue. The nurse can help parents to recognise the needs of siblings and, by her presence with the dying child, can enable them to spend time with the siblings. She can also help the parents to meet siblings' needs by accepting the siblings' involvement in the care of the sick child (Doyle, 1987). The parents may also need help to maintain as normal a family routine, including discipline, as possible for all members of the family. This helps the affected child and the siblings to feel secure (Cairns *et al.*, 1979; Cleary *et al.*, 1986).

Such enormous responsibilities for parents in these situations may cause break-up of the family (Gonda and Ruark, 1984). Hill (1993) shows how the strain of a terminal illness of a child upon a marital relationship can be destructive. The stress involved in coming to terms with the varied emotions described above, combined with the sheer physical exhaustion caused by trying to maintain normal work and family routines while caring for the dying child, may often cause conflict. The nurse should be aware of these potential tensions and, as far as possible, help parents to spend time together and give them time to express feelings separately or together. Kitchener (1993) suggests that the use of outside agencies such as social workers or 'CRUSE' may be helpful. Jennings (1992) suggests that mothers find it easier than fathers to express and work through their feelings. Nurses need to be alert to the possibility that this may be because mothers are more available, or that female emotions are easier for nurses to deal with. Consequently, it may be that fathers are given less opportunity to share their feelings, especially if their feelings are hidden as they strive to demonstrate strength.

Svavarsdottir (2005) found that mothers caring for children with cancer cited the most difficult aspect was providing emotional support for the affected child and the siblings. For fathers the difficult aspects were providing emotional support for the affected child and their partner.

Care of the Nurse

Caring for dying children is stressful. Vidovich (1980) found that the death of a child may cause the nurse to feel failure, guilt, anger or overwhelming sadness. Support for nurses caring for the dying child and

CRUSE
126 Sheen Road, Richmond, Surrey, TW9 1UR
Tel: 020 8939 9530
www.crusebereavementcare.org.uk
info@crusebereavementcare.org.uk

The Compassionate Friends
53 North Street, Bristol, BS3 1EN
Tel: 08451 20 37 85
www.tcf.org.uk
info@tcf.org.uk

Parent Lifeline
Volserve House, 14–18 West Bar Green, Sheffield, S1 2DA
Tel: 0114 272 6575
www.parentlifeline.org.uk

family is essential if burnout is to be avoided. Siedel (1981) suggests that a systematic approach to death education in nurse training may partly help to prepare nurses for meeting the needs of the dying. She also proposes that such a programme allows nurses to come to terms with their own beliefs about dying so that they are better able to cope with their own emotional needs.

Kitchener (1993) suggested regular support group meetings for nurses caring for dying children. This gives them the opportunity to acknowledge their feelings and discuss them with colleagues. It also allows them to discuss actions such as symptom control and talking with parents. Saunders (1982) suggests that a support group provides encouragement for many nurses and reassures them that they are doing the right things.

Nurses need to be informed of a child's death even when they have been off duty. They need to know what happened to cope with their own feelings and support the other children on the ward. Many nurses find it useful to be given time to attend the child's funeral to allow them to say their final goodbye.

Study activity

Find out what facilities are available to you to help you come to terms with stressful events on the ward.

Meeting Physical Needs

Pain relief

Pain is the most common feature of the dying and the feature that is most feared by children and their parents. Eighty per cent of dying children will experience pain (Hill, 1993). If it is not managed well, it can lower their morale and ability to cope. The first stage in relieving the dying child's pain is an accurate assessment of the severity, the type and the cause of the pain. Observing physiological changes can be a useful assessment of pain in infants who are less influenced by pain and stress. With toddlers, it is useful to listen to comments from parents who know their child well enough to recognise changes in behaviour that may indicate pain. In this way the nurse can begin to recognise the subtle changes in children that reveal their individual responses to pain. Objective ways of assessing pain using the child's own viewpoint are invaluable in planning and evaluating pain relief (*see also* Caring for children in pain p. 351 and Assessment of pain pp. 356–9).

The planning and implementation of pain relief should follow established models unless the child presents in severe pain. Generally the principle should be a gradual progression from a non-opioid analgesia to a weak opioid and finally a strong opioid (Hill, 1993). In her moving account of the care of a dying teenager Hunt (1990) describes the gradual progression from 30 mg dihydrocodeine daily to 300 mg twice daily of morphine slow-release tablets in the successful management of terminal pain. Unfortunately, there are still many myths about the use of opioids for children and the nurse may need to act as the patient's advocate to ensure that dying children receive the appropriate analgesia at the correct strength for their pain. If this is not achieved, the resulting negative effects of insufficient or overpowerful analgesia will cause the child and family further distress.

Pain in terminal illness is usually constant and for this reason analgesia should be given regularly so that the child can maintain a continuous level of pain relief. The adequacy of the relief should be reassessed regularly to ensure that this target is met. Oral analgesia is the route of choice for children, but is not necessarily accepted well by all children. The nurse may need to be imaginative in the use of play to ensure the acceptance of medicine on a regular basis. When nausea and vomiting do not allow oral medication, subcutaneous analgesia can be given using a syringe pump. This method has the advantage of enabling the child to remain mobile. Hill (1993) suggests that pain-free mobility should be one of the goals for pain relief. She suggests that the primary goal is to enable relief from pain during sleep. Secondly, the nurse should aim to provide sufficient analgesia to give the child relief from pain at rest. Finally, the child should be able to move around without pain.

Psychological methods of pain relief may also provide a useful adjunct to medication. Hypnosis, distraction techniques and the use of imagery and relaxation can all be helpful in the management of children's pain (Alder, 1991). They are relatively easy for children of all ages to use and have the advantage of giving them some control over their situation. The nurse should not forget the influence of fear upon pain and should aim to keep the child as relaxed as possible, with explanations of treatment and reassurance. Simple measures such as touch, being settled into a more comfortable position, or the presence of a nurse or parent may help to relax a frightened child and reduce the intensity of the pain (*see also* Coping strategies pp. 216 and 272).

Nausea and vomiting

Nausea and vomiting is a common problem for children who are dying and can cause them much distress. The commonest causes are constipation, raised intracranial pressure or excessive pharyngeal excretions (Hill, 1993). Prescribed anti-emetics should act on the site of the cause. When the cause is uncertain a combination of anti-emetics that act on different sites may be useful. When oral medication cannot be used, anti-emetics can be given rectally or via a subcutaneous infusion.

Nausea and vomiting are sometimes seen as side-effects of opioids but are usually only troublesome initially. Hill (1993) estimates that 25–30% of children will experience nausea or vomiting when opioids are first used but generally these symptoms are overcome in 5–10 days. She does not recommend the regular use of prophylactic anti-emetics and suggests haloperidol (25–50 mg/kg) or cyclizine (up to 75 mg daily) only if vomiting occurs.

Anorexia

Pain and/or nausea and vomiting may cause anorexia, which is often more a problem for the parents than the child. It may also be caused by offensive respiratory secretions or wounds. The child may be helped by small frequent snacks of favourite foods rather than two or three large meals a day. Parents may be reassured by understanding that the child's energy requirements are less because of his relative immobility. They may also feel that they are able to help the problem by bringing in favourite foods or drinks from home (*see also* Encouraging eating and drinking p. 365).

Dyspnoea

Dyspnoea in the dying child may be caused by secondary lung tumours, pleural effusion or direct respiratory centre invasion in children with malignant disease. It may be due to the primary disease process as in cystic fibrosis or due to respiratory muscle dysfunction in children with degenerative disease. Often a chest infection will exacerbate the primary cause.

Treatment of dyspnoea is often empirical. Dyspnoea is frightening for children and their parents, and their anxiety can often aggravate the problem. The nurse can often do much simply by providing a reassuring and calm atmosphere. Careful positioning of the child using a bean bag or elevating the head of the bed may increase comfort. A frightened child can be helped by being supported in an upright position on a parent's or a nurse's lap.

Excess secretions may be overcome by gentle physiotherapy or the administration of hyoscine. A dry cough which prevents rest and sleep can be overcome with simple linctus which is usually well accepted by children and will also act as a cough suppressant.

Constipation

Constipation is an inevitable consequence of opioid use and children who are prescribed strong opioids should also be given regular prophylactic laxatives. Constipation leads to abdominal distension, discomfort, nausea, vomiting and anorexia, and causes needless distress to the child and his parents.

Danthron (12.5–25 mg) is well accepted by children and can be given once at bedtime but it increases gut mobility and can cause abdominal cramps. It is not useful in children in nappies or those who have become incontinent as prolonged contact with the skin can cause discomfort and excoriation.

Lactulose (2.5 ml to 10 ml) acts by osmosis and softens stools by maintaining a volume of fluid in the bowel. It is a useful laxative when given regularly but children often dislike the taste and consistency and a twice-daily dose is recommended (*see also* Lactulose p. 486).

The nurse should be aware of the child's usual bowel habits and be alert to any changes in them so that the discomfort and distress of constipation does not occur.

Anxiety

If the anxiety of dying children and their families is not managed, it will aggravate the physical symptoms. Rodin (1983) has clearly shown that the anxiety of children is directly related to the anxiety of their parents. Harris's (1981) study showed that just having a child in hospital caused parents to become uncertain and frightened. It is easy to imagine how these feelings are magnified if the child has a terminal illness. Parental anxiety is reduced by having information about their child's treatment and the hospital routine, and being able to discuss the future (Sadler, 1988). They may also be helped by reassurance that their feelings are neither unusual nor silly (Kitchener, 1993).

Depression

Often, increasing physical deterioration in the child who is dying causes the child to become depressed. Children often demonstrate depression by psychological regression and they become very dependent and clingy to one parent. Depression may also cause a withdrawal and a loss of interest in normal activities such as play and watching television.

The nurse can help children by encouraging them to express their feelings. Such expressions of feelings may be initiated by the nurse's acknowledgement of them. Judd (1993) suggests that 'I know you are feeling sad' or 'This must be very hard for you' may be useful ways to open the discussion. The nurse may also help by enabling children to achieve control over their daily routine. The dying child often feels powerless and this can sometimes increase feelings of despair and dependence. The child should be encouraged to make decisions about care, and any efforts towards independent behaviour should also be encouraged.

Home or Hospital Care?

Goldman *et al.* (1990) consider that almost all children prefer to die at home in familiar surroundings. Caring for the dying child at home seems to reduce the long-term problem of guilt and depression experienced by bereaved parents and siblings (Lauer *et al.*, 1983). However, Bluebond-Langer (1989) disputes this and suggests that siblings can often feel confused, rejected and lonely when their home environment changes to care for the dying child. It would appear that there are both advantages and disadvantages of caring for a terminally ill child at home, and a positive outcome may relate to the amount of support available to the family.

Study activity

Consider the factors involved in considering whether home or hospital is the most suitable place for a child to die.

If the child has been in hospital, the parents will need clear instructions and advice. It has been shown that this is not always forthcoming. McDonald (1988) studied the discharge information given to mothers and found that many mothers left hospital with unclear or insufficient explanations.

It must also be recognised that not all parents will feel able physically and psychologically to care for their dying child at home. These parents should not be made to feel guilty at such a decision. Harris (1981) found that care at home sometimes fails because of lack of family resources and/or community support. The decision to care for the dying child at home needs careful assessment of all the factors involved in negotiation with the parents, siblings and the affected child. Provision should be made for alternatives if home care does fail, so parents recognise that they can return to hospital care without feeling inadequate.

An alternative to hospital care is the hospice, which will centre care entirely around the support of the family (Copsey, 1981). The nurse may be the person to discuss with the family the best option for them and their child.

Summary

Caring for the dying child and family is probably one of the most challenging roles of the children's nurse. The nurse needs to be sensitive to the needs, fears and anxieties of all the family members, and to try to enable them to maintain a normal family life. The aim of nursing in this situation becomes not to aid a cure but to help the child and family face the reality of death, and to enable the child to die with peace and dignity. It may also be to continue to support the family after the child's death and to help them cope with their grief. Inevitably, such experiences are stressful to the nurses involved with the family and they too need to share their feelings.

Key Points

1. Children's perceptions of death vary according to their stage of cognitive development and their individual experiences.
2. Children are usually only able to discuss death with the nurse in a secure atmosphere of trust and confidence.
3. Nurses need to have explored and confronted their own feelings and beliefs about death before being able to provide effective help for dying children and their families.
4. When a child is dying the whole family is affected and the nurse has to handle a variety of emotions, from fear, anxiety and guilt to despair, confusion and anger.
5. When their child is dying parents often need help to identify how they can best help their child.
6. The nurse has to recognise that this type of nursing is stressful and has to be able to access strategies which will help to overcome the effects of stress.

References

Abd-el-Maeboud, K., *et al.* (1991) Rectal suppository: common sense and mode of insertion. *Lancet,* **338** (8770), 798–800.
Action for Sick Children (1993) Planning paediatric home care. *At Home Newsletter,* **5**, 2.
Adams, J., *et al.* (1991) Reducing fear in hospital. *Nursing Times,* **87** (1), 62–64.
Ahmann, E. (1994) Family centred care: the time has come. *Pediatric Nursing,* **20** (1), 52–54.

Alder, S. (1991) Taking children at their word: pain control in paediatrics. *Professional Nurse,* **5** (8), 398–402.
American Academy of Pediatrics (1994) *Pediatric Advanced Life Support.* Dallas: American Heart Association.
Anderton, A., *et al.* (1993) A comparative study of the numbers of bacteria present in enteral feed preparation and administration in hospital and in the home. *Journal of Hospital Infection,* **23** (1), 43–49.
Angeras, M. H., Brandberg, A., Falk, A. and **Seeman, T.** (1992) Comparison between sterile saline and tap water for the cleaning of acute traumatic soft tissue. *European Journal of Surgery,* **158** (33), 347–350.
Atkinson, B., Glasper, E. and **Purcell, C.** (1996) Very sick children need children's nurses too. *Paediatric Nursing,* **8** (10), 10–11.
Atwell, J. and **Gow, M.** (1985) Paediatric trained district nurse in the community: expensive luxury or economic necessity? *British Medical Journal,* **291**, 227–278.
Audit Commission (1993) *Children First: A Study of Hospital Services.* London: HMSO.
Audit Commission (2003) *Services for Disabled Children: a Review of Services for Disabled Children and their Families.* London: Audit Commission.
Baillie, L. (1993) A review of pain assessment tools. *Nursing Standard,* **7** (23), 25–29.
Baker, C. and **Wong, D.** (1987) QUESTT: A process of pain assessment in children. *Orthopaedic Nurse,* **6** (1), 11–21.
Banco, L. and **Powers, A.** (1988) Hospitals; unsafe places for children. *Pediatrics,* **82** (5), 794.
Barry, P. and **Ralston, C.** (1994) Adverse events occurring during inter-hospital transfer of the critically ill. *Archives of Disease in Childhood,* **71**, 8–11.
Bastable, A. and **Rushford, H.** (2005) Parents' management of their child's post-operative pain. *Paediatric Nursing* **17** (10), 14–18.
Bates, T. and **Broome, M.** (1986) Preparation of children for hospitalisation and surgery: a review of the literature. *Journal of Pediatric Nursing,* **1** (4), 230–234.
Beaver, M. *et al.* (1994) *Babies and Young Children, Book 1. Development 0–7.* Cheltenham: Stanley Thornes (Publishers) Ltd.
Becker, R. D. (1972) Therapeutic approaches to psychopathological reactions to hospitalisation. *International Journal of Child Psychology,* **1**, 65–67.
Bedi, A. (1993) A tool to fill the gap. *Professional Nurse,* November, 112–118.
Beecroft, P. and **Reddick, S.** (1990) Intramuscular injection practices of pediatric nurses: site selection. *Nurse Education,* **15** (4), 23–28.
Benner, P. and **Wrubel, J.** (1989) *The Primacy of Caring: Stress and Coping in Health and Illness.* Menlo Park: Addison-Wesley.
Bennett, P. (1984) A care team for terminally ill children. *Nursing Times,* **80** (10), 26–27.
Beyer, J. (1989) *The Oucher: A User's Manual and Technical Report.* Denver: University of Colorado.
Beyer, J. and **Ardine, C.** (1988) Content validity of an instrument to measure young children's intensity of pain. *Journal of Pediatric Nursing,* **1**, 386–394.
Binnie, A. *et al.* (1988) *A Systematic Approach to Nursing Care.* Milton Keynes: Open University Press.
Bishop, J. (1988) Sharing the caring. *Nursing Times,* **84** (30), 60–61.
Bluebond-Langer, M. (1989) Worlds of dying children and their well siblings. *Death Studies,* **13**, 1–16.
Boge, E. (1910) The nurse on district. *Nursing Times,* **vi** (288), 916.
Bond, M. (1979) *Pain: Its Nature, Analysis and Treatment.* Edinburgh: Churchill Livingstone.
Booth, I. W. (1991) Enteral nutrition in childhood. *British Journal of Hospital Medicine,* **46**, 111–113.
Bowlby, J. (1953) *Child Care and the Growth of Love.* Harmondsworth: Penguin.
BPA (British Paediatric Association) (1991a) *Paediatric Medical Staffing in the 1990s.* London: BPA.
BPA (British Paediatric Association) (1991b) *Towards a Combined Child Health Service.* London: BPA.
BPA (British Paediatric Association) (1993) *The Care of Critically Ill Children: Report of the Multidisciplinary Working Party on Paediatric Intensive Care.* London: BPA.
Bradshaw, C. and **Zeanah, P.** (1986) Paediatric nurse assessments of children in pain. *Journal of Paediatric Nursing,* **1**, 314–322.
Bradshaw, E. and **Davenport, H.** (1989) *Day Care: Anaesthetics and Management.* London: Edward Arnold.
Bristol Royal Infirmary Inquiry (2001) *The Report of the Public Inquiry into Children's Heart Surgery at the Bristol Royal Infirmary 1984–1995: Learning from Bristol (The Kennedy Report).* London: The Stationery Office. Available at www.bristol-inquiry.org.uk (accessed 19 May 2006).
British Paediatric Association, British Association of Paediatric Surgeons, Casualty Surgeons Association (1988) *Joint Statement of Children's Attendances at Accident and Emergency Departments.* London: BPS.
Britto, J., Nadel, S., MacConochie, I., Levin, M. and **Habibi, P.** (1995) Morbidity and severity of illness during interhospital transfer: impact of a specialist retrieval team. *British Medical Journal,* **311**, 836–839.
Broome, M. and **Lillis, P.** (1989) A descriptive analysis of pediatric pain management research. *Journal of Applied Nursing Research,* **2** (2), 74–81.
Buckingham, S. (1993) Pain scales for toddlers. *Nursing Standard,* **7** (25), 12–13.
Budd, K. (1984) *Pain,* 2nd edn. London: Update Publications.
Burke, D. and **Bowden, D.** (1993) Modified paediatric resuscitation chart. *British Medical Journal,* **306**, 1096–1098.
Burrows, F. and **Berde, C.** (1993) Optimal pain relief in infants and children. *British Medical Journal,* **307**, 815–816.
Burton, L. (1975) *Family Life of Sick Children.* Boston: Routledge & Kegan Paul.
Burton, R. (1989) Parental perceptions of Accident and Emergency. *Paediatric Nursing,* **1** (3), 19–20.

Burton, R. (1994) How to bear the pain – a well teddy clinic as an educational tool. *Child Health,* **1** (6), 251–254.
Cairns, N., Clark, G., Smith, S. and **Lansky, S.** (1979) Adaption of siblings to childhood cancer. *Journal of Paediatrics,* **95**, 484–487.
Calne, S. (1994) Dehumanisation in intensive care. *Nursing Times,* **90** (17), 31–33.
Campbell, A. (1987) Children with ongoing health needs. *Nursing* (3rd series), **23**, 17–19.
Campbell, S. and **Glasper, A. (eds)** (1995) *Whaley and Wong's Children's Nursing.* London: Mosby.
Caring for the Children in the Health Service (1993) *Bridging the Gaps.* London: CCHS.
Carson, D., Gravely, J. and **Council, J.** (1992) Children's pre-hospitalisation conceptions of illness, cognitive development and personal adjustment. *Child Health Care,* **21** (2), 103–110.
Carter, B. (1995) A fundamental duty and right. *Child Health,* **3** (1), 4.
Casey, A. (1988a) A partnership with the child and family. *Senior Nurse,* **8** (4), 8–9.
Casey, A. (1988b) Developing a model of paediatric nursing practice. In Glasper, A. and Tucker, A. (eds), *Advances in Child Nursing.* London: Scutari.
Casteels-Van Daele, M. (1993) Reduction of deaths after drug labelling for risk of Reye's syndrome. *Lancet,* **341**, 118–119.
Catchpole, A. (1986) *Community Paediatric Nursing Services in England 1985.* Unpublished DN thesis.
Chawla, L. (2001) Evaluating children's participation: seeking areas of consensus. *PLA Notes 42. Children's Participation – Evaluating Effectiveness.* London: IIED
Child Accident Prevention Trust (1992) *Accidents to Children on Hospital Wards.* London: CAPT.
Children and Young People's Unit (2001) *Learning to Listen: Core Principles for the Involvement of Children and Young People.* London: HMSO.
Christenson, M. (2004) Do hospital personnel influence noise levels in an operating theatre and a post-anaesthesia unit? *Journal of Advanced Peri-Operative Care,* **2** (1), 19–25.
Cleary, J. *et al.* (1986) Parental involvement in the lives of children in hospital. *Archives of Disease in Childhood,* **61**, 779–787.
Cleeland, C. (1986) Behavioural control of symptoms. *Journal of Pain Symptom Management,* **1** (1), 36–38.
Clothier, C. (1994) *The Allitt Inquiry.* London: HMSO.
Clough, J. (2005) Using books to prepare children for surgery. *Paediatric Nursing,* **17** (9), 28–31.
Cohen, D., *et al.* (1984) The use of relaxation – mental imagery (self-hypnosis) in the management of 505 pediatric behavioural encounters. *Developmental and Behavioural Pediatrics,* **5** (10), 21–24.
Cole, R. (1995) When every second counts – reducing inaccuracy and delay in paediatric resuscitation. *Child Health,* **3** (2), 63–67.
Collinge, P. and **Stewart, E. D.** (1983) Dying children and their families. In Robbins, J. (ed.), *Caring for the Dying Child and the Family,* 1st edn. London: Harper & Row.
Collins, P. (1994) Knowledge and practice of CPR. *Paediatric Nursing,* **6** (2), 19–22.
Collins, P. (1995) Put the child first: paediatric attendance in A&E. *Child Health,* **2** (6), 225–228.
Conisbee, L. (1982) *A Bedfordshire Bibliography.* Bedfordshire Historical Record Society.
Copsey, M. K. (1981) Time to care. *Nursing Mirror,* **153** (22), 38–40.
Coulston, D. (1988) A proper place for parents. *Nursing Times,* **84** (19), 26–28.
Court, S. D. M. (1976) *Fit for the Future: Report of the Committee on Child Health Services,* vols 1 and 2. London: HMSO.
Couto, J., *et al.* (2004) Levels of neonatal care. *Pediatrics,* **114** (5), 1341–1347.
Cross, J. H., *et al.* (1995) Clinical examination compared with anthropometry in evaluating nutritional status. *Archives of Disease of Childhood,* **72**, 60–61.
Currie, M. (1982) *Hospitals in Luton: An Illustrated History.* Hitchin: Powis.
Curtis, K., *et al.* (2004) Consulted but not heard: a qualitative study of young people's views of their local health service. *Health Expectations,* **7**, 149–156.
Cutler, D. and **Taylor, A.** (2003) *Expanding and Sustaining Involvement – A Snapshot of Participation Infrastructure for Young People Living in England.* London: Carnegie Young People Initiative.
Darbyshire, P. (1994) *Living with a Sick Child in Hospital.* London: Chapman & Hall.
Davies, J. (1979) *Death of a Child.* London: Pitman Medical.
Davies, R. (2003) Establishing need for palliative care services for children/young people. *British Journal of Nursing,* **12** (4), 224–232.
De Courcey-Golder, A. (1996) A strategy for development of paediatric intensive care within the United Kingdom. *Intensive and Critical Care Nursing,* **12**, 84–89.
De Swiet, M., *et al.* (1989) Measurement of blood pressure in children. *British Medical Journal,* **299**, 497–498.
Dearmun, A. (1992) Perceptions of parental participation. *Paediatric Nursing,* **4** (7), 6–10.
DH (1998) *Paediatric Intensive Care: A Framework for the Future.* London: HMSO.
DH (1991a) *Welfare of Children and Young People in Hospital.* London: HMSO.
DH (1991b) *The Patient's Charter.* London: HMSO.
DH (1995) *Child Health in the Community: a Guide to Good Practice.* London: HMSO.
DH (1998) *Diana Community Children's Nursing Team HS (G) 95 Health Circular.* London: HMSO.
DH (2001) *High Dependency Care for Children: Report of an Expert Advisory Group.* London: HMSO.
DH (2002) *Seeking Consent: Working with Children.* London: The Stationery Office. Available at www.doh.gov.uk/consent

DH (2003a) *Copying Letters to Patients.* London: The Stationery Office.
DH (2003b) *Families and Post Mortems: A Code of Practice.* London: The Stationery Office.
DH (2003c) *Getting the Right Start: The Children's National Service Framework for Children, Young People and Maternity Services – Hospital Standard.* London: Department of Health.
DH (2004) *The National Service Framework for Children, Young People and Maternity Services – Hospital Standard.* London: Department of Health.
DHSS (1976a) *Fit for the Future (The Court Report).* London: HMSO.
DHSS (1976b) *Priorities for Health and Personal Social Services.* London: HMSO.
Dilworth, N. and **MacKellar, A.** (1987) Pain relief for the pediatric surgical patient. *Journal of Pediatric Surgery,* **22**, 264–266.
Doorbar, P. (1995) *Children's Views of Health Care in Portsmouth and South East Hampshire.* Portsmouth: Portsmouth and South East Hampshire Health Authority and Pat Doorbar & Associates.
Doorbar, P. (1996) *Well Now! The Report of the Second Stage of the Children's Views Project.* Portsmouth: Portsmouth and SE Hampshire Health Authority.
Doyle, B. (1987) I wish you were dead. *Nursing Times,* **83** (45), 44–46.
Eaton, N. (2001) Models of community children's nursing. *Paediatric Nursing,* **13** (1), 32–36.
Edge, W., *et al.* (1994) Reduction of morbidity in inter-hospital transport by specialist pediatric staff. *Critical Care Medicine,* **22**, 1186–1191.
Eland, J. (1985) Paediatrics. In Carey, K. (ed.), *Nursing Now: Pain.* Philadelphia: Springhouse.
Eland, J. (1993) Children with pain. In Jackson, O. and Saunders, R. (eds), *Child Health Nursing.* Philadelphia: J. B. Lippincott.
Eland, J. and **Anderson, J.** (1977) The experience of pain in children. In Jacox, A. K. (ed.), *Pain: A Source Book for Nurses and Other Health Professionals.* Boston: Little Brown.
Elander, G., Lindberg, T. and **Quarnstrom, B.** (1991) Pain relief in infants after surgery: a descriptive study. *Journal of Paediatric Surgery,* **26** (2), 128–131.
Ellershaw, J. and **Wilkinson, S.** (eds) (2003) *Care of the Dying: A Pathway to Excellence.* Oxford: Oxford University Press.
Ellet, M., *et al.* (1992) Predicting the distance for gavage tube placement in children using regression on height. *Pediatric Nursing,* **18** (2), 119–121.
Ellis, J. A. (1988) Using pain scales to prevent under medication. *American Journal of Maternal and Child Nursing,* **13**, 180–182.
Ellis, J. A. (1995) Administering drugs. *Paediatric Nursing,* **7** (4), 32–39.
ENB (English National Board) (1992) *A Survey of Students Gaining Nursing Experience in Children's Wards.* London: ENB.
Evans, M. (1991) Caring by parents. In Glasper, A. (ed.), *Child Care – Some Nursing Perspectives.* London: Wolfe.
Flavell, J. H. (1985) *Cognitive Development*: Englewood Cliffs, NJ: Prentice-Hall.
Foale, H. (1989) Healing the wound. *Paediatric Nursing,* **1** (5), 10–12.
Foxall, M., Zimmerman, S. and **Bene, B.** (1990) Comparison of frequency and sources of nursing job stress perceived by intensive care, hospice and medical-surgical nurses. *Journal of Advanced Nursing,* **12**, 281–290.
Fradd, E. (1990) Setting up a paediatric community nursing service. *Senior Nurse,* **10** (7), 4–5.
Fraser, J., Mok, Q. and **Tasker, R.** (1997) Survey of occupancy of paediatric intensive care units by children who are dependent on ventilators. *British Medical Journal,* **315**, 347–348.
Gadish, H., *et al.* (1988) Factors affecting nurses' decisions to administer paediatric pain medication post operatively. *Journal of Paediatric Nursing,* **3** (6), 383–390.
Galvani, J. (1997) Not yet cut and dried. *Nursing Times,* **93** (16), 88–89.
Garland, J., *et al.* (1987) Infectious complications during peripheral IV therapy with Teflon catheters: a prospective study. *Paediatric Infectious Disease Journal,* **6** (10), 918–921.
Gaskell, S., *et al.* (2005) Taking the sting out of needles. *Paediatric Nursing,* **17** (4), 24–28.
Gauderer, M., Lorig, J. and **Eastwood, D.** (1989) Is there a place for parents in the anaesthetic room? *Journal of Pediatric Surgery,* **24** (7), 705–707.
Gay, J. (1992) A painful experience. *Nursing Times,* **88** (25), 32–35.
Gillet, J. (1954) Domicillary treatment of sick children. *The Practitioner,* **172**, 281–283.
Gillies, M., Parry-Jones, W. and **Smith, L.** (1995) Post-operative pain in children under five years. *Paediatric Nursing,* **3** (1), 31–34.
Gillis, A. (1990) Hospital preparation: the children's story. *Child Health Care,* **19** (1), 19–27.
Glasper, A. (1990) Accompanying children: parental presence during anaesthesia. *Nursing Standard,* **4** (24), 6.
Glasper, A., Gow, M. and **Yerrell, P.** (1989) A family friend. *Nursing Times,* **85** (4), 63–65.
Glasper, E. R. (1993) Telephone triage: extending practice. *Nursing Standard,* **7** (15), 34–36.
Godfrey, K. (1997) Uses of leeches and leech saliva in clinical practice. *Nursing Times,* **26** (9), 62–63.
Godman, L. (1994) Case history – paediatric nursing training. *Paediatric Nursing,* **6** (1), 23.
Goldman, A., Beardsmore, S. and **Hunt, J.** (1990) Palliative care for children with cancer – home, hospital or hospice. *Archives of Disease in Childhood,* **65**, 641–643.
Gonda, T. and **Ruark, J.** (1984) *Dying Dignified. The Health Professional's Guide to Care.* Menlo Park, CA: Addison-Wesley.
Graham, P. (1987) *Child Health Ten Years after the Court Report.* London: NCB.
Griffiths-Jones, A. (1990) Prevalence of IV devices. *Nursing Times,* **86** (1), 6–7.
Haines, C. and **Childs, H.** (2005) Parental satisfaction with paediatric intensive care. *Paediatric Nursing,* **17** (5), 37–41.

Hall, C. (1996) The art of storytelling. *Paediatric Nursing,* **8** (1), 6–7.
Harris, A. C. (1993) *Child Development,* 2nd edn. Minneapolis: West.
Harris, P. (1981) How parents feel. *Nursing Times,* **77** (42), 1803–1804.
Hart, R. A. (1992) *Children's Participation: From Tokenism to Citizenship.* Florence: UNICEF, ICDC.
Hart, R. and **Bossert, E.** (1994) Self reported fears of hospitalised school-age children. *Journal of Pediatric Nursing,* **9** (2), 83–90.
Hazinski, M. F. (1992) *Nursing Care of the Critically Ill Child.* St Louis: Mosby.
Heaton, J. *et al.* (2003) *Technology Dependent Children and Family Life.* York: Social Policy Research Unit, University of York.
Hecker, J. (1988) Improved technique in intravenous therapy. *Nursing Times,* **84** (34), 28–33.
Hester, N. (1979) The pre-operational child's reaction to immunisation. *Nursing Research,* **28** (4), 250–255.
Hewitt, T. (1988) Prolonged contact with topical anaesthetic cream: a case report. *Paediatric Nursing,* **10** (2), 22–23.
Hicks, J. F., *et al.* (1989) Optimum needle length for diphtheria–tetanus–pertussis inoculation of infants. *Pediatric Nursing,* **84** (1), 136–137.
Higson, J. and **Bolland, R.** (2000) Telephone follow-up after paediatric day surgery. *Paediatric Nursing,* **12** (10), 30–32.
Hill, L. (1993) *Caring for Dying Children and Their Families.* London: Chapman & Hall.
Holden, C., *et al.* (1996) Enteral nutrition. *Paediatric Nursing,* **8** (5), 29–33.
Horgan, M., *et al.* (1996) Measuring pain in neonates: an objective score. *Paediatric Nursing,* **8** (10), 24–27.
House of Commons Health Committee (1997) *Hospital Services for Children and Young People.* London: Stationery Office.
Hughes, G. (1990) Tape measure to aid prescription in paediatric resuscitation. *Archives of Emergency Medicine,* **7**, 21–27.
Hughes, M., *et al.* (1994) How parents cope with the experience of neonatal intensive care. *Child Health Care,* **23** (1), 1–14.
Humphrey, G., *et al.* (1992) The occurrence of high levels of acute behavioural distress in children and adolescents undergoing venepuncture. *Pediatrics,* **90**, 87–91.
Hunt, J. (1990) Symptom care of the child with cancer. *Nursing Times,* **86** (10), 72–73.
Hutt, R. (1983) *Sick Children's Nurses. A Study for the DHSS of the Career Patterns of RSCNs.* Brighton: Institute of Manpower Studies.
Hynson, J. L. (2003) The dying child: how care is different. *Medical Journal of Australia,* **179** (6), 20–22.
Illingworth, R. (1975) *The Normal Child,* 6th edn. Edinburgh: Churchill Livingstone.
Jackson, K. (1995) The state we're in. *Child Health,* **3** (1), 14–17.
James, J. (1995) Day care admissions. *Paediatric Nursing,* **7** (1), 25–29.
Janes, S. (1996) Failure to thrive in children with chronic illness. *Paediatric Nursing,* **8** (3), 19–22.
Jennings, P. (1992) Coping strategies for mothers. *Paediatric Nursing,* **4** (9), 24–26.
Johnson, C., Stevens, B. and **Arbess, G.** (1993) The effect of the sight of blood and the use of decorative adhesive bandages on pain intensity ratings by pre-school children. *Journal of Pediatric Nursing,* **8** (3), 147–150.
Jolly, T. (1981) *The Other Side of Paediatrics.* London: Macmillan.
Jonas, D. (2003) Parents' management of their child's pain in the home following day surgery. *Journal of Child Health Care,* **7** (3), 150–162.
Judd, D. (1993) Communicating with dying children. In Dickenson, D. and Johnson, M. (eds), *Death, Dying and Bereavement.* London: Sage.
Kankkunen, P., *et al.* (2003) Parents' perceptions and use of analgesics at home after children's day surgery. *Paediatric Anaesthesia,* **13** (2), 132–140.
Kanter, R. and **Tompkins, J.** (1993) Adverse events during interhospital transport: physiological deterioration associated with pre-transport severity of illness. *Pediatrics,* **84**, 43–48.
Kelly, M., Ferguson-Clark, L. and **Marsh, M.** (1996) A new retrieval service. *Paediatric Nursing,* **8** (6), 18–20.
Kirby, P., *et al.* (2003) *Building a Culture of Participation. Involving Children and Young People in Policy, Service Planning, Delivery and Evaluation.* London: DfES.
Kirk, S. and **Glendinning, G.** (1999) *Supporting Parents Caring for a Technology-dependent Child.* Manchester: National Primary Care Research and Development Unit.
Kitchener, P. (1993) *Health in Bedfordshire.* Bedford: Bedfordshire Health Authority.
Kobran, M. and **Pearce, S.** (1993) The paediatric nurse practitioner. *Paediatric Nursing,* **3** (5), 11.
Koren, G., *et al.* (1985) Post-operative morphine infusion in newborn infants: assessment of disposition characteristics and safety. *Journal of Pediatrics,* **107** (6), 963–967.
Langdon, J. (1995) Neglect of an essential right. *Child Health,* **3** (1), 10–13.
Lansdown, G. (2001) *Promoting Children's Participation in Democratic Decision-Making.* Rome: UNICEF.
Lansdown, R. (1980) *More Than Sympathy.* London: Tavistock.
Lansdown, R. and **Benjamin, G.** (1985) The development of the concept of death in children aged 5–9 years. *Child Care and Development,* **11**, 13–20.
Lauer, D., *et al.* (1983) A comparison study of parental adaption following a child's death at home or in hospital. *Pediatrics,* **71** (1), 107–112.
Lawrence, A. (1993) Intraosseous infusion. *Nursing Standard,* **7** (4), 21–24.
Leask, A. (2005) Community nurses improve health of absentee pupils. *Paediatric Nursing,* **17** (4), 5.
Levy, D. (1960) The infant's earliest memory of inoculation. *Journal of Genetic Psychology,* **96** (3), 46–50.

Ley, P. and **Llewellyn, S.** (1995) Improving patients' recall satisfaction and compliance. In Broome, A. and Llewellyn, S. (eds), *Health Psychology: Processes and Applications*. London: Chapman & Hall.
Lightfoot, J. and **Sloper, P.** (2001) *Involving Children and Young People with a Chronic Illness or Physical Disability in Local Decisions about Health Services Development. Phase One: Report on National Survey of Health Authorities and NHS Trusts*. York: Department of Health.
Lightfoot, J. and **Sloper, P.** (2003) Having a say in health: involving young people with a chronic illness or physical disability in local health services development. *Children and Society*, **17**, 277–290.
Lightwood, R., *et al.* (1956) A London trial of home care for sick children. *Lancet*, **i,** 313–316.
Liossi, C. (2002) *Procedure-related Cancer Pain in Children*. Abingdon: Radcliffe.
Livesley, J. (1993) Reducing the risks. Management of paediatric intravenous therapy. *Child Health*, **1** (2), 68–70.
Llewelyn, M. (1991) A headache all over my body. *Paediatric Nursing*, **3** (7), 14–15.
Lloyd-Thomas, A. R. (1990) ABC of major trauma: primary survey and resuscitation. *British Medical Journal*, **301**, 334–336.
Logan, S. (1995) Commentary: evaluation of specialist paediatric retrieval teams. *British Medical Journal*, **311**, 839.
Lorenz, L., *et al.* (2005) The benefits of baby massage. *Paediatric Nursing*, **17** (2), 15–19.
Lous, J., *et al.* (2005) Grommets (ventilation tubes) for hearing loss associated with otitis media with effusion in children. *The Cochrane Database of Systematic Reviews*, Issue 4. Chichester: John Wiley & Sons.
Lucas, H. and **Attard-Montalto, S.** (1996) Central line dressings: study of infection rates. *Paediatric Nursing*, **8** (6), 21–23.
Mackowiak, P., Wasserman, S. and **Levine, M.** (1992) A critical appraisal of 98.6°F, the upper limit of normal body temperature. *Journal of the American Medical Association*, **286** (12), 1578–1580.
Mann, N., *et al.* (1986) Effect of night and day on pre-term infants. *British Medical Journal*, **293**, 1265–1267.
Marcoux, C., *et al.* (1991) Central venous access devices in children. *Pediatric Nursing*, **16** (2), 123–133.
Markovitch, H. (1991) Day case treatment for children. *Archives of Disease in Childhood*, **66**, 734–736.
Marriot, M. (1990) Parent powers. *Nursing Times*, **86** (34), 68.
Matthews, K., *et al.* (2006) Developing the Liverpool Pathway for the Dying Child. *Paediatric Nursing*, **18** (1), 18–21.
McCaffery, M. and **Beebe, A.** (1989) *Pain*. St Louis: Mosby.
McCaffery, P. (1983) *Nursing the Patient in Pain*. London: Harper & Row.
McConichie, I. (2005) UK accident & emergency departments failing children. *Paediatric Nursing*, **17** (3), 4.
McDonald, M. (1988) Children discharged from hospital – what mothers want to know. *Nursing Times*, **84** (16), 63.
McEvilly, A. (1993) Childhood diabetes. *Paediatric Nursing*, **5** (9), 25–28.
McGrath, P. (1990) *Pain in Children*. London: Guilford Press.
McInally, W. (2005) Whose line is it anyway? *Paediatric Nursing*, **17** (5), 14–18.
McMenamin, C. (1995) Making A&E less traumatic for children. *Professional Nurse*, **2**, 310–313.
Meakin, G., *et al.* (1987) The effects of fasting on oral pre-medication – pH and volume of gastric aspiration in children. *British Journal of Anaesthesia*, **59**, 687–682.
Metheny, N. (1998) Measures to test placement of naso-gastric and naso-intestinal feeding tubes: a review. *Nursing Research*, **37** (6), 324–329.
Metheny, N., *et al.* (1989) Effectiveness of pH measurements in predicting feeding tube placement. *Nursing Research*, **38** (5), 280–285.
Miles, M. and **Manthes, M.** (1991) Preparation of parents for the ICU experience: what are we missing? *Child Health Care*, **20** (3), 132–137.
Miller, S. (1991) Adolescents alone together. In Glasper, A. (ed.), *Child Care: Some Nursing Perspectives*. London: Wolfe.
MoH (1962) *A Hospital Plan for England and Wales*. London: HMSO.
MoH (1971) *Hospital Facilities for Sick Children*. London: HMSO.
Moore, A. (2004) The bigger picture. *Nursing Standard*, **19** (13), 18–19.
Morgan, E. (1990) *Siblings' reactions to short-term hospitalisation*. Unpublished dissertation, City University.
Morley, C., *et al.* (1992) Axillary and rectal temperature measurements in infants. *Archives of Disease in Childhood*, **67** (1), 122–125.
Morrison, L. (1997) Stress and siblings. *Paediatric Nursing*, **9** (4), 26–27.
Morrison, W., *et al.* (2003) Noise, stress and annoyance in a paediatric intensive care unit. *Critical Care Medicine*, **31** (1), 113–119.
Morton, R. J. and **Phillips, B. M.** (1992) *Accidents and Emergencies in Children*. Oxford: Oxford University Press.
Moules, T. (2005) *Whose quality is it? Children and young people's participation in monitoring the quality of care in hospital: a participatory research study*. Unpublished Doctoral Study, Anglia Ruskin University.
Moy, R. J., *et al.* (1990) Malnutrition in a UK children's hospital. *Journal of Human Nutrition and Dietetics*, **3**, 93–100.
Muller, D., *et al.* (1994) *Nursing Psychology: Research and Practice*, 2nd edn. London: Chapman and Hall.
National Pressure Ulcer Advisory Panel (1989) Pressure ulcers: incidence, economics and risk assessment. *Care – Science and Practice*, **7** (4), 96–99.
NAWCH (National Association for the Welfare of Children in Hospital) (1986) *NAWCH Update*, Autumn.
Nethercott, S. (1994) The assessment and management of post-operative pain in children by RSCNs. *Journal of Clinical Nursing*, **3**, 109–113.

New Opportunities Fund (2002) *Palliative Care for Children Programme – Guidance Notes.* London: New Opportunities Fund.
Newell, P. (1991) *The Convention of Children's Rights in the UK.* London: The Children's Bureau.
NHS Estates (2004) *Design for Health.* London: The Stationery Office.
NHS Executive (1998) *Evaluation of the Pilot Project Programme for Children with Life-threatening Illnesses.* London: The Stationery Office.
Nichol, J. (1909) The surgery of infancy. *British Medical Journal,* **2**, 753.
Nichols, K. (1993) *Psychological Care in Physical Illness,* 2nd edn. London: Chapman & Hall.
Nightingale, F. (1859) *Notes on Nursing.* London: Camelot Press.
Norris, E. (1992) Making the day bearable. *Paediatric Nursing,* **4** (3), 21–22.
NPSA (National Patient Safety Agency) (2005) Patient Safety Alert: Reducing the Harm Caused by Misplaced Naso-gastric Feeding Tubes. London: NPSA.
O'Brien, S. and **Konsler, G.** (1988) Alleviating children's post-operative pain. *Maternal and Child Nursing,* **13** (3), 183–186.
O'Malley, M. E. and **McNamara, S. T.** (1993) Children's drawings – a pre-operative assessment tool. *AORN Journal,* **57** (5), 1074–1089.
Oakley, P. (1988) Inaccuracy and delay in decision making in paediatric resuscitation. *British Medical Journal,* **97**, 1347–1351.
Orenstein, S., *et al.* (1988) The Santmyer swallow – a new and useful infant reflex. *Lancet,* **i** (8581), 345–346.
Oster, G. D. and **Gould, P.** (1987) *Using Drawings in Assessment and Therapy.* New York: Brunner/Mazel.
Paice, J. (1992) Pharmacologic management. In Watt-Watson, J. and Donavon, M. (eds), *Pain Management: Nursing Perspectives.* St Louis: Mosby.
Papadatou, D. (1997) Training health profesionals in caring for dying children and grieving families. *Death Studies,* **21** (6), 575–600.
Patel, N. (1990) The child with cancer in the community. In Thompson, J. (ed.), *The Child with Cancer.* London: Scutari Press.
Patel, R. I., *et al.* (1995) Complications following paediatric ambulatory surgery. *Ambulatory Surgery,* **3** (2), 83–86.
Peplau, H. (1952) *Interpersonal Relationships in Nursing.* New York: Putnam.
Perry, S. (1994) Communicating with toddlers in hospital. *Paediatric Nursing,* **6** (5), 14–17.
Peter, S. and **Flynn, A.** (2002) Advanced nurse practitioners in a hospital setting: the reality. *Paediatric Nursing,* **14** (2), 14–19.
Peterson, L. and **Toler, S.** (1986) An information seeking disposition in child surgery patients. *Health Psychology,* **5** (4), 343–358.
Peterson, L., *et al.* (1990) Preparing children for hospitalisation and threatening medical procedures. In Bellack, A. and Hersen, M. (eds), *Handbook of Clinical Behavioural Problems.* New York: Plenum Press.
Pfefferbaum, B., Adams, J. and **Aceves, J.** (1990) The influence of culture on pain in Anglo and Hispanic children with cancer. *Journal of the American Academy of Child and Adolescent Psychiatry,* **29** (4), 642–647.
Phillips, B. (2000) *The end of paternalism? Child beneficiary participation and project effectiveness.* Unpublished Masters dissertation, Institute of Social Studies, The Hague.
Platt, S. (1959) *The Welfare of Children in Hospital.* London: HMSO.
Pollack, S., *et al.* (1991) Improved outcomes for tertiary center pediatric intensive care. *Critical Care Medicine,* **19** (2), 150–159.
Pontious, S., *et al.* (1994) Accuracy and reliability of temperature measurement by instrument and site. *Journal of Pediatric Nursing,* **9** (2), 114–123.
Portman, R. and **Yetman, R.** (1994) Clinical uses of ambulatory blood pressure monitoring. *Paediatric Nephrology,* **8**, 367–376.
Pritchard, A. P. and **Davis, J. A.** (1990) *The Royal Marsden Hospital Manual of Clinical Nursing Procedures,* 2nd edn. London: Harper & Row.
Quershi, J. and **Buckingham, S.** (1994) A pain assessment tool for all children. *Paediatric Nursing,* **6** (7), 11–13.
Ramsay, J. (1990) *Parental knowledge and management of children with cystic fibrosis.* Unpublished MSc thesis, City University, London.
Read, J. V. (1994) Perceptions of nurses and physicians regarding pain management of pediatric emergency room patients. *Pediatric Nursing,* **20** (3), 314–318.
Redman, C. (1994) Handling with care. *Child Health,* **1** (5), 177–180.
Reilly, T., Hasazi, J. and **Bond, L.** (1983) Children's conception of death and personal mortality. *Journal of Paediatric Psychology,* **8**, 21–31.
Resuscitation Council (UK) (2005) Resuscitation Guidelines 2005. *Resuscitation,* **66**, 31–38. Available at www.resus.org.uk/pages/guidelmp.htm (accessed 19 May 2006).
Ring, F. and **Jones, M.** (2004) NHS Direct usage in a GP population of children under 5: is NHS being used by people with the greatest health need? *British Journal of General Practice,* **54** (500), 211–213.
Robertson, J. (1958) *Young Children in Hospital.* London: Tavistock.
Robertson, J. and **Robertson, J.** (1952) *A Two-year-old Goes to Hospital.* Ipswich: Concord Films.
Roche, J. (1999) Children: rights, participation and citizenship. *Childhood,* **6** (4), 475–493.
Rodin, J. (1983) *Will This Hurt*? London: RCN.
Rountree, D. (1991) The PIC catheter: a different approach. *American Journal of Nursing,* **91** (8), 22–26.
RCN (Royal College of Nursing) (1994) *The Care of Sick Children.* London: RCN.
RCN (Royal College of Nursing) (2000) *Children's Community Nursing – Promoting Effective Teamworking for Children and Their Families.* London: RCN.

RCN (Royal College of Nursing) (2004) *The National Paediatric Diabetes Audit.* London: RCN.
RCN (Royal College of Nursing) (2005) *The Directory of CCN Services.* London: RCN.
Royal College of Paediatrics and Child Health (2003) *Providing a Service for Children.* London: RCPCH.
Royal College of Surgeons of England (1992) *Guidelines for Day Case Surgery.* London: RCS.
Sadler, S. (1988) Being there. *Nursing Times,* **84** (34), 19.
Sahib el-Radhi, A. (2004) Management of paediatric pain in paediatric practice. *Nurse2Nurse Magazine,* **4** (4), 38–40.
Saunders, B. (1982) Staff support. *Nursing,* **1** (34), 1498–1499.
Schepp, K. G. (1991) Factors influencing the coping effort of mothers of hospitalised children. *Nursing Research,* **40** (1), 42–46.
Selwood, K. (2000) Integrated care pathways: an audit tool in paediatric oncology. *British Journal of Nursing,* **9** (1), 34–38.
Shapiro, C. (1989) Pain in the neonate: assessment and intervention. *Neonatal Network,* **8** (1), 7–21.
Shellabarger, S. and **Thompson, T.** (1993) The critical times: meeting parental needs throughout the NICU. *Neonatal Network,* **12** (2), 39–44.
Shields, L. and **Tanner, A.** (2004) Cost of meals and parking for parents of hospitalised children in Australia. *Paediatric Nursing,* **16** (6), 14–18.
Shier, H. (2001) Pathways to participation: openings, opportunities and obligations. *Children and Society,* **15**, 107–117.
Sidey, A. (1990) Cooperation in care. *Paediatric Nursing,* **2** (3), 10–12.
Siedel, M. (1981) Death education a contravening process for nurses. *Topics in Clinical Nursing,* **3** (3), 87–89.
Simon, K. (1993) Perceived stress of nonhospitalised children during the hospitalisation of a sibling. *Journal of Pediatric Nursing,* **8** (5), 298–304.
Simpson, K. (1977) Eighteenth John Snow Memorial Lecture: the anaesthetist and the law. *Anaesthesia,* **32**, 626.
Simpson, S. (1994) Paediatric basic life support – an update. *Nursing Times,* **90** (21), 40–42.
Sinclair, R. and **Franklin, B.** (2000) *A Quality Protects Research Briefing: Young People's Participation.* London: HMSO.
Slater, M. (1993) *Health for all our Children: Achieving Appropriate Health Care for Black and Ethnic Minority Children and their Families.* London: Action for Sick Children.
Smalley, A. (1999) Needle phobia. *Paediatric Nursing,* **11** (2), 17–20.
Smellie, J. (1956) Domicillary nursing service for infants and children. *British Medical Journal,* **i**, 256.
Smith, J. and **Kanagasundaram, S. A.** (2002) Nitrous oxide in alleviating pain and anxiety during painful procedures in children. In David, T. J. (ed.), *Recent Advances in Paediatrics 2002.* London: Royal Society of Medicine Press.
Smith, A. and **Wood, J.** (1998) Can some in-hospital cardio-respiratory arrests be prevented? A prospective survey. *Resuscitation,* **37** (3), 133–137.
Somes, J. (1991) Ventricular fibrillation in a 2-month-old infant. *Journal of Emergency Nursing,* **17** (4), 215–219.
Spence, J. (1947) The care of children in hospital. *British Medical Journal,* **i**, 125–130.
Spicher, C. and **Yund, C.** (1989) Effects on pre-admission preparation on compliance with home care instructions. *Journal of Pediatric Nursing,* **4** (4), 255–262.
Splinter, W. and **Schaeffer, J.** (1990) Clear fluids three hours before surgery do not affect gastric fluid contents. *Canadian Journal of Anaesthesia,* **37** (5), 498–501.
Stein, R. and **Jessop, D.** (1984) Does pediatric care make a difference for children with chronic illness? *Pediatrics,* **73** (6), 845–852.
Stiller, C. A. (1988) Centralisation of treatment and survival rates for cancer. *Archives of Disease in Childhood,* **63**, 23–30.
Svavarsdottir, E. (2005) Caring for a child with cancer: a longitudinal perspective. *Journal of Advanced Nursing,* **50** (2), 153–161.
Swanwick, M. and **Barlow, S.** (1993) A caring definition: defining quality care. *Child Health,* **1** (4), 137–141.
Thornes, R. (1991) *Just for the Day.* London: NAWCH.
Thornes, R. (1993) *Bridging the Gaps: An Explanatory Study of the Interfaces between Primary and Specialist Care for Children within the Health Services.* London: Action for Sick Children.
Thurgate, C. and **Heppell, S.** (2005) Needle phobia – changing venepuncture practice in ambulatory care. *Paediatric Nursing,* **17** (9), 15–18.
Torrance, C. (1983) *Pressure Sores: Aetiology, Treatment and Prevention.* London: Croom Helm.
Treseder, P. (1997) *Empowering children and young people: promoting involvement in decision making.* London: Children's Rights Office/Save the Children.
Tucker, A. (1989) Who cares for the child? *Nursing Times,* **85** (38), 34–35.
Tume, L. and **Bullock, I.** (2004) Early warning tools to identify children at risk of deterioration: a discussion. *Paediatric Nursing,* **16** (8), 20–23.
Turner, T. (1985) Which dressing and why? In Westaby, S. (ed.), *Wound Care.* London: Heinemann.
UKCC (United Kingdom Central Council) (1986) *Project 2000 – A New Preparation for Practice.* London: UKCC.
UKCC (United Kingdom Central Council) (1989) *Exercising Accountability.* London: UKCC.
Vessey, J. A. (1990) Parental participation in paediatric induction. *Children's Health Care,* **19**, 116–118.
Vetter, T. R. (1992) Pediatric patient controlled analgesia with morphine versus mepidine. *Journal of Pain Symptom Management,* **7** (4), 204.
Victoria Climbié Inquiry (2003) *The Victoria Climbié Inquiry: Report of an Inquiry by Lord Laming.* London: HMSO.
Vidovich, M. (1980) Caring for kids – death in the ICU. *Australian Nurses Journal,* **9**, 43–44.

Visintainer, M. and **Wolfer, J.** (1975) Psychological preparation for surgical patients – the effect on children and parents. *Pediatrics*, **56**, 187–202.
Vulcan, B. and **Nikulich-Barrett, M.** (1988) The effect of selected information on mothers' anxiety levels during their children's hospitalisation. *Journal of Pediatric Nursing*, **3** (2), 97–102.
Waterlow, J. (1988) Prevention is better than cure. *Nursing Times*, **84** (25), 69–70.
Watson, J. E. (1979) *Medical–Surgical Nursing and Related Physiology*. London: W. B. Saunders.
Wehbe, M. and **Moore, J.** (1985) Digital ischaemia in the neonate following IV therapy. *Paediatrics*, **76** (1), 99–103.
Weibley, T. (1989) Inside the incubator. *Maternal and Child Nursing*, **14**, 96–100.
Weinbaum, D. (1987) Nosocomial bacterias. In Faser, B. (ed.), *Infection Control in Intensive Care*. New York: Churchill Livingstone.
Whaley, L. and **Wong, D.** (2002) *Nursing Care of Infants and Children*. St Louis: Mosby.
While, A. and **Crawford, J.** (1992a) Paediatric day surgery. *Nursing Times*, **88** (39), 43–45.
While, A. and **Crawford, J.** (1992b) Day surgery: expediency or quality care. *Paediatric Nursing*, **4** (3), 18–21.
White, C. (1995) Life crises for children and their families. In Carter, B. and Dearman, A. K. (eds), *Child Health Care Nursing*. Oxford: Blackwell Scientific Publications.
White, J. (1997) Creating a Snoezelen effect in PICU. *Paediatric Nursing*, **9** (5), 20–21.
White, P., *et al*. (1988) Nausea and vomiting: causes and prophylaxis. *Seminars in Anaesthesia*, **6**, 300–308.
Whiting, M. (1989) Home truths. *Nursing Times*, **85** (14), 74–75.
Whiting, M. (1994) Meeting needs – RSCNs in the community. *Paediatric Nursing*, **6** (1), 9–11.
Willow, C. (1997) *Hear! Hear! Promoting Children and Young People's Democratic Participation in Local Government*. London: LGIU.
Wilson, K. (1993) Management of paediatric pain. *British Journal of Nursing*, **2** (10), 524–526.
Wong, D. and **Baker, C.** (1988) Pain in children: comparison of assessment scales. *Pediatric Nursing*, **14**, 9–17.
Woodward, S. (1994) A guide to paediatric resuscitation. *Paediatric Nursing*, **6** (2), 16–18.
Wright, B. (1991) *Sudden Death*. Edinburgh: Churchill Livingstone.
Wyckoff, P. M. and **Erickson, M. T.** (1987) Meditating factors of stress on mothers of seriously ill hospitalised children. *Children's Health Care*, **16** (1), 4–12.
Wyngaarden, J. and **Smith, L.** (1988) *Cecil Textbook of Medicine*, 18th edn. Philadelphia: Saunders.
Zideman, D. (1999) Paediatric life support. *Update in Anaesthesia*, **10**, 3–7.
Zideman, D. (2003) *Cardio-respiratory Arrest in Children*. London: Medicine Publishing Company.

Module 6

Specific Care of Sick Children

Joan Ramsay and Tina Moules

Learning Outcomes

The material in this module and the further reading/references should enable you to:

- revise your knowledge and understanding of applied anatomy and physiology
- develop an understanding of the pathophysiology of common disorders and problems of childhood
- appreciate the signicance of specific assessment for sick children and your role before, during and after medical investigations
- discuss some of the more common nursing interventions and how these could be applied to alternative situations
- have an awareness of appropriate health promotion advice for discharge

Introduction

The purpose of this module is to enable you to explore the problems associated with the structure and function of the body. It does not give detailed information about every disorder found in children but seeks to provide sufficient principles of care to enable you to apply these to any given situation. You are encouraged to add your own material and information as you meet different problems, so that you can build up a resource file that is specific to your own practice. Just as we have used our experience of nursing children to write this book, we would like to think that you might reflect upon children you have nursed. Each part of the module is arranged in a similar way:

- revision of structure and function
- common disorders with pathophysiology where relevant
- specific assessment (including medical investigations)
- nursing interventions (including drug administration)
- discharge advice

The module begins by examining the principles of care for a variety of disorders. There is no specific order in which this content has been arranged but you will find cross-references to other modules. The latter part of the module explores mental health in children, neonatal care, and the care of children receiving cytotoxic treatment and radiotherapy.

Chapter 37

Principles of Care – Children with Blood Disorders

Introduction

Due to the central importance of blood within the body, its normal function can be affected by primary conditions and as a result of problems in other systems. Many of the primary abnormal conditions of the blood give rise to chronic problems for children. Although advances in understanding and management of these problems have improved the quality of life for children, repeated treatment and care can detract from normality. In order to understand the causes and consequences of blood disorders and implement appropriate care you need to have a working knowledge of the haematological system and its functions, and the basis of genetics.

Study activity

Test your knowledge of the structure and function of the blood. Check your answers in an anatomy and physiology textbook. Read the sections on genetics in Module 2 (p. 54) and Module 3 (p. 128). If necessary freshen up your knowledge.

The most common disorders of the blood seen in children are anaemias (Table 37.1) and bleeding disorders (Table 37.2).

Assessment

Assessing the child with blood disorders requires the nurse to use her skills to examine a number of features alongside the general assessment process (Figure 37.1).

Test your knowledge

- List seven functions of the blood
- Plasma constitutes about ?% of the blood
- Apart from water what are the other constituents of plasma?
- Draw a diagram to show the life cycle of a red blood cell (RBC). What factors are essential for the formation of mature cells?
- What is the role of erythropoietin in the formation of RBCs?
- List the types of white cells in the blood and describe their function
- Identify the major steps in coagulation of the blood

Pathology of a bleed into a synovial joint

- Hypertrophy of the synovial membrane due to reabsorption of blood and absorption of iron pigments
- Synovium becomes a thickened seaweed-like substance, and begins to invade the articular cartilage and grow over edge of joint surface
- At the same time chemical action of the blood in the joint damages the cartilage which eventually begins to peel off leaving exposed bone
- With repeated bleeds and no treatment the bone becomes soft and joint's surface develops cysts leading to collapse of the joint

Table 37.1 Anaemias in children

Disorder	Description
Haemophilia	Sex-linked recessive disorder – deficiency of any of nine factors required for normal coagulation cascade – results in bleeding tendency – into joints, muscle and subcutaneous tissue
Haemophilia A (classic)	Deficiency of Factor VIII (80% of cases)
Haemophilia B (Christmas disease)	Deficiency of Factor IX (13% of cases)
Haemophilia C	Deficiency of Factor XI (6% of cases)
Von Willebrand's disease	Hereditary disorder – basic defect in ability of platelets to aggregate in the presence of normal platelet count (accompanied by deficiency of factor VII) leads to increased bleeding time and tendency towards purpura, epistaxis, ecchymosis, gastro-intestinal bleeding
Idiopathic thrombocytopenic purpura (ITP)	Decreased production of platelets leads to prolonged bleeding time and bleeding tendencies as above, plus petechiae and superficial bruising. A review of current guidelines is available regarding the investigation and management of ITP (British Committee for Standards in Haematology Transfusion, 2003)
Henoch–Schönlein purpura	Acquired of unknown aetiology – inflammation of small blood vessels and vasculitis of dermal capillaries – leads to extravasation of red blood cells – petechial skin lesions. Marks *et al.* (2005) and Shad *et al.* (2005) review current research and treatment strategies

Haemoglobin

Normal haemoglobin (HbA) consists of a red pigment haem and four polypeptide strands, two alpha chains and two beta chains. The difference between the two types of chains lies in the sequencing and kinds of amino acids which make up the strands. HbS is caused by the substitution of valine for glutamine at position 6 on the beta chain.

(Groer and Shekleton, 1979)

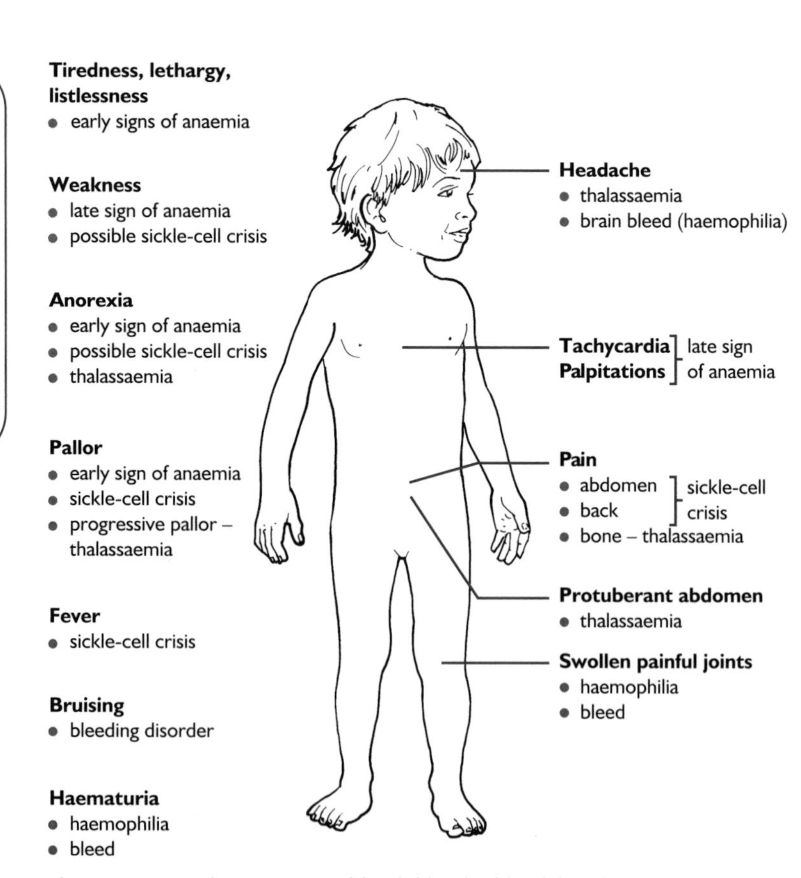

Figure 37.1 Specific assessment of the child with a blood disorder.

Table 37.2 Bleeding disorders in children

Disorder	Description
Iron deficiency anaemia	Infants store iron at birth sufficient for about 3–4 months. After this, additional iron is needed from the diet. Insufficient nutritional iron leads to deficient haemoglobin formation – red cells are hypochromic and microcytic. Eden (2005) explores a possible link between iron deficiency and impaired cognition in children. Levy *et al.* (2005) explore anaemia as a risk factor for infectious disease in infants and toddlers. See also http://whqlibdoc.who.int/hq/2001/WHO_NHD_01.3.pdf for further reading (accessed 25 May 2007).
Megaloblastic anaemia	Folic acid and vitamin B_{12} are essential for synthesis of nucleoproteins required for maturation of red blood cells; deficiencies of either interferes with this synthesis – red blood cells are immature and larger than normal (megaloblastic and macrocytic), the number of circulating blood cells is reduced and the total amount of haemoglobin is reduced
Aplastic anaemia: congenital, e.g. Fanconi, acquired	All formed blood elements are depressed simultaneously – the acquired type is caused by overwhelming infection, irradiation, drugs (chemotherapeutic agents) or chemicals (benzene); can be idiopathic. Fanconi – autosomal recessive condition. Locasciulli (2002) explores incidence, prognosis and treatment options
Haemolytic anaemia	Red blood cells have an abnormally short life span and are destroyed at an abnormally high rate – leads to increase in products of red blood cell (RBC) breakdown – jaundice results when the liver is unable to clear resulting pigment; bone marrow increases production to attempt to compensate – becomes hypertrophied. Norton and Roberts (2006) explore the management of Evans' syndrome
Sickle-cell anaemia	Abnormal haemoglobin (HbS) has reduced solubility within the RBC under conditions of hypoxaemia and hyperthermia – leads to the formation of a sticky gel-like substance in the Hb molecule, leading to the unusual sickle shape of RBCs. These abnormally shaped cells stick together easily, increasing blood viscosity and causing obstruction of blood flow, ischaemic tissue and pain (sickle-cell crisis). For recent advances in management of sickle-cell disease see Stinson and Naser (2003) for the management of pain; Anie (2005) for the psychological dimension; Hoppe (2005) for the risk of stroke and Okpala *et al.* (2002) for general issues
Thalassaemia	Deficiencies in the synthesis of beta-globulin chains in Hb – defective synthesis of Hb – structurally impaired RBCs (large and immature) with a short life span. Leads to compensatory bone marrow hyperplasia which produces overgrowth of facial and skull bones. Excess iron accumulates in tissues
Hereditary spherocytosis	Autosomal dominant condition – red cell membrane highly permeable to sodium, RBCs spherical in shape with increased osmotic fragility

Study activity

A toddler is admitted to your ward and on examination you find a number of bruises on his body. How do you differentiate between old and new bruises? What information might you need to ascertain from the child and his mother in order to conclude that the bruises may be a result of haemolytic disease?

Study activity

Pallor is a common sign of blood disorders. However it is also associated with many other serious chronic conditions. Find out which so that your assessment of the child with pallor can be more informed.

Table 37.3 Medical investigations (copyright is waived for the purpose of photocopying and enlarging this table)

Investigation	When and what for?	Role of the nurse
Blood count RBCs white cell count (WCC) platelets differential WCC reticulocyte count		
Hb		
Red cell indices		
Serum bilirubin		
Coomb's test: direct indirect		
Hb electrophoresis		
Serum iron		
Bleeding time		
Coagulation time		
Bone marrow aspirate		
Chest X-ray		

In assessing the child with a blood disorder the nurse may be required to assist in the implementation and interpretation of medical investigations. Table 37.3 shows the various investigations that may be carried out. See also Table 37.4. Find out in what circumstances each one might be used, what it might show and what the role of the nurse should be. Make notes in Table 37.3 for future reference.

Nursing Interventions

When caring for a child with a blood disorder you may be required to implement specific interventions. For the purposes of this section the following interventions will be examined:

- management of a sickle-cell crisis
- iron chelation therapy
- blood transfusion
- diet

Table 37.4 Normal blood values

	Infant	6–12 years	Adolescent
Haemoglobin (g/dl)	9–14	11.5–15.5	12–16
Haematocrit (volume fraction)	0.28–0.48	0.33–0.47	0.36–0.54
Red cell count	2.7–54	3.9–5.3	4.1–6.1
Platelet count (fl)	150–400	150–400	150–400
Red cell indices			
mean corpuscular volume (fl)	70–86	77–96	80–99
mean corpuscular Hb (fmol/cell)	0.39–0.48	0.39–0.54	0.39–0.54
mean corpuscular Hb concentration (mmol)	29–36	31–37	31–37
Reticulocyte count (%)	0.3–3.1	0.5–2.5	0.5–2.5
White blood count (× 10/l)	5.0–17.5	4.5–13.5	4.5–11.0
Differential WCC (number fraction)			
neutrophils	0.23	0.31–0.61	0.54–0.75
lymphocytes	0.61	0.28–0.48	0.25–0.40
monocytes	0.05	0.04–0.045	0.02–0.08
Bleeding time (minutes)	1–6	1–6	1–6
Clotting time (minutes)	5–8	5–8	5–8

Management of sickle-cell crisis

The factors that can precipitate a sickle-cell crisis include:

- infection
- dehydration
- hypothermia
- stress
- strenuous physical exercise
- acid–base imbalance

Children and their carers should be made aware of these factors so that they can take steps to avoid them wherever possible.

Study activity

What advice could you give a child with sickle-cell anaemia and her carers about how to avoid the factors that precipitate a crisis? Design a leaflet to back up your ideas.

The nursing interventions during a sickle-cell crisis are aimed mainly at relieving pain, promoting hydration and offering support and understanding to the child and family.

The pain that accompanies a sickle-cell crisis is classified as being mild, moderate or severe. Severe episodes require urgent and effective treatment. Explorations into pain management with sickle-cell disease suggest that current protocols are not sufficient (Chambliss *et al.*, 2002;

Additional aspects of management of sickle-cell crisis

- Administration of oxygen – helps to prevent sickling but will not reverse it.
- Bed rest at child's discretion – reduces oxygen consumption.
- Application of heat to affected areas (*not* cold as this enhances sickling and vasoconstriction).
- Antibiotics for infection.

(Hockenberry *et al.*, 2003)

For further information on sickle-cell disease see:

Bennett, L. (2005) Understanding sickle-cell disorders. *Nursing Standard*, **19** (32), 52–61.

Oxygen therapy

Oxygen therapy is considered not to be useful in vaso-occlusive episodes unless hypoxia is present (Charache *et al.*, cited by Whaley and Wong, 1995). It does not shorten the duration of pain or stop new pain.

(Zipursky *et al.*, 1992)

Stinson and Naser, 2003). Schecter *et al.* (1988) suggest that sickle-cell pain is often undertreated due to lack of knowledge, inappropriate attitudes about children with sickle-cell pain, concerns about addiction and lack of objective assessment criteria. As a result the child develops persistent pain with repeated requests for painkillers. This leads to the child being described as manipulative. It is therefore important to use an appropriate pain assessment tool before implementing treatment. The Children's Pain Assessment Project (Institute of Child Health, 2005) highlights current best practice guidelines in relation to the management of pain in children and young people. The use of patient-controlled analgesia devices has been advocated, as this enables the child to be in control. Non-pharmacological approaches to pain control should be considered alongside drug therapy. Children can be taught how to use self-hypnosis and imagery. They need to be taught about pain control so that they are informed when treatment becomes necessary. This will help to reduce fear and tension and will encourage the development of a trusting relationship with nurses and medical staff (*see also* Assessment and management of pain pp. 351–63 and Relaxation and imagery pp. 272–4).

Hydration therapy in the form of an intravenous infusion will be considered. This will help to dilute the viscous blood and reverse agglutination of sickled cells within the small blood vessels. At the same time, oral fluids should be encouraged.

Complications of iron overload

- Cardiac complications – cardiomyopathy occurs as a result of iron deposition in the heart; arrhythmias and pericarditis may also occur
- Hepatic complications – hepatitis B, cirrhosis
- Endocrine complications – retarded growth due to growth hormone deficiency; hypothyroidism; hypoparathyroidism caused by low levels of parahormone as a result of iron deposition in the parathyroid glands; diabetes mellitus

Iron chelation therapy

Children with thalassaemia require repeated blood transfusions every 3–4 weeks. Such frequent transfusions lead to an accumulation of iron that cannot be excreted or absorbed. Instead it is deposited in other body structures.

To prevent the build-up of serum ferritin, iron chelation therapy is usually administered about five to six times per week. The chelator of choice is desferrioxamine, which is given subcutaneously via a syringe pump over 8–12 hours (usually at night) (Roberts *et al.*, 1996). The nurse must be aware of the complications of chelation therapy:

- Local reactions – itching and rash – are common. Poor hygiene can result in skin infection and abscesses.
- Severe allergic reaction – the first dose must always be administered in hospital.
- Too rapid infusion of IV desferrioxamine can cause vertigo, hypotension, erythema and generalised pruritis (Roberts *et al.*, 1996).

Rahul, N., *et al.* (2005) Safety of oral iron chelator deferiprone in young thalassaemics. *European Journal of Haematology*, **74** (3), 217–220.

Where possible, home chelation therapy is implemented with the support of the community children's nurse. In this instance a teaching programme must be instigated that ensures that carers and children understand the theoretical background to the treatment and its practical management.

Desferrioxamine

Subcutaneous 20–50 mg/kg/day plus

Vitamin C 2 mg/kg daily on infusion nights (increases iron excretion in response to desferrioxamine)

Blood transfusion

It is likely that you will care for many children who require a blood transfusion for a variety of reasons. However, children with disorders of the blood are more likely to need this therapy and on a more regular basis. You therefore need to be familiar with the procedure and the role of the nurse in its administration (British Committee for Standards in Haemotology Transfusion, 2003; Bolton-Maggs and Murphy, 2004; Royal College of Nursing, 2004a; DH, 2005).

Children and carers may voice concerns about the transmission of hepatitis and HIV. They should be told that the risks are minimal and that this should be balanced against the effects of forgoing the transfusion. Information about how the blood has been collected and tested could help to reassure them.

The nurse should ensure safe administration of the correct blood. This requires careful checking of the blood and blood group against the child's identity band and notes. Administration of the blood should commence within 30 minutes of its arrival from the blood bank. Unused blood should be returned to the blood bank (*see also* Intravenous fluid therapy p. 344).

Study activity

Take an opportunity to donate blood. While you are there find out how donors are screened and what for.

Visit the blood bank to find out how the blood is stored and prepared ready for administration.

Study activity

Find out what your local policy says about monitoring children during a blood transfusion.

New blood safety and quality regulations came into force on 8 November 2005. For information see: http://www.dh.gov.uk/en/policyandguidance/healthandsocialcaretopics/bloodsafety/bloodsafetygeneralinformation/index.htm (accessed 31 May 2006).

The nurse must be aware of the potential complications of a blood transfusion (Table 37.5) and monitor the child according to local policy.

The need for repeated transfusions can be very disruptive. The child will be required to spend the day on the ward, perhaps missing school and all its attendant activities. Each child should therefore be allocated the same nurse (wherever possible) on each occasion so that a trusting relationship can be developed. The schoolteacher and play leader can be involved to encourage appropriate activities and help to reduce boredom.

Cultural perspective

According to Quintero (1993) the nurse must be aware of the alternatives to blood transfusion (e.g. albumin, Ringer's lactate) and the consequences of refusal.

Diet

Levy *et al.* (2005) state that anaemia due to iron deficiency is the most prevalent form of micronutrient malnutrition in the world. Children between the ages of 1 year and 5 years have high iron requirements due to rapid growth and the build-up of iron stores. A high proportion of preschool-age children in the UK has suboptimal iron intake, and iron-deficiency anaemia is common in this age group (Gregory *et al.*, 1997;

Table 37.5 Complications of blood transfusions and related nursing interventions

Complication	Features	Nursing interventions
Haemolytic reaction – severe but rare reaction caused by incompatible blood	Fever, chills, shaking Pain at needle site and along venous tract Nausea/vomiting Sensation of tightness in chest Red or black urine Headache Flank pain Progressive signs of shock and renal failure	Stop transfusion immediately in event of signs of reaction Notify doctor Monitor for shock
Febrile reaction – due to the presence of leucocyte, platelet or plasma protein antibodies	Fever and chills	Stop transfusion and notify doctor
Allergic reaction – recipient's blood reacts to allergens in donor blood	Urticarial rash, flushing Asthmatic wheezing Laryngeal oedema	Administer antihistamines as prescribed Stop transfusion immediately and seek help
Circulatory overload – due to too rapid transfusion or an excessive quantity of transfused blood	Precordial pain Dyspnoea Rales Cyanosis Distended neck veins	Take steps to ensure transfusion runs at the prescribed rate Stop transfusion immediately in event of signs of overload
Air emboli – due to blood transfused under pressure	Sudden difficulty in breathing Sharp pain in chest – apprehension	Ensure no air infiltration to administration set Stop infusion and seek help

Watt *et al.*, 2001). In a study by Gregory *et al.* (1997), 12% of children aged between one and a half and two and a half were described as being anaemic. Iron deficiency can have lasting effects on health and development (Grantham-McGregor and Ani, 2001) and Eden (2005) suggests that there may be a link between iron deficiency and impaired cognition in toddlers. Belton (2005) explores the Healthy Start initiative and analyses what measures have to be taken to rectify current deficiencies in the diet of children and young people. Children who present with iron-deficiency anaemia are managed by a combination of dietary modification and iron supplements. Carers need advice on:

- The sources of bioavailable iron. This describes the proportion of total iron in food that is absorbed and used for metabolism. Iron is most readily absorbed from foods rich in iron – liver, red meats, other meat (for example poultry) and meat products. Other sources of iron, although less well absorbed, include egg yolks, whole grains, fortified cereals and bread, legumes, green leafy vegetables, dried fruits and potatoes.
- Foods that enhance iron absorption – those containing vitamin C.
- Foods that reduce absorption of iron – cereals, plums, green beans, spinach, tomatoes and tea.

When weaning infants, parents should be encouraged to avoid giving too much milk but should ensure that adequate amounts of solid food are given. Milk (especially cows' milk, which is not advocated until after 12 months) is not a good source of iron.

anaemia

Anaemia is defined by the WHO as a haemoglobin of less than 11 g/dl.

(WHO, 1972)

Cultural perspective

Children who are being weaned as vegetarians need to have an adequate intake of vitamin C to enhance the absorption of iron.

Table 37.6 Education for discharge

Disorder	Education for discharge
Sickle-cell disease	Prevention of a crisis: • importance of maintaining hydration with a high fluid intake. Parents need to know how much to give per 24-hour period. They need to be aware of the signs of fluid loss – dry mucosa, weight loss, sunken fontanelle in the young baby • prevention of infection – importance of adequate nutrition to enable the child to fight infection, hygiene and the avoidance where possible of sources of infection. Prompt medical care should be sought if signs of infection are evident Details of support agencies
Thalassaemia	Parents and children need psychological support to enable them to deal with this chronic life-threatening disorder. Education for home management of iron chelation therapy
Iron-deficiency anaemia	Dietary advice (see above). It may not be sufficient just to tell parents what foods are rich in iron. The nurse may need to help with suggestions for recipes and buying the right foods. Paediatric dietician should be involved in education of family. Correct administration of iron supplements – as an increased stomach acidity reduces absorption of iron, supplements should be taken in between meals with a drink of citrus fruit juice to enhance absorption. Warn parents of effect of iron on stools – can make them tarry green. Liquid iron can cause temporary staining of the teeth – advise giving through a straw and cleaning teeth after administration. Warn parents that ingestion of large amounts of iron is dangerous so all preparations must be stored safely out of the reach of children
Haemophilia	Advise about regular dental care and good dental hygiene. Child should wear Medic-Alert identification. Teach parents and child how to recognise early signs of a bleed so that prompt treatment can be implemented – early signs of bleeding into a joint include stiffness, tingling, ache and reduced movement. Signs of internal bleeding include headache, slurred speech, loss of consciousness (bleed in the brain), black tarry stools, haematemesis (intestinal bleeding). Teach administration of Factor VIII/IX

Home Management for Children with Blood Disorders

Prior to discharge, the child and family must be familiar with all aspects of management of their particular problem. Table 37.6 highlights some of the important specific elements of care that must be taught to different children.

Study activity

Contact some of the support agencies identified on this page and in the Directory of British and Worldwide Sickle-cell Centres (http://www.sicklecellsociety.org/information/directory.htm, accessed 30 May 2006). Ask for copies of information sheets and analyse the advice available for children and their carers at home.

Many of the procedures and treatments needed by children with blood disorders can now be implemented at home with support from community children's nurses, and in ambulatory care settings such as outpatient clinics. In each case the child and carers need an individualised

Useful addresses

The Haemoglobinopathy Association of Counsellors
South-West London Sickle-cell and Thalassaemia Centre, Balham Health Centre, 120 Bedford Hill, London SW12 9HP
Tel: 020 8700 0615
Email: sicklethal.balham@swlondon.nhs.uk

The Haemophilia Alliance
http://www.haemophiliaalliance.org.uk/index.htm (accessed 30 May 2006)

Haemophilia Society
First Floor, Petersham House, 57a Hatton Gardens, London EC1N 8JG
Tel: 020 7831 1020
Fax: 020 7405 4824
Freephone helpline: 0800 018 6068 (Monday to Friday 10 a.m. to 4 p.m.)
Email: info@haemophilia.org.uk
Web site: http://www.haemophilia.org.uk/ (accessed 30 May 2006)

ITP Support Association
Synehurste, Kimbolton Road, Bolnhurst, Bedford MK44 2EW
Tel: 0870 777 0559
Email: shirley@itpsupport.org.uk
Web site: http://www.itpsupport.org.uk (accessed 30 May 2006)

Sickle-cell Society
54 Station Road, London NW10 4UA
Tel: 020 8961 7795
Email: info@sicklecellsociety.org
Web site: http://www.sicklecellsociety.org (accessed 30 May 2006)

UK Thalassaemia Society
19 The Broadway, Southgate Circus, London N14 6PH
Tel: 020 8882 0011
Fax: 020 8882 8618
Email: office@ukts.org
Web site: http://www.ukts.org/pages/contact.htm (accessed 30 May 2006)
Freephone advice line: 0800 7311109

teaching plan to ensure that they have the necessary knowledge and skills to carry out the procedures safely and effectively. For example, the administration of home treatment for haemophilia has developed considerably since the mid-1990s. Children are encouraged to learn self-administration of Factor VIII/IX before they reach senior school. Some require regular therapy, others can manage with intermittent use of Factor VIII/IX.

Study activity

Draw up a teaching plan to use with a 10-year-old boy with haemophilia to help him learn how to administer Factor VIII/IX. Give the rationale for your plan.

Chapter 38

Principles of Care – Children with Problems of Bones, Joints and Muscles

Introduction

Caring for children with problems of the bones and joints requires skill and patience. These problems can affect mobility, activity and almost every other activity of living to varying degrees. The child's appearance may be altered, giving rise to problems with body image. Many of the problems require long-term management and treatment, which can necessitate frequent visits to hospital and sometimes periods of immobility. It is important that you have an understanding of the structure and functions of the musculoskeletal system and its developments and maturation during childhood. A degree of prior knowledge is assumed, but you may need to refresh your memory (*see also* Maturation p. 65).

Study activity

Revise the structure and function of bones and joints. In doing this ensure that you understand:

- osteoblasts, osteocytes, osteoclasts
- the periosteum
- the role of parathyroid hormone, vitamin D, calcitonin
- the difference between types of joints

For the purpose of this text some of the problems likely to be faced by children are divided into congenital or genetic (Table 38.1) and acquired (Table 38.2).

Assessment

Some problems of bones, joints and muscles will be obvious to the eye (for example some fractures, congenital abnormalities). Others will require you to be able to assess movement and function of the musculoskeletal system.

Table 38.1 Congenital/genetic problems of bones, joints and muscles

Problem	Pathophysiology
Talipes:	
equinovarus	Foot is plantar flexed, the heel is inverted, the mid- and forefoot adducted. Interrelationships between bone, ligaments and muscle are disrupted. Often accompanied by neurological problems
calcaneovalgus	Foot is dorsiflexed and everted. Underlying structural deformity less profound – foot more amenable to manipulation
Congenital dislocation of the hip (Figure 38.1):	
unstable ('clicky hip')	Head of femur can be moved in and out of the acetabulum through manipulation. Head of femur and acetabulum are normal or near normal in shape
subluxed	Head of femur only in partial contact with acetabulum. Lack of development shape of acetabulum
dislocated	Head of femur lies completely out of joint. Shape and size of head of femur and acetabulum are abnormal. Will deteriorate if left
Scoliosis	Caused by failure of vertebral formation and segmentation. Lateral flexion of the spine causes trunk to shift from the midline, altering centre of gravity and shortening the spine. Spine rotates on its longitudinal axis; vertebra become permanently wedge-shaped; shape of rib cage alters
Marfan's syndrome	Autosomal dominant disease consisting of arachnodactyly, hypermobile joints, ocular abnormalities, high arched palate. Commonly associated deformities of spine and chest
Osteogenesis imperfecta (brittle-bone disease)	Autosomal dominant (occasionally recessive). Underlying failure in collagen metabolism resulting in multiple fractures of fragile bones, lax joints and thin skin. Other features include blue sclera, scoliosis
Duchenne muscular dystrophy (DMD)	Sex-linked recessive disease affecting male children. Progressive degeneration of groups of skeletal muscles and replacement of muscle by fibrous tissue leads to generalised wasting, kyphosis with thoracic deformity, hip and ankle contracture, inability to walk (usually apparent by 8–11 years), scoliosis and eventually cardiac muscle involvement. Gene has been mapped to p21 band of the X chromosome (Cree, 1997). Webb (2005) explores the information needed to cope with a child with DMD

Fractures

It is probable that you will have been made aware of children's fractures before they reach the ward. However, it is important that you know the features of fractures so that you can assess children in accident and emergency and at the scene of an accident, if necessary. The main features are:

- Pain – may be throbbing or localised, aggravated by passive or active movement.
- Loss of function – due to pain and instability of the fracture.
- Swelling – caused by oedema and effusion of blood. This takes time to appear, increasing over the first 12–24 hours after surgery.
- Deformity – a limb is bent or has a step in its alignment. There may be angular deformity, shortening of the limb, rotational deformity.

It is important that the child is systematically assessed for any other injury on admission to the ward.

Further reading

Craig, C. (1995) Congenital talipes equinovarus. *Professional Nurse*, **11** (1), 30–32.

Ryan, S., *et al.* (2003) *Core Paediatrics*. London: Arnold.

Thange, N., *et al.* (2005) *Pocket Essentials of Paediatrics*. London: W. B. Saunders.

Table 38.2 Acquired problems of bones, joints and muscles

Problem	Pathophysiology
Juvenile rheumatoid arthritis	Inflammation in joints; initially localised in joint capsule; tissue becomes thickened from congestion and oedema. Inflammatory response follows which invades interior of the joint; inflammatory tissue extends into interior of the joint along surface of articular cartilage; deprives the cartilage of nutrients; articular cartilage slowly destroyed. Growth plates may fuse prematurely; inflammatory changes may occur in tendons and sheaths; inflammation of muscle may occur
Osteomyelitis	Infection in metaphysis of long bones caused by bacteria – mainly *Staphylococcus pyogenes*. Resulting inflammatory reaction causes tissue necrosis, thrombosis of vessels leading to bone ischaemia; pus forms and spreads towards diaphysis, extending through cortex of bones; subperiosteal abscess forms raising periosteum from bone. Will either heal or progress to chronic condition
Idiopathic adolescent scoliosis	Affects mainly girls 10–14 years. See Table 38.1 for pathophysiology
Perthes' disease	Aseptic necrosis of the femoral head. Three stages: • *Stage 1* – avascularity; spontaneous interruption of blood supply to upper femoral epiphysis. Bone ceases to grow, swelling of soft tissue round hip • *Stage 2* – revascularisation; growth of new vessels – bone resorption and deposition take place; new bone is weak • *Stage 3* – reossification; head of femur gradually reforms, dead bone is removed, replaced with new bone which gradually spreads to heal lesion
Slipped upper femoral epiphyses	Posterior slipping of epiphysis of femoral head in relation to its metaphysis; results in shearing failure of growth plate. Further slipping can occur at any time – urgent treatment needed
Fractures – common ones seen in children include fractures of: • neck or shaft of humerus • supracondylar fracture of humerus • distal third of radius and ulna • distal radial physis • femoral shaft, tibia or fibula	Break in the continuity of a bone or cartilage usually caused by direct or indirect violence (Miller and Miller, 1985), by repeated stress and strain or by pathological processes (Pagdin, 1996). Children's bones are softer than adults' and can withstand a greater degree of deformity before breaking. Greenstick fractures are unique to children; bone breaks at one cortex and bends at the other – there is no complete loss of bony continuity. Injuries of the epiphyseal plate unique to children. Fractures heal more quickly than in adults
Bone tumours osteosarcoma	Occur mainly in adolescents; in the metaphysis of long bones (particularly around the knee). Highly malignant, destroying the cortex, extending into soft tissue and metastasising early via bloodstream to the lungs
Ewing's sarcoma	Highly malignant occurring mainly in diaphysis of long bones and flat bones of children and adolescents. Metastasises early to lungs and bone marrow

Assessing mobility

In assessing a child's mobility you should consider the following:

- Has the child reached the normal milestones in motor development? Delayed walking is sometimes evident in children with congenital dislocated hip (CDH).
- Watch the child walking. Is there a limp (Perthes' disease, CDH, bone tumour)? Is there an abnormal gait? A waddling gait is evident in CDH as is the Trendelenburg sign – note movement of the feet, legs, knees.

Module 6

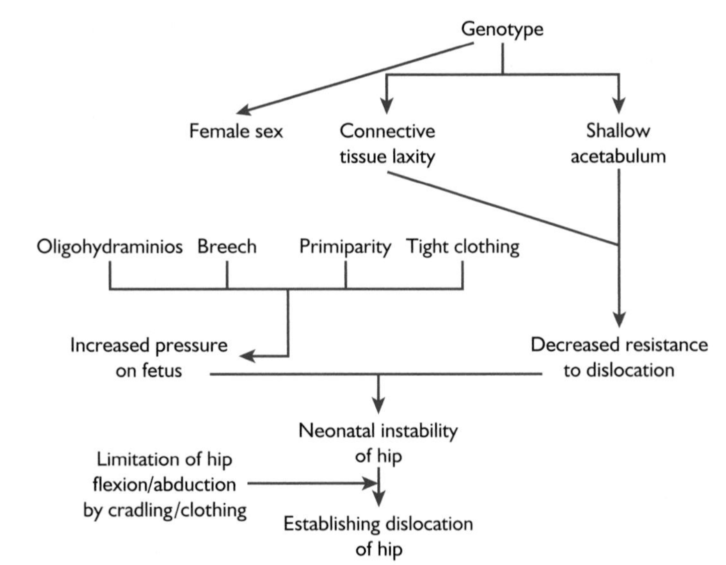

Figure 38.1 Developmental dysplasia of the hip, possible history (after Watson, 1990).

Okaro, T. (2006) *The Limping Child*, http://www.studentbmj.com/search/pdf/06/01/sbmj10.pdf (accessed 31 May 2006).

Trendelenburg's sign

The pelvis drops on the normal side when the child stands on the abnormal leg

Further reading

Anderson, J. E. (2002) Neonatal hip instability: results and experiences from ten years of screening with the anterior-dynamic ultrasound method. *Acta Paediatrica*, **91** (8), 926–929.

LeMaistre, G. (1991) Ultrasound and dislocation of the hip. *Paediatric Nursing*, May, 13–16.

A 1986 expert working party recommended that:

- all infants should have an examination within 24 hours of birth
- at the time of discharge or within 10 days of birth
- at 6 weeks
- at 6–9 months
- at 15–21 months
- the gait should be reviewed at 24–30 months and again at preschool examination

(Hall, 1996)

- Look at the child's posture. Is there any abnormality that might indicate scoliosis – poor posture, one shoulder higher than the other, one hip that seems more prominent, crooked neck, lump on the back?
- Is there any evidence of joint swelling, which may be indicative of arthritis? General swelling may accompany bone tumours.
- Is the child complaining of pain? Back pain is likely in scoliosis; pain in the hip referred to the knee, inner thigh and groin may accompany Perthes' disease; a reluctance to move a limb may be indicative of osteomyelitis. Pain can be a feature of bone tumours.
- Is the child generally unwell, showing signs of infection (reluctance to eat and drink, fever) linked to ostoemyelitis?
- Examine the child – limited abduction and internal rotation of the hip accompany Perthes' disease; asymmetry of the gluteal folds and leg length inequality are indicative of CDH (*see also* Motor development p. 68).

Other diagnostic tests may be used to determine potential problems (Table 38.3).

Study activity

Explore each of the tests/investigations in Table 38.3 and make notes in the boxes.

You should also become familiar with two screening tests used to diagnose CDH – the Barlow and Ortolani tests. Universal screening for CDH was first recommended in 1969 but since then debates about its role and effectiveness have been controversial (Leck, 1995). However, it is important to detect the condition early so that conservative treatment can be attempted, thus avoiding the need for surgery. Midwives, health visitors, general practitioners or community medical officers may carry out the screening tests.

Table 38.3 Diagnostic tests for bone, joint and muscle problems (copyright is waived for the purpose of photocopying and enlarging this table)

Investigation	When and what for?	Role of the nurse
Plain X-rays		
Bone scan		
Blood cultures		
Erythrocyte sedimentation rate (ESR)		
Leucocyte count		
Computed tomography		
Ultrasound (see LeMaistre, 1991)		

Study activity

Take an opportunity to observe someone carrying out screening for CDH. Discuss the use of the test with the person doing the screening and the implications of detection of a problem.

Nursing Interventions

You may be required to participate in implementing any one of a number of interventions for children with problems of bones joints and muscles. This section will address a few of the more common interventions. You are advised to explore each further as space precludes the inclusion of too much detail (*see also* Care of the child confined to bed p. 367).

Care of the immobilised child

For many children, treatment of problems will entail immobility for varying lengths of time. You need to have a clear understanding of the effects of immobility so that appropriate care can be implemented to avoid complications. The main effects and complications of immobilisation and associated care are:

- Decreased muscle activity and atrophy lead to weakness and loss of joint mobility – encourage both active and passive exercises; put joints through full range of movements where possible.

Further reading/Web sites for congenital dislocation of the hip (CDH)

Brown, J., *et al.* (2003) Efficiency of alternative policy options for screening for developmental dysplasia of the hip in the United Kingdom. *Archives of Disease in Childhood*, **88** (9), 760–766.

Contact a Family. For families with disabled children (CAF) http://www.cafamily.org.uk/home.html (accessed 2 June 2006).

Elbourne, D., *et al.* (2002) Ultrasonography in the diagnosis and management of developmental hip dysplasia (UK Hip Trial): clinical and economic results of a multicentre randomised controlled trial. *Lancet*, **360** (9350), 2009–2017.

Kamath, S. and Bramley, D. (2005) Is 'clicky hip' a risk factor in developmental dysplasia of the hip? *Scottish Medical Journal*, **45** (2), 56–58.

Kids for Health (The Royal National Orthopaedic Hospital). http://www.childrenfirst.nhs.uk/kids/hospital/england/theRoyalNatOrth/ (accessed 2 June 2006).

National Screening Committee (2005) Developmental dislocation of the hip. http://rms.nelh.nhs.uk/screening/searchResponse.asp?categoryID=1330 (accessed 31 May 2006).

Orthopaedic Surgery (Massachusetts General Hospital) http://www.massgeneral.org/ortho/ClubFoot.htm (accessed 31 May 2006)

STEPS http://www.steps-charity.org.uk/links.php (accessed 31 May 2006).

- Decreased metabolism – increase by encouraging activity within the child's limitations.
- Bone demineralisation, which can lead to high serum calcium levels – ensure increased hydration and active remobilisation as soon as possible.
- Disruption of normal elimination processes – adequate hydration promotes bowel and renal function. Enable the child to sit to use potty or bedpan wherever possible to encourage normal elimination. Provide privacy.
- Reduced integrity of the skin – change position frequently; keep the skin clean and dry; pay particular attention to prominent bony areas. Make use of sheepskins, avoid pressure on skin from equipment, tubes, tape, ensure adequate hydration and nutrition.
- Loss of appetite – offer small attractive meals, with nutritious snacks in between. Give preferred foods where possible.
- Psychological effects – make use of therapeutic play. Involve play therapists and teachers.

(*See also* Prevention of pressure sores p. 369.)

Processes involved in skin breakdown

Increased pressure on tissues leads to compression of small blood vessels. This, in turn, leads to infarction of soft tissues with a reduced supply of nutrients and reduced removal of waste. This results in cellular necrosis, which can cause open infected ulcers and the development of systemic infection.

Useful references

Hip Spica Casts – information leaflet. http://www.sheffieldchildrens.nhs.uk/patients/resources/134_hip_spica_caste.pdf (accessed 31 May 2006).

What is Developmental Dysplasia of the Hip? http://www.sheffieldchildrens.nhs.uk/patients/resources/020_development_dysplasia.pdf (accessed 31 May 2006).

Study activity

Explore the devices available to contribute to the prevention of pressure sores.

Study activity

Plan a day's activities for a 10-year-old boy confined to bed on traction. Give reasons for your decisions.

Principles of caring for children in plaster casts

A plaster cast is an immobilising device made up of layers of bandages impregnated with plaster of Paris (POP) (made from calcium sulphate dihydrate – gypsum) or synthetic lighter weight materials. Plaster casts are used to:

- immobilise and hold bone fragments in reduction
- permit early weight-bearing activities
- correct deformities

Nursing care is aimed at preventing complications and ensuring the child's comfort (Table 38.4). Specific care for certain types of cast may be needed (for example body cast or hip spica).

Many children can be discharged with a plaster cast and parents must be given adequate information about the care of the cast. The main points for inclusion should be:

Table 38.4 Nursing care for children in plaster casts

Potential complication	Nursing care
Plaster sores	Prevent irritation at edge of cast; avoid wetting the cast; do not place anything sharp down the side of the cast; monitor for signs – severe initial pain over bony prominence; increasing restlessness, fretful; (pain decreases when ulceration occurs); odour; drainage on cast. Report any of above
Circulatory disturbance – particularly after application of plaster	Elevate the body part to increase venous return; handle moist cast with palms of hands to avoid damage (dry POP sounds hollow when tapped); monitor for signs of inadequate tissue perfusion – swelling, blanching or discoloration of nail beds, tingling or numbness, inability to move fingers or toes, temperature change in skin – cold extremity may indicate ischaemia

- the plaster will take 2–3 days to dry out – do not write on it until it is dry
- keep the plaster dry
- keep fingers and toes moving
- do not cut or interfere with the plaster
- do not let child put small toys down the plaster
- return to hospital immediately if any of the following occur: the plaster feels tight or there is swelling; fingers/toes go blue/pale, cannot be moved, tingle or go numb; there is severe pain; there is an odd smell from the plaster; the plaster becomes wet or damaged

Types of plaster casts

- Short-arm casts – from below elbow to proximal palmar crease
- Gauntlet cast – extends from below elbow to proximal palmar crease including the thumb
- Long-arm cast – extends from upper level of axillary fold to proximal palmar crease (elbow usually immobilised at right angle)
- Short-leg cast – extends from below the knee to the base of the toes
- Long-leg cast – extends from junction of upper and middle third of thigh to the base of the toes
- Spica or body cast – incorporates trunk and an extremity
- Hip spica – extends from waist level to knees – holding the legs in the 'frog' position

Study activity

Design a handout to give to children using the points above. Give reasons for your choice of design. If you have an opportunity to do so, try it out and reflect on its effectiveness.

Managing traction

'When forces having both direction and magnitude act on an object at the same point simultaneously from opposite directions, the object either changes its state of rest or motion or remains in equilibrium' (Campbell and Glasper, 1995). Traction uses the direct application of these forces to produce equilibrium at a given site. The two essential components of traction are the forward traction (produced by attaching weight to the distal bone) and the countertraction (backward force of the muscle pull). There are two main types of traction:

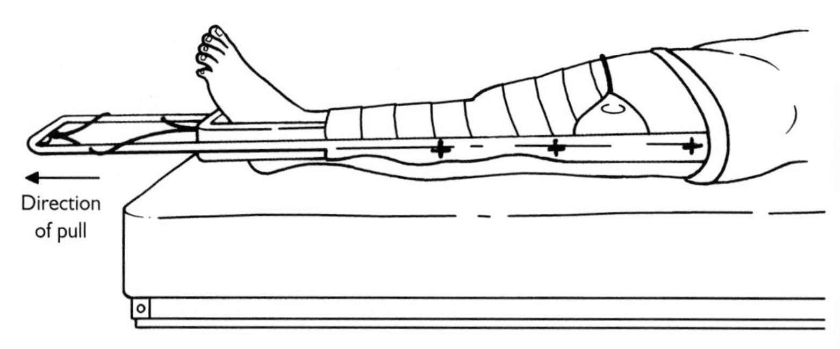

Figure 38.2 Thomas' splint: the traction works against the force of the child's body.

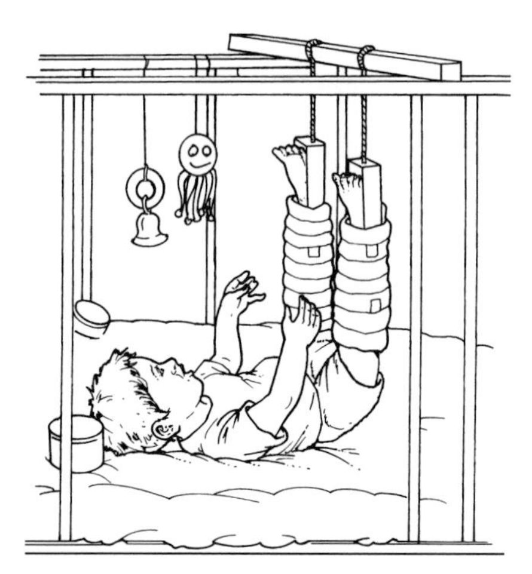

Figure 38.3 Gallow's traction: the child's weight serves as counter-traction to the vertical pull of the weights.

Indications for traction

- To relieve pain or muscle spasm
- To ensure rest of a limb during the healing period
- To maintain correct alignment
- To restore length where shortening after a fracture has occurred
- To reduce dislocation of joints
- To maintain the position of unstable fractures pre-operatively prior to external fixation
- To maintain good positioning after surgery

(Pritchard and David, 1990)

Further reading – pin-site care

Santy, J. (2000) Nursing patient with an external fixator. *Nursing Standard,* **14** (31), 47–52. http://www.nursingstandard.co.uk/archives/ns/vol14-31/pdfs/p4752w31.pdf (accessed 31 May 2006).

Temple, J. and Santy, J. (2005) Pin site care for preventing infections associated with external bone fixators and pins. *The Cochrane Database of Systematic Reviews,* Issue 4. http://www.mrw.interscience.wiley.com/cochrane/clsysrev/articles/CD004551/frame.html (accessed 31 May 2006).

- skeletal traction – the pull is applied directly to the skeletal structure by a pin inserted into or through the diameter of the bone
- skin traction – the pull is applied directly to the skin surface and indirectly to the skeletal structure

Adhesive strapping is applied to the skin with cords that can be attached to weights and/or pulleys, for example in the Thomas splint (Figure 38.2), or Gallow's traction (Figure 38.3).

Traction imposes degrees of immobilisation, so care aimed at preventing the complications of immobilisation should be considered. In addition you should implement care to:

- Maintain effective traction – check apparatus at regular intervals to ensure that ropes/pulleys/weights are in the right position and freely movable; maintain the child in the appropriate position; for example, in Gallow's traction the infant's buttocks should be elevated and clear of the bed.
- Maintain skin integrity – keep skin clean and dry; examine skin regularly. Remove bandages from skin traction and reapply daily; monitor skin for signs of soreness.

- Avoid infection at pin sites – Santy (2000) and Temple and Santy (2004) explore evidence-based care to prevent infection of external fixator sites and conclude that there is little evidence regarding which regime best reduces pin-site infections. Very often surgeons' preferences are the determining factor. Holmes and Brown (2005) provide a systematic analysis of the research literature on skeletal pin site care.

Study activity

Critically explore how pin-site care is managed in your area and compare with the ideas given here.

Traction is a very effective form of conservative treatment but generally has to be carried out in hospital because of the problems of accommodating traction equipment at home. Clayton (1997) describes the successful implementation of a 'traction-at-home' scheme. Care was shared between hospital and community staff. Caring for children on traction is not appropriate for everyone, but the scheme evaluated positively and this service is now offered to families.

Caring for children with juvenile idiopathic arthritis (JIA)

Although rare, the numbers of children diagnosed each year with JIA are almost equal to those with childhood diabetes. One child in every 1000 in the UK has JIA, and every year about one child in every 10 000 is diagnosed with the condition (ARC, 2003). 'Juvenile idiopathic arthritis' is a collective term that supersedes previous names such as juvenile chronic arthritis and rheumatoid arthritis. Leak (2002) identifies the problems in relation to treating a child diagnosed with JIA and suggests that treatment should relate to three main dimensions: pharmacological, physiotherapeutic and psychological. Children with JIA require support from their families and health professionals as the disease can affect almost every aspect of their lives. Current rheumatological research highlights evidence to support the need for more awareness to support children, young people and their families in relation to pharmacological management, the treatment regimen including the use and administration of etanercept (National Institute for Health and Clinical Excellence (NICE), 2002a) and methotrexate (Ramanan and Whitworth, 2003; Royal College of Nursing, 2004b); consideration of physical needs – given that JIA is a cause of varied growth disorders and may still be active into adulthood, giving rise to the need for consideration of living with potential long-term disabilities (Ravelli and Martini, 2005; MacRae *et al.*, 2006); with psychological considerations being tackled for all ages of sufferers (Britton, 2002; ARC, 2003).

Nursing care is aimed at:

- Relieving pain – using non-steroidal anti-inflammatory drugs (NSAIDs) including aspirin, ibuprofen, naproxen or mefenamic acid to help reduce pain and swelling in the joints.

Points to remember when applying skin traction

- Careful explanations should be given – it may be painful.
- Maintain privacy.
- Wash and dry the limb and check for any signs of injury or soreness prior to applying strapping.
- The use of solutions to enhance adhesiveness may be advocated.
- Keep the ankle free.
- Avoid folds and creases in the strapping.
- Check temperature and colour of skin after application to ensure that tension is correct.

Suggested process for planning and implementing home traction (adapted from Clayton, 1997)

- Involve community team.
- Inform all parents of possibility of home care from traction.
- Family must be committed to 24-hour care.
- Family must have been observed caring for the traction.
- Home circumstances should be assessed.
- All equipment is available before discharge.
- Transport home is arranged.
- General practitioner informed of discharge.
- Open access to ward should be allowed.

Further information

http://www.arc.org.uk/about_arth/booklets/6048/6048.htm (accessed 31 May 2006).

Britton, C. (2002) Views from the inside II: what the children said, and the experiences of mothers, fathers and grandparents. *British Journal of Occupational Therapy*, **65** (8), 1.

http://www.kidswitharthritis.org/articles/kwa_part2.pdf (accessed 31 May 2006).

Leak, A. M. (2002) Treatment of juvenile idiopathic arthritis. *CPD Rheumatology*, **3** (1), 3–7.

MacRae, V. E., Farquharson, C. and Ahmed, S. F. (2006) The pathophysiology of the growth plate in juvenile idiopathic arthritis. *Rheumatology*, **45** (1), 11–19.

National Institute for Health and Clinical Excellence (2002) *Guidelines on the Use of Etanercept for the Treatment of Juvenile Idiopathic Arthritis*. http://www.nice.org.uk/pdf/JIA-PDF.pdf (accessed 31 May 2006).

Ramanan, A. V. and Whitworth, P. (2003) Use of methotrexate in juvenile idiopathic arthritis. *Archives of Disease in Childhood*, **88**, 197–200.

Ravelli, A. and Martini, A. (2005) The long-term outcome of juvenile idiopathic arthritis. *Current Rheumatology Reviews*, **1** (2), 151–155.

RCN (2004) *Administering Subcutaneous Methotrexate for Inflammatory Arthritis*. http://www.rcn.org.uk/publications/pdf/administering-methotrexate.pdf (accessed 31 May 2006).

Goals of treatment for JIA

- To preserve joint function
- To prevent physical deformity
- To relieve symptoms without iatrogenic harm

(Campbell and Glasper, 1995)

Classification of juvenile idiopathic arthritis

- *Oligoarticular onset.* Affects less than five joints during the first 6 months of the disease. It is the most common and mildest form, affecting areas such the uveal tract in the eye. If unreated, it leads to uveitis and the possibility of blindness. It is for this reason that regular eye examinations are carried out.
- *Polyarticular onset.* Affects five or more joints during first 6 months, including small joints in the hands. Children are tested for the rheumatoid factor antibody (RF) and can be RF-negative or RF-positive. RF-positive polyarthritis is more common in girls over the age of 10 years.
- *Systemic onset.* Frequently starts in children under the age of 5 years and is associated with systemic features including high spiking fever, transient episodic erythematous rash, lymphadenopathy and hepatosplenomegaly. The familiarity of the symptoms with other childhood illnesses may mean that a diagnosis of this type of arthritis may be delayed, which may predispose the joints to problems later on. Some children may recover after a short period of illness with no lasting problems; some may have repeated episodic problems over the period of a few years.
- *Psoriatic.* Chronic arthritis, usually with asymmetric small and large joint involvement. It is more common in girls aged about 8 or 9 years and is linked with the development of psoriasis. It can involve particularly painful joints in the fingers and toes.
- *Enthesitis-related.* Previously known as juvenile spondyloarthropathy. It commonly affects the legs: it causes swelling where the tendons are attached to the bone, particularly in the feet and the knee. Children need regular eye examinations to monitor any redness, which may indicate iritis.
- *Unclassified* – any form of idiopathic chronic arthritis that does not fit into the above categories.

- Disease-modifying anti-rheumatic drugs (DMARDs) slow down and may stop the progress of arthritis. The most commonly used is methotrexate, usually taken weekly, by tablet, liquid or injection.
- Exercise – regular exercises are a vital part of treatment. Every child with arthritis will have a tailored programme of exercises designed by a physiotherapist.
- Promoting general health – well-balanced diet; weight control may be needed to avoid excessive strain on inflamed joints; regular rest periods.
- Maintenance of good posture and body mechanics – firm mattress to maintain good alignment of spine.
- Physiotherapy – focused on strengthening muscles, mobilising restricted joint movements, preventing or correcting deformities.
- Psychological care – helping the child to cope with the demands of the disease while attempting to reach their potential. May need counselling.

Support and Advice

Children with problems of bones, joints and muscles require support from a variety of sources.

Study activity

Some of the support agencies are listed below. Contact some of these to find out what information and support are available. Make up a resource pack for your ward/department.

- Arthritis Research Campaign, Copeman House, St Mary's Court, St Mary's Gate, Chesterfield, Derbyshire S41 7TD. Tel: 0870 850 5000. Web site: http://www.arc.org.uk/ (accessed 30 May 2006)
- Brittle Bone Society, 30 Guthrie Street, Dundee DD1 5BS. Freephone helpline: 08000 282459. Tel: 01382 204446. Fax: 01382 206771. Email: bbs@brittlebone.org. Web site: http://www.brittlebone.org (accessed 30 May 2006)
- Children's Chronic Arthritis Association, 47 Battenhall Avenue, Worcester WR5 2HN. Tel: 01905 763556. Web site: http://www.ccaa.org.uk (accessed 30 May 2006)
- Perthes' Association, PO Box 773, Guildford GU1 1XN. Tel: 01483 306637. Web site: http://www.perthes.org.uk/ (accessed 30 May 2006)
- Scoliosis Association (UK), 2 Ivebruy Court, 323–327 Latimer Road, London W10 6RA. Helpline: 020 8964 1166. Web site: http://www.sauk.org.uk/contact_us.htm (accessed 30 May 2006)
- STEPS, Warrington Lane, Lymm, Cheshire WA13 0SA. Tel: 0871 717 0044. Email: info@steps-charity.org.uk

Chapter 39

Principles of Care – Children with a Circulatory Disturbance

Causes of cardiac anomalies

Chromosomal anomalies

- trisomy 21
- Turner's syndrome
- Marfan's syndrome
- rubella syndrome

Environmental factors

- teratogens, e.g. thalidomide

Maternal health

- insulin-dependent diabetes
- alcoholism
- cytomegalovirus
- parental congenital heart disease

Maternal age

- > 40 years

Congenital cardiovascular defects

Of the thousands of babies born each year with congenital cardiovascular defects, the likelihood of the more common defects is:

- 4–10% atrioventricular septal defect
- 8–11% coarctation of the aorta
- 9–14% tetralogy of Fallot
- 10–11% transposition of the great arteries
- 14–16% ventricular septal defects

(American Heart Association, 2005)

Introduction

The common disorders affecting the heart can be categorised into congenital cardiac anomalies (Table 39.1) and acquired cardiac disease (Table 39.2). Congenital heart defects are anatomical defects that are present at birth and impair normal cardiac function. The incidence of congenital heart disease is 0.8 per 1000 live births (Holmes, 1996). Acquired cardiac disorders are those that develop after birth in response to infection, autoimmune disease, environmental and familial factors.

Common Cardiovascular Disorders

To understand the consequences of congenital and acquired heart disease it is important to have a knowledge of the anatomy and physiology of the heart before and after birth.

Study activity

Draw two large diagrams of the heart showing normal blood flow in the fetus and postnatally, and use these to identify the position and consequences of the anomalies described in Table 39.1.

The primary feature of impaired circulation is cyanosis and congenital anomalies are usually classified into cyanotic and acyanotic defects (Figure 39.1). Many of these congenital defects eventually lead to cardiac failure. Cardiac failure occurs when the heart is no longer able to maintain an adequate circulation of oxygenated blood to meet the body's metabolic demands. Cardiac failure can also result from myocardial failure. Cardiomyopathy, certain drugs and electrolyte imbalance can all weaken the contractability of the myocardium and cause cardiac failure. Failure of other body systems, especially the respiratory system,

Table 39.1 Congenital cardiac anomalies

Anomaly	Description
Acyanotic defects	
ventricular septal defect (VSD)	An opening in the ventricular septum. A small defect will allow blood to shunt from the left to right ventricle and into the pulmonary circulation. The increased pulmonary blood flow may cause pulmonary vascular disease
atrial septal defect (ASD)	A hole in the atrium which causes left-to-right shunting of blood because the right ventricle is more compliant than the left. The consequent volume overload of the right ventricle may not result in hypertrophy and heart failure until adulthood
patent ductus arteriosus (PDA)	Continued patency of the fetal ductus arteriosus which should constrict within hours postnatally. Blood shunts from the aorta into the pulmonary artery. A large shunt increases pulmonary blood flow, pulmonary venous return and a volume overload of the left ventricle. Left ventricular hypertrophy and heart failure results
pulmonary stenosis	The pulmonary valve is thickened and fused reducing the lumen of the valve. The increased resistance to blood causes an increase in the pressure generated by the right ventricle. Right ventricular hypertrophy and fibrosis ensues
aortic stenosis	Obstruction to the outflow of the left ventricle causes the left ventricle to generate greater pressure to maintain its flow. Consequently, left ventricular hypertension and hypertrophy occurs. Left coronary artery blood flow may be limited to diastole, causing tachycardia or angina on exercise
coarctation of the aorta	Aortic narrowing increases the resistance from the ascending to the descending aorta. The renal arteries which are served by the descending aorta receive a hypotensive flow and stimulate the release of renin which increases the aortic pressure above the coarctation. Collateral arteries may develop to allow the continuation of normal perfusion
Cyanotic defects	
tetralogy of Fallot	The association of four cardiac anomalies: VSD, pulmonary stenosis, right ventricular hypertrophy and dextroposition of the aorta. With mild forms of these defects resistance to pulmonary blood flow is usually equal to the resistance in the systemic circulation and minimal features are present. Right ventricular hypertrophy develops with larger defects to maintain a normal pulmonary blood flow. When this fails to prevent chronic arterial oxygen desaturation, a pulmonary collateral circulation and polycythaemia develops
tricuspid atresia	Absence of the tricuspid valve causes blood to leave the right atrium through some interatrial communication, usually a patent foramen ovale. If this is too small, right atrial hypertension and systemic venous congestion occur
transposition of the great arteries	Inappropriate septation and migration of the truncus arteriosus during fetal development causes the aorta to arise from the right ventricle and the pulmonary artery to arise from the left ventricle. Thus, the right side of the heart receives systemic venous blood and blood is returned to the systemic circulation via the aorta. Similarly, oxygenated blood circulates back and forth through the lungs and the left side of the heart. Signs of arterial oxygen desaturation are immediately present at birth unless some other defect allows shunting of blood to occur
truncus arteriosus	Inadequate division of the truncus arteriosus during fetal cardiac development. Instead of dividing to form the pulmonary artery and the aorta a single great vessel arises from the ventricles. This single vessel receives the output from both ventricles and mixed venous blood is circulated, resulting in cyanosis

also causes heart failure. Initially the body tries to compensate for a failing heart by using several compensatory mechanisms. This cardiac reserve includes hypertrophy and dilation of the cardiac muscle and stimulation of the sympathetic system. Hypertrophy of the cardiac muscle increases the pressure within the ventricle and dilation enables

Table 39.2 Acquired cardiovascular disorders

Primary cardiomyopathy	Idiopathic disease of the myocardium which becomes progressively more thickened around the ventricles. As a result the ventricles are significantly reduced in size and there is associated impairment of their dilatation and contraction. Cardiac failure will eventually result. Reduced pressure in the left ventricle may cause mitral valve regurgitation. Sudden death may also occur as a result of ventricular arrhythmia or complete obstruction of the ventricles
Primary hypertension	High arterial blood pressure forces the heart to pump harder to release blood against this resistance. As a result the heart muscle becomes enlarged and thickened. The increased demand for more oxygen may result in ischaemic changes. Increased pressure in the arterioles also causes thickening and narrowing of the lumen. Reduced renal perfusion stimulates the production of renin which exacerbates the high pressure
Subacute bacterial endocarditis	Microorganisms from any localised infection grow on a part of the endocardium which has been subject to some abnormal blood flow or turbulence. Areas of vegetation, fibrin deposits and thrombi develop which can break off and travel in the circulation to form renal, cerebral, splenic, pulmonary or skin emboli
Rheumatic fever	Inflammatory lesions develop in the heart, brain, pleura and joints from an autoimmune response to a group A, beta-haemolytic streptococcal sore throat. Lesions in cardiac tissue cause valvitis, myocarditis, pericarditis and endocarditis. Progressive valvular disease may eventually result in heart failure (rheumatic heart disease) and require surgery
Kawasaki disease	A microvascular inflammatory disease which progresses into myocarditis, pericarditis and sometimes valvitis. The myocardium is infiltrated with white cells, and the conduction system is impaired by oedema. Coronary artery dilatation may develop into aneurysms which may lead to coronary insufficiency, myocardial ischaemia and cardiac failure or infarction
Henoch–Schönlein purpura	Inflammation of small blood vessels causes widespread vasculitis of dermal capillaries, extravasation of red blood cells and a characteristic petechial rash. This inflammation and haemorrhage may also occur in the renal, gastro-intestinal or central nervous system

Common palliative operations for congenital heart defects

- *Pulmonary artery banding.* Performed for defects with a high pulmonary blood flow (e.g. VSD). A silk suture is tied around the pulmonary artery to reduce blood flow and reduce the risk of pulmonary vascular disease. Can be difficult to remove at the time of corrective surgery
- *Blalock–Taussig shunt.* End-to-side anastomosis of the subclavian artery to the pulmonary artery to increase pulmonary blood flow. Can occlude due to clotting
- *Modified Blalock–Taussig shunt.* A gortex tube is inserted between the subclavian and pulmonary arteries to increase pulmonary blood flow. Smaller shunts are likely to clot and prophylactic dipyridamole is usually administered
- *Waterson's shunt.* A direct side-to-side anastomosis between the ascending aorta and the pulmonary artery to increase pulmonary blood flow. Although less likely to clot it may cause distortion of the pulmonary artery making later repair difficult
- *Glenn procedure.* The azygos vein is ligated and the superior vena cava is resected and anastomosed to the transected right pulmonary artery to increase blood flow selectively to the right lung. It reduces the work of the heart but eventually causes damage to the pulmonary vessels within the right lung. It also makes it almost impossible to restore normal anatomy at the time of the corrective repair
- *Bi-directional Glenn procedure.* The azygos vein is ligated and the superior vena cava is transected and an end-to-end anastomosis is performed with the pulmonary artery to increase blood supply to both lungs. This procedure allows more chance of appropriate reconstruction at the time of corrective surgery

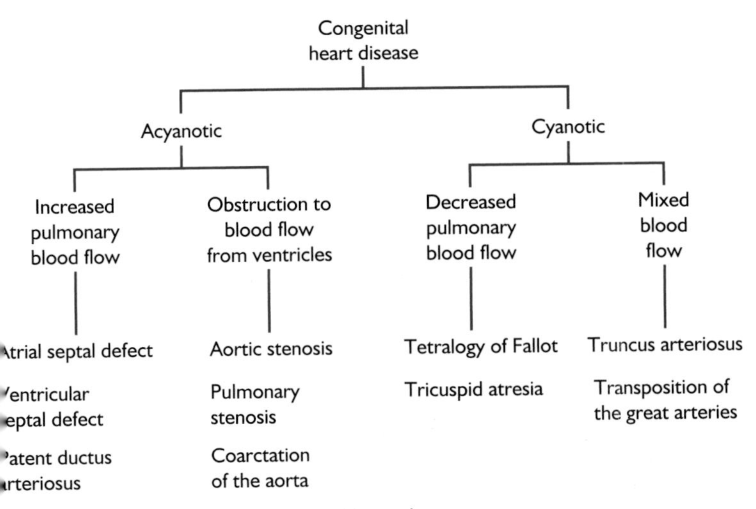

Figure 39.1 Classification of congenital heart disease.

the muscle to increase the force of each contraction, thus increasing cardiac output. However, these compensatory mechanisms can only benefit the situation temporarily. Eventually, compliance is lost from the hypertrophied ventricle and the increased muscle mass prevents adequate myocardial oxygenation. Additionally, there is a limit to the amount of possible dilation and beyond this limit the contractability force decreases. Cardiac failure accounts for 10% of paediatric cardiac transplants (Burch, 2002).

Stimulation of the sympathetic nervous system occurs in response to a reduced cardiac output. This stimulation is initiated by stretch receptors and baroreceptors in the blood vessels and catecholamines are released. Catecholamines increase cardiac contractions and also cause peripheral vasoconstriction, which results in increased peripheral resistance and venous return and reduced blood flow to the limbs, kidneys and abdominal organs. This increases blood flow to the vital organs but prolonged sympathetic stimulation reduces diastole, which impairs coronary artery circulation. Continued increases in peripheral resistance requires the myocardium to work harder and reduced renal perfusion activates the production of renin, angiotensin and aldosterone. Renin and angiotensin cause further vasoconstriction, which stimulates the production of aldosterone to cause retention of sodium and water. Sodium and water retention initially helps heart failure by increasing blood volume but this soon becomes excessive resulting in oedema and putting a further strain on the failing heart.

The most common cause of sudden death in previously healthy children is cardiac disease, especially cardiomyopathy. Very fit athletes often demonstrate an enlarged heart, but this is the result of fitness training rather than a pathological condition. Cardiopathy can be primary and idiopathic or secondary to other problems. Hohn and Stanton (1987) suggest that primary cardiomyopathy is linked to familial or genetic causes. Approximately one child in every 500 is affected, and in 1997 the first mass screening of children was introduced (Fletcher, 1997). Duchenne muscular dystrophy, Kawasaki disease, thyroid dysfunction and collagen diseases are all known causes of secondary cardiomyopathy (Purcell, 1989). Survivors of childhood cancer are also at risk of heart muscle disease, as around half of them will have been treated with an anthracycline (especially daunorubicin or doxorubicin), which causes irreversible cardiac myocyte necrosis. Damage is associated with high doses of these drugs, usually reserved for the treatment of solid tumours (Burch, 2002).

Hypertension can also be categorised as primary (essential) or secondary. Primary hypertension is more common in adolescents and appears to be related to genetic and environmental factors. Obesity, high salt intake, smoking and stress, which are often related to poor health behaviour in children, have all been identified as possible risks (Gillman *et al.*, 1993). Primary hypertension was traditionally thought to be a disease of adulthood, but now there is evidence of this disorder in children more emphasis has been made on routine screening of blood pressure. The American Heart Association (2005) recommends that all children over 3 years of age have an annual blood pressure check. Secondary hypertension is more common in younger children. The most common cause is renal disease (90%) but cardiovascular, neurological, metabolic and endocrine disorders and some drugs may also be responsible. The American Academy of Pediatrics (1987) suggests that children whose blood pressure measurements fall consistently between the 95th and 99th percentiles should be considered to have significant hypertension. They define severe hypertension as blood pressure that is consistently above the 99th percentile. Measurements recorded in a doctor's surgery may bear little relationship to the child's blood pressure during a normal day's activities, and Portman and Yetman (1994) recommend the use of the ambulatory blood pressure monitor to provide an overall profile of blood pressure patterns. Mild hypertension is usually controlled with non-pharmacological interventions (diet and regular exercise) as the long-term effects of anti-hypertensive drugs in children are not fully known (*see also* BP norms p. 287 and Recording children's health p. 282).

The cause of other forms of acquired cardiac disease, Kawasaki disease and Henoch–Schönlein purpura (HSP), are largely unknown. Kawasaki disease is seen in geographical and seasonal outbreaks, although there is no evidence for an infective cause. An environmental cause is supported by the evidence of its occurrence – it is most common in Japan. It has become the leading cause of acquired heart disease in children in the US, but it remains uncommon in the UK (Leung *et al.*, 1993). HSP often follows an upper respiratory infection or drug allergy and is nearly twice as common in boys as in girls.

Children with acquired or congenital cardiovascular disease are at risk of developing subacute bacterial endocarditis. Those particularly at risk are children with valvular disease and who have had recent cardiac surgery. Dajani *et al.* (1990) stress the importance of prevention, recommending individual prophylactic antibiotic therapy before and after any dental procedures or invasive procedures of the throat and respiratory, genito-urinary and gastro-intestinal tracts, which are known to increase the risk of bacterial contamination.

This prophylactic treatment is also recommended for children with rheumatic fever, who are subsequently susceptible to recurrent rheumatic fever for the rest of their lives. Rheumatic fever was a devastating problem and the leading cause of childhood deaths in the 1920s

(Bland, 1987). Its decline from 1920 to 1990 was explained by the development of antibacterial drugs but it now seems to be re-emerging in parts of America and the UK (Veasey *et al.*, 1994).

Assessment

Any critically ill child requires cardiovascular assessment. Severe illness in children tends to result in shock and hypoxia as well as being likely to induce heart failure and cardiopulmonary arrest. Shock is commonly associated with haemorrhage, infection, drug toxicity, fluid and electrolyte imbalances, hypoxia or trauma. Hypoxia may be a primary problem for children with respiratory problems or cyanotic congenital heart defects. Cardiac failure is also a problem for children with congenital cardiac problems as well as being secondary to myocarditis and cardiomyopathy.

Hazinski (1992) succinctly describes the child with severe circulatory failure as 'looks bad'. However, Figure 39.2 describes the features more objectively.

Study activity

Look at the features demonstrated by the child with cardiac failure listed in Figure 39.2 and determine the rationale for each feature.

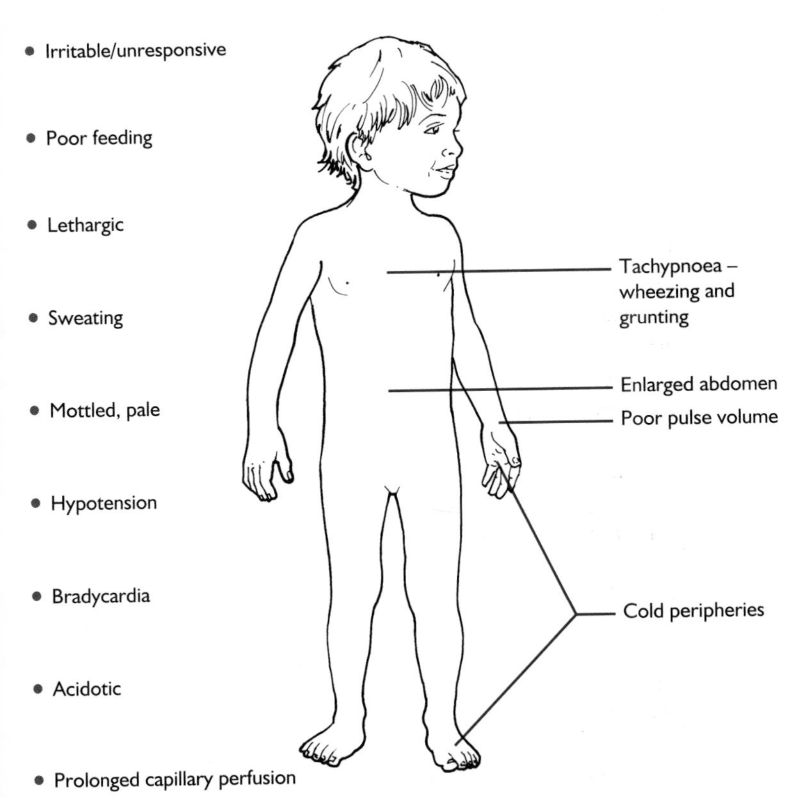

Figure 39.2 Assessment of the child with cardiac failure.

Table 39.3 Common investigations of the cardiovascular system (copyright is waived for the purpose of photocopying and enlarging this table)

Investigation	When and what for?	Role of the nurse
Chest X-ray		
Electrocardiography		
Echocardiography		
Cardiac catheterisation		
Exercise stress test		

In addition to these general features of cardiac disease there are some features that are characteristic of specific disorders. Clubbing of the fingers is thought to be the result of chronic tissue hypoxia and polycythaemia, which occur in cyanotic heart disease. Small children with unrepaired Fallot's tetralogy try to overcome this chronic hypoxia by squatting. This position reduces their desaturated venous return and diverts more blood into the pulmonary artery by increasing systemic resistance. Hypercyanotic spells occur in children with large ventricular septal defects or pulmonary stenosis whenever there is an unmet need for increased oxygen. They commonly occur in infancy during feeding, crying or defecation.

As well as making a nursing assessment of the child with a cardiac problem, the nurse will be involved in caring for the child before, during and after any medical investigations.

Study activity

Look at the common cardiac investigations listed in Table 39.3 and discover when and why these are performed. Make notes of the role of the nurse in each investigation.

Nursing Interventions

Specific nursing interventions that may be implemented for the child with cardiovascular disorder are:

- providing care to help reduce cardiac demands in the child with cardiac failure
- administering medication to improve cardiovascular function
- providing specific post-operative care following cardiac surgery

The child in cardiac failure needs to rest and save energy to reduce the demands made on the failing heart. Nursing activities should be organised carefully to enable the child to rest between interventions. Feeding the child in cardiac failure is a particular challenge. Increased heart and respiratory rates increase the metabolic rate, which needs to be met by a greater calorie intake. However, the breathless and exhausted child in cardiac failure has insufficient energy to suck.

Study activity

Taking the above comments into consideration, plan care for the child detailed in Table 39.4.

One of the most common medications given for cardiac disease is digoxin, but this is highly toxic and the nurse must be alert for signs of toxicity when administering it. As soon as toxic effects are noted, the next dose should be omitted. Once the therapeutic blood levels of digoxin (0.8–2.0 mg/l) are exceeded Opie (1991) suggests that it may be several days before they return to normal. Before administration of

Table 39.4 The child in cardiac failure: nursing care (copyright is waived for the purpose of photocopying and enlarging this table)

Alan is a 10-week-old infant who has been admitted to the ward in heart failure following a diagnosis of ventricular septal defect. On admission he is sweating, lethargic and irritable. His vital signs are: T 36: P 160: R 80. His mother reports that he is feeding poorly and that his hands and feet are always cold.

Problem	**Aim**	**Nursing actions**
Alan is having difficulty in breathing		
Alan has cold peripheries		
Alan is only able to suck for short periods		
Alan is at risk of skin breakdown due to poor perfusion		
Alan is at risk of renal failure due to poor renal perfusion		
Alan is irritable and tires easily		
Alan's parents are very concerned		

Post-operative care

Maintaining the airway

- ventilation for 24 hours
- continuous monitoring of respirations and O_2 saturations
- change of position and chest physiotherapy to promote lung re-expansion

Maintaining the circulation

- continuous ECG monitoring to observe for arrhythmias
- intra-arterial monitoring provides continuous BP measurements
- intracardiac monitoring gives constant readings of CVP
- measure chest drainage (Hazinski, 1992, indicates that drainage > 3 ml/kg/hour for more than 3 hours is indicative of haemorrhage)
- observe for complications of intra-arterial monitoring (arterial thrombosis, infection, air emboli or blood loss)
- observe for complications of CVP monitoring (dysrhythmias, haemothorax, pneumothorax)
- care of IV infusions (heparinised saline to keep vein open for intra-arterial line, IV fluids via CVP line)

Maintaining body temperature

- keep child warm for first 24 hours to allow gradual return of heat after hypothermia procedures
- pyrexia after 48 hours usually indicates infection

Provide rest and comfort

- continuous IV opioid infusion (Maguire and Maloney, 1988)
- plan care to allow adequate rest between procedures
- observe child for features of depression due to pain and stress

Maintain fluid balance

- measure all intake and output
- hourly urine measurements (< 1 ml/kg/hour is a sign of renal failure)
- daily weight
- nil by mouth for initial 24 hours or until extubation

Recognise complications of heart surgery

- mechanical trauma to red cells can cause haemolysis and anaemia
- haemorrhage may occur if clotting mechanisms are impaired by heparinisation
- impure blood entering the circulation can cause fat emboli, infection or thromboemboli
- neurological observations to identify cerebral oedema and/or neurological damage which can result from cerebral ischaemia or emboli
- pericardial and pleural effusions can occur 1–3 weeks after surgery

digoxin the apical pulse should be measured for a full minute to gain an accurate rate and rhythm, and the nurse should be aware of the prescribed pulse range within which the administration is considered therapeutic.

Care must be taken with the choice of analgesia for children with heart disease as there is now evidence that aspirin and other non-steroidal anti-inflammatory agents can exacerbate heart failure and may reduce the effect of diuretics, angiotensin-converting enzyme (ACE) inhibitors and beta blockers (Burch, 2002).

Study activity

Identify the uses, dosage/kg and side-effects of common medications used in cardiovascular disease (Table 39.5).

Table 39.5 Common medications used in cardiovascular disease (copyright is waived for the purpose of photocopying and enlarging this table)

Medication	Uses	Dose/kg	Side-effects
Digoxin			
Anti-arrhythmics propranolol			
Angiotensin-converting enzyme (ACE) inhibitors captopril			
Vasodilators hydralazine			
Diuretics frusemide spironolactone			

Many children with heart failure may eventually require mechanical support. For small children extracorporeal membrane oxygenation (ECMO) may be used but older children may require a pneumatic external pump such as the Berlin heart or the Medos. These can maintain the situation until a transplant becomes available. The number of child donor organs tends to match the number of children requiring transplant more closely than is the case with adults; however, in 2005 although 29 children received cardiothoracic transplants, seven died while waiting for the surgery. Child transplants have a 5-year survival rate of around 70% overall since 1982 (4419 cases) but Burch (2002) suggests that the current survival rate has increased in recent years with improvements in surgical technique, intensive care and mechanical support.

Cardiac surgery may be corrective or palliative. It may not be possible to undertake immediate corrective surgery due to the child's size or the severity of the condition. In such cases palliative surgery may be undertaken to stabilise the child until the corrective procedure can be performed. Immediate post-operative care following any cardiac surgery is undertaken in specialist intensive care units. The technology required to provide continuous observation of the child, including arterial pressure and central venous pressure (CVP) monitoring, usually requires critical care facilities. Rehabilitation and ambulation usually commence 48 hours after surgery, when ventilation, monitoring and drainage tubes can be removed and the child returned to the ward. Pain from thoracotomy incisions can limit lung expansion and remobilisation so it is important that regular assessment of pain and appropriate intervention is continued.

The Berlin heart

This device, which was invented in Germany and first used on adults in 1998, extends the time that children with life-limiting cardiac disease are able to wait for a transplant.

The external device has two tubes, which connect to the heart. One tube takes blood from the left ventricle and the other pumps blood back into the aorta. The tubes are inserted just below the rib cage.

A single external tube connects the device to the stationary driver computer, which powers and controls it and monitors the patient.

Education for Discharge

Discharge planning after cardiac surgery needs careful preparation. Parents need much reassurance and advice. Some cardiac surgery procedures can only be palliative and others may need repeating. Continued medical and emotional support is vital to help parents of children with such an uncertain prognosis. Holmes (1996) argues that this is the role of a cardiac liaison nurse.

Acquired cardiac disease such as hypertension may be preventable, and advice in childhood about the prevention of cardiovascular disease may prevent later problems in adulthood.

Cardiac surgery – advice on discharge

- Education about medication (e.g. anticoagulant therapy, digoxin)
- Restrictions to mobility
- Diet and nutrition
- Prevention of bacterial endocarditis
- Features of post-operative complications – recognition and reaction
- Follow-up appointments
- Wound care
- Medic-Alert identification (or similar) for children with a pacemaker, anticoagulation therapy
- Return to nursery or school
- Prognosis
- Effects on growth and development

Study activity

You are asked to talk to a group of primary school children about heart disease. Consider the best way to teach them about prevention of heart problems.

Chapter 40

Principles of Care – Children with a Metabolic or Endocrine Disorder

Introduction

Inborn errors of metabolism are relatively rare, but they include a large number of different disorders. The absence of, or deficiency in, a substance essential to cellular metabolism causes them all. It is becoming more possible to screen and detect these inherited disorders, and such processes enable early diagnosis and treatment. Prompt recognition and management of metabolic problems are essential if physical and mental retardation are to be avoided.

The most common endocrine disorder of childhood is diabetes mellitus (McEvilly, 1997). Diabetes UK (formerly the British Diabetic Association) (British Diabetic Association, 1996) reports that it occurs in:

- 1:50 000 infants
- 1:1500–2000 preschoolers
- 1:500 schoolchildren

In 2001 the Department of Health published the *Diabetes National Service Framework* because diabetes was so common amongst children and adults and its effective management is known to reduce long-term complications of the condition. This was followed in 2004 by the National Institute for Health and Clinical Excellence guidelines for best practice in diabetes care (NICE, 2004b). Recent statistics show that children are now developing type 1 diabetes at a younger age and that type 2 diabetes, once a disease of adulthood and associated with obesity, is now being seen in children. Shield (2006) reported that type 2 diabetes in children in the UK has risen tenfold in the past 10 years.

This section will therefore concentrate on the care and management of children with diabetes and only briefly discuss the principles of caring for children with metabolic disorders and other problems related to the endocrine system.

National Institute for Health and Clinical Excellence (NICE) guidelines for type 1 diabetes in children and young people

1. Management from diagnosis
   - Children and young people with type 1 diabetes should be offered ongoing integrated care by a multidisciplinary paediatric diabetes care team.
   - Members of the team should include staff with appropriate training in clinical, educational, dietetic, lifestyle, mental health and foot-care aspects of diabetes in children and young people.
   - At the time of diagnosis children and young people should be offered home-based or inpatient management according to clinical need, family circumstances and wishes and residential proximity to inpatient services.
2. Education
   - Children and young people should be offered timely and ongoing opportunities to access accurate and consistent information about the development, management and effects of type 1 diabetes to support informed decision making.
3. Monitoring glycaemic control
   - Care packages should be designed to achieve the target for long-term glycaemic control of an HbA_{1C} of less than 7.5% without frequent disabling hypoglycaemia.
4. Diabetic ketoacidosis
   - This should be treated according to the guidelines published by the British Society for Paediatric Endocrinology and Diabetes.
5. Screeing for complications and associated conditions
   - Coeliac disease at diagnosis and at least every 3 years thereafter until transfer to adult services
   - Thyroid disease at diagnosis and then yearly until transfer to adult services
   - Retinopathy annually from the age of 12 years
   - Microalbuminuria annually from the age of 12 years
   - Blood pressure annually from the age of 12 years
6. Psychosocial support
   - Children and young people should be offered timely and ongoing access to mental health professionals because they may experience psychological disturbances (anxiety, depression, behavioural and conduct disorders, and family conflict) which can affect the management of diabetes and well-being.

(NICE, 2004b)

Type 1 and type 2 diabetes

Type 1

- Occurs abruptly, most commonly in people under 20 years of age
- Absolute deficiency of insulin due to a marked decline in the number of insulin-producing beta cells of the pancreas
- Possibly caused by an autoimmunodestruction of beta cells
- Insulin receptors in the target cells are unaffected
- Termed 'insulin-dependent diabetes'

Type 2

- Less common form of diabetes in childhood
- Usually occurs in adults over 40 years who are overweight
- Sufficient or surplus amount of insulin produced by the beta cells
- Defects in the molecular machinery that mediates the action of insulin
- Many cells of the body, especially those in the muscles and liver, become less sensitive to insulin because they have fewer insulin receptors
- Termed 'non-insulin-dependent diabetes' (although some patients do require treatment with insulin)

Study activity

Complete Tables 40.1 and 40.2 to ensure that you can recall the principles of metabolism and the functions of the endocrine system.

Common Disorders of Metabolism and the Endocrine System (Table 40.3)

Phenylketonuria and galactosaemia are probably the two most commonly known errors of metabolism (Figures 40.1 and 40.2). Phenylketonuria is an autosomal recessive inherited absence of phenylalanine hydroxylase, an enzyme necessary for the metabolism of phenylalanine, an essential amino acid. The accumulation of phenylalanine in the bloodstream disturbs normal nervous system maturation by degeneration of grey and white matter and abnormal development of myelin and cortical lamination.

Table 40.1 The endocrine system (copyright is waived for the purpose of photocopying and enlarging this table)

Gland	Hormone	Function	Effect of hyposecretion	Effect of hypersecretion
Anterior pituitary	1 2 3 4 5 6 7 8			
Posterior pituitary	1 2			
Thyroid	1 2			
Parathyroid	1			
Pancreas	1 2 3			
Adrenals	1 2 3			
Ovaries	1 2			
Testes	1			

Table 40.2 Principles of metabolism (copyright is waived for the purpose of photocopying and enlarging this table)

Hormone	Effect upon the regulation of metabolism
Insulin	
Glucagon	
Epinephrine	
Human growth hormone	
Thyroxine	
Cortisol	
Testosterone	

Absorbed nutrients may be oxidised for energy, stored to provide heat and energy or converted into other molecules. The control of these different pathways is largely regulated by hormones.

Table 40.3 Common endocrine disorders

Disorder	Pathophysiology
Hypopituitarism	Growth retardation, absent or delayed puberty, hypothyroidism and adrenal hypofunction occur due to an impaired secretion of pituitary hormones. Usually due to pituitary or hypothalamic tumours
Congenital hypothyroidism (cretinism)	A deficiency of thyroid hormones which can be due to maldevelopment of the thyroid gland, pituitary dysfunction or abnormal thyroxine synthesis. Features of a decreased metabolic rate, which usually appear at 6 weeks of age when the maternal hormonal supply has ceased to have an effect, include bradycardia, hypothermia, lethargy and dry skin. If untreated normal nervous system maturation is impaired and mental retardation results
Lymphatic thyroiditis	The commonest cause of hypothyroidism in children aged 6–16 years. An autoimmune disorder in which lymphocytes infiltrate the thyroid gland and replace thyroid tissue with fibrous tissue, causing hyperplasia and enlargement of the gland
Hyperthyroidism	An autoimmune response of the thyroid stimulating hormone receptors causing an over-secretion of thyroxine. Irritability, hyperactivity, tremors, insomnia, tachycardia, heat intolerance, diarrhoea and vomiting can all result. Exophthalmos and visual disturbances are common although the exact rationale for these is unknown
Congenital adrenogenital hyperplasia	The commonest cause of adrenal hypofunction in children. An inborn deficiency of the enzymes necessary for the biosynthesis of cortisol causes an increased secretion of adrenocorticotrophic hormone. This causes hyperplasia of the adrenal cortex, reduced secretion of cortisol and aldosterone with the secretion of a large amount of immature steroids. These incompletely formed steroids have a masculising effect on the developing fetus

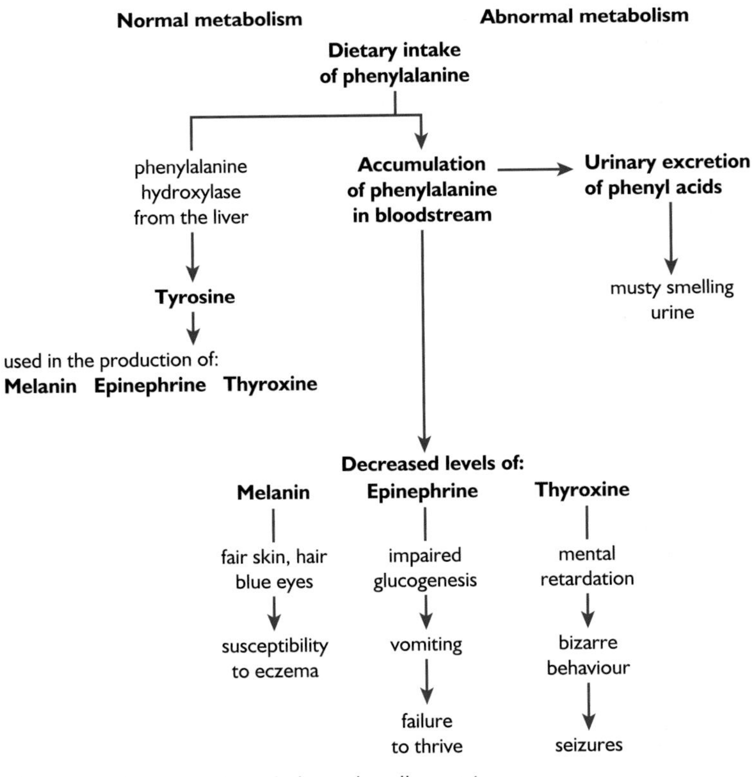

Figure 40.1 Disorders of metabolism: phenylketonuria.

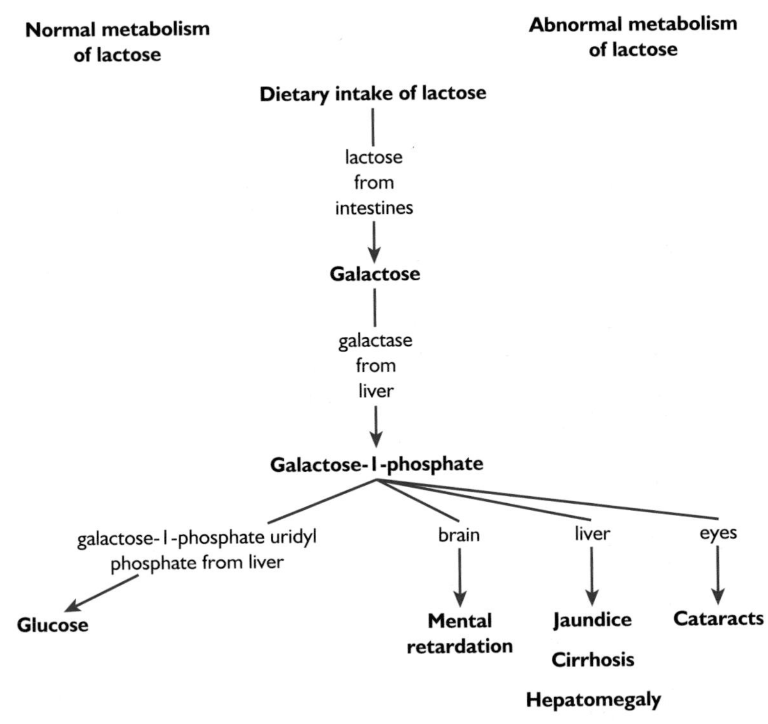

Figure 40.2 Disorders of metabolism: galactosaemia.

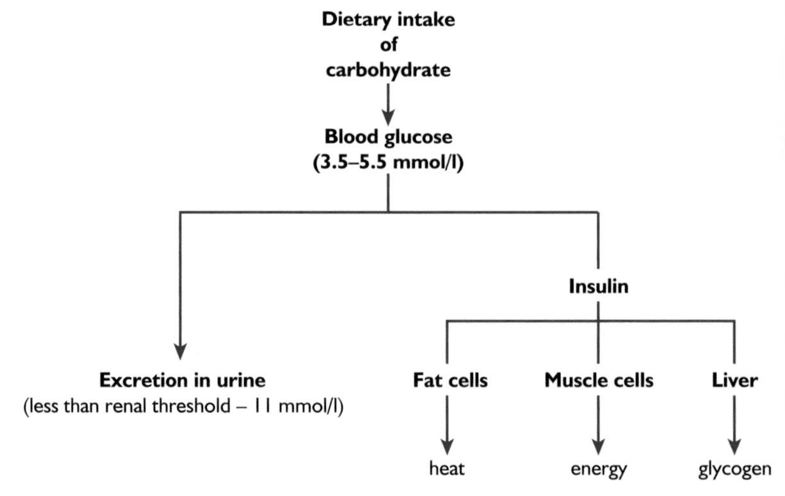

Figure 40.3 Normal carbohydrate metabolism.

Galactosaemia is also an autosomal recessive disorder and occurs in about 1 : 50 000 births. It affects normal carbohydrate metabolism by interfering with the normal conversion of galactose to glucose. The affected child is usually normal at birth but develops symptoms within a few days of commencing milk feeds. Vomiting, diarrhoea and weight loss are early signs, which quickly progress to drowsiness, lethargy, coma and sometimes death due to the accumulation of galactose in the bloodstream.

Module 6

Study activity

Identify the prenatal and neonatal screening processes for inborn errors of metabolism.

The incidence of insulin-dependent diabetes in infancy and childhood is increasing (Metcalf and Baum, 1991). It is thought to be an autoimmune disorder that is triggered by a viral, dietetic or environmental factor in children who have a genetic susceptibility to the disorder (see Figures 40.3 and 40.4). The mumps virus has been implicated as there appears to be a seasonal variation in the onset of diabetes in school-aged children. Karjalainen *et al.* (1992) identified cows' milk as a likely trigger factor. Environmental factors appear to be significant as the geographic distribution of the disorder is so variable. The incidence of diabetes in Sweden and Finland is three to four times the incidence in the UK and diabetes is almost unknown in Japan. The trigger factor initiates an autoimmune process in the beta cells of the islets of Langerhans in the pancreas. As a result, the beta cells are destroyed and no insulin is available to support carbohydrate metabolism.

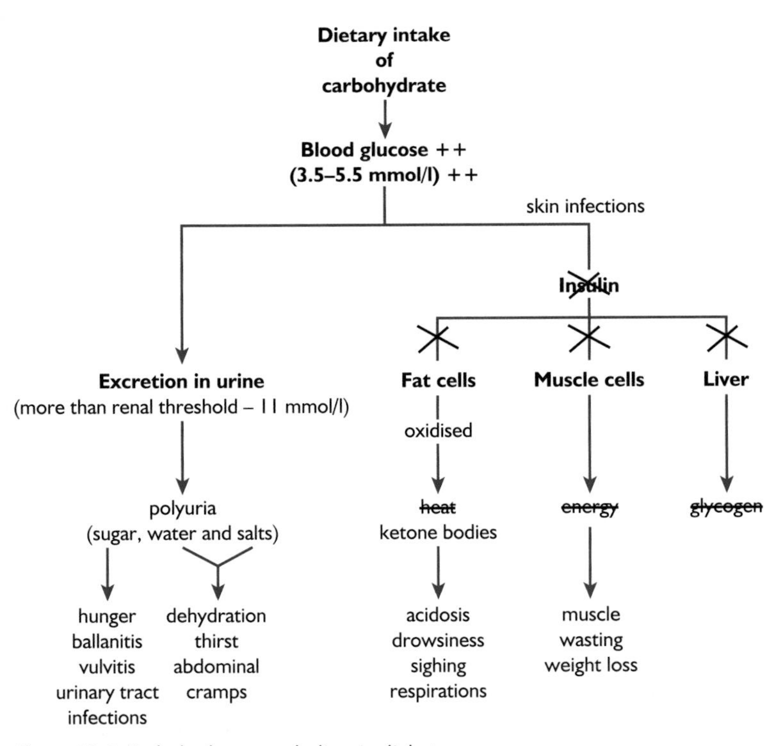

Figure 40.4 Carbohydrate metabolism in diabetes.

Specific Assessment of Metabolic and Endocrine Disorders (Figure 40.5)

Arn *et al.* (1988) report that there are certain characteristic clinical features that can be observed in any genetic or acquired metabolic disorders. If, moreover, the family history reveals a pattern of deaths in the neonatal period, the suspicion of a genetic metabolic problem is heightened.

It may be a family history of diabetes that first alerts parents to the possibility of this condition. The first features are often insidious and some children are not diagnosed until they present with ketoacidosis. The presence of excess glucose in the urine produces an osmotic diuresis and children who were previously dry at night may start bedwetting. This polyuria causes an extreme thirst and children may start to wake at night for a drink. Glycosuria may also cause a white sugary deposit around the toilet or urinary or genital infections. Repeated skin infections may also be apparent as the high blood glucose prevents the phagocytic action of white blood cells. Mature-onset diabetes in adults is often diagnosed by a glucose tolerance test but this has not been found to be a reliable diagnostic test for children. Instead, the diagnosis is confirmed by the presence of characteristic features:

- fasting blood sugar >6.7 mmol/l;
- random blood sugar >10 mmol/l (Higgins, 1995).

Assessment of diabetic control

Blood glucose

- spot check for hypoglycaemia
- spot check for hyperglycaemia
- 24-hour profile
- at least once a day, increase at times of illness

Urine testing

- for ketones when blood glucose > 17 mmol/l
- does not accurately reflect current blood glucose

Haemoglobin A

- glycosylated haemoglobin reflects control over previous 6–8 weeks

Monitor

- weight
- blood pressure
- eyesight

Specific assessment of metabolism

- Seizures
- Abnormal skin or hair
- Dysmorphic features
- Persistent vomiting
- Hepatomegaly
- Intractable diarrhoea
- Hypothermia
- Lethargy
- Abnormal eating patterns (aversion to certain foods, vomiting and/or diarrhoea after eating certain foods)

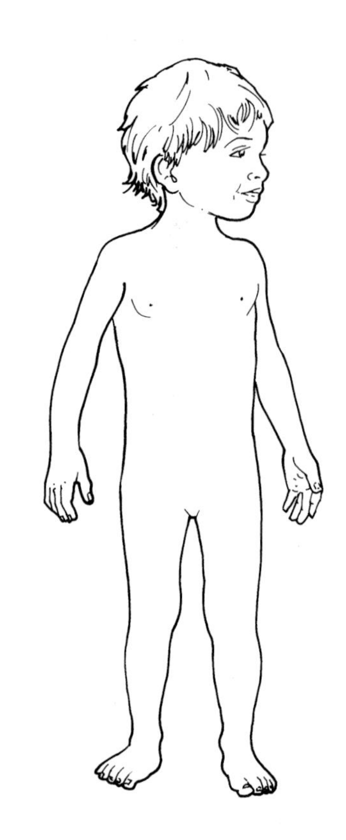

Specific assessment of the endocrine system

- Behavioural changes
- Excessive thirst
- Repeated skin infections
- Polyuria
- Signs of early puberty
- Weight loss *and* increased appetite
- Intolerance to changes of temperature

Figure 40.5 Specific assessment of the child with a metabolic or endocrine disorder.

Study activity

Find out how to use the blood glucose meter and measure your own blood glucose. Reflect on how you felt about this procedure and how you might react if you needed to repeat it every day.

Other specific investigations are commonly used to diagnose metabolic or endocrine problems. Use Table 40.4 to make notes about these tests and their uses. Check your role in the preparation for these and the care needed by the child during and after the tests.

Nursing Interventions

The main role of the nurse in the care of children with metabolic disorders is the education of the family about dietary restrictions. Dietary management in phenylketonuria aims to meet the child's nutritional needs for normal growth and development while maintaining phenylalanine levels within a non-toxic range (2–8 mg/dl). Brain damage occurs when levels exceed 10 mg/dl and protein stores are utilised for heat and energy, resulting in growth retardation if levels fall below 2 mg/dl.

Table 40.4 Metabolic and endocrine investigations (copyright is waived for the purpose of photocopying and enlarging this table)

Investigation	When and what for?	Role of the nurse
Bone scan		
Chromosome analysis		
Fasting/random blood glucose		
Guthrie test		
Thyroid function tests		
Thyroid scan and uptake		
Urinary catecholamines		

Therefore the low phenylalanine diet should contain 20–30 mg phenylalanine per kg body weight/day and be commenced as soon as possible unless the mother is breastfeeding. Normal breastfeeding may be possible as breast milk contains little phenylalanine (Lawrence, 1994). As the child grows older most high-protein foods must be avoided or restricted. Aspartame, the artificial sweetener, must also be restricted as it converts to phenylalanine once ingested.

Treatment of galactosaemia is a lactose-free diet. This includes the elimination of breastfeeding. Although this diet is easier to manage than the low phenylalanine diet, care must be taken to avoid medicines such as penicillin, which may contain lactose. Unfortunately, the outcome for children with metabolic problems, even with dietary control, is not good. The Medical Research Council (1993) reports that a high percentage of affected children demonstrate a degree of mental retardation.

Study activity

Assess the contents of your food cupboard for catering for a child with phenylketonuria and galactosaemia. When you next do your food shopping assess how easy it is to shop for these children.

Study activity

Study the list of drugs commonly used in endocrine disorders (Table 40.5) and find out their usual doses, uses, actions and side-effects.

Table 40.5 Drugs commonly used in endocrine disorders (copyright is waived for the purpose of photocopying and enlarging this table)

Drug	Dose (mg/kg)	Action/use	Side-effects
Aldosterone			
Cortisone			
Glucose			
Glycogen			
Growth hormone			
Hydrocortisone			
Sex hormones			
Thyroxine			

McEvilly (1997) states that the aims of care for the child with diabetes are initially to:

- correct dehydration and electrolyte imbalance
- stabilise the blood sugar
- educate and support the child and family in coming to terms with the diagnosis

Once these initial aims have been met the long-term objectives of care are to:

- achieve good control of carbohydrate metabolism
- reduce the risk of the acute and chronic complications of diabetes
- maintain near-to-normal blood glucose levels
- provide sufficient education and support to enable the transfer of care from the multidisciplinary diabetic team to the child and family

Swift *et al.* (1993) suggest that children with newly diagnosed diabetes are best managed at home rather than in hospital because it is so much easier to adjust their treatment around their usual routine and, as a result, subsequent hospital admissions are reduced. However, home management requires the support of a community diabetic team, which should include the paediatric diabetic nurse (British Diabetic Association, 1995) and be the most appropriate area for the individual child and family (National Institute for Health and Clinical Excellence, 2004a).

The majority of children with diabetes are treated with insulin, which should be administered 20–30 minutes before a main meal. Initially they will probably be given a mixture of short and intermediate acting insulin morning and evening. The child, if old enough, and the family need to be taught how to:

- obtain and store insulin and the injection device
- time their injections
- use an aseptic technique
- mix insulins
- choose injection sites
- inject insulin
- dispose of sharps

Study activity

Find out what to tell the child and family about the above.

Study activity

Reflect upon a child you have known with diabetes and how that child coped with injections.

Study activity

Find out the duration of action and the time of peak action for short, intermediate and long acting insulins. Then, using the list of insulins in Table 40.6, identify the length of action for different types of insulin.

Insulin treatment must be balanced with diet to promote a normal blood sugar level and maintain normal growth and development. There is a clear association between this control and the onset of chronic complications of diabetes in later life (Diabetes Control and Complications Trial Research Group, 1993). Ansell (1995) suggests that the dietician visit the child and family on the day of diagnosis to begin teaching the basic principles of dietary control. This should be followed by a series of short teaching sessions to expand and consolidate the information they will need.

However well controlled a child's diabetes is, it is likely that at least occasional hypoglycaemic attacks may occur (Ansell, 1995). At one time, hypoglycaemic attacks were induced as part of diabetic education. This is no longer thought to be good practice but the child and family should be taught how to recognise and manage an attack (Figure 40.6). Hyperglycaemia can occur as result of illness when stress hormones, produced to fight infection, cause a rise in blood sugar. The child and family should be aware that insulin should not be stopped during illness, even if the child is unable to eat normally. Instead carbohydrate should be given in the form of a snack or drink and if this is not possible medical advice should be sought. Blood glucose should be tested more frequently and the urine tested for ketones.

Complications of diabetes

Acute

- hypoglycaemia (insulin coma)
- ketoacidosis (diabetic coma)

Chronic

- diabetic retinopathy
- diabetic neuropathy
  - sensorimotor
  - autonomic
- diabetic foot
  - neuropathy
  - infection
  - ischaemia
- cardiovascular disease
  - coronary artery disease
  - cerebrovascular disease
  - peripheral vascular disease

Table 40.6 Types of insulin (copyright is waived for the purpose of photocopying and enlarging this table)

Insulin	Short action	Intermediate action	Long action
Human Actrapid			
Humulin S			
Humulin Insulatard			
Humulin I			
Human Monotard			
Human Ultratard			
Hypurin Bovine Isophane			
Insuman Basal			
Human Mixtard 30			
Human Mixtard 40			
Human Mixtard 50			
Novorapid			
Humalog			
Humulin M3			
Humulin M5			

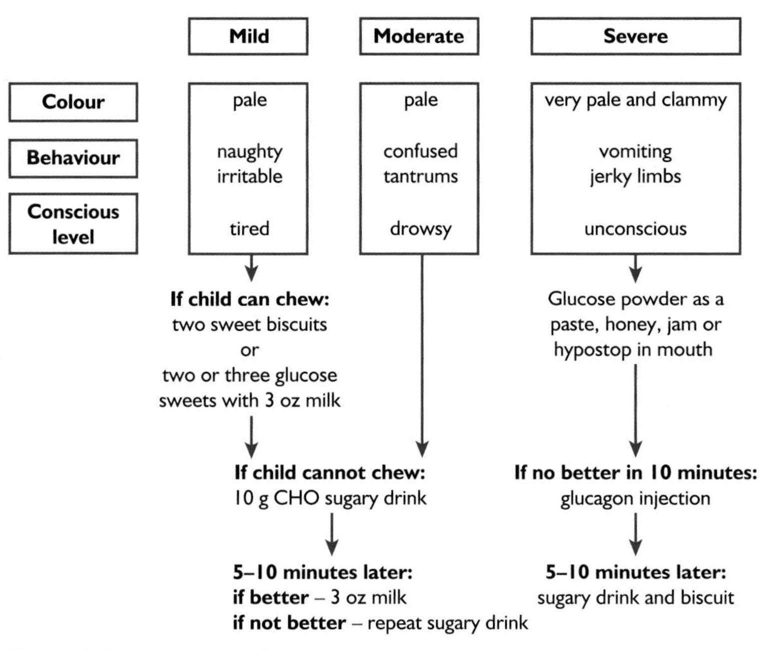

Figure 40.6 Management of hypoglycaemia.

Diabetic ketoacidosos (DKA) is a common acute complication of diabetes and is characterised by hyperglycaemia and acidaemia (pH < 7.30). It is rarely fatal if it is properly recognised and appropriately treated, but it is the most common cause of diabetes-related deaths in children (International Society for Pediatric and Adolescent Diabetes, 2000). In children with established diabetes, the risk of an episode of DKA is about 1–10% per child per year and many episodes occur as a result of poor compliance with treatment. The mortality rate of children with DKA in the UK is around 0.31%, the majority of these deaths occurring as a result of cerebral oedema (Edge *et al.*, 2001). Cerebral oedema is a serious complication of DKA treatment, which accounts for over half of DKA-associated deaths (Baunter, 2002). It usually occurs after 4–12 hours of treatment as biochemical abnormalities are improving. Risk factors appear to be: children under 5 years of age, those with newly diagnosed diabetes, more severe acidosis or dehydration at presentation, and administration of sodium bicarbonate (Glaser *et al.*, 2001). When caring for a child with DKA it is important to be aware of the features of cerebral oedema; changing levels of consciousness, bradycardia, hypertension, and decreasing respiration. To minimise neurological damage or death, cerebral oedema must be treated promptly with airway management (which may include 24–48 hours' intubation with paralysis and sedation), fluid restriction and intravenous mannitol 0.5 g/kg over 5 minutes.

Study activity

Consider what carbohydrate snacks or drinks you could offer a diabetic child who was feeling unwell and nauseous.

Management of hyperglycaemia

Correct hypoperfusion and shock

- IV infusion normal saline 20 ml/kg for first 2 hours
- IV infusion saline 0.45% + 4% dextrose 20 ml/kg for next 2 hours
- IV infusion saline 0.18% + 4% dextrose thereafter
- monitor pulse, respirations, fluid balance and oxygen saturations

Correct hyperglycaemia

- IV insulin (1 unit insulin : 1 ml saline)
- 0.1 unit/kg/hour initially
- 0.05 unit/kg/hour when blood sugar < 15 mmol/l
- discontinue 1 hour after first subcutaneous injection of insulin
- monitor blood glucose hourly for the first 4 hours

Correct electrolyte imbalance

- add potassium chloride (KCl) to infusion after 1 hour if serum K < 5 mmol/l
- if serum K 3.5–5 mmol/l add KCl 20 mEq/l
- if serum K < 3.5 mmol/l add KCl 40 mEq/l
- monitor urea and electrolytes hourly for first 4 hours

Recognise and treat possible cause

- IV antibiotics
- urine and blood specimens for culture
- chest X-ray
- swabs/specimens from any obvious sites of infection

Recent advances in the management of insulin-dependent diabetes

- Pancreatic transplantation
- Islet transplantation
- Insulin delivery systems
  - subcutaneous insulin infusions
  - implantable peritoneal pumps
  - implantable glucose sensors
  - intranasal insulin
  - insulin pens
- 'Designer' insulins

There are many situations that predispose to poor control of diabetes. The varying growth of children as well as their changeable levels of activity and emotions do not help diabetic control.

Study activity

Consider the particular problems of controlling diabetes in the

- infant
- toddler
- schoolchild
- adolescent

Study activity

Consider how to solve the problems of controlling diabetes outlined in the case histories in the box 'Problem solving in diabetes'.

Discharge Advice

The impact of being given the diagnosis of diabetes may be very stressful for some parents, especially if a grandparent has died from a long-term complication of diabetes. Common fears are dietary limitations, daily injections, and chronic invalidity. Teaching sessions and group discussions can sometimes help these fears. Diabetes UK (1997) emphasises the importance of consistent support for the child and family because there is so much to learn about diabetes and the growing child has changing needs. They also recommend at least an annual check of the child's development and the onset of any complications. The risks of complications occurring are known to be greater 5 years after the onset of puberty (McEvilly, 1997).

Problem solving in diabetes

1. David's mother has brought him to the clinic for a checkup. She is concerned that David has been having consistently high blood glucose levels although he is eating as usual and has not changed his insulin dose or level of activity. The diabetic nurse checks David's injection sites. Why?
2. Amanda, who is 15, is denying her diabetes and hiding it from her friends. When you ask her the reason for this she replies, 'They don't want to hang around with someone who is always ill'. How could you help Amanda to overcome these feelings about her condition?
3. Neil, aged 12, controls his diabetes fairly well with insulin and three meals and three snacks each day. He tells you that he has been chosen for his school football team and that he now needs to train with the team twice a week after school. What adjustments would you suggest he makes to maintain his control on these days?
4. Several months ago, Marie, aged 2 years, was diagnosed as a diabetic following convulsive hypoglycaemic reactions. Since then, her mother has been terrified of low blood sugars. At clinic, it is obvious that she is trying to keep Marie on a strict regimen to keep the diabetes under complete control 24 hours per day. How can you help Marie and her mother?
5. Michael, aged 15, is brought into the accident-and-emergency department by a friend. He has a fruity smell on his breath, flushed face, strong but slow pulse, and dilated pupils. He is sweating profusely and is confused about where he is. You discover a Medic-Alert bracelet stating that he is an insulin-dependent diabetic. What would you expect his diagnosis to be?

National Institute for Health and Clinical Excellence (2004a) guidelines stress the importance of children and young people with diabetes having timely and ongoing access to support. Baunter (2002) recognises that many children's diabetes services in the UK are understaffed, particularly with specialist paediatric diabetes nurses, dieticians and psychologists. This hampers diabetes control and many children in the UK with diabetes have suboptimal glycaemic control.

Study activity

Visit your local diabetic clinic and find out what support is available in your community for the diabetic child and family.

Study activity

Look at the practical problems of diabetes listed below and consider how these situations can be managed.

Practical problems for children with diabetes include:

- schooling/employment
- travel/holidays (for example, sickness, change of diet, time changes, storage of equipment, etc.)
- dental treatment
- surgery
- minor illness
- pregnancy

Diabetes is a long-term condition and at some point the adolescent needs to move to the care of an adult diabetic team. Adolesence is a difficult time for most children and moving from the sheltered atmosphere of a small children's service into an environment with older patients and less support can make this an even more traumatic time. There is evidence that properly planned transition programmes can result in better disease control and improved patient satisfaction. The Children's National Service Framework (NSF) (DH, 2004b) recommended that every paediatric general and speciality clinic should have a policy on transition to adult services, which should be the responsibility of a named person.

Study activity

Look at the arrangements in your hospital for the transition of adolescents with diabetes from paediatric to adult care. Do they meet the Children's NSF recommendations?

Useful address

Diabetes UK
Macleod House, 10 Parkway, London NW1 7AA
Tel: 020 7424 1000
Email: info@diabetes.org.uk
Web site: http://www.diabetes.org.uk (accessed 31 May 2006)

Transition to adult diabetic services

Policies on the transition to adult services should include:

- A flexible approach to the timing of transfer to take into account developmental readiness and other social transitions such as leaving school.
- A preparation period and education programme to enable the young person to identify and develop the skills necessary for smooth transfer to adult services.
- A coordinated transfer process with a named coordinator who can arrange personal introductions and visits to adult services. This may include coordination across health, social care, education and employment.
- An interested and capable adult clinical service which has close links with the children's service and has an understanding of the developmental needs of young adults.
- Administrative support to ensure smooth transfer of all records including a handheld summary for the patient's own use.
- Primary health and social care involvement to ensure continuity of care and to meet broader health needs.

(DH, 2004b)

Chapter 41

Principles of Care – Children with Eye, Ear, Nose and Throat Disorders

Introduction

After the first year of life upper respiratory tract infections are more common than infections involving the lower respiratory tract, and preschool children have about six upper respiratory tract infections per year (Valman, 1993). The pharynx and middle ear are so close together in these small children that infection in either area readily spreads to the adjacent organ. The most common disorder related to the nose is allergic rhinitis, affecting mostly older children.

Congenital problems affecting the upper respiratory tract are usually considered to be relatively minor defects, which can be corrected by surgery. They include cleft lip and palate and abnormalities of the larynx, trachea and the subglottal area. Although mostly not life-threatening conditions, these problems are often just as devastating for parents who may be disappointed, angry and rejecting of their 'abnormal' baby, especially when the defects are very obvious.

Visual impairment is a another common problem during childhood, which can cause emotional problems for parents and the child.

Test your knowledge of the structure and function of the eyes, ears, nose and throat

What is the normal process of vision?

What is the function of the:

- ciliary body?
- retina?
- lens?
- anterior cavity?
- vitreous chamber?

What structures lie close to the middle ear and are at risk from the spread of infection from otitis media?

What are the functions of the nose and the sinuses?

Why does the nose bleed readily?

Identify the position of the following:

- maxillary sinuses
- frontal sinuses
- ethmoid sinuses
- pharyngeal tonsils (adenoids)
- palatine tonsils

Where is a tracheostomy formed?

Study activity

Test your knowledge of the structure and function of the eyes, ears, nose and throat by answering the questions in the margin. Check your answers with your anatomy and physiology textbook.

Common Disorders of the Eyes (Table 41.1)

Visual impairment is the term used to describe children who are blind and partially sighted. There are many prenatal and postnatal causes of visual impairment, but the cause of most problems is unknown. Visual impairment can impair motor function and learning and prevention and early detection of problems is vital.

Table 41.1 Common disorders of the eyes

Disorder	Pathophysiology
Refractive disorders	
myopia	The eyeball is too long causing the image to fall in front of the retina. The individual only sees clearly when objects are close by (short-sightedness)
hyperopia	The eyeball is too short, causing the image to fall beyond the retina. The individual only sees clearly when objects are at a distance (long-sightedness)
astigmatism	Unequal curvatures in the cornea or lens cause light rays to bend in different directions resulting in blurred or distorted vision
anisometropia	Each eye has a different refractive strength causing the individual to avoid the use of the weaker eye
Amblyopia	Reduced visual acuity in one eye caused by a lack of stimulation and resulting in each retina receiving different images (double vision). Lack of use of visual cortex eventually results in loss of response and loss of vision in the affected eye
Cataract	Opacity of the lens prevents light rays from entering the eye
Conjunctivitis	Inflammation of the conjunctiva – usually bacterial in children – causing inflammation (pinkness) of the eyeball and the lining of the eyelids, pain and discomfort
Glaucoma	Increased intraocular pressure caused in children by a congenital defect in the flow of aqueous humour. The increased pressure eventually leads to atrophy of the optic nerve and blindness
Strabismus	A congenital defect, poor vision or muscle imbalance or paralysis results in unparallel visual axes causing the brain to receive two images

Table 41.2 Common disorders of the ears, nose and throat

Disorder	Pathophysiology
Otitis media	Obstruction of the Eustachian tube from the inflammation and oedema of upper respiratory tract infections, allergic rhinitis or hypertrophic adenoids, causes the accumulation of secretions in the middle ear (acute otitis media). If this fluid is not released, it thickens to develop a glue-like consistency which reduces the movements of the tympanic membrane and impairs hearing (secretory otitis media, 'glue ear')
Allergic rhinitis (hayfever)	Inhaled water-soluble allergens diffuse into the respiratory epithelium and react with antigen-specific immunoglobulin E on the susceptible child's nasal mast cells. As a result histamine is secreted causing vasodilation and swelling. Hypersecretion of nasal mucus and sneezing results
Tonsillitis	Infection of the palatine tonsils leads to inflammation and oedema. Obstruction of the passage of air and food results in difficulty in mouth breathing and swallowing
Infectious mononucleosis (glandular fever)	Infection by the Epstein–Barr (EB) virus causes mononuclear infiltration of lymph glands causing generalised lymphadenopathy and splenomegaly

Common Disorders of the Ears (Table 41.2)

Lous *et al.* (2005) suggest that few children escape childhood without some symptoms of secretory otitis media or 'glue ear'. Surgery to the middle ear is the most common cause of surgical admissions of children to hospital in the UK, at a cost of approximately £30 million per year, although there is increasing controversy about the benefits of such surgery (Lous *et al.*, 2005). The National Institute for Health and Clinical Excellence (NICE, 2002c) estimated that in 50% of affected children the effusion will resolve spontaneously within 3 months and within a year

95% will have recovered. The National Institute for Health and Clinical Excellence (2002c) recommended that most cases could be managed within primary care and therefore recommended 'watchful waiting' as the most appropriate treatment.

Because of the prevalence of otitis media much attention has been paid to possible causes. Strachan *et al.* (1989) indicate that passive smoking is a significant factor. They suggest that the inhalation of smoke impairs mucocilliary function and this causes congestion of the nasopharyngeal tissues, predisposing the child to upper respiratory infection and blockage of the Eustachian tube. Duncan *et al.* (1993) have found that breastfeeding appears to protect children from developing otitis media. They propose that breastfed babies are likely to be protected against respiratory allergies and viruses by maternal immunity and that the semi-prone position used for breastfeeding is less likely to cause reflux of milk into the Eustachian tube. The most common approach to the treatment of glue ear is surgical myringotomy and insertion of a grommet (incision into the tympanic membrane and the insertion of a small drainage tube). Some children gain little or no improvement from this surgical intervention and sometimes the grommet falls out too soon, necessitating repeat surgery (Lous *et al.*, 2005). The 'watch-and-wait' policy towards treatment has been criticised. Hogan *et al.* (1997) found that susceptible children develop frequent episodes of otitis media, which can result in hearing losses that can be as great as 50 decibels. In the young child hearing loss prevents normal development of speech and language, and the older child may fall behind in school and may be unfairly labelled as slow, backward, difficult or disobedient. However, Lous *et al.* (2005) did not find any evidence that grommets help speech and language development.

National Institute for Health and Clinical Excellence (NICE) guidelines for the management of glue ear

The majority of children can be managed by primary care. Referral to specialist services is advised if:

- there are atypical otoscopic features accompanied by a foul-smelling discharge suggestive of cholesteatoma
- excessive hearing loss suggestive of additional sensori-neural deafness
- proven hearing loss plus difficulties with speech, language, cognition or behaviour
- proven hearing loss together with frequent episodes of acute otitis media
- proven persistent hearing loss detected on two occasions separated by 3 months or more

(National Institute for Health and Clinical Excellence, 2002c)

Adenoidectomy may also be performed to relieve glue ear. The adenoids tend to hypertrophy in response to repeated upper respiratory tract infections and cause obstruction of the Eustachian tube, predisposing to glue ear. However, Widemar *et al.* (1985) express doubt that adenoidectomy prevents or treats glue ear and Flood (1989) warns that the longer hospital stay and risk of haemorrhage for such surgery may not outweigh the possible benefits.

Otitis media causes conductive deafness, which is the most common type of hearing loss, resulting from an impairment of the transmission of sound to the middle ear. Sensori-neural hearing loss or perceptive deafness is caused by inner ear and auditory nerve defects, which distort sound and prevent its differentiation. Hearing impairment is one of the most common disabilities of childhood and can vary from a slight deafness (below 30 decibels) to extreme deafness (above 90 decibels).

Common Disorders of the Nose (Table 41.2)

Hayfever or allergic rhinitis affects about 20% of the UK population and usually begins in childhood before the age of 10 (Rees, 1994). Dewers (1990) found that it is two to three times more common in first-born or only children and suggested that these children experienced less exposure to viral infections that prevent the development of allergies. Although not a serious disorder, hayfever causes extreme discomfort and affects sleeping and concentration. Both of these can have serious consequences for schoolwork. The major cause of hayfever is pollen. Pollen counts are now often given during weather forecasts to help hayfever sufferers determine the risk. These counts are measured in units of pollen per cubic metre. Symptoms usually occur at a count of 50 (Newman-Turner, 1992). Antihistamines are the preferred medication as they counteract the histamine secretion but their undesirable side-effects make them unpopular with all patients and may be the reason why most sufferers do not start treatment before symptoms appear. Rees (1994) stresses the importance of prevention and recommends the use of prophylactic nasal sprays. Topical sodium cromoglycate inhibits cell degranulation and can be used regularly. A corticosteroid spray reduces the responsiveness of the nose to allergens but is safest when used regularly on a short-term basis.

Clefts of the lip and palate are congenital malformations that occur to some degree in 1 : 700 births in the UK, affecting more females than males (Martin, 1995). These malformations are often associated with other chromosomal abnormalities but environmental factors and teratogens may also interrupt normal embryonic development of the palate. Clefts of the lips may be unilateral or bilateral and may range from a notch in the upper lip to complete separation of the lip extending to the base of the nose. They may or may not be associated with a cleft palate. Cleft palates are less obvious deformities but may have more serious consequences, such as inadequate nasal airways and malposition or missing teeth. It has been suggested that treatment outcomes for children in the UK with cleft lip and palate deformities did not compare well with those in Europe. As a result the 57 centres providing cleft care in England have now been reduced to nine main centres to enable the identification of standards of optimum care (Martin, 2005).

Causes of sensory loss

Deafness

- family history of hearing problems
- anatomical craniofacial malformations
- low birth weight (< 1500 g)
- significant deprivation of oxygen at birth
- maternal infection (cytomegalovirus, rubella, herpes, syphilis, toxoplasmosis)
- postnatal infection (meningitis, measles, mumps)
- chronic ear infection
- ototoxic drugs (e.g. gentamicin, streptomycin, tobramycin)
- syndromes known to include sensori-neural hearing loss

Blindness

- maternal infection (herpes, chlamydia, gonorrhoea, syphilis, rubella, toxoplasmosis)
- retinopathy of prematurity
- congenital defects causing glaucoma or cataracts
- meningitis
- trauma
- tumours (retinoblastoma)

Common Disorders of the Throat (Table 41.2)

Children have much larger tonsils than adults and this is thought to be a protective mechanism against respiratory tract infections. Tonsillitis is common in childhood and may be caused by a viral or bacterial infection. Putto (1987) found that viral tonsillitis, which should be treated symptomatically, was more common in children under 3 years of age. Bacterial tonsillitis usually responds to penicillin so tonsillectomy for chronic tonsillitis is controversial. Because of their protective function and the potential complications of this type of surgery, it is sometimes argued that they should not be removed unless they are hugely enlarged or causing other severe problems (National Institute for Health and Clinical Excellence, 2002c). In preschool children the tubal and lingual tonsils can enlarge to compensate for removal of the palatine tonsillar lymphatic tissue and pharyngeal and Eustachian tube obstruction continues. Alternatively, because recurrent bouts of tonsillitis may mean the child is consistently generally unwell and repeatedly missing school, surgery may sometimes provide significant improvement in health and social life. The National Institute for Health and Clinical Excellence (2002c) defines 'recurrent' as five or more episodes in the previous 12 months.

More severe obstruction of the upper airways, sometimes necessitating formation of a tracheostomy to bypass the obstruction and maintain a clear airway, may result from a number of congenital or acquired causes.

NICE guidelines for the management of recurrent sore throat in children aged up to 15 years

Almost all children can be managed by primary care. Children should be referred to a specialist service if they have:

- or are suspected of having, a quinsy
- tonsillar swelling which is causing acute upper airways obstruction
- tonsillar swelling which is interfering with swallowing, causing dehydration and marked systemic upset
- a history of sleep apnoea
- had five or more episodes of acute sore throat in the preceding 12 months documented by the parent or clinician, and these episodes have been severe enough to disrupt the child's normal behaviour or day-to-day activity
- guttate psoriasis which is exacerbated by recurrent tonsillitis
- a suspected serious underlying disorder such as leukaemia

National Institute for Health and Clinical Excellence (2002c)

Assessment

Hearing and visual impairment can severely affect the normal social, physical and psychological development of children and early detection and management of any problems can minimise these problems. Routine hearing and vision tests are carried out during developmental checks, but it is not always easy to test small children; sometimes their apparent inability to see or hear may be due to tiredness or boredom. Other testing may be necessary if developmental checks are abnormal or inconclusive.

Study activity

Find out in what circumstances and why the hearing and visual tests listed in Tables 41.3 and 41.4 are performed. Identify the role of the nurse in each test.

Table 41.3 Hearing tests (copyright is waived for the purpose of photocopying and enlarging this table)

Test	When and what for?	Role of the nurse
Developmental hearing tests		
Conduction test		
Audiometry		
Brainstem – auditory evoked response (BSAER)		

Table 41.4 Visual assessment (copyright is waived for the purpose of photocopying and enlarging this table)

Test	What for and why?	Role of the nurse
Developmental sight tests		
Snellen chart		
Peripheral vision test		
Colour vision test		

The nursing assessment of the ears, nose and throat can be gained largely by looking at and listening to the child (Figure 41.1). However, the nurse should be aware of strategies to restrain the child if more detailed medical examination of these structures is required (Figure 41.2). The child should be unable to suddenly move away as this could result in tissue damage. During otoscopic examination the ear lobe of the infant should be pulled down and back to straighten the upward

Tonsillectomy – yes or no?

Indications for surgery

- pus on the tonsils confirming bacterial infection more than three times in two consecutive years
- causative organism is found to be group A haemolytic streptococci more than three times in two consecutive years
- gross enlargement of the tonsils between infections, causing stridor or apnoea during sleep
- recurrent febrile convulsions related to repeated bouts of tonsillitis
- peritonsillar abscess (quinsy)

Contra-indications for surgery

- acute infections at the time of surgery; inflamed tissues are more likely to bleed
- bleeding disorders
- uncontrolled systemic disorders (e.g. asthma)
- cleft palate; tonsils help the escape of air during speech

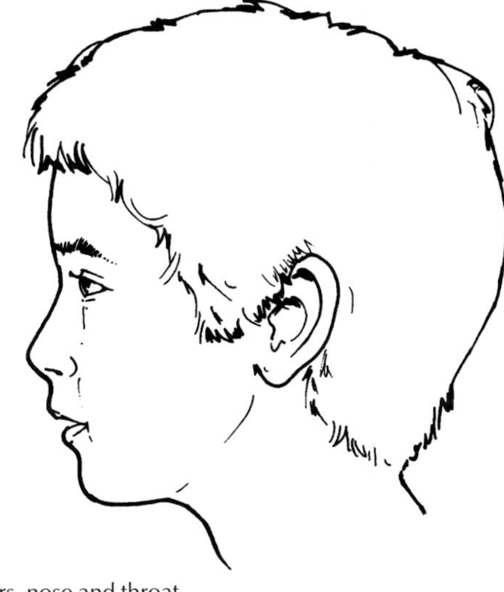

Figure 41.1 Assessment of the ears, nose and throat.

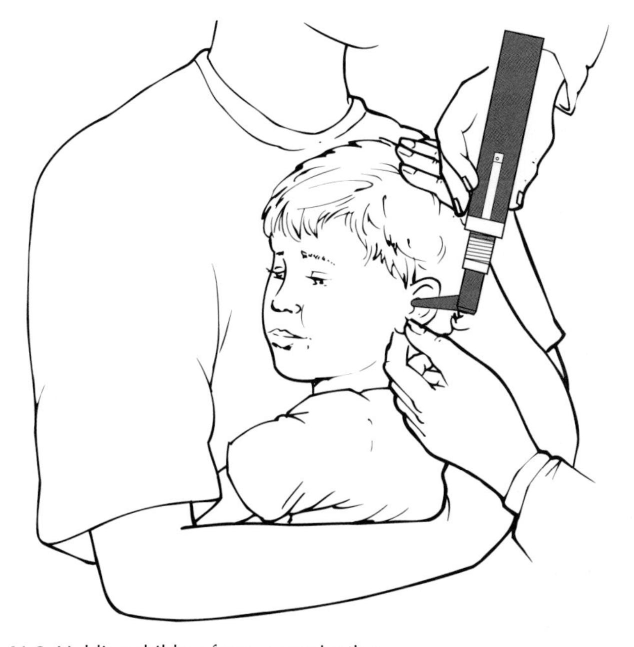

Figure 41.2 Holding children for ear examination.

Causes of stridor

Infection

- acute laryngitis
- epiglottitis
- croup
- bacterial tracheitis

Traumatic obstruction

- foreign body
- steam/smoke inhalation burns

Congenital abnormalities

- laryngocoele
- vocal cord paralysis
- subglottic stenosis
- subglottic haemangioma
- laryngeal webs, cysts
- tracheomalacia
- tracheal stenosis
- compression of the trachea by vascular anomalies

Stridor – types of sounds

- *Foreign bodies* – tend to change position with the airflow during respiration. Consequently, they create changing sounds according to their position
- *Fixed airway lesions* – produce nearly the same sound regardless of the phase of respiration
- *Superglottic airway abnormalities* – create noise in the initial phase of inspiration because the loose tissue in this area collapses inwards with inspiratory pressure. This, together with the abnormality, causes obstruction on inspiration which is relieved on expiration as the loose tissue returns to its normal position. These abnormalities also prevent normal air movement over the vocal cords and alter the sound of crying, speaking or coughing
- *Glottic and subglottic obstructions* – cause stridor on inspiration and expiration because the lumen of these areas is of fixed size

curving ear canal and visualise the tympanic membrane. In children over 3 years the canal curves downward and forward and the earlobe is pulled up and back.

As with respiratory problems, listening can provide useful information. Enlarged adenoids obstruct the passage of air from the nose to the throat and this affects the resonance of the voice, causing the child to talk nasally. Stridor is noisy breathing caused by obstruction in the pharynx, larynx or trachea. Most cases are due to acute laryngitis and are self-limiting (Valman, 1993), but stridor can also result from more severe infections, trauma and congenital defects. Valman (1993) warns that stridor is one of the most ominous sounds in childhood and recommends that, unless urgent treatment is required, all unpleasant procedures that may agitate the child and cause further hypoxia should be avoided. In non-emergency situations a detailed history of the development of the stridor should reveal the likely cause, as the type of sound is determined by the type of obstruction. Gilbert *et al.* (1993) suggest that the three most important questions are:

- Has the stridor been present since birth?
- Does the child cry, speak and cough normally?
- Is there any chance the child may have inhaled a foreign body?

Nursing Interventions

Nursing care of the visually or hearing impaired child aims to support the child and family and enables the child to achieve optimum independence. This will include teaching the child self-help skills, alternative methods of communication and helping them to come to terms with their disability. Children can become depressed by teasing about abnormalities such as squints, or the wearing of glasses and hearing aids (Swanwick, 1986).

Study activity

Find out what alternative methods of communication are available for deaf or blind children.

Susan, aged 10, who is blind, is anxious to go on the school holiday to France. How can you help her to identify colour-coordinated clothes?

Consider how you would explain pre-operative care to a deaf child.

Other nursing interventions for children with eye, ear, nose or throat problems in this section are related to specific pre-operative and post-operative care of:

- eye surgery
- ear surgery
- nasal surgery
- cleft lip and palate repair
- tonsillectomy
- tracheostomy

The most common type of eye surgery is squint repair, which may be performed if corrective lenses or patching the non-diverging eye are unsuccessful. This repair involves lengthening or shortening the appropriate muscles of the eye. This is usually performed as a day case and has no specific complications. The operated eye may be swollen and uncomfortable. Parents are advised to bathe the eye with cooled boiled water to remove any discharge or crusts. Intraocular surgery usually requires intervention to avoid:

- raised intraocular pressure, strain on the sutures and bleeding
- the child interfering with the dressing and causing injury or infection
- frightening the child whose eye(s) are bandaged
- causing discomfort or infection during dressing changes or instillation of medication

Study activity

Consider what care you would give to avoid the potential problems listed above.

As discussed previously the commonest type of ear surgery is myringotomy and insertion of grommets. This is also a day surgery procedure with no specific complications. Advice on discharge is a controversial issue. Some surgeons believe that water in the affected ear during hair washing and swimming poses an infection risk. Flood (1989) indicates that there is no evidence for this precaution and that the incidence of otorrhoea is the same for swimmers and non-swimmers. However, she warns against the entry of irritant soapy water and water entry under pressure when diving and swimming under water. Isaacson and Rosenfeld (1994) recommend that parents are shown a grommet so they can recognise it if it falls out, and know that this is normal. Grommets usually become blocked 6–9 months after insertion and are then gradually extruded from the ear. Other more complicated ear surgery is associated with the potential problems of giddiness and nausea due to interference with the inner ear.

Nasal surgery in children is usually relatively minor. Children may need reduction of a nasal fracture, removal of a foreign body or drainage of infected sinuses, which are mostly day cases. Post-operative care may involve the care and removal of a nasal pack. Nasal packs are very uncomfortable as they prevent nasal breathing, and interfere with normal speech, and eating and drinking.

Study activity

Consider how you could minimise the discomfort for a child with a nasal pack *in situ*.

Cleft lip and palate repair are performed at different times. The cleft lip is usually repaired during the first weeks of life. The palate repair is performed when the child is between 12 and 18 months old to make some allowance for the palate changes that occur during childhood, but

Tonsillectomy – advice on discharge

- Analgesia 30 minutes before meals
- Encourage rough foods to deslough wound and promote healing
- Seek GP advice if child seems feverish
- Some associated earache on swallowing is normal
- Avoid crowded places and contact with those who have coughs and colds for 10 days after discharge
- Stay away from school or nursery for 10 days post-operatively
- Call 999 for an ambulance if fresh bleeding from the throat occurs

also to correct the deformity before the development of speech is too impaired. Cleft palate often requires long-term treatment. Depending on the extent of the deformity, extensive orthodontic treatment may be needed for some time after the initial repairs and most children require some speech therapy. The only further treatment for cleft lip repair may be revision of the scar, although specialist centres usually have successful results (Martin, 1995). The immediate problems before the surgical repair are the support of the parents and the development of a feeding regime. Cleft lip and palate both impair the ability to suck, and feed taken into the mouth may escape through the cleft palate into the nose. Martin (1995) recommends assessment of the individual child to determine the most appropriate feeding technique. Breastfeeding is possible with the baby in an upright position, and a variety of teats and feeding devices are available to assist bottlefeeding. These methods help the baby to develop the sucking muscles as well as meeting sucking needs but cup feeding or naso-gastric tube feeding may be necessary if these do not ensure good weight gain.

Study activity

Identify the nursing actions to overcome the potential problems before and after cleft lip and palate repair (Table 41.5).

Tonsillectomy is beginning to be performed as a day case but is associated with asphyxia and haemorrhage because of the vascularity and position of the tonsils.

Table 41.5 Cleft lip and palate repair: specific pre- and post-operative care (copyright is waived for the purpose of photocopying and enlarging this table)

Problem	Aim	Nursing actions
Pre-operative care Risk of inadequate nutritional intake, choking and excessive wind	Feed/fluid chart shows adequate intake (ml/kg); no choking or excessive wind	
Risk of loss of parent–child attachment due to deformity	Parents demonstrate acceptance of child	
Post-operative care Risk of aspiration	Secretions and feed not aspirated	
Risk of trauma to site of repair	Site of repair remains undamaged	
Risk of inadequate nutrition due to feeding difficulties	Fluid/feed chart shows sufficient intake (ml/kg)	

Study activity

Identify the time of occurrence, causes and features of asphyxia, primary, reactionary and secondary haemorrhage.

Tracheostomy is often performed as a temporary measure to bypass an acute upper airway obstruction or provide access for long-term ventilation. Occasionally it is a more permanent treatment for a congenital obstruction of the airway. The use of tracheostomy to relieve respiratory distress is believed to have been first performed in 124 BC by a Greek physician. In the 21st century tracheostomies are becoming more commonplace in hospital and in the community (Serra, 2000). The child with a tracheostomy requires highly skilled care to maintain the airway and promote a normal lifestyle. Children with a tracheostomy require frequent suctioning during the initial post-operative period to maintain their airway. After this time they may still need periodic clearance of secretions. Suctioning is a potentially hazardous procedure with well-documented risks. Some associated procedures, such as the installation of saline prior to suctioning, are debatable practices (Table 41.6). Although saline may loosen secretions and facilitate their removal (Ridling *et al.*, 2003), we do not recommend its regular use and suggest that good hydration and humidification is a better way of ensuring loose secretions. The normal mechanisms of warming and humidifying air as it is breathed are bypassed by a tracheostomy. Dry gases can damage ciliary function so dry humidification, with the use of a device such as the 'Swedish nose', or wet humidification using a water bath is necessary for all children with a tracheostomy (Jevon and Ewens, 2001). Humidification also helps to minimise thick, tenacious secretions which may block the tracheostomy tube.

Table 41.6 Tracheal suctioning – potential risks

Risk	Prevention
Damage to the tracheo-bronchial mucosa (Sumner, 1990)	Perform suction when required – not at predetermined intervals Insert and withdraw the suction catheter gently Occlude suction pressure during catheter insertion
Hypoxia (Kerem *et al.*, 1990)	The external size of the catheter should not exceed half the internal diameter of the tracheostomy tube (Imle and Klemic, 1991) Duration of suctioning is ideally 15 seconds (Sumner, 1990) Limit suction pressure to 70–100 mmHg (Kusenski, 1978) Hyperoxygenate and hypoventilate with 100% O_2 before, during and after suction (Kerem *et al.*, 1990)
Cardiac arrhythmias	Only suction when necessary Do not suction for more than 30 seconds
Bacterial infection	Use clean or sterile procedure Change suction tubing and bottles at least daily Rinse suction tubing with sterile water between suctions

Indications for tracheostomy

Allergy

- angioneurotic oedema
- anaphylaxis

Prophylactic

- prolonged endotracheal intubation
- head and neck surgery

Degenerative

- vocal cord paralysis

Congenital

- choanal atresia
- microglossia
- Pierre Robin syndrome
- laryngomalacia
- laryngeal webs, cysts, stenosis

Trauma

- facial or oral injury/fractures
- facial burns/burn inhalation
- foreign body inhalation
- pharyngeal oedema

Toxic

- ingestion of corrosives

Infection

- epiglottitis
- croup
- diphtheria
- tetanus
- rabies
- retro-pharyngeal abscess

Neoplastic

- papillomatosis
- haemangioma
- lymphangioma

Study activity

Find out the following:

- What is needed at the bedside of a child with a tracheostomy?
- What are the procedures for changing tracheostomy tapes and tube?
- What nursing care is required to overcome the problems listed in Table 41.7?

If the tracheostomy is a temporary measure there is a gradual return to normal airway breathing. A smaller tube is inserted and if this does not cause respiratory problems the tube is occluded for 24 hours under close observation. If no problems occur, the tube is removed and the stoma occluded.

Table 41.7 Care of the child with a tracheostomy (copyright is waived for the purpose of photocopying and enlarging this table)

Problem	Aim	Nursing actions
Tracheostomy may become blocked or dislodged	Clear airway maintained	
Irritation of tube in stoma and nursing interventions may cause infection	Site remains free from infection	
Loss of function of upper respiratory tract	Air is filtered, warmed and moistened	
Air flow diverted from vocal cords	Child develops effective method of communication	
Bibs, dribbling may occlude airway	Child able to eat and drink without endangering airway	
Fluff from toys or small toys may be inhaled and obstruct airway	Child has no potentially dangerous toys	
Water and talcum, fluff from clothing may occlude airway	Washing and dressing avoids inhalants	
Small children reluctant to lie prone to learn to crawl	Child develops normal mobility	
Inability to call/cry for help at night	Strategies in place to monitor child at night	

Education for Discharge

Discharge advice following insertion of grommets and tonsillectomy have already been explored. Your answers to the previous activity should give you an idea of the tremendous responsibility the parents of a child with a tracheostomy at home have.

Study activity

Consider all the teaching needs of the parents taking home a child with a tracheostomy. Decide how you could sequence and organise this teaching to ensure they had the optimum preparation before discharge.

Chapter 42

Principles of Care – Children with Altered Gastro-intestinal Function

Processes related to gastro-intestinal function (eating, drinking and elimination) fill all aspects of our daily lives and are important physically, socially and psychologically. Indeed, much of the talk of young mothers centres around infant feeding and nappies. When a child has problems with elimination, the issues can cause psychological upset and can lead to a preoccupation with toileting. Problems of the gastro-intestinal tract are common in childhood. The nurse needs to understand the implications of such problems in order to help the children and their families cope with treatment and care.

Study activity

Before reading any further you should refresh your memory on anatomy and physiology of the gastro-intestinal tract. You should look at structure, the functions of digestion, absorption and elimination, and acid–base balance.

Some of the problems that children face (and related pathophysiology) are given in Tables 42.1 to 42.4.

Assessment

When assessing gastro-intestinal function the nurse needs to take into account more than just the physical signs. She must look at the whole child and his or her family and lifestyle. Familial problems may be identified or there may be psychological problems that might affect management and care of the child. As part of the assessment process (on admission and subsequently) the nurse should use her skills to ascertain information about a wide variety of aspects (Figure 42.2) (*see also* Cystic fibrosis pp. 513 and 532).

Table 42.1 Problems of motility

Gastro-oesophageal reflux	Incompetent/malfunctioning lower oesophageal sphincter; on inspiration stomach contents move into oesophagus which in turn leads to vomiting; oesophagitis; scarring; stricture. Can also result in aspiration pneumonia
Hirschsprung's disease	Absence of parasympathetic ganglion cells in intestinal muscle wall (usually sigmoid colon and rectum); no peristalsis as bowel is spastic and contracted; no faecal material can pass through; proximal bowel becomes distended and filled with faecal material and gas; internal sphincter fails to relax; no elimination; abdominal distension and constipation
Chronic constipation with soiling	Constipation caused by a variety of factors becomes so severe that the bowel becomes distended and eventually insensitive and unable to prevent soft faeces passing round the hard impacted masses and oozing out

Table 42.2 Problems of absorption

Coeliac disease	Changes in mucosal lining of small intestine caused by gluten; irregularity of epithelial cells; a reduction in normal villi which become flattened; disaccharide deficiency and depression of peptidase activity; malabsorption of fats, fat-soluble vitamins, minerals, some protein and carbohydrates
Short bowel syndrome	Diminished ability of the intestine to function normally following resection for bowel anomalies, inflammatory problems. Loss of more than 75% results in malabsorption (Campbell and Glasper, 1995)
Cystic fibrosis	Defective CFTR gene; disruption of normal electrolyte and water secretion by cells; increased loss of sodium and chloride in sweat; reduced hydration of secretions from exocrine glands (Cree, 1997); viscid secretions from pancreas and gastro-intestinal tract (and respiratory system); malabsorption

Table 42.3 Obstructive problems

Pyloric stenosis	Pyloric muscle is increased in length and diameter; there is marked increase in thickness in the circular muscle and attenuation of the longitudinal muscle (Cree, 1997); pyloric lumen is narrowed; stomach emptying is delayed causing distension; vomiting (often projectile) after feeds; dehydration and weight loss
Intussusception	'Invagination of a length of bowel into the succeeding bowel segment' (Cree, 1997:261); mesentery pulled into intestine as invagination occurs; intestine becomes curved; blood supply cut off; bowel begins to swell; complete obstruction may occur; necrosis

Table 42.4 Inflammatory problems

Appendicitis	Acute inflammation of the mucosa; inflammatory changes throughout wall of appendix; oedema compromises blood flow; ischaemia and ulceration of epithelial lining; necrosis and perforation; peritonitis
Meckel's diverticulum	Failure of obliteration of the omphalomesenteric duct; out-pouching of bowel wall close to ileo-caecal valve; lined by small intestine mucosa; presence of acid-secreting gastric mucosa can lead to ulceration; inflammation
Gastro-enteritis	Loss of water and electrolytes leads to dehydration, electrolyte imbalance and metabolic acidosis
Crohn's disease and ulcerative colitis	See Figure 42.1

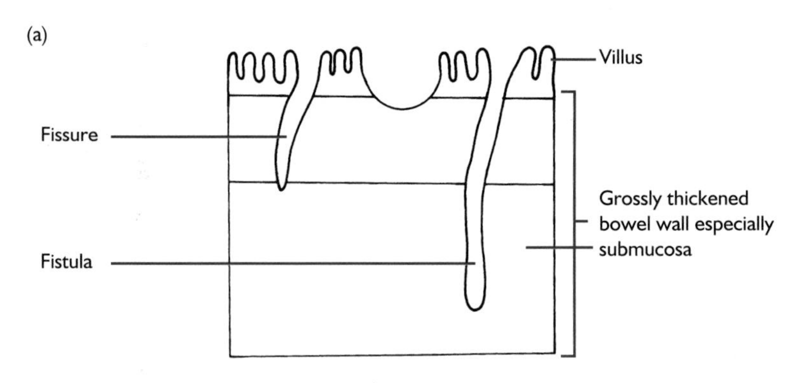

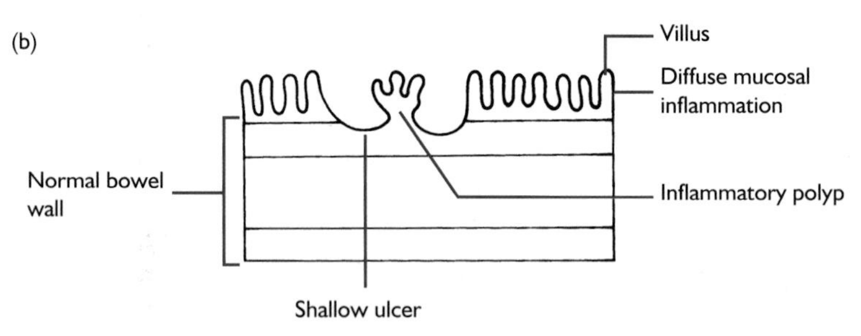

Figure 42.1 Cross section of small intestine to show comparison of pathology: (a) Crohn's disease and (b) ulcerative colitis (adapted from Cree, 1997).

Study activity

One of the most dangerous consequences of gastro-intestinal problems can be dehydration. Giving rationale, describe the possible effects of severe dehydration on a small child. Use information given in this book and other references to help you.

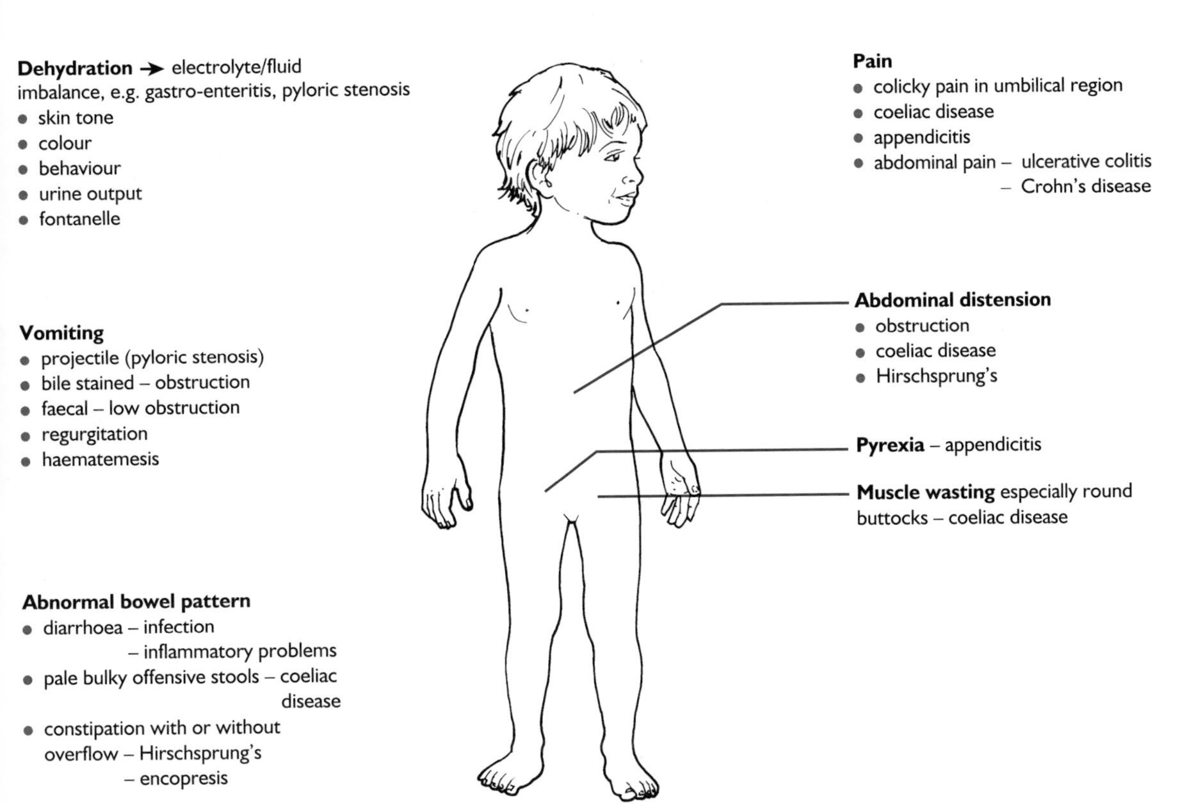

Figure 42.2 Specific assessment of the child with gastro-intestinal problems.

These observations, together with the results of medical investigations, will enable accurate decisions to be made about treatment and care. Table 42.5 shows the various investigations that may be done to diagnose problems of the gastro-intestinal tract.

> **Study activity**
>
> Find out in what circumstances each one might be used, what it might show and what the role of the nurse would be. Make notes in the boxes for future reference.

Interventions

This section concentrates on discussing care related to four of the specific interventions that may be implemented for children with gastro-intestinal problems. These are:

- specific pre- and post-operative care (Table 42.6)
- bowel retraining
- colostomy care
- drug therapy

> **Further reading**
>
> Rogers, J. (2004) Paediatric bowel problems. *Gastrointestinal Nursing*, **2** (4), 31–39.
>
> Royal College of Nursing (2005) *Perioperative Fasting in Adults and Children.* http://www.rcn.org.uk/publications/pdf/guidelines/perioperative_fasting_adults_children_full.pdf (accessed 31 May 2006).

Table 42.5 Medical investigations (copyright is waived for the purpose of photocopying and enlarging this table)

Test	When and what for?	Role of the nurse
Blood Hb haematocrit sodium potassium pH CO_2 WCC		
Biopsies jejunal rectal		
Manometry oesophageal rectal		
pH studies oesophageal stool		
X-rays plain barium		
Endoscopy		
Rectal examination		
Xylose absorption test		
Faecal fat excretion		

Module 6

- **Senokot** – a stimulant laxative – encourages bowel movement by acting on nerve endings in the wall of the intestine that trigger contraction of intestinal muscles. This speeds up the passage of faecal matter through the intestine therefore allowing less time for water to be absorbed. The faeces become more liquid and more frequent. Used as a short-term treatment. See the Senekot Web site for useful advice. http://www.constipationadvice.co.uk/index.html (accessed 30 May 2006)
- **Lactulose** – increases the amount of water in the large intestine and softens the stools. Used for long-term management

Study activity

Find out in what circumstances each of the above interventions may be implemented. Make notes in column 3 of Table 42.6.

Bowel retraining

The first step in managing encopresis, when there is found to be a severe degree of faecal retention, is to empty the bowel. This may be done by the short-term administration of a laxative such as Senokot. This is often accompanied by longer term administration of lactulose. This treatment can usually be given at home reducing the necessity for hospital admission. Where this conservative treatment does not work alternative therapies may be tried, including suppositories and/or enemas. These will often necessitate hospital admission. It is extremely important, if this is the case, to establish trusting relationships with

Table 42.6 Specific pre- and post-operative care (copyright is waived for the purpose of photocopying and enlarging this table)

Intervention	Rationale	Notes
Pre-operative care: V therapy	To restore fluid, electrolyte and acid–base balance; in conditions where there is metabolic alkalosis, superimposition of this on the respiratory alkalosis which follows mechanical ventilation can cause major problems in re-establishing spontaneous respirations (MacMahon, 1991)	
Naso-gastric tube – aspirated with possible gastric washout	To empty stomach contents to prevent vomiting and possible aspiration	
Bowel clearance using either rectal washouts with saline or via naso-gastric tube using a bowel cleansing preparation (e.g. Kleanprep)	To clear the bowel	
Low residue diet progressing to fluids only	To keep stools soft and complement bowel clearance	
Preparation for formation of colostomy	To identify most appropriate site; to prepare child/family psychologically	
Post-operative care: Naso-gastric tube on free drainage – aspirated as directed	To prevent abdominal distension	
Nil by mouth until bowel sounds return	To ensure that peristalsis has returned before reintroducing feeding	
Gradual reintroduction of oral feeding	Rate at which this is done will depend on operative procedure	
Care of colostomy observe drainage observe colour	 to ensure adequate bowel function to detect reduction in blood supply	

the child before administering the treatment. When there is no faecal retention management can move directly onto step two, which is a period of retraining using behaviour modification principles. Behaviour therapy is based on the principles of learning theory and on the belief that problem behaviours can be eliminated by the introduction of new learning experiences (Barker, 1995). However it has been recognised that behavioural and cognitive therapy alone may not have any benefit over conventional therapies as highlighted above.

It is important that a detailed assessment is carried out prior to developing an individual therapy plan for each child. In each case realistic goals need to be drawn up in discussion with the child and family. The context in which the family is operating must be taken into consideration and recognised as important in planning any treatment (Teris, 2001; McDonald *et al.*, 2004). (*See also* Family therapy p. 555 and Behaviour modification p. 556.)

Examples of positive reinforcers (rewards)

- *Tangible* – stars (on a star chart), points, money, food, sweets, treats such as trips out, small toys, privileges such as watching television
- *Intangible* – praise, attention, hugs, time with parent, smiles, words of thanks

Reinforcement must be immediate for young children. Delaying tactics will not act as a reinforcer

Patient information

Have a look at this site from Guy's and St Thomas's Constipation Clinic, which contains useful help for children:

http://www.bowelcontrol.org.uk/pdf/getgoing.pdf (accessed 31 May 2006).

According to Herbert (1987) there are two basic learning tasks:

- the acquisition of a desired behaviour in which the child is deficient – in this case bowel control
- the extinction of an undesired response – in this case soiling

These can be achieved using reinforcement, either positive or negative. Positive reinforcement is anything that will increase the likelihood of a previous behaviour being repeated. Therefore any desired behaviours (which should be agreed in the planning stage), for example clean pants, should be positively reinforced. Negative reinforcement is an alternative and occurs when attention-seeking behaviour is not reinforced. In this case, for example, soiled pants would be ignored. Dealing with the problem of bowel retraining requires patience and perseverance on behalf of the child and family. Family therapy may be required to help families cope with stresses and tensions, which may be an underlying factor (McDonald *et al.*, 2004). The nurse's role is to support and encourage adherence to the programme and to be aware of the distress this problem can cause.

Colostomy/ileostomy care

A colostomy/ileostomy may be temporary or permanent. In either case the child and family will need considerable support and education to manage at home. Time will be needed to adjust to the colostomy and to learn the principles of colostomy care. A study by Johnson in 1996 found that the support and advice given to children and families was often inadequate. Some of the concerns raised by parents/carers are highlighted. The principles of managing a colostomy are as follows:

- Hygiene and skin care – bathing can take place as normal, either with the appliance on or off. The skin around the stoma should be examined for signs of inflammation or excoriation whenever the appliance is changed. The skin around an ileostomy is particularly liable to become sore. Distal loop washouts may be required if the child has a colostomy. The purpose of these is to evacuate faeces and mucus from the distal bowel in order to minimise infection. They also assist in preparing the bowel for possible later surgery.
- Using appliances. The stoma therapist should be involved in choosing the most appropriate appliance and giving advice on changing the bags. Bags should be removed carefully and slowly. The skin around the stoma is washed and dried carefully and a barrier cream/gum applied. The bag should fit snugly round the stoma to prevent leakage.
- Observation of the stoma and its function. The stoma should be bright red. Signs of complications include a change in colour, ribbon-like stool, diarrhoea, bleeding, failure of evacuation of stool, prolapse, retraction and stenosis.
- Diet. There are no real restrictions to normal diet unless medically indicated. However, a low-residue diet may be advocated to decrease the stool bulk. As the risk of fluid loss is increased due to reduced colon absorption (particularly in hot weather) parents should be advised to ensure an adequate fluid intake. It is wise to avoid carbonated drinks as this increases flatus.

- Psychological aspects of care. The nurse must be aware of the effects of a change in body image and give support accordingly. Privacy and dignity must be maintained when dealing with the colostomy. Time must be set aside to discuss problems and concerns. Children and parents can be encouraged to contact support agencies as talking to families with similar difficulties can act as a powerful coping strategy.

Support agencies

British Colostomy Association
15 Station Road, Reading, Berkshire RG1 1LG
Tel: 0800 328 4257
Web site: http://www.colostomyassociation.org.uk (accessed 31 May 2006)

Digestive Disorders
PO Box 251, Edgware, Middlesex HA8 6HG
Tel: 020 7486 0341
Web site: http://www.digestivedisorders.org.uk (accessed 31 May 2006)

National Advisory Service for Parents of Children with a Stoma (NASPCS)
51 Anderson Drive, Valley View Park, Darvel, East Ayrshire, KA17 0DE
Email: john@stoma.freeserve.co.uk

National Advisory Service for Parents of Children with a Stoma
32 Sules Drive, Norwich, Norfolk NR8 6UU
Web site: http://www.patient.co.uk/leaflets/national_advisory_service_to_parents_of_children_with_a_stoma.htm (accessed 25 May 2007)

Rehydration therapy

This type of therapy is normally implemented for infants and young children who present with dehydration as a result of diarrhoea (with or without vomiting):

- Mild dehydration (5% or less) – give clear fluids for at least 24–48 hours. A range of formulas are available, which are based on the principle that oral rehydration works best when glucose or sucrose is added to an electrolyte solution. It is important that the solution is made up according to instructions on the packet. Young children often find the solution unpalatable and Moulai and Huband (1996) advocate the use of very weak fruit juice in this instance. Experience has shown that 'flat' fizzy drinks also work well. Milk should be avoided as it tends to prolong the diarrhoea and vomiting. After the initial period of 24 hours, intake can gradually be reintroduced according to local policy.
- Moderate to severe dehydration (more than 5%) – intravenous therapy with or without fasting. The type of fluid infused will depend on electrolyte results. The child's condition is monitored daily and, when appropriate, a regrading programme is introduced. (*See also* Calculation of IV fluid rates p. 345.)

Study activity

Find out the policy for rehydration therapy in your local children's ward or department. Make notes in the margin for future reference.

Concerns of parents regarding colostomies

- Will hurt him when I change the bag?
- Can he have a bath?
- How often do I change the bag?
- How will I manage if I want to go out?
- Can he go swimming?
- What will people say?
- Will it smell?
- Will people be able to tell that he has a colostomy?

Further reading

Black, P. (2000) Practical stoma care. *Nursing Standard*, **14** (41), 47–53.

McErlain, D., *et al.* (2004) Clinical protocols for stoma care: prolapsed stoma. *Nursing Standard*, **18** (18), 41–42.

Trainor, B., *et al.* (2003) Clinical protocols for stoma care: changing an appliance. *Nursing Standard*, **18** (13), 41–42.

Rehydration formulas

- Dioralyte
- Dextrolyte
- Pedilyte
- Rehydrat

Research suggestion

Explore the use of 'flat' fizzy drinks in the treatment of dehydration for young children with diarrhoea and vomiting

Further reading/advice – including WHO guidelines

Hand, H. (2001) The use of intravenous therapy. *Nursing Standard*, **15** (43), 47–52.

McVerry, M. (1999) Managing the child with gastroenteritis. *Nursing Standard*, **13** (37), 49–53.

Willock, J. and Jewkes, F. (2000) Making sense of fluid balance in children. *Paediatric Nursing*, **12** (7), 37–42.

Education for Discharge

Many children with problems of the gastro-intestinal tract can be managed at home. Others will need admission to hospital for surgical treatment, which may be followed up by many months of additional treatment. The community children's nurse plays a vital role in helping to plan for discharge, ensuring that support and advice is available in the community.

Children may go home with:

- total parenteral nutrition
- gastrostomy, jejunal, naso-gastric feeding systems
- stoma
- dietary restrictions
- drug therapy
- surgical wounds

In each case the nurse must ensure that an individual teaching plan is drawn up as soon after admission as possible to teach aspects of home care to the child and/or family.

Study activity

For each of the above, find out what specific care would be needed by a child on discharge. Make notes in the margin.

Study activity

A 10-year-old girl has been diagnosed as having colitis. Draw up a teaching plan to ensure that she can manage her diet and drug therapy correctly following discharge.

Chapter 43

Principles of Care – Children with Genito-urinary Problems

Introduction

Problems of the genito-urinary system are relatively common in childhood. One reason for this could be that the system has a high percentage of congenital and genetic abnormalities compared with other organ systems (Taylor, 1996). Some problems can improve with surgery or conservative treatment, others develop chronic disease and progress towards renal failure. Chronic disease invades all aspects of the child's life, with dietary and activity restrictions and altered elimination and growth patterns. To appreciate the impact that renal disease can have on a child and family, the nurse needs a clear understanding of the development and function of the genito-urinary system.

Study activity

Draw a labelled diagram of a nephron. Critically examine the functions of each part.

Problems of the genito-urinary system can be divided into:

- inherited and congenital anomalies (Table 43.1)
- acquired disorders (Table 43.2)

When the function of the kidney is compromised as a result of renal disease, renal failure may occur.

Causes of acute renal failure

Pre-renal – reduction of renal perfusion in a normal kidney:

- dehydration secondary to diarrhoea/vomiting
- surgical shock
- trauma

Renal – diseases which damage the glomeruli, tubules or renal vasculature

- glomerular disease
- ischaemia
- nephrotoxins

Post-renal

- obstructive lesions

Causes of chronic renal failure – end stage renal disease which occurs following progressive deterioration over months or years as a result of

- chronic glomerulitis
- recurrent pyelonephritis
- renal hypoplasia
- Alport's syndrome

Table 43.1 Inherited and congenital anomalies

Problem	Pathophysiology
Renal agenesis – unilateral or bilateral	In unilateral agenesis the remaining kidney becomes hypertrophied. Bilateral agenesis or Potter's syndrome, usually stillborn. May be associated with pulmonary hypoplasia
Renal hypoplasia – unilateral or bilateral	Kidneys are normally formed but small. Bilateral hypoplasia results in renal failure
Polycystic disease	Autosomal recessive disorder with gradual severity. The kidneys are grossly enlarged and renal function is impaired. There are cystic changes in the liver and other organs
Obstructive malformations ureteropelvic junction obstruction ureteric duplication posterior urethral valves	Obstruction to the flow of urine from the kidney or bladder results in backflow of urine into the kidney leading to hydronephrosis and impaired kidney function
Primary vesicoureteric reflux (VUR)	An inherited disorder where there is failure of the mechanisms which prevent reflux of urine; prevention of reflux is mainly due to the following process – when the pressure in the bladder is increased during micturition, the detrusor muscle contracts and the submucosal ureter is passively compressed increasing the resistance to reflux. Failure of this process is usually due to an inadequate length of the submucosal ureter. VUR predisposes to infection
Bladder extrophy	Failure of development of the anterior bladder wall and the overlying abdominal wall. The ureters open onto the exposed anterior wall mucosa which is prone to infection and metaplastic change. In boys the penis is up-turned, the pubic bone unfused and the lower limbs apparently rotated. In girls the genital tract is normal but with possible vaginal stenosis
Wilm's tumour – nephroblastoma	Originates from embryonal kidney – peak incidence age 3 years, more common in boys than girls, more often affecting the left kidney
Undescended testes	
incomplete descent	Testes follow normal descent route but fail to reach scrotum. May be impalpable. Testes often grossly abnormal with poor spermatogenesis
ectopic or maldescended	Testes follow abnormal route. Easily palpable and normal in appearance, normal spermatogenesis
Hypospadias	The urethra opens on the ventral aspect of the penis instead of at the end. Site of opening may be anywhere along the length of the penis. May be accompanied by ventral curvature or chordee of the penis distal to the abnormal urethra. Failure of fusion of the ventral part of the foreskin results in a redundant dorsal hood
Inguinal hernia and hydrocele	Caused by persistency of the processus vaginalis, the pouch of peritoneum which accompanies the descent of the testes

Manifestations of acute renal failure

- Oliguria (volume less than 0.5–1.0 ml/kg/hour)
- Scant bloody urine
- Lethargy
- Nausea and vomiting
- Diarrhoea
- Dry skin and mucous membranes
- Drowsiness, headache, muscle twitching, convulsions

Study activity

Consider the physiological explanations for the following manifestations of chronic renal failure:

- sustained metabolic acidosis
- significant bone demineralisation and impaired growth
- anaemia
- intractable itching
- loss of energy and increased fatigue on exertion

Then do the same for the manifestations of acute renal failure.

Table 43.2 Acquired disorders

Problem	Pathophysiology
Urinary infections	Caused by a variety of organisms – *Escherichia coli* most prevalent. May involve the urethra, bladder, ureters, renal pelvis, calyces or parenchyma. Ascension of organisms from perineal area is the most common scenario. Inflammation of the urethra can occur within 30 minutes of bacterial invasion (Wong, cited by Miller, 1996). Organisms then ascend into the bladder causing cystitis. A transient vesicoureteral reflux allows urine to ascend up to the kidneys causing pyelonephritis. Inflammatory changes can result in incompetence of the vesicoureteral valve leading to continuing reflux and renal scarring. Recurrent renal infections may lead to chronic renal failure
Acute post-streptococcal glomerulonephritis	Primarily affects early school-age children (6–7 years); more common in boys than girls. An immune complex disease with an onset 10–14 days after a beta-haemolytic streptococcal throat infection
Minimal change nephrotic syndrome (MCNS)	Idiopathic disease occurring mainly in preschool children. Cause is uncertain but the glomerular membrane becomes abnormally permeable allowing proteins (especially albumin) to pass through into the urine. This leads to a reduced serum albumin level which in turn decreases colloidal osmotic pressure in the capilliaries; fluid leaks out from the circulation into interstitial compartments (tissues and body cavities) leading to oedema; shift of fluid reduces vascular fluid volume (hypovolaemia)
Renal tubular acidosis	
proximal (type II)	Defect in bicarbonate absorption; hyperchloraemic metabolic acidosis; growth failure, tachypnoea; possible severe acidosis
distal (type I)	Inability of the kidney to establish a normal pH gradient between tubular cells and tubular contents. Inability to secrete hydrogen ions causes accumulation producing a sustained acidosis; retards growth, demineralisation of bone occurs, increased levels of calcium and phosphorus predispose to formation of stones
Renal disease associated with systemic disease	Diabetes mellitus, systemic lupus erythematosus, Henoch–Schönlein purpura, amyloidosis
Enuresis	Common problem in childhood – involuntary voiding of the bladder when there is no organic cause. It may occur by day (diuresis) or by night (nocturnal enuresis)
Phimosis	Stenosis of the preputial orifice mostly caused by recurrent balanitis or traumatic retraction of the foreskin. Leads to ballooning and a poor stream during micturition and further attacks of balanitis

Assessment

Skilled assessment of the child with potential renal problems is vital for prompt diagnosis. Problems may be difficult to identify as presenting symptoms are sometimes rather obscure, for example in the case of urinary tract infections. Many of the clinical manifestations of renal disease are common to a variety of other childhood disorders and therefore careful follow-up may be necessary. Figure 43.1 gives an indication of the specific aspects that should be addressed when assessing the child. Table 43.3 gives an indication of the signs of urinary tract infections in different age groups.

Further reading

Tomsett, A. and Watson, A. (1996) Renal biopsy as a day case procedure. *Paediatric Nursing*, **8** (5), 14–15.

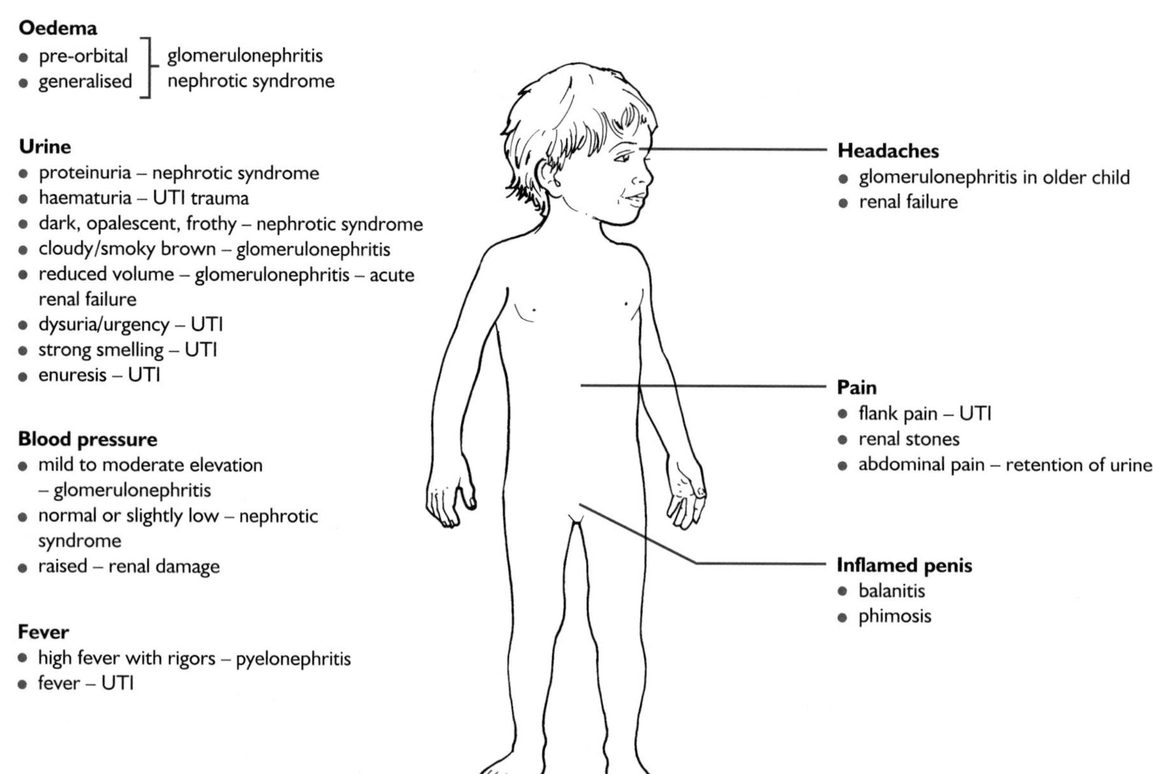

Figure 43.1 Specific nursing assessment of the child with renal problems.

In assessing the child you will be required to carry out a routine urinalysis. It is important that you are familiar with the various ways of collecting urine for this purpose and of the implications of your findings. The methods for collection include:

- Clean catch – this method is suitable for babies and young children who have not yet gained bladder control. The vulval area or penis should be cleaned with saline and the child left without a nappy. When the child micturates, the urine is caught in a sterile pot. Some suggest that this is an efficient method (MacFarlane *et al.*, 1999; Ramage *et al.*, 1999) but others report it being time consuming and technically difficult (Lewis, 1998; Feasey, 1999).
- Supra-pubic aspiration (SPA) – this is a reliable method of collecting an uncontaminated specimen from a child who is not toilet trained. However, it can be traumatic and needs to be carried out when the bladder is full. A needle is inserted through the skin into the bladder and urine aspirated through a syringe. The first few cubic centimetres should be discarded.
- Midstream urine (MSU) – a useful means of collecting urine from a cooperative child who has bladder control. The vulval area or penis should be cleaned as before and the child instructed to either retract the foreskin or hold the labia apart during micturition. Allow the

Table 43.3 Age-related signs of UTI

Neonates	Infants	Preschooler	School age	Adolescent
Unstable temperature				
Jaundice				
Apnoeic episodes				
Pallor	Pallor			
Sepsis	Sepsis			
Abdominal distension	Abdominal tenderness			
Nappy rash	Nappy rash			
Poor feeding	Failure to thrive	Anorexia		
Irritability	Irritability			
Lethargy	Lethargy			
Vomiting	Vomiting	Vomiting	Vomiting	Vomiting
Hypothermia	Fever	Fever	Fever	Fever
Diarrhoea	Diarrhoea	Diarrhoea	Diarrhoea	
		Strong urine	Strong urine	Strong urine
		Haematuria	Haematuria	Haematuria
		Frequency	Frequency	Frequency
		Urgency	Urgency	Urgency
		Dysuria	Dysuria	Dysuria
			Enuresis	
			Mood swings	
				Chills

child to pass some urine before collecting your sample. A young child will need assistance.

- Bag urine – the least reliable method of collecting an uncontaminated specimen especially in females (Miller, 1996) and fraught with complications (Al-Orifi *et al.*, 2000). Criticisms of this method include difficulty in application, leakage prompting reapplication, discomfort, high contamination rates, and cost.
- Urine collection pad – launched in 1994 (Vernon *et al.*, 1994). There is debate about this method. It is easy to use and relatively cheap. However, caution has been advised with regard to the filtering effect of the pad fibres and the high contamination rates of up to 68% (Farrell, 2002).
- Catheter specimen – used when a catheter is already *in situ* or if a child uses intermittent catheterisation for incontinence. This can also be used to collect urine from a stoma.

Observations of urine – the implications

- Smell – strong ammoniacal smell – urinary infection
- Appearance
  - red urine – frank blood usually due to renal trauma; dyes present in food, e.g. beetroot, and some drugs, e.g. rifampicin
  - pale urine – dilute
  - dark yellow – concentrated
  - deep orange – obstructive jaundice
- Urinalysis – in many cases there is no cause of urinary tract infection
  - proteinuria – small amount is normal; if present in large amounts may indicate renal disease, e.g. infection or glomerulonephritis
  - glucose – possible implications include diabetes mellitus, renal tubular disease (e.g. Fanconi's syndrome); can also occur as a result of total parenteral nutrition and steroid therapy
  - ketones – found in children who are fasting or on a weight-reducing diet, children who are pyrexial or those who have a metabolic disorder (e.g. diabetes mellitus)
  - pH – normal urine should have a pH greater than 5.5; a low pH means that the urine is very dilute. The pH is constant in renal failure

Further reading

Jadresic, L. (1993) Investigation of urinary tract infection in childhood. *British Medical Journal,* **307**, 761–764.

Taylor, C. M. and Chapman, S. (1989) *Handbook of Renal Investigations in Children.* Sevenoaks: Wright.

Interventions for children with genito-urinary problems

- Blood pressure monitoring
- Daily weight
- Catheterisation and catheter care
- Pre- and post-operative care
- Care of an ileal conduit
- Fluid restriction
- Administration of a salt-free diet
- Dialysis – peritoneal/haemo-dialysis
- Bladder training
- Management of oedema
- Administration of drugs

Study activity

You are asked to assist in an SPA on a 12-year-old girl who has severe spina bifida. The urine is wanted for a routine urinalysis – there is no specific reason to suggest the young girl has any renal disease. Consider your role as advocate in this instance.

Laboratory studies will help to identify renal problems, which can be further evaluated using radiological studies and renal biopsy (Thomsett and Watson, 1996). Table 43.4 shows the various investigations that may be done.

Study activity

Find out in what circumstances each of the investigations in Table 43.4 might be used, what it might show and what the role of the nurse would be. Make notes in the boxes for future reference.

In caring for children with genito-urinary problems you may be involved with implementing a variety of interventions. The following interventions will be discussed in more detail here:

- catheter care
- the administration of specific drugs
- the management of oedema
- peritoneal dialysis

Catheter Care

Urinary catheters are usually passed via the urethra into the bladder to allow drainage of urine. Some children will require an indwelling catheter, which is inserted on a short-term or long-term basis. An aseptic technique must be used when inserting the catheter and the following points noted:

- cleanse the area around the urethral meatus using an antiseptic solution
- avoid contamination of the surface of the catheter
- ensure the catheter is well lubricated (use packet of sterile lubricant)
- ensure that the catheter is the correct size (Smith, 2003) – use the smallest size capable of providing adequate drainage

Children who have indwelling catheters are prone to urinary tract infection and particular care should avoid this by:

- Keeping the area around the urethral meatus clean – normal bathing/showering should be sufficient. Too much cleansing around the meatus in boys can cause irritation and infection (De Sousa, 1996).
- Ensure that there is patency of the catheter with no kinking of tubes. If the child is ambulatory, ensure that the catheter and bag are strapped to the leg securely.

Table 43.4 Medical investigations (copyright is waived for the purpose of photocopying and enlarging this table)

Investigation	When and what for?	Role of the nurse
Glomerular filtration rate and creatinine clearance		
Laboratory urinalysis		
Urine culture		
Blood urea, creatinine, sodium, potassium, phosphate, haemoglobin, serum albumin		
ASO titre		
Radiologic studies: – micturating cysto-urethrogram – IV pyelogram – ultrasound – dimercaptosuccinic acid scan		
Renal arteriogram		
Radionuclide imaging		
Urodynamics		

- Ensure a high fluid intake to promote free flow of urine and prevent blockage of the catheter – monitor output.
- Observe urine regularly – check for colour and smell.

Some children will require intermittent catheterisation, which is often carried out by the child (self-catheterisation). The use of this type of catheterisation is indicated in children who have a neurogenic bladder (for example, in those with spina bifida). The catheters used are self-lubricating and can be washed and reused. The advantage of using this intervention is that children can learn to empty the bladder efficiently and therefore become dry by day and by night. This can promote self-confidence and allow the child to take a more active part in everyday life.

Reasons for use of indwelling catheter

Short term

- severely ill child requiring intensive care
- surgery to the renal tract
- surgery to the genital area
- reconstructive surgery

Long term

- unconscious child
- child with deteriorating/disabling condition
- to overcome obstruction to outflow of urine

Study activity

Some children may go home with a urinary catheter *in situ*. Devise a leaflet with details of the care needed. See if you can find any examples of leaflets from other hospitals.

Specific Drugs

Table 43.5 shows some of the more common drugs that would be used for children with genito-urinary problems. You should ensure that you are aware of the potential side-effects of each drug and of any particular role you should play in their administration.

Study activity

Consider the drugs listed in Table 43.5. Explore when each may be used, note normal dosage and any further important points regarding administration. Make notes in the margin and in the table for future reference.

Table 43.5 Specific drugs used for children with renal problems

Drug	Potential side-effects	Role of the nurse
Antibiotics (for UTI)		
sulphonamides	Nausea, vomiting, drug fever, rashes, photosensitivity	Keep child well hydrated – avoids crystallisation of drug in urine
gentamicin	Renal and auditory toxicity	Minimise toxic effects by using slow IV infusion Assist with taking blood for levels
cefalexin	Diarrhoea, nausea and vomiting	Must be taken with food
Immunosuppressives		
cyclophosphamide	Nausea, vomiting, hair loss, irregular menstruation, mouth ulcers	Encourage high fluid intake and frequent bladder emptying to prevent bladder irritation
Steroids		
prednisolone	Increased appetite, obesity, decreased resistance to infection, growth retardation, mood changes, adrenal suppression	
Antihypertensives		
hydralazine	Headache, dizziness, rapid heart beat; lupus erythematosus may occur with prolonged use	
nifedipine	Dizziness on rising, headache, flushing	
Diuretics		
frusemide	Dizziness; rare side-effects include noises in ears, cramps, rash	Ensure potassium-rich diet to combat reduction by the drug
metolazone		

Module 6

The Management of Oedema

Some children with renal problems may exhibit varying degrees of oedema. You need to take great care of the child's skin as oedematous skin is extremely susceptible to infection and breakdown. Keep the following points in mind when delivering care:

- keep skin clean and dry – skin folds are susceptible to thrush
- avoid friction between oedematous parts of the body by applying non-perfumed talcum powder or by using rolls of cotton, pillows
- support the scrotum with cotton pads held in place by a T-bandage
- avoid using tape on the skin as this can cause tearing when removed
- avoid bed rest other than in the acute phase; bed rest encourages venous stasis and can predispose the child to the risk of developing deep vein thrombosis and chest infections
- follow instructions regarding fluid restriction and salt restriction

Fluid restriction

Children with minimal change nephrotic syndrome should be allowed free access to fluids as fluid restriction can aggravate hypovolaemia, leading to serious complications such as venous thrombosis (Corlett, 1995).

Care of the child with nephrotic syndrome – further reading

Bell, F. (2002) Assessment and management of the child with nephrotic syndrome. *Paediatric Nursing*, **14** (1), 37–42.

Peritoneal Dialysis (PD)

This intervention uses the peritoneum as a semi-permeable membrane to filter and remove toxins and fluid. Sterile dialysis solution is instilled through a permanent silastic catheter into the peritoneal cavity. The solution is left to dwell (time will depend on method and reason for dialysis and can range from 30 minutes to 4–5 hours) and then drained off. Peritoneal dialysis may be implemented for children who are in acute renal failure where oliguria continues after 24–48 hours. In this case dialysis will be for a short period of time. Longer-term PD may be used for children with acute renal failure, where it gives more freedom than haemodialysis and can be done at home more easily. In the latter circumstances there are two main methods of implementing the process:

- *Continuous ambulatory peritoneal dialysis (CAPD)* – this method allows for continuous dialysis but does not necessitate bed rest or hospitalisation. Dialysis solution is left to dwell for specified time, allowing for four to five exchanges daily. During the dwell time, the bag is clamped and strapped to the child's abdomen leaving him to be relatively active. The dwell time can be lengthened overnight to allow for uninterrupted sleep.
- *Continuous cycling peritoneal dialysis (CCPD)* – a machine is used to deliver the desired exchanges automatically at night while the child sleeps.

Although this form of treatment has its advantages, it should be acknowledged that it is not necessarily that easy to cope with at home. Studies (MacDonald, 1995; Heaton *et al.*, 2005) have found that the time demands of the care routines and lack of compatibility with other social and institutional timeframes had some negative implications for the children and their families, limiting their participation in school, employment and social life in general.

When providing nursing care for a child receiving PD you should be aware of the complications of the procedure and take appropriate steps to prevent them (Table 43.6).

Principles of dialysis

PD removes water and electrolytes from the blood by virtue of the osmotic gradient that exists between the dialysate and the blood across the peritoneal membrane. By manipulating the concentration of the dialysis solution the quantity and speed of fluid movement can be altered.

(Hazinski, 1992)

Advantages of peritoneal dialysis

- Increased independence and freedom
- A steady blood chemistry is maintained
- A steady state of chemistries is maintained by the continuous method
- Enables home care more easily

Module 6

Further reading

Atkinson, D. (2001) Joseph Feinnes: continuous ambulatory peritoneal dialysis. In Sadik, R. and Campbell, G. (eds), *Client Profiles in Nursing. Child Health.* Cambridge: Cambridge University Press.

This is a case study that includes photographs or clear line diagrams where appropriate to illustrate key points. The case is also accompanied by timed, structured questions with comprehensive referenced model answers to enhance the book's use as a self-assessment tool.

Snethen, J. A., *et al.* (2001) Adolescents' perception of living with end stage renal disease. *Pediatric Nursing*, **27** (2), 159.

Table 43.6 Nursing care for a child receiving peritoneal dialysis

Complication	Nursing care
Peritonitis – mild to severe and ultimately resulting in loss of membrane integrity prohibiting further use of the peritoneum as a filter	Keep catheter exit site clean and covered with dry dressing; use aseptic technique throughout procedures; take care not to raise dialysate bottle above level of the bed as this allows reflux of drained solution; meticulous daily hygiene – showers not baths; monitor for signs of infection – cloudy dialysate, abdominal pain and tenderness, fever
Catheter problems	
obstruction	Ensure that the tubing hangs freely straight down from the bed to the collection bottle
leakage around catheter	Check for overflowing of abdomen – abdomen should not feel rigid; check insertion site; pack weighed, sterile dressings round site – weigh when changed to measure volume and notify doctor
Pulmonary complications – infusion of fluid into abdomen can cause abdominal fullness which can compromise movement of the diaphragm leading to hyperventilation and atelectasis	Assess breath sounds frequently, check effectiveness of ventilation. Encourage child to cough and take deep breaths; elevate head of the bed
Fluid and electrolyte imbalance	Maintain accurate records of all fluid in and out; implement fluid and sodium restrictions as prescribed. Monitor for signs of fluid and electrolyte imbalance – dehydration, peripheral oedema, blood sugar levels

Study activity

Explore the use of the other interventions. When might they be implemented and what would be your role?

Health Education for Discharge

Secondary education – preventing the reoccurrence of urinary tract infections

It is important to educate parents and children so that they understand the rationale for steps that can be taken to reduce the risk of urine infections. Begin by ensuring an understanding of the anatomy of the renal tract using pictures and diagrams and non-jargon terminology.

Study activity

Draw a labelled diagram of the renal tract that you could use to teach children and parents basic anatomy and physiology. Try it out and then critically evaluate.

Preventive measures are related to the factors that predispose to infection:

- In females the urethra is very short (about 2 cm in young girls, 4 cm in mature women). This means that there is an increased chance of contamination from a close proximity to the anus. Males are less susceptible due to the longer urethra and antibacterial properties of prostatic secretions. However, the presence of a foreskin is associated with an increase in periurethral bacteria that can easily ascend, particularly in the first year of life. It is important therefore to teach about basic hygiene and the need for frequent baths; clean from front to back when cleaning the vulval or anal area during nappy changing or toileting.
- Urinary stasis is perhaps the single most important predisposing factor for urinary tract infections (Miller, 1996). Normally regular emptying of the bladder flushes away any organisms before they can multiply. Incomplete emptying leaves urine in the bladder providing an ideal culture medium for bacterial growth. Teach to avoid 'holding on' and delaying micturition; encourage frequent voiding and complete emptying. Children are sometimes in a hurry to get back to play and may finish before the bladder is empty. Double voiding is useful and involves returning to micturate after a short time. Increased fluid intake encourages flushing of the bladder.
- Normal urine is slightly acidic with a pH of 5. This helps to hamper the multiplication of bacteria. However, alkaline urine predisposes to bacterial growth. Urine can be made more acidic by offering apple juice, cranberry juice or a diet high in animal protein.
- Essential oils in some bubble baths and soaps can irritate the urethra thereby predisposing to bacterial growth – use of these should be avoided.

Tertiary education – managing infections at home to reduce the risk of renal damage

Include the following points in a teaching plan:

- instructions regarding the administration of antibiotics
- specific guidelines on fluid intake – it is not sufficient to say 'encourage fluids' – offer a suggested amount, for example based on weight (100 ml/kg/day). Give ideas on how to encourage oral intake in reluctant children (use of bendy straws, frozen lollies, reward systems – for example stars). Give ideas on types of fluid to offer (for example, the child should avoid caffeine and carbonated drinks as these may irritate bladder mucosa; Miller, 1996).

Study activity

Design a teaching plan for a 4-year-old girl and her carers to prepare them for discharge following hospitalisation for a severe urinary tract infection.

Causes of incomplete emptying of the bladder

- Neurogenic bladder
- Obstructive lesions
- Anomalies in the urinary tract
- Constipation
- Infrequent voiding

Further reading

Avner, E. D., Harmon, W. and Niaudet, P. (2003) *Pediatric Nephrology*, 5th edn. London: Lippincott Williams & Wilkins.

A comprehensive reference on congenital and acquired kidney diseases and their therapies in children. Section One opens with an overview of the anatomy, physiology and biology of the paediatric kidney, critical to understanding disease. Section Two covers the evaluation, diagnosis and therapy of specific kidney disorders.

Thomas, N. (2002) *Renal Nursing*, 2nd edn. London: Bailliere Tindall.

This provides full coverage of all aspects of acute and chronic renal failure, including dialysis, transplantation, investigations, dietary management, children with renal problems and community nursing. It examines essential anatomy, physiology and psychology, cross-referencing between chapters and concluding with a handy, quick-reference appendix on drugs used in renal failure.

Helpful addresses

The British Kidney Patient Association
Bordon, Hants, GU35 9JZ
Tel: 01420 472021/2
Web site:
http://www.britishkidney-pa.co.uk/ (accessed 31 May 2006)

Enuresis Resource and Information Centre
32, Old School House,
Kingswood Foundation Estate,
Britannia Road, Bristol BS15 8DB
Tel: 0117 960 3060
Web site: http://www.eric.org.uk
(accessed 31 May 2006)

Chapter 44

Principles of Care – Children with Problems Related to the Immune System

Introduction

The body is protected from harmful agents by a complex system. The effects of dysfunction in this complex system can involve any or all of the body systems and, as such, can present the child with many varied problems. It is likely that you will meet the challenges presented by children with problems of the immune system and therefore it is essential that you have a working knowledge of the system's normal function and the mechanisms of dysfunction. Some aspects of anatomy and physiology are reviewed here for you but you will need to revise your knowledge more fully.

The organs that contribute to protection of the body are:

- Non-immunological host defences – skin, cilia, mucous membranes, tears and saliva.
- Inflammatory response – vascular and cellular changes that eliminate dead tissue, microorganisms, toxins, and inert foreign matter.
- Mononuclear phagocytic system (reticuloendothelial system) – removes pathogens from blood and tissue by phagocytosis – mainly by magrophages.
- Immune system – includes organs, tissue and cells circulating in the blood. Primary organs – bone marrow and thymus. Secondary organs – lymph nodes, spleen, tonsils, Peyer's patches and appendix. The main cells of the immune system are lymphocytes – T and B cells. There are two mechanisms by which the immune system responds to antigens – humoral and cell mediated (Figure 44.1). These usually work together to produce a combined response.

Definitions

The key to understanding the complex immune system is to have an understanding of the interactions of antigen and antibody:

- *antigen* – any substance capable of eliciting an immune response
- *antibody (immunoglobulin)* – serum proteins that bind to specific antigens and begin the processes that start lysis or phagocytosis of the antigen; produced by plasma cells

Study activity

Having read so far you should explore some aspects of anatomy and physiology further:

- the role of the complement system and cascade
- the role of macrophages
- the process of phagocytosis

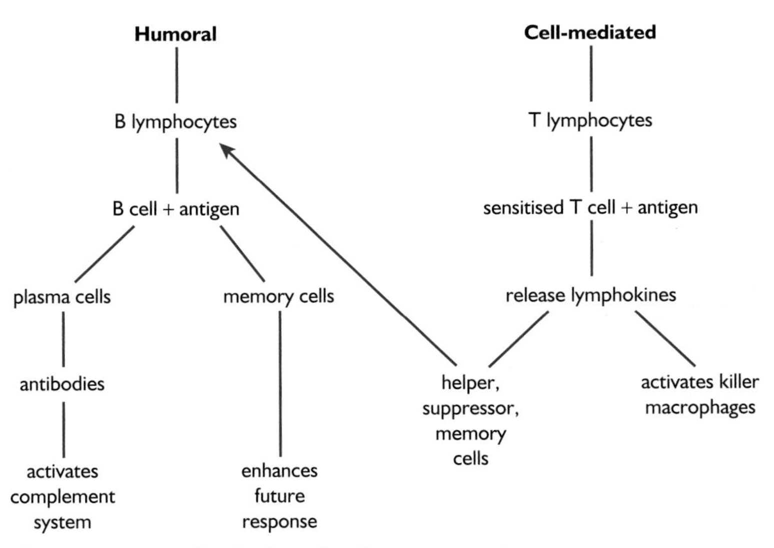

Figure 44.1 Humoral and cell-mediated response to antigens.

The immunoglobulins (Ig)

- **IgG** – major Ig (75%). Smallest. Only one that crosses the placenta; second Ig to respond to antigen in primary response BUT major one to respond on subsequent exposure. Activates the complement system
- **IgM** – found mainly in the blood. Largest Ig, first Ig to respond to an antigen. Binds with viral and bacterial agents in blood to activate complement cascade
- **IgA** – concentrates in exocrine secretions (colostrum, milk, tears, sweat, saliva), respiratory, gastro-intestinal and urogenital secretions. Provides specific protection
- **IgD** – found on surface of B cells; may be involved in differentation
- **IgE** – present in trace amounts normally. Elevated in allergic disorders

The problems associated with the immune system are numerous and are categorised here as:

- immunodeficiency disorders (Table 44.1)
- allergic disorders (Table 44.2)
- autoimmune disorders (Table 44.2)
- infectious diseases (Table 44.3).

Table 44.1 Immunodeficiency disorders

Problem	Pathophysiology
Congenital	
stem cell deficiency – severe combined immunodeficiency (SCIDS)	Early lack of stem cell which would normally give rise to lymphocytes resulting in striking lymphopenia. Absence of cellular immunity and antibody synthesis. Invariably leads to fatal infection
B cell deficiency – infantile X-linked agammaglobulinaemia	Humoral immunity is impaired; symptoms become evident at about 9 months of age when maternal immunity decreases. Leads to a susceptibility to severe infections caued by pyogenic organisms
T cell abnormality – DiGeorge's syndrome	Partial or total absence of the parathyroid and thymus glands.
T and B cell deficiency – Wiskott–Aldrich syndrome	Normal B cell humoral immunity but no cellular immunity. Immune system unable to initiate a response to antigens
Acquired iatrogenic: steroids, chemotheraphy, antibodies infections: transient (via infections); permanent (human immunodeficiency virus, HIV) antibody loss; nephrotic syndrome, protein-losing enteropathy	HIV virus targets helper T cells, enters them and uses them to reproduce. The virus then destroys the host cell, replicates and attacks other lymphocytes
Immunoproliferative disorders:	
leukaemia	Proliferation of abnormal white cells which accumulate in blood, bone marrow and body tissues
lymphoma – Hodgkin's disease and non-Hodgkin's disease	Abnormal proliferation of lymphoid stem cells

Lymphocytes

- *B cells* – precursors of antibody-producing plasma cells. Recognition of an antigen activates B cells to proliferate (to increase response) and differentiate into antibody-secreting cells (which synthesise immunoglobulin and memory cells able to respond more rapidly in subsequent attack)
- *T cells* – either promote (helper cells) or suppress (suppressor cells) the immune response, kill antigens directly or participate in other immune responses. Helper cells assist B cell proliferation

Further reading

Delves, P., Martin, S., Burton, D. and Roitt, I. (2006) *Essential Immunology*, 11th edn. Oxford: Blackwell Publishing

complement system

The complement system is 'composed of an interacting series of glycoproteins that, when triggered, are activated in an orderly sequence to produce biologically active substances that enhance the inflammatory reaction, promote removal of particular matter from the bloodstream, or possibly cause lysis of cells or microorganisms'.

(Shyur and Hill, 1996)

incubation period

The time between exposure to a pathogenic organism and the onset of symptoms of a disease.

infectious period

The time during which the infective agent may be transmitted (directly or indirectly) from the infected person to an uninfected person.

Table 44.2 Allergic and autoimmune disorders

Problem	Pathophysiology
Allergenic problems asthma hayfever eczema anaphylactic shock	Atopic individual combines certain antigens (allergens) with IgE. This complex then attaches itself to the surface membranes of basophils and mast cells. These cells respond by degranulation – the granules contain histamine which when freed causes weal formation, itching, bronchoconstriction and hypotension. Exact mechanisms are different for each type of reaction
Autoimmune disorders (immune complex disease) glomerulonephritis systemic lupus erythematosus (SLE)	Self-tolerance (i.e. tolerance of own cells and tissues) is thought to develop early in embryonic life. When this system fails autoantibodies are produced which become complexed with self-antigens resulting in a variety of reactions depending on which tissues are involved

Table 44.3 Infectious disorders

Infectious disease	Causative organism	Incubation period: infectious period
Chickenpox (varicella)	Varicella zoster	14–21 days after exposure: onset of fever until last vesicle has dried (5–7 days)
Diphtheria	*Corynebacterium diphtheriae*	2–6 days: 2–4 weeks untreated, 1–2 days with antibiotics. Child clear after two consecutive clear cultures
Roseola	Human herpes virus type 6	5–15 days: not known – probably not highly contagious
Measles (rubeola)	Measles virus, RNA-containing paramyxovirus	10–12 days: day 5 until 5–7 days after rash appears
Mumps	Mumps virus, paramyxovirus	14–28 days (average 18): until all swelling has disappeared, not less than 14 days from start of illness
Pertussis (whooping cough)	*Bordetella pertussis*	5–21 days: 7 days after exposure to 3 weeks after onset of paroxysms
Poliomyelitis	Enteroviruses, type 1, 2 + 3	7–14 days: not exactly known, virus is present in throat and faeces shortly after infection and persists for about 1 week in the throat and 4–6 weeks in faeces
Rubella (German measles)	Rubella virus	14–21 days: 7 days before rash – 5 days after rash
Scarlet fever	Group A beta-haemolytic streptococci	2–4 days (range 1–7 days): during incubation period and clinical illness, approximately 10 days

Assessment

Assessing children with potential immune problems can be confusing and requires you to keep many different aspects in your mind at once. Immune problems often produce multi-system effects and you need to take a thorough history and a general physical assessment. You need the ability to recognise immune-related signs and symptoms, keeping in mind the different types of immune dysfunction identified above. The first step in assessing the child is to talk to him and his carers. Ask questions about the following (try to get the child to answer wherever possible):

- Bleeding/bruising tendencies – this helps to identify platelet/clotting dysfunction, which can occur in some deficiencies and immune disorders.
- Any swellings that might have been noticed in the neck, armpits or groin. If so find out their nature (painful, tender, red). Swollen lymph nodes may be indicative of infection, inflammation, certain leukaemias or lymphatic tumours.
- Energy levels. Find out if the child has shown fatigue or weakness. Ask questions about normal energy levels and any noticeable changes. Relate to child's normal daily activities.
- Temperature. Has the child had a fever? If so, has it been constant or intermittent in nature? Frequently recurring fevers may indicate impaired immune system or increased cell proliferation.
- Joint pain – if so where and what has been the nature of the pain?
- Take a full immunisation history.
- Ask questions about general health.
- Does the child have any allergies?
- Is the child taking any medications? Steroids, some chemotherapy agents and some antibiotics can compromise the immune system.
- Take a family history – this may highlight any potential hereditary problems.

Study activity

You are taking a history from a 9-year-old boy who has been admitted with a possible immune problem. His mother is present and every time you ask him a question she answers for him. Think critically about this situation and explore ways in which you might encourage the mother to allow her child to answer. Why is it important that the child answers?

Your physical assessment of children should begin as soon as you meet them. You may pick up cues by just 'looking' before actually examining them or taking any vital signs. Figure 44.2 shows the specific signs that might alert you to an immune disorder.

During the assessment phase you may be required to assist in a variety of medical investigations. Many of the investigations are too complex to explain in detail here and some are listed in the margin for you to explore more fully at a future date. One of the initial tests will be a full blood count and differential, which provides quantitative values for haemoglobin, haematocit, platelets, RBCs and white blood cells.

Examples of investigations for immune disorders

- Immunohaematologic test
- Schick test
- Complement function
- Rosette test
- Delayed hypersensitivity skin test
- Immunoelectrophoresis
- Tests for antinuclear antibodies and anti-DNA antibodies
- Skin tests, food challenges, elimination diets
- Bone marrow aspirate and biopsy
- Lymph node biopsy
- Lymphangiography
- CT scan
- MRI scan

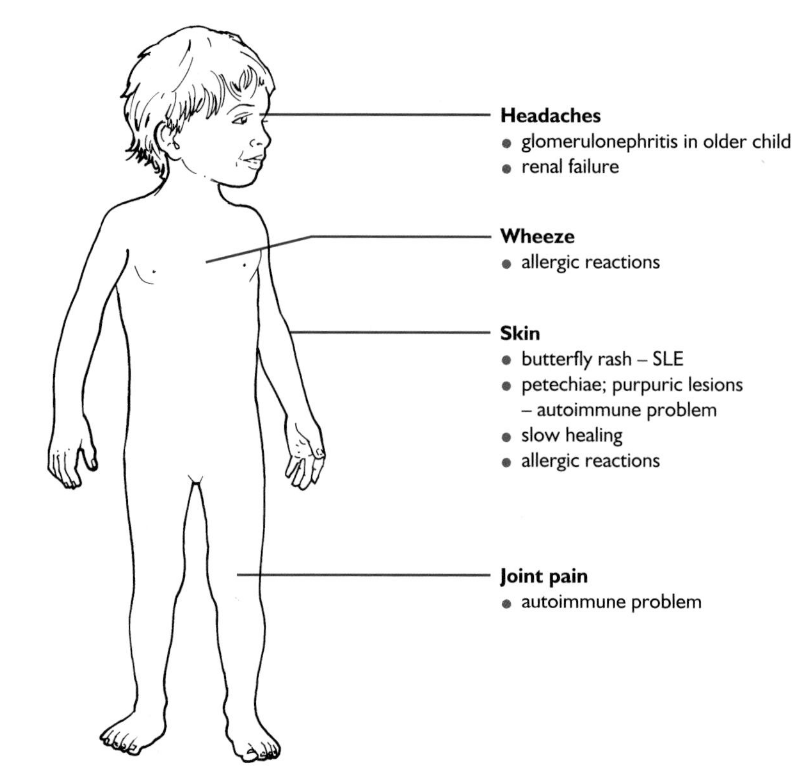

Figure 44.2 Specific assessment for immune disorders.

Table 44.4 shows the implications of an altered white cell count (*see also* Normal blood values p. 425).

Tests specifically related to the lymphocytes may be done:

- T and B cell proliferation tests – evaluate the mitotic response of T and B cells to foreign antigens. A lowered response implies decreased available cells or functional defect.

Table 44.4 Understanding the differential white cell count

Cell type	Increased by	Decreased by
Neutrophils	Infection, cancer, poisoning, stress, haemorrhage, myelocytic leukaemia	Chemotherahy, radiotherapy, deficiency of vitamin B_{12} or folic acid
Lymphocytes	Hepatitis, herpes simplex and zoster, mononucleosis, lymphocytic leukaemia	Wiskott–Aldrich syndrome; occasionally in SLE
Monocytes	Tuberculosis, cancer, anaemia, typhoid, myelocytic leukaemia	Rarely decreased
Eosinophils	Allergies, asthma, worm or parasitic invasion, inflammation plus many other conditions	SLE, stress, Cushing's syndrome
Basophils	Granulocytic leukaemia, basophilic leukaemia	Hyperthyroidism (occasionally), allergies

- T and B cell counts – these can help to diagnose deficiencies, evaluate immunocompetence in autoimmune disease and monitor response to therapy. An abnormal count suggests specific disease. However, a normal count does not necessarily rule it out.

Nursing Interventions

This section will concentrate on exploring:

- measures to prevent infection (standard precautions)
- care of children with HIV and AIDS
- the use of immunotherapeutic agents

Measures to prevent infection

One of the main principles in the control and prevention of infection is to halt transmission and contamination. Standard precautions underpin routine safe practice. These precautions include handwashing, which has been identified as being the single most important method of preventing the spread of infection if done properly (Lowberry, 1975; Taylor, 1978; Ayliffe *et al.*, 1992; Creedon, 2005; Royal College of Nursing, 2005). The areas that are most frequently missed during handwashing are the tips of the fingers, the thumbs, the wrist, the palms and the backs of the hands. Too much handwashing can cause sore skin, which in turn can lead to colonisation by pathogens. It is important therefore to wash your hands at the most appropriate times and avoid overwashing.

Study activity

Test your own technique. Before reading any further wash your hands as if preparing to enter the cubicle of a child who is immunosuppressed. Critically reflect on your technique. Could it be improved? The areas that are most frequently missed during handwashing are the tips of the fingers, the thumbs, the wrist, the palms and the backs of the hands.

Standard precautions (formerly known as universal precautions)

1. Achieving optimum hand hygiene.
2. Using personal protective equipment.
3. Safe handling and disposal of sharps.
4. Safe handling and disposal of clinical waste.
5. Managing blood and bodily fluids.
6. Decontaminating equipment.
7. Achieving and mantaining a clean clinical environment.
8. Appropriate use of indwelling devices.
9. Managing accidents.
10. Good communication with other health workers, patients and visitors.
11. Training/education.

RCN (2005) Good practice in infection prevention and control. Available at Web site: http://www.rcn.org.uk/resources/mrsa/downloads/Wipe_it_out-Good_practice_in_infection_prevention_and_control.pdf (accessed 31 May 2006).

Handwashing should be done before:

- entering or leaving an isolation area
- starting work, going for a break or leaving for home
- commencing any new cleaning operation
- reparing or handling food and drinks
- handling any catering equipment

and after:

- handling any soiled item
- handling linen, bedding or waste
- removing protective clothing, including gloves
- any cleaning operation
- using the toilet
- nose blowing

http://patientexperience.nhsestates.gov.uk/clean_hospitals/ch_content/cleaning_manual/infection_control.asp (accessed 31 May 2006)

Further reading

National Institute for Health and Clinical Excellence (2003) Infection Control: Prevention of healthcare-associated infection in primary and community care. Available at Web site: http://www.nice.org.uk/pdf/CG2fullguidelineinfectioncontrol.pdf (accessed 31 May 2006).

Clean Your Hands campaign

Low compliance with hand hygiene was identified by the NPSA in 2002 as a recognised safety concern for patients. The Clean Your Hands campaign aims to minimise the risk to patient safety of low compliance with hand hygiene by healthcare staff, through a national strategy of improvement. The campaign involves:

- near-patient disinfectant handrub for staff to use where they have patient contact
- poster displays and promotional materials to influence staff and patients
- patient involvement in improving hand hygiene by empowering them to ask staff if they have 'washed their hands'

A core component of the campaign is the requirement for all Trusts to implement near-patient disinfectant handrub following an NPSA patient Safety Alert.

Web site: www.npsa.nhs.uk/cleanyourhands (accessed 11 June 2006).

National Resource for Infection Control

National Resource for Infection Control (NRIC) is a project developed by healthcare professionals, aimed at being a single-access point to existing resources within infection control, for infection control and all other healthcare staff.

Web site: http://www.nric.org.uk/IntegratedCRD.nsf/NRIC_Home?OpenPage (accessed 31 May 2006).

Principles of handwashing

- use bactericidal solution
- use continuously running water
- position hands to avoid contaminating arms
- avoid splashing clothing or floor
- use friction on *all* surfaces
- rinse thoroughly with hands held down
- dry hands thoroughly

Categorising waste

Linen

- used (domestically dirty)
- foul or infested
- infected (used by child with infectious disease)
- high-risk (contaminated by blood, body fluids from child in high-risk category)

Waste

- household waste
- other clinical waste (includes dressings, nappies, stoma and urine bags)
- sharps
- glass

Study activity

Test your colleagues' handwashing techniques. How long do they wash for? Watch how well they wash. Do they use soap? Discuss the techniques together.

Protective clothing

Gloves should always be worn when handling or having contact with blood or body fluids (for example, when changing nappies or changing suction tubing). Gloves must be discarded after use – never washed and reused. The use of gloves should not preclude handwashing. Whereas Carter (1993) questioned the value of gowns in the prevention of cross infection, current consensus supports their use as an effective way of preventing infection (Rayner, 2003; Royal College of Nursing, 2005). The use of masks is usually indicated to prevent the spread of droplet infection. However, the effectiveness of this protection has been questioned (Romney, 2001). Filter masks and eye protection may be used for single use and only when clinically appropriate or when the carer is at risk from splashing (National Institute for Health and Clinical Excellence, 2003).

Correct disposal of waste

Guidelines for the disposal of waste and linen can be found in DH (2004c). Any waste that is contaminated with blood or body substances should be disposed of in yellow clinical waste bags and labelled according to department of origin. Examples of clinical waste include gloves, aprons, dressings and catheter bags. Clinical waste bags must be tied securely, not overfilled and stored in a designated disposal area prior to disposal. Non-clinical, or domestic, waste must be disposed of in black bags. Examples of domestic waste include flowers, packaging, newspapers and paper towels.

Study activity

Investigate your hospital's local policies for the management and disposal of waste and linen. Make notes in the margin for future reference.

Isolation techniques

There are also a number of isolation techniques:

- Source isolation – for children who are infectious and need to be nursed away from other children. The principle is not to take infection out of the cubicle.
- Protective isolation (sometimes called reverse barrier nursing) – for children who need protecting from infection. The principle is to keep infection out of the cubicle.
- Laminar airflow rooms – these provide a germ-free room for children at high risk. The room contains a high-efficiency air filter – filtered air flows across the room providing several hundred air exchanges per hour.

Study activity

Find out if your hospital has such rooms – make arrangements to visit and talk to staff about caring for a child.

Study activity

Make arrangements to spend time with members of the control of infection team. Discuss topical issues and find out about any new policies. Research which might affect nursing care.

Caring for children with HIV disease

The number of children with HIV disease is on the increase. In 1992, 403 children under 15 had been diagnosed as HIV positive (47 of whom had died) (Woodroffe *et al.*, 1993). By October 1996 this had increased to 450 reported cases (Public Health Laboratory Service – PHLS, 1996), and by the end of 2004 figures had risen to 1650 (Health Protection Agency, 2006). Of the 1650 children infected with HIV (Figure 44.3):

- approximately 40% of children who were infected from their mother were born abroad
- at the end of 2004 approximately 58 300 adults aged over 15 were living with HIV in the UK
- of that figure, 19 700 (34%) were unaware of their infection (Health Protection Agency, 2006)

Study activity

Find out the current figures and compare with those given here. What is the trend? Analyse the reasons for the trend.

The majority of children – 200 babies in 1993, 380 in 1996, 1119 in 2004 – are infected by vertical transmission of the virus from the mother before or during birth (PHLS, 1996; Health Protection Agency, 2006). Babies of mothers who are HIV positive before birth will test positive. However, maternal antibodies can persist until about 18 months when many will test negative, having seroconverted. Other sources of infection include:

- unprotected sexual activity – abuse or sexually active young people
- sharing of injections by drug users
- social contact (rare)
- no transmissions through blood products have been reported in the UK since viral inactivation of blood products was introduced in 1985 (Health Protection Agency, 2006).

We can now consider HIV disease a chronic illness in childhood with a range of complex problems that can affect the whole family, especially as the mother is also HIV positive in the majority of cases (Miah, 2004). Progression from HIV infection to AIDS occurs over an undefined time, which is different for every child. It may be that an infected parent will witness the deterioration and eventual death, which could forecast their own fate (Brown and Powell-Cope, 1991). Thus a family approach to care is vital. An in-depth qualitative study by Rehm and Franck (2000) found that families had three goals to establish normalcy and stability: staying healthy, facilitating children's participation in school and social activities, and enhancing social and emotional well-being of family members. Reidy *et al.* (1991) suggests that the role of the nurse in caring for a child with HIV disease can be based upon five needs, to:

- *Maintain physical integrity.* One of the most important aspects of care is infection control (a) to prevent the spread of the virus and (b) to protect the child from infection (which is particularly important when the child is admitted to hospital). Each hospital will have its own infection-control policies but you need to be aware of the principles of standard precautions.
- *Communicate.* Many difficult issues arise when considering this aspect of care. First, it is imperative that the family is given room and opportunity to communicate with healthcare staff. You should be aware of when to involve others who are perhaps more skilled at discussing feelings or concerns. The channels for communicating should be obvious and available to the child and family. One of the main concerns may be 'who to tell'. There is no legal requirement to divulge information about the child's HIV status and any decision to tell (school, nursery or playgroup) must rest with the family. All members of staff should give support for their decision.
- *Feel worthwhile and useful.* MacKenzie (1994) highlights the importance of developing a close relationship with the family based on trust and mutual respect. Acknowledgement of the caring skills of the family is vital so that you avoid making them feel inadequate.
- *Act according to a set of beliefs and values.* According to Friedemann (1989) it is important that the nurse and the family share the same goals. This may be difficult if the values and goals of the family are different from those held by the nurse. However, to maintain an effective

relationship the nurse must be able to set aside her own beliefs and respect those of the family. Nettleship (1994/5) highlighted the facing of personal prejudices as a factor when caring for children with HIV disease.

- *Learn.* Children with HIV or AIDS should be allowed to attend school. HIV infection or AIDS should not be a factor taken into account by local education authorities, governing bodies and head teachers in discharging either their various duties concerning school admissions, transfers and attendance or their powers of exclusion from school. You must ensure that families and children receive up-to-date information. The family need a sound understanding of the nature of HIV disease and its modes of transmission. In order to do this you need to keep up to date too and know where to send them for additional help and support.

Sources of support include:

- AVERT, 4 Brighton Road, Horsham, West Sussex RH13 5BA. Tel: 01403 210202. Web site: http://www.avert.org.uk (accessed 30 May 2006)
- Children with AIDS Charity, Lion House, 3 Plough Yard, London EC2A 3LP. Tel: 020 7247 9115; fax: 020 7247 9120. Web site: info@cwac.org
- Mildmay Mission Hospital, Hackney Road, London E2 7NA. Tel: 020 7613 6300. Web site: http://www.mildmay.org.uk/ (accessed 30 May 2006)
- National AIDS Helpline: 0800 567 123
- Paediatric Aids Resource Centre (PARC), Department of Child Life and Health, 20 Sylvan Place, Edinburgh, EH9 1UW. Tel: 0131 536 0806
- Positively Women, 347–349 City Road, London, EC1V 1LR. Tel: 020 7713 0222. Helpline for women living with HIV (Monday to

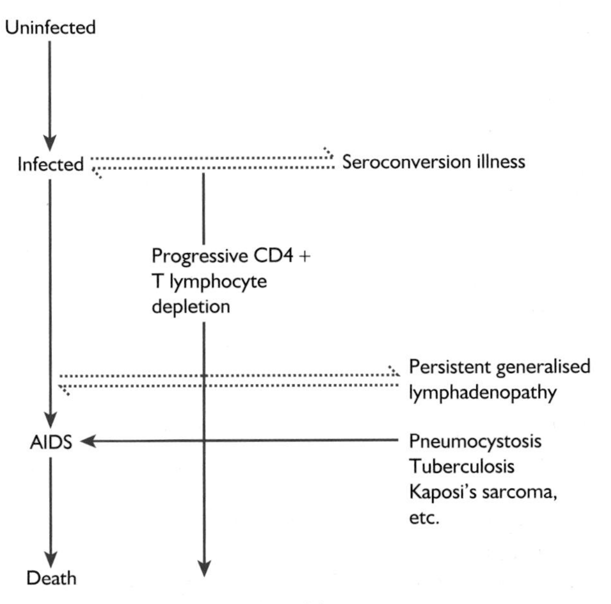

Figure 44.3 Course of HIV disease (adapted from Cree, 1997).

AIDS – acquired immune deficiency syndrome
The final phase of the chronic disease HIV infection. Characterised by a progressive decline in cell-mediated immunity and the consequent development of opportunistic infections, tumours and death.

(Cree, 1997)

Friday, 10 a.m.–4 p.m.). Web site: http://www.positivelywomen.org.uk (accessed 30 May 2006)

- Terence Higgins Trust, 314–320 Gray's Inn Road, London WC1X 8DP. Tel: 020 7812 1600. Email: info@tht.org.uk. Web site: http://www.tht.org.uk (accessed 25 July 2007)
- Waverley Care Solas, 2/4 Abbeymount, Edinburgh EH8 8EJ. Tel: 0131 661 0982; fax: 0131 652 1780. Web site: http://www.waverleycare.org (accessed 30 May 2006)

Study activity

First, consider your views towards HIV disease. Then draw up a short questionnaire asking about attitudes to caring for children with HIV disease. Give out to your colleagues and then analyse the results. Perhaps you might hold a meeting afterwards to discuss the points raised.

The use of immunotherapeutic agents

Table 44.5 shows some of the immunotherapeutic agents that may be used for children. Table 44.6 gives details of the current immunisation schedule (*see also* Aspirin, safety of the drug p. 317).

Study activity

Explore the use of these agents as and when you come across them, making your own notes with particular reference to dosages for children.

Module 6

Managing Infectious Diseases at Home

The majority of children with infectious diseases can be cared for at home. However, carers need adequate support and information to enable them to carry out appropriate care. Rickard and Finn (1997) surveyed 120 parents accompanying children to an accident-and-

Further reading

Miah, J. (2004) *Talking with Children, Young People and Families, about Chronic Illness and Living with HIV*. London: National Children's Bureau.

A Department of Health Web page giving answers to frequently asked questions about HIV in the UK: http://www.dh.gov.uk/PolicyAndGuidance/HealthAndSocialCareTopics/HIV/HIVFAQ/fs/en?CONTENT_ID=4039431&chk=IDUbeh (accessed 31 May 2006).

Weglarz, M. and Boland, M. (2005) Family-centered nursing care of the perinatally infected mother and child living with HIV infection. *Journal for Specialists in Pediatric Nursing*, **16** (4), 161–170.

Wood, S. A., Tobias, C. and McCree, J. (2004) Medication adherence for HIV positive women caring for children: in their own words. *AIDS Care*, **16** (7), 909–913.

Table 44.5 Immunotherapeutic agents (copyright is waived for the purpose of photocopying and enlarging this table)

Immunotherapeutic agent	Notes	Your notes/dosages
Anti-inflammatory drugs		
non-steroidal anti-inflammatory drugs (NSAIDs)	Care must be taken in the administration of aspirin	
corticosteroids	Oral preparations should be given with or shortly after meals to reduce gastro-intestinal side-effects. Warn not to discontinue without medical approval – can cause life-threatening adrenal insufficiency	
Immunosuppressive agents	Suppress immune responses to control disease activity. Major side-effects is bone marrow suppression and an increased susceptibility to infection (mouth sores and ulcers, fever, chills). Teach about side-effects and need to monitor for infection	
Antiallergic agents		
antihistamines	Block histamine receptors. Generally well tolerated but may produce drowsiness and dry mouth. Administer with food to avoid gastro-intestinal side-effects	
decongestants	Stimulate alpha-adrenergic receptors of vascular smooth muscle to constrict dilated blood vessels in nasal mucosa. May elevate blood pressure	
Immunoenhancing agents		
inteferon	Inhibit viral replication and tumour cell growth, enhance natural lymphocyte activity and phagocytosis. Side-effects include fever, pain at injection site, shivering and fatigue	
Immunisation		
active immunisation	Natural exposure to an infecting organism or use of vaccines and toxoids. May produce fever, malaise, soreness at injection site. Serious complications are rare. Caution with children allergic to eggs; live vaccines should not be given to children who are immunosuppressed; advise caution with live oral polio – inadequately immunised people can contract polio when exposed to viral excretions in stools	
passive immunisation	Administration of preformed antibodies to a non-immunised child. Animal serum can cause allergic reactions and life-threatening anaphylaxis; serum sickness reactions. Adverse reactions to human serum are rare, usually confined to injection site	
Other immunotherapies bone marrow transplant apheresis radiotherapy biological therapies	Space precludes giving details about these therapies. Investigate them if you come across them	

emergency department to explore parental knowledge of infectious diseases. The results indicated that lack of knowledge could lead to inappropriate use of medical time and resources. The research also found that some parents were unaware of potentially dangerous interventions (for example that aspirin should not be given to a febrile child). Finally, lack of knowledge about when to seek medical intervention could put the child at risk. Information about caring for children at home should therefore be made available from a variety of sources.

Table 44.6 Immunisation schedule (http://www.immunisation.nhs.uk/article.php?id=97 (accessed 30 January 2007))

When is the immunisation due?	Which immunisation?	Route
2 months	Diphtheria, tetanus, whooping cough, polio and *Haemophilus influenzae* type B (Hib). Pneumococcal conjugate vaccine	One injection
3 months	Diphtheria, tetanus, whooping cough, polio, *Haemophilus influenzae* type B. Meningitis C	One injection
4 months	Diphtheria, tetanus, whooping cough, polio and *Haemophilus influenzae* type B (Hib). Meningitis C. Pneumococcal conjugate vaccine	One injection
Around 12 months	*Haemophilus influenzae* type B (Hib) and meningitis C	One injection
Around 13 months old	Measles, mumps and rubella (MMR). Pneumococcal conjugate vaccine	One injection
3 years and 4 months to 5 years old	Diphtheria, tetanus, whooping cough and polio Measles, mumps and rubella (MMR)	One injection One injection
13 to 18 years old	Diphtheria, tetanus, polio	One injection

Following advice from the Joint Committee on Vaccination and Immunisation (JCVI) the current universal BCG vaccination programme delivered through schools will be replaced with an improved programme of targeted vaccination for those individuals who are at greatest risk. The new programme identifies and vaccinates babies and older people who are most likely to catch the disease, especially in those living in areas with a high rate of TB or whose parents or grandparents were born in a country with high prevalence of TB.

Information about infectious diseases

http://www.aap.org/healthtopics/infectiousdiseases.cfm (accessed 31 May 2006).

An American site but contains good fact sheets, brochures, books, audio files and policy statements about recognising, treating and caring for children with infectious diseases.

Leaflets and booklets could be made available in chemists, GP surgeries, wards and accident-and-emergency departments. The principal goals of care include:

- preventing the spread of infection to others
- prevention of complications
- maintaining comfort – including managing a fever and skin symptoms

Study activity

Using information given in this section and elsewhere in the book, draw up a leaflet or handout that will give appropriate guidelines for parents to enable them to care for a child with (a) chickenpox and (b) measles. Pilot the information and then critically evaluate its effectiveness.

Study activity

Check out the current immunisation schedule for infants and children. What advice would you give parents who ask you about the safety of the immunisations?

Chapter 45

Principles of Care – Children with a Neurological Problem

Introduction

Cerebral blood flow and oxygen consumption in children under 6 years of age is almost double that of adults, to meet the younger child's needs for rapid growth and development. The brain grows rapidly during the first 6 years of life, especially during infancy when half of its postnatal growth occurs. Consequently any problems occurring at birth or during early childhood that impair the cerebral circulation or oxygen consumption can have far-reaching effects on normal growth and development. The degree and type of impairment that result from such disturbances depend upon the function of the part of the brain involved. Therefore, the nurse needs an understanding of the structure and function of the central nervous system to be able to appreciate, recognise and implement appropriate care for the disorders that may occur.

Study activity

Answer the questions in the quiz about the structure and function of the nervous system. Check your answers with an anatomy and physiology text.

Neurology quiz

Identify the areas of the brain which control:

- temperature
- respiration, pulse and blood pressure
- posture and balance

Which cranial nerve is responsible for controlling pupil size?

Identify the sites of a:

- subdural haemorrhage
- subarachnoid haemorrhage

Where are the fontanelles and at what age do they close?

What is the position and function of the following:

- frontal lobes
- parietal lobes
- occipital lobes
- temporal lobes

Common Neurological Problems in Children (Table 45.1)

Febrile convulsions are one of the most common neurological disorders of childhood, affecting about 3% of children aged 6 months to 3 years. The cause of these seizures is not proven. Berg (1993) notes that the level of the temperature rather than the speed of the increase appears to be the significant factor. The pyrexia is usually over 38.8°C and the convulsion usually occurs during the rise rather than after it. Bethune *et al.* (1993) identify children at particular risk from febrile convulsions as those who meet all the following criteria:

Table 45.1 Common neurological problems of childhood

Problem	Pathophysiology
Cerebral palsy	A group of disorders caused by prenatal or postnatal anoxia. The consequences depend upon the area of brain deprived of oxygen but it usually involves impaired movement and posture due to disordered muscle tone and coordination. Sensory and mental impairment may also be present
Epilepsy	Spontaneous electrical discharges are initiated in the brain by hyperexcitable cells (epileptogenic focus) in response to a variety of physiological stimuli. These stimuli overcome the normal inhibitory mechanisms and the increased electrical activity is able to spread to normal cells via synaptical pathways. When the activity reaches the midbrain and reticular formation a generalised seizure occurs
Febrile convulsion	A pyrexia stimulates peripheral and central thermoreceptors in the skin and mucous membranes and impulses are sent to the pre-optic area of the hypothalamus. In children over 5 years this stimulates the heat-losing centre resulting in vasodilation, perspiration and decreased metabolism. In younger children this centre is too immature and its stimulation causes a convulsion
Head injury	Intracranial contents are damaged if the force of the injury is too great to be absorbed by the skull and diffuse swelling occurs. Cerebral oedema and increased intercranial pressure can result in hypoxia, hypercapnia and inadequate perfusion
Hydrocephalus	Impaired absorption or obstruction to the outflow of cerebrospinal fluid causes an accumulation of fluid in the ventricles which dilate, putting pressure on to cerebral tissue
Meningitis	Acute inflammation of the meninges caused by a variety of bacterial and viral agents. Organisms enter the cerebrospinal fluid via the bloodstream from infections or trauma of neighbouring sites and spread throughout the subarachnoid space. Inflammation, exudation and tissue damage to the brain result causing pyrexia and raised ICP. Septic shock and rashes may occur in severe infections

- have a family history of febrile convulsions
- are in full-time day care
- demonstrate delayed developmental milestones
- were nursed in special care units for at least 28 days

It may be that these criteria link with an increased risk and susceptibility to infection rather than any predisposition to seizures in relation to fever. Febrile convulsions are not associated with epilepsy: 95–98% of children recover with no lasting neurological damage.

Epilepsy (Table 45.2) affects about 1 in 200 people but its incidence varies greatly with age and the highest proportion of those affected are children (Shorvon, 1990). It has various causes but in around 80% of cases there is no obvious cause. It is associated with an excess mortality, two to three times that of the general population, and this excess is most apparent in children (National Institute for Health and Clinical Excellence, 2002b). An estimated 0.7–0.8% of schoolchildren are epileptic, equivalent to over 50 000 children in England and Wales. Epilepsy can be idiopathic (primary) or symptomatic (secondary) and can present as generalised or partial seizures. Until recently epilepsy in childhood was considered to be a progressive disorder, which required early treatment. This concept began to be questioned in 1997 with research findings that suggested that children may grow out of epilepsy, or that their convulsions decrease in frequency without treatment (Van Donselaar *et al.*, 1997). The National Institute for Health and Clinical Excellence (2002b) states that most children have a good prognosis, with 65–70% of affected children being able to be seizure free for 1–2

Table 45.2 Types of epilepsy

Type of seizure	Description
Generalised	Seizures which occur simultaneously in both cerebral hemispheres and cause a brief loss of consciousness at onset
Absence	Brief losses of consciousness lasting only seconds; onset and completion are sudden and the affected child may only appear to be briefly distracted
Myoclonic	Sudden, brief muscle contractions which result in sudden jerking movements of the limbs
Atonic	'Drop' attacks where the child suddenly loses muscle tone and falls to the ground
Tonic	Widespread muscle contraction which causes the child to fall to the ground due to muscle rigidity which prevents a coordinated posture
Clonic	Intense jerking movements of the limbs, trunk and facial muscles
Infantile spasms	Sudden repetitive limb flexion which causes the affected infant to fall backwards (Salaam attacks). Occurs in babies between the age of 3 and 12 months
Partial seizures	Seizures which arise in a specific area of the brain and therefore affect only one part of the body; ***simple partial (focal) seizures*** arise in the cerebral cortex and cause disturbances in sensation or movement without loss of consciousness; ***complex partial seizures*** cause impairment of conscious level, behaviour and memory
Secondary generalised	Partial seizures which develop into a generalised fit as the abnormal cerebral discharges spread from a localised area of the cortex to the subcortical areas of the brain

years with a single drug. However, up to 30% of children develop refractory epilepsy and require a combination of drugs, surgery or implants.

Epilepsy can be found with some types of acquired spastic cerebral palsy. Cerebral palsy (Table 45.3) is the most common permanent disability of childhood, although the degree of severity may vary from mild, when the child has impairment of only fine precision movements, to severe, when the child is unable to perform most of the daily activities of living independently. The incidence of cerebral palsy has risen by 20% since the 1960s and Bhushan *et al.* (1993) suggest that this increase is due to increased technology, which now enables the survival of very pre-term babies. Pre-term delivery is associated with a higher risk of cerebral palsy and Murphy *et al.* (1997) believe that an integrated approach to antenatal, intrapartum and neonatal care is the only way to reduce the incidence in these babies. They found that neonatal sepsis, pneumothorax and blood transfusion were all significantly associated with cerebral palsy, regardless of adverse factors antenatally and at delivery. It can also be acquired in association with meningitis or severe head injury.

Pre-term babies are also at risk from hydrocephalus as the result of intraventricular haemorrhage, but in most cases hydrocephalus results

Causes of epilepsy

In around 80% of cases the cause is unknown. In other cases, possible causes are as follows:

- malformations of the brain
- damage to the brain
    - infection
    - birth injury
    - head injury (associated with recovery for around 5% of children; Ghajar and Hariri, 1992)
    - brain surgery – post-operative complication
- cerebral tumours
- exposure to poisons
- low blood sugar
- low blood calcium
- meningitis/encephalitis

Table 45.3 Types of cerebral palsy

Type	Features
Spastic (50–60%)	Defect in the motor cortex of the pyramidal tract causes hypertonicity of certain muscle groups Hemiparesis is the most common form (30–40%), but quadriparesis is seen in 15–20% of children Hypertonicity causes poor posture, balance and coordination Unbalanced muscle tone predisposes to orthopaedic complications (scoliosis, contractures) Abnormal postures in movement and at rest Likely to include mental retardation
Dyskinetic (20–25%)	Defect of the extrapyramidal tract and basal ganglia causes uncontrollable movements of the affected muscle groups Athetosis (slow, writhing involuntary movements of the extremities) Stress may cause movements to become jerky or disordered Drooling and difficulty in speech can result from involvement of the pharyngeal, laryngeal and oral muscles Drooling may cause an increase in dental caries
Ataxic (1–10%)	Defect of the cerebellum impairs balance Wide-based gait Intention tremor Incoordination of gross and fine motor skills
Mixed type (15–40%)	Combination of spastic and athetosis

from congenital developmental defects, which cause obstruction to the flow of cerebrospinal fluid. Postnatal causes include cerebral tumours and infections or trauma.

Trauma in children often results in a head injury. The three major causes of head injuries in children are falls, road traffic accidents and bicycle accidents. Younger children are more prone to head injuries from falls and car accidents as their heads, which are relatively large and heavy compared with the rest of their bodies, tend to lead the fall. Valman (1993) reports that 40% of injuries at home to children under 5 years are due to falls. Great efforts have been made to promote the use of cycle helmets to prevent the number of head injuries in older children caused by bicycle accidents.

One of the complications of an open head injury is bacterial meningitis. Bacterial meningitis is considered to be a problem of childhood, with over 66% of cases occurring in children under 15 years of age and the peak incidence being between 3 and 12 months (Davies, 1996). The causative bacteria are also age related. Viral meningitis is less severe and the affected child usually recovers in 3–10 days without treatment. Certain predisposing factors appear to increase susceptibility to meningitis:

- maternal factors (premature rupture of membranes, maternal infection)
- immune deficiencies of the newborn
- pre-existing central nervous system anomalies
- open head injuries/neurosurgery
- upper respiratory tract infections before the development of acquired immunity

Bacterial meningitis – causative organisms

Neonates

- *Escherichia coli* and B streptococcus (acquired from maternal infection during birth or via umbilical cord or respiratory infection)
- *Listeria monocytogenes* – maternal listeria

>2 months

- *Haemophilus influenzae*, *Neisseria meningitidis* (meningococcus) and *Streptococcus pneumoniae* (pneumococcus) (droplet infection)

Rarer causes

- *Staphylococcus* – secondary to head wounds, upper respiratory tract infections
- *Mycobacterium tuberculosis* – primary TB or secondary to pulmonary TB

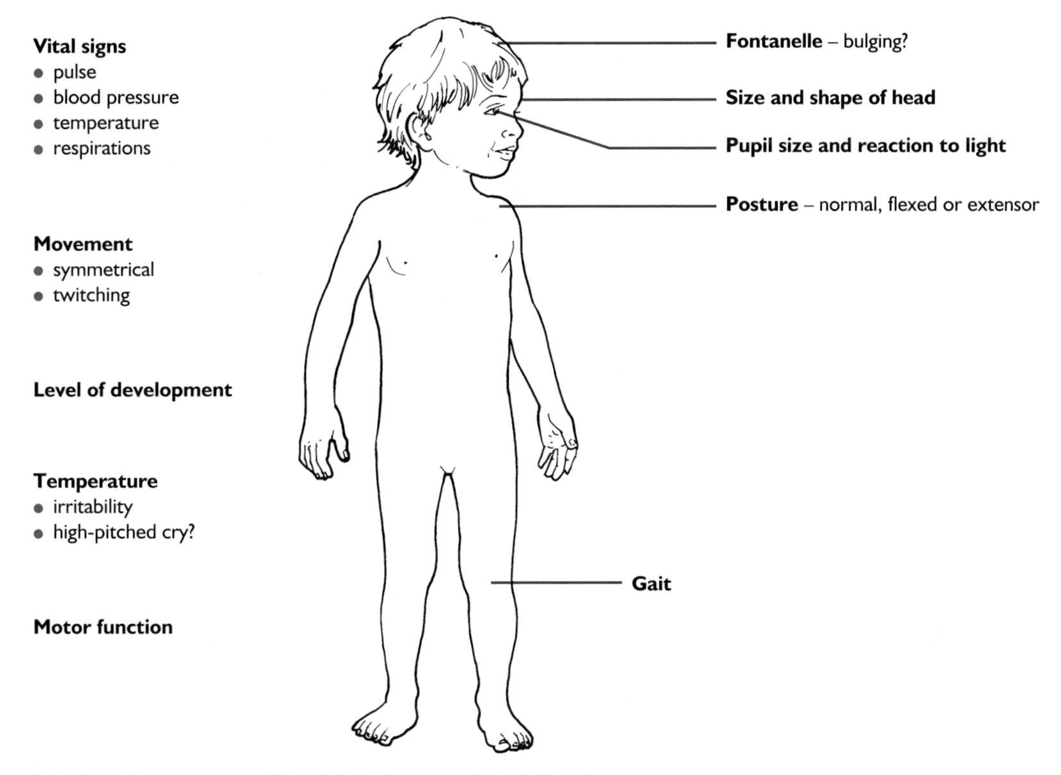

Figure 45.1 Specific assessment of the child with a neurological disorder.

Specific Assessment of the Child with a Neurological Disorder (Figure 45.1)

Specific neurological observations are important for almost any child with a neurological impairment. These observations include:

- level of consciousness
- pupil size and reaction to light
- vital signs
- motor function
- posture

(*See also* Assessment of consciousness level pp. 302–4.)

A decreasing level of consciousness is well known as an important initial sign of serious neurological damage. However, this is not always so in infants under 18 months of age. When the fontanelle is still open, any swelling of the brain, which would normally create raised intracranial pressure (ICP) and unconsciousness, can be accommodated by these open sutures, causing bulging of the fontanelle.

Assessing the level of consciousness in a child of any age is complicated by a child's lack of understanding and ability to respond appropriately to the common questions used to determine orientation to time and space. In addition, children commonly react to stressful situations by sleeping or non-communication (Reeves, 1989). The Glasgow Coma Scale (GCS) was introduced in 1974 by Teasdale and Jennet to meet clinical nurses' needs for a set of objective criteria to assess conscious level. The original scale was designed for use with adult patients and the need for an adapted version for children, which took account of the difficulties outlined above, was quickly recognised. In 1982 Simpson and Reilly produced a modification of the GCS for children. This recognised that young children may only verbalise by crying or making sounds other than recognisable speech. The type of cry is important to note, as raised ICP causes the young child to have a characteristic high-pitched cry. The modified GCS also accepted that fear may prevent a child from being able to demonstrate orientation. (See Figures 45.2 and 45.3; *see also* Neurological assessment pp. 513 and 302–4.)

The assessment of level of consciousness does not just involve verbal response but also eye opening and motor response, but these are also difficult to assess in young children. Assessment of children's pupil size and reaction to light is also complicated. Young children cannot always understand or obey the necessary instructions. Reeves (1989) suggests that nurses turn off the main lights and hand the child a pen torch. The natural response for most children is to turn the torch on and look at the light enabling the assessment to take place.

Study activity

Try out pupil assessment of healthy children and make a note of the normal pupil sizes and reactions in different lighting.

Motor responses are also impaired by immaturity. A 6-month-old baby has a best motor response of flexion whereas older children may obey commands and localise pain, although the ability to localise pain in preschool children is questionable. Frightened children may be unwilling and uncooperative to respond rather than unable to do so. Providing the child with appropriate toys and watching them play may prove a more successful way of assessing motor response than trying to push and prod the child.

Many authors recognise the importance of involving parents in the assessment of the level of consciousness. As Williams (1992) notes, parents' views are vital if an accurate assessment of the child is to be made. They should be asked about their child's:

- milestones in development
- language, hearing and visual abilities
- usual response to pain

The GCS is a useful predictor of outcome, and a score of 8 or less is generally accepted as a definition of coma and a sign of the severity of the neurological damage (Grewal and Sutcliffe, 1991). However, it should be remembered that it is not able to determine the responses of all children accurately. For example, a child with cerebral palsy may achieve a very low GCS because of physical inability rather than raised ICP. Together with the GCS score other neurological measurements are necessary to provide useful information about the site of involvement and the probable cause of the neurological damage. Changes in pulse

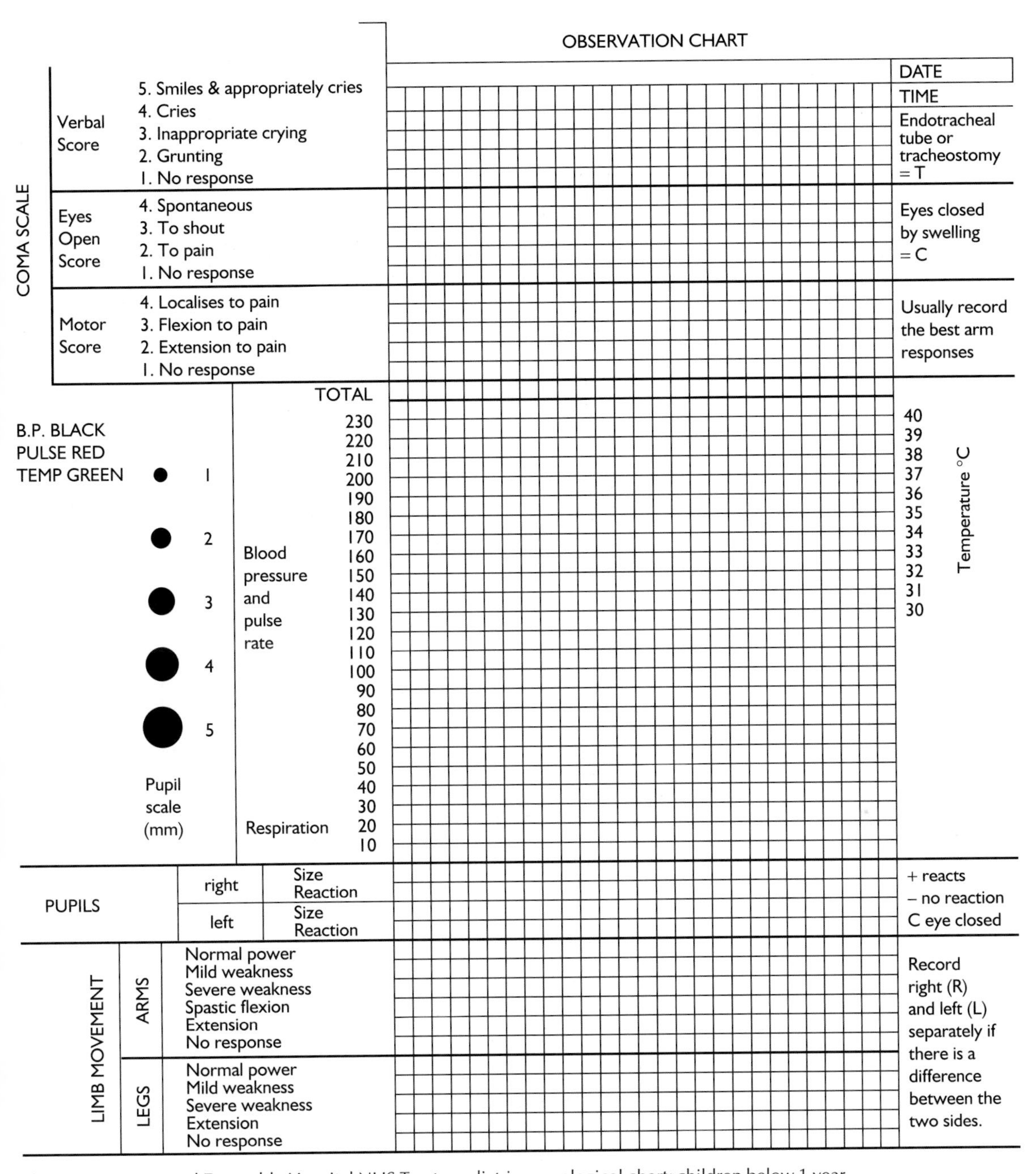

Figure 45.2 Luton and Dunstable Hospital NHS Trust paediatric neurological chart: children below 1 year.

and blood pressure are important indicators of disturbed autonomic activity that occurs in deep coma and brainstem lesions. The bradycardia and hypertension seen in adults in response to the inability of the cerebral arterial vessels to dilate further when the ICP is raised and maintain cerebral perfusion pressure, is rarely seen in children. When it occurs it is a very late sign. Respirations are slow and deep after seizures or in cerebral infections. Rapid, deep breathing may be the result of

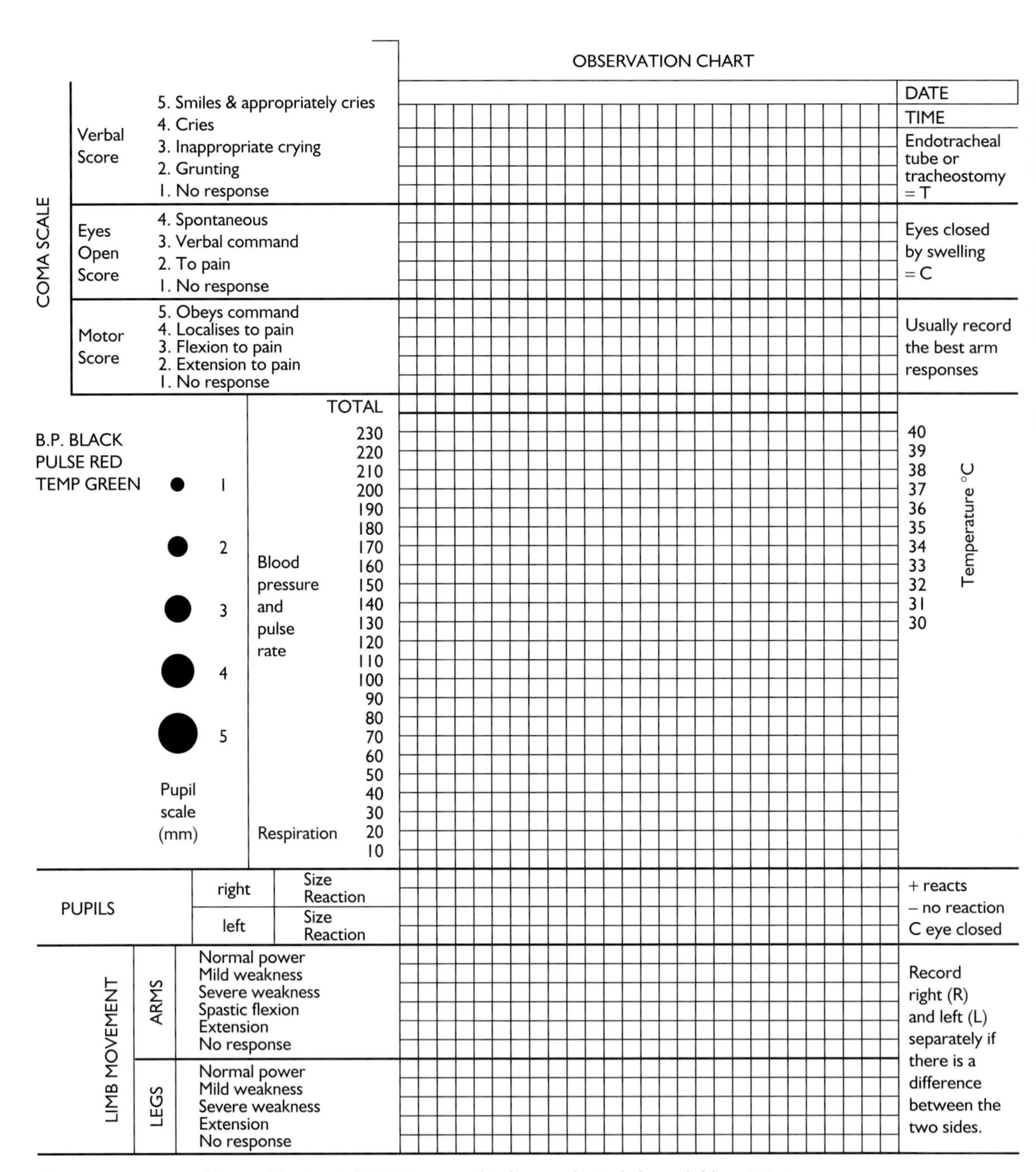

Figure 45.3 Luton and Dunstable Hospital NHS Trust paediatric neurological chart: children 1–2 years.

metabolic acidosis or poisoning. Damage to the brain stem usually produces irregular respirations. Hyperpyrexia, which is unresponsive to treatment, usually suggests a dysfunction of the hypothalamus.

Widely dilated and fixed pupils are indicative of paralysis of the oculomotor nerve due to pressure from herniation of the brain through the tentorium (coning). When this occurs in one eye only, the cerebral lesion is likely to be on the same side. When both eyes are affected,

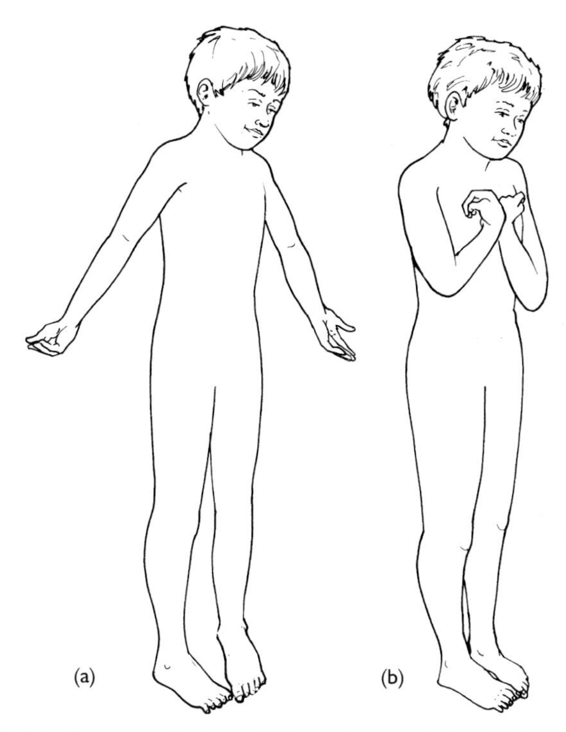

Figure 45.4 Primitive postural reflexes: (a) decerebrate posturing; (b) decorticate posturing.

brainstem damage is likely. However, such things as mydriatic drops, poisons and hypothermia also cause dilated, unresponsive pupils and a pre-existing strabismus also complicates accurate assessment.

Asymmetric movement or absence of movement suggests paralysis and dysfunction of the motor cortex or nerve pathway. Muscle tone may be flaccid or rigid and muscle tremors or twitching may occur. This hyperactivity is more likely to occur in acute febrile and toxic states than in association with raised ICP. When dysfunction of the motor cortex occurs or nerve pathways are lost, primitive postural reflexes occur. These reflexes demonstrate an imbalance between the central stimulating and inhibiting influences upon motor function, enabling stronger muscles to overcome weaker ones. When the lesion affects the motor cortex in the cerebrum, decorticate posturing is seen (Figure 45.4). Bilateral decerebrate posturing may be caused by tentorial herniation. Care should be taken to ensure that true postural reflexes are seen and not merely a flexion or extension of one limb in response to pain.

Posturing is not always evident until the administration of painful stimuli. Nurses need to ensure that they explain the purpose of this activity to parents and that they do not use methods that can cause tissue damage or bruising. Allan and Culne-Seymour (1989) advocate the use of nail-bed pressure by pressing the side of a pencil or similar object onto the proximal nail-bed.

As with adults, children can often suffer from headache with raised ICP but they are less skilled at vocalising their distress. Reeves (1989) suggests that restless irritability, immobility or rubbing of the head may

Case history – neurological observations

Liam O'Donnell, aged 6, had been playing on a swing in the playground and fell. He sustained a scalp wound which bled profusely. His mother reported that he had been unrousable 'for a couple of minutes' and she had rung for an ambulance.

On admission to A&E

Liam is conscious and able to give his name, age and address to the triage nurse. His mother gives the details of the accident as above, also adding that 'the ground was covered with blood'. The ambulance paramedic reports no change in conscious level during the journey to hospital.

On examination

Liam says he has a headache which is worse over the site of the injury. He has a 4-inch laceration over the right parietal area and, on examination, a small artery can be seen spurting blood. The Casualty officer immediately ligates the vessel and Liam is admitted to the paediatric ward.

On admission to the ward

Liam appears quite lucid and rational although he is uncertain of events in A&E. He appears in pain but is trying to be brave. Both parents are now present. The admitting nurse notes that Liam:

- is of average weight for his age
- appears rather pale
- has rather large pupils which respond briskly to light
- has cool, moist peripheries
- demonstrates a strong grip with both hands and motor power in both legs appears normal
- has a regular pulse 100/min, BP 100/70, respirations 22/min

be indicators of headache in small children. Vomiting due to raised ICP, especially as a result of a head injury, tends to occur more frequently in children than in adults (Reeves, 1989).

Study activity

Read the case history 'neurological observations' and analyse the information you are given. Consider the significance of this information and the implications for the nurse.

Study activity

Find out what chart is used for neurological observations in your area of work and critically evaluate (a) its appropriateness for children and (b) its ease of use.

It is essential that, whichever neurological chart is used, all practitioners should be aware of the significance of the observations taken and that each assessment should be documented in a simple, objective and easily interpreted manner. This enables an easy comparison of previous and current findings, which is especially important when nurses are changing over shifts.

Study activity

Complete Table 45.4 to ensure you know the common neurological investigations performed and the nurse's role in these.

Nursing Interventions

Nursing interventions for children with neurological problems often include:

- care of the unconscious child
- management of seizures
- care of the child with meningitis
- management of an intraventricular shunt
- administration of drugs used in neurology

Care of the unconscious child

Study activity

Using Roper's activities of daily living, plan care for an unconscious child.

Particular problems in the care of the unconscious child may include ICP monitoring, management of pain and fluid balance. Intracranial

Table 45.4 Specific neurological investigations (copyright is waived for the purpose of photocopying and enlarging this table)

Investigation	What for and why?	Role of the nurse
Computerised axial tomography (CAT) scan		
Electroencephalogram (EEG)		
Fundoscopic examination		
Lumbar puncture		
Magnetic resonance imaging (MRI) scan		
Skull X-ray		
Subdural tap		
Ventricular tap		

pressure monitoring is an intensive care procedure that was introduced in the 1960s but its value is now beginning to be questioned. Reynolds (1992) suggests that such monitoring does not reflect the degree of the initial cerebral damage, which is the most important factor in determining outcome. Intracranial pressure may be measured in different ways and the nurse caring for the child needs to be able to understand the type of monitoring used and be able to analyse the monitor readings. Nursing interventions may need adaptation to avoid increasing ICP further (*see also* Care of the child confined to bed p. 367).

Intracranial pressure may be increased by pain but the use of analgesia or sedation can complicate the assessment of level of consciousness. Codeine phosphate (0.5–1 mg/kg/dose 4 to 6 hourly) can be useful in such situations. The assessment of pain in the unconscious child is in itself a skill.

Study activity

Consider how you could assess pain in an unconscious child.

Fluid and electrolyte balance is particularly crucial in the child with raised ICP. Osmotic diuretics such as mannitol 20% 1–2 g/kg may be used but should be administered slowly unless herniation is occurring. An indwelling urinary catheter is necessary to monitor the urine

Intracranial pressure monitoring

Types of monitors:

- intraventricular catheters
- subarachnoid bolt
- epidural sensor
- anterior fontanelle pressure monitor

Specific nursing care

Care
Elevate head of bed 30° and maintain head position in the midline

Rationale
Compression of the neck veins impairs venous return and increases ICP

Care
Avoid causing the child pain and administer appropriate pain relief

Rationale
Crying raises ICP

Care
Minimise environmental stimuli

Rationale
Stress increases ICP

Care
Plan care to avoid overstimulation of child

Rationale
Stress increases ICP

Care
Use pressure-relieving/decreasing devices

Rationale
Turning side to side may compress the neck veins

Care
Prevention of constipation with regular use of laxatives

Rationale
Straining at stools raises ICP

output and assess the diuretic response. Intravenous fluids are indicated initially for any unconscious child, but the volume should be carefully calculated to two-thirds normal maintenance intake to avoid aggravating any cerebral oedema. Other means of providing fluid and nutrition will be necessary if there has been no improvement in conscious level in 48 hours.

Management of seizures

Treatment of a febrile convulsion is usually related to the treatment of the underlying cause. Rectal diazepam may be administered if the seizure continues until medical intervention. Environmental measures to reduce the temperature (opening windows, use of a fan) should be used with care as they often induce shivering. Shivering maintains the pyrexia as it increases the metabolic rate and thus produces heat. Tepid sponging is no longer recommended because it tends to cause shivering and also does not significantly reduce the temperature (Camfield and Camfield, 1993). Probably the most effective treatment is the use of an antipyretic (paracetamol or ibuprofen), although this can be disputed (*see* Module 5).

Epileptic seizures are a feature rather than a disease and children with epilepsy should be encouraged to lead as normal a life as possible. One of the roles of the nurse caring for the child with epilepsy is to teach the child and family to recognise trigger factors and auras and manage the seizure so that the child's safety is maintained.

Study activity

Find out how to care for the epileptic child:

- who complains of an aura
- during the clonic–tonic phase of a seizure
- after the seizure

Generally a seizure is self-limiting and the child will recover spontaneously. The British Epilepsy Association (1995) suggests that in a first-aid situation an ambulance need only be called if:

- the child is not a known epileptic
- the seizure follows a head injury
- the child is injured during a seizure
- the seizure is continuous and shows no sign of stopping after 4 minutes

Status epilepticus is a seizure in which the tonic–clonic phase is continuous for 30 minutes or more, or in which the child does not regain consciousness between bouts of tonic–clonic activity for this length of time. NICE (2002) recommends the use of rectal diazepam 0.3–0.5 mg/kg or buccal midazolam for pre-hospital treatment. McIntyre *et al.* (2005) suggest that buccal midazolam is more effective than rectal diazepam for children with acute febrile and epileptic seizures and does not have the side-effect of respiratory depression. In hospital, treatment is directed at the maintenance of vital functions, sedation and anti-epileptic drugs (Figure 45.5).

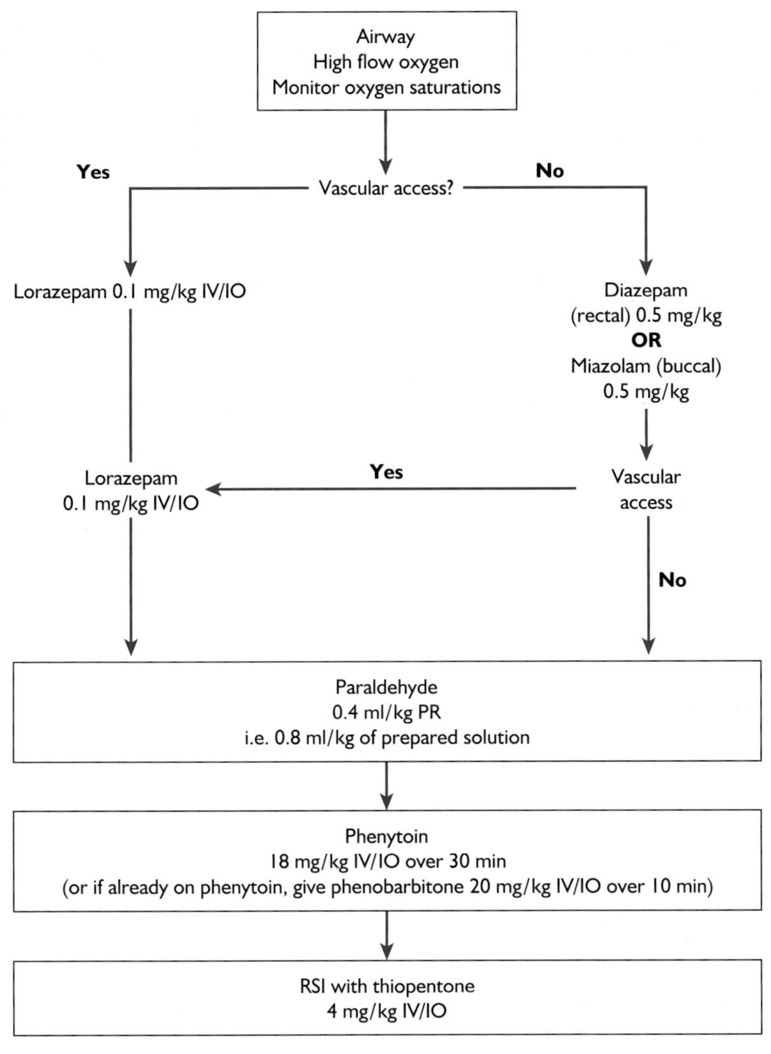

Figure 45.5 Status epilepticus algorithm (Advanced Life Support Group, 2005).

In most cases epilepsy can be controlled by medication but compliance and awareness of side-effects is crucial. To optimise this, the National Institute for Health and Clinical Excellence (2004a) recommend that any decision to start anti-epileptic drug treatment should only be made after a full discussion of the risks and benefits, taking into account the individual child's type of epilepsy, lifestyle and prognosis. Likewise, the decision to stop drug treatment, which may be possible after 2 years free of seizures, should be made jointly with the child and family. Any withdrawal of treatment should be carried out gradually over 2–3 months. For those children who are resistant to drug treatment, or as an adjunct to drugs, relaxation and cognitive behaviour therapy, vagus nerve stimulation and/or a ketogenic diet may be useful (National Institute for Health and Clinical Excellence, 2004a). Surgery is a relatively recent option for children who are drug resistant or suffer unacceptable side-effects of drug treatment and suffer repetitive uncontrollable seizures. Partial or full temporal lobectomy may benefit children whose lesions initiate in the temporal lobe and may prevent generalised seizures. Careful assessment is necessary to identify the children whose epilepsy is most likely to benefit from surgery, and the benefits of brain surgery must be weighed against the potential risks.

Study activity

Find out and make a list of the actual and potential problems after brain surgery.

Care of the child with meningitis

Meningitis is one complication of brain surgery but is more likely to be encountered as a childhood infection. It can be caused by a virus, a bacterium or a fungus. The three main causes of bacterial meningitis in the UK are:

- *Haemophilus influenzae* type B (Hib) – almost eradicated by the introduction of a Hib vaccine
- *Meningococcus* (in the UK groups B and C are the most common types)
- *Pneumococcus*

There is at present no vaccine for group B types of meningitis but the introduction of a vaccine for group C (MenC) in 1999 has significantly affected meningococcal disease. Prior to this vaccine meningitis C was the most common cause of meningococcal disease, accounting for about 1500 cases and with a 10% mortality. Currently, it accounts for fewer than 400 cases per year (DH, 2006). Group B disease now accounts for over 80% of cases. An improved childhood immunisation programme was introduced in 2006 to further improve protection against meningitis C and Hib.

As soon as meningitis is suspected the child should be hospitalised and a lumbar puncture performed unless the child shows features of raised ICP. If the child is shocked or has a petechial rash or if there is any suspicion of bacterial meningitis, the GP should start antibiotic treatment immediately with IV or IM benzyl penicillin (Markovitch, 1990). Cefotaxime is the treatment of choice once the diagnosis has been confirmed. IV dexamethasone 0.15 mg/kg, 6 hourly, for the first 4 days has been shown to hasten the reduction of meningeal inflammation (Schaad *et al.*, 1993) and to lessen the risk of permanent hearing impairment (Bhatt *et al.*, 1993).

Immunisation protection against meningitis

- Two months – pneumococcal vaccine*
- Three months – MenC vaccine*
- Four months – MenC plus pneumococcal vaccine*
- Twelve months – Hib/MenC
- Thirteen months – pneumococcal vaccine*

The most common side-effects are:

- Redness and swelling at the injection site (affects 2% to 4% of infants and toddlers)
- Mild fever (affects up to 5% of toddlers under 17 months)
- Irritability (affects up to 50% of infants, 19% of toddlers)
- Headaches

(DH, 2006)

* In addition to other routine vaccinations given at this time.

Study activity

Identify the specific nursing actions required to care for a child with bacterial meningitis (Table 45.5).

Bacterial meningitis may be the cause or effect of hydrocephalus. Hydrocephalus, or the accumulation of cerebrospinal fluid in the ventricles, can be the result of a congenital or acquired problem.

Table 45.5 Specific care of the child with bacterial meningitis (copyright is waived for the purpose of photocopying and enlarging this table)

Problem	Nursing action
Potential spread of infection to others in hospital and at home	
Altered conscious level due to raised ICP	
Pyrexial with cold, cyanosed peripheries due to septicaemic shock	
Potential development of: cerebral abscess ventriculitis hydrocephalus inappropriate anti-diuretic hormone secretion hearing loss motor or learning disability	
Unable to feed as usual due to alterations in conscious levels	

Drug treatment for bacterial meningitis

Neonates
3-week course of:

- cefotaxime
  100 mg/kg/24 hour
  12 hourly
- benzyl penicillin
  100 mg/kg/24 hour
  12 hourly
- gentamicin
  2.5 mg/kg/24 hour
  12–18 hourly

Infants and children
7–10 day course of:

- cefotaxime
  200 mg/kg/24 hourly

Prophylaxis for the immediate family
2–4 day course of:

- rifampicin
  5–10 mg/kg/12 hourly

Prophylaxis for other close contacts

- <6 years
  rifampicin 5–10 mg/kg × 1 dose
- 6–12 years
  ciprofloxacin 250 mg × 1 dose
- >12 years
  ciprofloxacin 500 mg × 1 dose

Maldevelopment of the central nervous system or maternal infection are the most common causes of congenital hydrocephalus. Causes of acquired hydrocephalus are infection, neoplasm or cerebral haemorrhage. When the accumulation of fluid occurs before closure of the fontanelles, the head enlarges as a result. If the accumulation is allowed to progress, the increasing ICP will eventually prevent brainstem functioning. The usual treatment is surgical removal of the ventricular obstruction or the insertion of a shunt to drain the excess fluid from the ventricles. A ventriculoperitoneal (VP) shunt is the preferred procedure for most children. The proximal end of the shunt is inserted into the lateral ventricle and the distal end is inserted into the peritoneal cavity. Although the insertion of a shunt significantly improves the survival rate of children with hydrocephalus, it may have complications and may not prevent mental retardation.

Management of an intraventricular shunt

Study activity

Look at the complications associated with shunts and consider how you would recognise these.

Complications of intraventricular shunts

Malfunction

- kinking of catheter
- plugging of catheter by tissue or exudate
- migration of tubing
- obstruction of the distal end of the catheter by thrombosis
- displacement of the distal end of the catheter due to growth

Infection

- septicaemia
- wound infection
- meningitis
- ventriculitis
- cerebral abscess
- peritonitis

Abdominal complications

- paralytic ileus
- perforation of abdominal organs at insertion of the shunt
- peritoneal fistulas

Administration of drugs used in neurology

Study activity

Identify the uses, usual dosages and side effects of the drugs used in neurology (Table 45.6).

Discharge Advice

Neurological problems such as head injury and meningitis can be prevented by good healthcare advice.

Study activity

Design two posters for your area of work to give parents advice about the prevention of:

- head injuries
- meningitis caused by *Listeria* or *Haemophilus influenzae* type B

Table 45.6 Medication used in neurology (copyright is waived for the purpose of photocopying and enlarging this table)

Drug	Dose/kg	Use	Side-effects
Carbamazepine			
Clonazepam			
Diazepam			
Gabapentin			
Lamotrigine			
Oxcarbazepine			
Paraldehyde			
Phenobarbitone			
Phenytoin			
Sodium valproate			
Tiagabine			
Topiramate			
Vigabatrin			

Febrile convulsions cannot always be prevented, but Miller (1996) suggests that parents need more information about the prevention and treatment of these seizures before they experience this traumatic and frightening event.

Study activity

Find out what information about febrile convulsions is available to parents in your area of work.

Families of children with epilepsy need information about the prevention of trigger factors and the management of the condition, as well as psychological support to help them overcome the prejudice others may have about this condition. The National Institute for Health and Clinical Excellence (2004a) states that health professionals have a responsibility to educate the public about epilepsy to reduce the stigma associated with it.

Study activity

- Look at the National Institute for Health and Clinical Excellence (2004a) guidelines for information to be given to the child and family with epilepsy. Find out what details are needed under each heading.
- Reflect on your first experience of witnessing a seizure and talk to some non-healthcare professionals about their perceptions of this condition. Talk to children with epilepsy and their families about others' reactions to their condition.
- Consider which day-to-day activities could pose risks for the child with epilepsy and the advice to be given in relation to them.

Information for children with epilepsy and their family and/or carers

- General information
  - What epilepsy is
  - Diagnosis
  - Reasons for tests, explanations of results
  - Seizure type
  - Prognosis
  - Sudden unexpected death in epilepsy (SUDEP)
  - Psychological issues
  - Managing risk
  - Self-care
- Seizures
  - Type(s)
  - Triggers
  - Control
- Treatment options
  - Anti-epileptic drugs – indications, side-effects, licence status
  - Action if dose missed or after a gastro-intestinal upset
  - Reasons for surgery
- Lifestyle
  - Independent living
  - Career options
  - Insurance issues
  - Driving
  - Alcohol
  - Recreational drugs
  - Sexual activity (and family planning if appropriate)
  - Sleep deprivation
- Safety
  - First aid
  - Safety in the home
  - Status epilepticus
  - Road safety
- Support
  - Support organisations and details
  - Claiming benefits
  - Support from social services

(National Institute for Health and Clinical Excellence, 2004a)

Useful address

Epilepsy Action
New Anstey House, Gate Way Drive, Yeadon, Leeds LS19 7XY
Tel: 0113 210 8800
Email: epilepsy@epilepsy.org.uk
Web site: http://www.epilepsy.org.uk (accessed 31 May 2006)

Chapter 46

Principles of Care – Children with Altered Breathing

Introduction

Acute problems affecting the respiratory tract are the most common cause of illness in infancy and childhood. Fifty per cent of illnesses in children under 5 years, and 30% of illnesses for children aged 5–12 years are due to respiratory problems. Respiratory problems can present as very mild illnesses, as the onset of chronic problems or can be life threatening. They can be the primary cause of the illness or they may occur as secondary complications to other problems. An adequate circulation relies upon an adequate oxygen intake, so they commonly affect the cardiovascular system.

Children are particularly prone to respiratory problems because of a number of differences between their respiratory tracts and those of adults.

The respiratory tract in children

Compared with the adult, the airway of the small child has:

- narrow nasal passages
- more anteriorly and cephalad positioned glottis
- longer epiglottis
- a 4 mm diameter larynx
- its narrowest portion at the level of the cricoid cartilage
- an upper airway which is funnel-shaped, pliable and may narrow with inspiration
- a very compliant chest wall
- increased resistance to airflow (16-fold) in the presence of 1 mm circumferential oedema
- a greater reduction (50%) in laryngeal radius in the presence of 1 mm oedema

Study activity

Test your knowledge of the structure and function of the respiratory system by answering the quiz overleaf. Check your answers with an anatomy and physiology textbook.

Common Disorders of the Respiratory Tract

Infection is the cause of most childhood respiratory disorders. The cause and the effect of the infection depends upon the individual child's age, medical history and environment. Most childhood respiratory infections (Table 46.1) are caused by viruses and tend to cause only a mild illness in older children but severe problems in the younger age group. The reason for this varied severity is partly due to the anatomical differences in the respiratory tract of the younger child but also to the older child's greater resistance to infection. Resistance to infection is influenced by

Table 46.1 Respiratory infections in children

Infection	Usual age range	Pathophysiology
Bronchiolitis	Infancy	Viral colonisation of the bronchiolar mucosa – spreads to bronchiolar epithelium causing necrosis of ciliated cells and proliferation of non-ciliated cells. Impaired clearance of secretions, increased mucus production and desquamation of cells leads to bronchiolar obstruction and lung collapse
Croup	6–36 months	Inflammation of the laryngeal and tracheal mucosa narrow the airways. The effort involved to inhale air past the obstruction causes an inspiratory stridor and sternal retractions. If air entry is insufficient, hypoxia will occur. Impaired exhalation of carbon dioxide will lead to respiratory acidosis and respiratory failure
Epiglottitis	2–5 years	Acute bacterial infection of the epiglottis and surrounding areas causing inflammation and swelling of the mucous membranes in this area which can completely obstruct the airway. Complete obstruction can be precipitated by stimulating the gag reflex by examination, manipulation or suctioning of the airway
Pneumonia	All ages	Inflammation of the pulmonary parenchyma, caused by viruses, bacteria, mycoplasmas and aspiration, involving: • lobar pneumonia – one or more lobes • bronchopneumonia – terminal bronchioles • interstitial pneumonia – within alveolar walls Inflammation impairs gaseous exchange and can lead to pulmonary effusion
Whooping cough	<4 years	The presence of *Bordetella pertussis* causes an inflammatory reaction in the mucosal lining of the upper airways. The bacteria adhere to the ciliated epithelial tissue in these areas inhibiting its function. As a result, cellular debris, mucus and pus collect and can cause plugging of the bronchial tree and necrosis of the bronchial epithelium. Stasis of secretions can lead to secondary infection. Paroxysms of severe coughing to expel secretions can increase ICP causing rupture of cerebral vessels, bradycardia, hypoxia and apnoea. If prolonged deprivation of oxygen occurs, permanent cerebral damage may result

the amount of lymphoid tissue, passive immunity developed by exposure to infective organisms, pre-existing chronic respiratory or cardiac problems, and the environment. Exposure to cigarette smoking by a child's main carer increases the likelihood of infection (Holberg *et al.*, 1993).

The most common of the chronic respiratory problems (Table 46.2) affecting children is asthma. Speight (1996) suggests that 20–25% of children will experience a significant degree of clinical asthma during childhood and that 5% of these will have frequent and severe problems, which will continue into adulthood. The cause of this increased incidence is debatable but it seems likely that environmental factors are implicated. Atmospheric pollution and home furnishings, which are favourable to the house dust mite, may be significant triggers. Hunt (1997) suggests that bronchodilator drugs used to treat asthma could be responsible for the rising incidence and severity of this condition.

Cystic fibrosis is the most common recessively inherited disease in the white population, affecting approximately 1 : 2500 (Davies, 1996). Although other organs are affected, the effects on the respiratory system are more likely to be the presenting feature and the cause of death. Ninety-five per cent of cystic fibrosis patients die from respiratory failure. Cystic fibrosis is due to various different mutations in the cystic fibrosis

Respiratory quiz

- Draw a diagram of the lower respiratory tract to identify the trachea, segmental bronchi, bronchioles and alveolar ducts.
- At what age do the lungs complete their development?
- Identify three conditions which can affect lung development.
- Explain the mechanism of inhalation and exhalation.
- How is respiration regulated?
- Identify the function of the following structures:
  - respiratory cilia
  - epiglottis
  - respiratory mucous membranes

Table 46.2 Chronic respiratory problems

Disorder	Pathophysiology
Bronchopulmonary dysplasia	Interstitial oedema and epithelial inflammation of the small airways results in fibrosis of the alveolar walls, reduced lung compliance, increased airway resistance and a severe reduction in expiration. This causes over-inflation and alveolar collapse leading to hypercapnia, and hypoxaemia. Chronic disease results in pulmonary hypertension and right sided heart failure
Cystic fibrosis	Thick viscous secretions predispose the individual to recurrent infections which cause chronic inflammation and oedema of the small airways. Excessive pooling of secretions leads to mucus plugging, increases the susceptibility to bacterial infections (*Staphylococcus aureus, Haemophilus influenzae* and *Pseudomonas aeruginosa*), and distorts the airways, causing bronchospasm and airway collapse. Abnormal secretions in other exocrine organs cause intestinal and bile duct obstruction, pancreatic enzyme deficiency, agenesis of the vas deferens. The primary defect causes elevated sodium and chloride levels
Asthma	Increased bronchoconstriction, oedema and hypersecretion of mucus occur in response to an allergen and result in narrowed resistant airways. Obstruction of exhalation causes wheezing, hyperinflation of the chest, air hunger and anxiety. Decreased ventilation causes insufficient oxygenation of blood

transmembrane regulator (CFTR) gene situated on chromosome 7. CFTR appears to function as a chloride channel and mutations affect chloride and sodium movement across epithelial cells, but it is still not clear how this affects the respiratory system (Koch and Hoiby, 1993).

Bronchopulmonary dysplasia (BPD) is a chronic iatrogenic respiratory disease that mainly affects babies who were born prematurely with lungs that were too immature to function independently. To support their inadequate respiratory function they are treated with high concentrations of oxygen and positive pressure ventilation. However, prolonged use of these treatments causes long-term pulmonary damage and many infants who survive are oxygen dependent, require repeated periods of hospitalisation and have increased susceptibility to respiratory infection (Northway *et al.*, 1990).

Factors affecting asthma

Allergic reactions:

- pollen, e.g. grass or birch
- animal fur or hair
- dust mites
- fungus

Triggers:

- cigarette or pipe smoke
- colds
- pollution and dust
- temperature change
- stress
- drugs such as beta blockers and aspirin-type pain relievers
- emotion, especially laughter
- exertion or exercise (however, this should not be avoided but encouraged, with asthma symptoms relieved by medication)

Effects of asthma

The National Asthma Campaign reported that asthma accounts for:

- 38% of schoolchildren missing more than 1 week from school per year
- 45% often missing physical education
- 34% staying indoors at break times
- 5% of all primary care consultations
- 14% of all hospital admissions for children

(National Asthma Campaign, 1999, 2002)

Assessment

Much information can be gained about a child's respiratory status merely by looking and listening (Figure 46.1). If the child is very distressed by the hospital environment, this is a useful method of assessment, allowing the nurse to make an immediate assessment of the severity of the child's condition and giving the child time to acclimatise to the situation. No observation is meaningful unless the nurse is

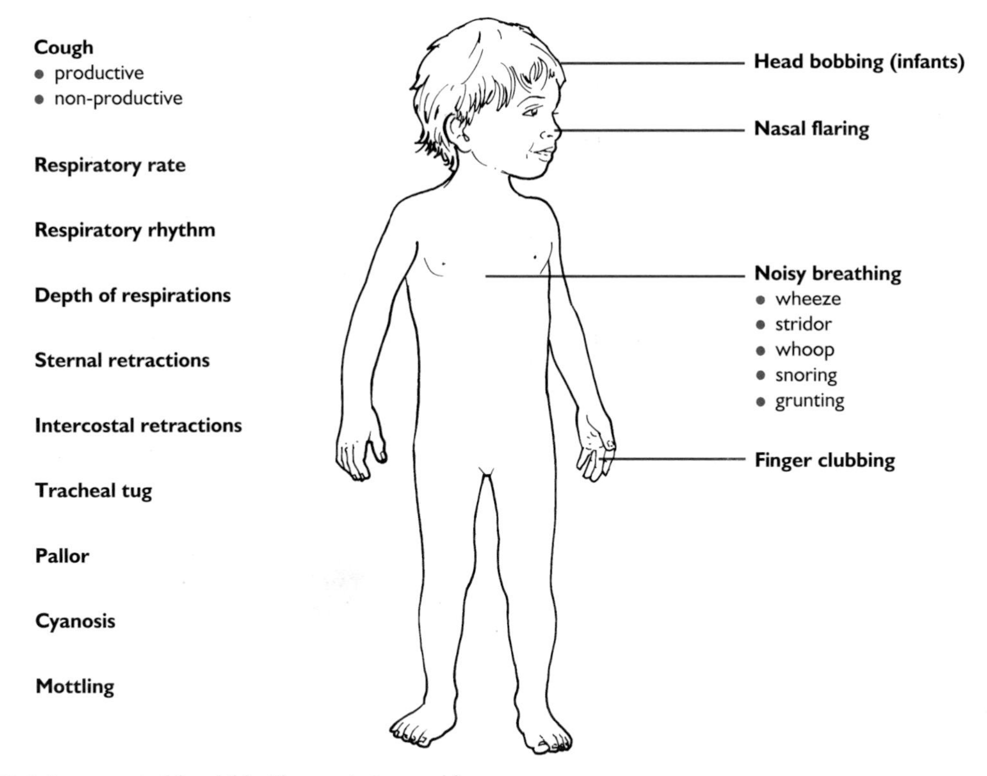

Figure 46.1 Assessment of the child with a respiratory problem.

aware of the normal parameters in children and the significance of any abnormalities (Table 46.3).

Older children may complain of chest pain related to respiratory disease. This pain may sometimes be referred to the abdomen, and abdominal pain can be the primary complaint of younger children with a respiratory problem. Infants often grunt to indicate chest pain, which is usually caused by inflammation of the pleura. Grunting can also be an indication of respiratory distress as it increases end-expiratory pressure prolonging the time available for alveolar exchange of oxygen and carbon dioxide (*see also* Normal respiratory rates p. 301 and Significance of respirations p. 284).

Accurate observations of children with respiratory problems enable the nurse to determine the most appropriate nursing interventions. The information provided by nursing observations may be enhanced by diagnostic tests. Table 46.4 details common medical investigations. An understanding of common diagnostic tests enables the nurse to appreciate their findings and also to help prepare and care for the child before, during and after the investigation. Some of these investigations (Table 46.5) are commonly performed by nurses. Pulse oximetry can be monitored at the bedside to give information about the need for, or the efficacy of, oxygen therapy. Although it can be measured intermittently, continuous monitoring will provide more information about the effect of activity upon oxygen consumption. Sensors should be covered to avoid ambient light interfering with the accuracy of the reading. The probe site should be changed every 4 hours to prevent pressure necrosis

Table 46.3 Blood gas analysis: normal values

Test	Normal value	Acidosis	Alkalosis
pH	7.35–7.45	<7.35	>7.45
pCO_2 (mmHg)	35–45	>45	<35
pO_2 (mmHg)	80–100	<80	>100
HCO_3 (mmHg)	22–26	<22	>26
Base	±2	More negative	More positive

Respiratory acidosis
Increased pCO_2, decreased pO_2 – caused by obstructive lung disease or hypoventilation

Respiratory alkalosis
Decreased pCO_2, increased pO_2 – caused by hypoxia or hyperventilation

Table 46.4 Medical investigations of the respiratory system (copyright is waived for the purpose of photocopying and enlarging this table)

Investigation	When and what for?	Role of the nurse
Pulmonary function tests spirometry peak flow		
Blood gas analysis		
Exercise tests		
Radiography CXR Ba swallow CT scan MRI scan		
Operative procedures bronchoscopy lung biopsy		
Sweat test		

Module 6

or burns from incompatible sensors and oximeters (Murphy *et al.*, 1990). Nurses should also be aware that using an extremity that is already being utilised for blood pressure monitoring or as the site for an arterial catheter will prevent the sensor from identifying pulsation and produce inaccurate readings. Movement of the child has the same effect, although with newer machines this is minimised.

Table 46.5 Nursing investigations

Capillary refill	Capillary refill is a quick and easy method for determining efficacy of respiratory function. A raised digit is pressed for 5 seconds and the time taken for blood to return to the area is estimated in seconds. A capillary rell time of over 2 seconds in a child (3 seconds in a neonate) is a sign of poor oxygenation
Oximetry	Determination of oxygen saturation (SaO_2) which can be a continuous or intermittent measurement. A light-emitting sensor and a photodetector are placed in an opposing position around a digit, hand, foot or earlobe. The diode emits red and infrared lights which pass through the skin to the photodetector. Oxyhaemoglobin absorbs more infrared light than deoxyhaemoglobin and a microprocessor measures the difference between the amount of absorption of red and infrared light and displays the percentage of oxyhaemoglobin
Peak expiratory flow rate (PEFR)	Peak flow measurement can be easily measured using a Wright's peak flow meter or a mini peak flow meter. Children can usually learn to use these from about 4 years. They need to be able to a take a deep breath and a fast and forced expiration. Peak flow rates are useful to monitor asthma and the efficacy of inhaled or nebulised medication. PEFRs vary with sex, age, height and race but a variation of up to 8% of normal values is acceptable
Naso-pharyngeal aspiration	Aspiration of the naso-pharynx is performed to identify the presence of respiratory syncytial virus (RSV) in infants with bronchiolitis

Study activity

Find out the rationale for using the investigations listed in Table 46.4 and determine the role of the nurse before, during and after each investigation.

Nursing Interventions

Specific nursing interventions which may be implemented for a child with a respiratory problem are:

- easing respiratory effort
- oxygen therapy
- chest physiotherapy
- administration of respiratory drugs
- care of chest drains

Easing respiratory effort is mainly achieved by ensuring maximum lung expansion. This is aided by positioning – breathless children will usually determine whichever position best enables them to breathe and the nurse can then use pillows to help them maintain this optimum position. Clothing and bedclothes should not constrict the neck or chest. Not only does this increase the child's comfort but it also makes observation of respiratory effort easier. Dyspnoea is a frightening symptom for both the child and the parents. For the child, the sympathetic nervous system reaction to fear leads to bronchodilation and an increased respiratory rate. This results in an increase in pCO_2 which produces bronchoconstriction and further breathlessness and panic. It is therefore important that the breathless child feels reassured by being treated in a calm and competent manner.

Oxygen therapy may be necessary to maximise respiratory efficiency (Table 46.6). Oxygen is a drug that should be prescribed by dose. Prolonged exposure to high percentages of oxygen causes complications and Higgins (1990) suggests that long periods of oxygen therapy above 50% should be avoided. Toxic effects include retrolental fibroplasia in premature neonates, lung collapse, increased destruction of red blood cells and carbon dioxide narcosis. Children with chronic respiratory disease are at risk from carbon dioxide narcosis, which occurs when they are given high percentages of oxygen. The principal respiratory stimulus for these children is a falling pO_2 (the hypoxic drive) because their diseased lungs and poor ventilation cause them to always retain carbon dioxide and to always be hypercapnic. High percentages of oxygen depress their respiration, leading eventually to unconsciousness and death. Oxygen may be given by a variety of methods, which all have their advantages and disadvantages (Table 46.6), but should ideally be accompanied by humidification. In health, the mucus-secreting cells of the naso-pharynx humidify the inhaled air and this process compensates for the loss of water, which occurs on expiration (Foss, 1990). This normal humidification process is often impaired in respiratory disease and added gas will exacerbate the dehydration of mucous membranes and pulmonary secretions. The method used for oxygen therapy should also suit the child. A method that distresses the child and causes crying will only cause further respiratory distress and it may be more effective to nurse the child sitting on a parent's lap with the oxygen administered through a funnel held as close to the child's nose and mouth as possible.

Table 46.6 The administration of oxygen

Method	Advantages	Disadvantages
Headbox	Delivery of high O_2% possible Enables observation of chest and control of O_2 concentration	High humidity – condensation can obscure child Needs removal to give most care Can rub infant's chin or shoulder
Nasal cannula	Enables care to continue Facilitates observation Ideal for low flow oxygen	Not always well tolerated Cannot attach to humidity Cannot give high flows of oxygen Difficult to control O_2 concentration
Oxygen masks	Different sizes available Known O_2 concentration	Not well tolerated by children Discomfort Interferes with talking and eating

Chest physiotherapy aims to remove retained bronchopulmonary secretions, reduces the airway obstruction and reinflates the areas of lung collapse caused by the excess secretions. It therefore improves ventilation and reduces the effort of breathing. The techniques of chest physiotherapy include:

- positioning
- postural drainage
- chest percussion
- chest vibrations
- manual hyperinflation
- breathing exercises

Study activity

Arrange to join a physiotherapist performing chest physiotherapy. Identify each of the techniques listed above, giving the rationale for each.

Children with cystic fibrosis must incorporate airway clearance methods into their lifestyle. Mechanical devices to aid this have been introduced to allow the older child more independence (George *et al.*, 2002). One such device is the positive expiratory pressure (PEP) mask, which helps to loosen secretions. Huffing and coughing can then be performed.

Study activity

Find a child with cystic fibrosis and find out the child's routine for chest physiotherapy. Reflect on the impact this has on his or her day-to-day activities.

In certain conditions chest physiotherapy may be inappropriate. Infants with acute bronchiolitis usually only have increased secretions in their upper airways, which is best managed by humidified oxygen and naso-pharyngeal suction (Prasad and Hussey, 1995). Chest physiotherapy may further impair respiratory embarrassment due to severe bronchospasm and is best avoided unless mucus plugging is evident. Inhaled foreign bodies are best removed by bronchoscopy; chest physiotherapy may only cause the object to move into a central airway or into the larynx, with disastrous results (Phelan *et al.*, 1990).

Medications for respiratory problems are often given by inhalation via inhalers or nebulisers. Common medications include bronchodilators, anticholinergics and anti-inflammatory agents, including corticosteroids (Table 46.7). While bronchodilators are useful for a range of respiratory problems, it is only children over 2 years who respond to such treatment. Only 50% of wheezy infants react to bronchodilators. Anticholinergics such as ipratropium bromide, which cause less hypoxaemia in young children, are recommended for children under 2 years (Wilson, 1996).

Table 46.7 Common repiratory medications (copyright is waived for the purpose of photocopying and enlarging this table)

Medication	Use	Route	Dose/kg	Side-effects
Bronchodilators salbutamol terbutaline salmeterol				
Anticholinergics ipratropium bromide				
Methylxanthines aminophylline				
Anti-inflammatory agents sodium cromoglycate prednisolone hydrocortisone				
Mucolytics rhDNase				
Virostatic Ribavirin				

The British Thoracic Society (1993) recommends the use of a 4- to 6-week course of cromoglycate as the primary anti-inflammatory treatment for asthma, and that steroids should only be given if this has no effect. Speight (1996) reports that 80% of GPs do not follow these recommendations and prescribe steroids straight away. There are concerns about children using inhaled steroids on a long-term basis, with fears about adrenal suppression, stunted growth and inhibition of normal lung development in preschool children. Speight (1996) indicates that the efficacy of inhaled steroids outweighs these potential and unproven complications. He suggests that asthmatic children are given steroids in doses which are high enough to control their asthma and administered via a spacer device to enhance lung deposition and to reduce the risk of systemic absorption. He also promotes a 'crash course' of oral steroids (prednisolone 1–2 mg/kg for 3–5 days) for acute episodes for children over 18 months. There is no evidence that such treatment is effective for children under this age (Wright, 1991). Prophylactic prednisolone 10 mg daily may also be useful to cover short periods such as holidays or examination times when an acute attack would be a major inconvenience (Speight, 1996).

Nebulised steroids in the form of budesonide have recently been found to improve the symptoms of children with severe croup, improving their symptoms in 2 hours and reducing their length of stay in hospital by one-third (Godden *et al.*, 1997).

Recent evidence shows that ibuprofen, a non-steroidal anti-inflammatory drug, given orally twice daily, provides a significant reduction in deterioration of lung function for children with cystic fibrosis (Konstan *et al.*, 1995) (but ibuprofen cannot be given to asthmatic children). Another relatively new treatment for cystic fibrosis, human recombinant DNase alpha (rhDNase) was introduced in 1994. RhDNase, administered via a nebuliser, breaks down the DNA strands in the respiratory secretions, thus reducing their viscosity, and has been shown to improve lung function and general health as well as reducing bacterial colonisation of the lungs (Scott, 1994).

Another relatively new medication is ribavirin, which is recommended by the American Academy of Pediatrics (AAP) for certain infants with respiratory syncytial virus bronchiolitis (American Academy of Pediatrics, 1993). Although it is used in some parts of the UK, not all British paediatricians are convinced that this is a beneficial treatment, and Rakshi and Couriel (1994) suggest that the cost and uncertain efficacy of ribavirin do not recommend it as the treatment of choice. However, they also recognise that there is no current evidence that any treatment reduces the severity or duration of viral bronchiolitis.

Study activity

Find out the uses, dosages/kg, routes of administration and side-effects of the common respiratory medications listed in Table 46.7.

Care of chest drains is a very specific intervention for children with respiratory disorders. Chest drains are inserted into the pleural or mediastinal space to drain air and/or fluid from a:

- pneumothorax
- haemothorax
- chylothorax
- empyema
- pleural effusion

Since interpleural pressure is normally subatmospheric, drainage of this space requires a special collecting system, which uses an underwater seal. For drainage to occur, the pressure in the collecting chamber must always be lower than the pressure in the interpleural or mediastinal space. This is achieved by the creation of a water seal in the collection chamber and the distal end of the chest tube is submerged in at least 2 cm of water. Increased amounts of water increase the resistance to drainage from the chest. Disposable chest drainage units are now common, which incorporate the collection chamber, water seal chamber and a suction control chamber in a closed system. Suction will facilitate drainage of viscous fluid. To ensure the drainage system is properly functioning the nurse should observe:

- the child for respiratory distress
- the chest drain for bubbling and fluctuation of water during respiration
- the quantity and appearance of drainage

Management of chest drains

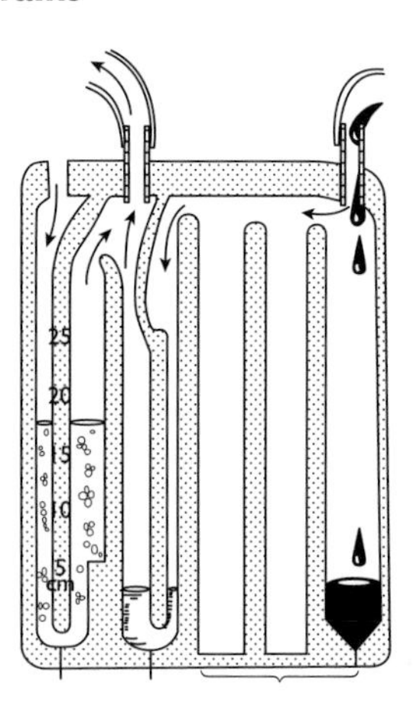

In the diagram above, identify the:

- water seal
- attachment to the child
- attachment for suction
- collection chamber

What fluid is put into chest drainage systems in your hospital?

Why is this fluid chosen?

How much fluid is put in?

Why does the nurse need to know how much fluid is in the system?

Which is more important and why? To have:

- a standard amount of fluid in the system?
- enough fluid to cover the end of the drainage tube?

What should you do if the chest drain:

- slips out of the child?
- becomes disconnected?

What is your hospital policy about clamping chest drains?

Table 46.8 Problem solving for the management of chest drains

Problem	Significance	Action
Cessation of drainage	Pressure on chest drain tubing may impede drainage	Check, straighten and secure tubing
No fluctuation of water	Re-expansion of the lung Tubing obstructed Tubing kinked Failure of suction	Chest X-ray to confirm Ask child to cough Dislodge clots or fibrin by 'milking' tubing Check, straighten and secure tubing Check connections
Constant bubbling	Air leak	Clamp drain close to chest wall – if bubbling stops, air leak is below chest level. If it continues leak is in pleural space – unclamp and call doctor
Child in respiratory distress	Tension pneumothorax	Report to doctor

Study activity

Study the box 'Management of chest drains' and answer the questions about the care related to chest drainage.

Two chest drain clamps should be kept at the child's bedside at all times in case of need. Hospital policies vary about their routine use. Some units advise clamping whenever the child is moved, while others believe that this routine clamping delays healing. However, if staff are unused to caring for chest drains, this may be the safer policy.

When the level of the water in the drain stops fluctuating the lung has probably re-expanded. A chest X-ray is taken to confirm this and the drain is then removed. The chest drain is stitched in place with a 'purse-string' suture. Following administration of analgesia it is removed by two nurses as one person is required to pull the suture tight while the other removes the tube to avoid air entry and tension pneumothorax from occurring. Older children can be asked to breathe in and hold their breath at the point of removal of the drain. This minimises the risk of air entry (Table 46.8).

Education for Discharge

Active involvement of asthmatic children and their families in the management of asthma seems not only to improve parental knowledge, skills and confidence, but also results in a significant reduction in the severity and frequency of acute attacks (Ramsay, 1994). Speight (1996) suggests that all families of asthmatic children should have a crisis pack of information and drugs to help them recognise and manage an acute attack. He found that 80% of childhood deaths (80–100 per year) could have been prevented by such a strategy. Harrop (2002) describes how self-management plans for children with asthma demonstrate positive results, but Price and Wolfe (2000) estimate that only 6% of families with asthma receive these plans. They give three possible reasons for this: lack of time, complicated plans and inappropriate plans. Harrop (2002) stresses the need for the active participation of the child and family in choosing a self-management plan if it is to be effective.

It seems appropriate that children and families living with chronic disorders are empowered in this way. The importance of this was highlighted on World Asthma Day in 2004 when *Living on a Knife Edge* (Asthma UK, 2004) was launched. This document explores the reality of living with asthma and promotes the philosophy that children with asthma should be able to live a normal life without symptoms. Module 4, Chapter 19 (pages 216–223) discussed how coping skills are enhanced by improved understanding of the problem.

Study activity

Find out what written information is available for children with asthma or cystic fibrosis and their families. Consider the helpfulness of this advice for managing acute problems.

Some children with chronic respiratory problems are oxygen dependent. Home oxygen therapy can promote family relationships and normal child development. It minimises healthcare costs and hospital-acquired infection, but it requires careful preparation and education. Usually certain criteria need to be met before discharge:

- child must tolerate nasal cannula
- infants must be feeding well and gaining weight
- O_2 requirements must be stable at 30% or below
- absence of other medical problems requiring medical treatment
- adequate community support, housing and telephone
- willing and able parents

Because oxygen supports combustion, it may be appropriate for parents to inform their insurance company and the fire brigade of the presence of oxygen in the home. An oxygen concentrator, which fits unobtrusively in the home, can manufacture oxygen from room air and eliminates the needs for the storage and delivery of bulky oxygen cylinders. It usually has two outlet points and ample tubing to maximise the child's mobility.

Benefits of self-management plans for children with asthma

- Improved quality of life
- Reduced morbidity and mortality
- Less frequent attacks
- Fewer GP/practice nurse/specialist consultations
- Decreased A&E attendances
- Fewer school absences
- Reduced cost to NHS services
- Empowers the child and family to take control of the disease
- Increases patient understanding of the disease and treatment

(Harrop, 2002)

Home oxygen therapy: parental teaching

- Changing nasal cannula
- Care of oxygen and cylinder
- Care of oxygen concentrator
- Setting up of low flow meter
- Discussion of anxieties
- Use of apnoea monitor*
- Recognition of hypoxia and appropriate action*
- Resuscitation*

* For parents of infants with bronchopulmonary dysplasia

Chapter 47

Principles of Care – Children with Skin Disorders

Introduction

Skin rashes and problems are common during childhood. They are rarely life threatening but they cause much physical and psychological distress for the affected child. Many conditions cannot be cured and their treatment is sometimes as psychologically upsetting as the disorders themselves. Parents are often embarrassed at their children's appearance and may be wrongly accused of not maintaining good standards of hygiene. Children's nurses need to be able to offer support and advice to parents and children that will overcome this teasing and these accusations by others. Lay people often shun children with obvious skin problems, believing all skin problems to be infectious. Nurses need to counteract this behaviour by always showing a positive acceptance of the child's appearance, while always remembering that some skin disorders are infectious or can be transmitted to other children and taking the necessary precautions against such transmission.

To recognise and care for skin disorders appropriately, nurses need to understand how the normal structure and function of the skin are impaired by various intrinsic and extrinsic factors.

The structure and function of the skin

Give five functions of the skin.

Explain how the skin helps to regulate body temperature. How does this differ in children?

Differentiate between the layers of the epidermis:

- stratum corneum (horny layer)
- stratum granulosum (granular layer)
- stratum spinosum (prickle cell layer)
- stratum basale (basal layer)
- stratum lucidum

What is the average life cycle for epidermal cells?

In which layer of skin do the hair follicles, sweat glands, nerves, lymph and blood vessels originate?

Where are the sebaceous glands found and what is their function?

Study activity

Test your knowledge of the structure and function of the skin by answering the questions in the box. Check your answers with an anatomy and physiology textbook.

Common Skin Disorders

Common skin disorders can be classified into problems in infancy, chronic disorders, infections and infestations of the skin (Tables 47.1 to 47.4). Chronic disorders include eczema, which has many causes

Table 47.1 Skin problems in infancy

Problem	Description
Milia	Distended sebaceous glands that appear as tiny white papules around the nose. They do not cause symptoms and disappear spontaneously
Mongolian spots	Irregular areas of deep blue pigmentation usually in the sacral and glutteal regions found in babies of African, or Asian origin. Can be mistaken for bruising
Congenital capillary malformations: port-wine stain	Flat, pink, red or purple 'stains' of the skin which often enlarge, thicken and darken as the child grows. The depth of colour varies according to whether superficial, middle or deep dermal vessels are involved. Goldman *et al.* (1993) recommend laser therapy to treat or minimise this deformity
Haemangiomas	Benign tumours consisting of closely packed small blood vessels which are sometimes apparent at birth or become noticeable within the first weeks of life ('strawberry mark'). They tend to enlarge during the first year of life and then resolve spontaneously
Cavernous haemangiomas	A less common type of birthmark. This benign capillary tumour has a soft spongy consistency and because of its fragility, which increases as it grows, it carries the risk of haemorrhage should injury occur. Early treatment by irradiation, surgery or injection of a sclerosing agent is recommended
Seborrhoeic eczema	Thick, adherent, yellowish, scaly and oily patches which usually appear within 2–8 weeks after birth. It mostly affects the scalp ('cradle cap'). Spowart (1995) indicates that the aetiology of this type of eczema is not well understood. Because the scalp has many sebaceous glands, it is thought to relate to a dysfunction of these glands. Although unsightly, this type of eczema does not disturb the baby and usually clears spontaneously within 3–4 weeks. Thick scaling can be relieved by the daily use of coconut or arachis oil massaged into the scalp followed by washing with a mild baby shampoo

Table 47.2 Common skin disorders of childhood

Disorder	Pathophysiology
Eczema	An inflammatory response of the epidermis which may be an innate response or a reaction to an external irritant. Erythema occurs and the burning sensations cause severe itching. Intercellular and intracellular oedema results in the formation of small vesicles and papules. The vesicles erupt and can become secondarily infected, especially if the skin is broken by scratching. Constant scratching produces dry, leathery and thickened skin which tends to exacerbate the irritation
Psoriasis	A familial loss of control of epidermal cells which causes epidermal hyperplasia and a rapid cell cycle of 37.5 hours as opposed to the normal 28 days. This results in thick scaly plaques of skin. The blood supply to the dermis is increased by the dilated capillaries causing marked erythema when the scales are shed
Acne	The formation of an excessive amount of sebum occurs as the result of increased androgen production in adolescence which stimulates the growth of the sebaceous glands and follicles. Alteration in the follicular lining prevents the excretion of sebum which accumulates and stagnates to form non-inflamed comedones or inflamed lesions which rupture to form papules, pustules, nodules and cysts

and can affect any age group. Eczema and dermatitis, which are interchangeable terms, may be caused by endogenous or exogenous factors or develop secondary to other disorders. One of the most common forms in children under 11 years (Kemp, 1999) is atopic eczema, which affects about 5% of the population (National Eczema Society, 2003). This form of eczema is an immunologically determined genetic disorder, often associated with asthma and hay fever, and its incidence appears to be increasing in the Western world (British Association of Dermatologists, 2005). The first clinical signs of atopic eczema usually

Table 47.3 Common skin infections of childhood

Disorder	Pathophysiology
Impetigo contagiosa	Bacterial infection caused by Gram-positive cocci causes an inflammatory epidermal reaction resulting in a papular erythema. This progresses into vesicles which weep seropurulent fluid and form yellow crusts
Herpes simplex	Type I herpes simplex virus causes inflammation of the epidermal cells which become inflamed and blistered
Verruca (warts)	Human papillomavirus causes epidermal inflammation and the epithelial cells react by proliferations
Tinea capitis	Fungal infection of the scalp. The fungus excretes an enzyme which digests the keratin of the hair. The dissolved hair breaks off to form the characteristic round areas of itchy, scaly skin or alopecia
Tinea corporis	Fungal infection which invades the stratum corneum layer of the skin of the body. The stratum corneum is dissolved by the action of the fungus and round or oval patches of erythematous scaly skin occur
Tinea pedis (athlete's foot)	Fungal infection of the feet involving the soles or between the toes. The dissolved stratum corneum in these areas causes itchy vesicles on the soles of the feet and maceration and cracking between the toes
Candidiasis (thrush)	The yeast-like fungus, *Candida albicans,* can affect the mouth or nappy area. In the mouth it causes white adherent patches on the tongue, palate and inner aspects of the cheeks. Infection of the warm, moist nappy area which encourages the infection, produces acute inflammation and redness. White patches may be visible in the genital area
Cellulitis	Inflammation of the skin and subcutaneous tissues from a staphylococcal or streptococcal infection often gained from a puncture wound which is no longer visible. Causes redness and swelling of the site, enlarged adjacent lymph nodes, pyrexia and malaise

Table 47.4 Common skin infestations of childhood

Infestation	Pathophysiology
Scabies	The scabies mite burrows into the stratum corneum of the epidermis usually in intertriginous areas. The affected child becomes sensitised to the mite and this initiates an allergic inflammatory response. As a result itching, redness and a papular, vesicular rash occurs around the area of burrowing
Pediculosis capitis (head lice)	The female head louse lays her eggs at the junction of the hair shaft and the skin and feeds by sucking blood from the host. The crawling insect and its saliva causes itching and scratching may cause secondary infection. The eggs (nits) may be visible as white areas attached to the hair shaft

occur between 3 and 6 months of age and are found on the cheeks. Flexural lesions appear within the next year. Acute exacerbations may be precipitated by secondary bacterial or viral infections. Children with atopic eczema seem particularly susceptible to virus infections, and staphylococci or streptococci infections are often caused by scratching. Childhood eczema can be very distressing for the child and parents, although its prognosis is usually good. Fifty per cent of children usually recover by the age of 6 years and 80% by the age of 10 years, but the years when the disorder is present are characterised by a miserable child who has severe itching and is constantly scratching, causing skin damage and bleeding. These areas heal to form crusts, which crack during movement causing further soreness and bleeding. The child cannot sleep because of itching and discomfort and the parents are unable to provide lasting relief. Often children with eczema fail to thrive because of protein loss from their inflamed skin, loss of sleep and poor appetite or restricted diet (Donald, 1995). Restricted diets are only recommended as the last line of treatment because results are disappointing and because of the risk of nutritional and growth problems. A strong family history of atopy, age of onset over 2 years and involvement of extensor skin surfaces are thought to be indicators of a prolonged disorder. Frank (1987) gives a harrowing account of the torture of incessant itching, the damage and disfigurement caused by constant scratching and the messy, repugnant treatments that plagued her childhood and early adulthood.

Nappy rash or dermatitis is a type of exogenous eczema, which is probably the most common skin disorder of childhood. The skin in this area can be in prolonged occlusive contact with urine and faeces. The warm, moist environment causes maceration of the skin and encourages bacterial conversion of the urine to ammonia. Ammonia is an alkaline irritant, which then produces a contact dermatitis reaction. Secondary infection can easily occur.

Study activity

How would you advise new parents about the prevention of nappy rash?

Psoriasis is thought to be due to hormonal and immunological factors as well as dermal factors (Buxton, 1993). It can appear at any age but usually presents during adolescence and affects about 2% of the population. It is very variable in its duration and course. In some individuals it may only affect knees and elbows, whereas others have widespread lesions. It appears to be a genetic tendency that can be triggered by injury, throat infections, certain drugs, and both physical and mental stress. Stress is often cited as a possible cause for skin disorders but this has to be considered carefully as stress is also an effect of skin disorders. Severe psoriasis is unsightly and leaves a trail of scales wherever the affected person has been. Ann, aged 10 years, was very depressed because no-one would sit next to her at school in case her psoriatic scales fell on them. She never wore skirts or short-sleeved shirts or dresses, so she could keep the affected parts out of sight. (The one advantage of psoriasis is that it rarely affects the face.) Craig, aged 14,

Types of childhood eczema

Endogenous eczema

- atopic eczema – flexural eczema associated with a familial tendency to hay fever, asthma or eczema
- discoid eczema – chronic oval or round areas of erythematous, itchy, and vesicular or dry and scaly skin; more common in coloured children than those of white origin
- seborrhoeic eczema – occurs in sites of increased sebaceous activity; commonly found on infants' scalps but can also affect any of the body folds in later life

Exogenous eczema

- irritant contact dermatitis – inflammation of the skin in response to an external irritant (e.g. nappy rash)
- allergic contact dermatitis – eczema arising from sensitivity to nickel, chrome, chemicals and medicaments; uncommon in children
- photodermatitis – an interaction of light and chemicals absorbed by the skin (e.g. drugs such as sulphonamides, cosmetics, chemical substances)

Secondary eczema

- lichen simplex (neurodermatitis) – areas of eczema that seem to appear secondary to itching. Often preceded by an insect bite or minor trauma which causes irritation. Persistent scratching damages the skin to produce redness, scaling and thickening. Rare in children
- pompholyx – intensely itchy vesicular lesions which occur on the palms and soles and between digits which occurs secondary to dysfunction of the eccrine sweat glands

Types of psoriasis

Guttate psoriasis

- widespread lesions are a few millimetres in diameter
- common in children
- often develops following an infection, especially a streptococcal sore throat

Plaque psoriasis

- commonest form of psoriasis
- coin-shaped and well-defined lesions all over the body
- scalp is also often affected

Flexural psoriasis

- confined to body folds
- erythematous inflammatory reaction which is often macerated and fissured at the centre
- no scaling

Pustular psoriasis

- lesions form pustules
- commonly affects palms and soles
- generalised type is very rare and causes an acute systemic illness

Psoriasis of the nails

- affects about 50% of individuals with psoriasis
- nails become thick and porous
- nail can detach from nail bed

Psoriatic arthritis

- seronegative arthropathy of the non-rheumatic type
- double normal incidence (2%) in individuals with psoriasis (Buxton, 1993)
- commonly involves distal interphalangeal joints
- familial psoriatic trait in 40% of those affected (Buxton, 1993)

was confined to his bedroom when his psoriasis worsened and his parents burnt his clothes because they were full of scales. These examples show how difficult it is to separate cause from effect.

Acne is another skin problem where the cause is not fully understood. It can occur on the faces of infants or be drug induced (by anabolic steroids, oral and topical corticosteroids) but these forms only last briefly and clear spontaneously. The usual age of onset is 12–14 years, with a peak severity occurring at 16–18 years in girls and 18–19 years in boys (Buxton, 1993). Its severity appears to be related to the genetically determined sebum secretion rate (Rothman and Lucky, 1993). Its high occurrence in families and identical twins seem to confirm a hereditary predisposition. At one time the cause was thought to be abnormal sebaceous glands but this has now been disproved. The abnormality seems to be in the sebum, the secretion of which is stimulated by androgens. Androgens are a likely causative factor as acne improves during pregnancy, is rare during young childhood and has a high occurrence in adolescent boys. It is also precipitated by androgen-producing tumours. However, some females experience a worsening of their acne premenstrually. Buxton (1993) suggests that this may be due to fluid retention which increases the hydration of the skin to cause swelling and hypersecretion of the sebaceous ducts. Another historical cause was fatty or oily food, especially chocolate and pork. It now appears that these are not implicated other than for certain susceptible individuals, but acne is known to be exacerbated by exposure to oily substances in the environment. Acne is of psychological concern for adolescents who are worried about their appearance. Unfortunately, constant fingering of the lesions tends to perpetuate the problems and may cause scarring.

Two very rare skin conditions are known to be inherited disorders. Epidermolysis bullosa (EB) is a group of disorders in which the skin is extremely fragile and blisters at the slightest touch. The tissues that attach each epidermal cell to the next are absent or dysfunctional, causing the cells to separate and fluid to fill the gap. At a touch, the thin upper layer can peel away to leave raw areas of sore and painful skin. Internal organs can also be affected. Congenital lamellar ichthyosis is almost always fatal due to loss of fluid, protein and electrolytes from the thick, inelastic and very permeable skin.

Assessment of Skin Disorders

The specific assessment of the child with a skin disorder involves:

- Listening to the history of the problem. A family history of a skin disorder or an onset related to another illness, medication or contact with plants, insects or animals may be very significant.
- Listening to symptoms. Alterations in feeling or sensation help to determine nursing interventions as well as helping the diagnosis.
- Looking at the lesions. The distribution, size and appearance of the lesions can help to identify allergic or irritant rashes, and differentiate between infections and other problems. It is useful to record your findings on a body outline. This helps to monitor progression or improvement.

Table 47.5 Dermatological investigations (copyright is waived for the purpose of photocopying and enlarging this table)

Investigation	When and why?	Role of the nurse
Skin scrapings		
Skin biopsy		
Patch testing		
Woods light		

In addition to this assessment, it may be necessary to carry out more detailed dermatological investigations.

Study activity

Find out when and why the dermatological investigations listed in Table 47.5 are performed. What is the role of the nurse in each investigation?

Nursing Interventions

Caring for children with a skin disorder involves relief of their physical and psychological distress. This distress is common to nearly all skin disorders so there are certain principles of care that can be applied regardless of the diagnosis.

Study activity

The common problems of children with skin disorders are identified in Table 47.6. Consider the aims of care and nursing actions for each of these problems.

As discussed above, the cause of many skin disorders is not clear. As a result, much of the treatment is symptomatic rather than curative. For this reason much work has been done to look at the efficacy of complementary therapies in the management of skin disorders. Traditional Chinese herbal treatments have been shown to be beneficial for the treatment of eczema but the long-term effects of this treatment are unclear and one study has shown that liver damage may ensue (Harper, 1994). Skin treatments usually involve some kind of local application, which is determined by the type of lesion involved and its site on the body. It

Skin disorders – terminology

- *Bullae* – large fluid-filled lesions
- *Burrow* – linear lesion caused by the scabies mite
- *Crusts* – dried areas of exudate (serum, pus, dead skin and debris) from lesions
- *Erythema* – reddened skin
- *Excoriation* – superficial loss of skin often caused by scratching
- *Fissure* – deep linear split through the epidermis into the dermis
- *Macule* – flat, round area of colour change less than 1 mm in diameter (e.g. freckle)
- *Nodule* – solid, round or ellipsoid raised area which originates in or below the dermis
- *Papule* – small, round, solid raised area less than 1 mm in diameter which lies mainly above the skin surface
- *Plaque* – large flattened disc-shaped raised area
- *Pustule* – pus-filled lesion
- *Vesicle* – small fluid-filled lesion
- *Scales* – flakes of dead tissue on the skin surface
- *Scar* – permanent dermal change formed by excess collagen in response to damage to the dermis

Specific assessment of the child with a skin disorder

Where?

- where are the lesions distributed?

When?

- when was the onset, did it relate to:
  - medication?
  - other illness?
  - changes in occupation?
  - changes in the home environment?
- when were there any previous episodes?

What?

- what symptoms are the lesions causing – itching, burning, scaling, blistering?
- what type and size of lesions are they?

Who?

- who else is affected?

How?

- how long have the lesions been present?
- how are the lesions now, compared with previous problems or since onset? (better or worse?)

Use of wet wraps

- Bathe and cleanse the skin
- Apply emollient liberally, so that it no longer sinks into the skin
- Soak tubifast bandages in warm water and then squeeze so they are not dripping wet
- Apply wet bandages to limbs and trunk
- Apply dry tubifast bandages to cover wet bandages, tying wraps together at the shoulders and tops of the legs

Table 47.6 The principles of caring for a child with a skin disorder (copyright is waived for the purpose of photocopying and enlarging this table)

Problem	Aim	Nursing action
Itching and irritation		
Potential risk of secondary infection due to scratching or rubbing		
Feelings of isolation and rejection due to altered body image		
Parental anxiety due to child's appearance		
Potential exacerbation of condition due to stress		

is important for nurses to wash their hands before and after the application of these topical treatments, not only to prevent cross infection, but to minimise the risk of absorption for themselves. The use of gloves for applications is debatable. Alderman (1988) argues that gloves may increase the child's feelings of being socially unacceptable. Topical treatments are usually drugs that have been suspended in a base. The choice of drug and base are both important and depend upon the disorder and state of the skin. Table 47.7 gives indications for uses of bases with their advantages and disadvantages. Most of these applications have to be covered by some kind of gauze body suit to help their adherence and absorption by the lesions. Other more specific interventions are bathing, wet dressings and occlusive therapy.

Bathing helps to remove scales, crusts and topical medications and provides hydration for dry skin. Donald (1995) recommends a lukewarm bath to avoid dilation of blood vessels and exacerbation of itching. Cleansing of old applications should be performed after the child has soaked in the bath for about 10 minutes and may be helped by soap, oils or colloidal oatmeal. The benefit of hydration is increased dramatically if topical applications are renewed immediately after the bath (Clark *et al.*, 1990). The benefit of hydration is also found with wet wraps, which are used to soothe weeping, crusting and purulent lesions. They cool the skin by relieving the inflammation and enhancing the absorption of the topical treatment. They are often used in acute eczema in conjunction with emollients.

Occlusive therapy is sometimes used to encourage penetration of topical steroids, but concern has been expressed about the use of such treatment in children because of the risk of systemic absorption (Hunter *et al.*, 1989). Steroids should therefore be used with care as under-use will not overcome the disorder and over-use may cause steroidal side-

Table 47.7 Types of topical treatments and their uses

Base	Uses	Action	Advantages/ disadvantages
Powder	Between flexures	Lessens friction	Can clump and irritate
Watery/shake lotions	Acutely inflamed wet and oozing lesions	Dries, soothes and cools	Tedious to apply; frequent changes needed
Creams	Moist and dry skin	Cools, moisturises and softens	Short shelf-life; fungal and bacterial growth possible
Ointments	Dry and scaly skin	Occludes and softens	Messy to apply; stains clothes
Pastes	Dry, scaly and lichenified skin	Protects and softens	Messy and tedious to apply; most protective
Sprays	Weeping, acutely inflamed skin	Drying, non-occlusive	Evaporate quickly; no need to touch inflamed, sore skin

effects. Hunter *et al.* (1989) recommend that nothing stronger than hydrocortisone 1% should be used on the face or for infants. Charman *et al.* (2000) recommend that steroid preparations are colour coded for different strengths to help reduce unnecessary parental anxiety about the safety of their use. Donald (1995) suggests that a blob of cream on the finger tip is about 0.5 g and that no more than 6 g should be used for a single application to the whole body for a small child.

Specific treatments are available for the treatment of infections and infestations of the skin (Table 47.8). Compliance with instructions for these is important if the problem is to be completely eradicated, and nurses should be aware of the instructions and advice to give parents using such treatments. Recent evidence appears to indicate that head lice are more prevalent because they have become resistant to popular treatments. Harper (1994) estimates that 10–20% of urban schoolchildren are affected by head lice. For this reason most health districts have a policy of rotating recommended treatments. There is also some concern that some preparations may be carcinogenic.

Study activity

Your local infant school asks you to give a talk to parents about the recognition and treatment of head lice. Prepare the content of your talk.

Table 47.8 Specific treatments for skin disorders (copyright is waived for the purpose of photocopying and enlarging this table)

Treatment	Uses	Dose/kg	Instructions for use/side-effects
Topical			
benzyl benzoate			
dithranol			
malathion			
Systemic			
aciclovir			
cyproterone acetate			
trimeprazine			
griseofulvin			
nystatin			
tetracycline			
Physical			
cryotherapy			
cautery			
phototherapy			

Advice on Discharge

Study activity

Consider all you have learnt about the problems and treatment of chronic skin disorders such as eczema and psoriasis. How would these disorders affect your normal lifestyle?

You will probably realise that such problems can affect every aspect of a normal lifestyle. Apart from a possible avoidance of mixing with others because of embarrassment, scaly skin disorders are not acceptable for some occupations, of which nursing is one example. Nurses with eczema of the hands often find that their skin cannot tolerate constant washing and contact with antibacterial lotions. The weather also affects the skin. Hot weather and sweating tends to increase the itching of eczema, and psoriasis tends to flare up in the winter due to the constriction of extra clothes. Work environments may therefore not be conducive to certain skin disorders. Environmental factors, including the dust mite, are thought to be as important as genetic factors in atopic asthma and controlling such factors may help to reduce itching. An allergic reaction to dust mite excreta may trigger eczema (Donald, 1995). Parents can be given advice about reducing dust mites in the home.

Support for the parents of children with skin disorders is important. Ben-Gashir *et al.* (2002) found that families of children with eczema

Avoidance of the dust mite: advice to parents

- Keep the child's bedroom cool
- Avoid the use of central heating and carpets in the bedroom
- Cover the mattress with an impermeable cover
- Vacuum the base of the bed and the room at least weekly
- Damp dust the room daily
- Wash all bed linen with a non-biological washing powder at 55°C
- Avoid soft toys or wash regularly

were distressed by disturbed sleep, tiredness and exhaustion, extra housework, restrictions on leisure activities and time required for skin treatments.

Study activity

Talk to a parent of a child with a chronic skin problem and find out how the problem affects family life.

Useful support agencies for parents are:

- National Eczema Society, Hill House, Highgate Hill, London N19 5N8. Tel: 020 7281 3553; Web site: http://www.eczema.org (accessed 11 June 2006); helpline@eczema.org.
- The Psoriasis Association, 7 Milton Street, Northampton NN2 7JG. Tel: 0845 676 0076; Web site: http://www.psoriasis-association.org.uk (accessed 11 June 2006); mail@psoriasis.demon.co.uk.

Chapter 48
Mental Health in Childhood

Introduction

According to the Office for National Statistics 1 in 10 children has a mental health problem. Their study, which investigated 10 500 5- to 16-year-olds in the UK, also found that 4% of children had an emotional disorder, 6% a conduct disorder, 2% a hyperkinetic disorder characterised by hyperactive and impulsive behaviour, and 1% had less common problems such as autism and eating disorders. Some children had more than one disorder (Office for National Statistics, 2004). The recognition, treatment and resolution of young people's mental health problems is vital to promote mental well-being in adulthood. The very nature of childhood exposes children to a wide variety of factors that can influence their development, and it is clear that emotional and behavioural problems are increasing as a result (Meltzer *et al.*, 2000). The role of children's nurses in promoting mental health is to be able to communicate with the child and family and be able to assess problems and needs, referring to the specialist team where necessary. The purpose of this section is to introduce you to the nature and management of mental health problems in children and young people, so that you will be able to take the appropriate steps to support and help them.

The Nature and Extent of Mental Health Problems in Childhood

Defining mental health

Study activity

Before reading on jot down your own definition of 'mental health'. Do you consider yourself to be mentally healthy? Why?

For many, mental health is linked to mental illness and therefore extreme states of incapacity. However, this is a very narrow view to take and one that fails to recognise the diverse nature of mental health problems, especially in childhood. Wilson (1995:90) suggests that mental health is essentially about emotional development and refers to 'the robustness, soundness and healthy functioning of the mind, consisting as it does of an individual's cognitive, emotional and volitional capacities'. Three further definitions are offered here for you to consider:

- 'The components of mental health include the following capacities: the ability to develop psychologically, emotionally, intellectually and spiritually; the ability to initiate, develop and sustain mutually satisfying personal relationships; the ability to become aware of others and to empathise with them; the ability to use psychological distress as a developmental process, so that it does not hinder or impair further development' (Health Advisory Service, 1995).
- 'Mental health problems in children and young people are said to occur when the child or young person fails to cope with, or adjust to, difficult or new life events and develops anomalies of emotions, behaviour or social relationships sufficiently marked or prolonged to cause disruption for the everyday life of the child or family' (Pearce, 2003).
- Mental health in young people is indicated by:
  - an ability to form and sustain mutually satisfying relationships;
  - a continuing progression of psychological development;
  - an ability to play and learn, achieving appropriately for age and intellectual level;
  - developing a moral sense of right and wrong;
  - a degree of psychological distress and maladapted behaviour within normal limits for the child's age and context (Wilson, 1995).

The extent of mental health problems in young people has been estimated by a variety of sources. Although the figures vary, there can be no doubt that many children and young people have behavioural and emotional problems that need help and, as a result, are failing to make the most of their potential:

- Meltzer *et al.* (2000) estimated that 10% of the child population had mental health problems, with boys being more likely to have a mental disorder than girls.
- Bone and Meltzer (1989) carried out a survey in 1988 and suggested that disabling emotional or behavioural problems were evident in 2.1% of all children in the United Kingdom.
- Mental Health Foundation (2006) – at least 1 in 15 young people harm themselves and some evidence suggests that rates of self-harm in the UK are higher than anywhere else in Europe.
- Health Advisory Service (1995) – between 10 and 20% of children may require help because of mental health problems at any one time.
- Various studies have attempted to estimate the prevalence of problems in different age groups (Table 48.1):
  (a) preschool – around 7% of 3-year-olds can be expected to show moderate to severe behaviour problems and a further 15% to exhibit mild difficulties (Stephenson and Goodman, 2001);

Table 48.1 Prevalence of psychiatric disorders in children aged 5–15 years (Office for National Statistics, 2004)

Disorder	Girls 5–10 years (%)	Girls 11–15 years (%)	Boys 5–10 years (%)	Boys 11–15 years (%)
Anxiety disorders	3	5	3	4
Depression	0.5	2	0.4	1.8
Conduct disorders	3	4	6.5	8.2
Hyperkinetic disorder	0.2	0.3	2.3	2.2
Less common disorders (tics, eating disorders)	0.1	1	1	0.7
Any disorder	6	9.8	10.3	13

Common behavioural problems of preschool children

- Bed wetting
- Soiling
- Waking at night
- Overactivity
- Poor appetite

Checklist of potentially serious symptoms

- Persistent deliberate destructiveness
- Aggression causing injury
- Deliberate self-harm
- Sexual behaviour that is inappropriate for age
- Arson
- Social disinhibition
- Persistent isolation and withdrawal
- Weird behaviour
- Hallucinations and delusions

(Pearce, 2003)

Disorders with a generally poor outlook

- Persistent aggression in children older than 7 years
- Hyperactivity together with other behavioural problems
- Severe, ongoing depression
- Low self-esteem due to abuse
- Persistent truancy, especially from primary school
- Repeated running away from home
- Repeated suicide attempts

(Pearce, 2003)

Module 6

(b) middle childhood – Office for National Statistics (2004) found that anxiety and conduct disorders were the most common problems for 5- to 10-year-olds;

(c) adolescence – all studies seem to indicate that a higher proportion of this age group (between 10 and 20%) suffers from mental health problems. Worrying statistics show that teenage suicide is on the increase. According to the 2001 mortality statistics, suicide rates among adolescents aged 15–19 years were 9.2%.

The classification of childhood mental health problems is complex but Goodman *et al.* (2002) identify the most common disorders as being:

- emotional disorders – depression, anxiety states, phobias and psychosomatic disorders
- conduct disorders – stealing, truancy, aggression, fire setting and persistent delinquency
- attention deficit disorder, with or without hyperactivity
- depressive disorder leading to suicide
- developmental disorders, for example language delay and autism
- severe eating disorders, for example anorexia nervosa
- elimination disorders, for example enuresis and encopresis

The Causes of Mental Health Problems in Childhood

There are various factors that interact to cause mental health problems in childhood. The result is that no two children react in the same way to the tasks associated with development. Some cope well with the demands placed upon them. Others do not cope so well with the same demands. Even children within the same family, with similar upbringings, can differ in their emotional development. The factors that seem to contribute to the development of mental health problems are grouped into four categories according to Barker (1995):

- Constitutional, including genetic factors, the effects of chromosomal abnormalities, the consequences of intrauterine injury and the results of birth injury.

- Physical disease and injury, including brain damage caused by injury, infection and tumours; chronic illness that can impose restrictions on children's lives leading to emotional problems.
- Temperamental factors. Pearce (2003) describes a difficult temperament as being a child risk factor for psychiatric disorders. However, he notes that there is often more than one single risk factor and that the interaction of each of the risk factors is more significant than the individual factor.
- Environmental factors. These include the influence of the family, school and the wider social environment.

Pearce (2003) identifies several situations in which there appears to be greater risk of mental health problems:

- in families where there is socio-economic disadvantage or family disharmony
- in families where there is a history of parental psychiatric illness, particularly maternal depression
- following child abuse
- in association with physical illness, especially chronic illness, very severe conditions and sensory deficit.

External factors that increase the risk of psychiatric disorder

- A school that has:
  - poor organisation and unclear discipline
  - lack of recognition of children as individuals
  - high teacher turnover
  - low morale amongst staff
- Peer group pressure
- Bullying
- Social deprivation
- Sociocultural influences

(Pearce, 2003)

Groups of children likely to have greater incidence of mental health problems

- Young offenders
- Children with a criminal background
- Children in the care of the local authority
- Children with learning disabilities
- Children with emotional and behavioural difficulties
- Abused children
- Children with a physical disability
- Children with sensory impairment
- Children who have parents with mental health problems
- Children with a chronic illness
- Children who experience/witness sudden extreme trauma
- Refugees

(DH, 1996)

Managing Mental Health Problems in Childhood

A range of interventions may be used for the treatment of mental health problems in childhood. Some may need the involvement of a specialised team on an inpatient or outpatient basis. The team may include a variety of professionals working within a multidisciplinary framework:

- psychiatrists
- social workers
- community psychiatric nurses
- child psychotherapist
- music therapists
- art therapists
- occupational therapists
- other medical staff

Other interventions may be implemented within the general paediatric area. For this reason you should become familiar with some of the variety of treatments available. Two examples of interventions will be considered here.

Factors that protect against psychiatric disorder

- Positive self-image
- Affectionate family relationships
- Supportive relationships with adults
- Stable personality
- Having a special skill or talent
- High IQ and academic achievement
- Parents who give high levels of supervision and clear discipline

(Pearce, 2003)

Family therapy

Module 1 examines the nature of the family and highlights its diversity and important role in the development of children. The family is a complex, ever-changing entity and factors that affect its function can affect family members in various ways. Family therapy aims to change the dynamics of the family system which inevitably leads to individual change (Goldberg and Hodes, 2003). The family group is the focus of treatment, not just the individual child. The therapist looks at the family as a whole and the dynamics within it, with the aim of establishing

The four-tier model of mental health services

Tier one
Primary care health professionals, especially general practitioners and health visitors. Also teachers and others in direct contact with children.

Tier two
Interventions by individual staff (psychologists, nurses or psychiatrists) within the Child and Adolescent Mental Health Service (CAMHS) providing an individual service in a health centre or in the community.

Tier three
Interventions by CAMHS provided in child and family psychiatric clinics.

Tier four
Specialist services such as those for children with attention deficit and hyperactivity disorder (ADHD) or eating disorders. This level includes specialist inpatient services for children and adolescents with mental health problems.

(Health Advisory Service, 1995)

National Service Framework for Children: standard 9

All children and young people from birth to their eighteenth birthday, who have mental health problems and disorders will have access to timely, integrated, high-quality multidisciplinary mental health services to ensure effective assessment, treatment and support, for them and their parents and carers.

(DH, 2004b)

healthy family functioning. Assessing the way the family functions is important in identifying areas in which the family may be experiencing difficulties. Steinhauer *et al.* (1984) give an example of a scheme for understanding families and how they function along six dimensions:

- task accomplishment (problem solving) – basic tasks, those which provide the essentials of life; developmental tasks, those which ensure the healthy development of family members; crisis tasks, those which must be dealt with in the face of unexpected or unusual events
- role performance
- communication
- affective involvement – the degree and quality of the family members' interest and concern for each other
- control – the influence family members have over each other – rigid, flexible, laissez-faire or chaotic
- values and norms

Study activity

Consider a child you have cared for/are caring for with behavioural or emotional problems. Using the six dimensions outlined above explore the possible difficult areas that the family may be experiencing.

Study activity

Arrange to talk to a family therapist about the different schools of thought and the use of family therapy for children with behavioural or emotional problems.

Behaviour therapy

This type of therapy is based upon work from the field of social learning theory and draws ideas from theorists such as Pavlov and Skinner. It focuses on the factors that maintain certain behaviours and how they can be altered. Assessment of the nature of the child's behaviour is paramount and includes ascertaining the:

- frequency of occurrence of the behaviour
- the developmental appropriateness of the behaviour – for example, temper tantrums are to be expected in the 2-year-old but would warrant more concern in an 11-year-old
- the social relevance of the behaviour
- the intensity and focus of the behaviour
- the costs and gains to the child (Varma, 1990)

(*See also* Bowel retraining pp. 494 and 556.)

Behaviour can then be categorised into that which is lacking or that which is in excess. Behaviourists are not concerned with exploring the nature and meaning of problem behaviour. Rather they believe that problem behaviours are learned and can be replaced by new learning experiences. Three main types of intervention are (Barker, 1995):

- operant and respondent conditioning – concerned with altering the conditions following (operant) or preceding (respondent) a problem behaviour
- cognitive behaviour therapy – attempts to teach the child to think differently about things so that their behaviour changes
- modelling – behaviour learned by observing and imitating another person; parents often do not realise how powerfully they can influence their child's behaviour in this way

Interventions for mental health problems

- Family therapy
- Behaviour therapy
- Psychotherapy
- Group therapy
- Pharmacotherapy
- Hypnosis and hypnotherapy
- Speech therapy

Study activity

Reflect critically on the management of a child you have cared for where this behaviour approach has been used. Consider the factors involved in influencing its outcome.

Suicide in Young People

The suicide rate among young people has risen alarmingly, especially among males, since 1980. In all developed countries, except the USA, suicide is now the second most common cause of death among young people aged 15–24 (Office for National Statistics, 2004). Official figures may underestimate the problem given that some deaths will be recorded as undetermined cause or accidental death. Parasuicide (attempted suicide) is also prevalent but is more common in young females than males. According to the Samaritans (2001) half of young suicides carry out an act of self-harm in the preceding year and many more young people contemplate killing themselves. Thus the prevention of suicide in young people is an important issue and one that should concern all who work with young people in whatever setting.

The cause of suicide is complex and arises from multiple factors acting together. Factors that have been shown to contribute to suicide and parasuicide in young people include:

- extreme and traumatic events (for example, physical and sexual abuse)
- alcohol and substance abuse – drugs and alcohol can 'affect thinking capacities and may act as a catalyst for suicidal thoughts by reducing inhibitions' (Borton, 1997)
- psychiatric illness – almost all young people who commit suicide were suffering from one or more (usually longstanding) mental health disorders (Shaffer and Gutstein, 2002)
- family dysfunction, for example, broken homes (through death or divorce), parental unemployment, poor support mechanisms

Although suicide can never be totally eradicated, the aim of prevention should be to reduce the number of suicides to the lowest possible level. The Department of Health (DH, 1992) set a target for reducing overall suicides by 15% by the year 2000, but the suicide rate actually increased steeply by 2000 (Office for National Statistics, 2004). A multi-agency, multifaceted approach to the three levels of prevention is essential in order to develop focused strategies.

Definitions of suicide

'. . . suicide is a conscious act of self-induced annihilation, best understood as a multidimensional malaise in a needful individual who defines an issue for which suicide is perceived as the best solution'.

(Shneidman, 1985)

'. . . suicidal behaviour in children can be defined as self-destructive behaviour that has the intent to seriously damage oneself or cause death'.

(Pfeffer, 1986)

Primary prevention – to prevent the contemplation of suicide:

- detecting and treating mental disorders in young people
- restricting access to alcohol and drug abuse
- reducing access to lethal means of suicide, such as firearms
- reducing media influences
- educating young people about the importance of talking through feelings and promoting mental health
- peer support schemes and anti-bullying strategies in schools

Secondary prevention – providing help for those who are already suicidal – includes:

- hotlines (for example, the Samaritans and Childline)
- identifying those at risk – children's nurses (particularly those working in schools and A&E) play a vital role here in picking up cues from young people in their care. Borton (1997) suggests signs of suicide to which we should be alert:
  - withdrawn behaviour
  - having definite ideas about how to kill themselves
  - talking about feeling isolated
  - losing self-esteem and expressing feelings of failure and uselessness
  - constantly dwelling on problems for which there seems to be no solution

The Samaritans are available on:
08457 909090
e-mail at jo@samaritans.org
Web site http://www.samaritans.org
and at: 10 The Grove, Slough, SLI IQP

Childline for children in trouble or danger
0800 1111

The risk is increased if there are any of the contributory factors mentioned above.

Tertiary prevention involves providing support for those who have attempted suicide. All young people who self-harm or attempt suicide should be referred. Diekstra (cited by Barton, 1995) suggests that only 1 : 4 cases lead to contact with medical or other professionals, and more recent studies suggest that this is because the young people do not feel that the professionals they deal with, and/or the services available, are recognising their need (Mental Health Foundation, 2006). According to Hawton and James (2005) ideally all young people should be assessed by a child and adolescent psychiatrist following a parasuicide attempt.

Self-harm

The National Institute for Health and Clinical Excellence (NICE) has defined self-harm as 'Intentional self poisoning or injury, irrespective of the apparent purpose of the act' (NICE, 2004b). Deliberate self-harm can occur at any age, but its peak incidence is seen in those aged around 15 years and the average age of onset is 12 years (Mental Health Foundation, 2006). Young people who self-harm mainly do so as an impulsive way of coping with emotional distress in their lives. This distress can range from bullying to family breakdown, and most affected children are not seriously distressed (Forrest, 2003). Self-harm can involve a range of harmful behaviour, which is often done in secret and can go on for a long time without being discovered. It can involve:

- cutting
- burning or scalding

- banging or scratching
- breaking bones
- hair pulling
- ingesting toxic or harmful substances or objects (such as glass)

The national inquiry into self-harm among young people found that multiple trigger factors (isolation, academic pressures, low self-esteem, poor body image) are more likely to induce self-harm than single significant events. Young people in the study

- described how self-harm 'gets out all the hurt, anger and pain'
- felt they had no alternatives: 'I don't know how to release my feelings in any other way'
- made them feel 'something – alive and real'
- said that 'if there had been people to talk to . . . then maybe I wouldn't have felt the need to start self-harming'

Of children who seek help for self-harm, 20% have made a previous attempt and the risk of suicide must always be assessed (Forrest, 2003). Children's nurses can help those who are admitted by trying to explore the background trigger factors, and admission to hospital is the ideal opportunity for secondary prevention. It also provides an opportunity for the young person and family to reflect on the situation. Because of the seriousness of self-harming behaviour, which can lead to suicide, it is essential that a risk assessment is undertaken on admission to the ward and appropriate care plans made to ensure the child's safety. The Mental Health Foundation (2006) advocates teaching coping strategies or distraction techniques to overcome self-harming behaviour. These must be individual to the child – different people find that different techniques work in different situations – and may take some time to establish. The Mental Health Foundation (2006) also suggests that young people urgently need the skills and support necessary to maintain positive mental health and emotional well-being to prevent the onset of this type of destructive behaviour.

Anorexia Nervosa

The most important eating disorder that can occur in prepubertal children as young as 8 years old is anorexia nervosa. Although it used to be seen as a disorder primarily affecting girls, it is now known that around 30% of anorexics are boys (Sharman, 1997). According to Lask and Bryant-Waugh (1998) it is characterised by determined food avoidance, profound weight loss or failure to gain weight during the adolescent growth spurt, and two or more of the following:

- preoccupation with body weight
- preoccupation with calorie intake
- distorted body image
- fear of fatness
- self-induced vomiting
- excessive exercising
- laxative abuse

Children with anorexia nervosa see themselves as grotesquely fat even when thin and emaciated. The anorexic young person sees starvation as a positive thing, helping to achieve the aim of being thin. The effects of starvation eventually lead to clinical signs. The youngster becomes weak and lethargic, with a slow pulse and low blood pressure; in girls, menstruation does not commence or ceases; and in severe cases heart failure can occur. Factors associated with the condition are depression, dissatisfaction with life and a poor self-image, perfectionism. According to Wright (1991) the death rate from complications arising from anorexia is about 4%. Important aspects of management include:

- The establishment of rapport with all concerned.
- A firm, accepting, non-punitive approach. Adults involved in care must be supportive towards each other and united. Non-eating is not negotiable, and privileges may have to be dependent on eating or preferably gaining weight. A clear contract of eating behaviour should be made together with the child.
- Behaviour away from the table should be observed so that food cannot be disposed of, for example down the toilet and vomiting, laxative abuse or excessive exercising can be prevented.
- Family therapy can lead to substantial benefits in terms of weight gain, attitudes to eating, reduced depression and an improved child and parent relationship (Eisler *et al.*, 2000).

Bulimia

- An eating disorder similar to, and often associated with, anorexia nervosa
- Word is derived from Greek and means 'ox hunger'
- Characterised by repeated episodes of binge eating followed by a variety of weight controlling activities:
  - self-induced vomiting
  - diuretics
  - laxatives
  - rigorous exercise
- Eating episodes are followed by periods of depression and self-deprecation

Promoting Mental Health in Children and Young People

A variety of measures have been identified that can contribute to the promotion of mental health and the prevention of problems (*see also* Levels of health promotion p. 133).

Primary level

This involves the prevention of problems particularly amongst those with a high potential for a mental health disorder:

- Developmental programmes – these concentrate on children at particular ages or stages of development.
- High-risk programmes – aimed at children believed to be at above-average risk for a disorder. These may include children admitted to hospital, children with chronic illness, bereaved children, abused children and those in the care of welfare agencies. Forrest (2003) encourages the use of positive steps to help children cope with crises, such as admission to hospital, involving anticipatory guidance (preparation) and preventive intervention (dealing with the here and now, understanding what is happening and developing coping skills).
- Community programmes – many factors associated with the community (such as economic factors, social class) in which the child lives can influence the development of a healthy emotional state and the development of mental health problems. Many controlled trials have shown that behaviourally based parenting programmes are effective in increasing child social behaviour (Scott, 2003).

Other high-risk programmes may include

- Self-help groups for children with chronic illness
- Bereavement counselling
- Child guidance clinics
- Counselling clinics

Module 6

Measures to promote mental health include:

- good obstetric and neonatal care to minimise the mental health problems associated with birth injury
- genetic counselling and screening
- parentcraft sessions
- development screening
- life skills sessions for children to help them communicate effectively
- school counselling services

Schools play a very important role in the promotion of mental health. Faulconbridge and Spanswick (1995) give an account of how school nurses were helped to provide counselling to adolescents. The scheme enhanced the school nurses' ability to deal with problems and recognise the need for early referral.

Study activity

Consider the potential role of the children's nurse in this level of mental health promotion. Design a programme to help your colleagues understand the need for mental health promotion.

Secondary level

This involves the early detection and treatment of mental health problems:

- Screening – screening for behavioural and emotional problems is not without difficulties but the important role of all those who work with children (particularly at preschool level) is recognised. In order to recognise behavioural and emotional problems in children, primary care staff need to be aware of normal development and the variations that can be expected.
- Treatment of problems will be dependent on the type of problem as discussed earlier. Some interventions, for example managing minor problems, can often be dealt with successfully by health visitors. Others can be managed through counselling and guidance services. Others will need referral to specialist services.

In preventing mental health problems and promoting mental health it is important to recognise the role of healthy public policy. Many of the factors that influence the development of mental health problems are outside the control of the individual. Consideration needs to be given to such issues as:

- poverty
- the environment
- child abuse
- the family and dysfunction within it
- unemployment
- homelessness
- education

Services for mental illness in children and young people

According to Kurtz (1992) the essential elements of service provision are:

- a multidisciplinary child and adolescent psychiatric service with a management team which coordinates the service and encourages liaison with other children's services
- an NHS base with appropriate secretarial and administrative support with access to database
- clearly identifiable budget within the control of the service manager
- a multidisciplinary team consisting of psychiatrists, psychologists, therapy staff, child psychiatry nurses and a specialist social worker
- a confidential service where information is only extended on a 'need to know basis'
- provided in a variety of settings other than health services – within social services, education and voluntary services

Study activity

Explore any policies that exist to deal with any of the issues cited above. How well do they reflect the needs of the population?

In conclusion, we must recognise the vital role of health promotion in the development of healthy minds as well as bodies. Children need to be encouraged to develop to their full potential and those who work with children and young people must be aware of the potential factors that can contribute to mental health problems in this age group.

Chapter 49

Care of the Sick and Preterm Newborn

Introduction

The advancement of medical technology and clinical interventions, together with the development of an evidence-based body of nursing knowledge particular to the newborn, has led to an improvement in the care of the sick neonate. The first 4 weeks following birth remain a vulnerable time for many babies, when a mortality rate of 3.5/1000 births compares with 1.6/1000 births for babies aged between 4 weeks and 1 year old (Office for National Statistics, 2004). Congenital disease and low birth weight are major contributors to the perinatal mortality rate. In recognition of this, a national antenatal screening programme is in place and public health initiatives to help the mother and baby share a healthy, full-term pregnancy.

If a baby is born sick or preterm, the impact on the family cannot be underestimated. The birth may bring anxiety and separation rather than celebration and the closer relationships that are usually associated with the birth of a baby. The care given to the baby and family must always take this into account and should aim to return the baby to a family that has been supported to its optimum health, as well as the baby. The baby needs to be nursed within an environment that provides it with a comfortable, secure place that not only allows the baby to recover to optimum health in the short term but will also prevent residual iatrogenic damage occurring that could affect child- and adulthood. The family will be experiencing the neonatal unit as a complete system of care and will be looking for their own individual needs to be met. It is not possible to fulfil these environmental needs of the baby and family without multidisciplinary partnership and cooperation. All members of staff must be aware of the disturbing effects that a poor environment of care can create for both babies and families, and work together to provide an excellent, therapeutic environment of care.

Table 49.1 gives an overview of some of the more common problems faced by the sick neonate. As there are too many to cover in detail, this section will concentrate on the main principles of managing care for the sick neonate.

Definitions

- Neonate – term given to describe baby from day 1–27.
- Preterm – a baby born before the 37th completed week of gestation.
- Post-term – a baby born during or after the 42nd completed week of gestation.
- SGA – small for gestational age; a baby whose birth weight is below the 10th centile. This may or may not be due to IUGR (intrauterine growth restriction) where growth of the fetus has been slowed down or interrupted.
- AGA – appropriate for gestational age.
- LGA – large for gestational age.
- LBW – low birth weight – a baby weighing less than 2.5 kg at birth.
- VLBW – very low birth weight – a baby weighing less than 1.5 kg at birth.
- ELBW – extremely low birth weight – a baby weighing less than 1.0 kg at birth.

Further reading

Crawford, D. and Hickson, W. (2000) *An Introduction to Neonatal Nursing Care*, 2nd edn. Cheltenham: Nelson Thornes.

Kenner, C. and McGrath, J. (2004) *Developmental Care of Newborns and Infants: A Guide for Health Professionals.* New York: Mosby.

Sparshott, M. (1996) *Pain, Distress and the Newborn Baby.* Oxford: Blackwell Science.

Table 49.1 Common problems of the sick neonate

Respiratory	Transient tachypnoea of the newborn Respiratory distress syndrome Congenital diaphragmatic hernia Choanal atresia Tracheo-oesophageal fistula Meconium inhalation Drug-induced respiratory depression Birth asphyxia: may also have an effect on all other systems
Gastro-intestinal	Oesophageal atresia Imperforate anus Meconium ileus Gastroschisis Exomphalos Necrotising enterocolitis
Renal	Acute renal failure Chronic renal failure Congenital abnormalities, e.g. ectopic vesicae
Cardiac	Cardiac failure Tetralogy of Fallot Tricuspid atresia Coarctation of the aorta Transposition of the great vessels Ventricular septal defect Patent ductus arteriosus
Blood	Jaundice ABO incompatibility Rhesus incompatibility
Nervous	Birth trauma Structural deformities, e.g. spina bifida Intracranial haemorrhage Recreational drug misuse by mother during pregnancy
Infection	Neonatal septicaemia Thrush Conjunctivitis Omphalitis HIV

General Principles of Care for the Sick Neonate

The environment of care

Even if a baby is born preterm, the world of the womb has given it a soft, warm, dark space in which it can grow. The womb has brought the baby into a good flexed position from which the baby can feel the barriers to its world, and against which the baby can flex and gain strength in its bones and muscles. The baby can bring its hands to its mouth to practise sucking and to self-comfort. Sounds are muted but the baby will gain comfort from his mother's and father's voices and the sounds of the mother's body. Once born, and having been taken to a neonatal unit, the baby may experience a very different world of bright light, loud, strange noise, varying temperature and the inability to be in a midline flexed position where it can continue to bring its hands to its mouth. Neonatal units now go to great lengths to replicate, as far as they can, the environment of care that the baby has experienced in the womb. Sick term babies will still need comforting surroundings but it is the preterm baby where it is essential that the baby continues to grow in womb-like conditions.

Study activity

Look around the neonatal unit and see what measures have been taken to make the environment right for the babies.

Developmental care

A preterm baby needs to grow and develop at a steady rate. The more of its limited resources that the baby can use for normal growth and development the less at risk the baby becomes of disease interrupting its path to maturity. If the baby becomes stressed, overstimulated or over-fatigued, it will use its limited physiological resources to try to maintain homeostasis, and in doing so divert resources from growth and development. Developmental care (Als, 1986) helps staff to recognise infant behavioural cues that indicate when it is an appropriate time to disturb the baby, when to leave the baby to sleep and when the baby is becoming stressed from handling and interventions. Developmental care gives the impetus of care to the baby, and staff need to plan care according to how the baby is behaving and responding. See Table 49.2 for factors that are important to the developmental care of the preterm baby.

Table 49.2 Essential factors of developmental care for the preterm baby

Environment of care	Gives uninterrupted deep sleep Does not overstimulate or stress the baby Minimal noise Lowest level lighting Lighting that creates a 24-hour cycle Odour free Thermoneutral to the baby Provision of comfort through non-nutritive sucking Pain free
Positioning of the baby	Able to observe behaviour and facial expression to assess when care is given Supported in a midline flexed position Supports to achieve rounded head shape Hands able to come to mouth Creation of close boundaries around the baby 'Skin to skin' care with parents, when appropriate
With the family	Positive touch from the mother and father Parents talking to the baby Close physical contact when appropriate Contact with the nipple and breast when appropriate

Study activity

Watch the responses and facial expression of a baby as it is being handled. What do the responses tell you about how the baby is coping with the activity? Discuss what you see with a senior member of the neonatal staff.

Assessing the neonate

Skilled observation and monitoring is essential. Some sick and preterm babies are sensitive to touch and handling and the process of assessment may induce a stress response that will alter physiological values. The practice surrounding assessment should incur minimal disturbance from touch, light, noise, pain or discomfort. The timing of clinical assessments and preparation of the baby must be carefully planned. Interventions should be performed when the baby is in a quiet, unstressed state.

Table 49.3 shows the types of observations that may be made and some of the possible associated problems.

Electronic measuring of vital signs using cardio-respiratory monitors allows continuous measurement of temperature, pulse, blood pressure and oxygen saturation. Arterial lines allow for regular blood sampling/monitoring without the need for traumatic venepuncture. These monitors provide essential information and give the baby long periods of undisturbed rest; however, the effectiveness of the technology often depends on the adhesion of sensors on the newborn skin. This can have a damaging effect, especially on the skin of the preterm baby. The removal of any adherent tape or electrodes must be carried out with extreme care as skin layers will also be removed and the integrity of the skin damaged.

Study activity

Make arrangements to visit a neonatal unit. Take time to find out about the different types of monitors available and what information they give.

Temperature control

Under normal circumstances neonates can control their body temperature within a small range. However, a poorly managed environmental temperature can significantly compromise the health of the baby. Underdevelopment or disease reduce the effectiveness of the vasomotor control of surface blood vessels, making vasoconstriction less effective and the skin will continue to lose heat. The large surface area of the body in relation to body weight increases the rate of heat loss from the body in proportion to the ability of the baby to generate heat from its body. The neonate's main method of heat production is non-shivering thermogenesis, which involves the metabolism of brown fat, found in the neck and abdomen. This fat has a high enzyme content and is capable of rapid conversion to heat and energy. This process is unique to infants and relies on the consumption of oxygen. Hypothermia will therefore increase babies' oxygen consumption as they attempt to raise

Table 49.3 Assessing the sick newborn: signs to observe

Behaviour	Irritability Lethargy Soundness of sleep The transition from sleep to wake Alertness when awake
Cry	Excessive crying/abnormally quiet – infection High-pitched cry – meningitis
Colour	Pallor Cyanosis Mottled skin Jaundice
Breathing patterns	Increased sternal recession and grunt – respiratory distress syndrome Asymmetrical chest movement – pneumothorax Tachypnoea – decreased circulating oxygen
Feeding	Not waking for feed Choking on feed – neurological disease Breathless during feed – respiratory disease Falls asleep before end of feed Milk returns down nostril – cleft palate Timing and type of vomit
Urine	Wet nappies or measured volume
Stools	Meconium passed Colour Consistency
Musculoskeletal	Hypotonia – neurological disorder Hypertonia – neurological disorder Abnormal body posture – neurological disorder Non-moving limb – bone injury Asymmetry of movement
Skin	Spots and rashes – infection Inflammation Birthmarks Texture
Neurological	Repetitive jittering movements Obvious fits 'Sunset' position of eye pupils – hydrocephalus Head circumference

their temperature. This will, in turn, accentuate any existing hypoxaemia. To avoid this, a neonate must be nursed in a thermoneutral environment. The aim should be to care for all babies in a thermoneutral temperature that is appropriate to their gestational age and state of health. Particular care must be taken with preterm and small for gestational age babies as they have less brown fat, little subcutaneous fat and a relatively larger surface area.

When the health of the baby allows, skin-to-skin contact with the mother and father is an excellent way of warming a baby or maintaining its temperature. The baby, wearing only a nappy, is placed on the

thermoneutral environment
The environmental temperature at which an infant can maintain his rectal temperature at 37°C with minimal oxygen consumption

The benefits of skin-to-skin (kangaroo) care

- Improves the emotional closeness between parents and baby
- Thermoneutral environment for the baby
- Improves lactation
- The baby can explore and suckle at the mother's nipple
- Good positioning for the baby
- Positive touch for both baby and the mother
- Has a regulating effect on the vital signs of the baby
- Reduction of infant stress, weight gain and sleep patterns of baby will improve

uncovered chest of the mother or father. The parents clothes are then wrapped around the back of the baby to keep the baby secure and warm (Brandon, 2003). The physiological response to this by the mother is a continual adjustment of her own temperature to maintain the temperature of the baby within a normal range. Skin-to-skin contact also increases the emotional attachment between the mother and the baby and helps to establish breastfeeding (BFI, 2006).

The risk of the baby becoming cold can be reduced by:

- Drying the baby immediately after birth and after washing or bathing. The baby should never be left wrapped in a damp or wet towel.
- A hat will reduce the amount of skin surface area through which heat can be lost. The use of other clothes will depend on where the baby is nursed – an incubator or open cot – and the need for access to the baby's skin or lines needed for assessment or therapeutics.
- The baby should never be laid on a cold surface. Warm towels or sheets must always provide a warm layer under the baby.
- The baby must not be nursed in a cold or draughty part of the room. Portholes of incubators should only be opened when necessary.

At the same time as preventing hypothermia it is important not to overheat neonates, who will then attempt to lower their temperature by increasing respiratory rate and fluid losses by evaporation. This in turn can increase weight loss, dehydration and jaundice (Morris, 1994).

Study activity

As you care for a baby, note which activities increase the risk of the baby becoming too hot or too cold. Consider how these risks can be minimised.

Infection control

The neonate is more prone to infection than older children and adults due to an immature immune system. The neonate will have some short-lived immunoglobulin G (IgG) that has passed through the placenta from the mother, but lacks previous other immunoglobulins that require the baby to have been exposed to infections as a precursor to their production (Boxwell, 2000). Premature infants will be even more deficient in IgG. Adult levels of IgG are not reached until about 4 years of age; adult levels of IgM are reached by about 2 years. Neonates have a reduced ability to make new antibodies and polymorphonuclear leucocyte function and stores are deficient during the first weeks of life (Wilson, 1986) (*see also* Children with problems related to the immune system p. 500).

The most effective way of reducing cross infection in neonatal units is the use of strict and rigid hand-washing routines. Disinfecting hand gel must also be used routinely. Parents and all staff must be taught the importance of thorough handwashing. Strict adherence to other infection control procedures must also be observed. Other aspects of care to prevent infection can include:

- isolating infected or potentially infected babies
- cots and incubators must be cleaned frequently

- a high standard of cleanliness in all parts of the neonatal unit
- breastfeeding should be encouraged
- a high standard of sterile technique when expressing and storing breast milk
- babies admitted from home should be regarded as potentially infected until proved otherwise
- babies must be examined daily for signs of infection
- visitors with active infections should keep away

It is important to note that neonatal infection is often difficult to assess and that, as there is not always accompanying fever, the baby may in fact become hypothermic. Other features are non-specific and include reluctance to feed, jaundice, lethargy, irritability and tachypnoea.

Study activity

Critically examine the infection control procedures in your nearest special care baby unit. How do they compare with those on the ward?

Skin care and handling

The skin of a newborn is delicate and easily damaged. The smaller and more premature the infant, the more the skin is prone to damage. Attention should be paid to minimising skin damage by careful cleansing and drying, regular change of position, and correct positioning of the lines required for therapy and clinical interventions. Babies who have very dry and cracked skin can be at increased risk of skin infection, for example post-mature babies. The advice of a pharmacist must be sought before a moisturing cream or oil is applied to a baby's skin. The skin is a large organ in comparison with the body mass in a baby, and all products absorbed through the skin of the baby will rise to high circulating values. This problem is compounded when applying creams to the less-developed skin of a preterm baby.

Nappy changing need not be carried out frequently unless the nappy area is reddened, sore or excoriated. The use of tapes to secure tubes, drains and vascular lines cannot be avoided and some damage is almost inevitable. Consideration should therefore be given to the type of tape used and its application and removal.

The umbilical cord, while still attached, should be left to dry in the air, using only water for cleaning when necessary. No other products should be used (Trotter, 2003). The umbilicus should be examined daily for signs of infection as it is particularly at risk when the infant is preterm or has an umbilical catheter *in situ*.

Positioning

Careful consideration should be given to positioning the preterm infant. The underdevelopment of the musculoskeletal system of the preterm baby gives weak resistance to the flattening effect of gravity as the baby lies in its cot. If this is not countered by positioning and supporting the baby correctly, the baby will remain in a frog-like position. Developmentally this will lead to pronounced extension and the inappropriate rotation of the hips and the retraction of the shoulders, creating problems with sitting and crawling. The baby may also develop 'toe walking' (Georgioff and Bernbaum, 1986). The skull of the preterm infant is usually thin, soft and rather pliable and therefore liable to postural deformity. Prolonged immobility can therefore result in a narrow, elongated head that can be quite distressing for parents (Cubby, 1991). The preterm infant should be nursed in supported positions with hip support recommended in all positions (Hallsworth, 1995). Support can be achieved through the use of specially designed, manufactured rolls or a roll of sheet or blanket. These supports should be extended laterally to create a womb-like barrier around the baby, a safe, comforting space.

Sick babies may be nursed prone, supine or on their side but no one position should be used for long periods of time. The reason for nursing the baby prone or on their side must be explained to the parents as this is against the advice given to prevent cot death (DH, 1996). It must also be explained that this would not be advised when the baby returns home, unless it was directly recommended by the clinical team.

Managing nutrition

Meeting the infant's nutritional requirements is an important part of care. As each baby must be treated according to its individual requirements only the principles will be considered here. Points to consider when planning and implementing feeding regimes include:

- Infants under 34 weeks' gestation have poorly coordinated sucking and swallowing reflexes. This makes them prone to reflux.
- Neonates have a small stomach capacity (reduced even more in preterm infants).
- Small babies have poor energy reserves and prolonged sucking will cause fatigue.
- An infant has a high metabolic rate, requiring more calories per kilogram of body weight than an adult.
- Gastric motility is reduced but gastric emptying is more rapid in neonates.

The method of feeding chosen will depend on the age, size and condition of the infant:

- Total parenteral nutrition (TPN) feeding – clinical indications for this method include the need for surgery, gut pathology such as necrotising enterocolitis (NEC) and an inability to tolerate enteral feeding due to gut immobility or immaturity (Dear, 1992).
- Trophic feeding is used when very preterm babies are fed parenterally. Each hour, 0.5–1 ml of preferably breast milk is given to the baby via a nasogastric or orogastric tube. The benefits this provides during the subsequent weeks are an increased rate of gut maturation and feeding tolerance. This leads to a more rapid transition to enteral feeding. Serum bilirubin values are also reduced (McClure *et al.*, 2000).
- Enteral feeding – babies will need enteral feeding through a nasogastric or orogastric feeding tube when they have difficulty sucking or cannot sustain the energy needed to take a full sucking feed. Feeds can be passed through a tube into the stomach, jejunum or duodenum.

Necrotising enterocolitis
The most commonly acquired gastro-intestinal problem among sick neonates (Hylton Rushton, 1990). The cause is unclear but it is thought that there is reduced blood flow to the gut due to hypoxaemia, hypoglycaemia or hypothermia. This in turn leads to mucosal oedema and ulceration allowing colonisation by Gram-negative organisms (e.g. *Escherichia coli, Klebsiella*)

Module 6

Although nasal tubes are easier to secure in place, they reduce the diameter of nasal air passages available for air entry, and this needs to be considered when a baby has respiratory difficulty and requires respiratory support. Bolus feeding is the preferred method of enteral feeding rather than feeds given by continuous infusion. Continuous infusion does improve feeding tolerance but the baby loses essential lipids as they adhere to the syringe and tubing. Bolus feeds seem to better prepare the digestive system for a more regular routine of feeding. When enteral feeds are used the stomach should be aspirated regularly to ensure that milk is not collecting there, as the risk of aspiration into the lungs is high.

- Oral feeding – breastfeeding or bottle feeding can be introduced whenever babies demonstrate an ability to suck and when their condition allows (for example, after surgery). Breastfeeding is always the preferred option and this is supported by the UNICEF Baby Friendly Hospital Initiative, which aims to promote beneficial breastfeeding practices and discourage detrimental ones. To help staff provide the mother with sound advice without conflicting approaches, WHO/UNICEF have published advice on supporting breastfeeding (World Health Organization, 1989). Although it is difficult, neonatal units need to provide an environment that helps the mother to express breast milk or breastfeed her baby. Patience and support will be needed for the mother who wishes to breastfeed, particularly when this has been delayed for some time. Encouraging mothers to express breast milk for their preterm and sick infants will help with the establishment of breastfeeding when the baby is ready. The use of breast milk for sick and preterm infants should be actively encouraged as it has long-term and short-term health benefits to the baby as well as helping the emotional closeness to grow between the mother and the baby. It may be feasible for some babies to alternate oral and enteral feeding to give an opportunity for the baby to rest, particularly if feeds are frequent (*see also* Enteral feeding p. 332 and Parenteral feeding p. 336).

Another method of supplementing breastfeeds for preterm babies is cup feeding. The milk is warmed and offered to the baby in a specially designed cup. It is held to the lips of the baby for it to lap the milk. The milk must never be poured into the mouth of the baby as the baby may aspirate the milk. For this reason correct training and supervision of staff and parents must be given for it to remain a safe process (Freer, 1999; Hedburg Nyqvist and Strandell, 1999). Cup feeding done by the mother may provide the additional effect of stimulating lactation and making the expression of breast milk easier. She will also gain confidence in holding and caring for the baby, endorsing her value as a full partner in the caring team (Ritchie, 1998).

Study activity

Arrange to visit a dietician to talk about the nutritional needs of preterm and small for gestational age babies.

Table 49.4 Signs of pain and distress in the newborn

Facial expression	Facial grimace, frown Tongue thrust Facial twitches Averted gaze Low level of alertness Look of panic or worry Eyes shut
Physiological changes	Abrupt change in skin colour Increase or decreasing heart rate and blood pressure Tachypnoea Apnoeic episodes Fall in oxygen saturation value Startle response Yawning, hiccoughing, gagging, vomiting
Body	Flaccidity Hypertonicity Splaying of fingers and toes Hand over face Arm extension
State	Crying and fussing Abrupt change to sleep or wake state

Managing pain and discomfort

Although much attention has been focused on pain in infancy and childhood there are still concerns about the management of pain in neonates. Appropriate tools to assess pain in the newborn have been developed, but difficulties remain when the assessment needs to be made on very preterm babies and babies with neurological dysfunction. Pain scales are usually based on the monitoring of behavioural signs and facial expression together with variations in physiological assessments such as increased heart rate (Table 49.4) (*see also* Caring for children in pain p. 351).

The use of drugs for pain relief in the newborn is problematic as few drugs are properly researched for use in this population. Non-pharmacological methods have been shown to reduce the babies' behavioural responses to pain – for example, positive touch and holding (Sparshott, 1997). Sucrose placed on the tongue of the baby provides a short-term, effective analgesic. As the baby is required to swallow the sucrose, its use must be restricted to babies who have established sucking feeds (Boyd, 2002). The timing of administration is crucial to its effectiveness and interprofessional planning is required prior to clinical procedures such as cannulation.

Minimising pain and discomfort for the newborn

- Be aware of and reduce environmental stressors, see Table 49.2
- Correct, comfortable positioning
- Thermoneutral environment
- Use baby behavioural cues to determine when it is appropriate to give care
- Do not wake the baby during deep sleep
- Use non-pharmacological methods to soothe the baby, i.e. crown–rump holding and positive touch
- Use good technique
- Allow periods of rest if the intervention needs to be repeated
- Care with the type of tape used and its removal
- Use appropriate analgesia
- Care when clinical monitors and other equipment need to be adhered to the body of the baby

Study activity

Find out if your local neonatal unit uses specific assessment tools for assessing pain in neonates. If they do, critically compare them with those used for older infants and children.

Managing unstable blood sugars

Newborn babies have high glucose needs and low glycogen stores. This makes them more at risk of hypoglycaemia if they use the available glucose to maintain homeostasis when they are distressed by disease or external stressors. In health there is no reason to monitor the blood glucose of the healthy term baby, even when breastfeeding is not fully established. Monitoring of blood glucose should only be done if the infant is ill, preterm, small for gestational age or born to a diabetic mother (National Childbirth Trust, 1997). Prolonged low blood glucose values can cause brain damage, leading to developmental abnormalities including cerebral palsy and severe mental retardation. The aim of management should be to prevent hypoglycaemia in all babies. This can be achieved by commencing breastfeeding immediately following birth. Falling blood glucose values in sick neonates can be counteracted by smaller, more frequent enteral feeds or intravenous infusion. A fall in body temperature and a reluctance to wake and feed may provide the first signs of hypoglycaemia before more serious signs of jitteriness, apnoea, respiratory 'grunting' or fits are seen.

Causes of hypoglycaemia

- Small-for-dates babies
- Infants of diabetic mothers
- Poor feeding/delayed feeding
- Severe birth asphyxia
- Sick babies where the illness is severe
- Haemolytic disease of the newborn
- Polycythaemia
- Inborn errors of metabolism

Study activity

What blood value does your unit/ward classify as hypoglycaemia in a term neonate? Note your findings in the margin for future reference.

Managing jaundice

The appearance of neonatal jaundice, typically on the third day of life, is normally a physiological response to the change from fetal to extrauterine life (physiological jaundice; Mupanemunda and Watkinson, 1999). The skin and sclera of the eye take a yellow discoloration. No treatment is necessary unless the serum bilirubin values rise to a very high value. Jaundice in the newborn can also be an important sign that the baby has an underlying disease (pathological jaundice). It is important to assess the baby when jaundice appears to determine which type of jaundice the baby is showing (Table 49.5).

Study activity

Before reading on, take time to refresh your knowledge of the metabolism of bile pigments. Figure 49.1 might help you.

Physiological jaundice. This appears from 2 to 5 days of age. Physiological jaundice is accepted as 'normal'. It occurs as a result of a temporary deficiency in the values of glucuronyl transferase, an enzyme in the liver that converts bilirubin to bile pigments for excretion. At the same time there is a rapid breakdown of fetal red cells after birth with a consequent rise in unconjugated bilirubin values. Serum bilirubin values return to normal by day 10 or 11. Circulating serum bilirubin will reach higher values if the baby is born with polycythaemia or has bruising to resolve from a birth injury.

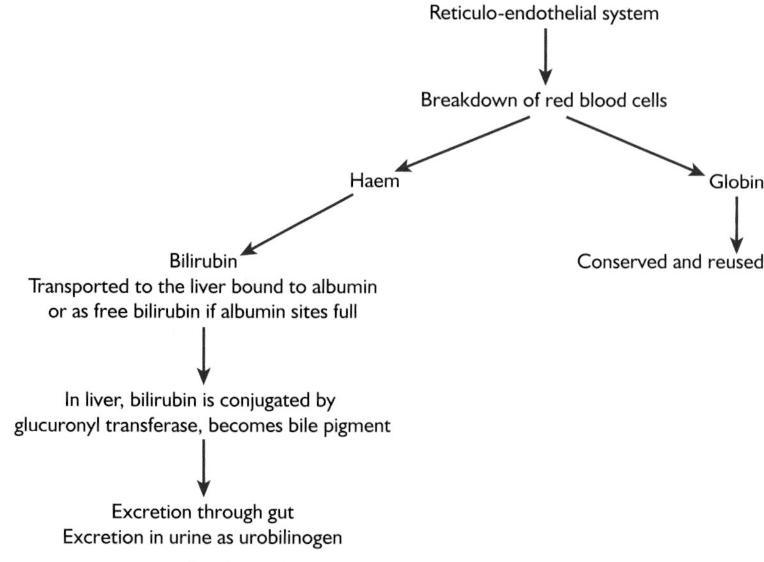

Figure 49.1 Normal pathway for red blood cell breakdown.

Pathological jaundice. Jaundice is associated with disease when it:

- Occurs at birth or within 24 hours due to haemolysis of red cells as a result of rhesus or blood group incompatibility with the mother. The level of unconjugated bilirubin rises and the cause should be investigated immediately.
- Is prolonged. In this cases there may be a rise in either conjugated or unconjugated bilirubuin or both.
- Appears as part of another neonatal disease.

It is important to assess serum bilirubin values particularly if there is a rise in unconjugated bilirubin. High levels of fat-soluble unconjugated bilirubin can pass across the blood–brain barrier and cause kernicterus – damage to the basal ganglia and brain stem. Clinical signs of kernicterus include opisthotonos, limb rigidity, tremors or convulsions and fever. Infants who survive kernicterus can present with mental retardation, deafness and other neurological problems. The values set as treatment criteria remain a matter of discussion and wide variations exist between neonatal units. Treatment criteria will also depend on the gestational age and weight of the baby.

Study activity

At what serum bilirubin value would your local neonatal unit treat neonatal jaundice? Note your findings in the margin for future reference. Compare this treatment value with values from other neonatal units.

Treatment for jaundice includes:

- *Phototherapy.* This treatment can often prevent unconjugated bilirubin from rising to dangerous levels. The infant is placed under

Table 49.5 Causes of jaundice

Jaundice occurring at birth or within first 24 hours – rapid treatment is essential	ABO incompatibility Rhesus incompatibility Congenital infection Haemolytic anaemia, i.e. sickle-cell anaemia
Causes of jaundice occurring between days 2 and 5	Physiological jaundice Some drugs Infection Polycythaemia at birth Bruising from birth injury Metabolic disease
Causes of prolonged jaundice	Breastmilk jaundice Liver disease Biliary atresia Cystic fibrosis

fluorescent light tubes, which emit blue light that converts bilirubin in the skin to harmless water-soluble metabolites. These are then excreted in the urine and bowel. Nursing management of babies having phototherapy must take account of the following:

- The baby must be nursed naked to maximise the area of skin exposed to the light. This makes the maintainence of a thermo-neutral environment important.
- The use of phototherapy looks uncomfortable for the baby and there can be a feeling that the baby is not accessible to the mother while treatment is continuing. This can cause parental anxiety, so full explanation and support must be given.
- Radiation from blue light has been shown to cause retinal damage. The baby's eyes must therefore be protected by the use of eye shields or a tinted screen. The protection must be checked regularly as small babies can often wriggle out from under the screen or push off eyeshields.
- There is often increased fluid loss from the skin during phototherapy. The treatment can also decrease bowel transit time, leading to diarrhoea. Jaundiced infants are often drowsy and do not always wake for feeds. Consideration must therefore be given to increasing fluid intake.

- *Exchange transfusion.* This is an effective rapid means of removing bilirubin from the blood, particularly if serum levels are near danger point. This procedure may now be done *in utero*.

Study activity

Investigate the types of phototherapy equipment used in your neonatal unit. Examine the advantages and disadvantages of each.

Planning for Discharge

Planning for discharge should ideally begin as soon as a neonate is admitted to the unit. Going home with a small baby or one that has been very ill can be a daunting prospect for any parent. Some hospitals have transitional care wards where the babies are cared for by their parents under supervision from the nurses. This can help to build confidence and allow the parents time to adjust to their baby. Each family is unique and will have unique needs, so a careful teaching plan should be drawn up to ensure that all aspects of the baby's care are covered. Some babies will go home with continuing care needs such as oxygen therapy, gastrostomy feeding, colostomies and wound dressings. In these cases parents will need support from community children's nurses. Some areas have special community nurses whose role is mainly to visit and support parents with special-care babies in the first few days and weeks at home. Whichever type of support is available, the nurse must take time to develop a trusting relationship with the family. Voluntary support agencies such as BLISS give valuable written information and are able to put parents in touch with other families with similar problems. Other voluntary organisations exist for other special problems such as tracheooesophageal fistula (TOF).

Preterm babies have an increased risk of cot death (SIDS). This is 12 times more likely to occur in babies born weighing between 1500 and 1999 g than in babies weighing more than 3500 g at birth (Office for National Statistics, 2001). Near-miss SIDS also occurs more frequently in low birthweight survivors. Before leaving the neonatal unit every parent must be taught resuscitation techniques and be given the advice prescribed by the Department of Health regarding the prevention of SIDS (DH, 1996) (*see also* Home oxygen therapy p. 541).

Study activity

Visit a neonatal unit and find out what resources are available to support parents and their babies on discharge from the neonatal unit.

Long-term Problems for Sick and Preterm Newborns

When a baby needs care in a neonatal unit at the beginning of its life, it will be separated from its mother and family, receive distressing and painful procedures, have multiple carers and experience a confusing range of sensations and experiences. The emotional impact of this on the growing child may overlie any other residual problems left by the condition that necessitated neonatal care.

The continuing EPIcure UK study (Costeloe *et al.*, 2000) gives a clear picture of the long-term effects of very preterm birth. Potential problems faced by these babies include:

- *Neurological problems*: cerebral palsy, developmental delay, severe learning difficulties, sensory, visual motor and attentional problems,

hydrocephalus, microcephaly, blindness, deafness and epilepsy. Some children display more subtle problems, such as lower than average IQ, clumsiness, poor hand–eye coordination, poor speech articulation and behavioural problems.
- *Respiratory problems*: bronchopulmonary dysplasia or chronic lung disease – a chronic inflammatory lung disease characterised by an increased oxygen demand. It occurs in preterm infants who have been mechanically ventilated.
- *Sensory problems*: retinopathy of prematurity – this normally occurs in babies who are born at an early gestational age and as a result of a variable partial pressure of oxygen in arterial blood where hyperoxic episodes have occurred. This damages the retinal blood vessel network, causing blindness.
- *Nutritional problems*: poor coordination and lack of stamina for sucking and swallowing, prolonged tube feeding, delayed weaning, poor weight gain, anaemia of prematurity, gastro-oesophageal reflux, and clinical interventions such as intubation and suction, giving the baby multiple negative experiences in and around the mouth.

All infants who have spent time in the special-care baby unit need close follow-up to:

- assess growth and development
- detect complications
- detect emergence of problems related to new treatments
- give continuing advice and support to the parents
- look for long-term effects of early care in the neonatal unit shown in social, educational and emotional development

Chapter 50

Principles of Care – Children Undergoing Cytotoxic Treatment and Radiotherapy

Introduction

Childhood malignancies are rare – cancers in those aged under 15 years account for only 1% of all cancers in industralised countries (Stiller and Draper, 1998) – and in 2005 NICE estimated that 75% of children in Britain who were diagnosed with cancer would survive. Over the past 30 years there has been a huge improvement in the survival rates of children with cancer, largely due to cytotoxic therapy. Chemotherapy for the treatment of childhood cancers really began in the 1970s and since then new, complex and multidrug regimes have evolved and contributed to the steady rise in cure rates. The most promising results have been demonstrated in children with acute lymphoblastic leukaemia (ALL), but solid tumours of childhood have also responded well to cytotoxic drugs when used in conjunction with radiotherapy and surgery (Hollis, 1997). Leukaemia is the most common cancer of children of all ages, accounting for 35.4% of all childhood cancers (NICE, 2005).

The acute leukaemias comprise over half of the leukaemias seen in clinical practice. Eighty per cent of leukaemias in children are of the acute lymphoblastic type. The incidence of ALL is highest at 3–4 years, falling off by 10 years. There is a low frequency after 10 years with a secondary rise after 40 years of age. Acute myeloid leukaemias (AML) occur in all age groups but are more common in adults and form only a fraction of childhood leukaemias.

The prognosis of acute leukaemia in children has been greatly improved by the use of chemotherapy, radiotherapy, better supportive therapy and the development of specialist leukaemia units:

- from 30 to 50% of children with ALL are now alive and have been off treatment 5 years from presentation
- relapsed disease is more difficult to treat, and has a worse prognosis
- progress in treatment of AML has not been as good as that of ALL

As drug therapy plays the main role in the treatment of many cancers, it is important to understand what action each drug has in order that nursing care can be given accordingly. The drugs fall into five main areas (Tables 50.1–50.4):

- cytotoxic therapy – the curative part of the treatment
- prophylactic drugs – to prevent or minimise the effects of cytotoxic therapy
- IV antibiotics – to treat isolated or suspected infections
- pre- and post-bone marrow transplant drugs – to prevent 'graft versus host' disease and to stimulate the action of the new bone marrow
- miscellaneous drugs – to correct or prevent the complications of the treatment or illness or given as part of the non-cytotoxic curative treatment

Risks of chemotherapy errors in children

- All doses have to be carefully calculated and prepared and fluid volume determined according to the size of the child.
- Weight loss or gain (often side-effects of the treatment) can significantly alter the correct dosage.
- Many drugs are not licensed for use with children, or are rarely used for children, and treatment regimens are complex.
- Oral preparations are not always available or palatable for children, making compliance difficult.
- Tablets may not be available in small dosages, requiring portions of tablets or small, regularly repeated doses to be given.

(NICE, 2005)

Cytotoxic Treatment

The aim of cytotoxic treatment is initially to induce a remission (absence of any clinical or laboratory evidence of the disease) and then to continue to reduce the hidden malignant cell population by repeated courses of therapy. Cyclical combinations of two, three or four drugs are given with treatment-free intervals to allow the bone marrow to recover. This recovery depends upon the differential regrowth pattern of normal haemopoietic and malignant cells. The delivery of chemotherapy to children is more complex with a greater potential for errors than in adults (NICE, 2005).

There are five types of cytotoxic drugs:

- Alkylating agents act on the nucleus of the cell and cause DNA strands to break or cross-link abnormally, preventing normal DNA replication and cell growth.
- Antimetabolites replace cell metabolites or inhibit their activity so that the normal cell growth is interrupted.
- Cytotoxic antibiotics are similar to alkylating agents as they break down the system of DNA/RNA replication and interfere with protein synthesis. They appear to increase sensitivity to radiation therapy.
- Vinca alkaloids – these inhibit cell division at the metaphase stage of chromosome separation and so have a growth-inhibiting action.
- Miscellaneous drugs – a group of ill-defined, unrelated substances that have a cytotoxic action.

Prednisolone, vincristine and asparaginase are the drugs usually used in ALL to achieve remission in over 90% of children in 4–6 weeks. Daunorubicin or doxorubicin (Adriamycin) is added to the regimen either in the induction phase or in the consolidation phase once remission has been achieved. The following carry a less favourable prognosis:

- males compared to females
- those with an initial high leucocyte count
- meningeal involvement at presentation
- very young (under 2 years) or older (adolescent or adult) patients

In all of these cases, more intensive induction regimens improve chances of long-term survival. Maintenance chemotherapy usually follows for 2–3 years with daily mercaptopurine and weekly methotrexate (vincristine, steroids and other drugs are added in some cases).

Table 50.1 Drugs used to treat childhood cancers

	Mechanism of action	Specific side-effects	Nursing care
Cyclophosphamide	Alkylating agent	Severe haemorrhagic cystitis, cardiomyopathy, alopecia	Mesna infusion runs concurrently (this inactivates the toxin acrolein) Give dose early morning to enable high fluid intake later Test all urine for blood, pH and sugar Ensure a high urine output is maintained
Methotrexate	Antimetabolite – inhibits the formation of folic acid, essential for metabolism and DNA synthesis	Severe gut toxicity, liver and renal damage, CNS toxicity, pneumonitis, mouth ulcers	Gut toxicity is reduced by the administration of 'folinic acid' (calcium leucovorin rescue); if this is not given after a high dose of methotrexate the toxicity may be fatal Observe for signs of neurotoxicity Avoid the use of folic acid-containing vitamins
Cytosine arabinoside (cytarabine)	Antimetabolite – a powerful depressant of bone marrow function	Hyperuricaemia, liver damage, gut toxicity, haemolytic anaemia, conjunctivitis	Observe for sore eyes, jaundice
G-mercaptopurine	Antimetabolite – has a valuable suppressive action in acute leukaemia and can produce a remission of the disease; however, response to a repeated course may be less dramatic and repeated treatment leads eventually to a refractory state unresponsive to further treatment	Unusual – hyperuricaemia, liver damage	None specific
G-thioguanine	Antimetabolite – similar to G-mercaptopurine, but mainly used in AML; a powerful myelo-suppressive drug	As for G-mercaptopurine	None specific
Doxorubicin (Adriamycin)	Cytotoxic antibiotic – binds with DNA to interfere with mitosis	Cardiac toxicity, causing tachycardia and arrhythmias, alopecia, colours urine red (but this is not significant)	ECG monitoring, warn child and parents of red urine up to 12 days after administration
Daunorubicin	Cytotoxic antibiotic – similar to doxorubicin	As for doxorubicin	As for doxorubicin
Vincristine	Vinca alkaloid	Neuropathy (peripheral, bladder or gut), abdominal colic, constipation and alopecia	Observe for signs of neurotoxicity, monitor bowel movements, administer stool softeners (e.g. lactulose)
Etanoside (VP16–231)	Miscellaneous – similar to the vinca alkaloids as it is a mitotic inhibitor	Alopecia, oral ulceration, hypotension, bradycardia, allergic reaction (rare)	Give slowly as IV infusion with emergency drugs available to treat anaphylaxis and/or shock
L-Asparaginase	Miscellaneous – an enzyme that depletes the cells of asparagine	Allergic reactions (urticaria, hypotension, anaphylaxis), fever, anorexia and weight loss, low albumin, pancreatitis, renal and liver dysfunction	Daily weight, emergency drugs available to treat anaphylaxis

Table 50.2 Prophylactic drugs – standard regimen

Mucosal infection

All patients are commenced on the following drugs on diagnosis and continue them throughout periods of chemotherapy:

- amphotericin suspension – anti-fungal prophylaxis of mouth
- Betadine/chlorhexidine mouthwash – for prevention of mucosal sepsis
- ciprofloxacin – used instead of neomycin in patients over 14 years old
- colistin – useful to prevent Gram-negative infection of the intestine
- fluconazole – an oral triazole anti-fungal used as prophylaxis against local and systemic candidiasis and cryptococcal infections
- neomycin – an aminoglycoside antibiotic used to prevent intestinal infection

Herpes

Aciclovir is given to all bone marrow transplant patients with pre-transplant IgC antibodies to the herpes simplex virus. It is given for 100 days from transplant. It is also used for patients who have had contact with chickenpox. It is an antiviral drug which is inactive until it enters a virus-infected site. It is then activated by a viral enzyme to form aciclovir phosphate, which blocks the replication of viral DNA

Tuberculosis (TB)

Prophylaxis with isoniazid is required for 6 months post BMT if there is a previous history of TB or an abnormal chest X-ray. Isoniazid is a highly selective antibacterial drug which has virtually no action against organisms other than *Mycobacterium tuberculosis*. It is rapidly absorbed and penetrates easily into the tissues and fluids, including the cerebrospinal fluid. As it is thought to interfere with normal pyridoxine metabolism, pyridoxine is also given

Pneumocystis carinii

Prophylactic treatment with Septrin is required for all BMT patients for 1 week prior to transplant and 6 months post transplant (or until counts increase). Septrin acts as an antibacterial agent by a combination of blocking the formation of folic acid and preventing its conversion to folinic acid

Other infections

Other than the specific treatments listed above, the following are the most commonly used prophylactic drugs:

- **amikacin** – a semi-synthetic aminoglycoside, effective against Gram-negative organisms and some staphylococcal infections
- **amphotericin B** – is the most effective drug for the treatment of deep fungal infections such as cryptococcosis, histoplasmosis and systemic candidiasis
- **azlocillin** – a broad-spectrum antibiotic with significant anti-pseudomonal activity
- **ceftazidime** – a bacterial cephalosporin antibiotic, active against a wide range of Gram-positive and Gram-negative bacteria
- **erythromycin** – effective against Gram-positive and a few Gram-negative organisms. Active against many respiratory infections, including *Mycoplasma pneumoniae*. Useful against penicillin-resistant organisms
- **metronidazole** – effective against anaerobic infections, e.g. peritonitis
- **vancomycin** – effective against many Gram-positive organisms and severe staphylococcal or streptococcal infections which do not respond to other antibiotics

Cytoxic therapy for AML is similar to that of ALL but with worse results. The most commonly used regimen for AML is cytosine, daunorubicin and 6-thioguanine. Compared with ALL:

- the remission rate is lower (60–80%)
- remission often takes longer to achieve
- myelotoxic drugs are of major value, with less selectivity between leukaemic and normal marrow cells
- marrow failure is severe and prolonged
- remissions are shorter and maintenance therapy is less effective

Central nervous system prophylaxis is not routinely given in AML although intrathecal methotrexate may be used as a prophylactic.

Table 50.3 Pre- and post-bone marrow transplant drugs

Anti-human granulocyte colony (ALG) stimulating factor
Used in haematology to treat severe aplastic anaemia or to treat 'graft versus host' disease post BMT. It is a purified solution of horse anti-human lymphocyte immunoglobulin. It is obtained by hyper-immunisation of horses with human lymphocytes. Thus, it acts by attacking lymphocytes and causes immunosuppression. It requires monitoring during infusion for signs of fever, hypotension, respiratory distress and urticaria. (ATG, which is a rabbit serum derivative, may be used where there is intolerance to horse proteins)

Campath
This an unlicensed investigational drug. It is used prior to bone marrow transplantation in order to prevent graft rejection or 'graft versus host'. It contains an antibody to human lymphocytes and monocytes which is produced in rats, and hence is an immunosuppressive. As it is a rat protein it may provoke hypersensitive reactions when the test dose is given, and monitoring is required during the infusion of further doses. Side-effects include fever, chills, rigors, nausea, urticaria, bronchospasm and hypotension

Cyclosporin 'A'
An immunosuppressive agent which will reduce the risk of 'graft versus host' disease. It has a selective action on the T lymphocytes (which react with foreign proteins), but unlike other immunosuppressive drugs it does not depress the general bone marrow activity

Human granulocyte colony stimulating factor (G-CSF)
Is a glycoprotein which regulates the production and release of functional neutrophils from the bone marrow. It is used post BMT or following a period of prolonged neutropenia post-chemotherapy. Marked increases in peripheral blood neutrophil counts can occur within 24 hours. G-CSF is usually restricted to non-myeloid leukaemia because of the possibility of its action causing an increase of malignant cells. However, this has not been established. Specific side-effects include mild or moderate musculoskeletal pain and dysuria

Drugs used for their cytotoxic action are not selective and therefore their effect on rapidly dividing malignant cells is duplicated on healthy cells that have a high rate of proliferation. These include the cells of the bone marrow, hair, skin and the epithelial cells of the gastro-intestinal tract. Problems caused by the destruction of these healthy cells are often more debilitating and traumatic to the child than the disease itself.

The actual administration of cytotoxic drugs is potentially dangerous. Many of these drugs are sclerosing agents that can cause severe cellular damage if extravasation occurs. The resulting inflammation and ulceration can progress slowly over several weeks. They should only be administered by specialist nurses using a patent vein that has been initially tested with isotonic saline. The injection site should be constantly observed for signs of infiltration and irrigated with saline after the administration to avoid leakage of the drug as the needle is removed. Suspected extravasation can be treated by:

- cessation of administration
- changing the syringe but leaving the needle in place and withdrawing as much of the drug as possible
- 100 mg hydrocortisone infiltrated into the surrounding tissue
- immediate application of warm compresses to the site to increase circulation and absorption of the drug into the bloodstream

Table 50.4 Miscellaneous drugs used in oncology

Allopurinol
Given post-chemotherapy to reduce uric acid formation which is produced by the breakdown of neoplastic cells. As there is mass cell destruction after a course of chemotherapy, increased uric acid may cause gout to develop. Allopurinol prevents this by inhibiting the action of an enzyme concerned with purine metabolism and so indirectly reduces uric acid formation

Amiloride
A potassium-sparing mild diuretic which is usually given to reduce potassium loss during a course of amphotericin

Analgesics
A variety are used according to the severity of the pain

Anti-emetics
Should be given regularly during courses of chemotherapy. Metoclopramide is used in children only for the severe nausea associated with cytotoxic therapy due to potential acute dystonic reactions. Ondansetron is a more effective, longer lasting anti-emetic, the action of which may be enhanced by dexamethasone

Azathiaprine
Has a marked depressant effect on the bone marrow and hence slows the disease process

Piriton and hydrocortisone
May be used prophylactically prior to the administration of blood derivatives when previous reactions have occurred. They may also be used to minimise reactions to ALG/ATG and campath

Prednisolone
A glucocorticosteroid which increases the resistance of the body to stress and shock and has the power of suppressing the inflammatory processes generally. It inhibits the development of lymphocytes and in leukaemia a high degree of remission of symptoms may result. Although it cannot prevent an ultimate relapse, as well as initiating a remission it may restore a sensitivity to other forms of treatment. Side-effects include delayed tissue repair, increased gastric acidity causing or exacerbating peptic ulcers, electrolyte imbalance, muscle wasting, loss of calcium, hypertension, Cushing's syndrome and diabetes

Ranitidine
May be used for either active or prophylactic treatment of peptic ulcers/mucositis. Unlike antacids which neutralise the gastric acid, ranitidine acts by inhibiting gastric acid secretion and pepsin output. This is done by blocking the histamine H_2 receptors which are chiefly found in the gastric parietal cells and are concerned with acid and pepsin secretion. Conventional antihistamines only block the H_1 receptors, hence cannot inhibit the acid secretion response to histamine

Vitamin and mineral supplements
Required to overcome the poor nutritional intake associated with the toxic effects of chemotherapy as well as the deficiencies caused by the intensive drug therapy. The commonly used supplements include pyridoxine (B_6), vitamin K, Parentrovite, folic acid, Sando-K, Sandocal and Sando-phosphate

- cold compresses after 1 hour to relieve pain and swelling
- referral to a plastic surgery team

(*See also* Intravenous fluid therapy p. 344)

In addition, many cytotoxic drugs may cause an anaphylactic reaction. After administration, the child should be observed for at least 20 minutes and emergency equipment must be close at hand. If a reaction is suspected, the administration should be discontinued and the line flushed with isotonic saline.

Many children have a surgically inserted indwelling intravenous access line to overcome the problems of repeated venous access required for intensive courses of cytotoxic therapy, blood analysis and the frequent administration of blood products. However, blood required to monitor antibiotic levels must be taken peripherally to ensure accuracy (Pinkerton *et al.*, 1996).

Skin care during radiotherapy

Do:

- use soft loose clothing
- keep the area clean, using only water to wash
- dress moist areas with non-adherent dressings, tubular bandages and non-allergic tape
- apply prescribed cream to area at least twice daily until the skin has returned to normal
- use sunscreen with a protection factor of 15 or more

Don't:

- rub or massage the area
- alter or wash off the indelible marks which delineate the area for treatment
- expose the area to the sun during treatment and for up to a year after treatment
- use perfumes, deodorants or perfumed toiletries on the area

Care of the pyrexial neutropenic child

Identify any potential sources of infection:

- central line site
- mucosal ulceration
- skin tears, abrasions
- blood, stool, urine and nasopharyngeal cultures
- chest X-ray

Treat the infection:

- IV administration of a combination of broad-spectrum antibiotics for a minimum of 10 days

Prevent further infection:

- protective isolation
- restriction of visitors with infection or history of contact
- varicella immunoglobin (ZIG) within 48 hours for children who have been exposed to chickenpox

Radiotherapy

Radiotherapy is normally used to treat or relieve childhood cancer in conjunction with chemotherapy and/or surgery. Whenever possible it is avoided for children under 3 years old because of the greater long-term effects. It may be beneficial in palliative care because its action shrinks tumours and thus reduces symptoms. It is the palliative treatment of choice for isolated bone secondaries as it relieves pain and prevents pathological fractures. Radiotherapy has a cytotoxic effect by:

- damaging the pyrimidine bases (cytosine, thymine and uracil) which are required for nucleic acid synthesis
- causing breaks in DNA or RNA molecules

During radiotherapy the child has to stay still for up to 25 minutes. In small children this may require anaesthesia and/or play therapy.

Side-effects of radiotherapy are mostly due to the cytotoxic effects of radiation but the specific problem is skin damage. The affected area of skin and mucous membranes can initially become blanched or erythematous. Later reactions include dryness, itching, peeling, blistering and loss of tissue. The area targeted for radiation should be monitored daily to enable early recognition and treatment of problems.

Side-effects of Cytotoxic Treatment and Radiotherapy

Cytotoxic treatment and radiotherapy have many side-effects but the most life threatening is bone marrow depression (Table 50.5). Overwhelming infection may occur secondary to neutropenia, and thrombocytopenia may cause haemorrhage. The child is most at risk from infection:

- at the time of diagnosis when the leucocytes have been largely replaced by malignant cells
- during immunosuppressive treatment
- after prolonged antibiotic treatment when resistant organisms may develop

The child undergoing cytotoxic treatment will often not show the usual overt features of infection and the first sign may be pyrexia. The care of neutropenic children is usually outlined in strict local protocols, which usually include protective isolation. However, research shows that such isolation neither decreases the infection risk nor improves survival (Frenck *et al.*, 1991). Reasonable precautions should be continued at home to protect the child from infection but this has to be moderated by the need for the child to resume a normal lifestyle which includes returning to school. Haemopoietic growth factors have recently been produced in the laboratory to stimulate the bone marrow and reduce the duration of high-dose cytotoxic therapy-induced neutropenia. Haemorrhage associated with thrombocytopenia can be prevented by the administration of platelets whenever the platelet count falls below 20. Packed red cells are usually transfused when the haemoglobin falls below 8 g/dl.

Table 50.5 Nursing care of children with cancer undergoing cytotoxic treatment or radiotherapy

Problem	Effect	Intervention
Due to bone marrow failure		
anaemia	Pallor, lethargy, dyspnoea	Blood transfusions
leucopenia	Fever, malaise, infections of mouth, throat, skin, lungs and risk of septicaemia	Isolation or clean care, antibiotics for specific infections, clean food
thrombocytopenia	Spontaneous bruising, purpura, bleeding gums and major haemorrhage risk	Platelet infusions, mouth care and mouth washes
Due to organ infiltration of		
bones	Joint pain, lytic bone lesions	Analgesia
lymph glands	Superficial lymphadenopathy	Analgesia
spleen	Moderate splenomegaly	Analgesia
liver	Hepatomegaly	Analgesia
gums	Gum hypertrophy	Action to minimise localised infection
bowel	Rectal ulceration	
skin	Skin involvement	
central nervous system	Headaches, nausea and vomiting, blurred vision diplopia, papilloedema, and haemorrhage	Intrathecal chemotherapy
testes	Swelling	Localised radiotherapy
Due to combined effect of above		
anorexia, nausea and vomiting	Loss of weight and muscle wasting	Anti-emetics, high calorie drinks and diet
long-term hospitalisation and effects of treatment (e.g. alopecia)	Delayed development, psychological problems of patient and parents	Involvement of psychosocial team, teaching staff and play leaders
long-term prognosis	Anxiety for family	Support of whole family

Nausea and vomiting are probably the most distressing side-effects of chemotherapy (Knapman, 1993) and the most difficult to control. A small study by Cook and Gallagher in 1996 revealed that chemotherapy-induced nausea and vomiting are poorly controlled and remain a challenge to children's nursing. The National Institute for Health and Clinical Excellence (NICE, 2005) suggested that non-pharmacological approaches (such as distraction techniques, relaxation or guided imagery) to the management of nausea and vomiting can be beneficial, especially if the symptoms are anticipatory. However, for the children themselves it appears that alopecia is the most traumatic side-effect of cytotoxic treatment (Reid, 1997). Wigs are available but most children prefer to wear hats, caps or scarves. Some kind of head protection is important to prevent hypothermia or overheating and sunburn. Children can be reassured that regrowth usually occurs in 3–6 months but should be warned that the new hair is often darker, thicker and curlier than before.

Porter (1994) suggests that 90% of children undergoing chemotherapy experience oral complications. The cause of this is not only the direct cytotoxic effect on the rapidly dividing cells of the oral mucosa but also the child's susceptibility to oral infections due to neutropenia, thrombocytopenia, anorexia and malnutrition. It may be also due to poor recognition of the problem. Campbell (1987) indicated that nurses did not have the knowledge to assess oral complications of cytotoxic therapy. Since then various assessment tools have been developed to assess and score the condition of the mouth (Table 50.6) and the

Table 50.6 Oral assessment scoring scale

	Scoring		
Assessment	**1**	**2**	**3**
Listening to child talking or crying	Normal	Deep or hoarse	Difficulty/pain when talking or crying
Observation of swallowing	Normal	Some pain	Inability to swallow
Looking and feeling the lips and corners of the mouth	Smooth, pink and moist	Dry and/or cracked	Ulcerated or bleeding
Looking at the tongue	Pink, moist with obvious papillae	Coated or smooth and shiny	Blistered or cracked

importance of prophylactic mouth care has been recognised. Pinkerton *et al.* (1996) recommend 6-hourly teeth cleaning with a soft toothbrush and toothpaste (and sterile water if neutropenic), Corsodyl mouthwash held in the mouth for 30–60 seconds and fluconazole (*see also* Dental hygiene p. 181).

Anorexia is often a side-effect of cytotoxic therapy. It may be related to a sore mouth, nausea and vomiting, constipation or anxiety and depression. It appears to distress parents more than the child (Brady, 1994). Steroids will sometimes alleviate anorexia but their side-effects often outweigh their benefits, especially if the anorexia is not concerning the child. An altered sense of taste may change the child's usual likes and dislikes and it may need some experimentation to restimulate the appetite. Small, frequent and varied snacks may help the child to eat. Poor nutrition not only affects the child's general well-being but also exacerbates children's susceptibility to infection and decreases their tolerance to cytotoxic therapy. Pinkerton *et al.* (1996) suggest that the vicious cycle of poor intake, poor appetite and weight loss is overcome by naso-gastric feeding until the child can return to normal eating. Total parenteral nutrition is usually only required by children on intensive chemotherapeutic regimens such as those required in AML, prior to bone marrow transplantation and for stage IV neuroblastomas.

Bone Marrow Transplantation (BMT)

Children who have malignancies that cannot be treated by other means may be given a bone marrow transplant. This involves the administration of lethal doses of chemotherapy, often in conjunction with radiation, to eradicate all the malignant cells and suppress the immune system to prevent rejection of the transplanted marrow. A transfusion of donor marrow cells can then be given to produce normal blood cells. Three types of BMT are possible:

- allogeneic – a match with a histocompatible donor (sibling or unrelated donor)

- autologous – uses the patient's own peripheral blood stem cells or marrow
- syngeneic – uses donated marrow from an identical twin

Study activity

Find out the procedure to become a bone marrow donor. Discuss this with friends and relatives to assess how many people outside the health service are aware of the bone marrow donor register. Consider how children's nurses could raise this awareness.

Allogeneic BMT is now used during the first remission with AML and in ALL patients who relapse and achieve a successful second remission after reinduction chemotherapy. It is also considered in poor prognosis ALL patients after the first remission.

Prior to BMT, intensive chemotherapy and total body irradiation (TBI) are given to kill all remaining leukaemic cells. Preliminary results of trials show 50% long-term survivors but the first month after transplant is potentially the most risky as the child is completely neutropenic and thrombocytopenic. In addition to the risk of overwhelming infection and life-threatening haemorrhage, the child is also at risk of graft-versus-host disease (GVHD). This is caused by the donor T lymphocytes, which perceive the host as a foreign protein and begin to attack the cells of the skin, gastro-intestinal tract, liver, heart, lungs lymphoid tissue or bone marrow. Treatment is by immunosuppressant drugs.

Place of Care

The major care for children with cancer usually takes place in one of the 17 specialist cancer centres in the UK. Inevitably, parents often live some distance away from these centres so it is common practice for other aspects of care to take place nearer home in hospitals that share care with the lead centre. There are only eight centres that are specifically designed for teenagers and very few paediatric services offer shared care for those over 16 years of age. Elements of specialised care (such as surgery or radiotherapy) may take place in other sites. Treatment usually spans 2–3 years, so much of the child's care is hopefully undertaken at home. Children's community services are not comprehensive and in some areas of the UK community care will be provided by general children's community nurses or district nurses, who may not have the skills to undertake all the necessary care and support for the child and family. In these cases outreach teams from the lead centre provide the necessary support, information and training for these staff to enable the child to remain at home as much as possible.

The National Institute for Health and Clinical Excellence (NICE, 2005) discovered that cancer services for children varied across the UK and made substantial recommendations for the investigation, treatment, rehabilitation and follow-up care of children with cancer in relation to the appropriate staffing and resources required by lead centres and shared care facilities.

Study activity

Find out the facilities in your area for the care of children with cancer.

Long-term Complications

Pinkerton *et al.* (1996) estimate that over 9000 young adults in the UK have survived childhood malignancy. Improved survival rates have made the late effects of successful treatment more apparent. As a result, long-term survivors are followed up yearly, both to monitor their long-term survival and also to identify and treat late effects of treatment (Table 50.7 and Figure 50.1). The National Institute for Health and Clinical Excellence (NICE, 2005) estimated that more than 1200 survivors of childhood cancer become eligible for long-term follow-up each year and this figure will increase steadily as the survival rates improve. As a result they recommend that each survivor has an individual follow-up care plan and an appropriate key worker to enable robust and effective surveillance.

Table 50.7 Potential long-term problems of radiotherapy

Site of radiotherapy	Potential problems
Central nervous system	Hypothalamic/pituitary dysfunction, psychological dysfunction, skeletal mass
Spine	Breast hypoplasia/malignancy, lung or gonadal dysfunction, adverse pregnancy outcome, bladder fibrosis, skeletal mass
Head	Cataracts, caries, hypoplasia of gums, dysfunction of salivary glands
Neck	Thyroid dysfunction/malignancy
Thorax	Breast hypoplasia/malignancy, lung dysfunction, cardiovascular disease
Liver	Dysfunction, fibrosis, malignancy
Gastro-intestinal tract	Dysfunction, fibrosis, malignancy
Kidneys	Renal dysfunction, hypertension, adverse pregnancy outcome
Bladder	Bladder fibrosis, adverse pregnancy outcome
Gonads	Infertility, hormone deficiency, adverse pregnancy outcome
Bone	Hypoplasia, pathological fractures, malignancy
Skin and soft tissue	Malignancy, pigmented naevi

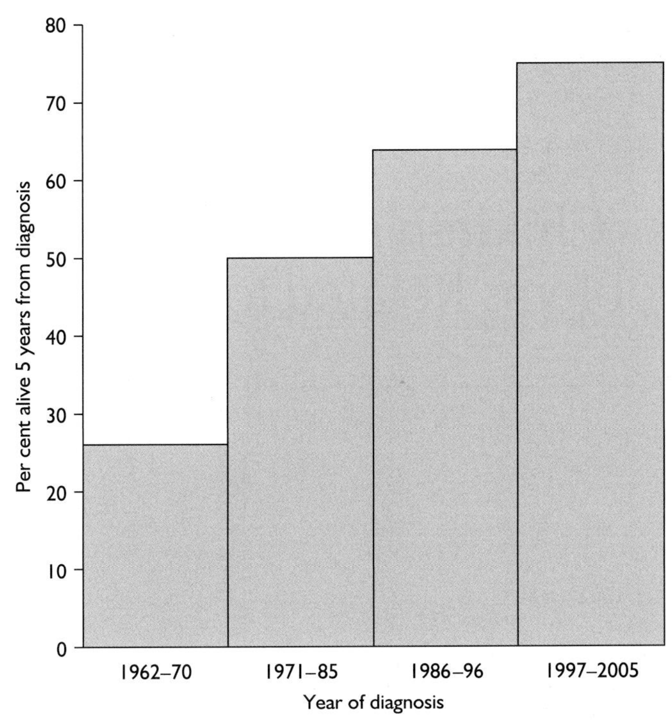

Figure 50.1 Five-year survival rates for childhood malignancy.

Study activity

Find out what follow-up arrangements are in place in your area for children who have been successfully treated for cancer.

Chapter 51

Principles of Care – Children and Adolescents with Problems Related to Sexuality

Introduction

Paediatric and adolescent gynaecology is a relatively neglected area of medicine and many healthcare professionals hesitate to explore problems related to sexuality or perform a gynaecological examination in children and adolescents (Amy, 2003). For this reason this chapter will concentrate mostly on gynaecological problems. The physical changes of puberty, which are occurring at a younger age each decade, are a cause of concern for many young people of both sexes. Although at times young people may be concerned about the physical changes they are experiencing, they often have little understanding of the related physiology. The biological events of puberty not only result in hormonal changes and the development of secondary sexual characteristics but also affect height, weight, strength and endurance. Young people who are confused about these changes may not be aware that they are normal and may find it a difficult topic to discuss. At this time the sexual drive emerges and the resulting outcomes of sexual experimentation in adolescents are a growing problem. The incidence of teenage pregnancies and sexually transmitted diseases continues to increase.

To help young people understand puberty and recognise and respond appropriately to problems, the nurse needs to be able to understand the normal structure and function of the male and female reproductive tract and the normal changes that occur at puberty.

Reproductive tract quiz

- Identify the function of the following hormones:
  - testosterone
  - oestrogen
  - progesterone
  - luteinising hormone
  - follicle stimulating hormone
- List the changes thar occur at puberty for boys and girls, in chronological order. At what average age do these occur?
- Explain the menstrual cycle.
- Describe the position and function of:
  - Bartholin's glands
  - prostate gland
  - ductus epididymis
  - Fallopian (uterine) tubes
- Explain how the ovaries are held in position in the pelvic cavity.
- List the signs that indicate that ovulation has occurred.
- Define the following:
  - vaginitis
  - smegma
  - leukorrhoea
- Explain why a neonate may bleed vaginally.

Study activity

Test your knowledge of the structure and function of the male and female reproductive tracts by answering the questions in the box. Check your answers with an anatomy and physiology textbook.

Common Gynaecological Disorders

Common gynaecological problems can be classified into problems related to menstruation, inflammation of the female genital tract and tumours (Tables 51.1–51.3). At the onset of menstruation cycles are anovulatory. The first ovulation does not takes place until 6–9 months later. Thus the first cycles tend to be irregular and symptom free. Chronic anovulation may be found in adolescents who exercise regularly, especially in girls who started intensive training before puberty (Greene, 1993). Much more is now understood about the problems associated with menstruation. When the author was a student nurse her class was told by the consultant gynaecologist providing their gynaecological lectures that dysmenorrhoea did not exist! Premenstrual tension was not even discussed. Amy (2003) recognised that adolescents with severe dysmenorrhoea tend to be anxious, stressed and depressed, but it is difficult to determine whether these features are the cause or effect of the pain. Dysmenorrhoea is often experienced by those with mothers or siblings who also had painful menstruation and it has been suggested that sufferers learn from their relatives' behaviour. However, Sundell and Milson (1990) suggested that there may be an inherited tendency to sythesise excessive amounts of prostaglandin.

adolescence
The period between puberty and maturity. In males this is around 13–24 years and in females 11–21 years.

puberty
The period during which the secondary sexual characteristics appear and the reproductive organs become functional. On average between 11 and 16 years.

menarche
The first appearance of menstruation.

Premenstrual syndrome (PMS) is a term that was first described in 1931 but it is still poorly understood. It describes the severe physical and emotional distress occurring late in the postovulatory phase of the menstrual cycle. Features such as weight gain, breast tenderness, abdominal distension, backache, irritability, crying and depression commonly increase in severity until the onset of menstruation and then abruptly disappear. The basic cause of PMS is unknown so treatments tend to depend on the type and severity of an individual's symptoms.

Study activity

Talk to some colleagues about their experiences of pain and other symptoms associated with menstruation. Try to identify some common ways of coping with these problems.

Toxic shock syndrome (TSS) was first identified in 1978 and although it can occur in adults, men and young children, it is primarily a disease of previously healthy young menstruating women who use tampons. It is characterised by a high temperature (40°C), sore throat, headache, muscle tenderness, abdominal pain, diarrhoea and vomiting, and rash. It can progress to septicaemia and hypovolaemic shock. Tampons that are highly absorbent enable the growth of bacteria (*Staphylococcus aureus*), which then produce toxins. TSS can also be a complication of the use of contraceptive sponges. Although the condition is rare, adolescent girls should be warned about TSS at the onset of menstruation and advised not to use superabsorbent tampons and always to change tampons every 4–6 hours.

Infections and inflammations of the reproductive tract are relatively common in children and young people. Children and toddlers tend to

Table 51.1 Problems related to menstruation

Primary amenorrhoea	No menstruation by the age of 16 years in the presence of normal secondary sexual characteristics
Secondary amenorrhoea	No menstruation for 3–6 months in previously menstruating females who have an established cycle and when pregnancy has been excluded
Primary (essential) dysmenorrhoea	Typically develops 1–3 years after the menarche. Caused by an excessive endometrial synthesis of prostaglandin during menstruation together with uterine hypertonicity and ischaemia. Lactic acid accumulates in the myometrium and within 1–4 hours of the onset of menstruation a spasmodic suprapubic pain develops, which lasts for 24–48 hours and may be accompanied by nausea, vomiting, fatigue, headache and dizziness. The pain sometimes radiates to the lower back, thighs or groin. It is extremely common and its prevalence tends to increase with age, usually declining after age 25 or childbirth
Secondary dysmenorrhoea	Arises more than 3 years after the onset of menstruation. Likely to be secondary to pelvic pathology. Commonest causes are endometriosis and pelvic inflammatory disease (PID). Usually cyclical but some adolescents experience acyclical or continuous pain
Menorrhagia	Menstrual loss exceeding 80 ml. In adolescents excessive bleeding is usually associated with the irregular cycles due to anovulation experienced at the onset of menstruation
Endometriosis	A benign condition where growths of endometrial tissue develop outside the uterus and swell during the menstrual cycle. The tissue migrates into the pelvis via the open uterine tubes and may be found on the ovaries, sigmoid colon, cervix, surface of the uterus, pelvic ligaments or peritoneum. Swelling of this tissue irritates nerve endings and can create adhesions between pelvic structures. Pain, which is not confined to the suprapubic area, is caused by the displaced tissue sloughing off as the normal endometrium is being shed during menstruation

Causes of vulvovaginitis

1. Bacterial

(a) Non-specific mixed infections caused by:
- Poor perineal hygiene
- Skin infections
- Respiratory infections (group A haemolytic streptococcus)
- Urinary tract infections
- Abrasion or maceration of the skin due to:
  - enuresis
  - ill-fitting underwear
  - sythetic fibres in underwear
- Foreign body (e.g. sand, marble)
- Local toxic reaction to detergent
- Local allergic reaction to soap, nylon, deodorant
- Eczema or other skin disorders
- Anal disorders
- Mechanical irritation (masturbation, sitting on heels)
- Sexual abuse

(b) Specific infections
- *Neisseria gonorrhoeae*
- *Chlamydia trachomatis*
- *Shigella flexneri*
- *Gardnerella vaginalis*
- Meningococcus, pneumococcus

2. Viral

- Herpes simplex
- Molluscum contagiosum
- Measles, varicella

3. Fungal

- *Candida albicans*

(Lammes, 2003)

have poor hygiene and frequently play in soiled areas. The natural curiosity of young children makes self-exploration of the genitalia common and this sometimes results in infection or foreign bodies being lost in the vagina. Although the cause is usually innocent, the possibility of sexual abuse in cases of vulvovaginal inflammation should always be considered. Vulvovaginitis in the adolescent is also very common. It is estimated that 75% of females experience at least one episode of vaginal candida.

Pelvic inflammatory disease (PID), which is a more serious problem and can have long-term effects, is sadly also very common. Cates *et al.* (1990) suggest that women under the age of 25 years are 10 times more likely to develop PID, with a 1 : 8 chance, due to their risky sexual behaviour.

Table 51.2 Inflammations/infections of the female reproductive tract

Vulvovaginitis	This is the most common gynaecological complaint in prepubertal girls. The skin of the vestibule is thin and barely protected by the labia majora and easily becomes irritated and contaminated by a number of causes. The irritation causes a foul-smelling discharge and itching. The commonest cause is poor perineal hygeine or a local reaction to an irritant. Treatment centres around the cause. In adolescents the commonest cause (apart from sexually transmitted causes discussed later) is a *Candida albicans* infection. This is usually the result of a proliferation of the fungus following antibiotic therapy for another condition. Predisposing factors include oral contraception, pregnancy, cortisone medications and diabetes. It causes extreme itching and a thick whitish-yellow discharge and is treated with topical or oral antifungal drugs
Pelvic inflammatory disease	A collective term for any excessive bacterial infection of the pelvic organs. It is commonly caused by sexually transmitted bacteria (*Neisseria gonorrhoeae, Chlamydia trachomatis*), and mostly affects the uterus, uterine tubes and ovaries. Features are fever, general malaise, and lower abdominal, cervical and uterine tenderness. It can spread to cause acute and chronic complications such as salpingitis, peritonitis, chronic abdominal pain, ectopic pregnancy and infertility. Treatment is with antibiotics. Adolescents with high-risk sexual behaviours are particularly at risk as the immature cervical mucus is more easily penetrated by bacteria
Dermatitis of genitals	Varieties of dermatitis involving the perineal area of children include mainly napkin dermatitis, seborrhoeic dermatitis, napkin psoriasis and atopic dermatitis. Lichenification results from constant rubbing or scratching the affected area and this sets up a vicious circle where the chronic inflammation, pruritus and epithelial hyperplasia are exacerbated by scratching. Treatment is with a topical corticosteroid and an oral antihistamine

Table 51.3 Tumours of the female reproductive tract

Sarcoma botryoides	The most common malignancy for girls under 10 years. It usually develops in the lower vagina but can appear in the upper vagina or cervix in older girls. It is a kind of embryonal rhabdomyosarcoma and causes prepubertal vaginal bleeding. Treatment is usually chemotherapy combined with radiotherapy and surgery
Clear cell adenocarcinoma	A cervico-vaginal tumour that occurs mostly in adolescents over 14 years with a prevalence of around 1:1000. Treatment is by radical surgery and radiotherapy but the 5-year survival rate is around 90%
Ovarian tumours	Ovarian masses are relatively common in childhood and adolescence. Functional cysts can be found during periods of hormonal imbalance, such as the neonatal period and puberty. Most ovarian tumours seen in childhood and adolescence are benign; malignant tumours account for only 1% of all malignancies in this age group. They tend not to cause specific features and are often found by chance in a child who is asymptomatic or has only non-specific complaints (nausea, vomiting, constipation). Rupture, torsion or bleeding of the mass may cause more acute symtoms. Treatment is by surgery
Polycystic ovary disease	This is a syndrome (cause unknown) that is defined as large ovaries with numerous small benign cysts arranged cirumferentially with elevated levels of luteinising hormone or testosterone. These abnormal hormone levels which become apparent at puberty cause acne, hirsutism and anovulatory infertility. Treatment centres around cosmetic measures and ovarian androgen-production inhibitors (such as oral contraceptives)

Common Problems of the Male Reproductive Tract

The common problems for boys relating to the male reproductive tract are given in Table 51.4. In addition to these, some uncircumcised boys may encounter problems of infection during adolescence, either due to a tight foreskin or not cleaning the area properly. Poor penile hygiene is an important predisposing factor for penile cancer. Trauma to the

Table 51.4 Problems affecting the male reproductive tract

Varicocele	The veins of the spermatic cord become elongated, dilated and tortuous. The condition is rare in young children but common around the age of onset of puberty. It presents as an asymptomatic unilateral scrotal mass or scrotal pain after exercise. The mass decreases when the boy lies down and becomes tense and distended when he is upright. Treatment for adolescents is usually surgical correction to avoid later infertility problems
Epididymitis	An inflammatory reaction of the epididymis to either infection or local trauma. Unilateral scrotal pain, redness and swelling usually starts gradually and may be accompanied by dysuria, pyuria and fever. Common infective causes in adolescence are chlamydia or gonorrhoea. Treatment consists of scrotal support, bed rest, analgesia and antibiotic therapy
Torsion of the testes	A condition that is comon in prepubertal and postpubertal males. The tunica vaginalis, which normally encases the testicle, breaks free allowing the testis to separate from its vascular structure. This results in a twisting of the vascular axis and a partial or complete occlusion of the testicular blood vessels. The affected organ becomes swollen and painful. The pain radiates to the groin and is accompanied by nausea, vomiting and abdominal pain. Emergency surgery is required to preserve the affected testicle
Undescended testicle	This condition occurs in about 3% of full-term infants and 30% of preterm babies. *In utero* the testes develop high on the embryo's abdominal wall. They usually descend into the scrotal sac via the inguinal canal during the seventh month of fetal development. In 80% of affected babies the testes will descend spontaneously during the first year of life. Surgical correction (orchidopexy) is performed in the remainder, usually around 5 years of age, to avoid the development of testicular cancer or fertility problems

foreskin can occur after retraction of the foreskin, masturbation or coitus. These injuries, although frightening, usually heal spontaneously.

Testicular cancer is the most common malignancy in young males and often goes undetected for some time as pain is a late symptom. It is often found accidentally as the affected testicle tends to hang lower and is more susceptible to trauma. Testicular cancer has a good outcome if treated early, so every adolescent male should be taught to perform monthly testicular self-examination.

Assessment of Reproductive Problems

The genital examination and history-taking of a child is not a common procedure and should be performed by a practitioner who uses a child-centred approach to ensure the experience is positive and to prevent future pelvic examinations causing anxiety and embarrassment. It is important to question the child first to allow control over the situation. Younger children must be accompanied by a parent but the adolescent should be given the choice of a supportive person to be present. Phillips *et al.* (1981) found that 71% of 12- to 13-year-old girls preferred their mother to be present, but older girls preferred a nurse rather than a relative to accompany them. In all cases it is useful to talk alone with an adolescent so any confidential information can be gained.

The sexual history is an essential component of the adolescent's consultation. It will reveal areas of concerns for the adolescent and alert the practitioner to potential sexual health risks. It also provides an excellent opportunity to give information about safe sex. Questions should be phrased carefully to avoid any hint of accusation, judgement or criticism. When assessing the child or adolescent with a reproductive tract problem ask about the following as appropriate to the situation:

- Vaginal discharge
  - type and amount
  - associated symptoms (itchiness, fever, abdominal pain)
- Menstrual history
  - age at menarche
  - menstrual cycle (usually expressed as the number of days of bleeding/frequency of menstruation)
  - blood loss (it is difficult to reliably assess loss but a history of passing clots, or having to change sanitary protection during the night, are associated with an abnormally heavy loss)
  - date of last menstruation
- Sexual activity
  - sexual experience
  - number of partners
  - contraception used
- Pregnancy history
  - number of pregnancies and outcomes

Ultrasound scanning is the most common investigation for reproductive problems in the young female. It is a non-invasive procedure that can detect anomalies and assess gestational age and fetal growth in pregnancy.

Indications for gynaecological examination in children

- Vulvovaginal discharge
- Anomalies of the external genitalia
- Suspicion of a foreign body in the vagina
- Genital bleeding
- Rectal or urinary bleeding
- Adominal pain
- Lower abdominal mass
- Precocious or delayed puberty
- Suspicion of sexual abuse

(Lammes, 2003)

Study activity

Find out the preparation necessary for an ultrasound and prepare a leaflet for the school-age child to explain this procedure.

Study activity

- A list of contraceptive methods is given in Table 51.5. For each method identified find out the percentage success rate and the advantages and disadvantages.
- Prepare a talk about safe sex for a group of 11-year-old children.

Sexually Transmitted Diseases

In 2004, the Department of Health revealed that more than 40 000 young people under the age of 20 years were seeking treatment for

Table 51.5 Methods of contraception

Method	Success	Advantages	Disadvantages
Withdrawal			
Rhythm			
Billings method			
Barrier methods:			
Condom			
Diaphragm			
Sponge			
Spermicides			
Oral contraceptives			
Depo-Provera			
Morning-after pill			

sexually transmitted infections (STIs) each year. The equivalent of 160 teenagers are seeking help each working day. The biggest increases are in London and the north-west where infection rates have doubled between 2000–2004. As many as 1 in 20 girls under 16 years could have chlamydia. Gonorrhoea rose by 30% in 16- to 19-year-old boys and by 29% in girls.

Although less than 1% of persons known to have AIDS are teenagers, this age group shows certain characteristics that increase their risk of becoming infected:

- Perceived invulnerability – adolescents characteristically believe that they are immune to disease, accidents and death.
- Development of personal identity – sexual orientation is clarified during adolescence. Remafedi *et al.* (1992) found that 1–2% of boys aged 16–19 years had experimented with homosexual relationships.
- Unprotected sexual intercourse – it is estimated that 70% of teenagers are sexually active, yet fewer than 50% use condoms.
- Drug experimentation – an individual's first experience with drugs is usually during adolescence. Although less than 1% use injectable drugs, experimentation with non-injectable drugs may impair reasoning and increase behaviour that carries the risk of HIV infection.

Increased sexual activity amongst teenagers may be influenced by environmental factors. Easy access to cars, increased unsupervised time at home as many parents are out at work, more explicit sexual behaviour shown in the media and the changing composition of families have all contributed to the sexual experimentation of teenagers. The resulting outcomes of such behaviour are teenage pregnancy and sexually transmitted diseases.

Study activity

- Use Table 51.6 to find out about the features and complications of the common sexually transmitted diseases for both sexes.
- Arrange a visit to your local clinic for sexually transmitted diseases. Consider how easy it might be for an adolescent to find out about the clinic. Discover how confidentiality is ensured and what information about sexual health is available for teenagers visiting the clinic.

Table 51.6 Common sexually transmitted diseases

Disease	Clinical features	Complications
Trichomonas vaginalis		
Chlamydia		
Gonorrhoea		
Syphilis		
Genital warts		
Genital herpes		

Teenage Pregnancy

The number of teenage pregnancies is steadily rising despite efforts to reduce it. The government set a target of reducing pregnancies in the under-18s by 50% by 2010. In 2006 it became apparent that this target was not going to be met. At this time figures for 2003/4 showed that the reduction had only been 1% in 17- to 18-year-olds, 6% in the under-16s, and the number of girls under 14 years old becoming pregnant had risen from 334 to 341 (Hall, 2006). The plan was then announced to lower VAT from 17.5% to 5% for the morning-after pill and condoms. This action was supported by many who consider condoms an essential item. However, it was criticised by the Family Education Trust who believed that any strategy that makes it easier for young people to access contraception would result in a rise in rates of sexually transmitted disease. As statistics show that around a third of teenagers tend not to use condoms, it is difficult to see what change this price reduction would bring amongst this age group. It is estimated that around 70% of pregnant teenagers choose to continue with their pregnancy.

With proper antenatal care, teenage pregnancy is no longer considered biologically disadvantageous to the baby but many studies have shown that it is socially, educationally, psychologically and economically disadvantageous to the mother. Poor school performance usually precedes adolescent pregnancy and for these girls pregnancy may be seen as an escape route from this failure and a 'fast-track' way to adulthood (Henderson, 1999). Adolescents with lower academic ability are also amongst those who are more likely to have further pregnancies. Teenagers who become pregnant may be isolated from their peer group, especially if they leave school, at a time when identity formation is closely linked with peer identification and acceptance. Adolescents tend to have unrealistic expectations of motherhood, and children of young mothers experience more developmental problems than children of adult mothers, as young mothers show less sensitivity and responsiveness to their baby. The amount of cognitive stimulation in the infant's early home environment has been shown to be linked with the child's level of cognitive achievement.

Most pregnancies in teenagers are unplanned so antenatal care is often lacking. This may be due to an unwillingness to accept the pregnancy or a rejection of care which is seen as 'humiliating and boring' (Black, 1986). Consequently, pregnancy problems such as hypertension, preterm labour, low birth weight and anaemia are more common in

Epidemiology of teenage pregnancy

- Teenage pregnancies are commoner in girls who have experienced:
  - physical abuse
  - psychosocial problems
  - regular use of cigarettes, alcohol, addictive drugs and solvents
  - a disadvantaged upbringing
- Genetic factors – pregnancy at a young age is often comon in some families
- Lower teenage pregnancy rates are found in countries with good school sex education and contraceptive services (e.g. Sweden)

(Garden, 2003)

this age group (Garden, 2003). Problems such as hypertension associated with pregnancy can only be detected by care provided antenatally. The creation of clinics which would be more acceptable to young mothers may help to overcome this problem.

Study activity

- Find out if there are any special arrangements for antenatal care for adolescents in your area.
- Organise a visit to an antenatal clinic in your area and consider how these facilities meet the needs of adolescents.

Preterm labour appears to be associated with biological immaturity in younger girls and social and lifestyle factors in older teenagers (Fraser *et al.*, 1995). Chlamydial infection is also a predisposing factor for preterm labour. However, it should be remembered that many teenagers present for care late in pregnancy and gestational age may be uncertain. Preterm and/or low birthweight babies are likely to need care in a special care baby unit and the consequent separation of mother and baby may add to the difficulties of accepting and providing appropriate care for the baby on discharge. Looking after these babies, who tend to require more attention, is likely to put mothers under extreme stress. Young mothers, preterm/low birthweight babies and separation of mother and baby in the first 24 hours after delivery are all predisposing factors for child abuse.

It seems likely that low birth weight is related to the mother's poor nutrition. Adolescents who become pregnant are more likely to already have inadequate nutrition (Garden, 2003). Adolescents have higher nutritional needs than adult women and pregnancy will increase these requirements. Teenagers' concerns about body image and food preferences, and eating habits that provide a diet low in vitamins and high in fat and sugar, probably contribute to their babies' low birth weights and their own anaemia in pregnancy. Anaemia in pregnant teenagers may also be more severe than in older mothers because their iron stores are depleted by the growth spurt in puberty and the heavy blood loss of initial menstruation (Lynch, 2000).

Labour in adolescents appears to have fewer problems than in the adult population. Labours are more likely to be spontaneous, shorter and not require Caesarean section (Garden, 2003). This may be partly due to the higher incidence of preterm and smaller babies. Postnatal care is not well accessed by teenagers unless they have received special care during the antenatal period (Quinlivan *et al.*, 2003) and without this opportunity for contraceptive advice could affect the likelihood of future pregnancy.

Termination of Pregnancy

Many children's nurses find termination a difficult topic to discuss but they have the specialist knowledge to care for teenagers. Although the specific care of pregnant teenagers is provided by midwives or gynaecological nurses, they are more used to older patients and may appreciate advice from children's nurses. Teenagers themselves are more likely to approach a children's nurse for advice, especially if they have had previous contact.

About 25% of teenage pregnancies are terminated, although this figure rises with younger girls. Hall (2006) reported that 60% of girls under 14 years undergo a termination. These figures do not take into account those potential pregnancies prevented by the morning-after pill. After a 2006 court case it became legal for a teenager to have a termination without the knowledge of her parents if she could be shown to be 'Gillick competent'. In cases where a competent underage girl refuses termination, it may be possible for a parent or guardian to authorise termination if it is believed to be in the girl's best interest. Termination is a controversial and emotional issue and there can be physical and psychological long-term effects of such a decision, even if at the time the teenager appears to have made an informed rational choice. It is therefore important that the teenager has access to counselling to consider all her options.

Study activity

Find out the advantages and disadvantages of termination of pregnancy for a teenager. Consider how you might advise a pregnant teenager who approaches you for advice.

Terminations of pregnancy can be undertaken as a medical or a surgical procedure. Medical termination of pregnancy (MTP) uses abortifacients (mifepristone, prostaglandin) to end an established pregnancy and is mostly used for early terminations (up to 9 weeks' gestation). Mifepristone, which is taken orally, blocks the action of progesterone, causing the uterine lining to thin and detach. Prostaglandin, which is given as a pessary 48 hours later, causes uterine contractions that expel the embryo and placental tissue. Medical termination of pregnancy is 97% effective and will cause bleeding (lasting up to 10 days) and cramping. Side-effects are nausea, vomiting, diarrhoea and headache. It should be undertaken under medical supervision to ensure all products of conception are removed. Surgical terminations can be undertaken up to 24 weeks' gestation. Suction aspiration terminations can be performed up to 7 weeks' gestation, conventional suction techniques and suction curettage are used for gestations between 7 and 15 weeks. Dilatation and curettage by specialist pracitioners is required for pregnancies of more than 15 weeks' gestation. In practice, less than 1% of terminations are performed after 20 weeks and in teenagers these late terminations usually occur when the young girl has concealed or not recognised the pregnancy. Most terminations are carried out as day cases but appropriate information about after-care and arrangements for adequate follow-up for any method of termination must be given before discharge.

Legal requirements for termination of pregnancy

The Abortion Act 1967 allows termination before 24 weeks of gestation if it:

- reduces the risk to the woman's life or
- reduces the risk to the woman's physical or mental health or
- reduces the risk to the physical or mental health of her existing children or
- the baby is at substantial risk of being seriously mentally or physically handicapped

There is no upper limit on gestational age if there is:

- risk to the mother's life
- risk of grave, permanent injury to the mother's physical/mental health (allowing for reasonably foreseeable circumstances)
- substantial risk that, if the child were born, it would suffer such physical or mental abnormalities as to be seriously handicapped

If the mother is under 16 years of age:

- Form HSA1 must be signed by 2 doctors
- these girls may make an informed decision independently of parents or guardians depending on their capacity to understand everything involved in the procedure
- if the girl is deemed unable to make an informed decision, a parent or guardian may given consent to or refuse the termination (GMC guidelines state that the court can be asked to overrule if the health professionals believe that it is not in the girl's best interests to consent or refuse)

Royal College of Obstetricians and Gynaecologists guidelines for terminations of pregnancy

- Any woman should have access to a clinical assessment.
- There should be arrangements to minimise delay – e.g. direct access from referral sources other than GPs.
- All women should be offered an assessment appointment within 2 weeks of referral (ideally within 5 days).
- All women should undergo an abortion within 2 weeks of the decision to proceed (ideally 7 days).
- No woman should wait longer than 3 weeks from the initial referral to the time of the termination.

(Royal College of Obstetricians and Gynaecologists, 2004)

Table 51.7 Caring for a teenager following surgical termination of pregnancy

Problem	Aim of care	Nursing care
Potential airway obstruction	The airway will remain patent	
Potential vaginal haemorrhage	Any excessive vaginal bleeding will be detected and managed as quickly as possible	
Potential specific post-op complications (infection, perforated uterus)	Any infection or perforation will be detected and managed as quickly as possible	
Abdominal pain	Pain will be kept within acceptable limits for the individual	
Potential distress	Any signs of distress will be noticed and the reasons discussed	
Unprepared and uninformed for discharge	The patient will be prepared for discharge and be given all the necessary information	

Study activity

- Look at the RCOG guidelines for termination services in the margin and find out how the facilities in your area match these.
- Find out about the care of a teenager following a surgical termination of pregnancy and complete the care plan in Table 51.7.

Promoting Sexual Health

Research shows that teenagers are less likely to experiment with sex and run the risk of acquiring a sexually transmitted disease or becoming pregnant if they are able to discuss sex openly. Children's nurses can help by talking to teenagers and also by helping to advise parents who may be unsure of how to approach these topics. It is useful to start to talk generally to children about sex and relationships from an early age – naming body parts for example. Most schools now teach sex education and it is useful to find out what topics are being included so any advice given consolidates and adds to this information.

Study activity

- Organise a visit to a local school and find out how and when sex education is being taught. See if you can observe a lesson.
- Consider what advice you could give to teenagers who are dealing with their first intimate relationships.

References

Advanced Life Support Group (2005) The convulsing child. In Resuscitation Council UK, *Paediatric Advanced Life Support.* London: ALS.
Alderman, C. (1988) Starting from scratch. *Nursing Standard,* 28 August, 36–37.
Allan, D. and **Culne-Seymour, C.** (1989) Paediatric Coma Scale. *Nursing Times,* **85** (20), 26–28.
Al-Orifi, F., *et al.* (2000) Urine culture from bag specimens in young children: are the risks too high? *Journal of Pediatrics,* **137** (2), 221–226.
Als, H. (1986) A synactive model of neonatal behavioural organization framework for the assessment of neurobehavioural development in the premature infant and for support of infants and parents in the neonatal intensive environment. *Physical and Occupational Therapy in Paediatrics,* **6** (3/4), 3–55.
American Academy of Pediatrics (1987) Report of the second task force on blood pressure control in children. *Pediatrics,* **79** (1), 1–25.
American Academy of Pediatrics (1993) Committee of Infectious Diseases: use of ribavirin in the treatment of RSV. *Pediatrics,* **92** (3), 501–504.
American Heart Association (2005) *Cardiac Disease in Children: Statistics.* http://www.americanheart.org
Amy, J. (2003) *Pediatric and Adolescent Gynaecology.* Amsterdam: Elsevier Science.
Anie, K. A. (2005) Psychological complications in sickle cell disease. *British Journal of Haematology,* **129** (6), 723–729.
Ansell, K. (1995) Let us show the way – dietary advice for children with diabetes. *Child Health,* **3** (2), 54–56.
ARC (2003) *When A Young Person Has Arthritis – A Booklet for Teachers.* http://www.arc.org.uk/about_arth/booklets/6048/6048.htm (accessed 11 June 2006).
Arn, P., *et al.* (1988) Inborn errors of metabolism: not rare, not hopeless. *Contemporary Pediatrics,* **5** (12), 47–63.
Asthma UK (2004) *Living on a Knife Edge.* http://www.asthma-uk.co.uk/asthma
Ayliffe, G. A. J., *et al.* (1992) *Control of Hospital Infection. A Practical Handbook,* 3rd edn. London: Chapman & Hall.
Barker, P. (1995) *Basic Child Psychiatry,* 6th edn. Oxford: Blackwell Scientific Publications.
Barton, J. (1995) A cause for public concern – suicide in children and young people. *Child Health,* **3** (3), 106–109.
Baunter, H. (2002) Advances in diabetes mellitus. In David, T. (ed.), *Recent Advances in Paediatrics.* London: Royal Society of Medicine Press.
Belton, N. R. (2005) Healthy Start – will it provide optimal infant and child nutrition? *Nutrition and Food Science,* **35** (2), 74–80.
Ben-Gashir, M., *et al.* (2002) Are quality of family life and disease severity related in childhood atopic dermatitis? *European Academy of Dermatology and Venereology,* **16**, 455–462.
Berg, A. (1993) Are febrile convulsions provoked by a rapid rise in temperature? *American Journal of Diseases of Childhood,* **147**, 1101–1127.
Bethune, P., *et al.* (1993) Which child will have a febrile convulsion? *American Journal of Diseases of Childhood,* **147**, 35–39.
BFI (2006) *Ten Steps to Successful Breast-feeding.* www.babyfriendly.org.uk
Bhatt, S., *et al.* (1993) Progression of hearing loss in experimental pneumococcal meningitis. *Journal of Infectious Diseases,* **167**, 675–683.
Bhushan, V., *et al.* (1993) Impact of improved survival of very low birth weight infants on recent secular trends in the prevalence of cerebral palsy. *Pediatrics,* **91** (6), 1094–1105.
Black, D. (1986) Schoolgirl mothers. *British Medical Journal,* **293**, 1047–1049.
Bland, E. (1987) The way it was. *Circulation,* **76**, 1190–1195.
Bolton-Maggs, P. H. B. and **Murphy, M. F.** (2004) Blood transfusion. *Archives of Disease in Childhood,* **89**, 4–7.
Bone, M. and **Meltzer, H.** (1989) *The Prevalence of Disability among Children. OPCS Surveys of Disability in Great Britain.* London: HMSO.
Borton, E. (1997) Young people at breaking point. *Nursing Times,* **93** (21), 32–33.
Boxwell, G. (ed.) (2000) *Neonatal Intensive Care Nursing.* London: Taylor & Francis.
Boyd, S. (2002) Sucrose analgesia: a realistic alternative to conventional pharmacology for pain relief in neonates. *Journal of Neonatal Nursing,* **8** (6), 184–190.
Brady, M. (1994) Symptom control in dying children. In Hill, L. (ed.), *Caring for Dying Children and their Families.* London: Chapman & Hall.
Brandon, E. (2003) Facilitating kangaroo care. *Journal of Neonatal Nursing,* **9** (3), inserted matter.
British Association of Dermatologists (2005) Atopic eczema. http://www.bad.org.uk
British Committee for Standards in Haematology Transfusion (2003) Guidelines for the investigation and management of idiopathic thrombocytopenic purpura in adults, children and in pregnancy. *British Journal of Haematology,* **120**, 574–596.
British Diabetic Association (1995) *The Principles of Good Practice for the Care of Young People with Diabetes.* London: BDA.
British Diabetic Association (1996) *Babies and Children with Diabetes.* London: BDA.
British Diabetic Association (1997) *What Care to Expect when Your Child has Diabetes.* London: BDA.
British Epilepsy Association (1995) *Living with Epilepsy.* London: BEA.
British Thoracic Society (1993) BTS guidelines. *Thorax,* **48**, S1–S24.

Britton, C. (2002) 'Views from the inside' II: What the children said, and the experiences of mothers, fathers and grandparents. *British Journal of Occupational Therapy*, **65** (8), 1.
Brown, M. A. and **Powell-Cope, G. M.** (1991) AIDS family caregiving: transition through uncertainty. *Nursing Research*, **40** (6), 338–345.
Burch, M. (2002) Heart failure in the young. *Heart*, **88**, 198–202.
Buxton, P. (1993) *ABC of Dermatology*, 2nd edn. London: BMJ.
Camfield, C. and **Camfield, P.** (1993) Febrile seizures: A treatment for parent fears and anxiety. *Contemporary Pediatrics*, **10** (4), 26–44.
Campbell, S. (1987) Mouthcare in malignancy patients. *Nursing Times*, **87** (29), 59–60.
Campbell, S. and **Glasper, A.** (eds) (1995) *Whaley and Wong's Children's Nursing*. St Louis: Mosby.
Carter, B. (1993) *Manual of Paediatric Intensive Care Nursing*. London: Chapman & Hall.
Cates, W., *et al.* (1990) Sexually transmitted diseases, pelvic inflammatory disease and infertility: an epidemiological report. *Epidemiology Review*, **12**, 199–220.
Chambliss, C. R., *et al.* (2002) The assessment and management of chronic pain in children. *Pediatric Drugs*, **4** (11), 737–746.
Charman, C., *et al.* (2000) Topical corticosteroid phobia in patients with ectopic eczema. *British Journal of Dermatology*, **142**, 931–936.
Clark, R., *et al.* (1990) *Principles and Practice of Dermatology*. London: Churchill Livingstone.
Clayton, M. (1997) Traction at home: the Doncaster approach. *Paediatric Nursing*, **9** (2), 21–23.
Cook, J. and **Gallagher, A.** (1996) Evaluation of an anti-emetic protocol. *Paediatric Nursing*, **8** (7), 21–23.
Corlett, S. (1995) Nephrotic syndrome. *Practice Nursing*, **6** (3), 36–37.
Costeloe, K., *et al.* (2000) The EPIcure Study: outcome to discharge from hospital for babies born at the threshold of viability. *Pediatrics*, **106** (4), 659–671.
Cree, I. A. (ed.) (1997) *Pathology*. London: Chapman & Hall.
Creedon, S. A. (2005) Issues and innovations in nursing practice. Healthcare workers' hand decontamination practices: compliance with recommended guidelines. *Journal of Advanced Nursing*, **51** (3), 208–216.
Cubby, C. (1991) Cranial deformities in premature infants. *Paediatric Nursing*, **3** (2), 19–21.
Dajani, A., *et al.* (1990) Prevention of bacterial endocarditis: recommendations by the American Heart Association. *Journal of the American Medical Association*, **264** (22), 2919–2922.
Davies, D. (1996) The causes of meningitis and meningococcal disease. *Nursing Times*, **92** (6), 25–27.
De Sousa, M. E. (1996) The renal system. In McQuaid, L., Huband, S. and Parker, E. (eds), *Children's Nursing*. London: Churchill Livingstone.
Dear, P. (1992) Total parenteral nutrition of the newborn. *Care of the Critically Ill*, **8** (6), 252–257.
Dewers, R. (1990) Rhinitis and intranasal fluticasone propionate. *Royal Society of Medicine Symposium*, 10 July 1990.
DH (1990) *Guidance for Clinical Health Care Workers: Protection against Infection with HIV and Hepatitis Viruses*. London: HMSO.
DH (1992) *The Health of the Nation: a Strategy for Health in England*. London: HMSO.
DH (1996) *Confidential Enquiry into Stillbirths and Deaths in Infancy*. London: HMSO.
DH (2001) *Diabetes National Service Framework: Standards*. London: HMSO.
DH (2004a) *Immunisation for Life*. London: HMSO. http://www.immunisation.nhs.uk (accessed 11 June 2006).
DH (2004b) *National Service Framework for Children, Young People and Maternity Services*. London: HMSO.
DH (2004c) *Healthcare Facilities Cleaning Manual*. http://patientexperience.nhsestates.gov.uk/clean_hospitals/ch_content/cleaning_manual/background.asp (accessed 11 June 2006).
DH (2005) Blood Safety General Information. http://www.dh.gov.uk/PolicyAndGuidance/HealthAndSocialCareTopics/BloodSafety/BloodSafetyGeneralInformation/fs/en (accessed 31 May 2006).
DH (2006) *Preventing Meningitis*. London: Department of Health.
Diabetes Control and Complications Trial Research Group (1993) The effect of intensive treatment of diabetes on the development and progression of long-term complications in insulin-dependent diabetes. *New England Journal of Medicine*, **329**, 977–986.
Donald, S. (1995) Atopic eczema: management and control. *Paediatric Nursing*, **7** (2), 30–34.
Duggan, C. (1996) HIV infection in children. *Paediatric Nursing*, **8** (10), 32–34.
Duncan, B., *et al.* (1993) Exclusive breast-feeding for at least 4 months protects against otitis media. *Pediatrics*, **91** (5), 867–872.
Eden, A. N. (2005) Iron deficiency and impaired cognition in toddlers: an underestimated and undertreated problem. *Pediatric Drugs*, **7** (6), 347–352.
Edge, J., *et al.* (2001) The risk and outcome of cerebral oedema developing during diabetic ketoacidosis. *Archives of Disease in Childhood*, **85** (1), 16–22.
Eisler, I., *et al.* (2000) Family therapy for adolescent anorexia nervosa: the results of a controlled comparison of two family interventions. *Journal of Child Psychology and Psychiatry*, **41**, 727–736.
Farrell, M. (2002) A method comparison study to assess the reliability of urine collection pads as a means of obtaining urine specimens from non-toilet trained children for microbiological examination. *Journal of Advanced Nursing*, **37** (4), 387–393.
Faulconbridge, J. P. and **Spanswick, S. M. L.** (1995) Back up when you need it. Teaching and support for school nurses involved in counselling. *Child Health*, **3** (3), 111–114.

Feasey, S. (1999) Are Newcastle urine collection pads suitable as a means of collecting specimens from infants? *Paediatric Nursing,* **11** (9), 17–21.
Fletcher, D. (1997) Sports day screening to curb heart risks. *Daily Telegraph,* 22 December.
Flood, J. (1989) Glue ear. *Nursing Times,* **85** (36), 38–41.
Forrest, G. (2003) Working with Paediatrics. In Garralda, M. and Hyde, C. (eds), *Managing Children with Psychiatric Problems,* (2nd edn). London: BMJ Books.
Foss, M. (1990) Oxygen therapy. *Professional Nurse,* **6** (4), 180–190.
Frank, G. (1987) Scratching the surface. *Nursing Times,* **83** (39), 19–21.
Fraser, A., *et al.* (1995) Association of young maternal age with adverse reproductive outcomes. *New England Journal of Medicine,* **332**, 1113–1117.
Freer, Y. (1999) A comparison of breast and cup feeding in preterm infants: effects on physiological parameters. *Journal of Neonatal Nursing,* **5** (1), 16–21.
Frenck, R., *et al.* (1991) Principles of total care: infections in children with cancer. In Fernbach, D. and Vietti, T. (eds), *Clinical Pediatric Oncology,* 4th edn. St Louis: Mosby.
Friedemann, M. L. (1989) The concept of family nursing. *Journal of Advanced Nursing,* **14**, 211–216.
Garden, A. (2003) Teenage pregnancy. In Amy, J., *Paediatric and Adolescent Gynaecology.* Amsterdam: Elsevier Science BV.
George, A., *et al.* (2002) Positive expiratory pressure (PEP) masks, flutter devices and other mechanical aids to physiotherapy in cystic fibrosis. In David, T. (ed.), *Recent Advances in Paediatrics.* London: Royal Society of Medicine Press.
Georgioff, M. and **Bernbaum, J.** (1986) Abnormal shoulder girdle muscle tone in premature infants during their first 18 months of life. *Paediatrics,* **77**, 664–669.
Ghajar, J. and **Hariri, R.** (1992) Management of paediatric head injury. *Paediatric Clinics of North America,* **39** (5), 1093–1123.
Gilbert, E., *et al.* (1993) Stridor in the infant and child. *American Operating Room Journal,* **58** (1), 23–41.
Gillman, M., *et al.* (1993) Identifying children at high risk for the development of essential hypertension. *Journal of Pediatrics,* **122**, 837–846.
Glaser, N., *et al.* (2001) Risk factors for cerebral oedema in children with diabetic ketoacidosis. *New England Journal of Medicine,* **329**, 977–986.
Godden, C., *et al.* (1997) Double blind placebo controlled trial of nebulised budesonide for croup. *Archives of Disease in Childhood,* **76**, 155–158.
Goldberg, D. and **Hodes, M.** (2003) Family work and family therapy in child mental health. In Garralda, M. and Hyde, C. (eds), *Managing Children with Psychiatric Problems,* 2nd edn. London: BMJ Books.
Goldman, M., *et al.* (1993) Treatment of port-wine stains with the flash-lamp-pumped pulse dye laser. *Journal of Pediatrics,* **122** (1), 71–77.
Goodman, R., *et al.* (2002) Mental health problems of children in the community: 18 month follow-up. *British Medical Journal,* **324**, 1496–1497.
Grantham-McGregor, S. and **Ani, C.** (2001) A review of studies on the effect of iron deficiency on cognitive development in children. *Journal of Nutrition,* **131** (2S-2): 649S–666S.
Greene, J. (1993) Exercise induced menstrual irregularities. *Comprehensive Therapies,* **19**, 116–120.
Gregory, J. R., *et al.* (1997) *National Diet and Nutrition Survey of Children Aged 1.5 to 4.5 Years.* London: HMSO.
Grewal, M. and **Sutcliffe, A.** (1991) Early prediction and outcome following head injury: an assessment of GCS score trends. *Journal of Paediatric Surgery,* **26**, 1161.
Groer, M. E. and **Shekleton, M. E.** (1979) *Basic Pathophysiology – A Conceptual Approach.* St Louis: Mosby.
Hall, C. (2006) Lower VAT on morning-after pill 'to reduce teenage births'. *Daily Telegraph,* 3 February 2006.
Hall, D. (1996) *Health for All Children.* Oxford: Oxford University Press.
Hallsworth, M. (1995) Positioning the pre-term infant. *Paediatric Nursing,* **7** (1), 18–20.
Harper, J. (1994) Traditional Chinese medicine for eczema. *British Medical Journal,* **308**, 409.
Harrop, M. (2002) Self-management plans in childhood asthma. *Nursing Standard,* **20** (17), 38–42.
Hawton, K. and **James, A.** (2005) Suicide and deliberate self harm in young people. *British Medical Journal,* **330**, 891–894.
Hazinski, M. (1992) *Nursing Care of the Critically Ill Child,* 2nd edn. St Louis: Mosby.
Health Advisory Service (1995) The commissioning role and management of child and adolescent mental health services: together we stand. *The NHS Health Advisory Thematic Review.* London: HMSO.
Health Protection Agency (2006) Epidemiology – HIV and AIDS. http://www.hpa.org.uk/infections/topics_az/hiv_and_sti/hiv/epidemiology/epidemiology.htm.
Heaton, J., *et al.* (2005) Families' experiences of caring for technology-dependent children: a temporal perspective. *Health and Social Care in the Community,* **13** (5), 441.
Hedburg Nyqvist, K. and **Strandell, E.** (1999) A cup feeding protocol for neonates: evaluation of nurses' and parents' use of two cups. *Journal of Neonatal Nursing,* **5** (2), 31–36.
Henderson, L. (1999) A survey of teenage pregnant women and their male partners in the Grampian area. *British Journal of Family Planning,* **25**, 90–92.
Herbert, M. (1987) *Conduct Disorders of Childhood and Adolescence: A Social Learning Perspective,* 2nd edn. Chichester: John Wiley.

Higgins, C. (1995) Pathology testing and blood glucose levels. *Nursing Times,* **91** (3), 42–44.
Higgins, J. (1990) Pulmonary oxygen toxicity. *Physiotherapy,* **76** (10), 588–592.
Hockenberry, M. J., *et al.* (2003) *Wong's Nursing Care of Infants and Children,* 7th edn. St Louis: Mosby.
Hogan, S., *et al.* (1997) Duration and recurrence of otitis media with effusion in children from birth to 3 years. *British Medical Journal,* **314**, 350–353.
Hohn, A. and **Stanton, R.** (1987) Myocarditis in children. *Pediatric Review,* **9** (3), 83–88.
Holberg, C., *et al.* (1993) Child day care, smoking by care givers, and lower respiratory tract infections in the first 3 years of life. *Pediatrics,* **91**, 885–892.
Hollis, R. (1997) Childhood malignancy into the 21st century. *Paediatric Nursing,* **9** (3), 12–15.
Holmes, A. (1996) The role of the cardiac liaison nurse. *Paediatric Nursing,* **8** (1), 25–27.
Holmes, S. and **Brown, S.** (2005) Skeletal pin site care. National Association of Orthopaedic Nurses guidelines for orthopaedic nursing. *Orthopaedic Nursing,* **21** (2), 99–107. http://www.orthonurse.org/images/PDF/PinCare2005.pdf (accessed 11 June 2006).
Hoppe, C. (2005) Defining stroke risk in children with sickle cell anaemia. *British Journal of Haematology,* **128** (6), 751–766.
Hunt, E. (1997) The big wheeze. *Nursing Times,* **93** (7), 32–33.
Hunter, J., *et al.* (1989) *Clinical Dermatology,* Vol. 3. Oxford: Glaxo/Blackwell Scientific Publications.
Hylton Rushton, C. (1990) Necrotising entero-colitis. Part I. Pathogenesis and diagnosis. Part II. Treatment and nursing care. *American Journal of Maternal/Child Nursing,* **15**, 296–313.
Imle, P. and **Klemic, N.** (1991) Methods of airway clearance: coughing and suctioning. In MacKenzie, C., *et al.* (eds), *Chest Physiotherapy in the Intensive Care Unit.* Baltimore: Williams & Wilkins.
Institute of Child Health (2005) Children's Pain Assessment Project, http://www.ich.ucl.ac.uk/cpap/ (accessed 31 May 2006).
International Society for Pediatric and Adolescent Diabetes (ISPAD) (2000) *ISPAD Consensus Guidelines for the Management for Type 1 Diabetes Mellitus in Children and Adolescents 2000.* Amsterdam: Medical Forum International.
Isaacson, G. and **Rosenfeld, R.** (1994) Care of the child with typanoplasty tubes: a visual guide for the pediatrician. *Pediatrics,* **93** (6), 924–929.
Jevon, P. and **Ewens, B.** (2001) Assessment of a breathless patient. *Nursing Standard,* **15** (16), 48–53.
Johnson, H. (1996) Stoma care for infants, children and young people. *Paediatric Nursing,* May, 8–11.
Karjalainen, J., *et al.* (1992) A bovine albumin peptide as a possible trigger of insulin dependent diabetes mellitus. *New England Journal of Medicine,* **327** (5), 302–307.
Kemp, A. (1999) Atopic asthma: its social and financial costs. *Journal of Paediatrics and Child Health,* **35**, 229–231.
Kerem, E., *et al.* (1990) Effect of endotracheal suctioning on arterial blood gases in children. *Intensive Care Medicine,* **16**, 95–99.
Knapman, J. (1993) Controlling emesis after chemotherapy. *Nursing Standard,* **7** (1), 38–39.
Koch, C. and **Hoiby, N.** (1993) Pathogenesis of cystic fibrosis. *Lancet,* **8852**, 1065–1069.
Konstan, M., *et al.* (1995) Effect of high dose ibuprofen in patients with cystic fibrosis. *New England Journal of Medicine,* **332**, 848–854.
Kurtz, Z. (1992) *With Health in Mind – Mental Health Care for Children and Young People.* London: Action for Sick Children.
Kuzenski, B. (1978) Effect of negative pressure in tracheobronchial trauma. *Nursing Research,* **27**, 260.
Lammes, F. (2003) Vulvo-vaginitis in children. In Amy, J. (2003), *Pediatric and Adolescent Gynaecology.* Amsterdam: Elsevier Science BV.
Lask, B. and **Bryant-Waugh, J.** (1998) Family therapy in eating disorders. In Hoek, H. (ed.), *The Neurobiology of Eating Disorders.* Chichester: John Wiley & Sons Ltd.
Lawrence, R. (1994) *Breastfeeding: A Guide for the Medical Profession,* 4th edn. St Louis: Mosby.
Leak, A. M. (2002) Treatment of juvenile idiopathic arthritis. *CPD Rheumatology,* **3** (1), 3–7.
Leck, I. (1995) Congenital dislocation of the hip. In Wald, N. (ed.), *Antenatal and Neonatal Screening.* Oxford: Oxford University Press.
LeMaistre, G. (1991) Ultrasound and dislocation of the hip. *Paediatric Nursing,* May, 13–16.
Leung, D., *et al.* (1993) Toxic shock syndrome toxin-secreting *Staphylococcus aureus* in Kawasaki syndrome. *Lancet,* **342**, 1385–1388.
Levy, A., *et al.* (2005) Anemia as a risk factor for infectious diseases in infants and toddlers: Results from a prospective study. *European Journal of Epidemiology,* **20** (3), 277–284.
Lewis, J. (1998) Clean-catch versus urine collection pads: a prospective trial. *Paediatric Nursing,* **10** (19), 15–16.
Locasciulli, A. (2002) Acquired aplastic anemia in children: incidence, prognosis and treatment options. *Pediatric Drugs,* **4** (11), 761–766.
Lous, J., *et al.* (2005) Grommets (ventilation tubes) for hearing loss associated with otitis media with effusion in children. *The Cochrane Database of Systematic Reviews,* Issue 4. Chichester: Wiley.
Lowberry, E. J. (1975) *Control of Infection. A Practical Handbook.* London: Chapman & Hall.
Lynch, S. (2000) The potential impact of iron supplements during adolescence on iron status in pregnancy. *Journal of Nutrition,* **130**, 448–451.
MacDonald, H. (1995) Chronic renal disease: the mother's experience. *Pediatric Nursing,* **21** (6), 503–507.
MacFarlane, P., *et al.* (1999) Pad urine collection for early childhood urinary infection. *Lancet,* **354** (9178), 571.
MacKenzie, H. (1994) HIV and AIDS: a family approach to care. *Paediatric Nursing,* **6** (10), 18–21.

MacMahon, R. A. (1991) *An Aid to Paediatric Surgery*, 2nd edn. Melbourne: Churchill Livingstone.
MacRae, V. E., *et al.* (2006) The pathophysiology of the growth plate in juvenile idiopathic arthritis. *Rheumatology*, **45** (1), 11–19.
Maguire, D. and **Maloney, P.** (1988) A comparison of fentanyl and morphine in neonates. *Neonatal Network*, **7** (1), 27–35.
Markovitch, H. (1990) Recognising meningitis. *The Practitioner*, **234**, 539–541.
Marks, M. K., Vadamalayan, B., Ekert, H. and **South, M. J.** (2005) Intended management of children with acute idiopathic thrombocytopenic purpura: a national survey. *Journal of Paediatrics and Child Health*, **41** (1–2), 52–55.
Martin, V. (1995) Helping parents cope. *Nursing Times*, **91** (31), 38–40.
Martin, V. (2005) Cleft care reorganisation six years on. *Paediatric Nursing*, **17** (4), 20–22.
McClure, J., *et al.* (2000) Randomised controlled study of clinical outcome following trophic feeding. *Archives of Disease in Childhood*, **82**, 29–33.
McDonald, L. A. B., *et al.* (2004) Constipation and soiling – outcome of treatment at one year. *Scottish Medical Journal*, **49** (3), 98–100. http://www.smj.org.uk/0804/const.htm (accessed 31 May 2006).
McEvilly, A. (1997) Childhood diabetes. *Paediatric Nursing*, **9** (3), 29–33.
McIntyre, J., *et al.* (2005) Safety and efficacy of buccal midazolam versus rectal diazepam for emergency treatment of seizures in children: a randomised controlled trial. *Lancet*, **366** (9481), 205–210.
Medical Research Council Working Party on Phenylketonuria (1993) Phenylketonuria due to phenylalanine hydroxylase deficiency: an unfolding story. *British Medical Journal*, **306**, 115–119.
Meltzer, M., *et al.* (2000) *Mental Health of Children and Adolescents in Great Britain*. London: The Stationery Office.
Mental Health Foundation (2006) *Truth Hurts – Report of the National Inquiry into Self Harm among Young People*. London: Mental Health Foundation.
Metcalf, M. and **Baum, J.** (1991) Incidence of insulin dependent diabetes in children under 15 years in the British Isles in 1988. *British Medical Journal*, **302**, 443–447.
Miah, J. (2004) *Talking with Children, Young People and Families, about Chronic Illness and Living with HIV*. London: National Children's Bureau.
Miller, K. L. (1996) Urinary infections: children are not little adults. *Pediatric Nursing*, **22** (6), 473–480, 544.
Morris, M. (1994) Nursing care of babies who are born too soon or too small. In Crawford, D. and Morris, M. (eds), *Neonatal Nursing*. London: Chapman & Hall.
Moulai, S. and **Huband, S.** (1996) Nutrition and the digestive system. In McQuaid, L. M., Huband, S. and Parker, E. (eds), *Children's Nursing*. Edinburgh: Churchill Livingstone.
Mupanemunda, R. H. and **Watkinson, M.** (1999) *Key Topics in Neonatology*. Oxford: BIOS Scientific Publishers.
Murphy, D., Hope, L. and **Johnson, A.** (1997) Neonatal risk factors for cerebral palsy in very pre-term babies: case-control study. *British Medical Journal*, **314**, 404–408.
Murphy, K., *et al.* (1990) Severe burns from a pulse oximeter. *Anesthesiology*, **73**, 350–351.
National Asthma Campaign (1999) *National Asthma Audit 1999/2000*. London: National Asthma Campaign.
National Asthma Campaign (2002) *Starting as We Mean to Go On. An Audit of Children's Asthma in the UK*. London: National Asthma Campaign.
National Childbirth Trust (1997) *Hypoglycaemia of the Newborn: Guidelines for Appropriate Blood Glucose Screening and Treatment of Breastfed and Bottlefed Babies in the United Kingdom*. London: NCT.
National Eczema Society (2003) Eczema: frequently asked questions. http://www.eczema.org
Nettleship, A. (1994/5) Do we have an attitude problem? *Child Health*, **2** (4), 150–153.
Newman-Turner, R. (1992) *The Hayfever Handbook*. London: Thorsons.
NICE (National Institute for Health and Clinical Excellence) (2002a) Guidelines on the use of Etanercept for the treatment of juvenile idiopathic arthritis. http://www.nice.org.uk/pdf/JIA-PDF.pdf (accessed 25 May 2007).
NICE (National Institute for Health and Clinical Excellence) (2002b) *Newer Drugs for Children with Epilepsy*. London: NICE.
NICE (National Institute for Health and Clinical Excellence) (2002c) Management of otitis media with effusion. http://www.nice.org.uk
NICE (National Institute for Health and Clinical Excellence) (2003) *Infection Control: Prevention of Healthcare-associated Infection and Community Care*. http://www.nice.org.uk/pdf/CG2fullguidelineinfectioncontrol.pdf (accessed 11 June 2006).
NICE (National Institute for Health and Clinical Excellence) (2004a) *The Epilepsies: Diagnosis and Management of the Epilepsies in Children and Young People in Primary and Secondary Care. Clinical Guideline 20*. London: NICE.
NICE (National Institute for Health and Clinical Excellence) (2004b) *Type 1 Diabetes: Diagnosis and Management of Type 1 Diabetes in Children, Young People and Adults, Clinical Guideline 15*. London: NICE.
NICE (National Institute for Health and Clinical Excellence) (2005) *Improving Outcomes in Children and Young People with Cancer*. London: NICE.
Northway, W., *et al.* (1990) Late pulmonary sequelae of bronchopulmonary dysplasia. *New England Journal of Medicine*, **323** (26), 1793–1799.
Norton, A. and **Roberts, I.** (2006) Management of Evans syndrome. *British Journal of Haematology*, **132** (2), 125–137.
Office For National Statistics (2001) *Health Statistics Quarterly and Population Trends*. London: HMSO.
Office For National Statistics (2004) *Mental Health of Children and Young People*. London: ONS.
Okpala, I., *et al.* (2002) The comprehensive care of sickle cell disease. *European Journal of Haematology*, **68** (3), 157–162.

Opie, L. (1991) *Drugs for the Heart.* Philadelphia: W. B. Saunders.
Pearce, J. (2003) Identifying psychiatric disorders in children. In Garralda, M. and Hyde, C. (eds), *Managing Children with Psychiatric Problems*, 2nd edn. London: BMJ Books.
Pfeffer, C. R. (1986) *The Suicidal Child.* New York: Guilford Press.
Phelan, P., *et al.* (1990) Pulmonary complications of inhalation. In Phelan, P., *et al.* (eds), *Respiratory Illness in Children*, 2nd edn. Oxford: Blackwell Scientific Publications.
Phillips, S., *et al.* (1981) Teenagers' preferences regarding the presence of family members, peers and chaperones during examination of genitalia. *Pediatrics*, **68**, 665–669.
PHLS (1996) *Communicable Diseases Report.* London: PHLS.
Pinkerton, J., *et al.* (1996) *Supportive Care – Guidelines for Shared Care Centres.* London: Great Ormond Street Hospital NHS Trust.
Porter, H. (1994) Mouthcare in malignancy. *Nursing Times*, **90** (14), 27–29.
Portman, R. and **Yetman, R.** (1994) Clinical uses of ambulatory blood pressure monitoring. *Paediatric Nephrology*, **8**, 367–376.
Prasad, S. and **Hussey, J.** (1995) *Paediatric Respiratory Care.* London: Chapman & Hall.
Price, D. and **Wolfe, S.** (2000) Delivery of asthma care: patients' use and views as determined by a nationwide survey. *The Asthma Journal*, **5** (3), 141–145.
Pritchard, A. P. and **David, J. A.** (1990) *The Royal Marsden Hospital Manual of Clinical Nursing Procedures*, 2nd edn. London: Harper & Row.
Purcell, J. (1989) Cardiomyopathy. *American Journal of Nursing*, **89** (1), 57–75.
Putto, A. (1987) Febrile exudative tonsillitis: viral or streptococcal? *Pediatrics*, **80** (6), 911–914.
Quinlivan, J., *et al.* (2003) Postnatal home visits in teenage mothers: a randomised trial. *Lancet*, **361**, 893–900.
Quintero, C. (1993) Blood administration in pediatric Jehovah's Witnesses. *Pediatric Nursing*, **19** (1), 46–48.
Rakshi, K. and **Couriel, J.** (1994) Management of acute bronchiolitis. *Archives of Disease in Childhood*, **71**, 463–469.
Ramage, I., *et al.* (1999) Accuracy of clean-catch urine collection in infancy. *Turkish Journal of Pediatrics*, **135** (6), 765–767.
Ramanan, A. V. and **Whitworth, P.** (2003) Use of methotrexate in juvenile idiopathic arthritis. *Archives of Disease in Childhood*, **88**, 197–200.
Ramsay, J. (1994) The psychology of childhood asthma. *Paediatric Nursing*, **6** (8), 17–21.
Ravelli, A. and **Martini, A.** (2005) The long-term outcome of juvenile idiopathic arthritis. *Current Rheumatology Reviews*, **1** (2), 151–155.
Rayner, D. (2003) MRSA: an infection control overview. *Nursing Standard*, **17** (45), 47–53.
Rees, M. (1994) The season of discontent. *Child Health*, **2** (1), 22–26.
Reeves, K. (1989) Assessment of paediatric head injury: the basics. *Journal of Emergency Nursing*, **15** (4), 329–333.
Rehm, R. S. and **Franck, L. S.** (2000) Long-term goals and normalization strategies of children and families affected by HIV/AIDS. *Advanced Nursing Science*, **23**, 69–82.
Reid, U. (1997) Stigma of hair loss after chemotherapy. *Paediatric Nursing*, **9** (3), 16–18.
Reidy, M., *et al.* (1991) Psychological needs expressed by the natural caregivers of HIV infected children. *AIDS Care*, **3** (3), 331–343.
Remafedi, G., *et al.* (1992) Demography of sexual orientation in adolescents. *Pediatrics*, **89** (4), 714–721.
Reynolds, E. (1992) Controversies in caring for the child with a head injury. *Maternal and Child Nursing*, **17**, 246–251.
Rickard, S. and **Finn, A.** (1997) Parental knowledge of paediatric infectious diseases. *Ambulatory Child Health*, **3**, 13–19.
Ridling, D., *et al.* (2003) Endotracheal suctioning with or without instillation of isotonic saline sodium chloride. *American Journal of Critical Care*, **12** (3), 212–219.
Ritchie, J. F. (1998) Immature sucking response in premature babies: cup feeding as a tool in increasing maintenance of breast feeding. *Journal of Neonatal Nursing*, **4** (2), 13–17.
Roberts, I., Dokal, I. and **Daly, P.** (1996) *Management Protocol for Patients with Beta Thalassaemia Major – Version 1.0.* London: Hammersmith Hospital.
Romney, M. G. (2001) Surgical face masks in the operating theatre: re-examining the evidence. *Journal of Hospital Infection*, **47** (4), 251–256.
Rothman, K. and **Lucky, A.** (1993) Acne vulgaris. *Advances in Dermatology*, **8**, 131.
Royal College of Nursing (2004a) Right Blood, Right Patient, Right Time. http://www.rcn.org.uk/members/downloads/rightblood.pdf (accessed 31 May 2006).
Royal College of Nursing (2004b) Administering Subcutaneous Methotrexate for Inflammatory Arthritis. http://www.rcn.org.uk/publications/pdf/administering-methotrexate.pdf (accessed 31 May 2006).
Royal College of Nursing (2005) *Good Practice in Infection Prevention and Control. Guidance for Nursing Staff.* London: RCN. http://www.rcn.org.uk/resources/mrsa/downloads/Wipe_it_out-Good_practice_in_infection_prevention_and_control.pdf (accessed 11 June 2006).
Royal College of Obstetricians and Gynaecologists (2004) *The Care of Women Requesting Induced Abortions.* London: RCOG.
Samaritans (2001) *Key Facts; Young People and Suicide.* London: Samaritans.
Santy, J. (2000) Nursing patient with an external fixator. *Nursing Standard*, **14** (31), 47–52.
Schaad, B., *et al.* (1993) Dexamethasone therapy for bacterial meningitis in children. *Lancet*, **324**, 457–461.
Schecter, N., *et al.* (1988) The use of patient controlled analgesia in adolescents with sickle-cell pain crisis: a preliminary report. *Journal of Pain and Symptom Management*, **3**, 109–113.

Schneidman, E. (1985) *Definition of Suicide.* New York: John Wiley.
Scott, M. (1994) A new treatment becomes reality. *CF News,* spring edition, p. 2.
Scott, S. (2003) Parenting programmes. In Garralda, M. and Hyde, C. (eds), *Managing Children with Psychiatric Problems,* 2nd edn. London: BMJ Books.
Serra, A. (2000) Tracheostomy care. *Nursing Standard,* **14** (44), 45–55.
Shad, A. T., Gonzalez, C. E. and **Sandler, S. G.** (2005) Treatment of immune thrombocytopenic purpura in children: current concepts. *Pediatric Drugs,* **7** (5), 325–336.
Shaffer, D. and **Gutstein, H.** (2002) Suicide in childhood and early adolescence. *Journal of Child Psychology and Psychiatry,* **23**, 136–141.
Sharman, W. (1997) *Children and Adolescents with Mental Health Problems.* London: Balliere Tindall.
Shield, J. (2006) Rising prevalence of diabetes related type 2 diabetes in the British Isles. Unpublished. Presented at the Royal College of Paediatric and Child Health 10th Spring meeting, University of York, April 2006.
Shorvon, S. (1990) *Epilepsy: A Lancet Review.* London: The Lancet.
Shyur, S.-D. and **Hill, H. R.** (1996) Recent advances in the genetics of primary immunodeficiency syndromes. *Journal of Pediatrics,* **129** (1), 8–24.
Simpson, D. and **Reilly, P.** (1982) Paediatric coma scale. *Lancet,* **ii**, 450.
Smith, L. (2003) Which catheter? Criteria for selection of urinary catheters for children. *Paediatric Nursing,* **15** (3), 14–18.
Sparshott, M. (1997) *Pain Distress and the Newborn Infant.* Oxford: Blackwell Science.
Speight, N. (1996) The changing face of childhood asthma management. *Paediatrics Today,* **4** (4), 78–80.
Spowart, K. (1995) Childhood skin disorders. *Paediatric Nursing,* **7** (3), 30–34.
Steinhauer, P. D., Santa-Barbara, J. and **Skinner, H.** (1984) The process model of family functioning. *Canadian Journal of Psychiatry,* **29**, 77–88.
Stephenson, J. and **Goodman, R.** (2001) Association between behaviour at age 3 and adult criminality. *British Journal of Psychiatry,* **179**, 197–202.
Stiller, C. and **Draper, G.** (1998) The epidemiology of cancer in children. In Voute, P., Kalia, C. and Barrett, A. (eds), *Cancer in Children: Clinical Management,* 4th edn. Oxford: Oxford University Press.
Stinson, J. and **Naser, B.** (2003) Pain management in children with sickle-cell disease. *Pediatric Drugs,* **5** (4), 229–241.
Strachan, D., Jarvis, M. and **Feyerabend, B.** (1989) Passive smoking, salivary cotinine concentration and middle ear effusion in 7 year old children. *British Medical Journal,* **298**, 1549–1552.
Sumner, E. (1990) Artificial ventilation of children. In Dinwiddie, R. (ed.), *The Diagnosis and Management of Paediatric Respiratory Disease.* London: Churchill Livingstone.
Sundell, G. and **Milson, I.** (1990) Factors influencing the prevalence and severity of dysmenorrhoea in young women. *British Journal of Obstetrics and Gynaecology,* **97**, 588–594.
Swanwick, M. (1986) The ugly duckling. *Nursing Times,* 3 December, 47–49.
Swift, P., *et al.* (1993) A decade of diabetes: keeping children out of hospital. *British Medical Journal,* **307**, 96–98.
Taylor, J. H. (1996) End stage renal disease in children: diagnosis, management and interventions. *Pediatric Nursing,* **22** (6), 481–490.
Taylor, L. J. (1978) An evaluation of handwashing techniques. *Nursing Times,* part 1, 54–55.
Teasdale, G. and **Jennett, W.** (1974) Assessment of coma and impaired unconsciousness. *Lancet,* **ii**, 81–84.
Temple, J. and **Santy, J.** (2004) Pin site care for preventing infections associated with external bone fixators and pins. *The Cochrane Database of Systematic Reviews,* Issue 4.
Teris, J. (2001) *Guidelines for the Management of Constipation.* London: Emergency Medicine Paediatric Interest Group.
Thomsett, A. and **Watson, A.** (1996) Renal biopsy as a day case procedure. *Paediatric Nursing,* **8** (5), 14–15.
Trotter, S. (2003) Management of the umbilical cord, a guide to best care. *RCM Midwives Journal,* **6** (7), 308–311.
Valman, H. (1993) *ABC of One to Seven,* 3rd edn. London: BMJ.
Van Donselaar, C., *et al.* (1997) Clinical course of untreated tonic–clonic seizures in childhood: prospective, hospital-based study. *British Medical Journal,* **314**, 401–404.
Varma, V. P. (ed.) (1990) *The Management of Children with Emotional and Behavioural Difficulties.* London: Routledge.
Veasey, L., *et al.* (1994) Persistence of rheumatic fever in the intermountain area of the United States. *Journal of Pediatrics,* **124**, 9–16.
Vernon, S., *et al.* (1994) Urine collection on sanitary towels. *Lancet,* **344** (8922), 612.
Watson, J. (1990) Screening for congenital dislocation of the hip. *Maternal and Child Health,* (October), 310–314.
Watt, R. G., *et al.* (2001) Socio-economic determinants of selected dietary indicators in British pre-school children. *Public Health Nutrition,* **4** (6), 1229–1233.
Webb, C. L. (2005) Parents' perspectives on coping with Duchenne muscular dystrophy. *Child: Care, Health and Development,* **31** (4), 385–396.
Whaley, L. F. and **Wong, D. L.** (1995) *Nursing Care of Infants and Children,* 5th edn. St Louis: Mosby.
WHO (1972) *Nutritional Anaemias.* WHO Technical Report Series 503. Geneva: WHO.
Widemar, L., *et al.* (1985) The effect of adenoidectomy on secretory otitis media. *Clinical Otolaryngology,* **10** (6), 345–350.
Williams, J. (1992) Assessment of head injured children. *British Journal of Nursing,* **2**, 82–84.

Wilson, C. B. (1986) Immunological basis for increased susceptibility of the neonate to infection. *Journal of Pediatrics,* **112**, 104.
Wilson, N. (1996) Early childhood wheezing. *Paediatrics Today,* **4** (4), 91–93.
Wilson, P. (1995) Which way forward? Provision of child and adolescent mental health services. *Child Health,* **3** (3), 90–94.
Woodroffe, C., *et al.* (1993) *Children, Teenagers and Health.* Milton Keynes: Open University Press.
World Health Organization (1989) *Protecting, Promoting and Supporting Breastfeeding: The Special Role of Maternity Services. A Joint WHO/UNICEF Statement.* Geneva: WHO.
Wright, S. (1991) Altered body image in anorexia nervosa. In Glasper, A. (ed.), *Child Care: Some Nursing Perspectives.* London: Wolfe.
Zipursky, J., *et al.* (1992) Oxygen therapy in sickle-cell disease. *American Journal of Pediatric Hematology Oncology,* **14** (3), 222–228.

Further Reading

Genito-urinary problems

Berry, A. C. and **Chantler, C.** (1986) Urogenital malformations and disease. *British Medical Bulletin,* **42** (2), 181–186.
Gartland, C. (1993) Partners in care. How families are taught to care for their child on peritoneal dialysis. *Nursing Times,* **89** (30), 34–36.
Jadresic, L. (1993) Investigation of urinary tract infection in childhood. *British Medical Journal,* **307**, 761–764.
Postlethwaite, R. J. (ed.) (1994) *Clinical Paediatric Nephrology,* 2nd edn. Oxford: Butterworth Heinemann.
Taylor, C. M. and **Chapman, S.** (1989) *Handbook of Renal Investigations in Children.* Sevenoaks: Wright.

Pathophysiology

Claxton, R. and **Harrison, T.** (eds) (1991) *Caring for Children with HIV and AIDS.* London: Edward Arnold.
Gibb, D. and **Walters, S.** (1993) *Guidelines for the Management of Children with HIV Infection,* 2nd edn. West Sussex: Avert.
Groer, M. E. and **Shekleton, M. E.** (1979) *Basic Pathophysiology: A Conceptual Approach.* St Louis: Mosby.

HIV disease

Orr, N. (ed.) (1995) *Children's Rights and HIV: A Framework for Action.* London: National Children's Bureau.

Family therapy

Anderson, T. (1990) *The Reflecting Team.* Broadstairs: Bergman.
Barker, P. (1992) *Basic Family Therapy,* 3rd edn. Oxford: Blackwell Scientific Publications.

Cognitive behaviour therapy

Murdoch, D. and **Barker, P.** (1991) *Basic Behaviour Therapy.* Oxford: Blackwell Scientific Publications.
Schaffer, D., *et al.* (1995) *The Clinical Guide to Child Psychiatry.* London: The Free Press, Collier and Macmillan.

Prevention of suicide

Jenkins, R., Griffiths, S., Wylie, I., Hawton, K., Morgam, G. and **Tylee, A.** (eds) (1994) *The Prevention of Suicide.* London: HMSO.

Psychological problems of 'surgical' babies

Ludham, L. (1992) Emotional development after major neonatal surgery. *Paediatric Nursing,* May, 20–22.

Part 3

Professional Issues in Child Care

Module 7
The Development and Process of Children's Nursing

Joan Ramsay

Learning Outcomes

The material in this module and the references should enable you to:

- explore the history of children's nursing
- examine the different roles of the children's nurse
- discuss the value of models of nursing
- assess the appropriateness of different models of children's nursing
- explore the meaning and practice of family-centred care
- consider the future of children's nursing

Introduction

This module is concerned with promoting children's nursing as a unique speciality that requires specific knowledge and understanding. It begins by looking at the history of children's nursing and considering how the speciality has developed. It discusses the different roles of the children's nurse in providing specific care for the sick child alongside caring, supporting and teaching the family. Children's nurses usually have a philosophy of family-centred care – this concept, and nurses' and families' understanding of it, are explored. Family-centred care is usually the basis of any model of nursing used in children's nursing but this module, while exploring how different models of nursing can be applied to children's nursing, also questions the usefulness of models. Finally the module discusses the future of children's nursing in the light of political changes to the health service.

Chapter 52

The History of Children's Nursing

Introduction

Children's nursing is a relatively new speciality that did not really appear until the mid-19th century. It began as a need to protect vulnerable children from disease and death and, although that fundamental concept has never been lost, it has developed into a service for the whole family, to enable the healthy growth and development of all children. In the beginning the nurses employed to care for the children were given no special training and were often less than satisfactory. Over the years children's nurse education has developed into a speciality with graduate and postgraduate programmes now available. There are also a number of recognised specialities within the field of paediatrics, which nurses can study at degree level.

The first children's hospitals were very basic and could cater for only small numbers of children, who were separated from their families during their stay in hospital. Nowadays, specialist children's hospitals have at least 300 beds, including facilities for intensive care, and cater for families as well as children. They employ a large number of medical and nursing staff but also other professionals important to children's welfare, such as nursery nurses, play therapists and teachers. Families of sick children, who were once rejected as a disturbance to the children and the ward routine, are now welcome to participate in the care of their children.

Despite these developments, there is still room for further improvement. Children's nursing has been fortunate to gain backing from various government reports since the 1940s but the recommendations contained within them must still be fully implemented. The number of registered children's nurses does not meet the growing demand for such specialist practitioners and their preparation needs review.

Hospitals for Sick Children

Children's hospitals in the UK date from 1739 when Captain Thomas Coram retired from a life at sea and returned to London. He was

Significant reports in the history of children's nursing

1959 *Welfare of Children in Hospital (Platt Report)*
A government report which recognised the adverse effects of hospitalisation for children and made recommendations to enable children to be nursed by specialist practitioners in a suitable environment

1976 *Fit for the Future: Child Health Services (Court Report)* (DH, 1976)
A government report which realised the disparity of health services for children and recommended a more coordinated integrated service which would shorten hospital admission and enable children to be nursed at home

1988 *Parents Staying Overnight with their Children* (Thornes, 1988b)
A recommended standard for the provision of overnight accommodation for resident parents produced by the consortium Caring for Children in the Health Services (comprising ASC, RCN, British Paediatric Association and the National Association of Health Authorities and Trusts)

1988 *Hidden Children – An Analysis of Ward Attenders in Children's Wards* (Thornes, 1988a)
A report from the Caring for Children in the Health Services group recommending good practice for the care of children who do not require a stay in hospital but still need to attend hospital

1989 *The Children Act: An Introductory Guide for the NHS* (DH, 1989)
Produced by the DH to clarify the provisions of the Children Act and the duty of NHS Trusts in providing services for children in need and their families

1991 *Just for the Day* (Thornes, 1991)
A report by the consortium Caring for Children in the Health Services which suggested ways of improving the quality of health care for children and produced a comprehensive set of standards for day care

1991 *Welfare of Children and Young People in Hospital* (Fish and Purr, 1991)
A government report reiterating the principles of the Platt Report and making more specific recommendations about staffing levels in areas where children are nursed and stressing the involvement of parents in the care of their children in hospital

1993 *Children First – A Study of Hospital Services*
The findings of the Audit Commissions's study into the hospital services for sick children, investigating why principles for good practice outlined in the Platt Report were not being met

1994 *The Allitt Inquiry (Clothier Report)* (DH, 1994b)
The findings of the independent inquiry team into the deaths and injuries of the children cared for by Beverley Allitt which includes recommendations aimed to tighten procedures for safeguarding children in hospital and prevent a repetition of the tragedy

1995 *The Children's Charter*
A government-produced charter to help children and their parents be aware of their rights in relation to health care

horrified by the numbers of sick and dying children he encountered in the streets of the capital and set about gaining support to fund a place to care for them. In 1739 he opened a foundling hospital to care for unwanted children. Yet he was still unable to stop the huge numbers of deaths amongst the children. During the next 20 years 15 000 children were admitted here, demonstrating the very great need at this time for a place of care for abandoned and unwanted children, but only 4400 of them managed to survive to adulthood (Besser, 1977). This high mortality rate of children in the 17th and early 18th century was mostly due to ignorance about childhood infections, their cause and the way in which they spread.

Coram also did not manage to change the attitudes to children of the time, which were largely influenced by John Wesley. Wesley believed that children were evil and could only be saved by physical punishment. In light of such widely held views it is not surprising that sick children were not catered for in hospitals and left to die. In 1843 the annual mortality rate was 50 000, yet children accounted for nearly half this figure. Of 2363 patients in the London hospitals, only 26 were children. At the London hospital, children under 7 years were actually prohibited unless they required an amputation or 'cutting for stone'. In 1831 Guy's hospital had 15 beds for children in a wooden building over some stables but this building was pulled down in 1850 and not replaced (De Mause, 1974).

However, as the Industrial Revolution progressed so did education and literacy and, gradually, with the help of such authors as Charles Dickens and Charles Kingsley who highlighted some of the worst child-care practices, attitudes towards children began to change. At the same time, Dr Charles West was taking an interest in childhood illnesses. He saw the children at local clinics or dispensaries where they were seen, treated and sent home. He put together his observations to form the first textbook on the diseases of childhood to be published in England. He also realised that the reason why most children did not recover from their illnesses was because they returned home to an overcrowded environment, poor sanitation and little or no healthy food. He resolved to open a children's hospital to overcome these problems.

Dr West had to battle to get his dream accepted. The arguments against a hospital for children were many. It would separate the children from their families and require one nurse for each child. The nurses would not agree with the mothers' care and the potential for the spread of infection would be great. However, Dr West did realise his dream despite these arguments and the Hospital for Sick Children, Great Ormond Street, was opened on 14 February 1852. Initially it had only 10 beds but the number gradually increased so that by 1858 the hospital could cater for 75 children.

Standards of Care

During the 1850s and for a long time afterwards it was believed that the child's parents should not be part of the child's care in hospital. This idea was partly due to the military philosophy of the Nightingale type of nurse training, which commenced in 1860. Parents were seen as amateurs in the care of sick children, who would distress themselves and the child if allowed to come into the hospital too often. Concern was also raised about the spread of infection and disruption to the hospital routine; consequently strict visiting hours for parents were imposed. Other members of the family were not allowed at all. Remember that at this time children were kept in hospital much longer than at present (*see also* Separation anxiety p. 201).

This state of affairs stayed unchanged for almost a century. For many years nurses used the fact that the children cried at the end of visiting time to support their beliefs that parental presence in hospital was upsetting and should not be encouraged. These beliefs began to be challenged in the post-war years. Concerned with the possible effects of the evacuation of children during the war and the consequence upon children of the changing role of women, psychologists began to study the effects of parental separation. Bowlby (1951) discovered that children formed an attachment with their parents from an early age and used this relationship as a source of comfort when distressed or stressed. The following year, evidence on film showed clearly the protest, despair and detachment that occurs in the child in hospital when parental separation occurs (Bowlby and Robertson, 1952). Later research by Robertson revealed that children in hospital who were separated from their mother took longer to recover from their illness and their development regressed (Robertson, 1958). As a result of this evidence, the government appointed Platt to report on the welfare of children in hospital. The report, published in 1959, revealed the restrictions imposed upon parents, the lack of proper facilities for children in hospital and the number of children being nursed in adult wards. It made several recommendations to change these bad practices. However, these recommendations involved a major change in current beliefs and practices and had financial and organisational implications. It is not surprising, therefore, that its implementation was slow and difficult. What is surprising is that more than 40 years later some of the recommendations of the Platt Report have still not been met (Audit Commission, 1993).

The Platt Report recommendations

- Hospitalisation only when absolutely necessary and for the minimum length of time
- Mothers to be resident in hospital with their sick child
- Unrestricted visiting
- Appropriately qualified children's nurses on all wards where children are nursed
- Children's usual home routine to be maintained in hospital
- Children should be nursed in an appropriate child-friendly environment
- Provision of play and education for all children in hospital
- Children's wards should have a strategy for preparing children for elective admission

(MH, 1959)

Study activity

Read the Platt Report recommendations and make a critical assessment of how your area of practice meets these.

Since the Platt Report, other government reports have highlighted the importance of special resources for the care of children. In 1961 the National Association for the Welfare of Children in Hospital (NAWCH) was established to campaign for the rights of sick children and their families. Now known as Action for Sick Children (ASC), this pressure group has done much to improve the quality of care for children in hospital. In other countries progress has been even slower. Stenbak (1986) revealed that in many parts of Europe parental visiting is still prohibited or limited. In 1988 the European Association of Children in Hospital (EACH) was established with the aim of producing a charter for children in hospital across Europe. Now representing 18 countries, EACH has agreed to focus its efforts on emphasising the importance of children being nursed on children's wards. Even in the UK, children are still admitted to adult ear, nose and throat, and ophthalmology wards (Audit Commission, 1993) (*see also* Allitt inquiry p. 262 and Number of registered children's nurses p. 251).

The 1990s saw a number of reports that highlighted the changes still to be met in order to comply with the Platt Report. These were particularly highlighted by the Beverley Allitt case in 1991. Allitt, a nurse working on a children's ward, murdered four children and attempted to kill at least eight others. The independent inquiry into the case recommended that there should always be a certain number of appropriately qualified children's nurses on a children's ward (DH, 1994a). While the rationale for such a recommendation may have been flawed – Allitt's mental state is surely unrelated to the absence or presence of a children's nursing qualification – the report's suggestions have not been acted upon. Over 10 years after the publication of the inquiry's report, 80% of children's wards were still lacking sufficient numbers of children's nurses.

Study activity

Study a month's duty roster in your own area and determine the numbers of appropriately qualified children's nurses on duty over a 24-hour period. Do these numbers meet with the Department of Health's guidelines of two registered children's nurses on duty at any time? Consider whether two such nurses are enough.

In 1995 the government followed their Patient's Charter with one for children. This was aimed to inform children and their parents of their rights in relation to health care. Surprisingly, it does not mention staffing issues other than to state that children can expect to have a named nurse in charge of their care. This was followed in 2004 by a series of three booklets for parents, older and young children, which explained 'what a really good hospital should look like' and set out the National Service Framework (NSF) standards for all children being treated in NHS hospitals in England. They state that all staff treating children should be trained to meet their needs. Perhaps, interestingly, they do not specifically mention registered children's nurses (*see also* Children's Charter p. 268).

Study activity

Read the summary of the standards in these and consider how your own area meets the standards.

Children's Nurse Education

At the time of Dr West's hospital for sick children there was no formal system of nurse education and most nurses resembled the notorious Sairey Gamp. Reports from visitors to the hospital in these early years state that everything seemed very satisfactory except for the nurses. Committee records make constant reference to nurses being found asleep, being 'dirty and disrespectful' and 'wholly incapable'. Consequently, Dr West decided to ensure that his hospital nurses were properly trained.

From 1862 Dr West employed sisters and recommended that they and the other nurses and probationers should reach a certain standard. He decreed that any nurse who hit a child should be dismissed immediately as this demonstrated an inability to keep children contented. He wrote a book entitled *How to Nurse Sick Children* and in 1878 he

What should a really good hospital look like?

- Children should not be alone
  - staff should treat them as individuals
  - parents should be able to stay and participate in care
- Children should be treated with respect
  - staff will consider any special needs – disability, religion, etc.
  - children should be given a choice of having a chaperone for examinations
  - they should be provided with privacy
- Children should have access to advice about
  - how to stay healthy
  - anything that worries them – bullying at school, drugs, etc.
- Children should be prepared for hospital by
  - arrangements to see the ward before admission
  - having written information
- Children should not be bored in hospital and should have access to
  - play specialists
  - television, radio and telephone at the bedside
  - hospital teachers
- Children can get the right food
  - food they like, when they want it
  - their family should be allowed to bring in their favourite food
- Children have access to information to enable consent
  - staff can help them to understand what is happening
  - they can ask as many questions as necessary
  - they are told their choices for treatment
  - time is made available to discuss options privately with their family
- Children are given have choice about:
  - times of nursing interventions
  - having a single room if available
- Children should be kept safe
  - the ward should have security to monitor people entering
  - they should be safe from dangers within the ward environment
  - the ward should be clean
- Children should be in control of pain by:
  - having medicine to control or reduce it
  - talking to staff about other ways of controlling it
- Children should have the best staff, treatment and facilities by access to:
  - up-to-date treatment and equipment
  - staff trained to understand children's needs and how these differ from adults'
  - suitable toilets and bathrooms
  - toys, games and books suitable for every age
  - specialist children's or adolescent units for mental health problems when necessary
  - all facilities even if disabled
- Children should be prepared for surgery
  - staff should explain what will happen and discuss any worries
  - be accompanied by a parent as far as theatre
  - a parent should be present in the recovery room
- Children should have a planned return home
  - the staff will organise any help or further treatment needed
  - the hospital will write to the family doctor (and school if necessary)
- Children will be helped to grow up
  - staff will help with the change to adult services
  - staff will explain individual children's needs to the adult service
  - staff will explain self-care to enable best care

(DH, 2004a)

Dr Charles West's standards of care for nurses and sisters

'The duty of attending on sick children calls not only for the ordinary amount of patience, gentleness and kindness necessary in the case of all sick persons, but also for the freedom from prejudice and a quickness of observation seldom found among the uneducated. No woman is to be admitted as a nurse who cannot read writing as well as printing, and who cannot repeat the Lord's prayer and the Ten Commandments and who is not acquainted with the principles of the Christian religion; and no-one is to be admitted as a Sister who is not able in addition to the above to write a legible hand. Further that it is to be the duty of every nurse not only to watch the children with care and to tend them with kindness, but also to try by all means to keep them cheerful and contented.'

appointed Miss Catherine Wood as Lady Superintendent of Nurses to arrange the training of all probationer nurses at the hospital. During her first year in post, Miss Wood also published her own textbook for nurses, *Handbook of Nursing*. Ten years later she produced a second book, *The Training of Nurses for Sick Children*. It is interesting to read excerpts from her work as she writes clearly about her philosophy of nursing children, revealing ideas that are still fundamental to children's nursing. However, these ideas must have been seen as revolutionary in 1888 bearing in mind the social climate of the time.

Although Miss Wood developed the first training programme for children's nurses in 1878, it was not until the 1920s that children's nurses became registered. Initially nurses were trained specifically to care for children. Applicants, who had to have their school certificate, were taken on unpaid probation for the first 1 to 2 months and then, if deemed suitable, undertook 3 years' training. Their lectures were given by doctors with practical sessions taught by a sister tutor or ward sister.

The training of nurses for sick children

'I commence by stating two propositions, first that sick children require special nursing; and second, that sick children's nurses require special training.

The child can give no reliable help in detailing his symptoms or in giving a detailed account of his bodily functions . . . He must not be left alone, his attendant must always be on the watch for any change in his physical condition as such changes for good or ill occur most unexpectedly and run their course with startling rapidity.

The child will thrive best who is best mothered by his own nurse, for little sick ones are quick to discern those who love them and that nurse will have most success who makes an individual study of her patients . . .

It will not be found that the same regularity and order can be maintained amongst the children as among the adults. Order and discipline there must be, or the child will not be happy; but the ward that is tidied up to perfection, in which the little ones look like well drilled soldiers . . . is hardly suggestive of the happy heart of a child. Toys and games are as much part of the treatment as physic, and the ceaseless chatter and careless distribution of toys are surely consistent with a well-ordered children's ward.'

(Wood, 1888)

The notion of nurses being trained only to nurse children then began to be considered rather narrow and it became accepted that a nurse should also have general nurse training to be able to manage a children's ward or hospital. Once parents became more involved in their children's care, this general qualification was also seen as necessary to appreciate and respond to parental needs. Obtaining two qualifications was difficult. The number of hospitals offering sufficient experience for children's nurse training was small and nurses who undertook their general training first were reluctant to return to student status on qualifying. As the numbers of registered sick children's nurses (RSCNs) declined and the government applied pressure to provide appropriately qualified practitioners to care for sick children increased, a further change was required.

This change has only occurred relatively recently. Children's nursing had always been considered to be less rigorous and significant than general training and, although Scotland retained and respected the single RSCN qualification, the rest of the UK was slow to accept that nurses wishing to care for children need only undertake a children's nursing course. In 1986, the United Kingdom Central Council (UKCC) for nursing, midwifery and health visiting proposed a new way of preparing nurses to practise (Project, 2000), which included an 18-month branch programme in the care of children. This new nurse education programme at diploma level proposed a move away from the traditional apprentice style of nurse training and proposed that students of nursing were supernumerary and should be paid on a bursary. It also proposed that students undertook an 18-month common foundation programme (CFP) where they would gain experience in a supernumerary capacity in all the nursing specialities. At the end of this time the students would choose their speciality for the branch programme and their future qualification. This innovation should have helped to overcome the shortage of qualified children's nurses as it enabled more colleges of nursing to offer children's nurse training.

However, other changes in the health service prevented the new diploma programmes from making these reforms. In 1989, when the pilot schemes for the diploma programmes were being initiated, Trust status for health services was being discussed, and the movement of nurse education away from health-service management and into the education sector was beginning. These changes may have improved the quality of patient service and given more academic credibility to nurse education but they may also have reduced the numbers of nurses entering the smaller branches of nursing, including children's nursing. Trust hospitals, responsible for their own budgets, had to consider carefully their need for trained nurses in the future to determine the number of students required for each speciality. The universities were then asked to meet these requirements. As a result, student nurses have to choose their speciality on entry and the ability to make an informed decision at the end of CFP is largely lost. The post-registration entry gate to children's nursing has also been largely lost. The placement experience has been given to diploma students and, because the original idea of PK2 was that the students chose their speciality, the need for a change of branch after qualification was not really considered and programmes were not developed. In addition, now that universities manage nurse education, most registered nurses wishing to change speciality have to return to a student bursary as well as finding funds to pay for the course. Funding for specialist qualifications in children's nursing has been drastically cut over the past 10 years and although there is no shortage of people wanting to train as children's nurses the limited availability of training places contributes to over two-thirds of applicants being rejected (Royal College of Nursing, 2002).

At present, therefore, there is still a lack of appropriately qualified children's nurses, especially in areas not specifically catering for children, such as general intensive care units and A&E units (Elston and Thormes, 2002). The Audit Commission (1993) discovered that most of the 31 children's wards studied were staffed with only one RSCN during the day and that 50% of the sample had no RSCNs on duty at night. Other areas, where children are the minority patient group, have no qualified children's nurses (DH, 1991). Nearly 10 years later this picture does not appear to have changed significantly. In 2002 Elston and Thornes found that 10% of district general hospitals had no registered children's nurses in general areas (theatres, A&E) where children were seen. In addition, 61.5% had insufficient registered children's nurses in children's wards to meet service requirements. Although the right of sick children to be cared for by appropriately qualified nurses who understand their special needs is not disputed and is supported by the government, the medical profession and pressure groups for the care of children (Colson, 1996), it appears that the argument is turning again, this time to consider the generic nurse. In 2005 the Department of Health recommended a set of generic skills for all persons involved with the care of critically ill or injured children in district general hospitals and minor injury units. The important debate would appear to be is this merely a financial solution that ensures the provision of a cost-effective qualified workforce rather than the best option for sick children?

Study activity

Consider the advantages and disadvantages of the generic nurse for children and their families.

It must be remembered that many nurses still believe that a general nurse qualification is fundamental for any speciality and many students wanting to nurse children are given the wrong career advice from registered nurses. The professional bodies have also been slow to adapt to the single qualification. In 2006 (17 years after the first diploma programmes commenced), advertisements for senior posts in paediatrics were still requiring general and paediatric qualifications. In addition, child branch students have difficulty entering health visiting and midwifery without a general nurse qualification, and recognition of the child branch qualification for those wishing to work abroad is not always easy. Glasper (1995) suggests that a generic registration could precede a specialist advanced qualification relating to the UKCC's 1995 recommendations. This would have the advantage of enabling children's nursing to become an academic subject in its own right, but would all nurses follow the specialist route? Would we be in danger of perpetuating a shortage of appropriately qualified children's nurses and recreating the second-level nurse?

In 2005 another threat to children's nursing as a separate speciality developed as many NHS Trusts found themselves in financial difficulty and began to consider the reconfiguration of the workforce to reduce expenditure. The new pay structure for health service employees, 'Agenda for Change', tended to reward specialist nurses with higher bandings. This recognised the extra skills of children's nurses but it also posed a threat to the number of these nurses that Trusts could afford. Workforce development plans suggest that assistant practitioner posts be created to overcome these problems, especially in areas where there are recruitment problems. Would these new posts also be recreating the enrolled nurse?

In view of these debates it is reassuring that the importance of specific children's nurses has been consistently recognised in the 1997 government reports, 'The Specific Health Needs of Children and Young People' and 'Health Services for Children and Young People in the Community: Home and School'. At the launch of these reports Mrs Marion Roe, chair of the Health Select Committee, said that: 'We recommend that all nurses for whom children comprise the focus of their work should be qualified children's nurses . . .' In 2004, the Chief Nursing Officer, Sarah Mullally, launched the results of a review into the nursing contribution to the health and well-being of vulnerable children. She stressed the importance of strengthening the role of children's nurses to ensure children and young people benefited from their skills. In 2004, the first children's hospital in Wales admitted its first patients. This new hospital aims to provide the environment, services and expertise to make it the centre of national and international excellence for the care of children (Davies, 2004). The RCN raised hopes that this quality care will illustrate the importance of ensuring that only registered children's nurses provide care for sick children (Royal College of Nursing, 2003). Hopefully, the future of children's nursing as a separate speciality can be assured by such support, allowing it to flourish and adding to its relatively short history.

Key Points

1. Services for sick children did not commence properly until the mid-19th century.
2. The first establishment to specifically care for sick children was established in the 18th century to look after unwanted children. Hospitals at this time had few or no facilities to care for children.
3. Hospital facilities for children arose initially in an effort to overcome their poor home environment, and parents were seen as an infection risk and not made welcome.
4. Psychological research in the 1950s showed that sick children needed their parents and gradually families have been more involved in the care of their sick children.
5. There are many recommendations about special care needed by sick children that have not yet been implemented.
6. Specific training for children's nurses commenced in 1878 but discussion has been ongoing through the years about the appropriateness of specialist versus generic training for the children's nurse.

Chapter 53

Roles of the Children's Nurse

Introduction

What is a children's nurse? What makes this type of nursing different from other branches of nursing? The following chapters about nursing models begin to explore the answers to these questions but the issue of the uniqueness of nursing children is so fundamental that it is worthy of further exploration. The history of children's nursing shows that government guidelines have always recommended that children should be cared for by registered nurses who have a children's nursing qualification (MH, 1959; DH, 1991, 1996a, b). *The Children's NSF* (DH, 2004b) stated categorically that:

- 'Children and young people should receive high quality evidence-based hospital care . . . delivered by staff who have the right set of skills'
- Staff treating and caring for children need to have the education, training, knowledge and skills to provide high quality care to deal with the highly specific problems of childhood

None of these reports really attempts to say what it is that children's nurses do that is so different from other nurses. Children's nurses care for every aspect of the growth and development of the children and their families. In developing a therapeutic relationship with the children and families their own individuality cannot be forgotten. In the present climate, which relies more and more on unqualified healthcare assistants, who are less costly than registered nurses, to carry out nursing care, it is important for children's nurses to be able to define exactly what they do and protect their important role.

These roles have been identified in various ways by nurse educationalists attempting to develop schemes of assessing children's nursing practice. Using these and Peplau's (1952) ideas about the roles of the nurse, it appears that children's nursing practice consists of nine roles, which link closely with each other:

- stranger
- surrogate

- technical expert
- advisor
- advocate
- resource
- teacher
- leader
- developing professional

The Stranger

Peplau (1952) talks about the role of the stranger as being the role in which the nurse may first meet the patient; in children's nursing practice the patient would be the child *and* family. It is in this role that the nurse makes an initial assessment of the child and family, remembering that this is also the time in which the child and family are making an initial assessment of the nurse. It is in this role that the nurse builds up the therapeutic relationship that is so crucial to quality care (Price, 1993). Darbyshire (1994) records several parents who talked about a special relationship with the nurse who had been present at admission. Nurses also spoke of their particular closeness to children and families whom they had admitted. In this study nurses relied heavily upon their first impressions of children and families in forming a relationship with them. As one nurse noted, 'we can't help it, we're only human'.

Nichols (1993) believes that a therapeutic relationship cannot be formed until the patient knows the nurse as a person. Children and families will not be able to share their feelings with a nurse until they have had time to trust that nurse. This trust is often built at the time of admission when the nurse has spent some time with the child and family. Enabling children and parents to discover the person behind the nurse and for them to accept that nurse as a caring, open and honest person is not easy. For many years nurses were taught not to get involved with patients and to maintain a professional distance from them. Close involvement with patients was considered to be too stressful for nurses, whose consequent anxiety would impair the care that they could give. Now it is accepted that nurses need to relate to their patients meaningfully while recognising their own needs and emotions. In an effort to define the characteristics of the therapeutic relationship, Barnsteiner and Gillis-Donovan (1990) outlined those behaviours that both aided and inhibited such a relationship. To enable the development of a therapeutic relationship, the nurse should be self-aware and be able to recognise and express personal emotions in an appropriate way (Nichols, 1993). Working alongside families within a therapeutic relationship is a fundamental principle of the Code of Professional Conduct (Nursing and Midwifery Council, 2004a) but it also warns about the need to maintain professional boundaries to avoid unhealthy involvement.

Behaviour that enables a therapeutic relationship

The nurse is able to:

- explore families' strengths and needs
- teach parents rather than doing everything for them
- separate the families' needs from personal needs
- recognise personal emotions arising from contact with different children and families
- demonstrate interpersonal skills as well as technical skills
- maintain clear, open communication with parents
- explore families' stressors and coping styles
- recognise own emotional overload and withdraw emotionally while remaining committed to the care of the child and family
- resolve conflicts and misunderstanding directly

(Barnsteiner and Gillis-Donovan, 1990)

Behaviour inhibiting a therapeutic relationship

The nurse:

- works overtime to care for an individual family
- spends off-duty time with families
- shows favouritism towards certain children
- competes with other staff or parents for the affection of certain children
- attempts to influence families' decisions
- is over-involved with children and under-involved with families
- is critical of families who cannot be resident with their child
- focuses on the technical aspect of care to the detriment of the emotional care

(Barnsteiner and Gillis-Donovan, 1990)

The Surrogate

Surrogate is a difficult word to define. The dictionary definition includes such synonyms such as 'substitute', 'replacement' and 'stopgap'.

RSCN competencies

- Advise on the promotion of health and the prevention of illness
- Recognise situations which may be detrimental to the health and well-being of the individual
- Carry out those activities involved when conducting the comprehensive assessment of a person's nursing requirements
- Recognise the significance of the observations made and use these to develop an initial nursing assessment
- Devise a plan of care based on the assessment with the co-operation of the patient, to the extent that this is possible, taking into account the medical prescription
- Implement the planned programme of care and, where appropriate, teach and co-ordinate other members of the caring team who may be responsible for implementing specific aspects of the nursing care
- Review the effectiveness of the nursing care provided and, where appropriate, initiate any action that may be required
- Work in a team with other nurses, and with medical and paramedical staff and social workers
- Undertake the management of the care of a group of patients over a period of time and organise the appropriate support services

Children's nurses are keen not to become replacement or substitute parents and Darbyshire's (1994) research reveals clearly that one of the parents' anxieties is that they (the parents) are incompetent and the nurses would take over their parenting role. Yet, nurses do act as a stopgap when family is not present. As discussed in Module 5 (*see* Role of the nurse as surrogate p. 364), the role of surrogate is to follow the usual home care routine when family cannot be present. It is not an opportunity for the nurse to replace the family and change the normal home practices if, in the nurse's view, they are not appropriate for that child.

The Technical Expert

Fundamental to all the roles of the nurse is the restoration of health. Although this includes meeting the psychological needs of the child and family, the nurse performs much of this activity by using specific technical skills. Nurses are largely responsible for monitoring the child's condition using their knowledge of growth and development and pathophysiology, and providing and initiating care that has a firm research rationale. It is interesting that the competencies of the registered children's nurse produced by the UKCC centre mostly on these skills and barely mention other roles. The body of knowledge required to fulfil this role is huge and is, of course, never static. Children's nurses have to know about the physical and psychological growth and development of the child from conception to adolescence. They have to understand all the factors that influence this growth and development and cause disease and disability. They also have to know how to meet the needs of the child with a specific problem.

The Advisor

Counselling is a highly complex activity that has little good research to support its effectiveness. There is a growing tendency for lay people to take on the role of counsellors without adequate training or preparation. Health professionals tend to see themselves as counsellors because they listen to families' problems and offer advice. This is not counselling and there is a danger of trivialising true counselling by calling it such. Counselling or personal-centred psychotherapy was founded in the 1940s by Dr Carl Rogers and is concerned with helping people to understand their personal perceptual world and to use this knowledge to move towards being able to direct their own lives. Most nurses' roles are more concerned with being an advisor and supporter.

In this advisory role the nurse encourages the child and family to share their feelings and thoughts and helps them to cope with or resolve problems. This involves some of the skills of counselling such as active listening, probing, reflecting, responding with empathy and helping the patient to explore their options. Davis and Fallowfield (1991) agree that nurses are not equipped to counsel patients but talk about nurses using basic counselling skills to improve communication with their patients.

The Advocate

As an advocate the nurse helps children and their families to make informed choices and act in the child's best interest (Rushton, 1993). Ellis (1995) believes that nurses are best placed to take on this role because their care is more holistic, and they have more opportunity to get to know the individual child and family than other healthcare professionals.

Some families are assertive and confident enough to act as their own advocates but many will have lost their usual abilities in the stress of the hospital environment (Darbyshire, 1994). In this situation the role of the nurse is to ensure that children and their families are informed and that they have the opportunity to express their opinions. It is a difficult role for nurses to undertake as there may be instances when they do not agree with the family about what action is in the child's best interests. Advocacy is not about overruling families' wishes but respecting and representing their beliefs. Another difficulty is when the child's wishes contradict those of the parents. Again, the nurse as an advocate must give both sides opportunity to express their wishes without imposing personal views.

Study activity

Identify occasions in your practice when either you have acted as an advocate or you have observed this role. What skills are needed?

Basic counselling skills

Make the situation safe

- use an open posture and manner
- avoid interruptions

Use active listening techniques

- let the parent or child talk freely
- use only short prompts or helping statements

Encourage the expression of feelings

- gently encourage emotions to be displayed
- accept displays of emotion calmly

Show empathy and understanding

- reflect back the expressed thoughts and feelings
- avoid giving instant advice
- do not overemphasise one's own experiences

Help resolve the problem

- aid with setting objectives, determining options

(Nichols, 1993)

To be an advocate the nurse needs the necessary knowledge to be able to explain all treatment and procedures and the available options in an unbiased manner. This enables the child and family to make informed choices. Advocacy also involves enabling parents of the appropriate way to change existing practice. Assertiveness is often required to speak out on behalf of children and families but care should be taken not to become aggressive and confrontational. On occasions advocacy will involve ethical decision making, so the nurse also needs to have an understanding of ethical theory and principles and skills in moral reasoning.

The Resource

A major part of any nurse's role is liaison with other members of the multidisciplinary team. The nurse, who tends to have most contact with the child and family, is ideally placed to coordinate the care. The nurse also knows the most appropriate personnel to refer the child and family to when their need is outside the nurse's usual practice. This may occur in hospital, for example when the nurse recognises the family's need for expert counselling, spiritual help or the specialist advice of a paediatric dietician. It may also occur on discharge when the nurse may be able to give families information and contact with community services or self-help groups.

Study activity

Create an annotated list for yourself of all the self-help groups with which you have contact during your practice. What benefits do these groups offer?

Nurses, through previous experience, can also act as valuable guides to mechanical resources, aids to living, dressings and medication. They are able to give a balanced view of the disadvantages and advantages of using one resource over another. Acting as a resource involves being able to answer questions about aspects of care or treatment.

The Teacher

As well as being able to answer questions, children's nurses also act as a teacher. They are required to teach parents and their children about health and they are often involved in teaching them about technical care so that the child and parents can continue this care independently.

Every children's nurse acts as a health educator. An increasing part of this role is health prevention, which needs a good understanding of the socio-economic factors in the families' environment that may affect their health. Health prevention in hospital has to be tackled with particular tact as often the accident or illness has already occurred. However, accidents often occur because parents do not recognise the children's abilities and the nurse is in a good position to discuss potential problems and advise preventive measures related to the child's stage of development. Health education posters, information leaflets and displays cannot change motivational or risk-perception factors but they can provide education when used imaginatively in the clinic or ward. This specific part of the teacher's role is discussed in more detail in Module 3 (*see* Role of children's nurses in health promotion p. 165).

Children's nurses teach children and their families and therefore need the skills to teach both age groups. It is important to assess their willingness to learn and not to make parents feel pressurised into taking on aspects of care. It is useful to teach more than one member of the family so that no one person feels that they carry sole responsibility for the care. Children learn best through play and the nurse can use this strategy to teach knowledge and skills. Teaching parents is often more difficult as they lack confidence because of their anxiety about their child and they often have the competing demands and fatigue caused by other children and other jobs. However, they are usually well motivated and are able to use their past experiences to aid new learning. In comparison to answering questions as a resource person, teaching is not a casual role and should be well planned beforehand to obtain the best results. Although education is not the sole factor in ensuring compliance, parents who are more knowledgeable about their child's condition are more likely to comply with treatment (Ley and Llewelyn, 1995). The nurse's relationship with parents should help in identifying the most appropriate way of imparting the knowledge: an American study found that 30–50% of mothers taught by doctors did not understand terms such as asthma, virus, vitamin or fever (Gablehouse and Gitterman, 1990) (*see also* Role of children's nurses in child health promotion p. 165 and Compliance p. 220).

Guidelines for teaching parents

Assessment

- what does the family already know?
- have they any immediate concerns?
- how do they learn best?

Planning

- consider what you have to teach
- break content into small steps, possibly into different sessions
- select your teaching method, using as much variety as possible
- choose a suitable time and place

Implementation

- use simple terms, avoid jargon
- introduce the most important issues first
- reiterate important points
- use verbal praise to reward learning but do not patronise
- have written material for parents to consolidate your learning

Evaluation

- allow time for parents' questions
- check learning has taken place

The Leader

Nurses may act as leaders in several ways. Care plans are best negotiated with the child and parents but there may be occasions when the nurse is more directive in determining care, such as after surgery. Being a primary nurse involves acting as a leader for other colleagues and ensuring continuity and consistency of care. Children's nurses also act as leaders for other nurses or healthcare professionals who are not used to caring for children. In this role, for instance, they may give specific advice to community staff or nurses in adult intensive care units about the care of children. The nurse in a multidisciplinary team is often the only member of the team with specific knowledge of the child and family and is likely to be the only member with the specific skills to care for children (Fradd, 1994). Nurses must feel confident and competent in their knowledge and skills to be able to share them in this way.

Study activity

Compile a list of the characteristics that you consider an effective leader should have.

At the 2005 Royal College of Nursing Congress, delegates were told that 'Now is a brilliant time to be involved in children's services. Never has been there such a high profile for children and young people; never has so much policy been focused on them'. The net result should be great opportunities for children's nurses to lead the way in developing services for children (Fradd, 2005). Leadership is about all practising children's nurses influencing every level of service because leadership has more to do with personal skills and attributes that one's position in the nursing hierarchy. Leadership skills are intrinsic to everyday nursing practice and are crucial if nurses are to initiate and implement change rather than have it imposed upon them (Sams, 1996).

Leadership skills

- time management
- delegation
- accountability
- assertiveness
- communication
- resource management
- inspires and motivates others
- team management

The Developing Practitioner

Discussion about Peplau's model of nursing (*see* Models of children's nursing p. 635) explains how Peplau believes that the nurse develops from each and every encounter with a patient. She believes that each nurse–patient relationship brings some new learning to the nurse. Benner (1984) recognised that nurses learn their intuitive knowledge by experience but that this experiential learning could not expand and develop unless they began to record what they learn from their experiences. Nurses are now beginning to recognise this valuable source of new knowledge and are using reflection to identify it in a more concrete way.

Study activity

Reflect upon a recent encounter with a child and family and identify what you have learnt from this occurrence.

Guidelines for reflection

- Briefly describe the experience, its context and any influencing factors
- Reflect upon what you did and why
- Examine the reactions of yourself and others
- Consider what influenced your behaviour and actions
- Think whether you could have behaved or acted differently
- Summarise what you have learned from this experience and how it will affect your future practice

Module 7

Reflection need not only be centred on professional practice. Personal incidents such as a bereavement, or a period of time as a patient, may be a valuable learning experience and affect the way in which you practise.

Nursing knowledge can also expand and develop through research. Nurses are now more involved in research, but this involvement tends to be confined to those in specialist roles. Clinically based nurses have greater opportunity to observe child and parental behaviour and children's responses to care and treatment, and often use innovative ways to encourage children to comply with treatment. They could be using this experience in an investigative way to challenge accepted practice or introduce new ideas (*see also* Research pp. 705, Reflective practice p. 652 and PREP categories of study p. 656).

The professional bodies in nursing also expect registered nurses to develop their practice. The NMC Code of Professional Conduct (Nursing and Midwifery Council, 2004a) states that registered nurses have a responsibility to maintain their professional knowledge and competence. Moreover, from January 2006 it became mandatory for all registered nurses, midwives and health visitors to provide evidence of their continuing post-registration development in order to reregister every year (Nursing and Midwifery Council, 2004b). This evidence must include:

- at least 5 days (35 hours) of study in every 3-year period relevant to the individual's role and area of practice, showing how the area of study has enhanced practice
- evidence that they have completed a minimum of 100 days (750 hours) of practice during the 5 years prior to renewal of registration
- a notification of practice form (or a statutory return to practice programme after a break of 5 years or more)
- a personal professional profile

Nurses also develop their practice by gaining increasing technical skills to meet the demand of technological advances. It is important that children's nurses keep abreast of new developments and continue to enhance their own practice if they are to maintain their identity and prove their unique contribution to child health.

Key Points

1. Although there is much support for the uniqueness of children's nursing, it is difficult but necessary to maintain the speciality to define exactly what this uniqueness means.
2. Children's nursing consists of nine interlinking roles: stranger, surrogate, technical expert, advisor, advocate, resource, teacher, leader and developing professional.
3. The children's nurse needs to be self-aware to be able to undertake many of these roles.
4. Effective communication is fundamental to all roles of the children's nurse.
5. Children's nurses need a wide knowledge base to carry out all the roles effectively.
6. Children's nurses owe it to themselves and their profession to develop their role as specialist nurses.

Chapter 54

Models of Nursing – Useless Theory or an Aid to Practice?

Introduction

Ever since organised nurse training began, nurses have been theorising about nursing. In the UK, early theories about nursing were communicated by Florence Nightingale in 1859. She described nursing as both an art and a science and her ideas provided the foundation of a knowledge base unique to nursing. After Nightingale, the emphasis moved from nursing to medical knowledge – although this was limited in the 1850s – and nursing began to focus on medical phenomena such as signs and symptoms, disease and medical and surgical procedures.

It was not until almost 100 years later that there was any effort to develop or define nursing. In the 1950s, with the advent of university education for American nurses, ideas about nursing began to develop that questioned both the nature of nursing and its traditional foundations. These ideas, which were called models of nursing, have had varied reactions. On the one hand, theory is seen as necessary if nurses desire a professional identity, wish to improve standards of care and consolidate, and want to increase and clarify the knowledge base of nursing. On the other hand, the continued production of multiple models of nursing is seen as elaborate waffle which does not relate to reality and is only indulged in by those academic nurses in teaching who never actually lay hands on a real patient. Thus, at the moment, nurses are divided in their opinions about the usefulness of models; Engstrom (1984) attempted to describe this situation: 'In all a portrait of the profession is one of confusion and lack of consensus'.

To discuss the values of models both from an historical viewpoint and as a means of progressing the discipline of nursing, the following questions need to be considered:

- What are models of nursing?
- Why did models develop?
- Were these reasons valid?
- What do models aim to do?
- Are they achieving their aims?

Nursing – what it is and what it is not

'. . . Nursing is occupied with the control of the patient's environment so that nature may act upon him or her.'

'It has been said and written scores of times that every woman makes a good nurse. I believe on the contrary that the very elements of nursing are all but unknown.'

Nightingale (1859)

Definitions of models of nursing

'. . . a collection of ideas, knowledge and values about nursing which determines the way nurses, as individuals and groups, work with their patients and clients.'

(Wright, 1990)

'. . . a descriptive picture of practice which adequately represents the real thing.'

(Pearson and Vaughan, 1986)

'. . . Representations of the reality of nursing practice. They represent the factors at work and how they are related.'

(Aggleton and Chambers, 1986)

Definitions of Models

Models of nursing have been defined in different ways by different authors but the common theme appears to be that models are expressing the reality of nursing and enabling nurses to be able to work towards common goals. This promotes continuity of care and benefits the nursing team and the patient.

Study activity

Discuss with your colleagues how you would define nursing. Look critically at some of the models of nursing you have seen in practice and assess whether you consider that your views have been incorporated.

The Emergence of Models

It appears that models of nursing emerged for several reasons. It is useful to consider whether these reasons are valid. One of the reasons given for the need to define nursing is nurses' constant bid to achieve professionalism. Professionalism is difficult to define and there appears to be no general consensus on one definition. One of the earliest writers in this field was Abraham Flexner (Flexner, 1915, cited by Jolley and Allan, 1989) who suggested that the attributes of a profession were:

- basically intellectual
- learned in nature because it is based on a body of knowledge
- practical rather than theoretical
- in possession of techniques taught through education
- well organised internally
- motivated by altruism

Several desirable consequences arise from the ability to claim professional status. These include monopoly of service, autonomy, public recognition, prestige, power and authority (Gruending, 1985). The benefits to nursing of professionalism would include relative freedom from supervision outside the discipline as well as monetary and status awards. However, Davies (1996a) suggests that nurses' desire for professionalism is outdated and instead of aiming for power, authority and mastery of a unique body of knowledge they should be aiming to develop supportive practice, empowerment of patients and knowledge gained by reflection.

Another of the reasons that models of nursing have developed is to provide the body of knowledge that can be applied to its practice – a dominant characteristic of a profession. However, in the obsession with the idea of professionalism, many models have been developed. Do these different theories about nursing, which all too often have not been proven, actually aid in the quest to be seen as a profession?

It may be argued that models of nursing emerged to improve standards of care. All thinking people process views of the world, their work and the subject of their work – in the case of nursing, the patient or clients. In nursing, the care given to patients or clients is influenced by the people who give the care. For example, in a team of nurses, one nurse may align the practice of nursing with that of medicine and aim for the efficient carrying out of medical treatment. Another may see the social activities as important in enabling the patient to function as an individual. One nurse may consistently do things such as washing and dressing for the patient because she sees doing things for people as an essential part of nursing. A second nurse may observe or support someone to do things for himself as she sees helping the patient to be independent as important.

All nurses are as individual as their patients and, consequently, their past lives and experiences, which influence their behaviour and values, are unique. Thus it is likely that each nurse has a slightly different image of what nursing is. It is the purpose of models to bring together these images so nurses have shared goals and can improve standards of care, as the alternative is a lack of direction and confusion not only for the patient but for other members of the healthcare team.

Obviously if models are to improve care by ensuring a consistent approach, they need to describe nursing as it is and not as some theoretical ideal. Opponents of nursing models suggest that models are unrealistic because:

- British nurses have tended to become dominated by American models. Are these theories realistic as their healthcare system is so different? Should developments in models of nursing from other countries be studied?
- Terms used are often obscure and incomprehensible. A *Nursing Times* correspondent comments that 'I suspect that many of us cannot understand it . . . I am sceptical whether "*consideration of supply of sustenal imperatives to the eliminative subsystem*" will do much to alert the nurse to a particular patient's need for brown bread for breakfast'. Models are more likely to be read and noticed if they are written in a clear, concise language.
- Most models have been developed by nursing theorists who see nursing as it ought to be rather than 'as it is'. Nursing is primarily a care-giving discipline so surely any model of nursing must be closely related to this practice?

Despite such criticisms, nursing needs to be able to measure its standards of care and prove its value to patients. A theoretical framework for care could be a useful tool in enabling nurses to manage their own budgets. Models of nursing have also emerged to meet the need to consolidate, increase and clarify the knowledge of nursing.

> Practice without theory is like a man who goes to sea without a map, in a ship without a rudder.
>
> (Leonardo da Vinci)

The model that traditionally guided nurses was the medical model, which concentrated information and decision making in the hands of doctors. As nurses have become more educated they have tried to emphasise the important role that nurses play in health and illness.

The traditional biomedical model

- Gives the doctor the power for decision making
- Devalues the role of nursing
- Loses sight of the patient as an individual
- Concentrates on the physical diagnosis
- Ignores the holistic view of health and illness
- Emphasises technology to the detriment of caring

The medical model centres around patients' diseases and the physical care needed to cure them. Emphasis is placed on routine and getting the work done. Knowledge is related to the physical sciences, and the nurses' role in such a model of care is centred on the achievement of tasks. This model saw the patient as a malfunctioning machine and, as in a factory, different people were given different jobs to correct the malfunction. This has allowed the emergence of nurse specialists (pain, TPN, IV therapy, etc.), which actually does not help the development of nursing models that see the patient as unique and advocate holistic care. Task-oriented care can confuse patients who may have several nurses attending to their needs, but it may also be reassuring to both parties. Nurses find they do not really know any patient well and this can protect them from becoming emotionally involved. Patients do not feel neglected if their nurse is not available and feel able to turn to other nurses for help (*see also* Specialist roles for children's nurses p. 673).

Study activity

Discuss the following issues with your colleagues:

- Does task orientation reduce stress?
- Do all nurses want to change the traditional handmaiden role?
- Do nurses really want to increase nursing knowledge?
- Does the specialist nurse practitioner role help individualised care?

While Project 2000 may have aimed to change traditional views, at the moment any nurse who achieves further knowledge and becomes skilled at bedside care is promoted away from the bedside or develops a speciality as above, which prevents the patient being seen as a whole person. Care often ends up being given by the unskilled and untrained. Will this be perpetuated by the emergence of healthcare assistants and assistant practitioners? Some nurses are already being managed at ward level by non-nurses – is this because nurses have not been able to clarify what nursing is? Models may add to nursing knowledge but do they really clarify it?

Aims of Models

Wright (1990) suggests that models may have a value for practice because they aim to define:

- the nature of the person and his/her environment
- the concept of health
- the concept of nursing

A model also aims to offer guidelines on:

- what kind of research is relevant to nursing
- how nursing should be managed
- the content and style of educational programmes
- the conduct of nursing practice to provide high-quality care (Figure 54.1).

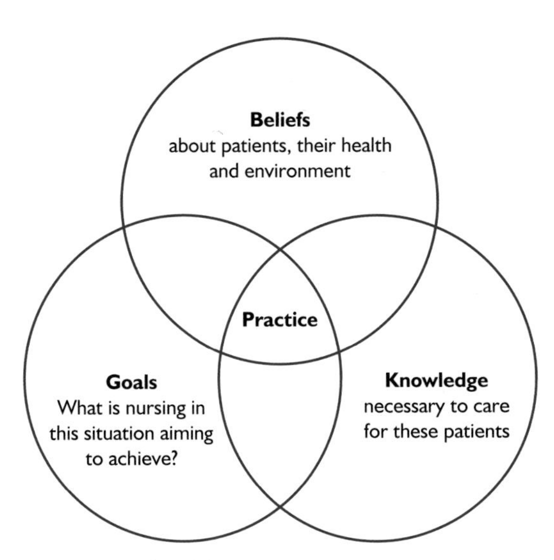

Figure 54.1 Components of models.

Study activity

Take a critical look at some of the models you have used in practice. Do they all achieve these aims?

On close inspection, many models of nursing omit large areas of detail. For example, Newman's model does not attempt to define nursing and even suggests that other healthcare workers can use the model! Much detail is given on the need to change but there is lack of advice on how to achieve the change. Nursing tends to impose change from above but this is inappropriate if the model is to reflect actual practice. Nurses who are ward based surely need to be helped to choose and develop a model which suits their area of practice otherwise it will be used in theory and not in practice. Wright (1990) agrees with this and advocates that if a model is to be applied realistically to a particular setting it should be created by those working in that area. Some nurses have created or adapted established models for use in their own setting. An example of this is the Burford model (Johns, 1994) (*see also* A reflective model of nursing p. 652).

Study activity

Opponents of nursing models consider that those models that originate outside the UK cannot accurately reflect nursing in this country. Discuss with some colleagues whether the nature of the patient and the concepts of health and nursing can be defined in universal terms.

Critics of nursing models appear to suggest that the administration of health care in different countries affects the delivery and thus the definitions of nursing care. If this is true, should nurses in this country be looking for different definitions of nursing now that health care is largely managed and commissioned by NHS Primary Care Trusts? Will the creation of Foundation Trusts make a difference?

Study activity

Talk to nurses of different generations. Do they have very different ideas about nursing?

Study activity

Consider if models of nursing should change to reflect changes in society and the Health Service.

If nursing is to remain as a recognised, independent and accepted discipline, the development of a unique knowledge base is essential. This knowledge base must be directly related to and useful in nursing practice. While there is still a lack of consensus and frustration about the relevance of models of nursing, consideration of how they can be developed, used and validated for nursing cannot progress.

Study activity

Discuss with colleagues their views about models of nursing and consider whether they are worth pursuit in the quest of knowledge about the uniqueness of nursing.

Key Points

1. Ideas about nursing began to become formalised in the 1950s when models of nursing were first created.
2. At present, nurses are divided in their views about the usefulness of nursing models for practice.
3. Models of nursing aim to define nursing, the nature of the patient and to offer guidelines on the knowledge, attitudes and skills necessary to maintain and develop nursing practice.
4. Opponents of nursing models believe that models are incomprehensible, unrealistic and unrelated to nursing in the UK.
5. Those in favour of nursing models argue that models help to clarify the uniqueness of nursing and enable nursing to be accepted as a profession.

Chapter 55

Models of Children's Nursing

Introduction

As discussed in the previous section, models of nursing aim to reflect the beliefs and values about nursing in specific settings. They aim to prevent disunity and conflict by clarifying these ideas and promoting a common philosophy of nursing.

In the UK, children's nurses generally share the philosophy of family-centred care, believing that parents should be enabled to participate in the care of their children at all times. This philosophy is supported by the children's NSF, which takes the view that parents should be closely involved in their children's health care (DH, 2004b). In other countries this philosophy has been slow to develop and Hostler (1992) reported that in 30 leading American hospitals there were no examples of nursing models that reflected family-centred care. Up until 1988 there were no specific models of nursing in the UK for the care of children, and children's nurses tended to use either Roper, Logan and Tierney's model of activities of living (Roper *et al.*, 1980), Orem's model of self-care (Orem, 1985) or Peplau's interpersonal relationships model (Peplau, 1952). In 1988, Casey developed the partnership model of nursing specifically for use in child care settings.

This section will summarise the concepts of each of these models, and explore their usefulness and effectiveness for paediatric practice, thus enabling children's nurses to take a critical look at the model used in their area of practice.

Roper, Logan and Tierney's Activity of Living Model

In the UK, this is probably the best known and most widely used model of nursing. It centres around the philosophy that an important part of living relates to the everyday activities which individuals regularly perform. They call these the 'activities of living'. The model is concerned with the individual's ability to carry out these activities independently,

Activities of living

- Maintaining a safe environment
- Communicating
- Breathing
- Eating and drinking
- Eliminating
- Personal cleansing and dressing
- Controlling body temperature
- Mobilising
- Working and playing
- Expressing sexuality
- Sleeping
- Dying

(Roper *et al.*, 1980)

recognising that physical, psychological, environmental, politico-economic and sociocultural factors may all affect a person's level of independence. It emphasises the individuality of each person's activities of living. The model recognises that fetal development, as well as physical, intellectual, emotional and social development in childhood and adolescence, affects the individual's ability to perform daily activities independently. It also discusses the impact of social relationships and the effect of the family upon the socialisation of children. It is these ideas, which relate to the care of children, that have made the model a popular choice for children's nursing.

The role of the nurse is seen as preventing, comforting and promoting maximum independence, the aim of nursing being to assess the individual's level of dependence in each of the activities of living, and planning how to help that individual move towards independence.

Study activity

Read the case study (Figure 55.1) describing Roper, Logan and Tierney's model in practice and identify:

- how Sarah's usual levels of dependence/independence have altered because of her illness
- how the roles of the nurse, as described by the model, will be used to help Sarah return to her usual dependence/independence

The activities-of-living model has been analysed and criticised by many authors. A popular criticism is that the model is medically biased because the activities of living relate to physiological systems (Aggleton and Chambers, 1986). Lister (1987) denies this claim because at least some of the activities of living have a strong psychological bias. Although many studies have been written about the use of this model, they do not examine its appropriateness to nursing practice (Fraser, 1996). Recent evidence appears to show that nurses find the model too simplistic (Parr, 1993) and Fraser (1996) could find no literature to describe its use outside the UK.

In relation to paediatrics, although the model recognises the importance of the family and developmental factors in shaping the individual, it does not consider the role of the family in helping the individual towards independence. This omission would appear to make the model difficult to use in any area where the philosophy was family-centred care.

Orem's Self-care Model

In contrast, Orem's model of nursing centres around the belief that all individuals have self-care needs, which they meet themselves whenever possible, but when unable to self-care they require help from others. The individual's ability to self-care depends upon the therapeutic self-care demand, which is affected by the individual's maturity, knowledge and life experience as well as their physical and mental health. The essential requirements for life are termed universal self-care requisites and these

Sarah was a 9-year-old who had been admitted to the ward as a newly diagnosed insulin-dependent diabetic. On admission, she was feeling ill due to hyperglycaemia and ketoacidosis.

Once Sarah's immediate medical problems had been treated a nursing assessment was carried out and Sarah's dependence/independence during health and illness was noted. When she was well Sarah was fairly independent at most activities. Her mother did say that she needed reminding to brush her teeth before bed and that she needed help to wash and dry her long hair. Her usual level of dependence/independence was thus assessed as follows:

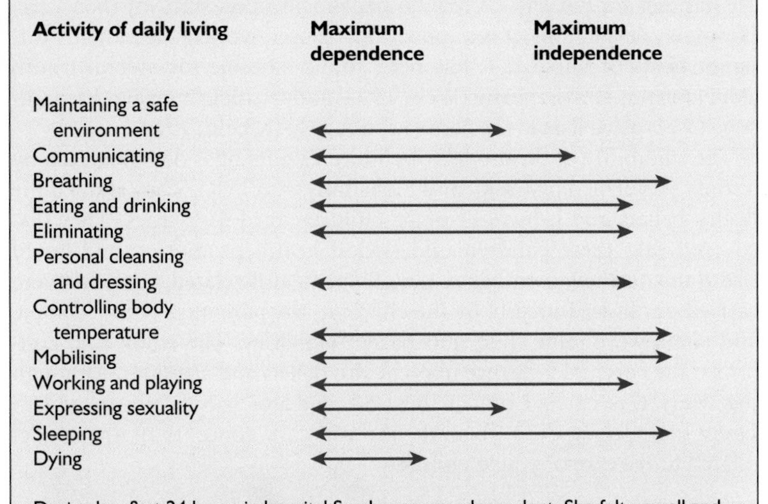

During her first 24 hours in hospital Sarah was very dependent. She felt unwell and had an IV infusion running to overcome her dehydration and was having sliding scale IV insulin. Although I explained all her care, she was not ready to eat and drink normally or to be taught how to test her blood and urine.

Figure 55.1 Roper, Logan and Tierney's model in practice.

needs may alter as a result of developmental or life changes. They also alter as a result of ill health or disability (health deviation self-care requisites). Individuals can often adapt their own care to meet deviations but intervention is required when the individual can no longer make these adaptations. Friends or family may make this intervention and it is only when their care becomes inadequate to overcome the deviation that nursing intervention is required. The role of the nurse, which may involve being wholly compensatory, partially compensatory or educative/developmental, is to use various types of helping methods to:

- eliminate any self-care deficits
- enable the client to decrease the self-care deficit
- help others to give dependent care
- meet the self-care needs directly

Orem defines nursing as being needed when the individual can no longer maintain the necessary self-care to sustain life and health. She recognises that nursing intervention is required in the care of children when the parent can no longer maintain the appropriate therapeutic amount and quality of care. Thus, this model appears to recognise some

Universal self-care requisites

- Sufficient intake of air, food and water
- Appropriate excretion of waste products
- Optimum balance between activity and rest
- Optimum balance between solitude and social interaction
- Avoidance of hazards to life and well-being
- Conformity with what is currently considered to be a normal lifestyle

(Orem, 1971)

Roles of the nurse

- Wholly compensatory to carry out all care for the patient, e.g. unconscious patient
- Partially compensatory to help the patient carry out care, e.g. helping a small child do up buttons and laces after the child has dressed independently
- Educative/developmental to teach the patient about care, e.g. showing the diabetic child self-injection technique

(Orem, 1971)

important concepts of nursing children. The developmental changes in self-care and the role of parents in meeting their child's needs are recognised. The nurse's role in teaching and helping parents to meet healthcare deviations is also made explicit.

Orem's language and writing style have been criticised as being very tortuous and jargonistic (Fraser, 1996). Other criticisms include the individual's desire for self-care. Lacey (1993) considers that some individuals have no desire or motivation to be involved in their own care. Lacey also suggests that some nurses, especially those in nursing homes, are happier for patients to remain dependent upon staff for their care. However, despite this, it is a model that is used worldwide in many different fields of nursing. It has been found suitable for mental health (MacDonald, 1991), theatre (Weir, 1993) and oncology nursing (Richardson, 1992) as well as in the care of the elderly (Kitson, 1986).

The suitability of the model for children's nursing is demonstrated by a study performed by Lasky and Eichelburger in 1985. They studied the health beliefs and behaviour of 75 children aged 4–6 years. They discovered that these children understood health promotion and could relate this to their own behaviour. Some health-related activities were carried out independently by the children, the parents performed some and some were joint child and parent activities. The study also confirmed the parental influence upon health beliefs and attitudes. Although the study was carried out in the USA and not specifically related to Orem's model, it does illustrate the self-care concepts of the model related to the care of young children.

Study activity

Read the case study in Figure 55.2 using Orem's model in practice and identify:

- examples of how the various helping methods are used
- the nursing roles used, with examples
- what knowledge and skills you would need to use this model

Peplau's Interpersonal Relationships Model

Hildegard Peplau was one of the first nurse theorists and she developed her model of nursing primarily for the field of mental health. Peplau believes that nursing is a significant therapeutic interpersonal relationship and is concerned with working in partnership with the individual to make health possible. The concept of stress is fundamental to this model. Peplau considers that all individuals have biological, psychological and social qualities that motivate them to live. When these qualities are impaired tension occurs. This tension can produce a positive reaction by the individual to overcome it and, as a result, to increase personal growth and development. Alternatively, the individual may react in a negative way and be unable to function effectively. At an extreme level this may cause regression. Using this model, the aim of nursing is to alleviate tensions and to help the individual to overcome problems in a positive way, thus increasing self-esteem. According to Peplau, the nurse

Edwin was a 15-year-old with cystic fibrosis. He was admitted to hospital for reassessment of his deteriorating respiratory function and treatment of a chest infection. Although Edwin was very breathless and had a high temperature, he was anxious to remain as independent as possible. On admission he and I made the following plan to meet his needs in hospital.

Universal self-care requisites

Sufficient intake of air	I would monitor his repiratory function 4 hourly. Edwin would perform his own chest physiotherapy.
Sufficient intake of water	Edwin would choose the time, content and amount of his food and meals according to his breathlessness. He would note down all his intake so that I could advise on calorie intake.
Balance of activity and rest, social activity and solitude	Edwin would determine this and put a note on his door when he required privacy. He had his own TV and computer games.
Elimination	Edwin would report any constipation.
Prevention of hazards	Edwin could meet his own needs. I would monitor his temperature 4 hourly.
Promotion of normal lifestyle	Edwin could go out to eat or meet his friends if he told a nurse first.

Developmental self-care requisites

Life cycle stage. As Edwin was an adolescent I needed to be aware of his need to assert his independence and establish his own personality. He wanted to take responsibility for himself and his illness, and I needed to respect that and allow him to make decisions about his care.

Life changes. Edwin was beginning to recognise that his lifespan could be shortened by his condition. He was concerned about his future and his employment/career prospects. He needed help and support to discuss these issues.

Health deviation self-care requisites

Edwin's chest infection required IV antibiotic treament which he was keen to learn how to do for himself. I would teach him how to do this.

Figure 55.2 Orem's model of nursing in practice.

uses six main roles to develop the necessary interpersonal relationship with the individual to be able to help in the resolution of problems. Central to the concepts of this model is the development of the nurse. Peplau believes that the nurse becomes more expert as a result of the knowledge, skills and attitudes gained by the therapeutic relationship with each patient.

Study activity

Consider your nursing experience to date. How do you think that you have developed as a result of your interaction with children you have nursed?

Peplau does not explicitly explore the use of her model for children's nursing but it is easy to make comparisons with the concepts of the model and the beliefs about nursing children. There is much research

Peplau's roles of the nurse

The nurse as a stranger

- accepts and treats the patient as an individual
- initiates the nurse–patient relationship
- orientates the patient to the care setting

The nurse as a surrogate

- helps the patient to become aware of the nurse as an individual
- is self-aware and presents her/himself to the patient
- promotes an interpersonal relationship

The nurse as a resource person

- provides specific answers to questions
- acts as a source of knowledge for improving health
- interprets prescribed care and treatment

The nurse as a teacher

- promotes the patient's interest in learning
- develops innovative teaching to meet individual needs
- uses individual outcomes

The nurse as a counsellor

- helps the patient to understand her/himself
- enables the patient to express feelings
- facilitates patient insight and discovery

The nurse as a leader

- encourages patient participation
- indicates new possibilities
- helps the patient to overcome problems
- develops patient independence

Bethany, aged 10 months, was readmitted to the ward for reassessment of her multiple physical disabilities. Due to problems caused by a rare genetic defect, she had a tracheostomy to help her breathe and was fed via a gastrostomy. She was also profoundly deaf and wore glasses to help her poor eyesight. Her facial features were very abnormal and she was small for her age.

During my assessment of Bethany using Peplau's model I needed to discover whether the physical stress of her disabilities was causing her mental and physical potential to develop or regress. Lisa, Bethany's mother, was resident during this admission, and I needed to find out if the stress of caring for Bethany's many problems was affecting her physically, psychologically and socially.

To achieve all of the above, I needed to get to know Bethany and Lisa (whom I had never met before) and help them both to gain from their situation by using my previous personal and professional experience. As a result of this relationship I would learn more about them as individuals as well as the stress of such situations. As Bethany's nurse, I also needed to:

- provide care in Lisa's absence
- coordinate the specialist services needed for Bethany's reassessment
- identify outside agencies and equipment which could help Lisa
- show Lisa nursing techniques to improve her caring skills
- enable Lisa to express any concerns

Figure 55.3 Peplau's model of nursing in action.

evidence to show that children do regress as a result of physical and psychological stress (Grey, 1993), and the role of the nurse is very concerned with minimising this stress and helping the child to cope with it. The nurse's relationship with the child and family is very crucial to the success of the treatment and most children's nurses would describe this as working in partnership with the parents. Nursing children is about accepting them as they are with their own home routine and it is also concerned with helping them develop and learn about health care. Some of the roles of the nurse described by Peplau may relate more to the nurse's relationship with parents, but they are very appropriate to the care of the older child. The role of surrogate carer has always been suspect when caring for children, as the nurse does not wish to replace the family, but Peplau views this as a temporary role until the patient is able to be independent again.

Study activity

Read the case study (Figure 55.3) of Peplau's model and identify:

- how Peplau's roles of the nurse are used;
- what knowledge and skills you would need to practise this model.

Casey's Partnership Model

Casey also centres her model around the concept of partnership but, because this model was developed for use in paediatrics, it clearly states that this partnership is one between the parents and the healthcare professional. This model maintains that the patient is both the child and family. It recognises that the child is an individual who is growing and developing physically, psychologically, spiritually and socially. It accepts that each family construction may be different and that in each situation the family must include anyone close to the child. It also believes that the role of the children's nurse is to support and strengthen the family's ability to care for their child. Casey's philosophy of children's nursing states categorically that the best people to care for the child are the family, with varying degrees of help from appropriately qualified healthcare professionals. She believes that this model can be applied in any setting where children are nursed.

To apply this model to practice, it is important to assess the child and family as an individual unit. What is the child's usual behaviour and how has the health problem changed it? Who is important to the child and how do they wish to be involved in the child's care? It is also necessary to discover the child's usual family care so that this can be followed as closely as possible. The child's plan of care can then, as far as possible, involve the child's usual carers and routine, while the nurse can work in partnership with the family to assess the child's return to health.

Casey's roles of the nurse

- *To provide family care* – when the child or family are no longer able to provide the care which they would normally carry out independently at home. This may be because the child is too ill or when parents cannot be resident
- *To administer nursing care* – the specific healthcare intervention required by the child
- *To act as a teacher* – by teaching parents to give family care and specific nursing care during their child's illness
- *To provide support* – by helping the family come to terms with their child's illness and treatment and to be available to enable the expression of concerns
- *To be a resource* – by providing specific answers to questions and liaising with other agencies to enable continuing care in the community

Study activity

Read the case study in Figure 55.4, using Casey's model. Identify how the roles of the nurse as described by Casey are used. Consider what knowledge, skills and attitudes are required to practise this model.

The concept of partnership has been the subject of much discussion. The Audit Commission (1993) discovered that many parents were unclear about their role when resident in hospital with their children and felt that their knowledge of their own children was often ignored. In this audit of hospital services for children both parents and children thought that they were not involved in care decisions. Campbell and Glasper (1995) point out that hospitals that provide meals for children but do not cater for resident parents can hardly be said to be enabling partnership. Similarly, many families are now being asked to pay car-parking charges and yet they need to be enabled to be the constant factor in the child's life in hospital, as would be the case at home. Darbyshire (1994) discovered that most children's units have difficulty offering adequate facilities for one parent and do not cater at all for other family members. Other impediments to providing a partnership philosophy of care are staff shortages, skill mix and other healthcare professionals' attitudes (Campbell and Clarke, 1992). Freidson (1970) argues that partnership is impossible if one member of the partnership has more knowledge and power than the other. Nurses practising the partnership model should take care to share their knowledge with the child and family. However, this does not remove the fact that the nurse is in a more powerful position because of this extra knowledge. Other writers suggest that some nurses avoid partnership with children and families as a means of avoiding the stress that such close relationships can bring (Ford and Turner, 2001) (*see also* Family-centred care p. 643).

Toby, aged 5, was admitted to the ward for elective surgery following recurrent severe episodes of vomiting, abdominal pain and diarrhoea. These episodes had been increasing to such a degree that it had now been decided to perform an ileostomy. Sue, Toby's mother, planned to be resident while grandparents looked after the rest of the family. It was decided that I would be Toby's named nurse, and when Toby was admitted I spent some time with him and Sue assessing and planning his care. Sue and Toby had been in hospital many times before and Sue knew that, while she wanted to be involved in Toby's care, she was not very good at it as she was frightened of hurting him. She also knew that since his illness Toby had become very clingy and she was anxious about leaving him.

Sue, Toby and I therefore agreed a plan of care which involved Sue but also gave her time alone for meals and to relax. In the pre-operative period I spent time with Sue and Toby getting to know them and their routines and answering questions about the surgery. During the post-operative period when Toby's nursing needs were at their greatest, I provided his specific nursing care and met his hygiene needs with Sue's help. I cared for the ileostomy until Toby started to mobilise when I helped Sue and Toby to learn how to do this. Each day when I arrived on duty, we would all plan the day so that Toby had either Sue or myself present. In the evenings when Dad visited, I would help them settle Toby for the night and then he was happy for them to go out together knowing I was available if he needed me. At the weekends we organised the day to allow Toby plenty of rest so that he could enjoy his late afternoon visits from his grandparents, siblings and the family dog.

Even when Toby and Sue were able to meet Toby's physical needs without me, I made sure I was available to talk, answer questions or just be there while Sue went for a break.

Figure 55.4 Casey's model in practice.

Study activity

Discuss with some colleagues whether nurses can ever truly work in partnership with all children and their parents. Discuss how you can make children and families feel valued and equal in their relationship with the nurse.

When partnership in care is achieved, its benefit is well documented. Families feel more confident and competent to care for their sick child and thus feel less stressed by the hospital environment. Nurses gain more job satisfaction and nurses and families develop more skills in the care of children (Curley and Wallace, 1992; Hawes, 2005).

Key Points

1. Most UK children's nurses have a philosophy of family-centred care, but this is a concept that is relatively new in other countries.
2. Family-centred care involves the acceptance of individual families' beliefs and values.
3. There are a number of models of nursing which encompass some of the concepts of caring for children but only Casey's partnership model was developed specifically for use in paediatrics.
4. Partnership is a difficult concept to achieve in practice.
5. More research is needed to validate the concepts of nursing models and their appropriateness for children's nursing.

Chapter 56

Family-centred Care

Introduction

Previous chapters have discussed the historical background to involving parents in the care of their sick child and the concept of partnership, as expressed by Casey's partnership model of nursing. Now it seems important to discuss the issues involved in practice when enabling parents to be with their sick children in hospital and to be active participants in their care. This idea of family-centred care, which is the basis of the children's NSF (DH, 2004b), is part of the philosophy of every paediatric unit and children's nursing course curriculum. However, Darbyshire (1995) warns that without careful consideration of the meaning of family-centred care it could become just an academic, abstract notion that is not actually practised.

There are three main principles for achieving family-centred care. First, children are admitted to hospital only if the care they require cannot be as well provided at home, in a day clinic or on a day-care basis in hospital (DH, 2004b). In this way they can be nursed at home mainly by the family with input from community staff and resources as required. Second, the philosophy is clearly explained to all the staff and family so they can understand and negotiate their roles. Finally, the philosophy has to be implemented in such a way as to take account of all the elements of family care.

Care at Home or in Hospital?

The concept of hospital admission only when there is no other suitable option appears to be in the best interests of the child and family. However, is it what parents want? I remember parents of children, referred by their general practitioner to a paediatrician, who have been sent home with medication and advice and who have been clearly unhappy at that decision because they felt unable to cope. All staff working with children need to be aware that not all parents feel able to care for their sick children. This may be because of work commitments, other dependent

Respecting parents and the family as a whole

A respectful partnership with a sick child's parents means recognising that:

- Parents are usually the experts in caring for their children.
- Parents may have other children to care for and will have to balance their needs against the needs of the child in hospital.
- Parents' time is valuable. They may need to take time off work to bring their child to hospital appointments and this may mean losing pay.
- Parents may have their own health or other problems to worry about. This may affect their ability to understand explanations and their ability or readiness to be resident or participate in their child's care.
- Health care can impose material hardship, for instance when a child is a long way from home.

(DH, 2004b)

family members or a lack of appropriate skills and knowledge. Remember, too, that not all parents feel at ease with sickness and simply feel unable to become involved in nursing care, and the children's community service has yet to develop to such a degree that it can offer a service to all sick children being nursed at home (*see also* Community nursing p. 375).

In North America, where community children's teams are not available, care-by-parent units have been developed to overcome this deficit. Cleary *et al.* (1986) argued that such units were surplus to requirements in the UK because of the development of children's community teams. On the contrary, such units may form a useful facility for parents who are frightened of being left alone at home to care for their child.

There is evidence to show that parents are taking on a greater role in the care of their sick children at home. The Audit Commission (1993) found that children now stay in hospital for a significantly reduced amount of time when compared with 30 years previously. In 1962, children's length of stay in hospital was an average of 13 days. In 2004 this had reduced to an average of 2 days, with most children only staying one night in hospital (DH, 2004a). This may not be entirely the result of complying with government guidelines, but could be a natural reduction caused by better treatments – a similar reduction is seen in the length of stay for adults. This reduced length of stay is helped by the expansion of day care for children, but the Children's NSF (DH, 2004b) noted that this facility is variable and could be developed further. Should this facility be developed further? Is it what parents want and are they offered a choice? Does family-centred care include the selection of a child for day surgery by diagnosis rather than by parental preference? The other reason for the reduced admission time is the development of home care, which has been shown to be more cost-effective than care in hospital (Chamberlain *et al.*, 1988). There is a danger that economics could take precedence over the family's wishes about home care and it is important to be clear that the choice is the family's. If care is truly family centred, the discharge from hospital should be when the family is ready and able to take over the care and not when the hospital is short of beds.

In spite of the reduced length of stay in hospital, shortage of paediatric beds remains a problem. Alongside the decreased inpatient stay is a marked increase in the number of children admitted to hospital. Since the 1970s the number of children admitted to hospital has more than doubled (DH, 2004b). This is unique to paediatrics and seems in opposition to the aims of the service to limit hospital admissions. The increase in admissions is matched by rising numbers of children being seen in outpatient and A&E departments. These increases may be due to changes in society as well as changing disease patterns, developments in medicine and GP services. In addition, although the shorter stay in hospital has increased paediatric bed availability, this has only caused a lowering of the criteria for admission and a continued bed shortage (Hill, 1989).

Study activity

Look at the causes of increased admissions of children to hospital and consider which of these may be pertinent to your area of work.

Gould (1996) suggests that family-centred care is more easily facilitated by the community nurse. The nurse is a guest in the child's home, which is a familiar and less threatening environment for the family. The institutional restrictions and regulations usually found in the hospital setting are also not present. However, this may be simplifying family-centred care. Unfortunately, community children's nurses have a caseload and have to prioritise their visits; their chosen time may not coincide with the family's needs. Families may feel that their home and usual routine is being judged or disrupted by the nurse and they may feel further threatened if a student is present. Strong (1997) found that parents of children with mental health problems trusted healthcare professionals but were then disappointed by the actual service available, promised visits that did not occur and cancelled appointments. Telemedicine is the new technology that has the potential to enable sick children to spend more time at home while giving help and support to parents. Guest *et al.* (2005) found that it helped parents to feel more reassured and less isolated, but the costs of their pilot project were met by fund raising. It remains to be seen if the NHS can fund this technology nationwide.

Causes of increased child admissions to hospital

Sociological changes

- increasing public awareness of health services
- geographical isolation of family members
- less experiential knowledge of home care
- increase in hospital births

Alteration of GP services

- increase in GP deputising service
- consultation only by appointment
- closer liaison with hospital services

Changes in disease patterns

- decrease in acute infectious diseases of childhood (Wyke and Hewison, 1991)
- increase in mental health problems in children (HAS, 1995)
- increases in childhood asthma and diabetes (Audit Commission, 1993)

Increased paediatric bed availability (Hill, 1989)

- day care developments
- shorter lengths of stay
- lower criteria for admission

Developments in medicine

- longer lifespan of children with disabilities and chronic illness
- increased survival rate for low birthweight babies but possibly at the cost of increased health problems during infancy and childhood

Communicating with Parents

The Audit Commission (1993) found that the root problem in relation to family-centred care was poor communication between staff and parents. Over half of the families involved in their study reported that their involvement in care was never made explicit and 32% felt that their role was to substitute for staff shortages. Parents in Ygge and Arnetz's study (2004) described their involvement in care as instinctive rather than planned or negotiated. He sensed that many parents felt a moral obligation to care for their children and help the nursing staff.

The Audit Commission (1993) also recognised that nurses play a major role in communicating the concepts of family-centred care. However, for nurses to be able to do this they must have a clear understanding of family-centred care. Evidence suggests that nurses do not have a clear idea of this concept (Callery and Smith, 1991; Gill, 1993; Darbyshire, 1994; Franck and Callery, 2004). Nurses appear to believe that parents have a duty to stay in hospital with their child and carry out the usual parenting care, whereas the more specific nursing care is left to the nurses. There is also the misconception that when parents are actively involved in their child's care that the nurse's role is no longer needed. Indeed, Casey has, in conversation, spoken of the 'dumping' model of nursing, which she says occurs when parents are giving all their child's care and are abandoned by the nurses.

These ideas may occur because nurses believe that their role gives them control over the provision of care in hospital and they are reluctant to release this control (Callery and Smith, 1991). Coyne (1996) believes that to understand the concept fully nurses should be more aware of parents' physical and psychological needs, so that the parents are not put under excessive stress. Darbyshire (1995) suggests that nurses need to appreciate what it means to be a parent of a sick child in hospital before they can begin to work with parents to provide real

Nurses' view about family-centred care

'Kids that are in overnight or two nights, I mean they [the parents] don't make much effort to have contact with us when it's not needed.'

'. . . after they've been in for a week, 2 weeks and things are stable then you start expecting the parents to participate in care.'

'I expect them to take care of the non-nursing duties of the child, like, you know . . . the feeding, changing, bathing and things like that, obviously, cos that's what they would do at home.'

'That's why they're there. I mean it's their child, even though they're in hospital. They would have to feed it at home . . .'

'We seem to expect that they will, if they're going to stay, help with the care . . . that they're not just going to sit there and be bystanders.'

'This woman didn't need our help because the acute stage had passed and she could do all the child's care herself . . . I haven't got a relationship with her at all . . . and that's because she doesn't need us.'

'I mean the normal things that they would do at home . . . the mothering-type things like washing and bathing and feeding . . . nothing medical like giving medicines or anything like that.'

'The longer that they're [the parents] in then the more you're able to . . . get a more relaxed relationship . . . a more friendly relationship with the person, you know, you get to know them and their family involvement.'

'I think that as they become more familiar with the nurses and . . . become part of the ward . . . I think that the rapport gets better.'

(Darbyshire, 1994)

'. . . tactfully encouraged her to try and get some rest, told her there was adequate staff to look after her son whilst in hospital and reassured her we were happy to care for him and did not think badly of her for going.'

'. . . talked to parents, constantly reassuring and encouraging them to try and carry out his care as they would at home.'

'. . . explained the importance and significance of the mother's continued involvement in the child's care . . .'

(Callery and Smith, 1991)

Family-centred care?

The principles of family-centred care

- parents cannot be partners in care because they do not have my specialist knowledge and skills and I am accountable for their child's care in hospital
- parents must be informed of what nurses are doing for their child but the final decision rests with the nurse
- each parent has the right to be involved in the nursing care to the extent of their or their child's wishes
- all parents must be given full information and their wishes must be met at all times

The principles in practice

- how much information are parents given on first contact, during any care given to the child and before discharge? What are parents not told? How is handover managed?
- can parents see their child's care plan? Is anything written about the child that parents cannot see? Do other members of the family have access to the care plan?
- how many choices does the parent have during their child's stay in hospital? In which areas do they not have a choice?
- if the care plans disappeared would it make any difference to the care given to that child? (i.e. how much of the care is routine and how much has developed from negotiation with the parents?)

(Adapted from Teasdale, 1987)

Module 7

family-centred care. He describes family-centred care as a valuable and meaningful connection with parents based upon genuine mutual respect.

Study activity

Discuss the concept of family-centred care with some children's nursing colleagues and parents of children in hospital. Compare their responses with those found in previous studies.

Another strategy for considering the meaning of family-centred care is for nurses to take a critical look at their own understanding of its principles and how they apply these to their practice (Teasdale, 1987).

When considering the principles of family-centred care, the nurse must not presume to be the expert in care or to make accountability the basis for the assumption that parents give up all responsibility for their child because they are in hospital. Teasdale (1987) considers that nurses permit involvement until it poses a problem and then they assert control. Equality should allow the nurse to give advice and should only prevent families' wishes when such choices would impair the care of other children and families. The parent is not always right but nor is the nurse, but parents do have the right to choose their level of involvement in care. The difficulty arises when their choice is not the choice of their child, which raises questions about responsible decision making.

Law *et al.* (2005) suggest that information should be given to parents, service providers and healthcare students to explain the main elements of family-centred care. Leaflets have been developed at many centres to provide families with this information but they are mostly designed and written by professionals (Glasper and Burge, 1992). Campbell *et al.* (1993) propose that families should be producing such advice. Now there is much more recognition of the need to use the views of children and families in health care, this should be a natural development. However, it is important to bear in mind that children's views do not always match those of their parents (Battrick and Glasper, 2004).

Study activity

Design a leaflet to explain family-centred care to parents and then discuss its suitability with some parents and children on the ward.

Parents' and nurses' misunderstandings of family-centred care may be overcome by improved nurse education, which emphasises not only communication and negotiation skills but family dynamics and psychology (Coyne, 1996). However, this may not help them to appreciate fully the role of the parent and the feelings of guilt, inadequacy, uncertainty, loneliness and anxiety that parents experience when their children are in hospital. One of the mothers in Darbyshire's study expressed this succinctly by saying, 'It's not like being a parent is it? . . . You're like a different parent' (Darbyshire, 1994). Nurses, therefore, have to be able to appreciate that parents in hospital can no longer perform as usual; all their intuitive parenting skills have been lost because of a range of emotions resulting from their child's hospitalisation. They need the nurses' help to overcome these feelings before they can return to normal functioning.

Study activity

Try to find the opportunity to discuss this altered role of parents with a child in hospital with a friend or relation who also has had the experience of being a parent with a child in hospital.

Implementation of Family-centred Care

Campbell *et al.* (1993) are among many authors who have attempted to define the elements of family-centred care. All these writers agree that the successful implementation of family-centred care involves not only the nursing staff but the entire healthcare system. The Children's NSF recognises that the implementation of effective policies of child and family-centred care requires a major change in attitudes on the part of managers, doctors, nurses and other staff involved in running the service. Baum *et al.* (1990) suggest that effective policies can only be achieved when parents are seen as essential and equal members of policy-making groups. These policies would also need to take into account the needs of different cultures but it is also important not to create cultural differences where none exist (Shah, 1994). Individualised care should cater for the individual and recognise any different needs regardless of ethnic background.

Fradd (1996) considers negotiated care plans to be essential for successful family-centred care and believes that families who have been given unbiased and complete information about their child's care are more likely to feel valued and supported. Negotiation is an interactive process and involves the sharing of ideas, which helps the nurse to appreciate families' beliefs and values as well as their ways of coping with the stress of having a child in hospital. In this way, the nurse is in a better position to offer appropriate support and to enable parents to provide support for their child in a way which best suits them. The negotiated care must be clearly expressed in the care plan to enable other nurses and members of the multidisciplinary team to continue care when the named nurse is not available. The Audit Commission (1993) recognises this communication of parents' wishes as an important part of the nurse's role in informing and changing others' attitudes to family-centred care.

Support for families often includes the care of the sick child's siblings. Siblings are often ignored in the caring process even though their emotional needs are similar to those of their parents (Walker, 1990). Most children's wards struggle to provide adequate facilities for parents and few are able to cater for siblings.

The elements of family-centred care

- Appreciation of the family as a constant factor within the child's life as opposed to the variation of health services and professionals with whom they come into contact
- Helping the liaison between parents and healthcare professionals to occur at all levels within the multidisciplinary team
- Imparting information to parents completely and openly
- Production and implementation of policies and procedures which ensure holistic care for the family as a whole
- Recognising families' individual reactions to, and methods of coping with, illness and hospitalisation
- Providing appropriate strategies to meet the developmental needs of siblings
- Enabling and empowering the parent–child relationship
- Designing healthcare facilities that are appropriate and accessible for families

(Campbell *et al.*, 1993)

Study activity

Explore the facilities for siblings in your hospital on the children's ward(s) and any other area where children are nursed. Talk to some resident parents to discover what facilities they would find useful for their other children.

Even if children are not being cared for as inpatients, the families' needs are often not met. Historically, health service facilities for outpatients have always been provided on a 9–5, Monday–Friday basis. This is never a good time for families; parents may have to take time away from work, children may miss school and younger siblings may need alternative care arrangements. Evening and weekend clinics may offer a more appropriate service.

Parental comments about family-centred care

'The only time we saw a nurse was in the morning to make the beds and take the temperatures. If the children who hadn't their mothers there wanted anything, one of the other mothers had to get it for them.'

(Callery and Smith, 1991)

'. . . I am not sure of their [the staff] attitude . . . they let me do it so that they don't have to do it . . .'

(Audit Commission, 1993)

'I dare say it takes a strain away from them [nurses] and they can spend more time with another child.'

'I find I'm feeding her, changing her, putting her down, sitting her up . . . all the time, and they're short-staffed sometimes . . . can't get a nurse to help you cos they're run off their feet.'

(Darbyshire, 1995)

'. . . they tend to expect you to stay. So it was just assumed that I would want to stay.'

'The mums told me where to find things – more help to me than any nurse . . . but they're very busy . . .'

'They want you to stay and it makes life easier if you do stay, because it's better for the nursing staff . . . but they don't encourage you to stay because you're not felt welcome or comfortable.'

'It helps me a lot when the staff sorta say do you want to do it? . . . and actually standing there watching me not going away and saying get on with it . . .'

'If I didn't want to do the care, then they would be there to do the care . . . I'm sorta sharing it with them . . .'

(Coyne, 1996)

'You know they didn't say, Right, change his nappy, and if at any time I don't want to, I can just say, No, I don't want to . . . it's a wee bit of give and take.'

'They [the nurses] were always friendly, but it's grown into a relationship now . . . that's my view anyway . . . they really have become friends . . . when I was at home I missed them.'

'. . . its not a nurse–patient or a nurse–parent [relationship] . . . you know, it seems to develop into us, I mean you can talk as if it's someone you've known for ages.'

'Some of these nurses, they just click. I don't feel I'm just here and no-one cares about me – I feel I'm part of the whole set-up.'

(Darbyshire, 1994)

Study activity

Explore how services in your own hospital meet family-friendly hours. Talk to colleagues to find out the support and the obstacles to introducing 'out-of-hours' services.

In conclusion, nurses need to have the support of management to be able to implement effective family-centred care. The Children's NSF (DH, 2004b) recommends that every hospital should have a specific management focus for children's services with appropriate managerial and financial support. Standards for family-centred care should be approved and monitored to ensure quality is maintained, and children, young people and parents should be routinely involved in the planning and improvement of services.

Key Points

1. Effective family-centred care involves the careful consideration of the criteria for the hospitalisation of children, improved communication between nurses and parents and the strategic implementation of all elements of family involvement.
2. Parents may not be given sufficient choice about day care or admission to hospital.
3. Despite changes in children's length of stay in hospital there has been an increase in the number of children admitted.
4. A major reason for the lack of family-centred care is the lack of communication between nurses and parents, mainly due to nurses' misunderstandings about the concept.
5. Parents have problems in functioning as normal parents because of the emotions involved in having a sick child in hospital.
6. Family-centred care relies upon a specific management focus for children's services.

Chapter 57

The Nurse as a Developing Professional

Introduction

Peplau (1952) believed that nurses continue to develop personally and professionally through encounters with different patients. This important aspect of the role of the nurse has only relatively recently been appreciated. Benner (1984) recognised that nurses gained their competence and intuitive grasp of situations from previous experience and she advocated the use of reflective practice to identify this learning in an explicit way. She believed that, while nurses continued to explain their actions as intuitive, the knowledge base for nursing would not expand and develop. Reflective practice is not an easy process as it may discomfort and challenge the reflector. Clinical supervision has developed as a means of guiding and supporting practitioners through the reflective process. The concept of exploring experiences to consider the thoughts, feelings and actions of those involved in the experience has been recognised by the UKCC as a useful way of providing evidence of continuing professional development (*see also* Guidelines for reflection p. 653).

In 1990 the UKCC recognised the importance of nurses being able to demonstrate the maintenance and development of their professional knowledge and competence and suggested that evidence of such progression was mandatory to maintain registration for practice. This reform was finally agreed and came into force in 1995. One of the post-registration and education (PREP) requirements is to maintain a comprehensive account of all learning and development in a personal profile. These PREP requirements were formal recognition of the need for lifelong learning. The idea of lifelong learning has developed in the UK as a result of changes in society. In the late 1980s the consequences of demographic changes became apparent. It was realised that the number of young people entering the job market between 1989 and 2011 would decrease by over 2 million. To counteract this there was a need for all employers to increase opportunities for mature employees. One way of doing this was to provide opportunities for training throughout an employee's working life and to recognise the value of experience. The UK also needed to be able to respond effectively to increased international competition and technological change by developing the skills of innovation, responsiveness and adaptability of its workforce. All employers have had to recognise the need to have a workforce capable of adaptation to the constantly changing social environment. The English National Board (1994) described lifelong learning as a process that helps nurses to be:

- innovative
- responsive to changing demands
- resourceful
- change agents
- adaptable
- challenging
- self-reliant
- able to share good practice

(*see also* PREP requirements p. 654).

Reflective Practice

Deliberate learning takes place in the formal college setting but a large proportion of learning takes place away from educational institutions.

Study activity

Consider all the activities you have done since getting out of bed this morning. Think about how you learnt to do these activities.

You will immediately realise that much of your learning has come from experience. For instance, how many of you, as children, made your first cup of tea without first boiling the water? Since then you have quickly learned through experience not only how to make a cup of tea but how to make it exactly as you like it. In the same way you will have learned through personal and professional experiences how to provide care in different situations. As a student, my class had to practise bed-bathing on each other. I still remember the embarrassment of that experience and how it felt not to be completely dried. This was a valuable learning experience that has affected the way in which I practise. I have learned so much from the many children and their families for whom I have cared, but one outstanding event was that of an abandoned child. This made me realise the importance of security for children, a need that even takes precedence over physiological needs. Later, the death of my father and my attempts to support my brother through his grieving highlighted the importance of making it clear to families that it is 'permissible' to share emotions.

The idea that reflection can enhance learning from experience is not new. Coutts-Jarman (1993) states that it was mentioned by Aristotle in his work on judgement and moral action. In the 1930s Dewey discussed reflective thought as a means of reconsidering experiences and linking theory to practice (Dewey, 1933). Although it may be argued that reflection is a subconscious activity, Boud *et al.* (1985) consider that it

Table 57.1 Traditional versus reflective practice

Traditional	Reflective
Importance of routine	Improvisation
Based on ritual	Research-based
Questioning discouraged	Spirit of enquiry
Didactic teaching	Experiential teaching
Displays of emotions discouraged	Feelings shared and explored
Skills explained by intuition	Knowledge-based skills

must become a more formal activity for learning to occur, and that there is a difference between thoughtful practice and reflective practice. Thinking about an incident does not usually involve the depth of exploration required to learn from the experience.

Historically, nurses were not expected to question practice or share their emotions, and nursing was associated with routine, authority and tradition (Table 57.1). Dewey (1933) describes this as practice that takes the everyday realities for granted. Reflection enables practitioners to question these realities and their reactions to them, 'to think on their feet, improvise, and respond to the uncharted and unpredictable' (Fish and Twinn, 1997). The aim of Project 2000 was to produce nurses who were enquiring, independent, critically self-aware and creative; 'knowledgeable doers' (United Kingdom Central Council, 1986). It would appear that reflection is the ideal tool to help to meet this aim and many universities now use reflection as part of their strategy for the assessment of practice. Johns (1996) believes that reflection in practice helps nurses to concentrate on the caring aspect of nursing and advocates the use of a reflective model of nursing.

Study activity

Assess a child and family using the adapted form of Johns' (1994) reflective model of nursing. Consider how the use of this model would affect the care of this child and family in comparison with the model you usually use.

It has been argued that reflection has become merely a rhetoric and that there are no accounts to demonstrate its benefit to patients (Newell, 1992). However, there are accounts of its beneficial effects upon child-care practice (Wooton, 1997), and Dearmun (1997) argued that this alone should be sufficient rationale for its continuation. Practice that is constantly under critical review is more likely to attract purchasers of health care than practice based on ritual and tradition.

Clinical Supervision

No one has ever suggested that reflection is easy. It is a process that requires self-examination of attitudes and behaviour, which may cause feelings of inadequacy and discomfort. Bond and Holland (1997)

Qualities required for reflection

- Having an open mind
- Being responsible
- Objectivity
- Ability to assess oneself
- Willingness to explore emotions
- Adaptability to change

A reflective model of nursing

Core question

- what information do I need to nurse this child and family?

Cue questions

- who is this child and family?
- what health event brings this child into hospital or care environment?
- how is this child and family feeling?
- how has this event affected this child and family's usual life patterns and roles?
- how can I help this child and family?
- what is important for this child and family to make the care environment comfortable?
- what support does this child and family have in life?
- how does this child and family view their personal future?

(Adapted from Johns, 1994)

Qualities of the clinical supervisor

The clinical supervisor should be able to:

- challenge thinking
- offer higher levels of skills and knowledge than those supervised
- provide a secure environment in which to share confidences
- offer constructive feedback
- motivate individuals to take responsibility for their own development
- assist with critical reflection
- raise clinical confidence and competence
- be supportive

suggest that practitioners, managers and educationalists can assist each other to learn in practice. Clinical supervision is one way of providing the time and opportunity for reflection and supporting and developing staff to provide a high standard of practice. Clinical supervision can also provide part of a package of staff development and support. It can be carried out on a one-to-one basis, usually with the line manager, or within a group. It has three main functions: to educate, support and manage. The educative or formative function involves the development of skills, knowledge and attitudes by helping the individual to reflect upon a clinical experience. Provision of support is required to help the individual accept the experience and learn from it, instead of becoming overwhelmed by negative emotions – the restorative function. The managerial or normative function, which acts as a quality control, enables the participants to review nursing policy or procedure in relation to the experience and plan for appropriate change (Butterworth and Faugier, 1992).

Study activity

Discover how clinical supervision is carried out in your area of practice. How do the participants feel about the process?

Clinical supervision should not feel threatening or become simply a managerial monitoring of progress. It should not become a forum for the discussion of general issues and non-specific complaints. It relies upon clear boundaries to ensure that participants feel valued and supported in their professional development. Webb *et al.* (2002) suggest that effective support systems are essential to prevent stress levels from becoming overwhelming. Clinical supervision and the work arising from it can be used towards meeting the PREP requirements for maintaining registration.

Maintenance of Registration

The basic requirements of PREP must be met for maintenance of registration. They include the need to undertake a minimum period of study equivalent to 5 days (35 hours) every 3 years. This study can include:

- attendance at lectures, courses, seminars, workshops
- distance learning, including the educational supplements in professional journals
- visits to other areas of practice
- personal study or research, including reflection of critical incidents

Any of the above mean little unless the practitioner can identify the objectives and outcome of the study. The UKCC firmly placed the responsibility of choosing appropriate study onto each individual nurse but Bagnall and Garbett (1996) criticise them for not being more specific about how the equivalent of 5 days' study may be calculated. However, by giving individuals the responsibility for their own development the UKCC can renounce any commitment for funding continuing education. There has probably been more discussion about the funding of the study requirements than any other aspect of PREP and the NMC have not changed these requirements for reregistration. It could be argued that compulsory study should be locally or nationally funded, especially as it aims to improve and develop practice. Alternatively, perhaps taking responsibility for self-development should include meeting the costs. Whatever the answer, it is clear that, at present, financial help available to nurses for study depends upon their employer and can vary tremendously.

Study activity

Find out what study leave and financial help is available to you in your current employment. How does this compare with that available to colleagues working in other healthcare areas (such as education or the private sector)? Also find out how it compares to employment outside health care.

The amount of continuing education available also seems to be unfairly distributed. Bagnall and Garbett (1996) believe that the provision for this is biased towards acute hospital trusts and that staff working in community areas have fewer opportunities and less access to further their education. It is clear from the categories of study (Table 57.2) suggested by the United Kingdom Central Council (1994a, b) that there are many ways of developing practice and meeting the requirements, which need not bear a financial burden. It would appear from this that staff need to be more innovative about their study and could be helped to explore such options by a preceptor.

Developing a Portfolio

The standards for maintaining an effective registration include the maintenance of a personal profile or portfolio to demonstrate the maintenance and development of knowledge. Apart from being necessary to reregister, profiling is a useful exercise as it:

- encourages you to reflect on all your past educational and practice experience
- clarifies those areas that you want to develop
- enables you to make comprehensive future plans
- provides you with an up-to-date record of achievements
- helps the discussion of achievements and developmental needs with current and future employers
- may help you to gain accreditation for further study

Study activity

Consider a recent achievement of which you are particularly proud. What did you learn from this experience and how can you provide evidence of this learning?

Developing your portfolio

Factual information

- personal/biographical information
- professional/academic qualifications
- positions held
- other activities/positions outside nursing
- record of your working hours

Self-appraisal of professional performance

- strengths and weaknesses
- achievements
- analysis of critical incidents
- areas of development

Personal aims and action plans

- goals for development
- action plans for achieving goals
- review of action plans
- outcomes from action plans

Record of formal learning*

- study days/seminars/courses/conferences attended
- visits to other areas
- time spent on other study (e.g. literature searching)

*Each entry in this category should discuss the relevance to your area of practice, your objectives, the outcomes of the activity and how it has contributed to the development of your practice

Table 57.2 PREP categories of study applied to children's nursing

Categories of study (UKCC, 1994a, b)	Examples of application
Reducing risk	
Identification of health problems	Noticing incorrect infant feeding
Protection of individuals	Teaching food hygiene to parents
Raising awareness of health risks	'Safety in the sun' poster for children
Health screening	Introducing BP check for all ages
Health promotion	
Care enhancement	
Developments in clinical practice	New treatment regimes
New techniques	Change of role
Innovative approaches to care	Introducing primary nursing
Standard setting	Writing standards of care for parents
Empowering consumers	Involving parents in policy writing
Patient, client and colleague support	
Counselling techniques	Care of bereaved siblings
Leadership in practice	Setting up a paediatric research group
Clinical supervision	Peer review of critical incidents
Practice development	
External/exchange visits	Visit to children's hospice
Personal study/research	Literature review – HIV in children
Clinical audit	Audit hospital safety for children
Changes in policy and procedure	Parental presence at resuscitation
Education development	
Teaching and learning skills	Teaching package for students
Educational audit	Audit of learning environment

Sometimes providing evidence of learning can seem difficult. However, attendance at a study day or involvement in a new activity does not necessarily mean that learning has taken place. You need to be able to consider ways of demonstrating your learning if you wish to include the activity in your portfolio to show your practice development. Thinking about providing evidence of learning will become more important with the knowledge and skills framework for annual performance reviews introduced by 'Agenda for Change'.

When the United Kingdom Central Council (1994a, b) introduced PREP it emphasised that the profile was personal property. It will undertake random audits of profiles but employers cannot demand to see them. If profiles are used as part of performance reviews, it is suggested that areas of the profile outside PREP requirements are kept separately (United Kingdom Central Council, 1996).

Preceptorship

Post-registration and education is not just about maintaining registration, although it may be argued that this area has the biggest impact for most nurses. It also introduced the idea of preceptorship. A period of support is recommended for newly registered nurses or those returning to practice after a break of 5 years or more. Benner (1984) describes newly registered nurses as advanced beginners who have yet to gain the experience to enable them to link theory and practice to actual clinical situations. Although Johnson (1996) disputes this, he does not take into account the feelings of uselessness and loss of confidence caused by the change in role that registration brings. This state of confusion is aptly described by Robinson (1996) in her reflection of her first 6 months as a newly registered nurse. Reading this account, one wonders if a preceptor would have eased this transition from student to staff nurse. Maben and Macleod Clark (1996) found that Robinson's experiences were common and that few nurses received a comprehensive programme of support during their first post as a registered nurse. A 2004 report into the careers of child branch diplomates showed that only 63% of newly qualified nurses had received preceptorship in the first 6 months after qualification and dissatisafction with preceptorship was ranked as the most important reason for leaving or considering leaving (Kings College Nursing Research Unit, 2004).

Study activity

Find out what support is available to newly registered children's nurses in your current area of work. Consider what support you would find most helpful.

Preceptors should be first-level registered nurses or midwives who have a minimum of 12 months' post-registration experience within the same or associated area of practice. The preceptor should:

- have sufficient knowledge of the preceptee's programme leading to registration (or return to nursing course) to be able to identify current learning needs
- help the preceptee to orientate to the new area of practice
- be able to help the preceptee apply theory to practice
- understand the potential problems associated with the transition from student to registered practitioner and assist the preceptee to overcome these
- act as a resource to facilitate professional development

The idea of support is not as simple as having a committed preceptor. The newly registered nurse also needs a supportive environment that provides approachable, forward-thinking, up-to-date staff, a good team spirit, trust, responsibility, feedback on progress and teaching. In addition, preceptors need preparation and support from the organisation to enable them to undertake this important role.

Levels of Nursing Practice

The PREP policy also includes standards for programmes of specialist preparation beyond initial registration. These standards are based on developing nurses beyond the fundamental knowledge, skills and attitudes gained in pre-registration programmes. The UKCC believed that after an initial period of practice with support following registration that specialist healthcare practice requires practitioners to have additional preparation to enable them to demonstrate higher levels of clinical judgement to:

Demonstrating learning – an example

Sally is a staff nurse on the paediatric intensive care unit. She recently went out with the retrieval team to collect a child from a district general hospital. She feels the transfer went well and wants to record her learning from this event in her portfolio. Maintaining confidentiality by the use of pseudonyms, she records:

- details of the child's condition and reason for transfer
- questions she asked the local nursing team
- actions she took before and during the journey to stabilise the child
- written summary of the child's nursing notes during transfer, dated and signed
- points she raised at handover on return to base
- feedback of her performance from the anaesthetist and receiving nurse
- account of her feelings during the incident, an analysis of what she learnt from it and actions for future practice

- monitor and improve standards of care
- undertake nursing audit
- develop and lead practice
- contribute to clinical research
- teach and support colleagues

Three levels of post-registration practice are identified. Primary practice meets the basic requirements of PREP and it is envisaged that most nurses will practice at this level. Specialist practice involves an additional post-registration specialist practitioner recordable qualification at degree level. Specialist qualifications are available for community and hospital nurses and include specific qualifications for children's nurses.

Study activity

Consider your future career plans and find out what specialist programmes are available to help you reach your goals after your period of primary practice.

Advanced practice is recommended for those who are specialist nurses and act as resources for others. This role, which requires a further recordable qualification, is envisaged as one in which the practitioner leads clinical practice either at local or national level. It is a clinically based post, which has direct accountability for practice. The PREP document suggests that these advanced practitioner posts are developed as consultant practitioner posts (United Kingdom Central Council, 1994a, b) (see Figure 57.1). Coyne (1997) suggests that experienced specialist nurses, who otherwise may reach the criteria for such a post, need to

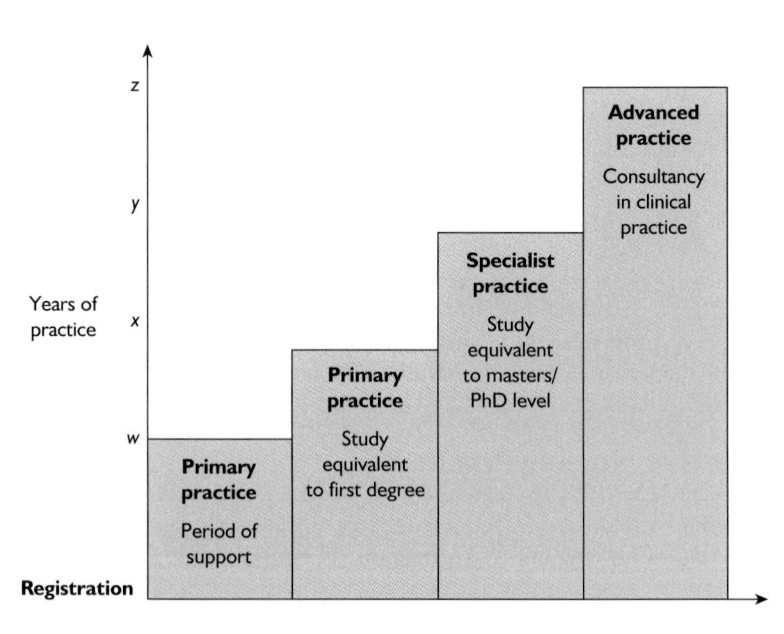

Figure 57.1 UKCC continuum of practice.

develop their marketing skills before being able to act as nurse consultants. He also points out that current pay scales for clinical posts do not provide appropriate remuneration for the complexity of advanced practice. However, the development of consultancy posts would finally give clinical nurses a chance to progress without having to move away from patient care. In particular, it would give children's nurses the credibility to influence the development of children's healthcare services, as recommended by the Audit Commission in 1993.

Key Points

1. Peplau (1952) and Benner (1984) believed that nurses' knowledge, attitudes and skills developed through their experiences with different patients and that this enabled them to practise at a higher level.
2. The NMC recognises the need for practising registered nurses to demonstrate this development of knowledge and skills.
3. Reflective practice is one way in which nurses can learn from their experiences and add to nursing knowledge.
4. Clinical supervision can educate, support and manage nurses' experiential learning.
5. Maintaining a profile can be a systematic way of recording professional development.
6. Preceptorship can support the newly registered nurse to gain confidence and ability in a new role.

Chapter 58

Children's Nursing in a Multicultural Society

Introduction

Effective nursing care of children and their families in any setting depends on an appreciation of that family's beliefs and values. In the UK there is an increasing diversity of cultures and there are many differences between the values and beliefs of the average British citizen and those of the minority groups. In 2004 over 3 million people (5.5% of the population) in Britain were from black or minority ethnic groups (Watt and Norton, 2004). The UK today is more culturally diverse than ever before, with 45% of non-white people living in London (Office of National Statistics, 2006). Children under 15 years of age comprise 33% of black and ethnic minority communities whereas only 19% of white communities are children (Watt and Norton, 2004). Some of the marked differences among different racial and ethnic groups are related to the attitudes and practices surrounding birth, pain and death and their specific susceptibility to certain diseases.

Generally, healthcare professionals in the UK and other Western countries have been taught according to the beliefs and values of a white, middle-class society, and only in recent years has transcultural education begun to identify that minority groups do not share these beliefs and values. Denial of these differences can create conflict and prevent children's nurses from working in a true partnership with children and families. Children's nurses need to accept that different health concepts and behaviour to their own are not necessarily better or worse – just different.

When discussing the needs of children and families with different concepts of health and related areas, it is important to appreciate the meanings of the terms used to identify why individuals from different backgrounds develop different attitudes and practices. 'Culture' is defined as the unique way of life a group of people has developed in specific physical and social circumstances, which acts as a frame of reference for their particular values and beliefs. The lifestyles of most cultures are influenced by religion, a particular system of faith and worship. Ethnicity refers to a specific group of people, usually a minority, who share the same cultural, linguistic or racial background. Race is described as a distinct group of people connected by common descent and identifiable by certain common characteristics such as colour. Individuals' values and beliefs are also influenced by the way in which they 'socialised' and learned the accepted behaviours of their cultural group as children.

The Children Act 2004 states that help provided for the child and family should be appropriate to race, culture, religion and language, and that regard should be paid to the different racial groups to which children and families belong. In addition, the NMC code of professional conduct (Nursing and Midwifery Council, 2004a) advises nurses that they 'must promote and protect the interests and dignity of patients and clients irrespective of their gender, age, race, ability, sexuality, economic status, lifestyle, culture and religious or political beliefs'. There is no doubt that healthcare professionals have a duty to provide care which takes into account the child and family's specific cultural needs, but Shah (1994) warns that cultural awareness training can sometimes reinforce stereotyping and racism. Nurses need to remember that all their patients are individuals regardless of race, ethnicity or culture.

Culture, race and ethnicity

Culture

- Learned from birth through the process of acquiring language and learning to socialise. The individual therefore fits into the social group's way of life.
- Shared by all members of the same cultural group.
- An adaptation to specific activities related to environmental factors.
- A dynamic, ever-changing process that determines the pattern by which individuals take on roles and responsibilities within the family, friendships and work.

(Andrews and Boyle, 1995)

Race

- Applies to biological features, such as skin colour, bone structure, hair type, which characterise a particular racial group.
- A contentious term in the light of genetic knowledge about biological variations.
- A social and political construct.
- Can be used to characterise specific health and disease problems in certain racial groups, such as thalassaemia among Greek and Cypriot populations.

(Watt and Norton, 2004)

Ethnicity

- A concept that refers to cultural practices and attitudes that are unique to a given group of people such as language, religion, ancestry.
- A system of shared attitudes, practices, values, and so forth, which members of different groups hold about themselves.

(Baxter, 1997)

Race and Ethnicity

Race and ethnicity cause specific differences in physical characteristics, predisposition towards certain disorders and susceptibility to disease. David (1990) found that Asian and black neonates are significantly smaller than white newborns. These findings had not changed in the 2001 census (Office of National Statistics, 2006). Black babies seem to overcome this difference quickly to become taller and heavier between the ages of 5 and 14 years than their white comparisons. Oriental children, however, are smaller throughout childhood. It is because of these differences that attention is now being given to the growth charts used to identify children who are outside the normal growth limits. These charts were first compiled in the 1960s, and revised in 1993 to take account of the increased height and weight of people in the UK since the publication of the first charts. However, they still do not take into account the multicultural variation in growth now seen in the UK (Fry, 1993).

Different racial and ethnic groups have a specific predisposition to certain disorders. Cystic fibrosis is one of the most common inherited disorders in white people but is rare in black and Oriental families (Dodge *et al.*, 1993). Tay–Sachs disease occurs mainly in Jewish children and sickle-cell disease is only seen in black Africans.

Race and ethnicity also affect the resistance to disease. Migrant families usually suffer more illness than the indigenous population. The first major immigrant mortality study in England and Wales was published in 1984 (Marmot *et al.*, 1984). Mortality rates vary according to the country of origin but all immigrants showed a higher mortality rate than the average for England and Wales for tuberculosis and accidents. They all had a lower than average mortality rate for chronic chest diseases. These inequalities have remained largely unchanged, as does the high

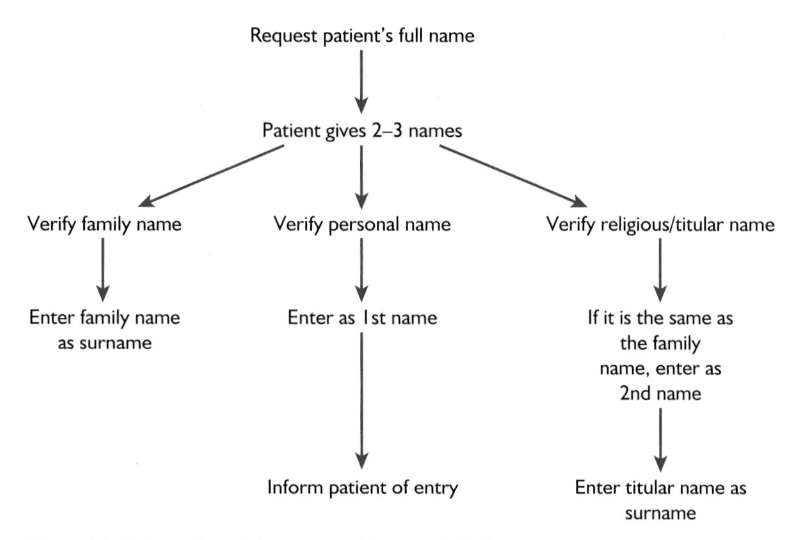

Figure 58.1 Recording Asian names (Mootoo, 2005).

mortality rate for babies of mothers born in Pakistan. It is difficult to know how much this is due to different immune factors or availability of health services.

Health care in the UK is mainly directed towards the needs of the white middle-class population (Whitehead, 1992). Immigrant families, particularly those who have just settled in this country, may lack the ability to access the appropriate services. In addition, their health beliefs and traditions do not tend to consider preventive health measures; instead they seek help only at the time of illness. Nurses have a responsibility to help them appreciate the value of preventive health care in a way that relates to their culture (Figure 58.1).

Beliefs and values

- What are your beliefs and values?
- What are your beliefs about death?
- What are your religious views? How important are they for you?
- Do you feel comfortable talking about religion and death?
- How would you describe your own culture?
- Do you think that health and illness is determined by fate, one's own behaviour or some other cause?
- What behaviour in others really upsets you? How do you react if you meet this behaviour?
- Do you believe that touch is important? Do you ever feel uneasy if a child or family gets too close to you (in a non-threatening manner)?
- How do you feel if others disagree with your beliefs and values?

Health Beliefs and Practices (Table 58.1)

Individuality is mostly determined by culture. Culture influences most of the way in which people live; their diet, their language, their mode of dress, their beliefs and values, and the accepted mode of behaviour for their cultural group. Variations in the growth and development of children are thought to be largely due to cultural factors.

Study activity

Consider your own beliefs and values (using the questions in the box), and think carefully about how these developed.

As well as family influences, subcultural influences such as ethnicity, religion, peer groups, social class and schooling can all affect the way in which children learn to socialise and the way they view health and illness. Nurses need to be aware of their own views and the reasons why these developed before they can truly appreciate others' beliefs.

The assessment of cultural beliefs is an important part of the nursing assessment process because compliance with treatment is influenced by the effect that treatment may have upon roles and lifestyles.

Different cultures have different views about health and the causation of illness. They differ in their beliefs about how much control individuals have over their health. Western cultures tend to believe that certain behaviours, such as overwork, stress, lack of exercise or sleep, are causes of illness. Other cultures believe that supernatural forces, 'the will of God' or fate cause disease and that health can only be restored by the same influence. These cultures may rely on wearing amulets or other religious symbols to protect them from disease. Asian, Oriental and Arab cultures believe that illness is caused by an imbalance of hot and cold forces. Health is regained by restoring the balance. For example, respiratory infections are thought to be caused by cold forces and must be treated by food or drugs considered to be 'hot'. For this reason children of these cultures who may have a pyrexia due to a respiratory infection will be overdressed to balance the cold force that caused the problem.

Beliefs about the cause of illness may also lead parents to try alternative medicine or homoeopathy. Provided these do no harm to the child they should be used in conjunction with conventional medicine. Complementary therapies can often reduce the pain and anxiety associated with illness and thus induce a feeling of well-being. Until more research becomes available about the use and efficacy of such therapies, it is worth considering their potential (*see also* Religious, cultural beliefs and diet p. 179).

Communication

Communication skills are important in nursing and usually have a prominent part in any nurse education programme but the skills taught are usually related to the Western culture. Apart from the different language used by many other cultures, Western communication 'rules' may have quite different interpretations for these people.

Communication with families who do not speak English is best carried out by a nurse who speaks their language. When this is not possible an interpreter should be used, ideally from within the family. Even this strategy has its drawbacks. If the interpreter is not familiar with medical terminology, or if there is no corresponding word in their language, confusion or misunderstanding may occur. The family may find it difficult and embarrassing to explore personal issues with an interpreter outside the family group. The nurse may find it difficult to know if the interpreter is relaying the exact information required. I have vivid memories of a crying baby clinic where the doctor was seeing a Turkish mother. The mother was obviously distraught by her baby who cried for about 20 hours a day. The doctor recognised and empathised with the mother's distress and showed great understanding of the mother's situation, wanting to admit the baby to give the mother some respite. However, the husband clearly believed that the mother should cope with the baby and it was difficult to know how much the male Turkish interpreter was able or willing to transmit the feelings of empathy from the doctor to the mother.

Table 58.1 Cultural and religious influences for nursing practice

Culture	Childbirth	Diet	General care	Death and dying
Buddhism	An astrologer provides the initial letter of the child's name and date of birth Birth control and abortion are condemned	Fasting days occur on religious days No alcohol Most are vegetarians	Analgesia or sedation may be refused as it may affect the ability to mediate	The dying patient should be visited by a Buddhist monk Cremation preferred
Christian Science	Contraceptive pill not generally used Abortion permitted only in life-threatening situations	No alcohol or tobacco	Surgery, prostheses and drugs may be refused Prayer is used for healing Not acceptable to donate or receive organs	Another Christian Scientist is usually welcomed as a support Only female staff should handle female bodies
Established and Free Church (of all denominations)	No special requirements	No special requirements	No special requirements	May require Holy Communion and/or the presence of their priest or minister
Hinduism	Special ceremony after birth Parents choose name from priest on 10th day	No meat (especially beef), fish, or dairy produce which contains animal fats	Married women cannot have their hair cut or consent for surgery without their husband's permission Patients prefer treatment from a doctor or nurse of the same gender as themselves Handwashing essential before and after eating Prefer to bathe in running water	Family (especially eldest son) should be at bedside Relatives prefer to wash the body Prefer to die at home
Islam	May refuse vaginal examination Baby must be bathed immediately after birth Family prefer to bury placenta 7th day – baby's head shaved (unless unwell), circumcised by family and named Birth control not permitted	Pork and pork products unacceptable All other meat must be ritually slaughtered (halal) Annual fast during sunrise for 1 month unless menstruating, following recent childbirth, old, weak or ill No alcohol	Prefer to be at home during religious festivals Exposure of body considered unacceptable After toileting, cleansing done with water and left hand Showers preferred to baths Washing of hands, neck, ears and feet, rinsing of mouth necessary before prayer five times a day	Family wash body prior to burial (without coffin) 24 hours after death Post-mortem not acceptable

Jehovah's Witness	Baptism not practised Abortion not acceptable	No tobacco No meat from animals that have been strangled (e.g. poultry) No blood products (e.g. black sausage)	Transfusion of blood and blood products is not acceptable Organ transplant not usually permitted	Support and prayers of fellow witnesses are appreciated
Judaism	Male circumcision at 8 days by a trained circumciser Men will attend and name the baby at this time	Meat only obtained from ritual slaughter Shellfish, pork and game forbidden	No drugs derived from the pig (e.g. porcine insulin)	Body should not be left unattended until burial (24 hours after death) and not touched by a non-Jew unless wearing gloves
Mormonism	Abortion opposed	No tea, coffee, cola drinks, alcohol or tobacco 24-hour fast 1st Sunday in the month unless undergoing medical treatment	White one or two piece underclothing not usually removed	Dying should be dignified and pain free Church elder gives blessing for the dying
Plymouth Brethren	Birth control not usually permitted	Eating with non-Brethren not always permissible	Patients may not be seen naked TV and radio may not be watched or listened to	No special requirements
Rastafarianism	Use of birth control unacceptable	No pork, shellfish, milk, coffee or tobacco	Most prefer not to cut hair or beards Blood transfusion from family members only Unacceptable to wear second-hand clothing, therefore disposable gowns should be used	Family prefer to be present at bedside
Roman Catholicism	Artificial birth control is unacceptable Natural birth control (e.g. rhythm method) may be practised	Some Catholics do not eat meat on Fridays	No specific requirements	Sacrament of the sick (previously known as the Last Rites) administered by the priest Family may wish to have holy water, rosary, or crucifix by the bed
Sikhism	Abortion not generally acceptable	Vegetarians No alcohol or tobacco	Showers preferred to baths Handwashing and rinsing of mouth before meals Males do not like to remove their turban or Sikh symbols (uncut hair, comb, bangle, sword or shorts) in public Women prefer a female present during examinations	Passages from the holy book read by a Sikh leader Family wash and dress the body before cremation

Adapted from Cracknell, R. and Cox, J. (1993) *Cultural and Religious Aspects of Caring Professionals.* Luton: University of Luton.

Study activity

Discuss with others from different cultures whether it is possible to interpret feelings as well as information.

We are all aware that if we do not understand someone or we have not quite heard what they said we just agree. Consequently, it is important that we ensure that families with poor or limited language really do understand when they smile or nod in agreement, so that they are enabled to give informed consent. Those from Oriental cultures sometimes believe in avoiding confrontation and these families may agree simply to avoid conflict (Weller, 1994). The lack of questioning by families does not always imply understanding as, in Asian cultures, questioning persons in authority is seen as disrespectful (Orque, 1983). In addition to these drawbacks it is important to remember that parents are already intimidated by a strange environment and bewildered by professional jargon and medical terminology.

In Western cultures avoidance of eye contact is seen as disrespectful or a sign of disinterest, boredom or deceitfulness. In other cultures the reverse is sometimes true and some cultures avoid looking directly at the nurse as a sign of respect.

Emotions are also expressed differently in different cultures. In Western cultures public displays of emotion are viewed as embarrassing and inappropriate, but in Jewish and Latin cultures people are expected to share their emotions openly and loudly with others.

Dietary Customs

Food preferences for different ethnic groups tends to originate from the easy availability of such food in their native environment. Most children's wards allow parents to bring food in for their children and the family may prefer to do so as they can be sure that it is appropriate to their beliefs and the child's appetite. However, hospitals should be able to provide a variety of meals for different cultures and not put added pressure on parents who may feel obliged to bring in suitable foodstuffs (*see also* Religions, cultural beliefs and diet p. 179).

Study activity

Take a critical look at how your own area of practice caters for the dietary needs of different cultures. If changes are necessary what would you recommend?

Nurses should be careful not to impose their dietary values upon other cultures. Baxter *et al.* (1990) found that disabled Asian children in the UK are often taught to eat with cutlery because staff do not realise that eating with fingers is an important part of the Asian culture.

Child-rearing Practices

Nurses should be aware that different cultures have different beliefs about raising their children so that their assessment of needs, and the planning, implementation and evaluation of care, are appropriate for that family. Generally, Asian families value conformity, respect for elders, obedience and sexually appropriate behaviour more than indigenous white British families, who value self-sufficiency and independence (Stopes-Roe and Cochrane, 1989). Second-generation immigrants continue to be influenced by their traditional values, but also take on some of the values of the host culture. These values affect the way in which families raise their children. American mothers encourage their babies to socialise by stimulating them with active chatting. Japanese mothers believe that babies should be quiet and contented babies and they soothe and lull their infants to produce this relaxed state (Swanwick, 1996).

Religion

Religion is an important part of most cultures. It determines families' wishes in relation to practices concerning birth and death, and there may be other important rituals to be performed during childhood or illness. It is not enough for the nurse to ask the family's religion on admission. Burnard (1988) discovered that the majority of British people call themselves Christian although they do not formally belong to a church. Bradshaw (1996) warns that the same may be true for other cultures and that it may be dangerous to assume that Sikhs, Jews and Muslims take their religion seriously. The nurse's assessment should ascertain if there are any special religious practices or needs that are important to the family and should not make assumptions from their given religion. Some families, regardless of culture, turn to religion in times of stress for support, and may appreciate talking to the hospital chaplain or a member of their own religious group. Others find that severe illness in the family challenges their previous beliefs and find it difficult to gain support in this way.

Not everyone may have religious beliefs but they do have a spirituality (Burnard, 1988). Spirituality has been defined as the meaning, value and purpose of life, which may have nothing to do with religion (McSherry, 1996). Bradshaw (1996) argues that meeting families' spiritual needs are an intrinsic part of providing holistic care and should not need to be separated out as a specific topic. It is about helping families to express their feelings and emotions about their child's condition, and how that condition has challenged the meaning, value and belief that a disabled child is punishment for sins from their previous life (Baxter *et al.*, 1990). Disability in the family reduces the marriage prospects for the rest of the family in a culture where arranged marriages are the norm and it often causes shame, particularly if the disabled child is male. Language problems often make it difficult for Asian families to find out about their children's disability and the community support available. Voluntary support groups for the disabled are usually set up and run by white middle-class families and tend not to cater for cultural differences (Shah, 1992). Shah (1992) also discovered that Asian families found it difficult to accept respite care because they were uncertain that their religious beliefs would be upheld. It is important for children's nurses to appreciate that Asian families coping on their own with a disabled child may not be doing so because they do not want help but simply because they are not aware of the help available.

Key Points

1. The UK is a multicultural society with Asians comprising the main ethnic minority group.
2. It is important not to make assumptions about people's beliefs; individuality is more important than race, ethnicity or culture.
3. Health care in the UK is mainly directed towards the needs of the white middle class and is difficult for ethnic minority groups to access.
4. People from different ethnic origins often have different beliefs and practices in relation to health, illness, diet and religion. They have a different physical appearance and are likely to experience different diseases.
5. Nurses should care for all children and their families in the same way regardless of their ethnic origin but they should take care to appreciate and respect individual beliefs and values.
6. Nurses need to be aware of their own beliefs and values and the origin of these before they can fully appreciate the beliefs and values of others.

Chapter 59

The Future of Children's Nursing

Introduction

> The secret balance of life's current paradox is to allow the past and future to coexist in the present.
>
> (Handy, 1994)

If Charles Handy's philosophy is to be believed, children's nurses need to demonstrate insight and a wider vision to recognise future trends, and to develop children's nursing to meet innovations in practice. Unless nurses are able to react in this way they will find that the government will impose reforms upon the profession from outside. Nurses cannot be content to let this happen and should be exploring how their current knowledge and skills can be used to influence their future.

In 1988, when Anne Casey was developing her family-centred care model of nursing, she questioned over 300 practising children's nurses about their beliefs regarding children's nursing and its future. The most common responses related to the development of:

- recognition of children's nursing as a speciality
- research-based evidence for paediatric practice
- specialist roles within children's nursing
- family-centred care
- children's community nursing
- children's nurses' role as health educators
- technology in children's nursing

These seem useful headings to use to explore current knowledge and skills and to discuss how their development may affect the future of children's nursing. However, children's nursing is part of the wider field of nursing and its developments cannot be explored without also looking at the future of nursing as a whole.

Children's Nursing as a Speciality

The future of nursing as an independent profession began to be questioned in the 1990s and the possibility of nursing being phased out has to be considered before discussing the development of children's nursing as a speciality. In 1990, managers began to consider that nurses were too expensive to be employed to perform fundamental caring and that less qualified, less expensive healthcare assistants should be used instead. This idea was steadily accepted by post-NHS reforms and many Trusts now employ a large percentage of unqualified support workers. These changes cannot be considered without comparison with previous trends. Before the advent of Project 2000, wards were largely staffed by student nurses and enrolled nurses who were a relatively inexpensive work force. Once student nurses started to become supernumerary and the second-level nurse was deemed inappropriate it was too expensive to replace them all with registered nurses. Thus the healthcare assistant (HCA) came into being. Initially, the HCA role was created to assist the registered nurse in non-nursing duties but shortages of staff have led nurses to allow HCAs to take on more and more of the nursing role until nursing has become difficult to define.

Study activity

Take a critical look at the work of unqualified staff in your own area. How much of this would you define as nursing? Why is it not being done by nurses?

Many HCAs consider that qualified staff are unaware of their role and training needs. Uncertainty about this role can lead to HCAs being used inappropriately (Reeve, 1994) and if these unqualified staff are used to give bedside care, it is they who spend more time with patients and develop a relationship with them. Is that what nurses really want? In 1997 the Health Department increased intakes of student nurses and the benefit of this should have been apparent in 2000. However in 2002 Elston and Thornes were reporting:

- an estimated shortfall of 2769 (whole time eqivalents) registered children's nurses
- 27% of Trusts had difficulty recruiting registered children's nurses in A&E, 24% in neonatal units and 18.8% in children's wards
- 66% of staff in neonatal units and children's wards were registered children's nurses
- 35% of nurses working in paediatric oncology had an appropriate specialist oncology qualification
- limited availability of training places contributed to over 66% of applicants for child branch courses being rejected

To ensure an adequate workforce these shortfalls in children's nurses will have been replaced with HCAs or adult branch nurses. Over the past 10 years many children's wards have consistently not been able to meet government recommendations of a minimum of two registered children's nurses per shift, and children continue to be nursed in adult wards (DH, 1991, 1996a, b; Clothier, 1994; Elston and Thornes, 2002). There is a danger that those providing the care will be treated as if they have the skills of the registered children's nurse and the specialist nurse will be seen as unnecessary. The problem is worse in areas other than children's wards – where children are the minority group.

In 1996 a report from Manchester University (University of Manchester Health Services Management Unit, 1996) proposed the creation of a generic healthcare worker. The lowest grade of this post would perform the bedside nursing as an entry gate into specialities such as physiotherapy or occupational therapy. This is effectively stating that nursing is not a specific speciality that needs a particular body of knowledge, skills and attitudes. Glasper (1993) has suggested that a generic nurse may appear a more cost-effective option and that specialist nurses who are unable to gain work in Europe, America and Australia may support this idea. He proposes that, if nursing does return to the generic route, children's nursing becomes a postgraduate qualification. However, this is an expensive option that may only be taken up or available to a few very motivated nurses (*see also* Generic nurse p. 619).

In this climate of uncertainty, what is the future of children's nursing? Campbell (1995) recognises that the speciality could be in danger and warns that if registered children's nurses wish to retain the title 'children's nurse' a concerted effort needs to be made to ensure that the role is uniquely identifiable from that of other health professionals and discrete from other roles (*see also* Number of registered children's nurses p. 619).

Study activity

Discuss with some colleagues how these dangers can be overcome to enable children's nursing to remain as an important speciality.

Several authors have attempted to address this issue. Campbell (1995) believes it important to be able to define the nature of children's nursing. Colson (1996) advocates greater collaboration between service and education managers to develop flexible yet rigorous post-registration programmes to help those nurses, working with children, who do not possess a children's nursing qualification.

The future of children's nursing may not be bleak. Children have different needs from adults, and these needs are both complex and demanding. It has been clearly established that admission to hospital can cause children psychological trauma. There is research to support the importance of maintaining the child and family relationship and the value of working in partnership with parents. These principles are strongly supported by the Children's NSF (DH, 2004b). This body of evidence helps children's nurses to be able to define the nature of their role. The 1996 Royal College of Nursing Society of Paediatric Nursing presented evidence that children's nurses do make a difference and that children's nurses were aware of the need to assert their role and were reacting to current pressures. If government support for children's nurses is to remain, nurses themselves must continue to prove their worth as specialists and not allow their role to be taken over by unqualified staff.

Research-based Evidence for Paediatric Practice

The movement of nurse education into higher education has aided nursing research. However, because nursing had no research history, the first nurse researchers were forced to rely upon established methodology for healthcare research. This has not helped nursing research to gain credibility and the 1992 Higher Education Funding Council (HEFC) research assessment placed nursing research at the bottom of their leagues of excellence. In addition, funds for healthcare research are much in demand and other healthcare professionals, who are more experienced and respected as researchers, find it easier to gain this funding. This situation is slowly changing. The 1997 HEFC assessment showed that the quality of nursing research had significantly improved, with 10 of the 36 institutions assessed improving their rating since 1992. In 1992, 30 Nursing Development Units (NDUs) were established by the Department of Health to provide optimum client care through the development of practice. The number of NDUs is gradually increasing and, led by Campbell in 1993, now includes paediatric units. Nurses within NDUs are encouraged to question practice and use evidence-based knowledge to plan care (Vaughan and Edwards, 1994). These units have firmly ensured that nursing research is linked to practice. Now it is important that nurses react to the research findings. Benner (1984) described the expert nurse as one who 'has an intuitive grasp of the situation' but her work must not become an excuse for experienced children's nurses to continue to use intuition to assess and plan care. Practitioners who cannot express their rationale for care are in danger of perpetuating a ritualistic and unproved approach to children's nursing. As Walsh and Ford (1994) noted, rituals are dangerous because they give a feeling of security and decrease the acceptability of change. Equally dangerous is the enthusiastic implementation of research without questioning its value.

Study activity

Take a critical look at the care plan of a child you have nursed. Can you give a research-based rationale for all the care prescribed?

Traditionally nurses have tended to cling to routines and have not been good at reacting to research findings. I still meet nurses who tell me that pressure sores are best prevented by massaging the areas at risk. Changes in practice are often painful because they involve an acceptance that earlier beliefs are now outmoded and devalued but if children's nursing is to develop, children's nurses must be prepared to question practice and accept change. Although all nurses cannot lead change or be researchers, it is important that all nurses appreciate research (DH, 1993). By appreciating the value of research, all children's nurses can support the development of practice to ensure that children receive the optimum care. Research appreciation may be defined as a critical questioning approach to one's work, the desire and ability to find out the latest research in that area and the ability to assess its value to the situation and apply it as appropriate (Macleod Clark and Hockey, 1989).

There has been considerable debate on the ethical dilemmas and legal issues surrounding research involving children and their families. Jolley (1995) accepts that paediatric nursing research involves some difficulties but argues that a lack of research may lead to unsafe practice. Research may be defined as a careful search or enquiry that aims to discover new facts. Nurses have always done this in an informal way by evaluating their care and by using their past experience to adapt or create innovative ways of caring for specific children's problems. Unfortunately, nurses have tended not to record or analyse their evaluations and their changes to care remain largely unknown. Reflective practice is now helping nurses to question their practice in a more systematic way but they need to be more active in sharing their findings (*see also* Research p. 705).

UKCC (1992) guidelines for critiquing research reports

The research question

- are the aims clearly stated?

The rationale for the study

- is the importance of the study made clear?
- is any similar work noted?
- is there a comprehensive literature review?

Methodology

- is this appropriate to the study?
- is it explained fully?
- is the sample unbiased?
- are the reliability and validity of the method proven?

Results

- are these clearly expressed?
- is there discussion of the findings?
- are limitations to the study recognised?
- do they add to nursing knowledge?

Specialist Roles for Children's Nurses

The role of the qualified nurse in the UK has expanded tremendously in the past decade. In many areas the nurse is now recognised as a specialist and is an autonomous practitioner. The UKCC advisory document *Scope of Professional Practice* (1992) gave nurses guidelines on which to base their decisions about developing their role in response to the changing needs of society. Specialist roles for nurses have also arisen because of the reduction in junior doctors' hours. In 1991 the NHS Management Directive proposed a new deal to improve junior doctors' hours and change their conditions of service. This led to an investigation of the junior doctor role and it was suggested that many duties were inappropriate and could be performed by others, including nurses (Hopkins and Hodgson, 1996). These developments have enabled children's nursing to grow.

The scope of professional practice – the principles

- Putting the needs of patients and clients first at all times
- Updating and developing your knowledge, skills and competencies
- Recognising limitations in your personal knowledge and skill and taking action to address these deficiencies
- Ensuring that you do not compromise standards of care by new developments to your practice and taking on new responsibilities
- Acknowledging your own personal professional accountability
- Refusing tasks for which you are not competent

Study activity

Find out what specialist roles are available to children's nurses. Consider how these roles enhance the care of children.

Nurse specialist posts within children's nursing have developed considerably in recent years. Just a few examples of these specialist posts are listed below:

- infant care/feeding advisor
- adolescent oncology and haematology
- asthma care
- cystic fibrosis
- HIV and AIDS
- dermatology

- pain control
- plastic surgery

(*see also* Emergence of nurse specialists p. 673).

In addition to specialist posts, individual children's nurses' roles have widened to include specialist skills. One example of the developing scope of practice is the role of the children's nurse practitioner. In children's A&E departments these experienced children's nurses are able to assess, diagnose and treat some specified children without referral to a doctor. In Nottingham there are nurse-led clinics for children with asthma and enuresis where nurses assess and monitor the child's condition, giving additional advice and support as necessary (Fradd, 1994). From October 1984 community nurses began to prescribe certain drugs and this initiative has gradually developed to include acute paediatric care. Specialist roles can be seen to be recreating the task aspect of nursing, but Fradd (1994) believes that such developments add credibility and increase respect, trust and confidence in the role of the children's nurse. However, she warns that any role development should in the best interests of children and not evolve merely to make other healthcare workers' jobs easier.

Will this role development continue? General developments in the NHS appear to favour the expansion of the GP role with perhaps a return to GP hospitals for minor surgery. Children's nurses could play a vital role in such developments especially as children comprise over 30% of a GP's workload and the number of children with complex medical problems are increasing. However, it is worth noting that nurses without a general nurse qualification were only able to access practice nursing and health visiting from 1995, so there are few children's nurses with these qualifications. It must also be remembered that the Health Service is also very cost conscious at present and very experienced, specialist nurses may be too expensive. There is a need to prove the cost-effectiveness of such roles if they are to continue.

Family-centred Care

There is no doubt that the family will always be an important part of children's nursing and that this philosophy of care will continue to develop. Darbyshire's research in 1994 gave valuable information about the reality of family-centred care for nurses and families but further research is now needed into the:

- nurses' perspectives of parental participation
- social implications of parental participation
- definition of 'family'
- nature of being a parent of a sick child
- implications of participation for parental control and autonomy
- effects of participation upon parental anxiety levels

Campbell *et al.* (1993) suggest that family-centred research could represent the way forward for the development of children's nursing. They suggest that family-centred care should be broadened to enable parents to be involved in all decision-making about children's nursing, including deciding research priorities.

Community Children's Nursing

With evidence of the increasing number of children at home with chronic and complex disorders, it is likely that the community children's nurse service will continue to develop. From April 1996, GP fundholders were able to purchase specialist nursing services and it is known that many GPs and district nurses admit that they lack the confidence, experience and skills to care for sick children at home (Brocklehurst, 1996). Unfortunately, being a relatively new speciality, community children's nursing is poorly understood by GPs. Community children's nurses need to be able to market their expertise and justify the need for such skills and experience to be certain of their survival.

One area of community children's nursing that could help to justify the need for such a service is in the care of children with mental health problems. In 1995 the Health Advisory Service reported that between 10 and 20% of children required help because of mental health problems and recommended the development of primary health mental health services for children. The Department of Health has recognised that care of these children should take priority, as failure to do so may cause increased demands on the social and educational services as well as leading to continued problems in adulthood. Few psychiatric nurses have qualifications in child and adolescent mental health (McMorrow, 1995) but children's nurses have been taught to appreciate the stresses of childhood and ways of helping children to cope with their problems (*see also* Mental health in childhood p. 120).

However, there are still very few community children's nurses. Courses to prepare children's nurses to work in the community are hampered by the lack of suitably qualified practitioners to act as teachers, mentors and placement supervisors. At the same time, those suitably qualified practitioners have to appreciate families' privacy and confidentiality and not endanger their relationship with them by always being accompanied by students. There is a need for innovative ways of teaching nurses how to care for sick children at home. Perhaps one way of overcoming this issue is to link with families and other healthcare professionals working with children in the community.

The Role of Children's Nurses as Health Educators

The importance of health education for children is gradually being recognised. While most health education used to be aimed at the adult population, there are now specific strategies for health promotion for children. Attitudes and behaviour are established during childhood, so it makes sense to influence these at an early age. There has been much debate about whether health education is the role and responsibility of the parent, the teacher or the healthcare professional, but many adults have already developed unhealthy behaviour and may be confused about the right information to give children (*see also* Role of children's nurses in child health promotion p. 165 and Developing strategies for health p. 148).

Whitehead (1995) points out that healthcare behaviours are not intrinsically rewarding and that environmental influences often make it difficult for children to comply with health education. Children's nurses are taught what health education to give and are aware of children's perceptions of health and illness. They can adapt the health message according to the age of their target group. Initiatives that have provided sexual health education for teenagers have shown a reduction in under-16s registering at family planning clinics (Jackson and Plant, 1996). Other specific health education programmes have been developed to teach primary school children about diet, dental hygiene, smoking and skin cancer.

Health education has tended to be based in the community rather than the hospital. This is slowly changing and needs to continue to do so in the future. Children's nurses working in any field are in the best position to use their influence and experience with children to provide and reinforce the relevant health education to help children to attain both mental and physical well-being, without antagonising parents whose beliefs may be different. This is yet another area where children's nurses should exploit their expertise in family-centred care and make good use of their close relationship with the children and families in their care.

Study activity

Choose a specific hospital ward or department and consider what health education programmes would be most suitable for the children and families in this area.

Technology in Children's Nursing

Technology in all branches of nursing has increased tremendously over the past 10–20 years. There has been an increase in the number and types of transplantations performed, and this type of surgery is no longer a rare event. Nurses have needed to increase their technological skills to care for these highly dependent children. Extracorporeal membrane oxygenation (ECMO) is one example of how technology has developed to care for seriously ill children who previously would have died. It provides pulmonary or cardiopulmonary support for children with reversible respiratory or cardiac failure and ECMO specialists have been appointed to complement the existing staff and provide the specific knowledge and skills to maintain and monitor the ECMO process. These specialists are often children's or neonatal nurses.

Community children's nurses are supporting families of children with special needs who are likely to have quite complicated care at home, such as total parenteral nutrition, tracheostomies, gastrostomies and even ventilation. As the resuscitation of infants becomes more sophisticated, this type of situation can only develop further. It is likely that development in general practice care will increase the amount of technology in the community still further. Alongside this, it is likely that children in acute hospitals will require even more highly dependent care.

The reduction in junior doctors' hours has also given nurses responsibility in areas they were not previously familiar with. For instance, children's nurses have now become the experts in the care of implantable

IV devices, while many doctors may have had little experience of such devices.

Children's nurses will need to react proactively to these changes. They need to be certain of their role and not take on extra responsibilities that may result in the reduced provision of nursing care of children and families. It is worth considering how extra responsibilities affect the concept of partnership in care. Perhaps the philosophy of Great Ormond Street Hospital for Children, 'children first and always', should be remembered when considering any change in practice.

Key Points

1. Children's nurses need to be proactive in their response to change to ensure they maintain their role as specialists in the care of children and their families.
2. If generic nurse education develops, children's nursing may become a postgraduate speciality and children's nurses may be less common.
3. Developments in the HCA role and the inability of many children's wards to meet minimum staffing requirements for qualified children's nurses may lead hospital managers to abandon the attempt to gain these more expensive nurses.
4. To maintain the speciality, children's nurses must be able to:
   — define their role and justify its continued existence
   — demonstrate an appreciation of research findings
   — only take on new areas of practice that are in the best interests of the child
5. More research into family-centred care and involving families is needed to strengthen this concept of care.
6. Future developments to the role of the children's nurse include:
   — health education in hospital care
   — mental health care of children and adolescents
   — children's practice nurses
   — continued initiatives in nurse-led clinics, nurse prescribing and specialist roles

References

Aggleton, P. and **Chambers, H.** (1986) *Nursing Models and the Nursing Process.* Basingstoke: Macmillan Education.

Andrews, M. and **Boyle, J.** (1995) *Transcultural Concepts in Nursing Care,* 2nd edn. Philadelphia: Lippincott.

Audit Commission (1993) *Children First – A Study of Hospital Services.* London: HMSO.

Bagnall, P. and **Garbett, R.** (1996) Continuing education: how well is PREP working? *Nursing Times,* **92** (7), 34–35.

Barnsteiner, J. and **Gillis-Donovan, J.** (1990) Being related and separate: a standard for therapeutic relationships. *Maternal and Child Nursing,* **15** (4), 223–228.

Battrick, C. and **Glasper, A.** (2004) The views of children and their families on being in hospital. *British Journal of Nursing,* **13** (6), 328–336.

Baum, D., Sister Francis Dominica and **Woodward, R.** (1990) *Listen, My Child has a Lot of Living to Do.* Oxford: Oxford University Press.

Baxter, J. (1997) Cultural relativism and cultural diversity: implications for nursing practice. *Advances in Nursing Science* **20** (1), 3–11.

Baxter, J., *et al.* (1990) *Double Discrimination.* London: King's Fund Centre.

Benner, P. (1984) *From Novice to Expert: Excellence and Power in Clinical Nursing.* Menlo Park, CA: Addison-Wesley.

Besser, F. (1977) Great Ormond Street anniversary. *Nursing Mirror,* **144** (6), 31–33.

Bond, M. and **Holland, S.** (1997) *Skills of Clinical Supervision for Nurses.* Milton Keynes: Open University Press.
Boud, D., Keogh, R. and **Walker, D.** (1985) *Reflection: Turning Experience into Learning.* New York: Kogan Page.
Bowlby, J. (1951) *Maternal Care and Mental Health.* Geneva: WHO.
Bowlby, J. and **Robertson, J.** (1952) *A Two-year Old Goes to Hospital. Mental Health and Infant Development.* London: Routledge & Kegan Paul.
Bradshaw, A. (1996) The legacy of Nightingale. *Nursing Times,* **92** (6), 42–43.
Brocklehurst, N. (1996) Selling children's community nursing. *Paediatric Nursing,* **8** (9), 6–7.
Burnard, P. (1988) The spiritual needs of atheists and agnostics. *Professional Nurse,* **4** (3), 130–132.
Butterworth, C. and **Faugier, J.** (eds) (1992) *Clinical Supervision and Mentorship in Nursing.* London: Chapman & Hall.
Callery, P. and **Smith, L.** (1991) A study of role negotiation between nurses and the parents of hospitalised children. *Journal of Advanced Nursing,* **16**, 772–781.
Campbell, S. (1995) What makes a children's nurse? *Child Health,* **2** (5), 117.
Campbell, S. and **Clarke, F.** (1992) Ethos and philosophy of paediatric intensive care. In Carter, B. (ed.), *Manual of Paediatric Intensive Care.* London: Harper Row.
Campbell, S. and **Glasper, A.** (eds) (1995) *Whaley and Wong's Children's Nursing.* St Louis: Mosby.
Campbell, S., Kelly, P. and **Summerskill, P.** (1993) Putting the family first. *Child Health,* **1** (2), 59–63.
Casey, A. (1988) A partnership with child and family. *Senior Nurse,* **8** (4), 8–9.
Chamberlain, T., *et al.* (1988) Cost analysis of a home intravenous antibiotic programme. *American Journal of Hospital Pharmacy,* **45** (2), 2341–2345.
Cleary, A., *et al.* (1986) Parental involvement in the lives of children in hospital. *Archives of Disease in Childhood,* **61** (8), 779–780.
Clothier, C. (1994) *The Allitt Inquiry.* London: HMSO.
Colson, J. (1996) Creating opportunities for children's nurses. *Paediatric Nursing,* **8** (10), 6–7.
Coutts-Jarman, J. (1993) Using reflection and experience in nurse education. *British Journal of Nursing,* **2** (1), 77–80.
Coyne, I. (1996) Parent participation: a concept analysis. *Journal of Advanced Nursing,* **23**, 733–740.
Coyne, P. (1997) Developing nurse consultancy in clinical practice. *Nursing Times,* **92** (33), 34–35.
Cracknell, R. and **Cox, J.** (1993) *Cultural and Religious Aspects of Caring Professionals.* Luton: University of Luton.
Curley, M. and **Wallace, J.** (1992) Effects of the mutual cooperation participation model of care on parental stress in the paediatric intensive care unit. *Pediatric Nursing,* **7** (6), 377–385.
Darbyshire, P. (1994) *Living with a Sick Child in Hospital.* London: Chapman & Hall.
Darbyshire, P. (1995) Parents in paediatrics. *Paediatric Nursing,* **7** (1), 8–10.
David, R. (1990) Race, birthweight and mortality rates. *Journal of Pediatrics,* **116** (1), 101–102.
Davies, C. (1996a) Cloaked in a tattered illusion. *Nursing Times,* **92** (45), 44–46.
Davies, C. (1996b) A new vision of professionalism. *Nursing Times,* **92** (46), 54–56.
Davies, R. (2004) The first children's hospital in Wales. *Paediatric Nursing,* **16** (6), 24–25.
Davis, H. and **Fallowfield, L.** (1991) *Counselling and Communication in Health Care.* Chichester: Wiley.
Dearmun, A. (1997) Using reflection to assess degree students. *Paediatric Nursing,* **9** (1), 25–28.
De Mause, L. (1974) *The History of Childhood.* London: Souvenir Press.
Dewey, J. (1933) *How We Think.* Boston: D. C. Heath.
DH (1976) *Fit for the Future – Child Health Services.* London: HMSO.
DH (1989) *The Children Act – An Introductory Guide for the NHS.* London: HMSO.
DH (1991) *Welfare of Children and Young People in Hospital.* London: HMSO.
DH (1993) *Research for Health.* London: HMSO.
DH (1994a) *The Allitt Inquiry. Report of the Clothier Committee.* London: HMSO.
DH (1994b) *The Children's Charter.* London: HMSO.
DH (1996a) *The Children's Charter.* London: HMSO.
DH (1996b) *Services for Children and Young People.* London: HMSO.
DH (2004a) *What Should a Really Good Hospital Look Like?* London: Department of Health.
DH (2004b) *Children's NSF – Standard for hospital services.* London: Department of Health.
Dodge, J., Morrison, S., Lewis, P., *et al.* (1993) Cystic fibrosis in the UK 1968–1988: incidence, population and survival. *Paediatric and Perinatal Epidemiology,* **7**, 156–166.
Ellis, P. (1995) The role of the nurse as the patient's advocate. *Professional Nurse,* **11** (3), 206–207.
Elston, S. and **Thornes, R.** (2002) *Children's Nursing Workforce: A report to the Royal College of Nursing and The Royal College of Paediatrics and Child Health.* London: RCN.
English National Board (1994) *Creating Lifelong Learners: Partnerships for Care.* London: ENB.
Engstrom, J. (1984) Problems in the development, use and testing of nursing theory. *Journal of Nursing Education,* **23** (60), 245–251.
Fish, D. and **Purr, B.** (1991) *The Evaluation of Practice-based Learning in Continuing Education in Nursing, Midwifery and Health Visiting.* London: ENB.
Fish, D. and **Twinn, S.** (1997) *Quality Clinical Supervision in the Health Care Professions. Principled Approaches to Practice.* London: Butterworth-Heinemann.

Ford, K. and **Turner, D.** (2001) Stories seldom told; paediatric nurses' experiences of caring for children with special needs and their families. *Journal of Advanced Nursing*, **33** (3), 288–295.
Fradd, E. (1994) A broader scope to practice. *Child Health*, **1** (6), 233–238.
Fradd, E. (1996) The importance of negotiating a care plan. *Paediatric Nursing*, **8** (6), 6–9.
Fradd, E. (2005) Leading the future. *Paediatric Nursing*, **17** (6), 3.
Franck, L. and **Callery, P.** (2004) Re-thinking family centered care across the continuum of children's healthcare. *Child Care, Health and Development*, **30** (3), 265–277.
Fraser, M. (1996) *Conceptual Nursing in Practice*, 2nd edn. London: Chapman & Hall.
Freidson, E. (1970) *Profession of Medicine*. New York: Dodds, Mead & Co.
Fry, T. (1993) Charting growth. *Child Health*, **1** (3), 104–107.
Gablehouse, B. and **Gitterman, B.** (1990) Maternal understanding of commonly used medical terms in a pediatric setting. *American Journal of Diseases in Children*, **114**, 419–425.
Gill, K. (1993) Health professionals' attitudes toward parent participation in hospitalised children's care. *Children's Health Care*, **22**, 257–271.
Glasper, A. (1993) Back to the future. *Child Health*, **1** (3), 93–95.
Glasper, A. (1995) The value of children's nursing in the third millennium. *British Journal of Nursing*, **4** (1), 27.
Glasper, A. and **Burge, D.** (1992) Developing family information leaflets. *Nursing Standard*, **6** (15), 24–27.
Grey, M. (1993) Stressors and children's health. *Journal of Pediatric Nursing*, **8** (2), 85.
Gruending, D. (1985) Nursing theory: a vehicle for professionalism? *Journal of Advanced Nursing*, **10**, 553–558.
Gould, C. (1996) Multiple partnerships in the community. *Paediatric Nursing*, **8** (8), 27–31.
Guest, A., Rittey, C. and **O'Brien, K.** (2005) Telemedicine helping neurologically impaired children to stay at home. *Paediatric Nursing*, **17** (2), 20–22.
Handy, C. (1994) *The Empty Raincoat*. London: Hutchinson.
Hawes, R. (2005) Therapeutic relationships with children and families. *Paediatric Nursing*, **17** (6), 15–18.
HAS (Health Advisory Service) (1995) *The Commissioning Role and Management of Child and Adolescent Mental Health Services*. London: HMSO.
Hill, A. (1989) Trends in paediatric medical admissions. *British Medical Journal*, **298** (6686), 1479–1480.
Hopkins, S. and **Hodgson, I.** (1996) Junior doctors' hours and the expanding role of the nurse. *Nursing Times*, **92** (14), 35–36.
Hostler, S. (1992) Personal communication. In Johnson, B., *et al.* (eds), *Caring for Children and Families: Guidelines for Hospital*. Bethesda: Association for the Care of Children's Health.
Jackson, P. and **Plant, Z.** (1996) Youngsters get an introduction to sexual health clinics. *Nursing Times*, **92** (21), 34–36.
Johns, C. C. (ed.) (1994) *The Burford NDU Model: Caring in Practice*. Oxford: Blackwell Scientific.
Johns, C. C. (1996) The benefits of a reflective model of nursing. *Nursing Times*, **92** (27), 39–41.
Johnson, M. (1996) Student nurses: novices or practitioners of brilliant care? *Nursing Times*, **92** (26), 34–37.
Jolley, J. (1995) Forging the way ahead. *Child Health*, **2** (5), 202–206.
Jolley, M. and **Allan, P.** (1989) *Current Issues in Nursing*. London: Chapman & Hall.
King's College Nursing Research Unit (2004) *Careers of Nurse Diplomates: Child Branch Diplomates*. London: King's College NRU. http://www.kcl.ac.uk/nursing/nru/child2.html.
Kitson, A. (1986) Indicators of quality in nursing care – an alternative approach. *Journal of Advanced Nursing*, **11**, 133–144.
Lacey, D. (1993) Using Orem's model in psychiatric nursing. *Nursing Standard*, **7** (29), 28–30.
Lasky, P. and **Eichelburger, K.** (1985) Health related views and self-care behaviours of young children. *Family Relations*, **1**, 13–18.
Law, M., Teplicky, R. and **King, S.** (2005) Family-centred care in practice: moving ideas into practice. *Child Care, Health and Development*, **31** (6), 633–642.
Ley, P. and **Llewelyn, S.** (1995) Improving patients' understanding, recall, satisfaction and compliance. In Broome, A. and Llewelyn, S. (eds), *Health Psychology*, 2nd edn. London: Chapman & Hall.
Lister, P. (1987) The misunderstood model. *Nursing Times*, **83** (41), 40–42.
Maben, J. and **Macleod Clark, J.** (1996) Making the transition from student to staff nurse. *Nursing Times*, **92** (44), 28–31.
MacDonald, G. (1991) Plans for a better future. *Nursing Times*, **87** (31), 42–43.
Macleod Clark, J. and **Hockey, L.** (1989) *Further Research in Nursing*. London: Scutari Press.
Marmot, M., Adeelstein, A. and **Bulusu, L.** (1984) *Immigrant Mortality in England and Wales* (OPCS 47). London: HMSO.
McMorrow, R. (1995) The role of the community psychiatric nurse in child psychiatry. *Child Health*, **3** (3), 95–98.
McSherry, W. (1996) Raising the spirits. *Nursing Times*, **92** (3), 48–49.
MoH (1959) *Welfare of Children in Hospital (The Platt Report)*. London: HMSO.
Mootoo, J. S. (2005) *A Guide to Cultural and Spiritual Awareness*. Harrow: Nursing Standard.
Newell, R. (1992) Anxiety, accuracy and reflection: the limits of professional development. *Journal of Advanced Nursing*, **17**, 1326–1333.
Nichols, K. (1993) *Psychological Care in Physical Illness*, 2nd edn. London: Chapman & Hall.
Nightingale, F. (1859) *Notes on Nursing*. London: Harrison.
Nursing and Midwifery Council (2004a) *The NMC Code of Professional Conduct*. London: NMC.
Nursing and Midwifery Council (2004b) *Registration Fee Rises*. London: NMC.

Office of National Statistics (2006) *Focus on Ethnicity and Identity.* London: HMSO.
Orem, D. (1971) *Nursing: Concepts of Practice.* New York: McGraw-Hill.
Orem, D. (1985) *Nursing: Concepts of Practice,* 3rd edn. New York: McGraw-Hill.
Orque, M. (1983) Nursing care of South Vietnamese patients. In Orque, M., Bloch, B. and Monrroy, L. (eds), *Ethnic Nursing Care.* St Louis: Mosby.
Parr, M. (1993) The Neuman Health Care Systems Model: an evaluation. *British Journal of Theatre Nursing,* **3** (8), 20–27.
Pearson, A. and **Vaughan, B.** (1986) *Nursing Models for Practice.* London: Heinemann.
Peplau, H. (1952) *Interpersonal Relationships in Nursing.* New York: Putnam.
Price, P. (1993) Parents' perceptions of the meaning of quality nursing care. *Advanced Nursing Science,* **16** (1), 33–41.
Reeve, J. (1994) Nurses' attitudes towards health care assistants. *Nursing Times,* **90** (26), 43–46.
Richardson, A. (1992) Studies exploring self-care for the person coping with cancer: a review. *International Journal of Nursing Studies,* **29** (2), 191–204.
Robertson, J. (1958) *Young Children in Hospital.* London: Tavistock.
Robinson, R. (1996) A state of confusion. *Paediatric Nursing,* **8** (7), 6.
Roper, W., Logan, N. and **Tierney, A.** (1980) *The Elements of Nursing.* Edinburgh: Churchill Livingstone.
Royal College of Nursing (2002) *Lack of Training Places Causes Chronic Shortage of Children's Nurses.* RCN Press release, 13 December.
Royal College of Nursing (2003) *Children and Young People's Services.* London: Royal College of Nursing.
Rushton, C. (1993) Child/family advocacy; ethical issues, practical strategies. *Critical Care Medicine,* **21** (9), 387–388.
Sams, D. (1996) The development of leadership skills in clinical practice. *Nursing Times,* **92** (28), 37–39.
Shah, R. (1992) *The Silent Minority.* London: National Children's Bureau.
Shah, R. (1994) Practice with attitude. *Child Health,* **1** (6), 245–249.
Stenbak, E. (1986) *Care of Children in Hospital.* Geneva: WHO.
Stopes-Roe, R. and **Cochrane, R.** (1989) Traditionalism in the family: a comparison between Asian and British cultures and between generations. *Journal of Comparative Family Studies,* **21**, 141–158.
Strong, S. (1997) Peripheral parents. *Nursing Times,* **93** (4), 20–21.
Swanwick, M. (1996) Child rearing across cultures. *Paediatric Nursing,* **8** (7), 13–17.
Teasdale, K. (1987) Partnership with patients? *Professional Nurse,* September, 17–19.
Thornes, R. (1988a) *Hidden Children – An Analysis of Ward Attenders in Children's Wards.* London: Caring for Children in the Health Services Consortium.
Thornes, R. (1988b) *Parents Staying Overnight with their Children.* London: Caring for Children in the Health Services Consortium.
Thornes, R. (1991) *Just for the Day – Children Admitted to Hospital for Treatment.* London: Caring for Children in the Health Services Consortium.
United Kingdom Central Council (UKCC) (1986) *Project 2000 – A New Preparation for Practice.* London: UKCC.
United Kingdom Central Council (UKCC) (1990) *The Report of the Post-registration Education and Practice Project.* London: UKCC.
United Kingdom Central Council (UKCC) (1992) *The Scope of Professional Practice.* London: UKCC.
United Kingdom Central Council (UKCC) (1994a) *PREP – Government Support for UKCC Proposals.* London: UKCC.
United Kingdom Central Council (UKCC) (1994b) *PREP – Standards for Post-registration Education and Practice.* London: UKCC.
United Kingdom Central Council (UKCC) (1996) PREP – putting the record straight. *Register,* **18**, 6–7.
University of Manchester Health Services Management Unit (1996) *The Future Health-care Work Force.* Manchester: University of Manchester.
Vaughan, B. and **Edwards, M.** (1994) *The Research Practice Interface.* London: King's Fund Centre.
Walker, C. (1990) Siblings of children with cancer. *Oncology Nurses Forum,* **17** (3), 355–360.
Walsh, M. and **Ford, P.** (1994) *New Rituals for Old: Nursing through the Looking Glass.* Oxford: Butterworth-Heinemann.
Watt, S. and **Norton, D.** (2004) Culture, ethnicity, race: what's the difference? *Paediatric Nursing,* **16** (8), 37–42.
Webb, Y., *et al.* (2002) Nursing the nurses: why staff need support. *Nursing Times,* **98** (16), 36–37.
Weir, L. (1993) Using Orem's model. *British Journal of Theatre Nursing,* **3** (6), 19–22.
Weller, B. (1994) Cultural aspects of children's health and illness. In Lindsay, B. (ed.), *The Child and Family: Contemporary Issues in Child Health.* London: Balliere Tindall.
Whitehead, M. (1992) *The Health Divide.* Harmondsworth: Penguin.
Whitehead, N. (1995) Behavioural paediatrics. In Broome, A. and Llewelyn, S. (eds), *Health Psychology,* 2nd edn. London: Chapman & Hall.
Wood, C. (1888) *The Training of Nurses for Sick Children.* London: Great Ormond Street Hospital for Sick Children.
Wooton, S. (1997) The reflective process as a tool for learning: a personal account. *Paediatric Nursing,* **9** (2), 6–8.
Wright, S. (1990) *Building and Using a Model of Nursing,* 2nd edn. London: Edward Arnold.
Wyke, S. and **Hewison, J.** (eds) (1991) *Child Health Matters.* Milton Keynes: Open University Press.
Ygge, B. and **Arnetz, J.** (2004) A study of parental involvement in pediatric hospital care: implications for clinical practice. *Journal of Pediatric Nursing,* **19** (3), 217–223.

Module 8
Legal and Ethical Issues

Judith Hendrick

Learning Outcomes

The material contained within this module and the references should enable you to:

- understand the legal and ethical principles that underpin children's nursing
- evaluate critically the relationship between law and ethics, in particular their interaction in resolving problems that arise in practice
- consider the limitations of legal intervention
- explore the way in which legal and ethical aspects of children's nursing differ from those of adult nursing
- analyse critically the extent to which children's rights are upheld in a variety of practice settings.

Introduction

The 1989 United Nations Convention on the Rights of the Child has been described as a landmark in the history of childhood, not least because it was so universally welcomed. In fact, the response to it was so enthusiastic that more countries signed up to it more rapidly than was the case with any other international instrument. Closer to home, the Children Act, which was also passed in 1989, received similar support. Hailed as a children's charter, it went further than any other previous legislation in highlighting children's autonomy, acknowledging their independent status and legitimating them as persons rather than objects of concern. Its fundamental principle, however, is the paramountcy of children's welfare. All its provisions, in one way or other, aim to ensure that children's best interests are always at the forefront. The impact for health professionals of this basic premise cannot be overestimated as it affects every aspect of children's health care and includes both legal and ethical principles.

This module will begin by examining the nature and scope of the law of consent and the extent to which it enhances children's autonomy. It will examine the complex legal and ethical issues that arise when children, or those who care for them, refuse life-saving treatment. The next section will explore those aspects of the Children Act 1989 and subsequent legislation such as the Human Rights Act 1998, which increase children's involvement in decision making – in particular their participation and independence rights. The concept of parental responsibility will also be examined. Other sections in this module look at children and confidentiality, the legal and ethical principles underpinning research, the role of law in allocating resources and the extent to which it can be used in guaranteeing access to health care. The relationship between law and ethics in regulating and maintaining standards of professional practice is examined. Finally, the issue of children's rights and their implementation in practice is explored.

Ethical issues terminology

- Beneficence – doing that which will produce benefit.
- Non-maleficence – doing that which will cause no harm.
- Justice – doing that which respects and acts upon a person's rights. Fairness.
- Autonomy – the quality of having the ability to function independently.
- Deontology – concerned with duty, focusing on the actions rather than their consequences.
- Consequentialism – concerned with the nature of the outcome of one's actions.

Chapter 60

Legal and Ethical Issues

Consent to Treatment

The right to consent to (or refuse) treatment is one of the most well established and cherished of 'medical rights', which has long been protected by the law – at least in relation to adults. Recently described as a 'basic human right' (*Yf* v. *Turkey* 2004 39 EHRR 34) it was first expressly recognised in a 1914 American case (*Schloendorff* v. *Society of New York Hospital* 105 NE 92 (NY, 1914)) when the judge said: 'Every human being of adult years and sound mind has a right to determine what shall be done with his own body; and a surgeon who performs an operation without the patient's consent commits an assault'.

Since then the English courts have repeatedly confirmed that the unauthorised invasion of bodily integrity can give rise to a civil action for damages and may even result in criminal liability. The right to bodily integrity is, of course, also enshrined in almost all medical and research codes of ethics. However, why is the right to consent (which is usually referred to as 'informed consent') regarded as inviolable? Several reasons are usually advanced. One is that it protects health professionals from legal action even if the touching of a patient is designed to 'help' her. Another is its therapeutic benefit, namely that it helps secure the patient's cooperation and trust. A third reason is that it enables individuals to be responsible for their own choices. In short, it is the way patients exercise autonomy. As Mason and Laurie (2006) state: 'the seriousness with which the law views any invasion of physical integrity is based on the strong moral conviction that everyone has the right of self-determination with regard to his body'.

The word 'autonomy' is commonly defined very broadly as 'self-determination', 'being your own person' and 'self-rule'. It is highly valued in modern Western society and many of the legal requirements of consent are based on this principle. But autonomy is a complex concept with ancient roots. Our modern understanding of the concept, however, is more recent and dates mainly from the works of two great philosophers – Immanuel Kant (a deontologist) and John Stuart Mill (a

The United Nations Convention on the Rights of the Child

This assures respect for a child's view under **Article 12**, which states that: 'the child who is capable of forming his or own views [has] the right to express those views freely in all matters affecting the child, the views of the child being given due weight in accordance with the age and maturity of the child'.

It should be noted that **Article 12** does not guarantee autonomy but refers to consultation and participation rights.

utilitarian). Its basic idea can, none the less, be summed up in the phrase 'freedom of thought, will and action'. Put simply this means that individuals should have the right to do whatever it is they want to do with their lives (live out their 'life plan'). In other words, they should be able to control their lives by thinking for themselves, deciding what to do (or not to do) and acting on their decisions.

Few would disagree, too, with the general principle of respect for autonomy (which basically means treating people as persons with rights and not as objects of care) given the benefits it is said to confer. These include not just increasing personal well-being by enabling people to lead happier, more fulfilling lives but also by treating people never simply as means to ends but as ends in themselves – preventing coercion, exploitation and oppression. However, when applied to children and young people, these benefits are commonly questioned. This is partly because of the obvious developmental differences between children and adults (which cannot be ignored) but also because of the myths and assumptions about the nature of childhood (likewise the proper role of parents and health professionals) and misconceptions about children's abilities, needs, and desires for autonomy. It is claimed, for example, that children lack the developed sense of self that an autonomous person requires, or that they lack the ability to make rational choices or the experience to make wise ones. As such they do not have a will of their own but must rely on others to make decisions for them. However, as Fortin (2003) notes in her review of research on the way children and young people think and reason, there is now clear evidence that, as children mature, they become increasingly able to cope with abstractions and so can think and plan for the future. Research also makes it clear that although the typical 12- or 13-year-old cannot appreciate that there may be more than one solution to a problem and that actions are not necessarily absolutely right or wrong, by the age of 14 or 15 the average adolescent is not just more self-reflective but is also able to think more critically and pragmatically.

This does not mean that all children should be forced to make decisions against their will or always have the final say, because respect for autonomy is not an absolute principle but is a matter of degree. Thus, if treatment is complex and carries serious risks, respecting autonomy may involve no more than letting the child express his or her wishes freely. It may even be appropriate to refer the decision to someone else. However, if the treatment is relatively minor a child's wishes could be determinative despite opposition (parental or otherwise).

Study activity

Consider the extent to which children ought to be allowed to take responsibility for decisions regarding treatment. Child C, for example, is an average 13-year-old. Giving your reasons, identify those medical treatments for which you feel he or she should be (a) solely responsible and (b) never responsible.

It seems self-evident, then, that autonomy is not an absolute principle. This raises several questions – for example, what kinds of things can undermine a person's autonomous choices? And to what extent do they justify paternalism? These are important questions, especially in relation to children when paternalistic interference (making a decision for someone else that involves either overriding their expressed wishes or not even consulting them) is not uncommon in practice.

People's capacity for autonomous action can be undermined because they are unable to make or communicate their decisions (this category would include, for example, unconscious patients, newborn babies and very young children). As such, there is no doubt that their autonomy is limited. But in other situations patients' autonomy may be limited because of serious doubts about whether they are competent. These kinds of concerns about capacity typically arise in respect of children and adolescents. Finally, there are those patients whose ability to make decisions is impaired because of short-term factors such as sedative medicine, pain, stress or fear.

Other factors that can limit autonomy include the need to balance the autonomy of health professionals with that of the patient. Case law has established, for example, that doctors are not obliged to give treatment that is against their better judgement. In other words, the courts have made it clear that they will not dictate to health professionals what treatment they should give. This important principle was first clearly established in the early 1990s in a series of cases involving severely brain-damaged babies. In *In Re J* [1992] 4 All ER 61, for example, doctors wanted to withhold life support from a profoundly handicapped baby who was microcephalic, had cerebral palsy, cortical blindness and severe epilepsy. J's mother wanted treatment to be continued as long as possible but the court rejected her claim. In more recent cases (for example, *A National Health Service Trust* v. *D* [2003] 2 FLR 677), although the courts have continued to refuse to order health professionals to provide treatment they consider to be futile, they have nevertheless displayed much more sensitivity to distressed parents than in the past. That said, these cases do highlight the potential for tension that exists between autonomy and the principle of beneficence. Beneficence, which basically means doing good for others, requires health professionals and parents to do whatever is necessary to promote and safeguard the welfare of child patients.

Despite this tension there is, none the less, increasing interdependence between the autonomy of health professionals and that of all patients. In relation to consent, this focuses in particular on the issue of information disclosure. To make informed choices patients need information – about the risks and benefits of proposed treatment, for example, and alternative options. Health professionals have a key role not only in deciding how much and what information to provide, but also in helping patients interpret and evaluate that information. This may mean, if the patient is young, ensuring that the information is given in an age-appropriate way, possibly with the help of dolls, storybooks, drawings and other aids (Alderson and Montgomery, 1996).

It should perhaps be evident by now that obtaining consent involves the application of both legal and ethical principles. The central concept is, however, that of competence (or capacity as it is also called). Yet, like terms such as 'maturity' and 'understanding', the concept of competence is essentially meaningless unless reference is made to the body of

Barriers to listening to children

- *Attitudes* – the greatest obstacles arise from prejudices about children's abilities, and beliefs that it is unwise or unkind or a waste of time to listen to children.
- *Scarce time and resources* – practical problems such as lack of time, or of a quiet place to talk, lack of pictures or of cards in other languages.
- *Lack of confidence* – professionals need to believe that it is possible and valuable to listen to children and that many children can cope with bad news and hard decisions.
- *Lack of skill* – failure to hear what young people have to say can result from adults' unwillingness to listen rather than children's inability to form and express their views.
- *Language barriers* – parents may act as two-way interpreters for younger children; explaining the child's terms and views to professionals and translating the technical language into words more familiar to the child.
- *Beyond words* – it is helpful to encourage children to express themselves in non-linguistic ways.
- *Collusion between adults and children* – professionals tend to communicate mainly with the parents and to young people this may appear like a collusion between adults.
- *The need for adults to feel in control* – adults may fear seeming to renege on their responsibility.

(Alderson and Montgomery, 1996:58)

The NMC Code of Professional Conduct: Standard for Conduct, Performance and Ethics (2004) states:

Clause 3.1

all patients have a right to receive information about their condition. You must be sensitive to their needs and respect the wishes of those who refuse or are unable to receive information about their condition. Information should be accurate, truthful and presented in such a way as to make it easily understood.

Clause 3.9

in relation to obtaining consent for a child, the involvement of those with parental responsibility in the consent procedure is usually necessary, but will depend on the age and understanding of the child. If the child is under 16 in England and Wales, 12 in Scotland and 17 in Northern Ireland, you must be aware of legislation and local protocols relating to consent.

research on children's developmental processes. That said, in practice the following questions are usually raised when a child's or adolescent's capacity is in issue:

- Is the child 'Gillick' competent?
- Who assesses competence?
- If a child is not competent, who has the right to make a decision on the child's behalf?
- What if there is a disagreement?

Before looking at these aspects in detail it is important to outline the general legal elements of consent.

General Legal Principles

Consent must be effectively obtained

With very few exceptions, the law does not prescribe what form consent to medical treatment should take. This means that it can either be express or implied, written or oral. For routine minor procedures consent is usually obtained verbally and may well be implied, such as when patients roll up their sleeves for an injection. More serious procedures, especially involving surgery, will normally be preceded by written consent using a standard NHS consent form. Whatever the form of consent, it can be withdrawn at any time before or even during the relevant medical procedure. If this happens a fresh consent must be obtained.

Consent must be voluntary

To be legally valid consent must be freely given. In other words it must be given without force, undue pressure or influence. This aspect of consent has been described as one of the foundation stones of consent, which imposes on professionals a high ethical obligation. In practice, whether or not consent is genuine will depend on several factors including the effect of pain, tiredness, drugs and so on. The relationship of the 'persuader' to the patient may also be crucial, especially if he or she is a parent. Note, too, that the notion of voluntary consent is more subtle than might first appear because, although arm twisting and overt threats are not part of medical practice, patients, especially children, can be subject to more complicated forms of pressure. They may be overanxious, for example, or easily embarrassed.

Sufficient information must be given

The importance of exercising choice is acknowledged by the requirements the law imposes in respect of information disclosure. Although no precise legal test has ever been established, broad guidelines were set out in *Sidaway* v. *Bethlem Royal Hospital Governors* [1985] 1 All ER 643. Briefly, this case established that patients need only be told what health professionals think they should be told. This means that it is the medical profession itself that decides what should (or should not) be revealed. Until recently, this so-called 'professional standard' of disclosure was favoured by English courts. But there are signs that this may be changing as, in more and more cases (for example, *Smith* v. *Tunbridge Wells HA* [1994] 5 Med LR 334; *Pearce* v. *United Bristol Healthcare Trust* [1999] 48 BMLR 118; *Chester* v. *Afshar* [2005] 1 AC 134), they have adopted a more patient-friendly approach, which obliges professionals to disclose what 'reasonable' patients would want to know.

Legal definition of treatment

Surgical, medical or dental treatment as well as examination, investigation and diagnostic procedures (and any other procedure which is ancillary to such treatment such as anesthesia).

(S.8, Family Law Reform Act 1969)

Legal definition of voluntary consent

. . . the real question in each case is: 'Does the patient really mean what he says or is he merely saying it for a quiet life or to satisfy someone else or because the advice and persuasion to which he has been subjected is such that he can no longer think and decide for himself?' In other words 'Is it a decision expressed in form only, not in reality?'

(Lord Donaldson in *In re T* [1992] 3, WLR 782, p. 797)

Study activity

What information does the current standard DH/NHS Consent Form No. 2 (used to document consent to a child's treatment, where that consent is being given by a person with parental responsibility) require health professionals to give?

The combined effect of case law and current advice from the DH is that:

- Patients must be given enough information to make a balanced judgement – that is, they should be told in broad terms about the nature and purpose of the procedure, its likely risks – in particular those that are 'material' or 'significant' (those that would affect the judgement of a reasonable patient) – any alternatives to proposed treatment and the risks incurred by doing nothing.
- Patients who ask direct questions should be answered truthfully. As Lord Wolfe said in *Pearce* v. *United Bristol Healthcare NHS Trust* [1999] 48 BMLR 118: 'it is clear that if a patient asks a doctor about a risk, then the doctor is required to give an honest answer'.
- In some circumstances it is lawful to withhold information. This is known as 'therapeutic' privilege and is justified when revealing certain facts would merely serve to distress or confuse the patient (Mason and Laurie, 2006).
- Information for children should be given in a way that is appropriate for their age and understanding.

Study activity

Do you think 'therapeutic' privilege is more likely to be relied on in respect of child patients? If so is it justified? Can you think of examples in your practice?

Patients must be mentally competent

This aspect of the law of consent is still controversial because, even though it was assumed that the Gillick case (1986) and the Children Act 1989 had settled once and for all the question of when children could or could not consent to treatment, developments in the law since then have shown that the law's commitment to children's autonomy is far from strong. To explain how the law operates it is necessary to distinguish between children of various age groups and whether they are giving or refusing consent.

16- and 17-year-olds

Giving consent

The Family Law Reform Act 1969 (Section 8) applies to this age group. It sets a presumptive standard in that 16- and 17-year-olds are presumed (like adults) to be competent unless the contrary is shown. The current test for capacity is set out in *Re. C* [1994] 1 All ER 819. This states that an adult (a person over 16) is competent if he or she can (a) understand and retain information, especially as to the likely consequences of having or not having the treatment, and (b) use and weigh up this information in reaching a decision. This approach to assessing capacity has now been enshrined in the Mental Capacity Act 2005 – although the Act is not expected to come into force until 2007 at the earliest. But even if 16- and 17-year-olds are competent, the courts (but not parents) retain their protective role and can veto their consent. If young people in this age group are not competent, consent can be given by a proxy – usually a parent or someone with 'parental responsibility'.

Refusing consent

Although some might think it illogical to distinguish between a young person's ability to consent to treatment and the ability to refuse, in that 'the right to say yes must carry the right to say no', the courts are content to make such a distinction. Thus even though they are competent, 16- and 17-year-olds can have their 'informed refusal' overridden. This was established in *Re. W* [1992] 4 All ER 627 in which a 16-year-old girl suffering from anorexia nervosa had her refusal of treatment overridden by the court. Her weight was dangerously low and without treatment her reproductive organs were likely to be damaged. Her life was also in danger. The court held she was not competent because her condition had affected her ability to make a decision about treatment. More controversial, however, were the general principles it laid down about how future cases involving refusal of treatment by young people under 18 should be resolved. Briefly, these were that even if they were competent, their refusal could be overridden – not just by a court but by parents (or anyone else with parental responsibility) as well. In other words health professionals could rely on the consent of a proxy.

Several reasons are usually advanced to justify the courts' paternalistic interference in cases like *Re. W*. A common one is that refusing consent may close down the options. Another is 'that while consent involves the acceptance of an experienced view, refusal rejects that experience – and does so from a position of limited understanding' (Mason and Laurie, 2006:372).

But when parents or the court override a competent young person's consent they must act in his or her 'best interests'. This phrase is essentially a subjective term and has yet to be defined precisely. It is nevertheless clear from case law that it includes: (a) medical interests – the nature of treatment, chances of success, suffering and risks, quality of life; and (b) general interests – family relationships, educational benefits, financial benefits. Reference should also be made to the 'welfare checklist' in s.1(3) of the Children Act 1989. Clearly then the 'best interests' test would include therapeutic treatment. Whether other treatment, such as cosmetic surgery, would be in a child's best interests would depend on the particular circumstances of each case.

Study activity

It has been suggested that an adolescent forced to undergo treatment may be able to invoke the Human Rights Act 1998 and claim that Articles 3 and 5 have been breached. What do you think?

Under-16s – 'Gillick' competent

Giving consent

The right of competent under-16-year-olds to give consent was established in the Gillick case. This landmark decision acknowledged the independent right of mature young people to control their own health care and introduced the concept of Gillick competence. Within a short time the concept was applied to all medical treatment, not just contraceptive care. However, despite being widely used both in the literature and in practice there is still some debate about what the concept means and what level of competence the law requires children to achieve in individual cases. In short, it is a very imprecise and flexible concept. Perhaps this is not surprising as competence for decision making in medical contexts will vary enormously, depending on a variety of factors, such as the nature of the proposed treatment, peer pressure and family environment. That said, research on the way children and young people think and reason suggests that, bearing in mind the elements required for competent decision making (namely choice, comprehension, creativity, compromise, consequentiality, correctness, credibility, consistency and commitment), the majority of older adolescents are equipped with developmental skills for relatively sophisticated decision making (Fortin, 2003:73).

Study activity

Read *Re. P (a minor)* [1986] 1 FLR 272, in which the court agreed that a schoolgirl aged 15 should be allowed to have an abortion despite her parents' opposition. Do you agree with the court's decision?

Deciding when a parent's right to decide should yield to the child's right to make his or her own decisions can, in practice, of course, be very difficult. None the less, respecting a young person's autonomy means at the very least finding out whether a child agrees with his or her parents' wishes. Finally it is important to note that a court (but not parents) can veto a Gillick-competent child's consent.

Refusing consent

It was assumed, following the Gillick case, that young people under 16 who were competent to give consent were also legally entitled to refuse it. However, recent case law has shown that respecting the autonomy of mature under-16-year-olds does not entitle them to refuse treatment – at least not if it is life saving and offers the child a chance, however slim, of surviving. This means that Gillick-competent children under 16 years old can have their informed refusal overridden (until they are 18) by a

Human Rights Act 1998

Article 3: Prohibition of torture
No-one shall be subjected to torture or to inhuman or degrading treatment.

Article 5: Right to liberty and security
Everyone has the right to liberty and security of person.

The Gillick case

In *Gillick* v. *West Norfolk and Wisbech Area Health Authority* [1985] 3 All ER 402, the House of Lords held that young people under 16 could give consent to contraceptive advice without their parents' knowledge or consent providing they had 'suffcient maturity and intelligence' to understand the proposed treatment. Points to note about the Gillick test include:

- It applies to all medical treatment, not just contraception.
- Although there is no automatic age-based cutoff, capacity will normally increase with age.
- The level of competence required will vary depending on the nature of the proposed treatment.
- Competence, according to *In re R.* [1991] 4 All ER 117 (a case involving fluctuating capacity), is a developmental concept that must be assessed on a broad long-term basis, taking into account a child's whole medical history, background and mental state. As such, no child who is only competent on a good day can pass the Gillick test.

court or any person with parental responsibility and so may be lawfully treated against their will. In the few cases to reach the courts when parents, their children or health professionals have disagreed about treatment, the courts have, nevertheless, stressed how important it is to consider the young person's views. It is also clear from these cases that the courts have demanded a very sophisticated level of maturity. Note, too, that, as with 16- and 17-year-olds, it is only lawful to override refusal of consent if the proposed treatment is in the child's best interests. In *Re. E* [1993] 1 FLR 386, for example, a Jehovah's Witness boy aged nearly 16 was refusing (as were his parents) a life-saving blood transfusion urgently needed to treat his leukaemia. The judge imposed a very strict competency test, which few adults could have achieved – it required him to consider the manner in which he might die and the extent of his and his family's suffering. Accordingly he was not competent and so he could be treated despite his opposition.

Study activity

Fortin (2003:134) suggests that society has an interest in protecting young people from their own mistakes and that it might be more honest to accept that a patient is Gillick competent but to override his or her wishes all the same. Do you agree?

Children under 16 – not 'Gillick' competent

Permission for treatment for children in this group must come from a proxy – normally a person with parental responsibility or, exceptionally, someone who is temporarily looking after the child. If there is no such person, or if they are refusing to give consent, an application should be made to court to resolve the issue. The guiding principle is, of course, the child's best interests. In the vast majority of cases this is not problematic. However, what if, in the opinion of health professionals, they chose an option that is contrary to the child's welfare? This is when a court may be involved, as happened in the controversial case of *Re. T* [1997] 1 All ER 906. In this case parents of a child suffering from biliary atresia, a life-threatening liver defect, refused a liver transplant. In an unprecedented ruling the court upheld the parents' refusal even though medical opinion supported a transplant (which would have given the child a number of years beyond his current prognosis).

Consent and the Children Act 1989

When the Children Act 1989 was passed it was hailed as a children's charter not least because several of its provisions, enshrined the spirit of Gillick, appeared to give mature young people an absolute right of informed refusal to medical, psychiatric examinations (and exceptionally also treatment). It was not long, however, before the courts intervened and showed their willingness to override those provisions. This was in the case of *South Glamorgan CC* v. *B and W* [1993] 1 FLR 574 (see box). The Glamorgan decision was a controversial one – but has since been followed (see *Re. C (Detention: Medical treatment)* [1997] 2 FLR 180 p. 00) – in that it undermined the clear intention of the Children Act 1989. It is therefore not surprising that some commentators, for example Fortin (2003), have argued that it is doubtful whether such a decision would now survive a challenge under the Human Rights Act 1998.

Before concluding this section on consent it is worth noting the position in Scotland which, unlike the rest of the UK, has yet to litigate the issue of competent young people refusing treatment. It is suggested that certain historical factors and Scottish legislation may give young people greater control over medical decision making.

Key Points

1. Obtaining consent involves the application of both legal and ethical principles.
2. Assessing children's competence is a complex process, which requires consideration of their ability to understand that there are choices, and a willingness to make such choices.
3. Definitions and assessments of competence vary widely but good practice requires clear guidance as to the factors that should be considered as relevant or irrelevant to the assessment of legal competence.
4. In some circumstances it may be justifiable to override the wishes of a competent child.
5. The ultimate forum for resolving disputes about a child's medical treatment is the court and children should have the opportunity to explain to a judge the reasons for their refusal of consent.

Provisions in the Children Act 1989 concerning examinations

Children with sufficient understanding to make an informed decision can refuse to submit to medical, psychiatric examinations or other assessments:

- interim care order
- interim supervision order
- full supervision order (this order also covers treatment)
- child assessment order
- emergency protection order

The facts of *South Glamorgan CC* v. *B and W* [1993]

A 15-year-old girl with severe behavioural problems had refused to undergo various medical and psychiatric examinations under the Children Act 1989. She had confined herself to the front room of her father's house with the curtains drawn for approximately 11 months and had hardly had any contact with the outside world. If her family refused to obey her instructions, she threatened to commit suicide or harm herself. Despite being assessed as competent, her informed refusal was overridden by the court because without being examined it felt that she was likely to suffer serious harm.

Chapter 61

Children Act 1989

There is little doubt that the Children Act 1989 is the most comprehensive and far-reaching reform of child law of the past century. The legislation replaced a confusing and complex system with a simpler and much more comprehensive code. Most importantly, the Act attempted to bring about a new beginning to the philosophy and practices of the childcare system. In particular it was designed to strike a 'new' balance between the role of the state, the rights of children and the responsibilities of parents. The Act was built on several fundamental principles. These include the following:

- The welfare principle. This is a 'golden thread' running through the Act. It emphasises that children come first and that their interests must be the paramount consideration whenever a court makes a decision about their upbringing.
- The primacy of the family. Many of the Act's provisions reflect the belief that the best place for children to grow up is with their families. Overall these provisions aim to ensure that the state should only intervene in family life when it is absolutely necessary – when it is the only way to protect a child. Local authorities are therefore expected to do all they can to keep families together and children living at home.
- The child's voice. Throughout the Act there are sections that aim to enhance children's legal status and capacity for independent action. This is achieved mainly by giving them greater rights than in the past to have their views taken into account.

The Children Act was hailed as a children's charter because, unlike previous legislation dealing with children, it relied far less on notions of paternalism, which viewed children as defenceless and vulnerable objects of welfare in need of protection. Instead, although there is no specific reference to children's rights in the Act itself, it did seem to be the first statute to take the notion of rights seriously in relation to children and young people. As such they were no longer possessions over whom power was exercised but individuals to whom duties were owed.

Children Act 1989

1. Welfare of the child

(1) When a court determines any question with respect to

(a) the upbringing of a child; or

(b) the administration of a child's property or the application of any income arising from it, the child's welfare shall be the court's paramount consideration

(2) In any proceedings in which any question with respect to the upbringing of a child arises, the court shall have regard to the general principle that any delay in determining the question is likely to prejudice the welfare of the child.

However, not all commentators agreed with this assessment of the Act even if, as Bainham (2005:30) points out, the Act remains the most important single source of child law. Thus Fortin (2003), for example, argues that despite an attempt to liberalise the parent–child relationship by a change of language, the Act essentially adopted a non-interventionist approach to family life. Indeed, she claims the Act reflected an exaggerated legislative 'hands off' approach to family democracy (Fortin, 2003:9). Freeman (2000) similarly questions whether the Act can be considered 'successful' in so far as it seems to have failed in practice to put children's interest sufficiently to the fore (see also Bainham, 2005:Chapter 2). Concerns such as these reflect fears that the Children Act 'privatised' the family and thus could not provide adequate protection for all children 'in need'. This is perhaps why the child protection framework put in place by the Act has been significantly amended by the Children Act 2004.

As regards children's autonomy, the main provisions in the Act, which are particularly significant, are (a) those that increase their involvement in decision making (participation rights) and (b) those that recognise their capacity for independent action (independence rights). However, the concept of 'parental responsibility' is also worth noting in this context, largely because it reflects the tension between children's autonomy and their welfare and so also has implications for the exercise of their rights.

Study activity

How does s.17 of the Children Act 1989 define a 'child in need'?

Participation Rights

Participation rights have several advantages. First, they are relatively unconditional in that children do not have to pass any competency test before they express their wishes. Secondly, even very young children can be informed and involved. Thirdly, children can avoid the burden of being blamed for wrong decisions despite having their say. However, participation rights also have their disadvantages, notably being used to deny children the greater status of autonomous individuality. An unequivocal commitment to autonomy could have been assured by making the wishes of mature young people determinative. But, except in relation to medical and psychiatric examinations and assessments (which, as was shown in the previous section, the courts have since eroded), the Act did not adopt this approach. Instead it gives children the 'right' to be consulted – to be heard and so have the opportunity to express their wishes and feelings. In practice what this should mean is that there is less chance that children's views will be ignored.

The main vehicle for the child's voice in the Act is the 'welfare checklist'. Introduced to improve and standardise the way court decisions are made, the checklist requires the courts to have regard to 'the ascertainable wishes and feelings of the child concerned (considered in the light

Welfare Checklist Section 1(3) Children Act 1989

Ascertainable wishes and feelings of the child (considered in the light of his age and understanding), his physical, emotional and educational needs, the likely effect of any change in circumstances, his age, sex, background and any personal characteristics which the court considers relevant, any harm which he has suffered or is at risk of suffering, how capable each of his parents (or any other person in relation to whom the court considers the question to be relevant) is of meeting his needs, the range of powers available to the court under the Act in the proceedings in question.

Paramountcy test: Section 1(1) Children Act 1989

When a court determines any question with respect to

(a) the upbringing of a child; or
(b) the administration of a child's property or the application of any income arising from it, the child's welfare shall be the court's paramount consideration.

of his age and understanding)'. This factor is the first in a list of seven. Its prominence suggests that it is the most important one, but this is misleading because they all carry equal weight. More importantly the child's wishes do not have to be followed, even though they can strongly influence the outcome of a case and, in some cases, they may well be decisive, provided the court agrees that the child's best interests are thereby promoted. In practice, of course, the weight to be attached to a child's views will depend on the child's maturity and the nature of the issue in question. But, as Herring (2004) points out, even if a court thinks a child's views to be mistaken, it may still be appropriate to follow such views. There are two main reasons why a judge may do this. First, practical considerations may be very persuasive. Thus teenagers could simply ignore a court order that they oppose. Secondly, a judge may consider it beneficial for a child to learn from his or her mistakes. As Butler-Sloss LJ, a leading family court judge, famously said: 'nobody should dictate to mature minors, because one is dealing with their emotions, their lives, and they are not packages to move around. They are people entitled to be treated with respect' (*Re. S (Access: Religious Upbringing)* [1992] 2 FLR 313).

The Act also significantly increases children's rights to be consulted when they are in the public care system – being cared for away from home, for example by foster parents or a children's home. Hence, local authorities now have to find out children's views both before making a decision about their future care and when their case is reviewed. Changes introduced by the Children Act 2004 also stress the importance of considering a child's wishes before services are provided (under s.17 of the Children Act 1989).

Importantly, though, despite the fact that children's participation rights are at least specifically acknowledged in the welfare checklist, they are still subject to the so-called 'paramountcy test' enshrined in s.1(1) of the Act. This is essentially a paternalistic formula that can be used to override a child's autonomy. As a consequence, so Diduck and Kaganas (2006:610) claim, the ability of young people to participate effectively is limited – not least because the courts seem uncomfortable with the notion of a child as an active participant in decision making. Whether the establishment of the office of Children's Commissioner (by the Children Act 2004) will ensure a voice for children at national level remains to be seen.

Independence Rights

Other provisions appear to acknowledge children's capacity for independent action. As such they arguably create the possibility that children can, in practice, enforce their own substantive rights. Thus children now have the right to initiate court action by, for example, challenging an emergency protection order or asking for a care (and supervision) order to be discharged. Perhaps even more significant is their 'right' to seek the court's permission to apply for a so-called Section 8 order – one relating to their own health care, for example, or with whom they should live. But these (and other Section 8 orders) can only be sought if the court considers that the child has 'sufficient understanding to make an application'. Designed to filter out inappropriate applications, this leave requirement has been restrictively interpreted and in practice it is rare for children to bring applications successfully before the court (Herring, 2004). In other words by linking children's empowerment to competence the courts can (by requiring a relatively high degree of understanding) deny young people the right to be treated as autonomous individuals, at least in this context.

Section 8 orders (Children Act 1989)

- Contact – regulates contact between a child and another person, usually a parent with whom the child is not living.
- Residence – settles with whom the child lives.
- Prohibited steps – prevents something being done without the court's permission.
- Specific issue – settles a single issue that has arisen in respect of a child's upbringing.

Study activity

- Which Section 8 order could be applied for to prevent controversial medical treatment such as sterilisation of a child?
- Find out which Section 8 order health professionals can apply for in respect of a child patient and how they might go about doing this.

Parental Responsibility

This term is a central concept in the Act. It describes the legal authority parents have over their children and replaces the phrase 'parental rights' in earlier legislation. According to Diduck and Kaganas (2006) this change of terminology – from rights to responsibilities – was no surprise in that it reflected the direction in which the law was already developing even before the Act was enacted.

The Act does not define parental responsibility in any detail nor does it list the things parents can or cannot do. This is an omission that has been criticised because 'it suggests a misplaced complacency over the existing state of family values' and re-emphasises the privacy of the family (Fortin, 2003:276).

Definition of parental responsibility Section 3(1)

'All rights, duties, powers, responsibility and authority which by law a parent of a child has in relation to the child and his property.'

Furthermore, detailed legislative guidance would have been useful not just to parents but also childcare practitioners. The absence of written rules means that the scope and nature of the concept remains uncertain. Nevertheless it is usually accepted that those with parental responsibility can take the following decisions:

- Providing a home – deciding how to meet a child's physical needs and emotional needs. It thus includes making major decisions such as where a child lives as well as more mundane ones, such as what he or she should eat.
- Contact. This is especially important for parents who are not living with their children because it entitles them (subject to any court order to the contrary) to see and spend time with them. In some cases contact can be limited and consist of telephone calls or letters. It is generally assumed, however, that children benefit from continued contact with both parents.
- Discipline. Disciplining a child includes using corporal punishment and other forms of punishment. The law on hitting children has been modified by s.58 of the Children Act 2004, which came into effect in January 2005. But because the new law continues to give parents a legal defence of 'reasonable punishment' the NSPCC is campaigning for further reforms, claiming that the law still sends out the wrong message – that hitting children is lawful. Note, too, that corporal

punishment is banned in most schools and whenever children are being looked after by a local authority and living away from their families.

- Religious upbringing. Parents have the right to decide what religious faith their child should follow, if any. But, parental choice will not prevail over the strongly held religious views of a mature child.
- Name. Although it is usual, it is not obligatory for a child of married parents to take the father's surname.
- Education. Parents have a wide discretion in deciding how to educate their children, although some form of education is compulsory for school-age children (between 5 and 16). Most parents fulfil this obligation by sending their children to school (state or private). However, some opt out of the school system and educate their children themselves at home.
- Marriage. A child under 16 cannot get married. Those between 16 and 18 need parental consent.
- Consent to medical treatment. Subject to the rights of competent 16- and 17-year-olds and 'Gillick'-competent under 16-year-olds, those with parental responsibility have the right to consent and refuse medical treatment.

Who has parental responsibility?

The combined effect of the Children Act 1989 and the Adoption and Children Act 2002 is that the following have parental responsibility:

- both parents, if they are married
- the mother, even if she is not married to the father
- the father who has made a parental responsibility agreement, has been granted a parental responsibility order or who has registered the birth jointly with the mother
- a step-parent (by agreement or court order)
- adoptive parents
- 'special' and ordinary guardians
- other people who have parental responsibility because of a court order, for example a residence order granted to grandparents or a care order granted to the local authority

How parental responsibility can be obtained by non-parents

Relatives, step-parents and local authorities can acquire parental responsibility through court orders such as residence orders, emergency protection orders and care orders.

Section 3(5) Children Act 1989

A person who (a) does not have parental responsibility for a particular child; but (b) has care of the child may (subject to the provisions of this Act) do what is reasonable in all the circumstances of the case for the purpose of safeguarding or promoting the child's welfare.

Limits to Parental Responsibility

Although the scope of parental responsibility is very broad, giving parents (and anyone else who has acquired it) extensive control over children's lives, it is not absolute. It is, in practice, subject to two major restrictions. The first is the welfare principle. In applying this principle the courts have made it clear that unless parental responsibility is exercised in accordance with that principle it can be challenged and even overridden. The second restriction is that parental responsibility diminishes as children mature and become more capable of making their own decisions. As the courts stressed in the Gillick case, the legal right of a parent ends at the eighteenth birthday, and even before then it is a dwindling right, which the courts will hesitate to enforce against the wishes of children the older they are. It starts with a right of control and ends with little more than advice.

Other People who may be Involved in a Child's Care

Foster parents

Foster parents look after children but do not have parental responsibility. They may have been appointed by a local authority or be caring for a child as a result of a private arrangement. Foster parents have no legal rights over children but they can make decisions about their day-to-day care by virtue of s.3(5) of the Children Act 1989.

De facto carers

This group covers a wide range of people who may be temporarily caring for a child, such as childminders, teachers, babysitters, relatives and so on. *De facto* carers do not have parental responsibility, but s.3(5) of the Children Act 1989 applies to them so they, too, can make day-to-day decisions. These are unlikely to be more than minor ones, however, and would cover such matters as discipline, and what the child eats and wears.

Study activity

A child of 3 years is brought into an A&E department by a nursery teacher and needs stitches on a leg wound. Her parents cannot be contacted. Who can give consent for the medical treatment?

Step-parents

Step-parents do not have parental responsibility even though they have been living with their step-child. However, again by virtue of s.3(5), they have the legal authority to make day-to-day decisions about a child's care, which given their parental role, are likely to more significant than those taken by temporary carers. Step-parents can acquire parental responsibility through, for example, a parental responsibility agreement or court order (or adoption).

Adoptive parents

Adoptive parents replace a child's biological parents and thus acquire parental responsibility. For legal purposes they are then treated as the child's legal parents and have all their rights and duties.

Special guardians

The status of special guardians was created by the Adoption and Children Act 2002. Special guardians engage in a form of foster-plus parenting. As such they are mainly designed for children looked after by a local authority (see s.14 A–G of the Children Act 1989).

Age-related Activities

Children acquire certain rights and powers at various different ages. Below are listed some of the most important. At any age children can:

- initiate proceedings under the Children Act 1989 (if they have sufficient understanding and maturity)
- choose their own religion (unless it is harmful)
- change their name (if they have the maturity to understand the implications of that decision)
- seek advice and counselling (if they are 'Gillick' competent)
- give consent to surgical, dental and medical treatment (if they are 'Gillick' competent)
- apply to see most personal files (whether on computer or held in manual form) provided they understand the nature of their request

- sue in court (through a 'litigation friend')
- borrow money
- inherit property
- make a complaint about discrimination (on the basis of race, colour, ethnic or national origin, or nationality; or on grounds of sex or marital status)
- make a complaint against the police
- have their bodies pierced
- babysit
- smoke cigarettes (but they cannot buy them until 16)
- enter a bingo club (but not take part in the game)
- take flying lessons

At 5 years children

- can drink alcohol in private
- must pay a child's fare on trains as well as buses and tubes
- must receive full-time education

At 7 children can

- open and draw money from a National Savings account or Trustee Savings Bank account

At 10 children can

- open a bank or building society account
- be convicted of a criminal offence
- in certain circumstances be searched, fingerprinted, have samples taken by the police
- if boys, be capable of committing any sexual offence, including rape

At 12 children can

- buy a pet
- be trained to participate in dangerous performances

At 14 children can

- obtain a part-time 'light-work' job (subject to several restrictions)
- ride a horse on a road without wearing protective headgear

At 16 children can

- buy aerosol paints
- enter a bar on their own, but only buy soft drinks
- leave school
- work full time (subject to certain restrictions)
- leave home
- marry with parental consent
- register as blood donors
- apply for their own passports (but one parent must give written consent)
- buy cigarettes, tobacco, liqueur chocolates, fireworks, premium bonds
- be street traders
- sell scrap metal
- enter or live in a brothel
- if young men, join the armed forces with parental consent

At 17 young people can

- hold a licence to drive certain vehicles (such as a car or small goods vehicle);
- donate blood without parental consent
- buy or hire any firearm or ammunition

At 18 young people reach the age of majority and can do most things, such as

- vote
- marry
- serve on a jury
- make a will
- own land, buy a house or flat or hold a tenancy
- buy and drink alcohol in a bar
- be tattooed
- donate their bodies or organs
- pawn goods at a pawn shop
- enter a betting shop and bet
- apply for a passport without parental consent

At 21 young people can

- adopt a child
- stand in a general or local election
- hold a licence to drive a lorry or bus

Further information about age-related activities can be obtained by contacting the Children's Legal Centre: www.childrenslegalcentre.com

Key Points

1. The key principles underpinning the Children Act 1989 are the paramountcy of the child's welfare, the empowerment of children, and the primacy of the family.
2. The Act's overall objective is to strike a new balance between the protection of children, the integrity of the family and the role of the state.
3. The welfare checklist emphasises the importance of consulting children.
4. The concept of parental responsibility emphasises the duties of parents rather than their rights.

Chapter 62
Confidentiality

To control their health care children need not only the right to consent to (or veto) medical treatment (see above) but also a right of control over personal health information. Laws on confidentiality help secure this control but, whereas the principle of confidentiality is one of the oldest in medical ethics and is also widespread in professional codes, research has shown that many teenagers are deterred from seeking professional help for personal and sexual issues because they fear a lack of confidentiality.

The duty to respect confidential information comes from several sources but what is its precise nature and scope? Put very simply, the duty of confidentiality means that health professionals must respect their patients' secrets. Rules of confidentiality are usually justified on two main grounds. One (the utilitarian or consequentialist argument) claims that unless patients feel that they can trust health professionals with potentially embarrassing information and are confident that it will not be divulged, they will fail to reveal certain details about themselves (which may be medically very important) or may be deterred from seeking medical care altogether. As a consequence their health may suffer, for without full information from patients health professionals cannot make accurate diagnoses and prognoses or recommend the best course of treatment.

The second common justification derives from the deontological school of philosophy. This claims that confidentiality should be respected because it is inherently right to do so. In other words, irrespective of welfare considerations, there are strong moral grounds for keeping information private and secure, notably respect for personal autonomy and fidelity (or promise keeping).

NMC Code of Professional Conduct: Standards for Conduct, Performance and Ethics (Clause 5.1)

You must treat information about patients and clients as confidential and use it only for the purposes for which it was given.

Consequentialist (or utilitarian) philosophy

This seeks to judge the morality of an act by its consequences. In simple terms, this means the right act is that which gives the greatest happiness to the greatest number.

Deontological philosophy

This holds that there are rules that govern actions and which tell us whether acts are inherently right or wrong irrespective of the consequences.

Study activity

Read the Confidentiality Code of Practice for NHS staff (DH, 2003a).

- How does it define confidentiality?
- Does it make any special reference to children in relation to confidentiality?

The principle of medical confidentiality is universally acknowledged even though no specific statute in English law defines when precisely a confidential relationship arises (but see the Human Rights Act 1998, Article 8, which protects respect for private life). That said, it is generally accepted that a duty of confidence arises where confidential information (for example, private health information) comes to the knowledge of a person (the confidant), in circumstances where that person has notice, or has agreed, that the information is confidential, with the effect that it would be just in all the circumstances that he or she should be stopped from disclosing the information to others. Confidential relationships can be either formal or informal. The most obvious formal confidential relationships arise between health professionals and their patients (likewise lawyers and their clients). Other relationships that could similarly be confidential arise in more informal settings, such as when a person uses a counselling service.

Legal duty of confidentiality

The law recognises a duty of confidentiality when:

- information is of a private or intimate nature
- information is given in a situation where it is obvious that it is expected to be kept secret
- protecting the information is in the public interest or the patient would suffer if the information was revealed

(Hendrick, 2004:116)

Human Rights Act 1998, Article 8

Everyone has the right to respect for his private and family life, home and correspondence.

Children and Confidentiality

Once an obligation to maintain confidentiality has arisen in law it is owed as much to young people under 18 as it is to any other person sufficiently mature to form a relationship of confidence. What this means is that, irrespective of a child's competence to consent to (or veto) treatment, they are none the less in principle legally owed a duty of confidence if they understand what it means to trust someone with secret information. This is, however, subject to any relevant exception (see below). Note, too, that even if the requested treatment is refused, the confidentiality of the consultation should still be respected. Put simply, competence and the duty of confidentiality are not necessarily connected. In some cases – for example, very young children – they will be neither competent nor mature enough to understand what keeping a secret means.

Study activity

Find out:

- whether children under 16 years old have to visit their own GP for contraceptive advice
- if a child under 16 years old receives contraceptive advice from another GP, whether his or her own GP has to be informed
- if it is lawful for community nurses, nurses, midwives and health visitors to give contraceptive advice to young people under 16
- where young people under 16 can obtain contraceptive advice and supplies

Exceptions to the Duty of Confidentiality

This section outlines the exceptions to the duty of confidentiality that are most relevant to children and young people. In other words we consider when it is both lawful and ethical to breach confidentiality. What this means is that, in some circumstances, the duty of confidentiality is

The NMC code of professional conduct: standards for conduct performance and ethics (2004)

Clause 5.3
If you are required to disclose information outside the team that will have personal consequences for patients or clients, you must obtain their consent. If the patient or client withholds consent, or if consent cannot be obtained for whatever reason, disclosures may be made only where:

- they can be justified in the public interest (usually where disclosure is essential to protect the patient or client or someone else from the risk of significant harm)
- they are required by law or by a court order

Clause 5.4
Where there is an issue of child protection, you must act at all times in accordance with national and local policies.

not absolute (as all professional codes of practice acknowledge). Any health professional who decides to breach a patient or client's confidence must, of course, justify that breach.

Consent of the patient

Consent can be expressed or implied, but in all cases must be freely given. If patients are too young or too immature, consent of a parent is acceptable providing it is in the child's interests. When a child is 'Gillick' competent then he or she has the independent legal right to consent to disclosure, providing he or she understands the consequences of information being revealed.

Disclosing information between health professionals (and others in the multi-agency team) on a need-to-know basis is usually justified on the assumption that patients realise that their welfare depends on relevant information being passed back and forth between all those involved in their care. It is therefore assumed that they have given their implied consent to such disclosure.

Disclosure in the patient's best interests

The ethical principle underpinning such disclosures is paternalism. In other words, limiting a person's autonomy for his or her own sake. In this context it means disclosing information obtained in confidence (to a parent or third party) without consulting the patient (or even despite his or her expressed wishes to the contrary) in order to protect the child's health, safety or welfare. To prevent child abuse, for example, disclosure is almost certainly likely to be necessary (Dimond, 2005:174). Hence, a health professional who suspects that a child has been abused will, by reporting his or her suspicions to a third party, technically break confidentiality but, by doing so, is almost always going to be acting in the child's interests.

More problematic, however, are cases involving 'Gillick'-competent young people who do not want confidential information about their health revealed to a parent. According to Mason and Laurie (2006:273) the situations most likely to raise concerns about confidentiality are when drugs are prescribed and when sexual matters are in issue. In deciding how to balance the duty to respect the young person's confidentiality against his or her interests in disclosing the information, a health professional might also have to consider what is in the public's interest (see below). The spread of the HIV virus, for example, has, not surprisingly perhaps, raised many problems relating to confidentiality.

Study activity

Critically reflect on examples from your practice, when, in relation to a child, you considered it appropriate to breach confidentiality.

Disclosures in the public interest

Legally this exception is the most controversial, mainly because its scope is so uncertain – it can be invoked to justify any disclosure that is thought to be for the 'good of society'. Case law suggests that this means when there is a 'real' or 'genuine' risk of danger to the public even though that danger does not have to be imminent. Furthermore, the 'risk' must usually be to the public's physical safety – injury or disease. In one case, *W* v. *Edgell* [1990] 1 All ER 836, an independent psychiatric report commissioned by a patient detained in a hospital secure unit was disclosed (to a hospital and the Home Secretary) despite his opposition. The psychiatrist (Edgell) disclosed his report because the patient had applied to be discharged. However, Edgell considered that he continued to have an abnormal interest in firearms and home-made bombs (10 years previously the patient had been convicted of the manslaughter of five people) and was still a threat to the pubic. The Court of Appeal rejected the patient's claim for breach of confidentiality on the basis that the duty owed to him was outweighed by the overriding public interest in public safety.

More recently the courts have revisited the question of public interest in the important case of *Campbell* v. *Mirror Group Newspapers* [2004] AC 457. Here the House of Lords had the opportunity to consider the impact of the Human Rights Act 1998 (in particular the relation between Articles 8 and 10). But as Mason and Laurie (2006:264) observe, despite an extensive discussion of the public interest exception by the Law Lords the exception remains frustratingly ill defined. The Campbell case involved a famous supermodel who had been treated for drug addiction and brought an action for breach of confidence in relation to the publication of details of her therapy and of photographs taken of her (secretly) in the street as she left the clinic. Campbell claimed that these acts interfered with her right to respect for private life (Article 8). The newspaper's defence relied on freedom of expression (Article 10) and on the public interest in publishing the materials in order to correct the model's previous statements. The House of Lords held that Campbell's privacy had been infringed. Public interest did not extend to the publication of the additional details about her therapy or the photographs and captions drawing attention to her problems.

Other exceptions to the duty of confidentiality include:

- those required by statute, for example to combat terrorism or report notifiable diseases
- civil proceedings and court orders

Human Rights Act 1998, Article 10

Everyone has the right to freedom of expression. This right shall include freedom to hold opinions and to receive and impart information and ideas without interference by public authority and regardless of frontiers.

Examples of when it is lawful to breach confidentiality in the public interest

To prevent, detect or prosecute:

(a) serious crime
(b) a threat to national security
(c) risk of harm (e.g. child abuse or neglect)

Children and Rights of Access to Health Records

Children and young people who have a confidential relationship with a professional may seek access to their health records at a later date. Young people are entitled to gain access to their records, whether kept manually or computerised, under the Data Protection Act 1998. A request for information should be made in writing. There is no set age at which a child can make an application for disclosure of data held. Note, too, that if the data controller decides that a child is not sufficiently mature to have access to his or her records, a request can be made on behalf of the child by anyone who is legally entitled to act on the child's behalf (for example, those with parental responsibility). If a request for

Data Protection Act 1998

The Data Protection Act 1998 allows patients to be:

- informed whether personal data is processed
- given a description of the data held, the purposes for which they are processed and to whom the data may be disclosed
- given a copy of the information constituting the data
- given information on the source of the data

information is ignored or refused, the child may complain to the Data Protection Commissioner.

Under the Act a health record (which includes both NHS and private records) is defined very broadly as a record consisting of information about the physical or mental health or condition of an identifiable individual made by or on behalf of a professional in connection with the care of that individual. The term 'health professional' is also defined very broadly and so includes nurses, doctors, dentists, midwives, health visitors, occupational therapists, physiotherapists, art and music therapists and so on.

Study activity

Go to the DH Web site at http://www.dh.gov.uk/PolicyAndGuidance/InformationPolicy/PatientConfidentialityAndCaldicottGuardians/fs/en (accessed 17 July 2006) and answer the following questions:

- Describe the various ways health records can be recorded.
- What provisions are made for access by child patients?
- In what circumstances can information be withheld?

Key Points

1. To control their health care children need a right of control over personal health information.
2. Exceptions to the duty of confidentiality are justified in certain circumstances, in particular when abuse or neglect is suspected.
3. The relationship of trust and confidence between patients and health professionals is a two-way process. One element is the patient's right to know what information has been compiled and the other is the health professionals' duty of confidentiality.

Chapter 63

Research

As Mason and Laurie (2006:685) persuasively state:

> A child is by no means a miniature version of an adult. Children respond differently to drugs, as they do to a number of other treatments, and it is impossible to say that the effect of a particular therapy on an adult will be mirrored when applied to a child. Medical research on children is, therefore, necessary before a treatment can be approved for paediatric use.

Yet, even though it is now widely accepted that research involving children is a vital means of promoting their health and well-being, numerous surveys have indicated that there is a worrying dearth of such research (Smyth, 2001).

Research can be classified in two ways:

- Therapeutic research. This type of research (sometimes called clinical research) aims to benefit a particular group of patients by improving available treatment. It is therefore research that is related to patients' health status and so combines research with their care and treatment.
- Non-therapeutic research. This aims only to gain new knowledge and so is unlikely to confer any benefit on participants who may be healthy subjects or existing patients.

How is Research on Children Regulated?

Guidance on research derives from several sources. These include advice from the Department of Health (see below), ethical codes and professional guidelines issued by (amongst others) the Medical Research Council (2004), the British Medical Association (2001) and the Royal College of Paediatrics and Child Health (2000). In the European context an Additional Protocol to the Council of Europe Convention on Human Rights and Biomedicine (1997), specifically relating to biomedical research, was opened for signature in January 2005. All these codes support research on children in principle but emphasise how it can be justified only if certain principles are observed:

Clinical Trial Regulations (2004) and minors

Clinical Trial Regulations (2004) on research involving minors state that the following four principles must be observed:

- the interests of the patient always prevail over those of science and society
- informed consent should be given by a person with parental responsibility or a legal representative to a minor taking part in a clinical trial, and this shall represent the minor's presumed will
- the clinical trial has been designed to minimise pain, discomfort, fear and any other foreseeable risk in relation to the disease and the minor's stage of development, and
- the risk threshold and the degree of distress have to be specially defined and constantly monitored

- research involving children is important for the benefit of all children and should be supported, encouraged and conducted in an ethical manner
- children are not small adults; they have an additional, unique set of interests
- relevant information cannot be gained by comparable research on adults
- legally valid consent must be obtained

In addition to these basic principles, the Department of Health guidance (DH, 2005) makes it clear that research involving patients, their organs, tissues or data must undergo prior independent scrutiny to ensure that ethical standards are met. Reinforcing the importance of this requirement is the fact that it is now a criminal offence under the 2004 Clinical Trial Regulations to commence a clinical trial of an investigational medicinal product (CTIMP) without such approval.

The Department of Health Research Governance guidance sets out principles for good research governance applying to all research conducted within the remit of the Secretary of State. It lays out principles, requirements and standards of acceptable research, mechanisms to meet these criteria, methods of monitoring compliance and issues concerning the proper protection of research participants and the wider public. Overall, however, as Mason and Laurie (2006:656) point out, the Research Governance framework makes it clear that consent is the linchpin to ethically acceptable research.

Finally, it is important to outline the role of research ethics committees in regulating research. Official local research ethics committees

Declaration of Helsinki (last revised in 2000)

Key provisions:

A. Introduction
   4. Medical progress is based on research that ultimately must rest in part on experimentation involving human subjects.
   5. In medical research on human subjects, consideration related to the wellbeing of the human subject should take precedence over the interests of science and society.

B. Basic principles for all medical research
   11. Medical research involving human subjects must conform to generally accepted scientific principles and should be based on a thorough knowledge of the scientific literature, other relevant sources of information, and on adequate laboratory and, where appropriate, animal experimentation.
   18. Medical research involving human subjects should only be conducted if the importance of the objective outweighs the inherent risks and burdens to the subject.
   22. In any research on human beings, each potential subject must be adequately informed of the aims, methods, sources of funding, any possible conflicts of interests, institutional affiliations of the researcher, the anticipated benefits and potential risks of the study and the discomfort it may entail.
   25. When a subject deemed legally incompetent, such as a minor child, is able to give assent to decisions about participation in research, the investigator must obtain that assent in addition to that of the legally authorised representative.

(LRECs) are set up by health authorities to scrutinise research involving patients. The composition of ethics committees in the UK, the procedures they are required to follow and the principles underpinning research projects are governed by guidelines issued by the Department of Health (DH, 2006). In addition, nationwide guidance contained in Standard Operating Procedures (SOPs) issued in 2004 must be followed (available at www.nres.npsa.nhs.uk/).

Study activity

What does the current 2001 DH guidance to LRECs say about research involving children?

As was noted above, consent is the linchpin of ethical research. In the absence of any specific legislation covering research (nor is there any case law in the UK where the legality of research involving children has been the central issue), there is common law relating to research. The law of consent was discussed in a previous section and will only be outlined here.

Under-18s – Gillick competent

Doubts as to whether the Family Law Reform Act 1969 covers research have led most legal texts to advise that only if children under 18 pass the Gillick competency test can they independently consent to research. Applied to research, this means they must understand:

- the nature and purpose of the research, any possible risks and how great or small those risks are
- what will happen to them if they agree to enter the trial
- whether the trial will directly benefit them (whether the research is therapeutic or non-therapeutic)

Other important points to note are:

- a relatively high level of understanding and maturity would normally have to be reached (especially if the research is non-therapeutic)
- if a competent young person under 18 refuses to participate in research, it is wise not to rely solely on parental consent; this means that either the mature minor's refusal should be respected or the court's approval should be sought
- many legal texts advise against carrying out research (especially if it is non-therapeutic) unless parents also consent

Under-18s – not Gillick competent

As to children who are not Gillick competent, consent must be obtained by a proxy – usually a parent or anyone else with parental responsibility, or a court. A proxy's powers in relation to research are wide but do have limits. Thus if the research is therapeutic the proxy's consent will be lawful if it is in the child's best interests. The term 'best interests' has been discussed previously (briefly it includes both medical interests and general interests). Thus applying the test to a child with a serious illness, it may be reasonable for the proxy to consent to research even if the risks are significant – assuming, of course, that the child could benefit (either in the long or short term) (Montgomery, 2003:364).

As regards non-therapeutic research, in applying the best-interests test it seems that a proxy's consent is only lawful if the risks to the child are minimal. The term 'minimal' has been defined (in Federal regulations in the US, 1997) as 'the probability and magnitude of harm or discomfort anticipated in the research are not greater in and of themselves than those ordinarily encountered in daily life or during the performance of routine physical or psychological examinations or tests'. Mason and Laurie (2006:687) suggest that a risk ceases to be minimal where there is a risk that makes one stop and think.

It is also important to note that even when children are not mature enough to make their own decisions about participating in non-therapeutic research, most professional guidelines recommend obtaining their assent or agreement (in addition to the proxy's consent). As the current guidelines on research involving children issued by the Medical Research Council (2004) make clear: 'A child's refusal to participate or continue in research should always be respected . . . [i]f a child becomes upset by a procedure, researchers must accept this as a valid refusal.' It seems therefore that although a proxy's consent is undoubtedly important, it is not determinative.

Key Points

1. Research on children is justified if relevant knowledge cannot be gained by research on adults.
2. Research on children is an important means of promoting child health and well-being.
3. When a choice of age groups is possible, older children should be involved in preference to younger ones.
4. Legally valid consent must always be obtained before research is undertaken.

Chapter 64

Resources and Rationing

'Health care resource allocation troubles patients, the public, doctors, NHS managers, and government yet we have no stable principle on which to respond to it' (Newdick, 2005:1). This short statement, which introduces Newdick's important book on rights, rationing and resources in the UK, neatly sums up the fact that however health care is organised or funded, there will always be a gap between supply and demand. The legal and ethical dilemmas raised by the gap are well illustrated by one of the most poignant cases to reach the courts in recent years, namely *R* v. *Cambridge Health Authority, Ex Parte B* [1995] 2 All ER 129. It concerned a 10-year-old girl suffering from leukaemia, with a life expectancy of 6–8 weeks, who was refused a second bone marrow transplant and a third course of chemotherapy costing approximately £75 000 because there was only a small chance of the treatment being successful. In taking the health authority to court B's father hoped to force it to fund the treatment. He failed, but the case generated an enormous amount of publicity, much of which was critical given the health authority's apparent 'inhumanity' in denying a child's only chance to live on grounds of cost.

rationing

Rationing (also called priority setting and prioritisation) – a process or mechanism for setting priorities in health care, bearing in mind that resources cannot be provided to everyone who demands them; it involves deciding (a) who should get treatment, (b) what treatments should be provided and (c) how these decisions should be made.

Study activity

Read the case of *R* v. *Cambridge HA, Ex parte B*. Do you think the health authority's refusal of treatment was justified? Give reasons for your answer.

As we shall see below, other court cases about rationing have similarly generated a great deal of public debate. That these types of cases attract such media attention is not surprising. It is also very likely they will continue to do so for several reasons. First, advances in medical technology and knowledge – for example, our understanding of the role genetics plays (through the Human Genome Project) – are likely to revolutionise our ideas about sickness and health. Such developments will almost certainly increase pressures on the health service. Secondly,

Protection of the right to life and health care

- Article 24 of the United Nations Convention on the Rights of the Child requires states to recognise the right of the child to the enjoyment of the highest attainable standard of health and to facilities for the treatment of illness and rehabilitation of health, and to strive to ensure that no child is deprived of his or her right of access to such healthcare services.
- Article 2 of the European Convention of Human Rights states that everyone's life shall be protected by law. No one shall be deprived of his life intentionally.

although access to health care has always been rationed in the past, the process was less open. Now the mechanisms and processes of the NHS are much more transparent. As a result, the allocation of resources is more visible and open to public scrutiny. Another factor that explains the media's interest in rationing debates is that healthcare expectations – expectations that the state will provide a 'good' heath service and guarantee access to health care – are much higher than in the past. This, in turn, fuels an ever-expanding demand for health care. It is therefore not surprising that the importance attached to health care is reflected in both the United Nations Convention on the Rights of the Child and Article 2 of the Human Rights Act 1998.

If we accept that health care must be rationed, it then becomes crucial to find a 'fair' way of distributing scarce financial and medical resources to satisfy the competing claims of patients. In addition, difficult decisions have to be made not just about what categories of illness and so forth should have priority, but also about which technologies or procedures to prioritise.

As Newdick (2005:1) asks: 'if hard choices have to be made, should we focus more on acute care to make people better, chronic care to make them more comfortable, or preventive care to stop people becoming sick in the first place? Do we need more clinicians, more medicines or hospitals? Should children have greater priority than adults?'

There are several different approaches that can be taken to ensure that scarce resources are distributed fairly. Here are some:

- Needs theory. Put simply, this approach is based on the view that some patients are more 'needy' than others and so should have a special claim on resources. This approach initially seems one of the fairest approaches to allocating scarce resources, not least because it corresponds most closely with the founding principles of the NHS (a tax-funded service providing universal health care, free at the point of use to those in need). However, what does the term 'need' mean in this context? Despite being widely used, there is very little agreement as to what it means. Perhaps this is not surprising in that our perceptions of need are subjective and value laden. Furthermore, whereas medical need may well be a necessary criterion for the distribution of resources, it does not make choosing between competing candidates (who are agreed to be 'in medical need') any easier.
- Medical criteria. This is another value-laden concept in so far as it presupposes (wrongly) that there is a consistent and scientific set of criteria measuring the outcome (probability of medical success) of treatment. However, as with the needs theory, there are problems in defining what is meant by medical success. How should the concept be measured, bearing in mind that there is no objective yardstick by which medical effectiveness can be assessed? In other words, it too is a subjective term and so one that is influenced by our perceptions of illness and health, which vary not only from person to person but also in the same person, from time to time. It has been suggested, however, that the practice of evidence-based medicine (EBM) will result in practice being much less driven by subjective clinical instinct. But as Newdick (2005:19) points out, there will always be areas in which the evidence is ambiguous, incomplete or inconsistent.

- Maximisation of welfare. Another way of dealing with the gap between supply and demand for health care has been developed by health economists. It is the theory called 'quality adjusted life years' (QALYs). Often described as 'scientific', it adopts a cost–benefit analysis. As such it measures healthcare outcomes by evaluating the cost of treatment and the extent to which, and for how long, it will improve a patient's quality of life. Very crudely, the QALY principle is that a year of healthy life expectancy scores 1 and a year of unhealthy life is taken as less than 1, its value diminishing as quality of life decreases in the unhealthy. The QALY principle compares the cost (in financial and other terms) of different treatments, procedures and health 'problems'. Not surprisingly, the most efficient are those treatments that are the cheapest yet achieve the best quality of life over the longest period of time. Several objections have been made to QALYs. A common one is that they discriminate against older people (because the elderly have a shorter life expectancy). Another is that the QALY concept does not take into account the personal response of individuals to their illnesses and their views of medical treatment.

For further reading see Newdick (2005:Chapters 1 and 2).

Study activity

- Which approach to rationing do you think is the 'fairest'? Why? Do you think children should be given priority? If your answer is yes, why?
- Do you think individuals should forfeit the 'right' to health if they have a lifestyle or 'habit' such as smoking which adversely affects their health? If so, which kinds of behaviour should 'count' and why?

Finally, before concluding this section it is necessary to outline the law's role in allocating health resources. Provision of health care is governed by the National Health Service Act 1977. The Act imposes very comprehensive duties on the Secretary of State for Health and has been the central issue in several high-profile cases. The general principle that the courts will not intervene in resourcing issues of the NHS appears to continue to be accepted by the courts, but there have been two recent cases where health authorities have been held liable for failure to provide services and a third where the patient won the principle that the NHS should pay for treatment (Dimond, 2005:91).

In *R* v. *North Derbyshire Health Authority* [1997] 8 Med LR 327 the health authority refused to prescribe beta-interferon for patients in its catchment area (because it had not yet been proved to be effective treatment for multiple sclerosis). A patient with the disease challenged this refusal and succeeded on the grounds that the authority had failed to follow the relevant Department of Health Guidance (NHS Executive Letter, EL(95) 97).

In *North-west Lancashire Health Authority* v. *A, D and G* [1999] Lloyd's Rep Med p. 399, a health authority refused to fund gender reassignment treatment (other than general psychiatric and psychological services) for three transsexuals. This decision was based on the

National Health Service Act 1977

Section 1(1) imposes a duty on the Secretary of State to continue the promotion in England and Wales of a comprehensive health service designed to secure improvement in:

- the physical and mental health of the people
- the prevention, diagnosis and treatment of illness and for that purpose to provide or secure the effective provision of services in accordance with the Act

Section 3(1) imposes a duty on the Secretary of State to provide throughout England and Wales, to such extent as he considers necessary to meet all reasonable requirements:

- hospital accommodation
- other accommodation for the purpose of any service provided under this Act
- medical, dental, nursing and ambulance services
- such other facilities for the care of expectant and nursing mothers and young children as he considers are appropriate as part of the health service
- such facilities for the prevention of illness, the care of persons suffering from illness and the after-care of persons who have suffered from illness as he considers are appropriate as part of the health service
- such other services as are required for the diagnosis and treatment of illness

authority's policy that gender reassignment treatment should be given a very low priority (except if there was overriding clinical need or exceptional circumstances). The claimants challenged the decision and ultimately the Court of Appeal ruled (amongst other things) that the health authority's policy was flawed in two respects. First, it did not treat transsexualism as an illness, but as an attitude of mind that did not warrant medical treatment. Secondly, in effect the health authority operated a 'blanket policy' against funding treatment for the condition because it did not believe in such treatment. As such the health authority was not genuinely applying the policy to the individual exceptions.

In the third case, *R (Watts)* v. *Bedford Primary Care Trust and Another* [2003] EWHC 2222, the patient was told she could not have a hip replacement for a year. She therefore went abroad for treatment. She won the principle that the NHS should pay for treatment overseas.

It is, of course, the 'life or death' decisions that generate the most public debate, especially when urgent decisions have to be made about the withdrawal or withholding of life-sustaining treatment for babies and children. But although scarce resources undoubtedly influence decision making, other factors are equally relevant. Thus, for example, in the case of *In Re J* [1990] 3 All ER 930, the court, although recognising a strong presumption in favour of prolonging life, none the less allowed treatment to be withheld. This was because it was necessary to perform a 'balancing exercise' – a process that involved judging the quality of life a child would have to endure if given treatment and then deciding whether in all the circumstances such a life would 'be so afflicted as to be intolerable to that child'.

J was born 13 weeks premature, weighing 1.1 kg at birth. By the time the case came to court he was 5 months old but had suffered recurrent convulsions and had been ventilated twice for long periods. Despite being able to breathe independently his long-term prognosis was very poor: he was unlikely to survive into his teens and would almost certainly develop serious spastic quadriplegia and be blind and deaf. He would, however, experience the same pain as a normal baby. J was not dying or near the point of death. Nevertheless, the Court of Appeal decided that it would be lawful not to reventilate him if he suffered a further collapse (although he should be treated with antibiotics if he developed a chest infection and hydration should be maintained). In other words the court allowed life-saving treatment to be withheld because this course of action was – given the hazardous and invasive nature of reventilation and the risk of further deterioration – in J's best interests.

It is also worth assessing the impact of the Human Rights Act 1998 in that it has been suggested that this Act might be used by aggrieved patients who have been refused treatment more successfully than the NHS legislation. According to Newdick (2005:127), however, a cautious note must be sounded. He argues that although the Human Rights Act might make primary care Trusts think more carefully about their procedures and the manner in which they make decisions – to make sure their discretion has been exercised in a reasonable and proportionate manner – it is unlikely that Human Rights legislation will be helpful in individual cases.

Key Points

1. Setting healthcare priorities is a complex process that involves finding a fair way of distributing scarce financial and medical resources.
2. The National Health Service Act 1977 imposes very comprehensive duties on the Secretary of State for Health to provide a comprehensive health service.
3. The reality of scarce resources undoubtedly influences the courts when they are involved in urgent life-or-death disputes.
4. Demand for health care is increasing but the role of law in guaranteeing access to healthcare is limited.

Chapter 65

Standards of Care

The right to receive a reasonable standard of medical care has, like the right to consent, long been recognised as a legal right. It is also enshrined in several clauses of the NMC *Code of Professional Conduct: Standard for Conduct, Performance and Ethics* (2004).

The 'duties' imposed in the Code do not have legal force. However, they are expected to be followed given that they aim to establish, maintain and improve standards of professional practice. Furthermore, several of them are linked with the law of negligence, as they replicate, albeit in broad terms, well-established legal rights.

NMC *Code of Professional Conduct: Standards for Conduct, Performance and Ethics* (2004)

Key provisions

1.3 You are personally accountable for your practice. This means that you are answerable for your actions and omissions, regardless of advice and directions from another professional.

1.4 You have a duty of care to your patients and clients, who are entitled to receive safe and competent care.

6.1 You must keep your knowledge and skills up-to-date throughout your working life. In particular, you should take part regularly in learning activities that develop your competence and performance.

6.3 If any aspect of practice is beyond your level of competence, you must obtain help and supervision from a competent practitioner until you and your employer consider that you have acquired the requisite knowledge and skill.

Disciplinary action

Nurses who fail to achieve the professional standards set out in the Code may be the subject of the following action:

- professional accountability – proceedings before the professional conduct committee
- accountability to employer – in failing to act with care and skill the nurse is likely to have breached her contract of employment

Notwithstanding the similarities between the legal and ethical positions on negligence, there are important differences. Thus the ethical duty of care is wider than the legal duty. In other words nurses may, for example, have a moral and professional duty to help strangers, but legally they have no responsibility for them. Similarly, the standard of care, which aims to set a minimum level of competence below which practitioners must not fall, is lower than the ethical standard, which aims for the best possible level of care (Hendrick, 2004:93).

The ethical principles which inform the standards of care set out in the Code are briefly: the principle of non-maleficence (the duty not to harm patients) and that of beneficence (of positively helping patients by promoting and safeguarding their interests). However, both in practice and in theory there are problems in applying them, mainly because all medical treatment involves balancing risks and harms.

Turning now to legal principles, the standard required by the law is best described as a minimum one – one that is concerned primarily with guaranteeing a basic level of competence. Practitioners who fall below that standard may be sued and found liable in negligence. The law of negligence (which is another name for medical malpractice) has two broad aims. These are:

- Compensation. This is the main function – damages awarded are intended to put victims in the position they would have been in if they had not been injured. Compensation can include lost earning potential and higher living expenses.
- Deterrence. Here the aim is to reduce the number and seriousness of accidents by making health professionals personally liable. In other words the threat or fear of legal action and potential damage to professional reputations is a powerful incentive to achieve high standards and ensure that greater care is taken.

The three elements that a patient needs to establish to win a negligence case are set out below. These elements will now be analysed, although the focus will be on the second – breach of duty.

Elements in a negligence action

- Duty of care – this means that the health professional was responsible for the patient.
- Breach of duty – this means that the health professional failed in his or her responsibility.
- Damage – this means that the health professional's action (or inaction) caused the patient's injuries.

Duty of Care

In almost all healthcare settings it is easy to establish whether a duty of care exists, in that any patient a health professional is currently treating will be owed a duty. So, for example, patients in hospital (whether as inpatients or outpatients), likewise those seeking treatment in A&E departments, are owed a duty of care, as are those on GPs' lists. Less clear, however, is the duty owed to colleagues or patients' relatives. In such cases, whether or not a legal duty is owed depends on applying the so-called 'neighbour test'.

The 'neighbour' test

Establishes when a duty of care exists, i.e. whenever (a) the damage is foreseeable; (b) there is a sufficiently 'proximate' (near) relationship between the claimant and the defendant; and (c) it is just, fair and reasonable to impose a duty.

Note that a duty of care is owed to child patients whether they have sought medical services independently or not. Thus 16- and 17-year-olds and young people under 16 who are 'Gillick' competent have the right to apply for inclusion on a GP's list and to seek treatment from other health professionals irrespective of their parents' knowledge or permission. As for children under 16 who are not 'Gillick' competent – the request for medical services must come from someone else, usually a parent.

Study activity

You are off duty and shopping in a supermarket. A young child has an accident and is bleeding profusely. Are you obliged to offer medical assistance? Is there a difference between your legal and ethical duty?

Breach of Duty

Proving breach of duty is usually much harder than establishing a duty of care. The starting point for establishing a breach of duty is the Bolam test (set in the famous case of *Bolam* v. *Friern Barnet Hospital Management Committee* [1957] 2 All ER 118). The case held that doctors are not negligent 'if they have acted in accordance with a practice accepted as proper by a responsible body of medical men skilled in that particular art'.

The Bolam test (which essentially means that health professionals set their own standards) now applies to all health professionals, and basically means that practitioners are judged by their peers – sisters by sisters, specialist nurses by other specialist nurses, midwives by midwives, and so on. In other words, legal liability can be avoided if a health professional can show that other reasonably competent (reasonably skilled and experienced) practitioners would have acted in a similar way. This does not mean they would have done exactly the same, but rather their actions were within an acceptable range.

Note that in recent years the Bolam test has been challenged not just by clinical guidelines but also by the so-called Bolitho approach. The Bolitho approach derives from the case of *Bolitho* v. *Hackney Health Authority* [1998] AC 232. In this case all five law lords said that 'the judge, before accepting a body of opinion as being responsible, or respectable, will need to be satisfied . . . that the experts have weighed up the risks and benefits and have reached a defensible conclusion'.

The new approach strongly suggested that the courts would be more willing than in the past to question professional opinion – even perhaps setting the standard of care themselves. But what seems to have happened in practice is that although the courts are now certainly more willing to scrutinise professional practice more critically, they will only very rarely reject it (Montgomery, 2003).

Study activity

Read Hendrick (2004:87) and then consider which clinical guideline has most changed your practice in the past year.

Other important issues, which the courts have dealt with in establishing what amounts to a breach of duty, are given below.

Several schools of thought

No liability arises just because a health professional chose to act in one way rather than another, providing that he or she acted in accordance with accepted practice. Put simply, the law recognises medical differences of opinion.

Departing from accepted practice

Deviation from standard practice is by no means conclusive evidence of negligence and may well be acceptable providing the unconventional treatment can be justified – given the circumstances, innovative or unusual procedures were appropriate.

Trainees and inexperience

It is now well settled that the law does not accept a defence of inexperience, lack of ability or knowledge. In short, students and other trainees are expected to perform to the same standard as their trained, more experienced colleagues. None the less, those 'learning on the job' are expected to know their limitations. They should therefore ask for help (which should be available) rather than undertake a task they are not competent to carry out. In so doing they would normally have a defence to any subsequent negligence claim should a mistake occur. This approach explains the outcome of *Wilsher* v. *Essex AHA* [1986] 3 All ER 801 in which a junior doctor who mistakenly inserted a catheter into a vein rather than an artery escaped liability (because he consulted a registrar). However, the registrar who repeated the mistake was found liable because he should have known better.

The facts of the Wilsher case

Martin Wilsher was born prematurely, suffering from various illnesses including oxygen deficiency. His prospects of survival were poor and he was placed in the 24-hour special care unit. A medical team, consisting of two consultants, a senior registrar, several junior doctors and trained nurses, looked him after. He needed extra oxygen to survive and one of the inexperienced doctors monitoring the oxygen in Martin's bloodstream mistakenly inserted a catheter into a vein rather than an artery, but then asked the senior registrar to check what he had done. The registrar failed to see the mistake and some hours later, when replacing the catheter, did exactly the same thing himself. In both instances the catheter monitor failed to register correctly the amount of oxygen in Martin's blood, with the result that he was given excess oxygen. Martin claimed that the excess oxygen in his bloodstream caused an incurable condition of the retina resulting in near blindness. But notwithstanding the registrar's negligence Martin failed to win compensation because he could not prove causation (the third element in a negligence claim).

When standards are judged

The facts of the Bolam case: Mr Bolam claimed that the broken pelvis he sustained during electroconvulsive treatment could have been avoided had he been given relaxant drugs and been properly restrained. He also complained that he was not warned of the risks of treatment. The court rejected his claim because at the time there was evidence that different doctors used different techniques and methods – some used relaxant drugs, other did not. Since both approaches were equally acceptable, the doctor was not negligent in choosing one method over another.

The law accepts that standards change as current medical knowledge and skills develop. Standards are therefore judged at the time treatment was carried out and not when the case comes to trial (which is typically several years later).

Causation

This is the third hurdle a victim of medical negligence has to overcome, and in practice it is one of the hardest. It requires proof that the defendant's conduct caused (or materially contributed to) the victim's injury. In simple terms this means that it was more than 50% probable that the injuries were caused by the negligence. In some cases the link is self-evident, such as when a foreign body is left in a patient after surgery. However, in other cases, proving a link is much more difficult – the injuries may have been caused by natural causes or the patient's underlying illness. Sometimes the victim's case collapses because his or her

Breaches of duty most likely to involve children

Case law and textbooks on medical negligence have shown a clear pattern of when breaches of duty are most likely to occur in relation to children. These include:

- High technology – developments in medical technology have increased the likelihood of litigation, in particular claims arising from progress in medical treatment, new or quasi-experimental treatment and unproved treatments.
- Failures in communication – this includes, for example, inadequate instructions to nurses and failure to organise follow-up arrangements. Lack of communication with parents is also a factor.
- Pain relief – children and parents now have higher expectations in respect of pain relief due to progress that has been made in assessing and measuring pain in children.
- Drug-induced and prescribing errors – these are commonly due to a breakdown of communication between the practitioner who prescribed the drug and the one who administered it.

injuries could have been caused by several factors. This is why Martin Wilsher lost his case because, even though it was admitted that the registrar had negligently administered excess oxygen (which was well known as a cause of blindness), there were at least five other possible causes of blindness in premature babies. With so many potential competing causes the evidence linking the negligence with Martin's blindness was inconclusive.

Once a victim has proved that the practitioner's conduct caused the injuries, he or she will be entitled to compensation (which is normally paid by the health professional's employer). In medical cases damages (the legal term for compensation) consist of several categories including pain and suffering, loss of earnings and earning capacity.

Reform of the Law of Negligence

This section discusses the most common criticisms of the law of negligence as a system of paying compensation, and current reform proposals.

The most common criticisms are that the law

- is complex
- is unfair because apparently similar cases may reach different conclusions
- is slow – cases on average take 4 years from time of claim to settlement
- is costly – in legal fees, diversion of clinical staff time from clinical care, staff morale and public confidence
- undermines health professional–patient relationships (DH, 2003b)

Many of these criticisms (and others) have now been addressed in the NHS Redress Bill 2005. Although the Bill does not propose a no-fault scheme (of the sort that exists in New Zealand, for example) it is an important step to a far less confrontational and more efficient scheme than the present one.

Key Points

1. The right to receive a reasonable standard of care is a long-established legal right.
2. The NMC code of professional conduct enshrines both legal and ethical principles of good practice.
3. Failure to reach the required standard of practice can result in legal proceedings.

References

Alderson, P. and **Montgomery, J.** (1996) *Health Care Choices: Making Decisions with Children.* London: Institute for Public Policy Research.
Bainham, A. (2005) *Children: The Modern Law,* 2nd edn. Bristol: Jordan.
British Medical Association (2001) *Consent, Rights and Choice in Healthcare for Children and Young People.* London: BMA.
DH (2003a) *National Health Service Confidentiality Code of Practice.* London: HMSO.
DH (2003b) *Making Amends: A Consultation Paper Setting Out Proposals for Reforming the Approach to Clinical Negligence in the NHS.* London: HMSO.
DH (2005) *Research Governance Framework for Health and Social Care.* London: HMSO.
DH (2006) *Report of the Ad Hoc Advisory Group on the Operation of NHS Research Ethics Committees.* London: HMSO.
Diduck, A. and **Kaganas, F.** (2006) *Family Law, Gender and the State,* 2nd edn. Oxford: Hart Publishing.
Dimond, B. (2005) *Legal Aspects of Nursing,* 4th edn. Harlow: Pearson Longman.
Fortin, J. (2003) *Children's Rights and the Developing Law,* 2nd edn. London: Lexis Nexis Butterworths.
Freeman, M. (2000) The future of children's rights. *Children and Society,* **14**, 277–293.
Hendrick, J. (2004) *Law and Ethics: Foundations in Nursing and Health Care.* Cheltenham: Nelson Thornes.
Herring, J. (2004) *Family Law,* 2nd edn. London: Longman.
Mason, J. K. and **Laurie, G. T.** (2006) *Mason and McCall Smith's Law and Medical Ethics,* 7th edn. Oxford: OUP.
Medical Research Council (2004) *Medical Research Involving Children.* London: MRC.
Montgomery, J. (2003) *Health Care Law.* Oxford: OUP.
Newdick, C. (2005) *Who Should We Treat: Rights, Rationing and Resources in the NHS.* Oxford: OUP.
Nursing and Midwifery Council (NMC) (2004) *Code of Professional Conduct: Standards for Conduct, Performance and Ethics.* London: NMC.
Royal College of Paediatrics and Child Health (2000) Ethics Advisory Committee: guidelines for the ethical conduct of medical research involving children. *Archives of Diseases in Childhood,* **82**, 177.
Smyth, R. L. (2001) Research with children. *British Medical Journal,* **322**, 1377.

Module 9
Managing Professional Practice

Joan Ramsay

Learning Outcomes

The material contained within this module and the references should enable you to:

- examine the discharge planning process
- discuss the role of the children's nurse as leader
- explore standard setting and the audit cycle
- evaluate the different methods of organising work
- consider how to plan staffing levels and determine patient dependency
- describe ways of maintaining patient safety by managing risk

Introduction

One of the most important roles of the children's nurse is that of leader, especially for children's nurses working in a general hospital environment. These nurses need to be able to promote the importance of children's nursing as a speciality and the unique needs of children. This module looks particularly at this leadership role, and explores issues such as skill mix for children's nursing and methods of calculating patient dependency to enable the nurse to justify claims for appropriate staffing levels. It also examines the organisation of work on a children's ward and the advantages and disadvantages of task or patient allocation, and team or primary nursing. In the current market forces of health care the provision of safe and quality care is essential, and this module discusses the management of risk to maintain safety, and standard setting and audit as a means of monitoring quality. The importance of cost-effective health care, as well as the need to minimise the length of hospital stay for children who are particularly stressed by being in this strange environment, has meant that the need for careful discharge planning has never been so important. The module looks at how this can be best achieved in conjunction with other members of the multidisciplinary team.

Chapter 66
Discharge Planning

Introduction

Since the Platt Report in 1959 (MoH, 1959) much has been written about the effects of hospitalisation on children. Most of the resulting recommendations suggested that children should only be admitted to hospital if absolutely necessary and this stay should be kept to a minimum. Although the development of community nursing services for children has been slow, there has been a significant reduction in the average length of their hospital stay (DH, 2003a). This move towards community care has given impetus to the need for good discharge planning. Good discharge planning not only improves patient care and outcomes of care but minimises readmission due to inadequate aftercare.

Discharge planning must begin with an assessment of the family's wishes, resources and abilities to undertake the care of their child at home. It also involves education of the family and identification of the community and support services available. As discharge planning is often very complex, government recommendations since 1989 have stated that it should begin as early as possible, ideally during the assessment process at admission and, for booked admissions, before the child is even admitted to hospital (DH, 1989b). Another important guideline was that the family should be at the centre of the planning process. This is reiterated strongly in the National Service Framework (NSF) for children (DH, 2003a).

Tierney *et al.* (1994) found that the majority of families were not consulted about discharge arrangements and that one-fifth of patients had probably been discharged too soon. This latter point was supported by the fact that more than a quarter of the patients were readmitted within 3 months of their discharge. The psychological benefits and economic advantage of discharging children into the community as soon as possible must be balanced against the risks of discharging highly dependent children into an unsuitable environment with insufficient support mechanisms.

Coordination of Discharge Planning

The coordination of discharge is a complex multidisciplinary and multi-agency process. It involves various members of the hospital team, social services, community services and GPs as well as the family. Gatford (2004) recommends that a named member of the multidisciplinary team should be given the responsibility of coordinating the discharge arrangements. This named individual, ideally someone who has the relevant knowledge and experience of local services, should be responsible for recording all information relating to the discharge, including the results of any assessments and the services contacted, on a specific discharge plan used by all staff involved in the discharge. A comprehensive discharge planning document, placed either in the child's medical records or at the bedside with the nursing notes, allows all members involved in the discharge, including the family, to be able to see at a glance the progress with the arrangements. This process was supported by the UKCC in 1995 following a report on a survey of current discharge practices in acute hospitals. They recommended that:

- every ward should have a written discharge policy, discharge standards and discharge plans
- each patient should have a named member of staff designated to take responsibility for the discharge coordination
- patients and families should know which member of staff is responsible for coordinating their discharge arrangements, they should be regularly and fully involved in the discharge planning, and they should be given written information about all arrangements
- GPs and community nurses should be involved early in the discharge planning process and community/hospital liaison should be improved
- improvements should be made in the content and speed of delivery of the discharge letter
- each ward should have an audit system for discharge procedures
- patients should not be discharged at times that were inconvenient for community services
- wards should receive regular statistical information relevant to discharge planning to enable evaluation of the process

Discharge planning – the multidisciplinary team

The family

- education, advice and support

Community nurse/health visitor/GP

- liaison and continuity of care
- ongoing education, advice and support
- clinical input
- maintenance of treatment

Social services

- home/financial assessment

Occupational therapists

- activities of daily living
- home assessment
- equipment

Physiotherapists

- mobility and mobility aids
- respiratory care

Speech and language therapy

- communication skill/aids

Dietician

- enteral feeding
- special dietary needs

School nurse

- continuing care/treatment at school

Study activity

Investigate how the discharge planning in your current area of practice meets these recommendations (see Figure 66.1).

In 2003, it was evident that these principles were still not being acted upon. Smith and Daughtrey (2000) illustrate how frustrating planning for discharge can be for parents. In response to these failings the Department of Health produced a document to provide practitioners with guidance and practical tools to achieve best practice in discharging patients from hospital. Although concerned primarily with adults with physical ill health, it recognised that many of the principles and practices apply equally to children. It supported the above recommendations and stressed that coordination and continuity of discharge planning is

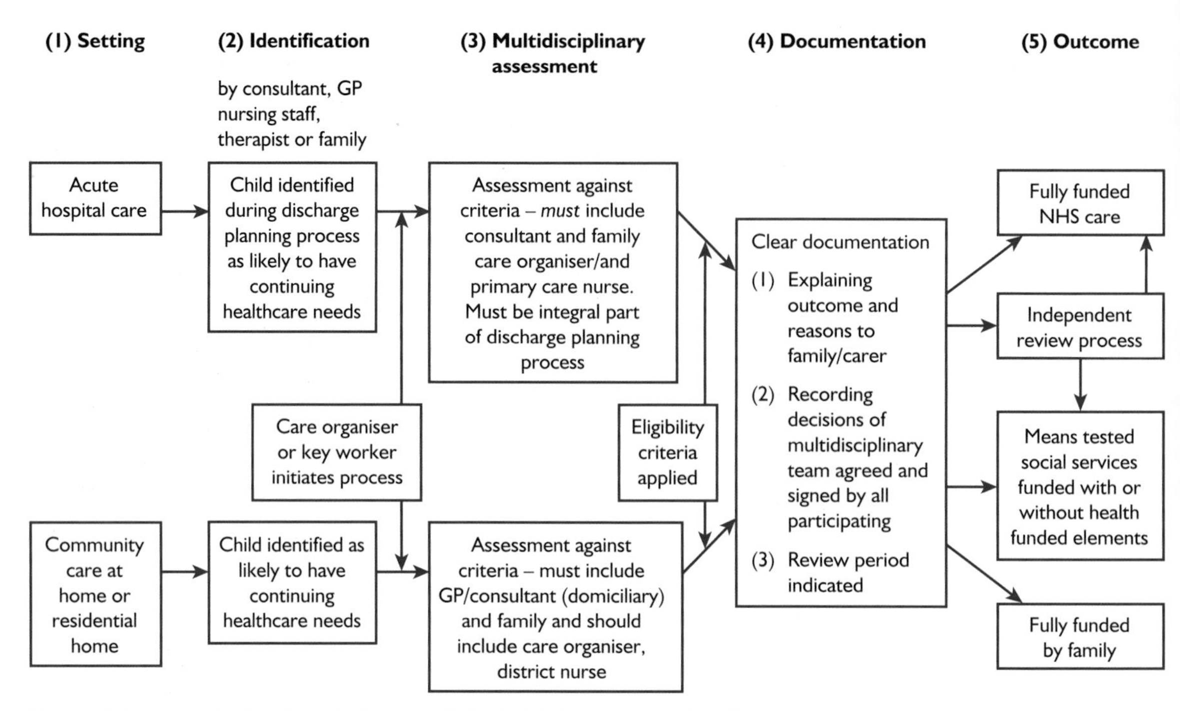

Figure 66.1 Process for deciding whether a family is eligible for continuing health care.

only as effective as the communication within and between the different agencies and disciplines involved. This is facilitated by a clear understanding of the funding arrangements and the roles of all participants (DH, 2003b).

NHS Funding of Community Care

In 1995 the government required each health authority to agree eligibility for continuing health care, which would be fully funded by the NHS with its local social services department(s). Continuing care is the provision of care over an extended period of time to meet physical and mental health needs due to a long-term condition. It can be provided in a range of settings, from an NHS hospital, residential home, hospice or the child's own home.

Study activity

Find out the criteria in your own area for fully funded health care.

The NHS and local authorities with responsibilities for social services are required to work together to meet the needs of all patients with continuing health and social care needs: 'Strategic health authorities and local authorities have to agree joint continuing health and social care eligibility criteria and set out their respective responsibilities for the

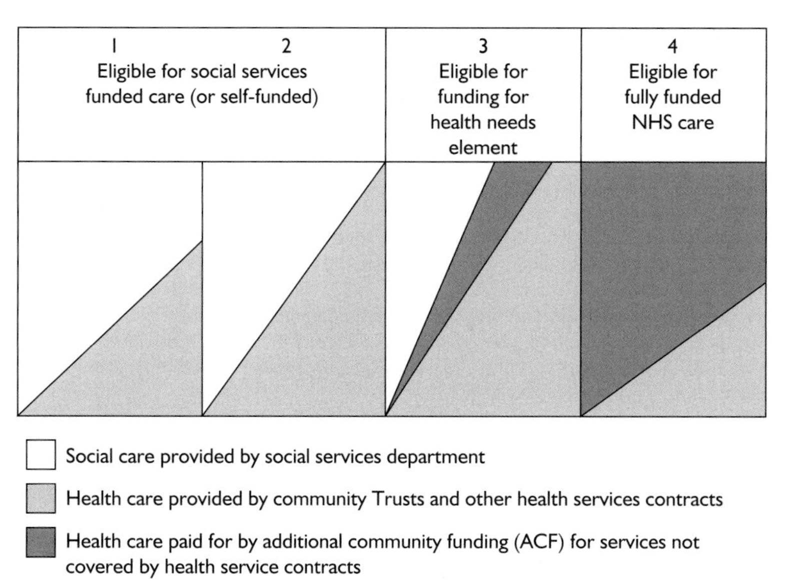

Figure 66.2 The continuum of health and social care.

provision of the full range of health and social care services, regardless of age' (Royal Commission on Long-term Care, 1999). The eligibility for continuing healthcare funding does not stand alone. It should be seen as part of the continuum of community care with social services (see Figure 66.2). At the lower end of the continuum, chronically ill children may need a minimal amount of health care but a high level of social care. Depending on their financial status, families may be required to contribute to the cost of the social care element. At the opposite end of the continuum, children requiring a high level of health care would meet the criteria for fully funded NHS care. At this level families would not be expected to contribute financially for any part of the care their child receives, even if some of this care is provided by social services. At all levels the biggest responsibility for the care of the sick/disabled child falls upon the family, and their views about their needs is essential.

The multidisciplinary team is responsible for deciding if a patient is eligible for fully funded NHS continuing health care. The underlying principles for assessing this are that the assessment:

- is part of the care management process
- involves the child (if appropriate) and family
- is not initiated until a sufficient period has been allowed for recovery and rehabilitation
- is multidisciplinary, involving all those providing care or therapy
- involves a consultant or GP
- decision is fully and clearly documented and signed by all those involved

Most health authorities have additional community funds to pay for a patient's care in the community where this care is not provided under contract with an NHS Trust or other provider. Application for this funding should be part of the multidisciplinary team's assessment.

Discharge planning – points to remember

- Involve the family from the time of admission
- An estimated date of discharge facilitates the support process
- Families may have unrealistic expectations and may not remember all information (see p. 729)
- Discharge is easier to postpone than arrange urgently
- Inform the appropriate therapist on admission when children need to practise skills (e.g. walking with crutches) before discharge
- Ensure family have practised and feel competent in any care they will be giving
- The amount, as well as the frequency, of support should be clearly identified
- If the child needs a key discharge item of equipment (e.g. wheelchair) it should be ordered on admission
- Equipment and/or home alterations may take time and the family should not be given false hopes
- Do not assume that the child's and family's needs on admission will be the same at the time of discharge

Example criteria for continuing NHS-funded health care

Families will be eligible for care paid for by the NHS if their child:

- is totally dependent (i.e. where withdrawal or unavailability of help threatens survival) AND has specific additional needs *such as* one of the following:
  - complex methods of feeding
  - care of large pressure sores (grade 4–5)
  - supervision and monitoring of the last stage of cardiac, respiratory, renal or other major organ failure
  - permanent tracheostomy requiring frequent changes and suction
  - skilled lifting and handling needing two or more people
  - unstable or unpredictable medical/psychological conditions requiring specialist clinical intervention
- is terminally ill and needs specialist nursing supervision or support when death is expected within about 3 months
- is in need of ongoing supervision to prevent self-harm or harm to others (e.g. challenging behaviour with a learning disability or severe behavioural problems arising from a brain injury)
- has needs which individually would not be of sufficient severity to meet the above criteria, but when put together their complexity requires high levels of care
- is in need of phased or intermittent respite care and fall into the above categories
- needs a programme of rehabilitation following an episode of illness or an accident and before long-term needs can be assessed
- will require transport to and from the GP, hospice, healthcare facilities which is above contracted levels and falls into one of the above categories

(Bedfordshire Health Authority, 1996)

The Social Services Perspective

The NHS and Community Care Act (1990) promoted the collaborative working of health, housing, education and social services for the provision of care in the community, which included the private and voluntary services. The Act stated that any member of staff could act as the named discharge organiser but, in practice, this role is often undertaken by the social worker. The named social worker interviews the family to ascertain its wishes and its current resources, including support networks. Other agencies become involved when the amount of care needs are not all within the remit of social services. Any care that involves health needs is put forward to the health authority or GP fundholder to finance. A case conference may need to be arranged when discharge needs are particularly complex.

When a family is not eligible for fully funded NHS care, it may qualify for support from social services. Social services usually assess the priority of the situation to determine whether families qualify for this support. Only high-risk and medium-risk priorities are eligible for services (see Table 66.1).

- *High priority* – children in this category require radical intervention to change or ameliorate their situation. They are, or may be, exposed to significant harm. They may be dependent on others for protection and/or their own family cannot care for them.
- *Medium priority* – when children need continued support to prevent deterioration of the situation. Their relationship with their family may have broken down and they are unsupported and exposed to risk. This category also includes families with consistent financial problems or substandard accommodation and children in need.

Table 66.1 Social services and health input to different levels of care

	Level of need			
	1	**2**	**3**	**4**
Lead care planning agency	Social services	Social services	Social services	Social services and healthcare staff
Lead funding agency	Social services	Social services	Social services and NHS	NHS
Social services priority	Medium–high	High	High/more than social service provision	More than social service provision
Example of health input	General medical services (GP, CCN, etc.)	General medical services and specialist nurse	Clinical input above usual PHCT remit	Specialist input from nursing and medicine
Example of social services input	Home care or residential care	Extensive home or residential care	Extensive home and specialist care	Advice to health staff

- *Low priority* – when the child's quality of life could be enhanced and/or the risk of deterioration could be significantly reduced.

The Nursing Perspective

On admission to hospital the named nurse and medical team should initiate post-discharge care and determine the approximate length of the child's stay. If parents are actively involved in the child's care planning during hospitalisation it is relatively easy to adapt these care plans for home use. Marland (1994) suggests that sharing nursing care plans with parents in this way not only supports a shared holistic approach to caring for the individual child, but also enables the nurses to assess how parents are coping. The family's named nurse needs to undertake a thorough assessment of the family and the home environment to ensure that the family's emotional and physical resources are able to support the responsibility of home care. This assessment should take the child and family's learning needs into account to enable a planned approach to teaching them any new knowledge and skills well in advance of discharge. This gives them an opportunity to practise the care before going home, and sometimes it may be appropriate to arrange a trial period at home to ensure they can transfer their skills to the home environment. Ideally, more than one member of the family should be taught so that the burden of this responsibility can be shared. A written plan of teaching that itemises learning goals is helpful for the family and members of the multidisciplinary team to identify progress. This approach is also advocated by Casey and Mobbs (1988), who suggest that it helps clarify the legal implications of parents providing health care (*see also* Community nursing p. 375).

Written homecare instructions should be available not only to remind parents of salient points but to facilitate continuity of care for other professionals involved in the child's home care. These should include a list of useful telephone numbers to enable the family to seek help when

Assessment of the family and community services for home care

Physical environment

- safe and adequate housing
- telephone in the home
- space for equipment

Psychological status

- firm marital status or alternative support mechanisms
- knowledge of this illness/disability or motivation and ability to learn
- realistic perceptions of the effects of the child's illness/disability upon the family

Available resources

- appropriate equipment available
- appropriate healthcare personnel available
- home renovation possible
- peer/parent support group available
- appropriate transport available

Providing resources for discharge

Equipment

Social services

- long-term equipment
- aids and adaptations for the home

Occupational therapy/hospital or community short-term loan stock

- short-term equipment (3 months or less)

Red Cross/self-help groups

- loan equipment for social need only

Prescription items

Dressings, medication, needles and syringes, and feeds provided by the hospital on discharge and then by repeat prescription from the GP

Human resources

Community trust

- community children's nurse
- health visitor
- school nurse
- therapies

Specialist services

- MacMillan nurse
- hospice care

Social services

- home help
- night sitter
- advice about available allowances

Ambulance trust

- transport arrangements

needed. Parents should also be advised to discuss their child's home care with their insurance company. If, for instance, their child requires home oxygen, this may alter their fire risk. Local emergency services should also be aware of such home situations to enable them to respond appropriately in case of emergency.

The RCN (2000) suggests that good communication between the named hospital nurse and the community children's nurse (CCN) is the most important factor in transferring care to the home environment. Early liaison with the community nurse also benefits the child and family, who can begin to get to know their new nurse before discharge. The key principle for any discharge planning is that it should commence on admission to hospital. This is even more crucial if the child has complex needs (Stephens, 2005). Once the referral to the CCN service has been made, a discharge planning group should be set up with the parents and all the professionals involved in the discharge. Stephens (2005) suggests that their meetings should include:

- introducing the parents to the multidisciplinary team
- joint understanding of the current nursing, medical and social needs
- anticipating the child's level of nursing and support needs at home
- developing an action plan of responsibilities and roles
- identifying the key worker to coordinate the discharge and be the main contact for the family
- establishing funding

Study activity

Arrange to observe a discharge planning meeting and identify how the multidisciplinary team work together to facilitate a smooth discharge process.

The named nurse should be alert to the fact that home care may not be appropriate in all cases. In addition, even if home care seems initially appropriate, changing circumstances may delay or prevent this option. The nurse may need to help parents come to terms with these changes and make the appropriate alterations to the discharge plan.

The Physiotherapy and Occupational Therapy Perspective

Discharge planning is essential from the perspective of the physiotherapist and the occupational therapist. The physiotherapist needs time to ensure that:

- the child is fitted with the appropriate equipment
- the child and family know how to use and fit the equipment
- the family know exactly what the child is able to do
- the equipment will be suitable in the home environment

The occupational therapist (OT) is concerned with promoting independence in the activities of daily living and will identify the appropriate equipment to help with this. The key worker and OT will undertake a home assessment for children with complex needs. Hospitalisation may need to be prolonged if the home is inadequate or inappropriate and requires major adaptations (Noyes, 2002). Having made the assessment of any adaptations and/or equipment that is required, the OT will then make a referral to social services OTs for delivery of the equipment. The social services usually need substantial notice for any long-term equipment before they can arrange for its delivery.

Written instructions for home care

Healthcare needs

- care plan to identify the child's routine of specific healthcare needs
- list of regular observations required and child's individual norms
- telephone numbers of healthcare team for advice
- specific information about the child's condition

Equipment

- care of equipment
- problem solving for malfunctions
- telephone numbers of equipment providers in case of failure

Support

- frequency and amount of home support organised
- names and telephone numbers of support agencies involved in home care
- information about self-help groups

Emergency care

- explanation of emergency procedures
- emergency telephone numbers

Study activity

Organise a visit to your hospital's OT department and discuss the OT's views on discharge planning and identify the range of equipment available to help children with special needs.

Key Points

1. Hospitalisation is traumatic for children and should therefore be kept to a minimum for this group of patients.
2. Effective discharge planning improves patient care and minimises the need for readmission.
3. Discharge planning should begin before or during the assessment process, on admission to hospital.
4. The family must be at the centre of the discharge planning process which must include all the multidisciplinary team.
5. A named individual should be responsible for coordinating, planning and evaluating discharge for each individual child.
6. Each child's named nurse should be aware of the criteria used to determine eligibility for continuing healthcare funding and be able to apply for such funding on behalf of the child and family.

Chapter 67

The Nurse as a Leader

Introduction

As discussed previously, the role of the children's nurse as a leader involves the direction of other nurses or healthcare professionals who are not used to caring for children. It may also involve influencing those outside the healthcare field who have some control over health services for children. All children's nurses can act as leaders in this way to ensure the rights of children are maintained and improved.

As families become more aware of children's rights in relation to health, nurses can expect to be involved with the handling of complaints. The acceptance and sensitive handling of complaints about the service can be influential in improving the quality of the service. On occasions the quality of the service can be linked with the available resources to provide that service, and all nurses can be instrumental in helping to ensure the best use of the available resources within the budget restraints.

The work of children's nurses can never be context free. It often takes place within healthcare settings where conditions exist, such as restricted budgets, which influence nurses' actions (Figure 67.1). Nurses clearly need to understand and manage these conditions if they are to achieve effective practice. These contexts of practice can be seen within the immediate environment of health care where nursing takes place and in the wider environment outside this setting. The wider context of practice includes such issues as government policy and how this is interpreted. Salvage (1985) stresses the importance of nurses becoming aware of political issues if they are to act effectively to respect the autonomy of individual patients and clients and safeguard the health of the wider community (Nursing and Midwifery Council, 2004).

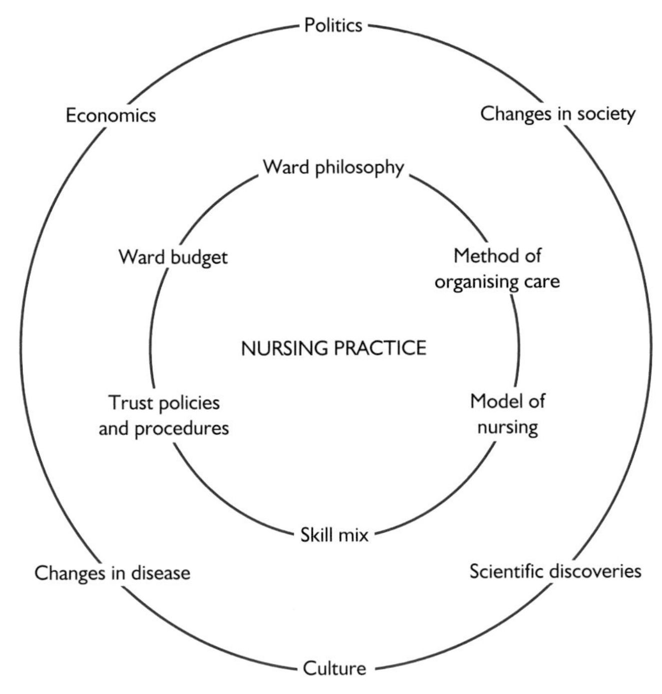

Figure 67.1 Contexts of nursing practice.

Political Influences

Study activity

Identify the political influences upon the community and hospital care of children.

Children's nursing in the community has changed dramatically since the 1970s. The move from hospital to community care has been very much influenced by government policy. As a result of a series of reports, the government White Paper *Caring for People* (1989) aimed to provide care in an environment which encouraged a normal lifestyle. This was followed by the NHS and Community Care Act 1990, which gave primary responsibility for the organisation of community care to the local authorities. This move towards community care has changed the practice of nursing; children in hospital tend to be more acutely ill and community nurses are caring for children who are more dependent and need more resources for their care. Hospital care has also been affected by the NHS and Community Care Act. Hospitals are now gradually changing into Foundation Trusts, which are autonomous bodies and can introduce their own policies and conditions of service. This could drastically alter the way in which nurses work. Some Trusts are already offering financial incentives for children's nurses to overcome a shortage of these specialist practitioners. This may benefit those Trusts with the money to offer such incentives to the detriment of others with less available cash.

The government White Paper *Working for Patients* aimed to give more power to the consumers of health care and representation in healthcare decision making. Additionally, the Children's Charter (DH, 1996), and more recently the Children's NSF (DH, 2003a), aimed to make children and parents more aware of their rights in relation to health care. Parents may now be more questioning as a result of this knowledge.

As people become more aware of their rights in relation to health care they begin to demand that their healthcare needs are met. Unfortunately, this is not always possible as economic restraints sometimes interfere with the provision of health care. Similarly, nurses, as advocates for children and their families, strive to provide the best resources but are sometimes hindered by economic factors (*see also* Children's Charter p. 268).

Managing Material Resources

The NHS is almost totally funded by the government and must compete for its funds with other government departments, such as Defence and Education. Eighty-eight per cent of NHS funds arise from general taxation, which means that the NHS relies upon the country's economic growth. It also means that health authorities have an obligation to function effectively within their budget. Increasing technology and greater demands and expectations of care have set a pattern of financial restrictions. Nurses have an important role to play in managing resources and providing high quality care within set budgets. The NHS and Community Care Act (1990) aimed to promote a closer relationship between services and cost by increasing the responsibility for budget management at ward level. It is important for nurses to play a leading role in agreeing these clinical budgets because only they can identify their nursing needs. As nursing becomes more autonomous and involved with technical advances, nurses become concerned with choosing medical stores, supplies and equipment. Although nurses are not usually involved in prescribing drugs, their knowledge of the effectiveness and acceptability of certain medications may influence the doctors' choice.

Study activity

Consider ways of encouraging nurses to be more cost conscious in the use and ordering of stores and pharmacy.

Staff cannot be encouraged to budget wisely unless they are aware of the cost of clinical supplies. Marking the prices of items in the store cupboard can raise the staff's awareness of costs but after a time this may be less effective. Monthly information about the usage and expenditure may help staff to appreciate wasteful practices. My own unit was spending so much money on Tempadots that these were no longer a cost-effective way of taking temperatures. However, when staff became aware of the high expenditure, they identified that they were taking handfuls of Tempadots at the beginning of their shift and keeping them in the pockets of their tabards. At the end of their shift any remaining ones either ended up in the washing machine or had to be discarded as they had changed colour by contact with the nurses' body heat. As a result this practice stopped and the unit made an immediate significant saving.

Savings can also be made by an effective means of stock control. Many areas now use a top-up system so that items in constant use are replaced regularly and the practice of stockpiling is prevented. This system still benefits from nurses' appreciation of costs and the identification of any actual or predicted change in the use of supplies.

Study activity

Imagine you are thinking of buying an expensive piece of equipment for yourself (e.g. computer, video recorder, dishwasher). The department store has a range of different makes of this equipment. What factors would determine your choice?

The management of material resources is not just concerned with the ordering process. Just as you would do when buying equipment for yourself, the ward manager must consider the following:

- How do the costs of various makes compare?
- Does it perform all the functions required?
- How easy will it be to use? How much training would staff require to use it?
- How soon is it likely to be replaced by a better model?
- Is it easy to store?
- What are the maintenance costs?
- Does it require special equipment to be used with it or can existing equipment be used?

Study activity

Take a critical look at the way in which stores and equipment are ordered in your current area of practice. Is it a cost-effective way of managing material resources?

Cost-effective material resource management

- Stores ordered in a way which prevents stockpiling but ensures a ready supply of items used most frequently
- Authorisation of orders by named staff allows budget control but should not be so restrictive that stores can only be ordered by one person
- A strategy for ensuring a constant turnover of stock so items do not become unusable because of date or condition
- Clear understanding of the length of time orders take to be dispatched to enable planning of the stock required
- A clear strategy for identifying, reporting and removing obsolete or faulty equipment which is known by all staff
- All staff are aware of the cost and usage of stores and the monthly budget report and know how to report concerns or changes in relation to these

The Provision of Health Care

Unfortunately, like resources, the provision of health care, especially in relation to specialist care, is not equally distributed across the UK. Access to certain care is often determined geographically and although this was formally recognised by the government in 1993 in the Tomlinson report, changes have been slow.

Study activity

Compare the specialist services available in your nearest major UK city with those in a more rural area known to you.

Rural areas often have limited access to specialist services. Some big cities in the UK have a helicopter emergency medical service (HEMS), which significantly improves mortality rates for trauma victims by being able to provide expert care within the first hour (the golden hour) of the incident. Specialist care for children may only be available in selected centres and transfer to these centres inevitably takes time and may affect outcome. In 1996 the tragedy of a child who died while being transferred to the only available paediatric intensive care bed highlighted the shortage of such specialist care outside the major UK cities (NHS Executive, 1996). As a result of this, the Department of Health set up a national coordinating group to report on the best way to provide paediatric and intensive care services. This report (DH, 1997) described how all hospitals should be part of a unified paediatric intensive care (PIC) service, with a lead PIC unit. The lead PIC unit should provide a retrieval service supporting a network of hospitals, each of which will ensure the provision of high-dependency care and be able to initiate intensive care and stabilise the child while awaiting retrieval. This model has recently been reviewed (DH, 2003a) and found to be effective in managing this level of care and the peaks in demand for critical care (*see also* The demand for paediatric intensive care p. 393 and Resources and rationing p. 709).

The alternative argument relates to the success of these leading specialist centres. Some childhood illnesses are very rare and the special skills needed to care for and treat such children may only be available at major centres where sufficient numbers of these children have been seen. For instance, neonates have a better prognosis if treated in specialist units than if treated by district hospitals (Confidential Enquiry into Stillbirths and Deaths in Infancy, 2003), and the mortality of children with some types of cancer is lower at tertiary centres (National Institute for Health and Clinical Excellence, 2005). Edge *et al.* (1994) noted that adverse events are more likely to occur if a child is transported to specialist centres by non-specialist staff and recommend that a dedicated specialist paediatric team transfers children.

Different purchasers of health care may discriminate against children who need costly treatments. General practitioners may be reluctant to register children who will use much of their budget on expensive medical treatment. Even relatively inexpensive treatments may not be available to children as NHS Trusts are forced to make financial savings. In some areas routine surgery, such as tonsillectomies and insertion of grommets, have been curtailed. This surgery has no proven effect for all children, but it is recommended that paediatricians and ENT surgeons jointly determine which children would benefit from surgery (National Institute for Health and Clinical Excellence, 2001). The access to specialised services for children with special needs and mental health problems also varies widely according to geographical area (*see also* Ear surgery p. 469).

As leaders, nurses who are aware of such discriminatory practices should help families to make an informed choice about the available care and the possible options. Although this may raise questions about the availability of expensive or sophisticated forms of treatment, people are entitled to this knowledge. In the 21st century the emphasis in health care has been on competition and all areas of health care are rated by their achievement of various standards and targets. Increased patient choice, payment by results and the creation of Foundation Trusts mean that providers of health care now have to ensure their care is of the highest quality if they are to attract patients and receive the necessary funding to survive. They have to be able to 'market' their successes. Casey (2006) indicated that quality improvements do not always reach the media and listed some successes related to children's nursing for that year:

- rates of MRSA bacteria in children's hospitals are amongst the lowest in the NHS
- accidents in children, requiring hospitalisation, decreased from 2.5 million in 1997 to 2.01 million in 2002
- the proportion of breastfed babies in the UK rose by 3%
- numbers of community nursing teams in the UK rose to 240 from just 47 in 1987

Study activity

Discuss with some colleagues the marketing strategy you could use to 'sell' your area of children's nursing.

The NHS can no longer provide for everyone and there is often a partnership between it and the voluntary sector. Many areas of children's nursing, such as hospices and cancer nursing services, are funded by charities. As members of the public become aware of this they are often motivated to set up pressure groups and raise money themselves to provide the necessary resources. In 1997, a specialist children's ward was saved from closure because parents organised a series of protests to make sure their concerns were heard (Payne, 1997). As you can see, nurses and families can influence the provision of care but fundraising is only one way of doing this.

Influencing the provision of health care

Nurses can influence the provision of health care by:

- negotiation with senior managers
- raising local awareness
- appealing to the local league of friends of the Trust
- research to provide clear evidence of the need

Families can influence the provision of health care by:

- drawing up a petition
- obtaining support of the local MP
- writing to the local press
- appealing to the health service commissioner
- involving rotary clubs
- informing the Community Health Council

Study activity

Consider other ways in which you, and the families you care for, can influence healthcare services.

The effectiveness of such measures will depend upon the continuing motivation of those involved and their access to influential people and organisations. Obviously, nurses have to be careful not to compromise their professional code of conduct and must be able to present their case objectively with valid and reliable evidence to support their argument. Families who are trying to improve services may use the complaints procedure, among other strategies, to highlight a problem.

Handling Complaints

Although praise, thank-you letters and congratulatory notes are offered more freely than complaints (DH, 1994a), it is only the latter that attract publicity and need investigation. The incidence of complaints, however, does provide an indicator of the quality of care for purchasers of health care who can obtain copies.

Study activity

Find out what complaints have been received during the past year in your current area of practice. Who is the complainant in these cases and at what point in the child's care was the complaint received? Consider how you would handle complaints such as these.

Common areas of complaints include:

- inadequate explanations about care
- misunderstandings about discharge arrangements
- inedible or unsuitable hospital food
- care or treatment omitted
- poor staff attitude

The value of complaints

- Improving the standards of service
- Providing the encouragement to improve communication
- Emphasising the importance of accurate, timed and dated record keeping
- Reflection upon words and actions
- Ensuring a clear rationale for practice

(Reid, 1996)

All these complaints may seem trivial but they are all potentially serious. The first two complaints are related to a lack of communication between healthcare professionals and families. This is the most common reason for complaints and is usually the easiest to remedy. The omission of care may be due to negligence and have potential legal implications for the Trust and accusations of professional misconduct for the member of staff involved. The complaint about hospital food may reflect upon the quality of care offered by the Trust, especially as evidence shows that nutrition is related to healing and immunity to infection (Westwood, 1997). Families also have a right to expect that appropriate food will be part of children's care in hospital as this aspect is part of the Children's NSF (DH, 2003a). Complaints are often the result of anxieties and feelings of guilt which parents have not been able to express in any other way.

The most likely complainants are the parents but occasionally a relative will complain on their behalf. Most people prefer not to complain while the child is still receiving attention. Many reasons are given for this, such as 'I know you are always busy' or 'I didn't like to bother you', but a more disturbing reason is that of fearing victimisation. Obviously, people who believe this have lost their trust and confidence in the nursing profession. Others may simply want to avoid confrontation. Consequently, most complaints are received after the child has gone home.

The management of complaints will vary according to the type and severity of the complaint but each Trust should have guidelines for handling complaints with which you should make yourself familiar (see Figure 67.2). As stated previously, the most common cause for complaints is lack of communication, therefore complainants should initially have an opportunity to discuss their problems and feel that their concerns are being listened to. In the majority of cases, complaints start as concerns and are made orally. It is important to try to resolve them on the spot (DH, 2004). This can often be done easily by acknowledging

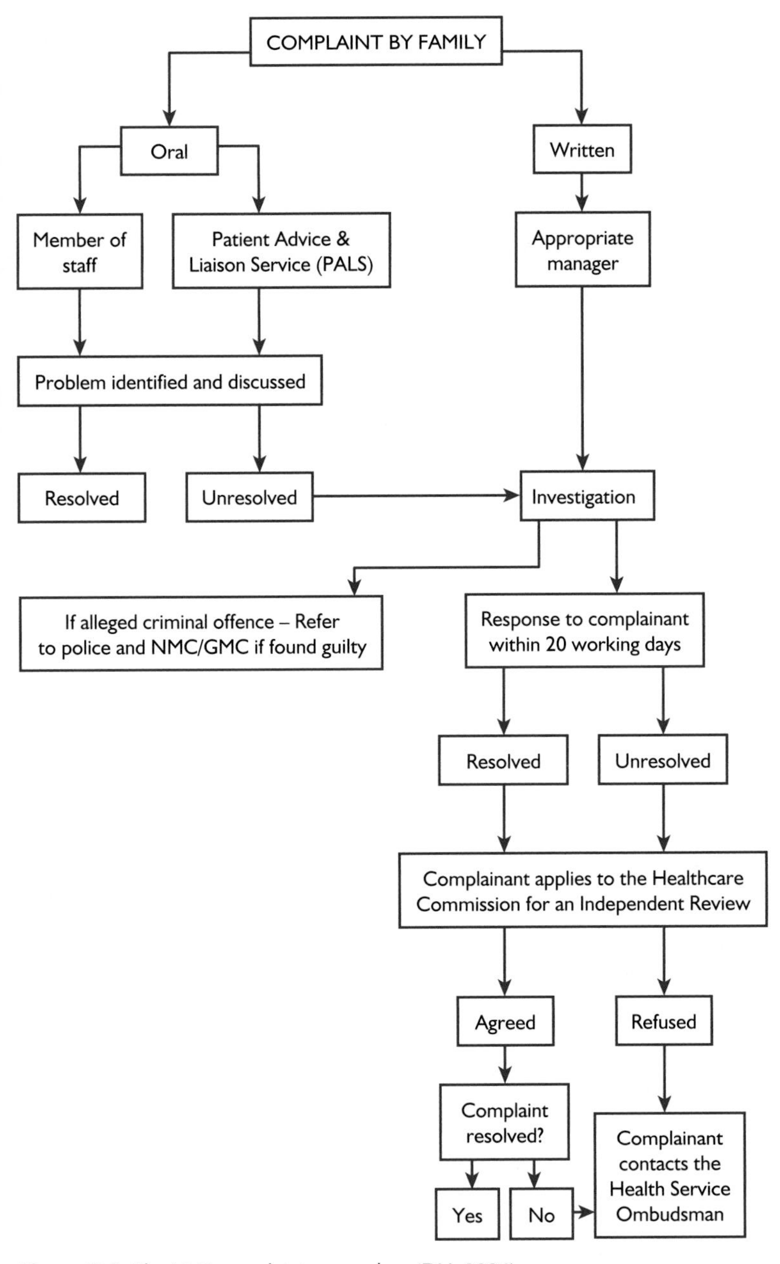

Figure 67.2 The NHS complaints procedure (DH, 2004).

the concerns and outlining any subsequent action to prevent a reoccurrence of the problem. The Ombudsman has noted that a significant number of complainants do not pursue their complaints when they are satisfied that action has been taken (Blackshaw, 1994). Complaints can be seen as a way of improving services and the Department of Health (2004) suggests that nurses look at complaints rationally and honestly and advises that an explanation and apology can be very reassuring to a concerned parent.

Key Points

1. All children's nurses should act as leaders to ensure that the rights of children are heard and acted upon.
2. Political influence on healthcare provision for children is great but nurses can also have an effect upon this provision.
3. The provision of healthcare services for children is unequally distributed across the UK and families may need help to identify the availability of services for their child's needs.
4. Nurses attempting to influence the provision of services for children should do so in a constructive way that will not bring themselves or their profession into disrepute.
5. The management of material resources is one way in which nurses can influence the quality and effectiveness of care.
6. Complaints should be seen as positive as they promote a way of reflecting upon and improving practice.

Chapter 68

The Organisation of Patient Care

Introduction

There are various ways of organising the care of children in hospital, which have evolved over the years to meet the needs of those managing the care and to respond to changes in nursing. These changes have occurred as nurses have become dissatisfied with their image as doctors' handmaidens and have sought ways of raising the profile of nursing. As one result of this dissatisfaction, models of nursing have evolved. These models redefine the traditional nurse–patient relationship and promote the care of patients as individuals. If patients are to be cared for as individuals, the system of delivery of care must enable nurses and patients to be able to relate to each other as individuals and be flexible enough to enable nurses to develop innovative ways of meeting individuals' unique needs.

Although models of nursing and ways of organising patient care have lost popularity in recent years, they are likely to be important again now the issues of workforce redesign and individualised care have emerged as the key themes in the health service of the 21st century. The children's NSF (DH, 2003a) sends out a strong message about working in partnership with the child and family to plan all aspects of care. This principle has always been linked with primary nursing but this is not the only way to organise care with a named nurse providing individualised care. As with all methods of organising care, primary nursing has its advantages and disadvantages and nurses need to look carefully at their individual areas of work and identify the method that can offer the best quality of care for their patient group. Shaw (1986) has suggested a framework for measuring quality assurance, which enables an impartial discussion of these various organisational methods:

3Es: Efficiency – producing results with minimum effort.
Effectiveness – capable of producing the desired results.
Equity – capable of being impartial.

3As: Accessibility – easiness of availability.
Appropriateness – degree of suitability for the job.
Acceptability – endorsement from those involved.

Task Allocation

In this system the child's care is broken down into a hierarchy of tasks, mostly concerned with physical needs. Traditionally, more senior nurses carried out the more complicated tasks and junior staff did the more fundamental care. This, of course, immediately tends to suggest that the fundamental care is less important. Such care may not be life saving, but it is often important for the child and family, and often better illustrates the concept of caring than the more technological care. Fundamental care can take some time to deliver, and in this organisational system the least experienced staff are with the child and family longer than the qualified staff. Thus these inexperienced staff are in the best position to develop a therapeutic relationship but lack the knowledge and skills to develop and use this partnership. Alternatively, task allocation may mean that the child and family come into contact with a large number of nurses but do not relate to any of them well.

However, task allocation has been shown to be an efficient way of using resources (Huczynski and Buchanan, 1985). With an increasing HCA work force in health care whose NVQ training is task centred, task allocation may be the most cost-effective method of managing care. Cost-effectiveness is a powerful argument for NHS Trusts, which aim to provide value-for-money quality care. This quality is often measured by standards that reduce care into measurable tasks. However, the question of what constitutes quality in care must be considered. Does the fragmentation of care into tasks provide quality of care?

Huczynski and Buchanan (1985) have also shown that task allocation is effective. It clearly delegates responsibility and is easy to allocate staff whatever the skill mix of those on duty. Task allocation ensures equity by matching highly skilled care to the most experienced staff. It is much less stressful for junior staff who may be anxious about carrying out care in which they lack experience. This argument may be counteracted by the fact that children and families may rely more on them because they are at the bedside for the longest time. While task allocation supports Benner's (1984) ideas about the development of nursing skills, it can hinder personal development if nurses remain only performing tasks in which they have the most practice.

Task allocation gives children and families more access to more staff. This enables them to identify the nurse with whom they feel most comfortable and gives them the choice of the nurse with whom they wish to develop a relationship. Adult patients endorse this method as they find the access to more nurses reassuring and less stressful than relying on one nurse. There is no reason to think that children and families would react differently. Nurses are involved in the care of more children and families and can develop more nursing knowledge as a result of the varied experience available in task allocation. However, it is this increased accessibility which seems to be in direct opposition to the concept of family-centred care. Is it possible for several nurses to create a therapeutic relationship with one child and family? In addition, sociologists have found that this method of work organisation in industry produces boredom, frustration and a sense of alienation and powerlessness amongst workers (Blauner, 1964).

Task allocation appears very acceptable for nursing today. It matches the increasing unqualified workforce, so general managers may see it as a way of saving money on qualified, experienced and expensive staff. It may also be attractive to some nurses who find close relationships with children and families too stressful. Its acceptability may be shown by the number of specialist posts in paediatrics that have tended to be task related. For example, a child with Crohn's disease may be cared for by the stoma nurse, the nutrition nurse, the pain control nurse and the nurse providing the day-to-day care.

Study activity

Read the above section on task allocation again and consider the individualised care questions in the box. Then discuss with some colleagues the future of this method of organising care.

Individualised care – questions to ask

- Does the organisation of care promote an individualised approach to care?
- Does it provide nurses with opportunities to develop relationships with children and their families?
- Does it encourage such opportunities?
- Does it enable the recognition of nurses as individuals?
- Does it give nurses the opportunity to be creative and innovative in meeting individual needs?
- Does it help nurses to gain knowledge and skills about providing individualised care to help future children and patients by enabling (a) an insight into their own feelings and (b) feedback about the care they gave?

Patient Allocation

In this organisational method each nurse is allocated a group of patients. This nurse provides all the care for these patients for a specific length of time, which can vary from the duration of a shift, or for a week, or whenever the nurse is on duty. Patient allocation is efficient because it makes best use of the skills of each nurse to be matched to the patients' needs. However, just because a child and family do not need highly skilled nursing care does not also mean that they do not need a high degree of support or teaching. It is an effective way of delivering care because it clearly defines areas of responsibility and accountability for each shift. It is less effective over a period of time because a number of nurses will have been involved in the care. It is equitable because it assigns patients according to the skills of each nurse on duty and this can be less stressful for junior nurses who may be less confident about caring for acutely ill children.

Patient allocation appears to give children and families optimum access to a number of nurses if it is practised over a period of time. The families are not dependent on one nurse alone, but they do have the continuity of carers by having access to a few named nurses across their period of hospitalisation. This depends on careful planning of off-duty rotas, to match nurses who have just had time off, and are then on duty for several days, with new admissions. If patient allocation is only practised for the duration of a shift, the child and family, as well as the nurse, may not have time to establish a therapeutic relationship. This may suit some nurses who find such relationships stressful.

Patient allocation appears to be an acceptable way of organising care because nurses have the satisfaction of being able to meet all the needs of their children and families who have fewer nurses with whom to relate.

Team Nursing

Although patient allocation ideally gives children and families three nurses with whom to relate over a 24-hour period, it can also mean several nurses if the child is in hospital for 7 days or longer. Team allocation tries to overcome this. The ward staff are divided into teams and each team is responsible for the total care of a certain number of patients. The patients are usually grouped in one geographical area of the ward. The team's hours of duty are organised to ensure that at least one nurse from the team is on duty at any time. Kron (1981) suggests that a small group of nurses working together, guided by a nurse leader, is more efficient than nurses working alone, but also warns that without good leadership this method of working can lead to fragmentation, a return to task allocation and lack of accountability. It can be an effective way of working as individual nurses can receive help, support and supervision from the rest of the team and therefore feel more confident (Reed, 1988). Thomas *et al.* (1992) found that nurses within a team considered that they had a greater knowledge of their patients and families and that, as a result, they could provide more security for them. This method of working also gives equal status to team members and promotes a democratic view. Children and families have access to a group of named nurses, one of whom will always be on duty. This can provide the child and family with a degree of choice in whom they choose to share their problems with, while maintaining continuity of care. However, team nursing can pose problems with skill mix. The amount of care an unqualified team member on duty can safely provide is limited. However, that individual can still provide continuity for the child and family even if other nurses may be required to help with specific aspects of care. Good communication and flexible off-duty rotas are key issues in the success of team nursing.

Team nursing is appropriate for an area where the skills and qualifications of staff are different. It also incorporates part-time staff much more easily than other systems of managing care. It enables these staff to recognise their limitations within the security of a supportive team. It is also an appropriate way of meeting the government requirement for a named nurse. The team leader is the experienced and appropriately qualified registered nurse but the family knows the other team members when the leader is not present. Thomas *et al.* (1992) found that most staff accepted team nursing well, experiencing greater job satisfaction than with previous organisational methods.

Primary Nursing

Primary nursing was developed by a group of American nurses in the 1970s who were concerned by the fragmentation of care and responsibility provided by other systems of patient care organisation (Manthey *et al.*, 1970). A primary nurse is responsible and accountable for the total care of a group of patients from admission to discharge (and any subsequent readmissions). The original idea was that this nurse retained responsibility and accountability even when off duty. When off duty, the care is delegated to an associate nurse who works according to the primary nurse's prescribed care. Any alteration in care, except in emergency situations, is discussed with the primary nurse. Primary nursing is an efficient method of organising care because it makes the optimum use of qualified staff. The appropriately qualified and experienced nurses act as primary nurses, with other qualified staff as associate nurses. Unqualified staff take over responsibility for housekeeping duties and are not involved in direct patient care. This is a much more cost-effective use of staff, as found in the University of York's study into the effectiveness of the nursing workforce (Carr-Hill and Jenkins-Clarke, 2003). This system is also effective in producing good results. Gahan (1991) found that continuity of care was facilitated and there was consistency in the approach to care and the information given to families. She found that it enabled a holistic approach to care, with the role of the family being better negotiated, clarified and documented than previously. Primary and associate nurses provide support for each other and can experience increased job satisfaction with the increased responsibility and autonomy provided by this way of nursing (Gahan, 1991).

Primary nursing is equitable as it uses the expertise of all staff members. It completely alters the traditional hierarchical roles within nursing and the ward sister develops a clinical specialist and support role. This equity of roles and the destruction of the hierarchy of nursing may have a negative influence unless staff are well prepared and motivated towards primary nursing. Robinson (1991) warns that this type of nursing can lead to the development of an elite core of nurses and this should be prevented by supporting and developing all staff to make the best use of their abilities. Care must be taken in considering the roles of part-time and night staff. Gahan (1991) describes how healthcare assistants' roles changed from providing direct care to ordering supplies and catering for families' hotel needs. This change gave them a clearer identification of their role and its contribution to the total care of the child and family.

Primary nursing gives the child and family close access to a highly skilled children's nurse. The families are in no doubt which individual nurse is responsible for their child's care. Primary nursing is very suitable for paediatrics, as it provides families the opportunity for partnership in care in a much more structured way than other methods of organising care. It has been shown to be well accepted by nurses (Fradd, 1988) and children and families (Rogers *et al.*, 1992). Binnie (1987) suggests that it is also acceptable to managers as it provides good value for money and, although it usually means a change in staff establishment to increase the number of registered nurses, this change improves the quality of nursing care. This idea does not fit well in today's NHS where the predictions for health care in 2010 show a tendency to substitute lower paid support workers to provide small numbers of highly qualified staff (Browne and Odell, 2004). However, there is increasing recognition of studies that show that hospitals with higher proportions of registered nurses give better care outcomes (Aitken *et al.*, 2002).

Study activity

- Consider how well each method of care described above promotes individualised care.
- Consider an area in which you have worked and rationalise which method of organising care is most suitable for that specific setting and patient group.

Primary nursing – nurses' roles

The primary nurse

- is usually a registered children's nurse
- has the responsibility for the total care of a group of children and families from admission to discharge
- acts as an advocate for the child and family
- coordinates and ensures continuity of care
- has accountability and autonomy in decision making
- requires support and help
- acts as an associate nurse for other primary nurses
- acts as a link nurse for student nurses

The associate nurse

- is a first or second level nurse
- works with the primary nurse to carry out agreed care
- provides support and help for the primary nurse
- may also be a primary nurse for other children and families

Primary nursing – changes to the ward sister role

- Devolves autonomy to primary nurses
- Facilitates a supportive environment
- Helps nurses to assess their own practice
- Provides expert advice and teaching
- Organises workloads and shift systems to enable:
  - close nurse/child/family relationships for primary nurses
  - continuity of care
  - even distribution of primary and associate roles
- May act as role model by taking on primary and associate nurse roles
- Helps the multidisciplinary team to understand primary nursing

Potential problems for the implementation of primary nursing

Attitudes of nursing staff

- willing and motivated to undergo change
- able to manage close relationships with children and families
- real knowledge and understanding of primary nursing

Attitudes of medical staff

- willing to accept loss of ward sister as controller
- able to accept in-depth knowledge of the family by the primary nurse

Grades of nursing staff

- need for appropriately qualified and experienced staff

Shift patterns

- need to allow the primary nurse to be on duty for the majority of the child's and family's stay in hospital, or enable the community nurse to be present for the main part of the agreed care

Nature of nurse education

- preparation for the autonomous practitioner
- clinical placements enable the primary nurse role to be appreciated

Unit and hospital policies

- should take into account the autonomy of the primary nurse

Key Points

1. There are four main ways of organising patient care: task allocation, patient allocation, team nursing and primary nursing.
2. Whatever method of care organisation is used it should meet Standard 8 of the Patient's Charter and provide the child and family with (a) a named nurse and (b) individualised care.
3. The care organisational method should provide the optimum care for that specific care setting and group of patients.
4. The method of organising care may be evaluated by testing its efficiency, effectiveness, equity, accessibility, appropriateness and acceptability.
5. Changing care organisational methods requires motivation and commitment from all staff as roles may undergo considerable change.

Chapter 69

Standard Setting and Audit

Introduction

Developing practice using clinical audit is a challenging and complex task. It should be concerned with improving the quality of care provided for children and their parents but it is sometimes viewed with scepticism and suspicion. If it is not performed appropriately, it can be seen as a government cost-cutting exercise or a regulatory mechanism (Morrell, 1996). Used properly, it provides a tool that contributes to the monitoring of quality, quantity and resources and leads to an improvement in the care provided for patients (see Figure 69.1).

Changes in the health service in the 21st century have made clinical audit a necessity. The commissioners of health care require all service providers to define the service they can expect. Increasingly, patients also expect to know the kind of service they can expect of their chosen healthcare provider. Just as you do your main shopping in the store that you believe gives the best quality and value for money, purchasers of health care will opt to place contracts with the service provider who can offer the highest quality, most cost-effective care. Patients are likely to choose hospitals that can provide high-quality patient-focused and evidence-based care. The development of NHS Trusts has meant that hospitals are in direct competition for the services they offer, so the demonstration of quality is essential.

Nursing and midwifery account for nearly half of an acute hospital's pay budget and this proportion rises in non-acute and community services. The NHS Management Executive (1991) argue that this gives nursing the greatest potential for improving the quality of patient services.

Study activity

Consider your usual choice of supermarket and jot down your reasons for shopping in this particular store.

Clinical audit

'. . . the systematic and critical analysis of the procedures used for diagnosis, care and treatment, the associated use of resources and the effect care has on the outcome and quality of life for the patient.'

(DH, 1993)

'. . . a multi-professional, patient-focused audit, leading to cost-effective, high-quality care delivery in clinical teams.'

(Batstone and Edwards, 1994)

'Nursing audit is part of the cycle of quality assurance. It incorporates the systematic and critical analyses by nurses, midwives and health visitors, in conjunction with other staff, of the planning, delivery and evaluation of nursing and midwifery care, in terms of their use of resources and the outcomes of patients/clients, and introduces appropriate change in response to that analysis.'

(NHS Management Executive, 1991)

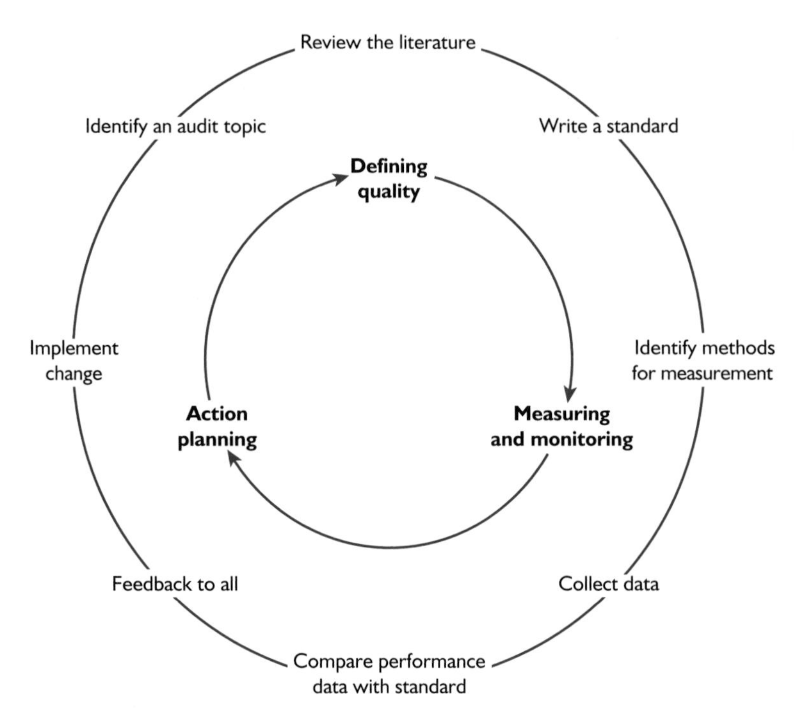

Figure 69.1 The audit cycle.

Individuals, as consumers of a service, have very firm ideas about what they expect from the people who provide that service. The usual reasons for choosing a specific service are:

- value for money
- accessibility
- clean and hygienic surroundings
- friendly, knowledgeable and helpful staff
- best quality, up-to-date products

It is easy to see how these qualities can be applied to healthcare services. Patients' charters have helped people to realise that they can expect these qualities in the provision of health care as well as in other areas of their lives. Purchasers of health care are given the responsibility of choosing the best healthcare providers for their customers. Purchasers are either fundholder general practitioners or county community councils.

Study activity

Imagine that you are a buyer of clothes for a large chain store. What criteria will you have for purchasing stock?

Purchasers have the responsibility for spending a large amount of money in the wisest way, so their choices are crucial. It is likely that some of the criteria you selected are:

- goods able to be delivered on time
- quality finish
- best deal for money in comparison with rivals
- effective and harmonious communication networks with providers
- good reputation
- meets the needs of your customers
- discount for bulk orders

These factors can be easily translated into health care, and in the same way that businesses only remain solvent when they maintain a quality service which ensures a regular income and prevents bankruptcy, healthcare Trusts now also have to achieve these aims.

Setting Standards

Managers of supermarkets and chain stores and chief executives of healthcare Trusts have to consider how to ensure that their staff are aware of the criteria that indicate the quality of their service. One of the criteria for choosing to shop in a particular store is that staff are approachable and knowledgeable. What does this really mean? If you were asked to demonstrate these qualities would you really know what was expected of you? It is also likely that different people would interpret these qualities differently.

One of the main reasons for setting standards in health care is to let everyone know exactly what is expected of them in order to provide care at the highest level. It also provides an objective way of measuring this high-quality care. Nursing standards, which should be written in discussion with all those involved in any particular aspect of care, are usually written using the following headings:

- *Standard statement* – a broad aim which states the intention to provide an optimum level of care.
- *Structure* – the physical, social and psychological environment and resources necessary for the care to be given.
- *Process* – how the nursing care will actually be performed.
- *Outcome* – the anticipated effect of the care in measurable terms (see Table 69.1).

The DH (1994b) recommends that standards are a multidisciplinary activity to form a consistent and collaborative approach to improving the quality of patient care. Much of the original work on standard setting was said to be patient centred but patients were not usually involved; in 1995 the NHS Management Executive funded work to develop the involvement of service users. This has resulted in local initiatives where patients have become actively involved in standard setting and monitoring. The children's NSF (DH, 2003a) stresses the importance of including parents and children in setting and measuring standards of care. Children are keen to be involved in monitoring quality of care and most children's nurses want to include children in all stages of the audit cycle 'because they are the service users' (Moules, 2004). Once written, standards must be agreed by line managers and made available to all staff.

The audit process for nursing

- *Objective/standard setting* – a precise definition of what is to be achieved and why which reflects the overall objectives of the service
- *Implementation* – the introduction of clinical, operational and management policies, procedures and guidelines to enable staff to deliver the agreed standards
- *Measuring and recording* – the process of measuring and recording appropriate data in a valid, systematic and objective way
- *Monitoring and identifying an action plan* – the interpretation and use of the data to make any changes in any of the previous stages and/or revise standards as appropriate

Study activity

Study the standards used in your current area of practice and find out who was involved in writing them. Identify how the involvement of members of the multi-disciplinary team and children and their parents could further contribute to these standards.

Standards cannot be set in isolation from the organisation. They should reflect the overall aims of the service, which are usually found in the Trust's annual business plan where key objectives are set to provide a framework for the following year. If standards are to be effective and valuable they should also be:

- based on the best available research
- subdivided into discrete, observable items of practice
- capable of being measured
- realistic and able to be achieved
- unambiguous and clearly understood by all
- readily available to all.

Implementing Standards

'Standards do not implement themselves.' The Department of Health (2006a) warns that standards will only improve care if the organisation provides the appropriate policies and resources support the standard. Clinical, operational and management polices, procedures and guidelines and the appropriate human and medical/nursing resources should be in place or introduced to enable the standard to be met and to be audited.

Managing the audit process

- *Organisational arrangements* – determine how the audit process operates within the organisation and who will take overall responsibility for acting upon audit findings
- *Leadership* – is required to ensure that staff feel supported and are aware of their role and responsibility
- *Coordination* – to ensure that all those involved in the audit topic are involved and informed
- *Expertise* – in research methodology to make appropriate use of measurement tools
- *Education* – of all staff to provide the appropriate awareness, knowledge and skills to enable them to accept and participate in the audit process
- *Resources* – sufficient funding and/or resources are needed to support the audit process
- *Prioritisation* – of issues to be audited by comparing the desirability and impact of the audit with the feasibility of being able to undertake it and/or act upon the results

(NHS Management Executive, 1991)

Study activity

Reread some the standards you studied in the previous activity and identify the policies required to implement them.

Measuring and Recording Standards

Study activity

Study the example standard given in Table 69.1 and consider how you could measure and record the outcomes of this standard.

There are numerous techniques for measuring and recording standards, with certain techniques being more appropriate to particular aspects being audited. It is particularly difficult to measure outcomes that relate to feelings and emotions and, for this reason, most standards

Table 69.1 Pressure sore risk assessment: example of a standard

Standard statement		
All patients who are admitted to the Unit shall have a pressure sore assessment chart completed on admission, and reviewed at appropriate intervals, thus providing an individual approach to prevention of skin breakdown in patients.		
Structure	**Process**	**Outcome**
Assessment charts to be available in admission packs	On admission, the allocated nurse will complete the Waterlow risk-assessment chart for each individual patient	Patients will be individually cared for in relation to prevention of skin breakdown
Information on how to use assessment charts available in each clinical area	The admission and subsequent Waterlow scores will be documented on the individual patients' care plans and referred to at report time	Assessment of skin breakdown will be based on current research findings
Nurses who can demonstrate a knowledge of wound assessment	New nurses will be oriented by the ward sister to wound assessment charts	A multidisciplinary involvement in pressure sore risk assessment will enhance communication and understanding in this field
Availability of 'aids' within the clinical areas to prevent skin breakdown	The child's care team will review effectiveness of assessment charts on a monthly basis	Reduction in pressure sores will reduce patient's stay in hospital and overall costs A nursing team committed to and competent in relation to managing individual patients' risk assessment

are best measured using a variety of measuring tools. These tools should follow research rules, procedures and best practices or the audit findings may be invalid (DH, 2006a). The Audit Commission's audit of children's services in 1992/3 included an assessment of the quality of care using objectively measured data, the views of children and parents and staff, and observations made by the auditors (Table 69.2).

Questionnaires

There are many patient satisfaction questionnaires that cover a range of issues such as the approachability of staff and the availability and quality of facilities. These questionnaires can be used during or after the patients' stay. Clearly, only older children can use questionnaires and, although parents can be asked about their satisfaction with their children's care, it is difficult to involve younger children in this way.

Questionnaires can also be used to ask staff how standards are being maintained, but they cannot be used reliably to evaluate the effectiveness or competence of practitioners. The NHS Management Executive (1991) suggests the use of the Slater Nursing Competency Rating Scale to assess competence. This audit tool uses retrospective ratings on care plans and direct observation of nurse performance.

Observation

An impartial observer from another area, or a healthcare auditor, can observe the service given and report their findings. Self-recording can be

Table 69.2 Auditing the quality of children's services: examples of measurements (Audit Commission, 1993)

Area of care	Objective data	Child/parent view	Staff view	Auditor observation
Named nurse	Identified on care plans?	Do they know who this is?	How does the system work?	Is this made obvious?
Pain relief	Are pain assessment forms in place?	Are they involved in assessment?	How do they assess pain?	Do pain charts show evidence of assessment?
Information	Is a range of information leaflets available?	Have they been given appropriate information?	How do they provide information?	Are leaflets readily available?
Registered children's nurses	Do duty rosters show a minimum of two per shift?		How does the senior nurse maintain the skill mix?	How many RSCN/RN (child) are on duty?
Facilities for parents	What facilities are available?	What do parents think about the facilities?	Can they offer facilities to all parents?	What are the facilities like?

used as an alternative to observers who can be expensive in terms of their time.

Internal monitoring/peer review

Teams of nurses can measure their own standards and this method is probably more reliable than self-monitoring and less threatening than using outsiders. It is still difficult to avoid the subjectiveness of this type of measurement.

Record audit

Spot checks of records provide a way of examining the relevance and quality of nursing practice.

Clinical indicators

Indicators such as measures of health, infection rates or the incidence of pressure sores or accidents provide objective data about clinical care.

Benchmarking

Agreed standards of best practice (benchmarks) can be used by practitioners to compare and share practices to ensure that quality care is delivered in a fair and consistent way (DH, 2001a). Benchmarking can be undertaken with other wards in the same or different hospital, regionally or even nationally.

Study activity

Find out how the area in which you are working measures parents' and children's views on the quality of care. How do they use their findings? How do they provide feedback for staff and the families?

Another way of using the patient's viewpoint is to use the patient story technique. This can be done by the practitioner joining a child and parent for the day and trying to experience the event as part of the family. Alternatively, practitioners can put themselves into the patient role and try anonymously to appreciate the patient's experience. This is an objective and powerful way of seeing what areas of practice may need improving.

Study activity

Find a family who are willing to let you tell their story. Accompany them through a hospital experience (outpatient visit, day surgery, trip to the X-ray department, and so forth) and see how this changes your perspective of the care provided.

Monitoring the standard and planning further action

The monitoring stage of clinical audit processes the information gathered during the measurement of the standard. Once all the information has been collated and reviewed the resulting data should be compared with the standard. Then an action plan can be formulated to identify any further steps that may need to be taken to enhance the area of practice under review. If the standard is shown to have been met, it may be appropriate to raise the standard or simply to set the next review date. It is important to remember that a negative outcome may not always mean that the quality of care is poor. At this stage of the audit the validity of the previous steps should be considered:

- Was the measurement tool valid and reliable?
- Was the sample size sufficient?
- Was the implementation of the standard made possible (was the standard supported by appropriate resources and policies)?
- Was the initial standard appropriate?

One outcome of the audit process is a better understanding of appropriate standards (NHS Management Executive, 1991), so if the audit identifies that the standard requires modification, the audit should not be considered a failure.

The outcome of the audit process should be clearly summarised to all those involved and any need for change discussed before implementation and remeasurement. The process is repeated as often as necessary to ensure the maintenance and development of clinical excellence (Nursing and Midwifery Audit Information Service, 1996).

Essence of care – fundamental aspects of care

- Privacy and dignity
- Personal and oral hygiene
- Food and nutrition
- Pressure ulcers
- Continence and bladder and bowel care
- Safety of clients with mental health needs in acute mental health and general hospital settings
- Record keeping
- Principles of self-care

(DH, 2001a)

Essence of care – promoting health

- Empowerment and informed choice
- Education for practitioners
- Assessment of health promotion needs
- Opportunities to promote health
- Engagement of individuals, groups and communities
- Partnership with partner organisations to promote health
- Access and accessibility to health promotion information, services and support
- Environments which promote health and well-being
- Outcomes of promoting health

(DH, 2006a)

Essence of Care

The Department of Health issued *Essence of Care* in 2001 to help nurses measure the quality of the fundamental aspects of care. The eight aspects of care considered important for patients were chosen from an analysis of complaints, Health Commissioner reports, professional conduct committee hearings and patients' views. Each area was given an overall statement of best practice, which expresses what patients want from practice and is supported by a list of factors that have been identified to achieve the outcome. In 2006, a further nine standards were added to reflect health promotion (Table 69.3 and Figure 69.2).

Study activity

Look at the essence of care standards measured in your own area and choose one to benchmark with another area in which you have worked.

Research, Audit or Evaluation?

There is often confusion about what is audit and what is research or evaluation. This confusion is not helped by the fact that all three words can have 'to examine' as part of their definition and the terms tend to be used interchangeably. However, in the context of health care, the purpose of each is quite different with specified criteria (Table 69.4).

Table 69.3 Essence of care: diagrammatic presentation of benchmark statements (DH, 2001a)

0		5	10
Worst practice statement	Statements of practice that step towards best practice	Statements of practice that step towards best practice	Best practice statement

Table 69.4 Clinical audit and research

	Clinical audit	Research
Purpose	Compares practice against agreed indicators, improvements	Contributes to knowledge about health care using scientific principles
Process	Uses criteria-related studies, surveys, case note analysis, adverse incidents	Uses experimental studies, surveys, case studies, descriptive accounts
Results	Results are compared with agreed standards or guidelines to see if these have been achieved	Results provide new knowledge to verify a hypothesis or generate a new hypothesis
Implications	Implications only relate to the service being audited	Implications for the whole field of health care
Reporting	Usually only reported locally	Reported publicly, open to scrutiny

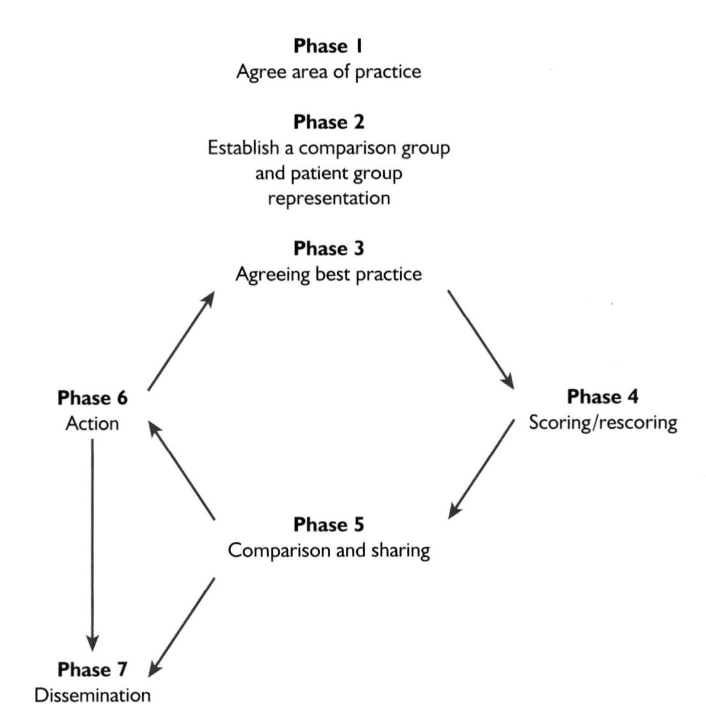

Figure 69.2 Essence of care – phases of benchmarking (DH, 2001a).

Scientific and social research is concerned with advancing understanding through the acquisition of new knowledge, establishment of facts or perceptions and the development of new methods. The findings from the new knowledge should be generalisable to similar problems elsewhere. Generally research is directed at achieving one or more of the following objectives:

- understanding the causes of diseases and how they can be detected or prevented
- developing improved interventions to promote health, treat ill health or improve social care
- providing information on improving quality, access and efficiency for health and social care
- producing reliable evidence of what works best to meet health and social care needs

Clinical audit is a quality improvement process that seeks to improve patient care and outcomes by a systematic review of care against explicit criteria and, as a result of the review, implements change. The criteria used are found by the use of good-quality guidelines, integrated care pathways, literature reviews or local consensus.

If research establishes the best way of practising, and audit checks and establishes that this is being practised correctly, evaluation may be undertaken to assess its impact. Evaluation is the way to determine the effectiveness, efficiency and acceptability of a planned intervention in achieving its stated objectives. In summary:

- *Research* – what are the causes and extent of the condition and what is the right thing to do?
- *Audit* – having established the right thing to do, are we doing it correctly?
- *Evaluation* – if we are doing it correctly, is it having the desired effect?

Key Points

1. The audit process critically examines clinical effectiveness and identifies areas for change.
2. Since the development of NHS Trusts and patient charters, healthcare policy has placed an increasing emphasis on the audit of care.
3. The first step in the audit process is standard setting. Standards should be evidence based and produced by all those involved in that specific aspect of care.
4. Implementation of standards relies upon the support of appropriate policies and resources.
5. Methods of measuring standards should be valid and reliable.
6. The audit process is cyclical and the comparison of performance data with the standard should identify changes and/or dates for remeasurement.

Chapter 70

Workforce Allocation

Introduction

Appropriate staffing levels to meet the care of children depends on many variables such as the dependency of the children, the ward layout, the number of support staff, the shift system and the availability of appropriate staff. Traditionally, nurses believed that their areas of work were understaffed but had no objective method of substantiating their claim. The argument used tended to relate to the care the patients received compared with the ideal care that the nurses perceived they should be providing. Unfortunately, this subjective view did little to sway management and has been shown to be a flawed argument (Giovannetti, 1979). Historically, staffing levels tended to be determined in an arbitrary way and nurses have not always had the most appropriate skills for the area in which they worked (Giovannetti, 1984).

This situation eventually prompted nurses to search for an objective planning tool that would enable them to develop a formula to identify the number of staff required to achieve a desired quality of care. Unfortunately, these tools did not help specialist areas such as paediatrics. Historically, most strategies for setting staff establishment levels were designed for acute hospital wards (Hancock, 1980) and do not allow for the uniqueness of nursing children. More recently tools have been developed to manage capacity and workload in children's services (Burr, 1992; Smith and Valentine, 1999; Royal College of Nursing, 2000; Wyatt and Healey, 2005).

Calculating staffing

For one nurse on duty at any time:

No. of nurses = (length of each shift × no. of shifts per week) ÷ hours worked per week

For example:

No. of nurses = (8 hours × 3 shifts) × 7 days ÷ 37.5 hours
= 24 × 7 ÷ 37.5
= 168 ÷ 37.5
= 4.48 nurses

i.e. to provide one nurse per 8-hour shift each day of the week, 4.48 nurses are required to ensure each nurse only works 37.5 hours per week. This does not allow for sickness, study or maternity leave

Skill Mix

Skill mix is the term used to ensure that staff with the most appropriate skills are available to meet the needs of the service in the most cost-effective way. It is obviously inappropriate for highly skilled nurses to be performing housekeeping activities, yet nurses allow themselves to be used in this way (Carr-Hill and Jenkins-Clarke, 2003). On the other hand, it is also inappropriate for unqualified staff to be providing unsupervised hands-on care. Research is available to show the cost-effectiveness and improved quality of care provided by qualified staff (Aitken *et al.*, 2002; Healthcare Commission, 2005). To appreciate the complex role of the qualified nurse it is important to analyse the array of skills used when carrying out any aspect of care.

Factors to be considered when reviewing nursing establishments

- Political, local, regional and national influences – changes in commissioning processes, models of care, other local staffing levels.
- Human resources – changes in the workforce profile, roles and responsibilities, mandatory training requirements.
- Working patterns – changes to support the efficient use of resources and create flexibility to improve recruitment and retention.
- Activity and service levels – the dimensions of the service to be sustained, including strategic priorities, service developments and the increasing dependency of children in hospital.
- Learning environment – requirements to teach, support and mentor students and support the education and ongoing training of permanent staff.
- Clinical grading and pay structures.
- Safety issues – the need to ensure a safe and secure environment for children, families and staff.
- Clinical environment – layout of ward and ability to observe and staff all areas.

(Smith and Valentine, 1999)

Study activity

Brainstorm and note down typical aspects of nursing care specific to your current area of practice.

Carr-Hill and Jenkins-Clarke (2003) note that qualified nurses have difficulty in defining their specific roles. Often nurses first think of manual skills when responding to this activity. In nursing, manual skills are often referred to as basic nursing care or fundamental nursing skills. However, such a response would be supported by the *Collins Dictionary and Thesaurus*, which defines a skill as 'something requiring special training or manual dexterity'. This definition implies that these skills require knowledge and understanding. Without an underlying rationale, a skill becomes the ability to perform a meaningless task. In nursing, as in any occupation, it is easy at first to concentrate on the individual components of a skill and forget the subject as a whole. It is only when the nurse becomes proficient at a skill that the actual performance becomes almost automatic and other factors can be considered during the procedure.

Study activity

Consider the task of bed bathing and list the knowledge, skills and attitudes that are required to perform this aspect of care proficiently.

When any fundamental nursing task is considered in this way it can be seen that the nurse uses many different skills apart from that of performing the actual task. When nursing is considered in this way, the notion of manual skills can be broadened to include specialist competencies specific to a particular area of practice. This process of identifying and defining specific skills is important if nurses are to justify their employment. When nurses accept doctors' roles and delegate some parts of their role to unqualified staff they are in danger of eroding the role of the qualified nurse and making it more difficult to define and justify. Budget-conscious service managers, who are not always nurses, could decide to employ more unqualified staff for patient care at the expense of qualified staff if their role cannot be clearly identified. Indeed, in 1991, the Audit Commission's report *The Virtue of Patients* described cost savings of up to £40 million if healthcare assistants were used to carry out some of the duties currently performed by qualified staff.

Service managers have the responsibility to ensure a cost-effective skill mix. In other words, each area should employ the right number of qualified and unqualified staff to meet the varying need of each shift during the week. To make decisions about skill mix it is important to know:

- patient dependency levels
- times of increased workload
- skills available from each member of staff
- available hours of duty of staff

In many areas, information technology has helped to analyse the above information and determine skill mix. Sometimes an emphasis on grading is placed on skill mix but, although this is relevant, it is probably more important to look at individuals' different skills and experience. This may be done by an observer who statistically analyses the activities carried out by various nurses in one particular area of practice over a 24-hour period.

Study activity

Analyse your own activities for a shift. Construct a spreadsheet to jot down the time spent on each activity during a shift. At the end of the shift you can add up the time spent on each activity and determine the time spent on non-nursing tasks such as portering and domestic or secretarial duties.

Skill mixing is an important part of workforce planing within the NHS. In the current financial crisis in the NHS it is essential that cost-effective, appropriate care is provided for all patients. In most Trusts, nurses represent the largest part of the workforce and therefore have a huge impact on the pay budget. Trust finances can therefore be hugely affected if the skill mix is poorly planned. The Healthcare Commission acute hospital review of ward staffing across England and Wales 2005 raised concerns about the considerable variations in both skill mix and staffing levels in wards of a similar type in different Trusts. They concluded that those Trusts that employed more staff and spent more on staffing the wards were more likely to have better outcomes for patients than those Trusts that spent more per staff member. This means that children's nurses need to rise to the challenge of considering the role of support workers in caring for children. The children's NSF (DH, 2003a) clearly states that to ensure there are sufficient numbers of appropriately trained and motivated staff there needs to be an: 'Increase in workforce capacity and productivity through skill mix and continuing professional development: moving work from doctors and to other healthcare professionals and from other healthcare professionals to the support workforce . . .'

This should be done with caution as there is evidence to show that care can be demonstrably poor if proportions of registered nurses are too low (Healthcare Commission, 2005) and the higher the grade of nurse the better the quality of care (Smith and Valentine, 1999). Naish and Tassa (2006) found that improved patient satisfaction and clinical outcomes (incidence of pressure ulcers) are linked to the number of skilled and experienced nurses rather than simply higher numbers

Bathing a bed-ridden child – task analysis

Knowledge

- areas at risk of pressure sores
- characteristics of healthy skin
- child's disorder and treatment
- prevention of cross infection

Skills

- not causing pain or discomfort during the procedure
- observing: skin colour and condition, temperature and respirations, child's mental state, improvement/deterioration in child's condition
- using play appropriately
- adapting procedure to take account of any medical equipment

Attitudes

- relating to the child appropriately
- talking to the child and family
- explaining/teaching the procedure to the family
- sharing of knowledge in an appropriate way
- negotiating parents' role

of registered nurses. Reduced skill mix can correlate with an increase in complaints, critical incidents and staff turnover (Smith and Valentine, 1999).

Study activity

Using the results of your findings from the above activity, and in discussion with colleagues, identify the role of a support worker in children's nursing. What specific training would you consider appropriate for this role?

With consideration being given to core training in the care of children for all professionals who work with children, it may be that the foundation part of such generic training could be the entry for a support worker in children's nursing in the future.

Time and Staff Management

Part of ensuring an appropriate skill mix is securing round-the-clock expertise. For this reason, nurse managers have had to consider a more flexible approach to shifts. Most areas now practise internal rotation (when staff rotate from day to night shift) to provide continuity of care and facilitate a team approach. Many areas have also considered variations in shift patterns to reduce the numbers of nurses needed, provide family-friendly hours of work and at the same time produce a more cost-effective service.

The numbers of nursing staff required mainly depends on five factors (Roscoe, 1990):

- staffing requirements
- contracted hours of duty
- number of shifts per week
- length of each shift
- average time absent due to holiday, sickness, study or maternity leave

Traditionally, nurses have worked two types of daytime shift, which overlap in the afternoon. This overlap is often not used to its best advantage and can be seen as a waste of resources to have double the number of required staff for this period of time. Consequently, various initiatives have taken place to counteract this problem.

Shift work inevitably causes problems to humans who have evolved as a diurnal species. Northcott and Facey (1995) note that there is little published work to substantiate the efficacy of any of the various shift patterns available to nurses. Probably the most researched shift is the 12-hour 'long day', which has been introduced in some acute clinical areas. However, Todd *et al.* (1991) suggest that the evidence that these long shifts are beneficial for staff and patients is invalid. In 1995, Barton was commissioned by the Department of Health to identify the shift system that suited most nurses. She recognised that shift work can affect nurses' psychological health, quality of sleep, cardiovascular and digestive functioning, social and domestic life and job satisfaction. Barton

Advantages and disadvantages of 12-hour shifts

Advantages

- 14 shifts/month reduces travel time and expenditure
- increased number of days off per month improves leisure time
- improved continuity of care, especially for short-term patients
- only two handover periods per day
- reduced absenteeism (McKillick, 1983)
- improved opportunities for staff education (McColl, 1983)

Disadvantages

- fall-off in nurses' performance at the end of the shift (Underwood, 1975)
- overall lower quality of care (Todd *et al.*, 1991)
- continuity of care difficult for patients who stay longer than 3–4 days
- possibly contravenes 1974 Health and Safety at Work Act by giving nurses hours which are detrimental to their health and performance
- poor accumulative effect of three to four 12-hour shifts
- reduced communication by ward team members as contact is less

found that flexible rostering, which enabled individuals to cater for their preferences, also appeared to reduce some of the health problems and job dissatisfaction associated with shift work. Flexible working is seen as an effective way of recruiting and retaining the workforce, especially when the workers are predominately women.

Flexibility may also mean allowing a number of staff to work permanently on day or night shifts. Managers tend to prefer internal rotation to night duty, believing that it prevents animosity between day and night staff, facilitates professional development for all staff and promotes primary nursing across all shifts. The cost-effectiveness of internal rotation has not been proven, but research has shown that night duty disturbs circadian rhythms and for some individuals this is too stressful to be acceptable (Sadler, 1990).

Northcott and Facey (1995) warn that the European Union treaty contains a clause, yet to be agreed, which could enforce all shifts to be a maximum of 8 hours long to minimise the harmful effects of shift work upon staff. For the same reason, this clause would also enforce a maximum 48-hour working week and prescribe a maximum length of time between shifts, which may affect the late shift followed by an early shift that is common practice in many rosters. He suggests that nurses should examine their own shift patterns and produce rotas that are safe and acceptable to staff and patients before legalisation forces changes upon them.

Shift patterns

- *Regular* – a fixed roster over a period of time which is repeated when each cycle is completed. Minor variations may occur to meet special requests or to cover annual leave and sickness
- *Irregular* – a duty roster where there is no pattern of shifts and individual preferences are not taken into account; shifts are planned to meet the service need
- *Flexible* – no regular fixed hours or shift patterns. Individuals are consulted about their preferred hours of work and these are matched with the needs of the service

Study activity

Look critically at the shift patterns in your own area of work. Are these the most suitable for the staff and the type of work? Is there an even distribution of skills across the 24 hours? Are more staff available for the busiest periods? What suggestions for change could you make?

Nursing Workforce Planning

Unfortunately, there is no single formula available for assessing staffing for a typical children's ward (Royal College of Nursing, 1999). First, there is no such thing as a typical children's ward and many influencing factors for determining skill mix and numbers of staff vary across different wards. The following four techniques tend to be used, each with its own disadvantages and advantages:

- professional judgement method
- nurses per occupied bed
- timed nursing interventions
- dependency and activity analysis

Professional judgement method

This method uses the previous knowledge and experience of senior clinical and managerial staff to estimate staffing numbers and skill mix in relation to the number of beds and the predicted activity. It is quick and easy to use and is well accepted by the nursing team as it takes local practices into account. The disadvantages are lack of scientific credibility as it is using subjective data. It is therefore difficult to gain support outside nursing for findings using this method.

Nursing per occupied bed

Staff to patient ratios are calculated by using actual staffing levels from historical or current nursing data that are judged to be appropriate. This methodology is seen as more credible and it can be reassuring to some staff to be measuring staffing levels against regional 'norms'. The main disadvantages is that there is no consideration given to local services, variations in activity and the dependencies of the children.

Timed nursing interventions

This method measures the frequency of nursing interventions. Each child's direct care nursing needs for the day are recorded on a specifically designed checklist. Each intervention is matched with a previously agreed time frame. The amount of time needed to provide nursing care for all the children and the number of nurses required to provide the care can then be calculated. The advantage of this method is the ease of use once the tool has been designed. It is easily transferable to other settings and can be easily changed if activity changes. The disadvantage is the time needed to create the tool and the fact that it tends to reduce the holistic nature of nursing into tasks.

Patient dependency and activity analysis

The necessary numbers and skills of staff required in any area are determined by measuring the dependency of the patients in that area. Many scoring systems are available to determine patient dependency but they are often not useful for paediatric areas. For instance, highly dependent, severely ill patients are allocated a high score because they require a lot of highly skilled care, and self-caring patients rate a minimal score. In paediatrics, a toddler without parents present may require almost the same one-to-one nursing care as an acutely ill child. Children with parents present could be rated as self-caring but this would ignore the support and teaching required by the family, which may be a highly skilled and time-consuming process. This method is criticised as it fails to take into account the time required for psychological care and is usually a retrospective analysis (Royal College of Nursing, 1999).

Another system of determining the necessary resources for specific patients is the case management model. Patients are assigned to a case type according to their presenting problems and the services they require. Each case type has a prescribed pathway of care, which describes the patient's expected outcomes within a given time scale. The predetermined care involves all aspects of the patient's care and all personnel involved in that care. As these plans identify the care and resources required for each patient, they enable the nurse to spend more time on direct patient care and improve the continuity of care (Mosher *et al.*, 1992). Despite these advantages it does not seem appropriate for the care of children. With this type of pre-planned care the partnership philosophy of children's nursing may become lost unless the care mapping system is altered to take this into account (Finnegan, 1996). Such systems may also prevent nurses from using their autonomy to plan individualised care.

Study activity

Use the patient dependency system to determine the dependency of the children in your current area of work on one specific day. Calculate whether the number and grade of staff are appropriate for these dependency levels. Finally, look critically at your findings. Are they valid? Does the method used take account of all the variables in determining dependency?

Examples of non-nursing activities

- Making empty beds
- Trips to pharmacy, stores, etc.
- Looking for notes or X-rays
- Ordering stores, pharmacy
- Moving beds
- Telephone calls unrelated to patient care

Patient dependency studies cannot be considered in isolation from other issues. The available skill mix is important. Some care can be given more quickly by experienced staff than by newly qualified staff but more experienced staff may also have management duties as part of their role. Other staff may require time to teach and assess students.

Study activity

Look back to your activity analysis (above) and note the time you spent on non-nursing activities. Multiply this figure by the number of staff on duty during your dependency study (presume that each nurse on duty also used this amount of time for non-nursing). How does this affect your dependency figures?

Wyatt and Healey (2005) state that workforce planning is a complex calculation that needs to take into account all the variables, including intensity, urgency, expertise, probability and the extent of the facility. They suggest the use of 'STEAM', a paper-based tool developed for a

An example of patient dependency levels

- *Minimal dependency* – 4 hours of nursing care in 24 hours; < 10 minutes' direct care/hour (e.g. child having 4-hourly observations, 4-hourly oral/nebulised drugs, ready for discharge, baby with 4-hourly feeds)
- *Low dependency* – 6 hours' care in 24 hours; 10–15 minutes of direct care per hour (e.g. child having 2–4-hourly observations, 4-hourly BM stix, 4-hourly pain assessment, child with parents intermittently resident, baby with 2–3-hourly feeds, routine admission, 48 hours after major surgery)
- *Medium dependency* – 12 hours' care in 24 hours; 15–30 minutes' direct care/hour (e.g. child with IV fluids/analgesia/blood, babies and toddlers with no resident parent, acutely ill admission, child/parents requiring psychological support, children with feeding problems, hourly neurological observations, day 1 following major surgery)
- *High dependency* – 24 hours' care in 24 hours; active and intensive nursing care for 30 minutes/hour (e.g. child with special needs or requiring isolation with no parent resident, child with airway problems (unconscious, croup, severe asthma, tracheostomy), critically ill/multiple injuries child, immediate care after major surgery, care of child and parents following death/emergency transfer to another hospital)

neonatal unit, to record the level of intensity of care provided to each patient. These measurements are then used as a basis for a risk assessment of the capacity of the department and communicated using a traffic-light system to indicate whether staffing meets requirements and, if not, what action to take.

Key Points

1. Nurses must be able to give managers firm evidence of the need for appropriate numbers and skills to meet the requirements of the workload.
2. Fundamental nursing activities require specific knowledge, skills and attitudes and cannot be delegated to unqualified staff.
3. Decisions about skill mix depend upon many variables, e.g. workload, availability and experience of staff. Children's nurses must be able to analyse these variables if they are to convince management of the need for an appropriate nursing establishment.
4. Providing a 24-hour/day service for the care of sick children requires a flexible and innovative approach to shift planning.
5. Patient dependency systems do not always take the uniqueness of children's nursing into account.

Chapter 71

Risk Management

Introduction

Advances in healthcare knowledge and technology have increased the complexity of providing patient care over the past few decades. With this increase in complexity comes the associated potential for risk. Health care usually brings patients great benefits but when things go wrong it can also cause great harm. Not only does the patient suffer physical and psychological harm but the cost to the NHS is huge in monetary terms, in adverse publicity and in the distress experienced by the staff involved. Historically, the NHS has had a blame culture and the focus when things went wrong was on individual actions (DH, 2000). This can encourage people to cover up mistakes for fear of reprisal and also does not take into account the huge number of interacting factors that usually influence any incident. The Department of Health (DH, 2000) argues that a safety culture, where open reporting and analysis of incidents is encouraged, can have a positive impact on the performance of the organisation. One of the recommendations of the Bristol Royal Infirmary Inquiry in 2001 into the increased number of deaths in the paediatric cardiac unit stated that: 'For the future, the NHS must root out unsafe practices. It must remove barriers to safe care. In particular it must promote openness and the preparedness to acknowledge errors and to learn lessons.'

The Children's NSF (DH, 2003a) is also very clear about the need to maintain the safety of children in hospital by thoroughly investigating all serious events and near misses and using the findings as learning opportunities in a non-threatening multidisciplinary setting. It is only in this way that Trusts can prevent similar incidents reoccurring in their own Trust and throughout the NHS. The Department of Health (DH, 2000) recognises that many incidents in health care could have been avoided if only the lessons of experience had been learnt and shared. Yet, in 2001 a teenager died after the accidental intrathecal injection of vincristine, which should have been administered intravenously. This was the fifteenth incident of this kind in the United Kingdom since 1975 and

Why is risk management an issue in health care?

Every year in the NHS:

- Four hundred people die or are seriously injured in adverse events involving medical devices.
- Nearly 10 000 people are reported to have experienced serious adverse reactions to drugs.
- Around 1150 people who have been in recent contact with mental health services commit suicide.
- Nearly 28 000 written complaints are made about aspects of clinical treatment in hospital.
- £400 million is paid out in settlement of clinical negligence claims.
- £2.4 billion is the potential cost of existing and expected claims.
- Hospital-acquired infections (around 15% of which are avoidable) cost nearly £1 billion.

(DH, 2000)

Clinical governance

'A framework through which NHS organisations are accountable for continously improving the quality of their services and safeguarding high standards of care by creating an environment in which excellence in clinical care will flourish.'

(DH, 1998)

An organisation with a memory: recommendations for the NHS

1. Introduce a mandatory reporting scheme for adverse health events and specified near misses.
2. Introduce a scheme for confidential reporting by staff of adverse events and near misses.
3. Encourage a reporting and questioning culture in the NHS.
4. Introduce a single overall system for analysing and disseminating lessons from adverse healthcare events and near misses.
5. Make better use of existing sources of information on adverse events.
6. Improve the quality and relevance of NHS adverse event investigations and inquiries.
7. Undertake a programme of basic research into healthcare events in the NHS.
8. Make full use of NHS information systems to help staff access learning from adverse healthcare events and near misses.
9. Act to ensure that important lessons are implemented quickly and consistently.
10. Identify and address specific categories of serious recurring adverse healthcare events.

(DH, 2000)

in almost all the previous cases the patient (usually a child or teenager) eventually died. Why is it so difficult to learn lessons from such incidents?

To help fulfil its duty to maintain quality, every NHS Trust is required to have a system of clinical governance. Clinical governance should ensure that the organisation and all its staff are focused and coordinated to deliver high standards of care and service. This kind of culture should put patient safety at the top of the agenda and ensure the implementation of an effective risk management process. It is important that nurses understand the whole process of risk management as 'promoting children's wellbeing and safeguarding them from harm is the responsibility of all staff' (DH, 2003a).

Incident Reporting

Incident reporting is the foundation of effective risk management. An incident is defined as any event that causes, or may cause, physical or psychological injury, patient dissatisfaction, or loss or damage to property. This definition encompasses all accidents, ill health, dangerous occurrences and near misses. A near miss is an occurrence that, but for luck or skilful management, would in all probability have become an incident. A serious incident is any event arising from the delivery of health care that has, or could have, adversely affected more than one patient and/or is likely to attract the attention of the media.

Formal guidance on reporting untoward incidents was first issued in 1955 by the Ministry of Health: 'a brief report should be prepared by the secretary of the Board of Governors or Hospital Management Committee as soon as possible after any occurrence of the kind in question, giving the name of the person injured, the names of all witnesses, details of the injuries and the full facts of the occurrence and of the action taken at the time . . .' (MoH, 1955).

Despite these guidelines from over 50 years ago, the evidence suggests that, historically, incident reporting has been haphazard (DH, 2000). The Clinical Negligence Scheme for Trust (CNST) was established in 1995 to provide a means for NHS Trusts to fund the costs of clinical negligence claims, and almost all NHS Trusts are members. Member Trusts receive a 10–30% discount on their scheme contributions when they can demonstrate compliance with the CNST standards at level 1, 2 or 3. The clinical risk management standard includes the requirement for a local incident reporting system.

Study activity

- Find out what level of CNST is held by your NHS Trust.
- Find out how your Trust complies with the recommendations from *An Organisation with a Memory* (DH, 2000).

Even though most hospitals have some form of incident reporting, there is substantial variation in the coverage and efficacy of these reporting systems. In 1999, Dineen and Walsh reported that:

- 20% of NHS Trusts do not have reporting systems covering the whole organisation
- less than 50% of NHS Trusts provide specific training on risk management or incident reporting
- under 33% provide guidance to staff on what to report
- around 30% do not expect clinicians to report unexpected complications or events
- rates of reporting vary widely

In 2000 the Department of Health issued 10 recommendations to address the problems and weaknesses in the NHS relating to risk management. Their first recommendation included the need for the establishment of: 'sound, standardised local reporting systems'. To some extent the 1955 guidelines about reporting incidents remain useful for today's NHS. Incidents should be reported promptly and the facts, rather than suppositions, recorded clearly and concisely. Details of the person affected and any witnesses will aid any later investigation. Immediate and later actions should also be recorded and one of the most important aspects, missing from the original guidance, is an explanation of the actions taken to prevent a recurrence of the incident.

Study activity

Find out the policy for reporting incidents in your Trust and what guidelines are available to you.

The Bristol Royal Infirmary Inquiry (2001) found that the fear of being victimised, labelled a 'troublemaker' or being seen as disloyal had prevented staff from speaking out earlier about their concerns. The Public Interest Disclosure Act 1998 gives significant protection to employees who disclose information appropriately and in the public interest. After this Act became law in 1999 the NHS Executive issued guidance to NHS Trusts on 'whistleblowing' and suggested that every NHS Trust and Health Authority should have local policies and procedures to ensure an open and fair culture. These policies should include as a minimum:

- a designated senior manager with specific responsibility for addressing concerns raised in confidence
- guidance to help staff who have concerns about malpractice
- a clear commitment that such concerns will be taken seriously
- an unequivical promise that staff who raise such concerns will be protected against victimisation (NHS Executive, 1999)

Study activity

Find out the 'whistleblowing' policy for your Trust and discuss with colleagues if you would feel able to raise concerns about malpractice. Consider how you would do this.

Effective risk management

An organisation that has an effective risk management system should:

- rarely have serious failures of standards of care
- not have reoccurrence of serious events of a similar kind
- not have serious incidents similar to those experienced elsewhere in the country
- have systems in place to reduce to a minimum the likelihood of serious failures of care
- be actively monitoring and reducing levels of less serious incident

(DH, 2000)

Reporting incidents

Minimum information required for reporting incidents and near misses:

- When did it happen? (Date and time)
- Where did it happen? (Location/speciality)
- What happened? (Event/near miss description, severity of actual or potential harm, people or equipment involved)
- What impact did the incident have? (For the patient, staff, others, organisation)
- What immediate action was taken?
- What later actions were taken, including those taken to prevent a recurrence? (For example, patient/family informed, clinical records updated, risk assessment undertaken?)

Reporting adverse drug reactions

The reporting of adverse drug reactions is an essential part of establishing the safety of medicines. The Medicines Control Agency (MCA) has operated a 'yellow card' scheme since 1964 for reporting potential drug safety problems. Since 1964, more than 350 000 reports of suspected adverse reactions to medicines used in the UK have been sent to the MCA (DH, 2000).

Reporting adverse incidents involving medical devices

Adverse incidents involving medical devices are reported to the Medical Devices Agency (MDA). The MDA logs the information received onto a central database which contains details of over 48 000 incidents. Each incident is investigated at a level that correlates with the degree of risk involved. When an investigation reveals a device-related safety problem the MDA issues a hazard or safety alert bulletin (SAB) to all healthcare organisations. Hazard notices are used in the most serious cases, when either a patient's health or life has been put at risk or the safety of staff has been compromised. Healthcare organisations are required to take immediate action on receipt of these notices to ensure no further incidents occur.

Safety alert bulletins are sent to all healthcare organisations when a potential safety problem has been found with a medical device. Organisations have to respond within a given time scale to explain the action taken to avoid the potential problem. This may involve alerting staff about the risk, or altering procedures for the use or maintenance of the device.

Study activity

Explore what recent SABs have been received in your Trust. Find out how the information is cascaded and what actions were taken in response to the risks identified in the bulletin.

The MDA has found that not all medical device incidents are related to manufacturing problems. They report that out of 6610 adverse incidents:

- 37% were manufacturing problems related to design, quality control, packaging and so forth
- 27% related to faults that developed during use of the device
- 12% were user error
- 24% had no link to device failure (Medical Device Agency, 1999)

Nurses should take note of the latter 36%. It is vital that all nurses are trained to use the medical equipment commonly used in their area of work and that their competency is assessed annually. They should not be afraid to state that they need help to use an unfamiliar device. It is also important that the prime cause of incidents that involve medical devices is identified before presuming that the device is at fault. If there is any doubt, the device must be labelled and taken out of use until it can be checked and serviced by a medical technician (Clothier, 1994). The Clothier Report also highlighted the need for all healthcare professionals to be alert to the possibility of malpractice as a cause of unexplained clinical incidents. This advice is supported by the Department of Health in association with the Health and Safety Executive and the association of Chief Police Officers who stress the need to involve the police at the earliest suspicion of unusual or unexplained incidents. If this had happened in the case of Beverley Allitt (who murdered four children and attempted to kill at least eight others) or that of Dr Harold Shipman (who murdered 15 of his patients), perhaps there would not have been so many deaths.

Grading Incidents (Figure 71.1)

Once an incident has been reported it is usually the responsibility of the person in charge to consider the severity of the consequences and the chance of the incident happening again. The CNST risk management standards require that:

- incidents should be graded for severity as soon as possible after the event
- the time scales for reporting incidents should be linked to the initial severity grading and to external reporting requirements
- the level of investigation should be linked to the incident grading

All incidents should be investigated at some level. Incidents that are near misses or that have little consequence may be the start of a larger problem if the root cause is not explored. Research suggests that for every serious incident there are likely to be several hundred 'near misses' (DH, 2000) (Figure 71.2). It is also useful to look at incident trends because many similar minor incidents are likely be a warning of a system failure that requires attention. More serious incidents warrant an in-depth investigation by individuals who have had extra training to undertake this role.

Investigating Incidents

The purpose of any incident investigation is to determine:

- the full facts
- what exactly happened

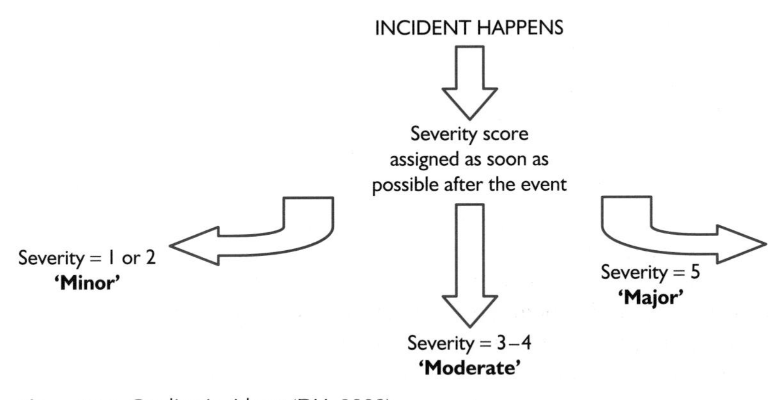

Figure 71.1 Grading incidents (DH, 2000).

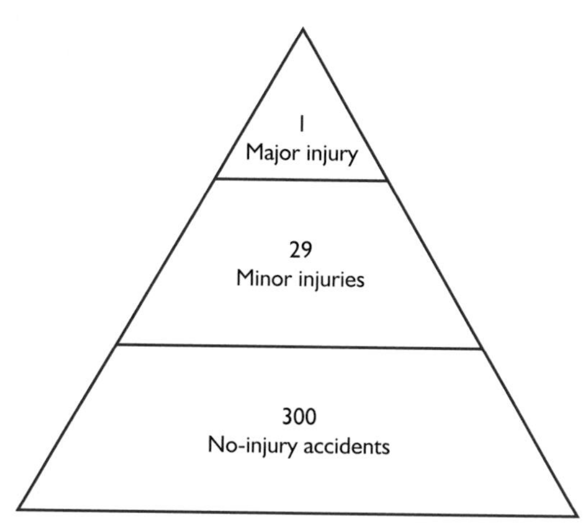

Figure 71.2 The Heinrich ratio (Heinrich, 1941).

- how, why and what can be learnt from the incident
- what went well
- the root cause of any error, omission or concern
- actions required to prevent recurrence
- persons responsible for implementing actions

Incidents generally occur because of a combination of human factors: slips, lapses, mistakes, violations, active failures and latent failures. Slips, lapses and mistakes arise primarily from informational problems (forgetting, inattention). Violations are more often associated with motivational problems, such as low morale, poor examples from senior staff, inadequate management. Behind these error-producing conditions may lie a further set of wider organisational problems such as conflict between meeting targets and safety, inadequate communication and deficient training. Latent failures stem from unsound management, which promotes incompatible goals (for example, conflict between available resources and clinical need), a blaming culture that discourages learning and lacks support, a closed culture that covers up incidents, negative unchallenging attitudes, inadequate communication and consultation. Any investigation into an incident needs to take all these potential causes into account (Figure 71.3).

The key to successful learning from adverse events is the use of an investigation process that includes a meaningful analysis to establish the underlying or root cause of the incident. The philosophy of root cause analysis can be used to underpin the investigation of all incidents and near misses and is favoured by the NHS (DH, 2001b). Its methodology can be used more formally to investigate incidents graded as serious. The term 'root cause analysis' originates from industry and has been criticised as being misleading. It can imply that there is a single root cause for an incident rather than a chain of events and a wide variety of contributory factors (Taylor-Adams and Vincent, 2004). Taylor-Adams and Vincent recommend the use of the London protocol, an approach that has been refined and developed in the light of experience and research into healthcare incident investigation. They suggest that this

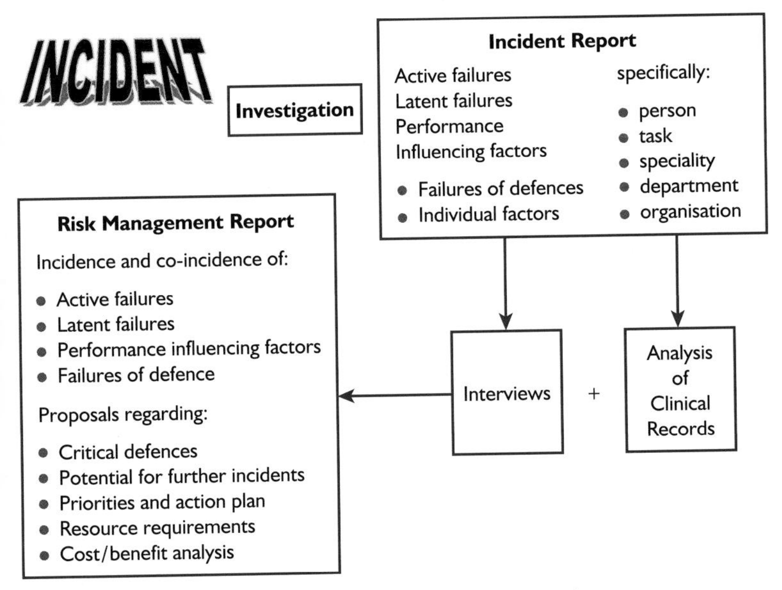

Figure 71.3 The incident investigation process (Healthcare Risk Resources International, 2001).

protocol enables a more comprehensive and thoughtful investigation of the incident, and have extended the framework of contributory factors described above (Table 71.1).

Defences and barriers are created in any organisation to protect against hazards and to reduce human or equipment failure. These barriers may be physical (such as gates), natural (distance), human actions (checking) or administrative (protocols). The first step in any incident investigation is to identify how these barriers would normally operate and why they were breached.

Study activity

Consider what defences and barriers are in place to prevent nurses from making drug errors.

Generally, people do not deliberately practise outside safety measures, procedures and standards, but lapses in judgement, forgetfulness and carelessness are all human characteristics. In certain conditions, such as at times of stress or high workload, these types of errors are more likely. Taylor-Adams and Vincent (2004) call these types of active failures 'care delivery problems' as they believe that a problem in health care can occur over time and is not easily described as a specific unsafe act. The identification of care delivery problems is the next step in the investigation process. These are problems that arise in the process of care. They are usually acts or omissions by members of staff, which have two essential features: first, care deviates beyond safe practice and, secondly, the deviation has contributed directly or indirectly to the adverse outcome.

The incident investigation flowchart

- Identify incident and decide to investigate
- Select people for investigation team
- Organise and gather data from documentation and interviewing those involved
- Establish a detailed chronology of the incident
- Identify the care management problems
- Identify the contributory factors
- Make recommendations and develop an action plan

(Taylor-Adams and Vincent, 2004)

Table 71.1 Framework of contributory factors influencing clinical practice (Taylor-Adams and Vincent, 2004)

Factors	Contributory influences
Patients	Condition (complexity and seriousness) Communication (language or other barriers) Personality and social factors
Task and technology	Task complexity Availability and use of protocols Availability and accurarcy of test results Decision-making tools
Individual staff	Knowledge and skills Competence Physical and mental health
Healthcare team	Verbal and written comunication Supervision and ability/culture for seeking help Structure (consistency, leadership, etc.)
Work environment	Staffing levels and skill mix Workload and shift patterns Availability and servicing of equipment Administrative and managerial support General environment (space, temperature, etc.)
Organisation and management	Financial resources and constraints Organisational structure Policies, standards, objectives Health and safety culture and priorities
Institutional context	Economic and regulatory context Links with external organisations

There may be more than one care delivery problem involved in one incident. Having identified these, the investigator then considers the conditions in which the incident occurred and the wider organisational context. These are known as contributory factors, which influence performance and may precipitate errors.

A variety of methods can be used to match each care delivery problem with contributory factors and Taylor-Adams and Vincent (2004) suggest the use of the fishbone technique or a chronology map (Figures 71.4 and 71.5). Once these have been determined, the next step in the investigation is to decide upon recommendations to tackle the weaknesses that have been identified.

Study activity

Reflect upon some mistakes you have made (in your personal or work life) and consider:

- what personal influences played a part
- what contributory factors were present
- how you could prevent yourself from making the same mistake again

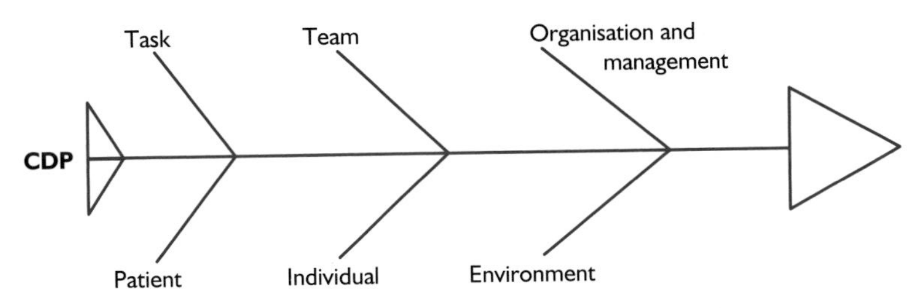

Figure 71.4 Fishbone technique.

TIME	CHRONOLOGY OF INCIDENT		
Care delivery problems			
Contributory factors			
Recommendations			

Figure 71.5 Chronology map.

Even if an incident has been shown to be the result of a chain of influencing factors rather than the fault of one or two individuals, most staff involved in an incident will feel personally responsible. It is important to recognise this and help staff to talk through the event and be involved in any action plan to prevent further incidents.

Learning from Incidents

It is important to gather and analyse information about an incident, but this alone will not bring about change and prevent a recurrence of the incident. The final step of any investigation must include a set of recommendations to prevent problems from arising again. The action plan should include:

- prioritisation of contributory factors
- actions to overcome the contributory factors
- those responsible for implementing the actions
- a time scale for completion of the actions
- identification of any resources to implement the changes
- criteria for evidence of completion
- a date to evaluate the effectiveness of the action plan

Study activity

Look at the scenarios of actual incidents and for each one consider:

- What questions you would ask to find out more about the incident and to try and determine the cause(s).
- How they might have been prevented.

Scenarios

- In a 3-week period, two young children received double the dose of medication in a hospital X-ray department, prior to having a scan. In both cases their weight had been recorded in pounds rather than kilograms.
- A baby in a neonatal intensive care unit died after being given an excessive dose of morphine – 15 mg instead of 0.15 mg – due to a miscalculation of the dosage. The dose was calculated by the SHO, checked by a nurse and administered by a registrar.
- A 5-month-old baby was accidentally given an overtransfusion of 60 ml of blood. The staff nurse caring for him did not think that this amount was significant so did not report the subsequent tachypnoea or inform a doctor until 6 hours later at the end of the night shift.
- A teenager admitted after an overdose was found unconscious and heavily sedated after managing to take a further overdose of her prescribed sedatives.
- A child received a head injury after getting out of bed after surgery (tonsillectomy) to go to the toilet and fainting. He hit his head on the bathroom sink as he fell.
- In 1996, four babies contracted the same type of serious infections. Two died and one had part of a limb amputated. The organism was traced to wooden tongue depressors, which were being used as splints to immobilise limbs for the stabilisation of intravenous infusions.

Table 71.2 An example of a severity score

1	Minor injury/damage (or none)
2	Some treatment required
3	RIDDOR[a] reportable or equivalent
4	Major injury
5	Death

[a] Reporting of Injuries, Diseases and Dangerous Occurrences Regulations – Health and Safety Executive (1995) requiring formal reporting to the HSE of any incidents that result in staff unable to work for at least 3 days or the equivalent effect for patients.

Prevention of Incidents

Ideally, incidents would not happen, and serious incidents and failures of services are uncommon in relation to the high volume of health care provided throughout the NHS. Nevertheless, they do occur and can have disastrous consequences for patients and their families. It should be possible to reduce the likelihood of failure of care if all staff understand their contribution to providing high-quality care and can identify and act upon opportunities for improving quality and safety.

There are always areas of risk within health care but it is possible to eradicate dangers or reduce them to a minimum by being proactive and undertaking a risk assessment.

Once a potential risk is identified, the potential hazard should be analysed to understand fully who is at risk (patient, staff, others) and the likelihood of the risk occurring. This can be measured in a similar way to severity scoring for an incident (Table 71.2). Current control measures (which are already in place to prevent the hazard) should be identified, together with any extra measures that can be put into place to reduce the likelihood to a minimum.

The price of failure

Failure to learn from adverse incidents results in:

- Around 425 000 adverse events each year in the NHS hospital sector might be avoidable (DH, 2000).
- £400 million in clinical litigation claims in 1998/9 with a further potential liability of about £2.4 billion from existing and unsettled claims – many cases show potentially avoidable causes (National Audit Office, 2000a).
- Nearly 28 000 complaints about aspects of clinical care in hospitals in 1998/9 (DH, 2000b).
- Since 1985 at least 13 patients were paralysed or killed by a drug wrongly administered intrathecally (DH, 2000).
- Over 6600 adverse incidents involving medical devices were reported to the MDA in 1999, resulting in 87 deaths and 345 serious injuries (MDA, 1999).
- Hospital-acquired infections costs the NHS nearly £1 billion per year and about 15% are regarded as preventable (National Audit Office, 2000b).

Study activity

Consider the admission to your ward of a disturbed teenager who has taken an overdose. Undertake a risk assessment to identify:

- the risk of further self-harm or absconding
- the control factors in place on the ward already to prevent these risks
- extra controls that could be put in place to increase these safety measures

Key Points

1. The increase in the complexity of health care has increased the potential risks for children receiving it.
2. Harm to children receiving health care causes unnecessary additional physical and psychological distress for them and their families. As a consequence there are additional costs for the NHS in increased length of stay and compensation.
3. Safety of children in healthcare settings should be maintained by thorough investigation of all adverse events and near misses with a blame-free, multidisciplinary approach.
4. Learning from incidents should be disseminated locally and nationally to prevent further recurrences.
5. The whole process of risk management promotes children's safety and well-being and is the responsibility of all staff.
6. Nurses should recognise their responsibility in promoting safety and effective risk management in their work area to minimise the likelihood of harm.

References

Aitken, L., *et al.* (2002) Hospital nurse staffing and patient mortality, nurse burnout, and job satisfaction. *JAMA*, **288** (16), 1987–1993.
Audit Commission (1991) *The Virtue of Patients: Making the Best Use of Ward Nursing Resources.* London: HMSO.
Audit Commission (1993) *Children First. A Study of Hospital Services.* London: HMSO.
Barton, J. (1995) Is flexible rostering useful? *Nursing Times*, **91** (7), 32–33.
Batstone, G. and **Edwards, M.** (1994) Clinical audit: 'how do we proceed'? *Southampton Medical Journal*, **10** (1), 13–18.
Bedfordshire Health Authority (1996) *Do you Qualify for Continuing Health Care?* Luton: Bedfordshire Health Authority.
Benner, P. (1984) *From Novice to Expert: Excellence and Power in Clinical Nursing.* Menlo Park, CA: Addison-Wesley.
Binnie, A. (1987) Structural changes. *Nursing Times*, **83** (39), 36–39.
Blackshaw, D. (1994) Problems that just refuse to go away. *Nursing Management*, **1** (4), 20–21.
Blauner, R. (1964) *Alienation and Freedom: The Factory Worker and his Industry.* Chicago: University of Chicago Press.
Bristol Royal Infirmary Inquiry (2001) *Learning from Bristol.* London: Department of Health.
Browne, A. and **Odell, M.** (2004) A review of nursing skill mix to optimise care in an acute trust. *Nursing Times*, **100** (6), 34–39.
Burr, S. (1992) *Staffing Issues in Paediatric Nursing.* London: RCN.
Carr-Hill, R. and **Jenkins-Clarke, S.** (2003) *Improving the Effectiveness of the Nursing Workforce.* York: The University of York, Centre for Health Economics.
Casey, A. (2006) Accentuate the positive. *Paediatric Nursing*, **17** (10), 3.
Casey, A. and **Mobbs, S.** (1988) Partnership in practice. *Nursing Times*, **84** (44), 67–68.
Clothier, C. (1994) *The Allitt Inquiry.* London: HMSO.
Confidential Inquiry into Stillbirths and Deaths in Infancy (2003) *Project 27/28.* Norwich: The Stationary Office.
DH (1989a) *Caring for People.* London: HMSO.
DH (1989b) *The Children Act: An Introductory Guide for the NHS.* London: HMSO.
DH (1993) *Clinical Audit: Meeting and Improving Standards in Healthcare.* London: HMSO.

DH (1994a) *Being Heard. The Report of a Review Committee on NHS Complaints Procedures.* London: HMSO.
DH (1994b) *The Evolution of Clinical Audit.* London: HMSO.
DH (1996) *The Children's Charter.* London: HMSO.
DH (1997) *Paediatric Intensive Care: A Framework for the Future.* London: Department of Health.
DH (1998) *A First Class Service: Quality in the New NHS.* London: Department of Health.
DH (2000) *An Organisation with a Memory.* London: Department of Health.
DH (2001a) *Essence of Care; Fundamentals of Care.* London: HMSO.
DH (2001b) *Building a Safer NHS for Patients.* London: Department of Health.
DH (2003a) *Getting the Right Start: the National Service Framework for Children and Young People – Standard for Hospital Services.* London: Department of Health.
DH (2003b) *Discharge from Hospital: Pathway, Process and Practice.* London: Department of Health.
DH (2004) *Handling Complaints in the NHS – Good Practice Toolkit for Local Resolution.* London: Department of Health.
DH (2006a) *National Audit Projects – Establishing the Successes and the Lessons Learnt.* London: Department of Health.
DH (2006b) *Essence of Care: Promoting Health.* London: Department of Health.
DH (2006c) *Memorandum of Understanding.* London: Department of Health.
Dineen, M. and **Walsh, K.** (1999) *Incident Reporting in the NHS.* Health Care Risk Report, March 1999. London: HMSO.
Edge, W., *et al.* (1994) Reduction of morbidity in inter-hospital transport by specialist pediatric staff. *Critical Care Medicine,* **22**, 1186–1191.
Finnegan, A. (1996) Managing cost and quality in case management. *Paediatric Nursing,* **8** (8), 25–26.
Fradd, E. (1988) Achieving new roles. *Nursing Times,* **84** (50), 39–41.
Gahan, B. (1991) Changing roles. *Paediatric Nursing,* **3** (10), 22–24.
Gatford, A. (2004) Time to go home: putting together a package of care. *Child Care, Health and Development,* **30** (3), 243–246.
Giovannetti, P. (1979) Understanding the patient classification system. *Journal of Nursing Administration,* **9** (2), 4–9.
Giovannetti, P. (1984) Staffing methods – implications for quality. In Willis, L. and Linwood, M. (eds), *Measuring the Quality of Care.* Edinburgh: Churchill Livingstone.
Hancock, C. (1980) Finding the right level. *Nursing Mirror,* **150** (2), 37–38.
Hancock, C. (1992) Nurses and skill mix. *Senior Nurse,* **12** (5), 9–12.
Healthcare Commission (2005) *Acute Hospital Portfolio Review: Ward Staffing.* London: Healthcare Commission.
Heinrich, H. (1941) *Industrial Accident Prevention: A Scientific Approach.* London: Prentice Hall.
Huczynski, A. and **Buchanan, A.** (1985) *Organisational Behaviour.* London: Prentice Hall.
Kron, T. (1981) *The Management of Patient Care – Putting Leadership Skills to Work.* London: Saunders.
Manthey, M., *et al.* (1970) Primary nursing – a return to the concept of my nurse and my patient. *Nursing Forum,* **9** (1), 65–83.
Marland, J. (1994) Back where they belong: caring for sick children at home. *Child Health,* **2** (1), 40–42.
McKillick, K. (1983) Modifying schedules makes jobs more satisfying. *Nursing Management,* **14** (1), 53–55.
Medical Device Agency (1999) *Annual Report.* London: MDA.
MoH (1955) *National Health Service – Reporting of Accidents in Hospitals.* London: HMSO.
MoH (1959) *The Welfare of Children in Hospital (Platt Report).* London: HMSO.
Morrell, C. (1996) Clinical audit makes progress in care and teamwork. *Nursing Times,* **92** (30), 34–36.
Mosher, C., *et al.* (1992) Upgrading practice with critical care pathways. *American Journal of Nursing,* **99** (1), 41–44.
Moules, T. (2004) Whose quality is it? *Paediatric Nursing,* **16** (6), 30–32.
Naish, J. and **Tassa, B.** (2006) Our level best. *Nursing Standard,* **20** (18), 13–15.
National Audit Office (2000a) *NHS Summary Accounts 1998/9.* London: National Audit Office.
National Audit Office (2000b) *The Management and Control of Hospital Acquired Infection in Acute NHS Trusts in England.* London: National Audit Office.
National Institute for Health and Clinical Excellence (2001) *Referral Advice.* London: NICE.
National Institute for Health and Clinical Excellence (2005) *Improving Outcomes in Children and Young People with Cancer.* London: NICE.
NHS Executive (1996) *Paediatric Intensive Care Report from the Chief Executive to the Secretary of State.* London: NHS Executive.
NHS Executive (1999) *The Public Disclosure Act 1998 – Whistle Blowing in the NHS.* London: NHS Executive.
NHS Management Executive (1991) *Framework of Audit for Nursing Services.* London: HMSO.
Northcott, N. and **Facey, S.** (1995) Twelve hour shifts: helpful or hazardous to patients? *Nursing Times,* **92** (7), 29–31.
Noyes, J. (2002) Barriers that delay children and young people who are dependent on mechanical ventilators from being discharged from hospital. *Journal of Clinical Nursing,* **11** (1), 2–11.
Nursing and Midwifery Audit Information Service (1996) *Evidence-based Practice and Clinical Effectiveness.* London: NMAIS.
Nursing and Midwifery Council (2004) *The NMC Code of Professional Conduct: Standards for Conduct, Performance and Ethics.* London: NMC.
Payne, D. (ed.) (1997) This week. *Nursing Times,* **93** (16), 7.
Reed, N. (1988) A comparison of nurse-related behaviour, philosophy of care and job satisfaction in team and primary nursing. *Journal of Advanced Nursing,* **13**, 383–395.
Reid, W. (1996) Righting wrongs. *Nursing Standard,* **10** (24), 19.

Robinson, K. (1991) A primary flaw? *Nursing Times,* **87** (42), 36–38.
Rogers, M., *et al.* (1992) Looking forward. *Paediatric Nursing,* **4** (2), 23–25.
Roscoe, J. (1990) Planning shift patterns. *Nursing Times,* **86** (38), 31–33.
Royal College of Nursing (1999) *Skill-mix and Staffing in Children's Wards and Departments.* London: RCN.
Royal College of Nursing (2000) *Children's Community Nursing.* London: RCN.
Royal Commission on Long Term Care (1999) *With Respect to Old Age – Rights and Responsibilities.* London: The Stationary Office.
Sadler, C. (1990) Beat the clock. *Nursing Times,* **86** (38), 28–31.
Salvage, J. (1985) *The Politics of Nursing.* London: Heinemann.
Shaw, C. (1986) *Introducing Quality Assurance.* London: King's Fund.
Smith, F. and **Valentine, F.** (1999) Value added decisions. *Paediatric Nursing,* **11** (7), 9–10.
Smith, L. and **Daughtrey, H.** (2000) Weaving the seamless web of care: an analysis of parents' perceptions of their needs following discharge of their child from hospital. *Journal of Advanced Nursing,* **31** (4), 812–820.
Stephens, N. (2005) Complex care packages. *Paediatric Nursing,* **17** (7), 30–32.
Taylor-Adams, S. and **Vincent, C.** (2004) *Systems Analysis of Clinical Incidents.* London: Clinical Safety Research Unit.
Thomas, D., *et al.* (1992) Team nursing. *Nursing Times,* **88** (52), 40–43.
Tierney, A., *et al.* (1994) Older patients' experiences of discharge from hospital. *Nursing Times,* **90** (21), 36–39.
Todd, C., *et al.* (1991) The impact of 12 hour shifts. *Nursing Times,* **87** (31), 47–50.
Underwood, A. (1975) What a 12 hour shift offers. *American Journal of Nursing,* **75** (7), 1176–1178.
Westwood, O. (1997) Nutrition and immune function. *Nursing Times,* **93** (15), i–vi (supplement).
Wyatt, M. and **Healey, K.** (2005) Managing capacity and workload in children's services. *Paediatric Nursing* **17** (6), 31–34.

Index